Dementia

Dementia

Comprehensive Principles and Practice

Edited by

Bradford C. Dickerson, MD

Associate Professor of Neurology, Harvard Medical School
Director, Frontotemporal Disorders Unit
Co-Investigator, Alzheimer's Disease Research Center
Department of Neurology, Massachusetts General Hospital
Boston, MA

and

Alireza Atri, MD, PhD

Instructor in Neurology, Harvard Medical School
Assistant in Neurology, Massachusetts General Hospital
Director, Outpatient Memory Disorders & Dementia Units
Associate Director, Clinical, GRECC, ENRM VA Medical Center
Boston, MA

OXFORD
UNIVERSITY PRESS

OXFORD
UNIVERSITY PRESS

Oxford University Press is a department of the University of
Oxford. It furthers the University's objective of excellence in research,
scholarship, and education by publishing worldwide.

Oxford   New York
Auckland   Cape Town   Dar es Salaam   Hong Kong   Karachi
Kuala Lumpur   Madrid   Melbourne   Mexico City   Nairobi
New Delhi   Shanghai   Taipei   Toronto

With offices in
Argentina   Austria   Brazil   Chile   Czech Republic   France   Greece
Guatemala   Hungary   Italy   Japan   Poland   Portugal   Singapore
South Korea   Switzerland   Thailand   Turkey   Ukraine   Vietnam

Oxford is a registered trademark of Oxford University Press
in the UK and certain other countries.

Published in the United States of America by
Oxford University Press
198 Madison Avenue, New York, NY 10016

© Oxford University Press 2014

All rights reserved. No part of this publication may be reproduced, stored in
a retrieval system, or transmitted, in any form or by any means, without the prior
permission in writing of Oxford University Press, or as expressly permitted by law,
by license, or under terms agreed with the appropriate reproduction rights organization.
Inquiries concerning reproduction outside the scope of the above should be sent to the
Rights Department, Oxford University Press, at the address above.

You must not circulate this work in any other form
and you must impose this same condition on any acquirer.

Library of Congress Cataloging-in-Publication Data
Dementia (Dickerson)
Dementia : comprehensive principles and practice / edited by Bradford C. Dickerson & Alireza Atri.
   p. ; cm.
Includes bibliographical references.
ISBN 978–0–19–992845–3 (alk. paper)
I. Dickerson, Bradford C., editor of compilation.   II. Atri, Alireza, editor of compilation.   III. Title.
[DNLM: 1. Dementia. WM 220]
RC521
616.83—dc23
2014004364

The science of medicine is a rapidly changing field. As new research and clinical experience broaden our
knowledge, changes in treatment and drug therapy occur. The author and publisher of this work have
checked with sources believed to be reliable in their efforts to provide information that is accurate and
complete, and in accordance with the standards accepted at the time of publication. However, in light of
the possibility of human error or changes in the practice of medicine, neither the author, nor the publisher,
nor any other party who has been involved in the preparation or publication of this work warrants that the
information contained herein is in every respect accurate or complete. Readers are encouraged to confirm
the information contained herein with other reliable sources, and are strongly advised to check the product
information sheet provided by the pharmaceutical company for each drug they plan to administer.

The writing and production of this book have been conducted during early mornings, late nights, weekends,
and several "vacations." Dr. Atri's contributions to this book were conducted both outside his VA tour of
duty and his Massachusetts General Hospital/Harvard University/National Institutes of Health research
and clinical time. The contents of this book do not represent the views of the Department of Veterans Affairs,
the United States Government, Massachusetts General Hospital, or Harvard Medical School.

9 8 7 6 5 4 3 2
Printed in the United States of America
on acid-free paper

Dedication

To my mother and father, Jeannae and John Dickerson, who showed me the value and joy of a lifelong love of learning; and my grandmother, Gladys Jastram, and my great-grandmother, Tillie Sorensen, whose strength and kindness inspired me to try to be compassionate in every interaction with patients and families.
—*Brad C. Dickerson*

To my father Seyed Ali Atri, who showed me that "giving is the greatest joy in life" and that optimism, resilience, and forgiveness are necessary choices; my uncle, A. Hamid Ghodse, M.D., Ph.D., whose character, integrity, and humanity shine as an eternal beacon to guide and emulate; and my aunt, Zahra Daneshmand, whose unconditional kindness, generosity and love sustained and taught me what matters.
—*Alireza Atri*

To all patients, families, caregivers, and colleagues who suffer from and continue to battle these devastating conditions.
—*Brad C. Dickerson and Alireza Atri*

Contents

Foreword ix
   Creighton H. Phelps

Preface xi

Contributors xvii

Part I. Functional Neuroanatomy and Cognitive Neuroscience of Dementia

1. Cognitive Functions and the Cerebral Cortex 3
  David Caplan

2. Neuroanatomy and Behavioral Neurology of Subcortical Systems 32
  Jeremy D. Schmahmann and Deepak N. Pandya

3. Executive Control, the Regulation of Goal-Directed Behaviors, and the Impact of Dementing Illness 71
  Kirk R. Daffner and Kim C. Willment

4. Memory Systems in Dementia 108
  Andrew E. Budson

5. Motor Programming Disorders in Dementia 126
  Kenneth M. Heilman

Part II. The Dementias: The Major Diseases and Clinical Syndromes

6. The Neuropathology of Neurodegenerative Dementias 145
  Etty P. Cortes Ramirez and Jean-Paul G. Vonsattel

7. Chronic Traumatic Encephalopathy 160
  Ann C. McKee

8. Frontotemporal Dementia 176
  Bradford C. Dickerson

9. Primary Progressive Aphasia: A Language-Based Dementia 198
  Marsel Mesulam

10. Posterior Cortical Atrophy 208
  David F. Tang-Wai, Alison Lake, and Neill Graff-Radford

11. Progressive Supranuclear Palsy and Corticobasal Degeneration 220
  Stephanie Lessig and Irene Litvan

12. Dementia With Lewy Bodies and Parkinson's Disease Dementia 231
  Haşmet A. Hanağası, Başar Bilgiç, and Murat Emre

13. Vascular Cognitive Impairment 260
  Charles DeCarli

14. Cerebral Amyloid Angiopathy and Cognitive Impairment 274
  Ellis S. van Etten, Steven M. Greenberg, and Anand Viswanathan

15. The Differential Diagnosis of Rapidly Progressive and Rare Dementias: A Clinical Approach 291
  Jeremy D. Schmahmann

16. Alzheimer's Disease and Alzheimer's Dementia 360
  Alireza Atri

17. Mild Cognitive Impairment 432
    *Meredith Wicklund and
    Ronald C. Petersen*

18. Preclinical Alzheimer's Disease 448
    Reisa A. Sperling

Part III. Assessment, Diagnosis, and Comprehensive Treatment: From Principles to Practice

19. Dementia Screening and Mental Status Examination in Clinical Practice 461
    Meghan B. Mitchell and Alireza Atri

20. Neuropsychological Assessment of Dementia: A Large-Scale Neuroanatomical Network Approach 487
    Sandra Weintraub

21. Neuropsychiatric Symptoms of Dementia 508
    Haythum O. Tayeb, Evan D. Murray, and Bruce H. Price

22. Neuroimaging, Cerebrospinal Fluid Markers, and Genetic Testing in Dementia 528
    Bradford C. Dickerson

23. Pharmacological Therapies for Alzheimer's Disease: Clinical Trials and Future Directions 563
    Michael Rafii and Paul Aisen

24. Management of Agitation, Aggression, and Psychosis Associated With Alzheimer's Disease 575
    Clive Ballard and Anne Corbett

25. Management of Depression, Apathy, and Sexualized Inappropriate Behavior in Dementia 588
    *James M. Ellison and
    Cynthia T. Greywolf*

26. Nonpharmacological Approaches to Managing Behavior Symptoms in Dementia 600
    Sumer Verma

27. The Role of the Family in the Care and Management of Patients With Dementia 609
    Licet Valois and James E. Galvin

28. Mental Competence and Legal Issues in Dementia Care 622
    Barry S. Fogel

Index 639

About the Editors 667

Foreword

The concept of dementia, defined originally as "without mind" or "madness," has existed since ancient times. The term referred to many mental disorders, including schizophrenia, which was originally termed *dementia praecox*. Gradually dementia became more associated with old age and was often termed *senility* or *senile dementia* and was considered by many to be a normal consequence of the aging process. However, it became more apparent late in the 19th century and early 20th century that many dementias occurred earlier in life and were "presenile." Others were reversible or sometimes preventable such as the dementia caused by syphilis, if treated early. In the mid-1970s Robert Katzman proposed that presenile dementia and senile dementia due to Alzheimer's disease (AD) pathology very likely represented variations of the same syndrome differing only in age of onset. The term *dementia* as it is used now refers to progressive and severe loss of cognitive abilities that prevent affected persons from functioning normally in society no matter what their age or the underlying cause. Since AD is the most common form of dementia, research in recent years has focused more on AD than other dementias, even though they are sometimes closely related or even overlapping with AD.

Because clinical differentiation among the dementias is sometimes difficult in practice, especially in early stages and, often, more than one underlying cause may contribute to the clinical presentation, diagnosis has been difficult for many clinicians. In recent years guidelines for diagnosis have been developed for many of the dementias caused by neurodegenerative diseases, and they have helped to distinguish among the various dementias. The diagnostic guidelines for dementias due to frontotemporal lobar degeneration, Lewy bodies, vascular changes, and Alzheimer's-related pathologies are discussed at length in this volume by respected experts. In addition, the American Psychiatric Association has issued a new version of the *Diagnostic and Statistical Manual of Mental Disorders* (*DSM-5*) in which they present neurocognitive disorders as major and minor, and have reclassified the dementias as major neurocognitive disorders.

In 2011, US President Obama signed the National Alzheimer's Project Act (NAPA), which prescribed the development of a National Alzheimer's Plan. To that end, a National Advisory Council on Alzheimer's Disease was established and developed the plan, which was issued in May 2012 by the Secretary of the Department of Health and Human Services. The United States is now one of about twelve nations that have issued national plans. In addition, there are a number of subnational plans in various countries, including many state and provincial plans. The US National Plan, while focusing on Alzheimer's disease, does include language addressing "Alzheimer's disease–related dementias." To support implementation of the National Plan, the National Institutes of Health (NIH), private foundations, and interest groups, as well as corporate groups, have sponsored a series of meetings to address various aspects of the plan. An Alzheimer's Summit was convened by the National Institute on Aging (NIA) in 2012, where scientific leaders gathered to develop recommendations for how to implement the scientific directives in the national plan. In 2013 the NINDS convened another meeting to address the related dementias resulting in another series of recommendations. Stemming from these recommendations, the NIH has issued a series of new initiatives and milestones have been developed to measure success in meeting these recommendations with the goal of preventing and effectively treating Alzheimer's disease (and related dementias) by 2025.

This is an exciting time in dementia research and the editors of this volume have done a superb job in bringing together a diverse set of experts to summarize current thinking regarding underlying brain mechanisms, including the spectrum of diseases and syndromes resulting in dementia, assessment and diagnosis, and care and management issues in all of its manifestations. With better understanding of the basic pathobiology of the various neurodegenerative dementias and the development of more sensitive diagnostic tools such as better measurement of subtle cognitive decline and the advent of biomarkers such as amyloid and tau imaging, the prospect for better diagnosis and treatment of the dementias at earlier stages has never looked brighter.

Creighton H. Phelps, PhD
Deputy Director, Division of Neuroscience
Director, Alzheimer's Disease Centers Program
National Institute on Aging
National Institutes of Health
Bethesda, MD

Preface

Dementia: Comprehensive Principles and Practice is a clinically oriented book that has blossomed from the annual *Dementia: A Comprehensive Update* continuing medical education course offered by Harvard Medical School. Now, in its eighteenth year in 2014, this 3- to 4-day course is organized by faculty who specialize in the care of patients with cognitive and behavioral disorders at Massachusetts General Hospital, Brigham and Women's Hospital, McLean Hospital, and Edith Nourse Rogers Memorial Veterans Administration Bedford Hospital. We are also fortunate to include a number of internationally renowned guest faculty from other major institutions. This course was begun by Drs. David Caplan, Jeremy Schmahmann, and Kirk Daffner in 1997; we are immensely indebted to all of them for their mentorship as we enter our fourth year of codirecting the course. Motivated by the care of our patients and their families, and inspired by the integrative review of these topics by faculty and the thought-provoking discussions generated with attendees and colleagues, we developed this book by working with course faculty and selected additional experts.

Why do we need another book on dementia? Alzheimer's disease (AD) and other dementias are increasingly recognized as a scourge of our time. Few of us will be spared the personal or professional effects of these conditions. As medical care continues to lengthen life span, these largely age-related illnesses become more prevalent. AD, the most common cause of dementia, is thought to affect more than 5 million people in the United States, nearly 1 million people in the United Kingdom, and similar numbers in other developed nations. In 2010, low estimates for dementia-related costs accounted for greater than 1% of the world gross domestic product. Without major "cures," projections—in the United States as well as globally—estimate potentially crippling dementia-related costs for world economies in the coming decades. But since the authors of chapters in this book are all clinicians, we look beyond statistics; the devastation wrought by these illnesses upon each patient and family is immeasureable. Unfortunately, even today with growing public awareness, dementing illnesses often escape early diagnosis and appropriate clinical care, adversely impacting the patients, their families and caregivers, health care–related costs, and public health in a variety of ways, as discussed in detail in the following pages.

This book is designed to improve knowledge about dementia and competence in its clinical management, hopefully translating into improved early detection, accurate diagnosis, and compassionate comprehensive care. Written primarily for clinicians, this volume takes a multidisciplinary approach to understanding dementia and is aimed toward neurologists, psychiatrists, geriatricians, psychologists, nurse specialists, internists, primary care physicians, social workers, occupational therapists, clinical pharmacists, research scientists, and other health professionals involved in the diagnosis, management, and investigation of disease states causing dementia. The organization of the book takes an integrative approach by providing three major parts that (1) establish the neuroanatomical and cognitive framework underlying disorders of cognition and behavior, (2) provide fundamental as well as cutting-edge material covering specific diseases associated with dementia, and (3) discuss approaches to the diagnosis and treatment of dementing illnesses that are pragmatic and highly relevant to clinical practice.

Part I provides the basic cognitive and anatomical foundation upon which the book builds in subsequent sections. A conceptual framework of the functional and anatomical organization of the cerebral hemispheres and their systems is provided by Caplan and Schmahmann, and then specific domains of function are reviewed by Budson, Daffner, and Willment, and Heilman, including memory, executive, and motor control systems of the brain.

Part II provides comprehensive reviews of the major dementing diseases, starting with Cortes Ramirez and Vonsattel on the neuropathology of dementias and McKee on chronic traumatic encephalopathy. We then continue with new clinical and basic science concepts of frontotemporal dementia and primary progressive aphasia by Dickerson and Mesulam; posterior cortical atrophy by Tang-Wai, Lake, and Graff-Radford; "parkinsonian dementias" by Lessig, Litvan, Hanagasi, Bilgic, and Emre; vascular dementias by DeCarli; and cerebral amyloid angiopathy by Etten, Greenberg, and Viswanathan, concluding with rare and rapidly progressive dementias by Schmahmann. Finally, a comprehensive update is presented by Atri, Wicklund, and Petersen, and Sperling on the AD spectrum from dementia to mild cognitive impairment and preclinical AD. This part contains a particular emphasis on the highly contemporary issues, including the new diagnostic criteria for many of these disorders published in the last few years.

Part III concludes the book with chapters focusing on evaluation and management, including a clinical approach to cognitive screening and the mental status exam by Mitchell and Atri; neuropsychological testing by Weintraub; the neuropsychiatry of dementias by Tayeb, Murray, and Price; and imaging and biomarkers in clinical diagnosis by Dickerson. A thorough review of management issues concludes the volume with chapters on future directions in pharmacologic management of AD by Raffi and Aisen; management of behavioral and psychological symptoms of dementia by Ballard and Corbett, and Ellison and Greywolf; nonpharmacological approaches to symptom management by Verma; social service and caregiver/family-centered approaches by Valois and Galvin; and medico-legal issues by Fogel.

We hope that readers find value in not only the cutting-edge discussions and evidence-based reviews of the literature by leaders in the field but also appreciate the clinical wisdom conveyed by many highly experienced investigators and compassionate clinicians. The topics relating to clinical neurology, psychiatry, geriatrics, psychology, and neuroscience research discussed here directly bear on present and future approaches to the diagnosis and management of dementia. Specialists will find the book to be an up-to-date reference work; generalists will obtain valuable principles useful in daily clinical practice; and trainees will be treated to a "one-stop" source for learning the scientific basis of the field of dementing diseases, and clinical methods and pearls on how to effectively and compassionately care for patients and caregivers who are affected by these highly challenging diseases.

Appropriate dementia care takes a village—a village of well-informed and interested multidisciplinary clinicians and caregivers. We have endeavored in this book to collate the essential and latest information and tools to allow our colleagues to better affect this comprehensive care in the relentless battle against the havoc wreaked by the effects of the dementias. It is a battle that is not only worthy and noble but is also an imperative derived from our responsibilities as clinicians to adhere to the principles of medical ethics: nonmaleficence, beneficence, autonomy, and justice. It is a battle, which when properly waged, can allow major victories in a small minority, minor victories in the majority, and meaningful benefits by ameliorating suffering in all. Until we can cure, we will care and help in anyway we can, and this book is part of our small contribution to this ongoing effort.

We greatly appreciate the work by our coauthors, who took time out from their usual activities to contribute to this volume. The efforts of Craig Panner and Marni Rolfes at Oxford University Press were invaluable in helping us to transform the materials here from a course syllabus into the book you are reading. A number of our friends and members of our laboratories were kind enough to provide expert assistance in reviewing and editing drafts of chapters, especially Lynn (Lili) Shaughnessy, Meghan Mitchell, Steven Shirk, and Jessica Dodd. More broadly, we thank our mentors whose guidance and encouragement provided formative influences on our thinking and approach to patient/family care. Brad Dickerson extends special thanks to the following mentors and colleagues: Tony Phelps, Sheryl Williams, Bill Greenough, Theresa Jones, Leyla deToledo-Morrell, Frank Morrell, Marsel Mesulam, Sandy Weintraub, Martin Samuels, Marilyn Albert, Reisa Sperling, Kirk Daffner, Deborah Blacker, Brad Hyman, John Growdon, David Caplan, Bruce Price, Merit Cudkowicz, Bruce Rosen, Janet Sherman, Dorene Rentz, Keith Johnson, Barbara Maxam, Diane Lucente, Rudy Tanzi, Matthew Frosch, Bruce Miller, Bill Seeley, David Wolk, Lisa Feldman Barrett, and Anne Young. Dr. Dickerson also thanks Liz and George Krupp for their generous support. Ali Atri offers special thanks the following mentors and colleagues: John Growdon, Reisa Sperling, Martin Samuels, Daniel Lowenstein, John Engstrom, Cheryl Jay, Joseph Martin, James Sneyd, Carol Newton, David Caplan, Jang-Ho Cha, Merit Cudkowicz, Kirk Daffner, Steven M. Greenberg, Fran Grodstein, Michael Hasselmo, Albert Hung, Michael Irizarry, Joseph Locascio, Barbara Maxam, Dorene Rentz, Bruce Rosen, Janet Sherman, Chantal Stern, Nagagopal Venna, Liang Yap, Anne Young, Steven DeKosky, Rachelle Doody, and Dan Mungas. Most important, for their love, support, and positive influences in our lives, we thank our families. Brad Dickerson thanks Allison Berger, Molly Dickerson, Lilly Dickerson, Jeannae Dickerson, John Dickerson, Jim Dickerson, Sarah Dickerson, Lewis Berger, Ileana Berger, and Stacie and the Siebrecht family. Alireza Atri thanks his family and friends, particularly Natalie Atri, Taraneh Atri, Bijan Atri, Seyed Ali Atri, Nasrin Daneshmand, Ali Atri, Erik, Karine, Lukas and Caroline Alexander, Abbas Atri, Mehrnaz Atri, Glen and Betsy Chatfield, Wayne and Grace Chatfield, Wayne D. Chatfield, Ramin and Homa Daneshmand, Zahra Daneshmand, Tim Duffy, Hamid, Barbara, Hossein, Nassrin and Ali-Reza Ghodse, Mansour, Shahnaz, Ellie and Arie Farahabadi, James Ford, Jessica Ford, Ian Fullmer, Andrew Kayser, Jennifer Harris, Jeff and Brenda McConathy, Sally Miller, Tracey and Jeff Milligan, Mahin Moeinazad, Mary Norman, Homa, Vahid and Hamid Noshirvani, Michael Opre, Tahereh Shirvani, and Abbas Taheri. We also thank each other for the inspiration, encouragement, and wise counsel during this process—the process and product would not have been nearly as fun or fruitful without the balance, motivation, and support we provided each other. Last but not least, we acknowledge, with great humility, a deep gratitude for the privilege of being entrusted, by thousands of our patients, their families and caregivers, the awesome responsibility of counseling and caring for them. We have learned immensely from listening and caring for you, and will unfailingly carry forth this inspired legacy to help others, regardless of their circumstances, to live their lives better and to diligently work towards treatments and cures.

Human beings are members of a whole,
In creation of one essence and soul,
If one member is afflicted with pain
Other members uneasy will remain.
If you have no sympathy for human pain,
The name of human you cannot retain
—Saadi Shirazi *(Persian/Iranian poet, 1184–1283)*

No man is an island, entire of itself. . .
Any man's death diminishes me, because I am involved in mankind;
and therefore never send to know for whom the bell tolls;
it tolls for thee
—John Donne *(English poet, 1572–1631)*

To cure sometimes
To help often
To console always
Medical proverb of unknown origin—has been attributed
to several physicians including Trudeau, Pare' and Hippocrates
—Hippocrates *(Greek physician, 460–370 b.c.)*

Contributors

Paul Aisen, MD
Director, Alzheimer's Disease
Cooperative Study
Professor, Department of Neurosciences
UC San Diego School of Medicine
San Diego, CA

Alireza Atri, MD, PhD
Instructor in Neurology
Harvard Medical School
Assistant in Neurology
Massachusetts General Hospital
Director, Outpatient Memory Disorders &
Dementia Units
Associate Director, Clinical, GRECC
ENRM VA Medical Center
Boston, MA

Clive Ballard, MD, MRCPsych
Professor of Age-Related Diseases
Wolfson Centre for Age Related Diseases
King's College London
London, UK

Başar Bilgiç, MD
Associate Professor of Neurology
Istanbul University
Istanbul Faculty of Medicine
Department of Neurology
Behavioral Neurology and Movement
Disorders Unit
Istanbul, Turkey

Andrew E. Budson, MD
Professor of Neurology
Boston University School of Medicine
Boston University Alzheimer's Disease Center
Department of Neurology
Associate Chief of Staff
VA Boston Healthcare System
Lecturer on Neurology
Harvard Medical School
Boston, MA

David Caplan, MD, PhD
Professor of Neurology
Harvard Medical School
Director, Cognitive Behavioral Neurology Unit
Massachusetts General Hospital
Boston, MA

Anne Corbett, PhD
Lecturer in Dementia Research Communications
Wolfson Centre for Age Related Diseases
King's College London
London, UK

Etty P. Cortes Ramirez, MD
Assistant Director
New York Brain Bank
Taub Institute for Research on Alzheimer's
Disease and the Aging Brain
College of Physicians and Surgeons
Department of Pathology and Cell Biology
Columbia University Medical Center
and the New York Presbyterian Hospital
New York, NY

Kirk R. Daffner, MD
J. David and Virginia Wimberly Professor
of Neurology
Harvard Medical School
Chief, Division of Cognitive and Behavioral
Neurology & Director
Center for Brain/Mind Medicine
Brigham and Women's Hospital
Boston, MA

Charles DeCarli, MD, FAAN
Professor of Neurology and Director of
Alzheimer's Disease Center
Department of Neurology
University of California at Davis
Sacramento, CA

Bradford C. Dickerson, MD
Associate Professor of Neurology
Harvard Medical School
Director, Frontotemporal Disorders Unit
Co-Investigator, Alzheimer's Disease Research
Center
Tom Rickles Endowed Chair in Primary
Progressive Aphasia
Department of Neurology
Massachusetts General Hospital
Boston, MA

James M. Ellison, MD, MPH
Associate Professor of Psychiatry
Harvard Medical School
Director, Geriatric Psychiatric Program
Department of Psychiatry
McLean Hospital
Boston, MA

Murat Emre, MD
Professor of Neurology
Istanbul University
Istanbul Faculty of Medicine
Department of Neurology
Behavioral Neurology and Movement
Disorders Unit
Istanbul, Turkey

Ellis S. van Etten, MD
Philip Kistler Stroke Research Center
Department of Neurology
Massachusetts General Hospital and Harvard
Medical School
Boston, MA

Barry S. Fogel, MD
Clinical Professor of Psychiatry
Harvard Medical School
Brigham Behavioral Neurology Group
Brigham and Women's Hospital
Boston, MA

James E. Galvin, MD, MPH
Professor of Neurology, Psychiatry
Nutrition and Population Health
Director of Clinical Operations
Comprehensive Center on Brain Aging
Director, Pearl Barlow Center for Memory
Evaluation and Treatment
Alzheimer Disease Center
New York University Langone School
of Medicine
New York, NY

Neill Graff-Radford, MBBCh
Professor of Neurology
Department of Neurology
Mayo Clinic College of Medicine
Jacksonville, FL

Steven M. Greenberg, MD, PhD
Professor of Neurology
Harvard Medical School
Director, Hemorrhagic Stroke
Research Program
John J. Conway Endowed Chair in Neurology
Philip Kistler Stroke Research Center
Department of Neurology
Massachusetts General Hospital
Boston, MA

Cynthia T. Greywolf, DNP-PMHNP, BC
Assistant Professor & AGNP Program Director,
Department of Nursing
University of Hawaii at Manoa
School of Nursing and Dental Hygiene
Honolulu, US

Haşmet A. Hanağası, MD
Professor of Neurology
Istanbul University
Istanbul Faculty of Medicine
Department of Neurology
Behavioral Neurology and Movement
Disorders Unit
Istanbul, Turkey

Kenneth M. Heilman, MD
The James E. Rooks Jr. Distinguished Professor
of Neurology and Health Psychology
University of Florida College of Medicine and
GRECC-Malcom Randall VAMC
Gainesville, FL

Alison Lake, OT
University Health Network Memory Clinic
Department of Occupational Therapy
University Health Network
Toronto, Canada

Stephanie Lessig, MD
Associate Professor, UCSD Neurosciences
Acting Chief of Neurology
VA Medical Center San Diego
UC San Diego
Department of Neurology
San Diego, CA

Irene Litvan, MD
Tasch Endowed Professor in Parkinson Disease Research
Director of the Movement Disorders Program
UC San Diego
Department of Neurosciences
San Diego, CA

Ann C. McKee, MD
Professor of Neurology and Pathology
Boston University School of Medicine
Director of Neuropathology
NE VA Medical Centers
Center for the Study of Traumatic Encephalopathy
Alzheimer's Disease Center
Departments of Neurology
Pathology
Boston University School of Medicine
Boston, MA

Marsel Mesulam, MD
Ruth Dunbar Davee Professor of Neuroscience, Neurology and Psychology
Northwestern University Feinberg School of Medicine
Director
Cognitive Neurology and Alzheimer's Disease Center
Chicago, IL

Meghan B. Mitchell, PhD
Neuropsychologist, Geriatric Research, Education and Clinical Center (GRECC)
ENRM Bedford VA Hospital
Research Fellow
Department of Neurology
Massachusetts General Hospital
Harvard Medical School
Boston, MA

Evan D. Murray, MD
Instructor in Neurology
Harvard Medical School
Assistant in Neurology
McLean Hospital/Massachusetts General Hospital
Director
Traumatic Brain Injury Service
Manchester VA Medical Center
Manchester, VA

Deepak N. Pandya, MD
Professor
Department of Anatomy and Neurobiology
Boston University School of Medicine
Boston, MA

Ronald C. Petersen, MD, PhD
Cora Kanow Professor of Alzheimer's Disease Research
Director
Mayo Alzheimer's Disease Research Center
Division of Behavioral Neurology
Department of Neurology
Mayo Clinic
Rochester, MN

Bruce H. Price, MD
Associate Professor of Neurology
Harvard Medical School
Chief, Department of Neurology
McLean Hospital
Boston, MA

Michael Rafii, MD, PhD
Medical Director, Alzheimer's Disease Cooperative Study
Director, Memory Disorders Clinic
Assistant Professor
Department of Neurosciences
Director, Residency Program
UC San Diego School of Medicine
San Diego, CA

Jeremy D. Schmahmann, MD
Professor of Neurology
Harvard Medical School
Director, Ataxia Unit
Director, Laboratory for Neuroanatomy and Cerebellar Neurobiology
Cognitive Behavioral Neurology Unit
Department of Neurology
Massachusetts General Hospital
Boston, MA

Reisa A. Sperling, MD
Professor of Neurology
Harvard Medical School
Director, Center for Alzheimer Research and Treatment
Department of Neurology
Brigham and Women's Hospital
Massachusetts Alzheimer's Disease Research Center
Harvard Aging Brain Study
Department of Neurology
Massachusetts General Hospital
Boston, MA

David F. Tang-Wai, MD
Assistant Professor of Neurology and
Geriatric Medicine
Division of Neurology
Department of Medicine
Co-Director
University Health Network Memory Clinic
University of Toronto
Toronto, Canada

Haythum O. Tayeb, MBChB, FRCPC
Assistant Professor and Consultant in
Neurology, Neuropsychiatry, and Clinical
Neurophysiology
Faculty of Medicine, King Abdulaziz
University
Jeddah, Saudi Arabia

Licet Valois, LMSW, MPS
Comprehensive Center on Brain Aging
Departments of Neurology, Psychiatry
Nursing, Nutrition and Population Health
New York University Langone Medical Center
New York, NY

Sumer Verma, MB, BS, MD
Associate Clinical Professor Psychiatry
Boston University School of Medicine
Boston, MA
Medical Director, Alzheimer's Program
Briarwood Healthcare and Rehabilitation
Center
Needham, MA

Anand Viswanathan, MD, PhD
Assistant Professor of Neurology
Harvard Medical School
Philip Kistler Stroke Research Center
Department of Neurology
Massachusetts General Hospital
Boston, MA

Jean-Paul G. Vonsattel, MD
Professor of Pathology
College of Physicians and Surgeons, and
Department of Pathology and Cell Biology
Director
New York Brain Bank
Taub Institute for Research on Alzheimer's
Disease and the Aging Brain
Columbia University Medical Center
and the New York Presbyterian Hospital
New York, NY

Sandra Weintraub, PhD, ABPP-CN
Professor of Psychiatry, Neurology and
Psychology
Director, Clinical Core
Northwestern Alzheimer's Disease Center
Cognitive Neurology and Alzheimer's Disease
Center
Northwestern University Feinberg School
of Medicine
Chicago, IL

Meredith Wicklund, MD
Assistant Professor of Neurology
University of Florida
Gainesville, FL

Kim C. Willment, PhD
Instructor in Psychology
Department of Psychiatry
Brigham & Women's Hospital and
Harvard Medical School
Boston, MA

Part I

Functional Neuroanatomy and Cognitive Neuroscience of Dementia

1

Cognitive Functions and the Cerebral Cortex

David Caplan

This chapter presents a brief overview of human cognitive functions and the organization of the cerebral cortex that supports them. It begins with a discussion of cognitive functions and then discusses their neural basis. It is focused on cortical organization and mentions subcortical mechanisms only briefly; Chapter 2 discusses the contribution of subcortical mechanisms and white matter connectivity to cognition and behavior in greater detail. The discussion in this chapter is at the "systems" level. Molecular and genetic processes that underlie the cognitive processes described here are only mentioned in relation to organizational features of the cortex.

Though the presentation is not clinically oriented, the material presented here has direct clinical applications as discussed elsewhere in this book. To the extent that cognitive functions are localized, the regional topography of different diseases associated with dementia, and progressive changes in the topography of neurodegenerative or other lesions over time, produce characteristic deficits that are critical to diagnosis and evolution of symptoms. From the point of view of management, understanding the cognitive deficits that give rise to symptomatology is essential to formulating an approach to monitoring of the effects of treatments.

Cognitive Functions

Overview

Like many terms, the word "cognitive" has an intuitive meaning for most educated laypersons and professionals, but it is hard to say exactly what it means or refers to. This chapter begins with a descriptive overview of cognition in an attempt to place it in a framework of factors that affect human behavior, and to say something about what it is.

One place to start is with the observation that cognition determines aspects of behavior in a way that differs from how other factors do. A fairly standard view of how cognition affects behavior is through "propositional attitudes"—beliefs (propositions) that constitute the contents of "attitudes" (e.g., desires), also called belief/desire psychology. Many of us take it for granted that believing something is true is being in a cognitive state. Consider believing the proposition that a train from Boston to New York leaves South Station at 9:14. That belief might affect behavior in the following way. A person wants to go to New York and also believes that it will take 90 minutes to wash, get dressed, have coffee, and to get to South Station. The combination of beliefs about departure time, preparation time, the need to leave a margin for the unexpected, and so on leads the person to the conclusion that, in order to satisfy the desire, she should get up at 7:15. This leads to the behavior of setting an alarm clock for 7:15.

Contrast this way of affecting behavior with other determinants of behavior, such as biological states (e.g., being hungry) and emotional states (e.g., being sad). Biological states lead to behaviors that one might characterize as resetting biological parameters: being hungry leads to eating, and being sleepy leads to sleeping. Emotions affect what are here called "attitudes." Being sad (or happy) may affect your desire to go to New York. Neither biological states nor emotions affect behavior by constituting the content of beliefs or by determining the relations between the contents of beliefs that enter into the chains of logic and association that underlie the relation of beliefs to behaviors. Emotions may affect the *formation* of beliefs (e.g., if a person is afraid of dogs, he may find it harder to believe that Fido is harmless), but they do not constitute the content of beliefs.

These intuitions suggest that there are different types of "forces" that affect behavior, but they do not provide a general answer to the question of what cognitive processes are. One way to put the question is: What is it about a belief that makes having one being in a "cognitive" state, as opposed to an emotion, being affected by which does not put one in a cognitive state? One possible answer is that cognitive processes are processes that operate on representations. The second is that cognitive processes are processes that operate on categories. Although both of these definitions/descriptions may be inadequate in part because they may not delineate a set of processes that fall together in a justifiable taxonomy of psychological/neurological states and processes, they will nonetheless frame the discussion because they provide insight into elements of cognition.

A representation is an expression that has two components: It conveys information about something else, and it is possible to perform operations on it that preserve the information that it conveys. In philosophical terms, it is semantically evaluable (it is possible to determine its reference, extension, truth) and it enters into a computational system by virtue of its syntactic features. For instance, a word is a representation. Put very informally, the *word* "table" represents the *concept* "TABLE" and the concept TABLE represents real tables. Put somewhat more formally, it is possible to evaluate whether the use of "table" to refer is satisfied by a particular item. The word "table" also enters into computations that retain the information "table" conveys, based upon its form (not based on what it represents). The rules of language allow the word "table" to be modified by the word "red," itself a representation of the concept of the color red, to produce the phrase "red table," a representation that retains a connection to both redness and tables. This view of representations is the one expressed in Fodor (1998); readers familiar with Turing's (1936) work will recognize his seminal idea of the computational roles of items being determined only by their syntactic properties.

The second way of defining/describing cognitive processes is as processes that operate on categories. A category is a substantive (as opposed to logical) term in a theory of some domain (i.e., "understanding of the workings of" that domain). "Lightning" is a category because it is a substantive term in a theory (i.e., in a person's understanding) of climate.[1] Seeing a flash of light as a bright white irregular form is a sensory response to a particular stimulus, but seeing a flash of light as a lightning bolt is an act of perceptual identification that categorizes the sensory information. What makes categories special is that we know things about them that we can exploit for other purposes. Having perceived a flash of light as a lightning bolt, a person knows a lot about the event, and this knowledge can result in behavior in the same way as what was described previously regarding setting an alarm. A person can think "lightning is a prelude to rain; I will count the seconds until I hear thunder and know when rain will start," which will lead to taking cover at a particular time.

These definitions/descriptions of representation and category have some desirable features. For instance, the description of representations excludes items such as smoke as a representation of fire, or rings of a tree as representations of the age of the tree. These items are semantically evaluable (smoke and tree rings convey information about fire and tree age, respectively, with some degree of reliability), but they do not enter into computational systems based on their forms. The description of cognitive processes as operating on categories as defined draws a line at points that seem reasonable. For instance, if the output of on-center off-surround retinal ganglion cells can be described as a "circle," and "circle" is a category in theories of object recognition, the process of transforming the output of rods and cones to the output of retinal ganglion cells is cognitive.[2] This would imply that operations that occur very early in the perceptual process and some that operate very late in motor execution are cognitive. This seems to be a perfectly reasonable conclusion, insofar as it allows many operations that are part of specific cognitive domains to be considered cognitive. However, not all operations are cognitive: Transduction of energy at sensory receptors is not a cognitive process, even though it is the first step in a process that eventuates in categories, because the output of a receptor is not itself a category.[3]

This effort to define "cognition" likely raises more questions than it answers, but it may be useful to review some of the considerations that arise when we try to determine what we mean by the term; this introduces concepts such as representation, category, and computation based on formal properties of an item that are ubiquitously associated with cognitive functions.

Moving on from these abstract considerations to actual practice, the term "cognitive" is applied to a wide set of functions. A partial list includes the abilities to categorize elements in the world, to relate categories to one another, to consciously retrieve events and facts from memory, to reason, to communicate, to set criteria for acting, to plan actions, and to estimate and monitor the consequences of one's actions on the physical and social world. Cognitive processes rank among the most important of the determinants of human behavior, are the most important factor in determining the success of the human species as a whole, and are arguably the most important factor in determining the success of the individual in his or her social setting in modern industrial and postindustrial societies.

At the psychological level, we can distinguish two main types of cognitive operations: "primary" and "control" operations. Primary operations are the basic processes that activate, transform, store, and retrieve information. They operate in sets that constitute perceptual, motor, memory, and language systems. Control operations set primary operations into action, stop and inhibit them, and shift the mind/brain to other operations. Control and primary operations work in tandem on a time scale of at least hundredths of a second.

Covering all cognitive systems, or even one in any depth, is not possible. The operations of the system that recognizes objects will be outlined next as an example of a primary cognitive system; then a simple task will be described in which object recognition is required to illustrate the nature of control.

Perceptual Identification, Recognition, and Categorization of Visually Presented Objects

When compared to other cognitive processes (e.g., thinking logically, making decisions about major life issues, writing a paper), perceptual identification and categorization of visually presented objects appear to be very simple. However, this process is more complex than one might think, and it illustrates how complex even the simplest cognitive processes are. The description that follows outlines the major aspects of this process.

The process of perception of visually presented objects begins with transduction of light by cones and rods in the retina. This first step has two properties that determine much of the process of perceptual identification. The first is that visual features of the object are segregated at the visual receptors: Cones are sensitive to color and rods are not; this requires that later operations integrate these separated visual elements into a single item. The second is that a three-dimensional object in the world is projected onto the two-dimensional retinal surface; this requires that later operations reconstruct the three-dimensional object from its two-dimensional projection.

Neurologically, the separation of visual features of objects continues through lateral geniculate, visual koniocortex (V1), and unimodal visual association cortex, in the selective sensitivity of magno- and parvo-cellular neurons, blobs, interblobs, and other anatomically identifiable groupings of neurons. Visual features are derived from complex

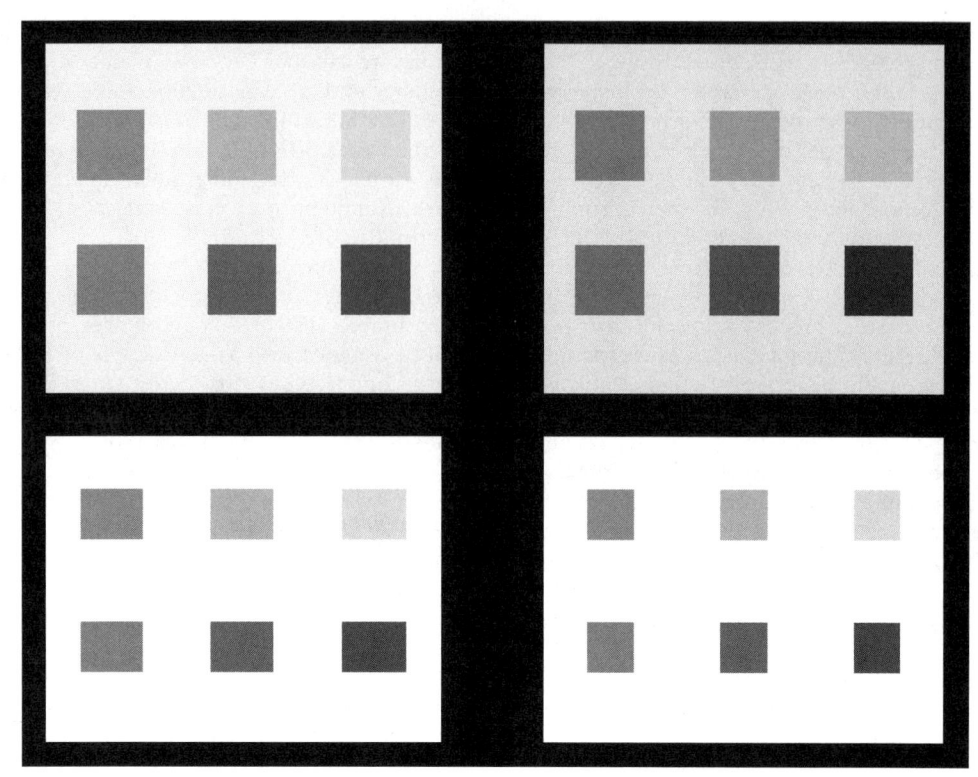

Figure 1.1 Color constancy. The color patches in the top and bottom figures are the same but are matched differently across the left and right rectangles as a function of the color of the background. (See color plate section)

interactions of sets of neurons. Lines, for instance, result in part from topographic projections of retinal on-center-off-surround and off-center-on-surround neurons onto lateral geniculate nucleus and from topographic projections of neurons in lateral geniculate nucleus onto individual neurons in V1, and in part from sensitivity of V1 neurons to first derivatives of luminance (see Fig. 1.1). Perceived color results from integration of the wavelength of the attended item with wavelengths throughout the visual field. Figure 1.1 shows patches of identical colors, which are matched differently depending upon the color of their context. This integration of local wavelength with wavelengths in a broader part of the visual field is the reason that colors are perceived in environments such as jungles, in which most of the light is in the green portion of the spectrum. It requires integration of retinal receptors with cortical neurons, hence the name "retinex theory" (Land, 1974).

Features such as lines, color, and texture are regrouped into retinotopic objects—two-dimensional reconstructions of the objects that produce retinal responses. A large number of mechanisms have been proposed to apply at this stage of processing on the basis of physiological and psychological studies. Examples of mechanisms are the Gestalt laws of closure, proximity, good continuation, and others (Fig. 1.2) and the use of texture to produce shape (Fig. 1.3), of shading to produce contour (Fig. 1.4), of angles to produce surfaces (Fig. 1.5), and of completion to produce shape (Fig. 1.6). In one model, a critical aspect of this process is the activation of a limited set of basic shapes ("geons") that are constituents of objects (Fig. 1.7).

Retinotopic objects are situated in retinal-, head-, and body-centered coordinates, and are therefore useful for navigation and manipulation. However, they need to be related to items in long-term memory to access the rich array of information that a viewer has about the object. Most theories maintain that accessing this information includes a step of activating an object-centered visual representation of the object, known as its "structural

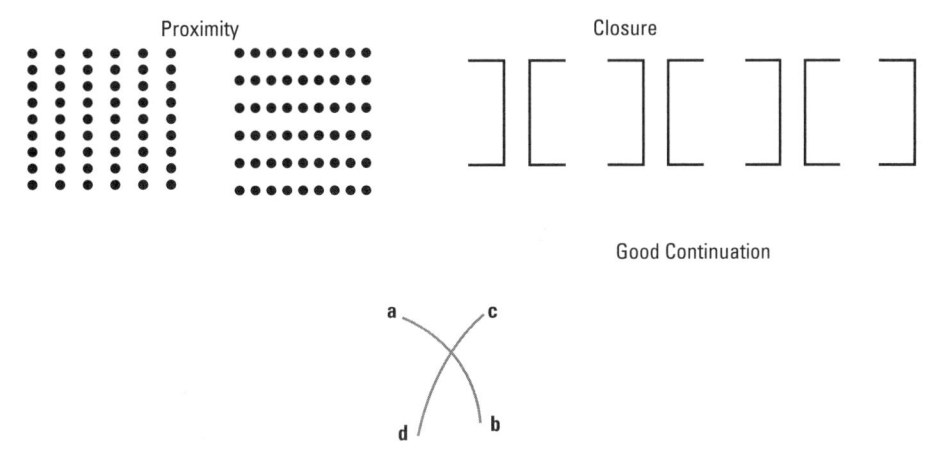

Figure 1.2 Gestalt principles of proximity, closure, and good continuation. Dots spaced closer together are seen as lines; lines that form closed shapes are seen as related; lines that are slowly curved (*a-b; c-d*) are seen as continuous, while lines that form sharp angles (*a-c; b-d*) are not.

description." A structural description can be thought of as the equivalent, in the domain of visual object recognition, of a long-term memory of the form of a word. Just as it is necessary to recognize a written or spoken item as a word to access the meaning and other features of that word, it is necessary to recognize the form of a visually presented object to access other features of that object. This process may be called "perceptual identification."

There is considerable debate about what structural descriptions of objects consist of. Neuropsychological data have been interpreted as suggesting that structural descriptions are idealized object-centered depictions of objects in a "canonical" projection in which the principal axes of symmetry and elongation and distinctive visual features are displayed, and that objects displayed in other projections are mentally rotated to match these canonical representations (Fig. 1.8) (Humphreys & Riddoch, 1987).

Structural descriptions must be sufficiently general to allow visually different items of the same sort to be perceptually identified as instances of the same type of an object, and, at the same time, sufficiently constraining to exclude items that are similar but not of the same sort. For instance, each snowflake is unique and the structural description of a snowflake must be sufficiently broad to allow all snowflakes to be mapped onto it but also sufficiently constraining to stop items with certain similarities to snowflakes from being recognized as snowflakes (e.g., tiny paper

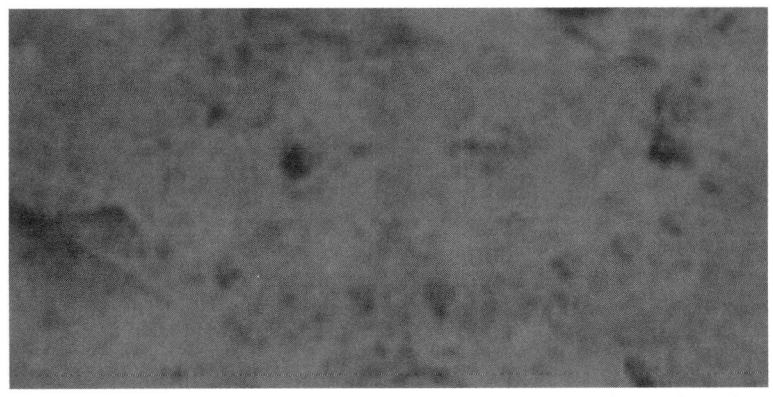

Figure 1.3 Shape derived from texture cues. The picture shows a camouflaged flounder.

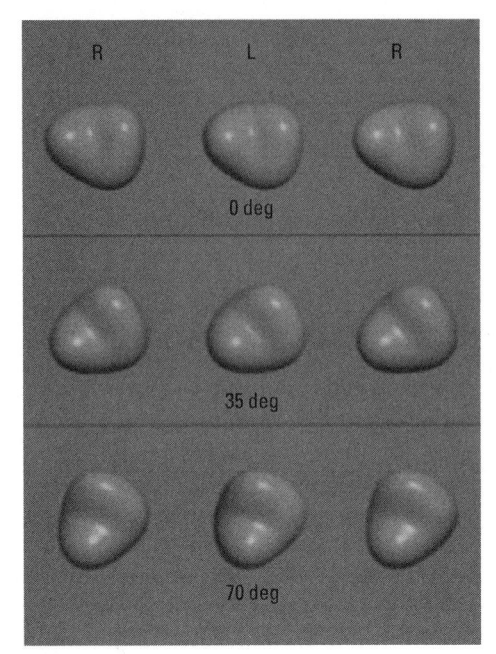

Figure 1.4 Depth derived from shading.

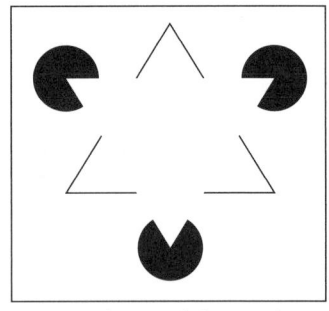

Figure 1.6 Completion of shape. The boundaries of the perceived triangle are largely physically absent.

snowflake cutouts). In models in which there is a single structural description for an object, that memory must be an abstract schema that specifies possible visual properties of objects.

No matter how they are represented, structural descriptions are distinguished from one another in a way that corresponds to object categories, which depend on the way a person divides the world into concepts. A structural description is one aspect of an object concept—an object-centered schema or amalgamation of its visual features—that is used to access the concept from visually presented instances (in this respect it differs from the form of a word, which is not part of the concept that it allows access to). Activating a structural description is the step in the visual process that maps visually presented items into concepts. It is also the last purely visual step in that process; further processing deals with properties of concepts that are not purely visual.

Accessing a concept from its structural description can be called "object recognition." Although object recognition is closely related to perceptual identification, there is neuropsychological evidence that it is a separate step in processing (Humphreys & Riddoch, 1987). Patients with "apperceptive agnosia" have a variety of problems mapping visual items onto structural descriptions (Fig. 1.9). In contrast, patients with "associative agnosia" have trouble describing features of objects despite being able to activate structural descriptions (as evidenced, for instance, by being able to match different instances of an object, or an object presented from different viewpoints).

Object recognition unlocks the door leading to information about the object concepts that structural descriptions are part of. Recognizing a visually presented item as a car informs the viewer about items that are likely to be in certain locations within the percept (a transmission under the hood; seats behind a steering wheel), functional properties of the percept (it will move in certain ways under certain conditions), social and utilitarian properties of the percept (its cost; its role in commuting), and others. Several features of these properties are worth noting. First, some of them are visual, and some are not; some psychologists

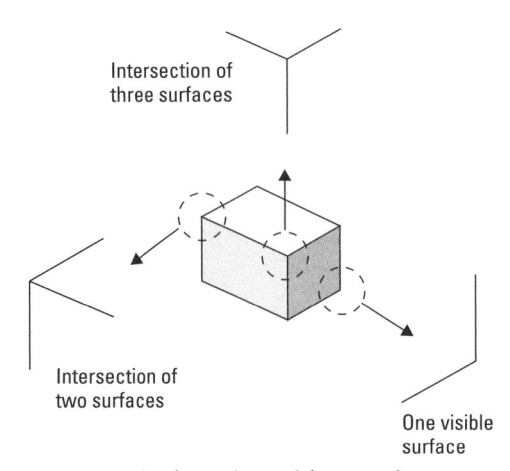

Figure 1.5 Surfaces derived from angles.

(A) Geons

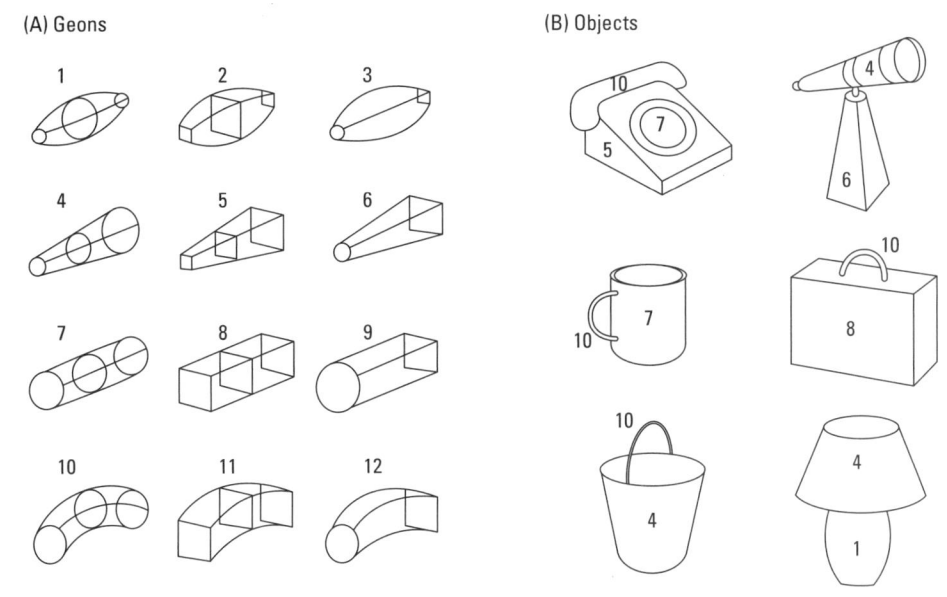

(B) Objects

Figure 1.7 Postulated geons and their relation to shapes of objects.

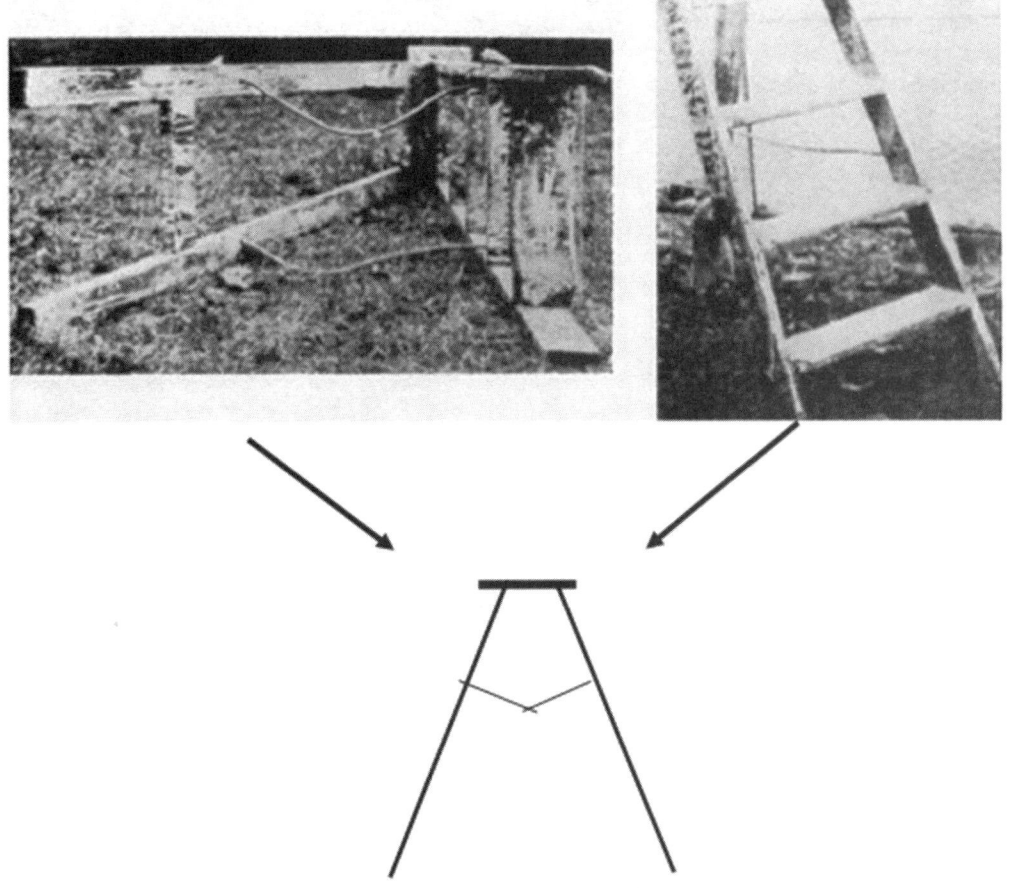

Figure 1.8 Cartoon of a structural description of a stepladder, showing orientation invariance.

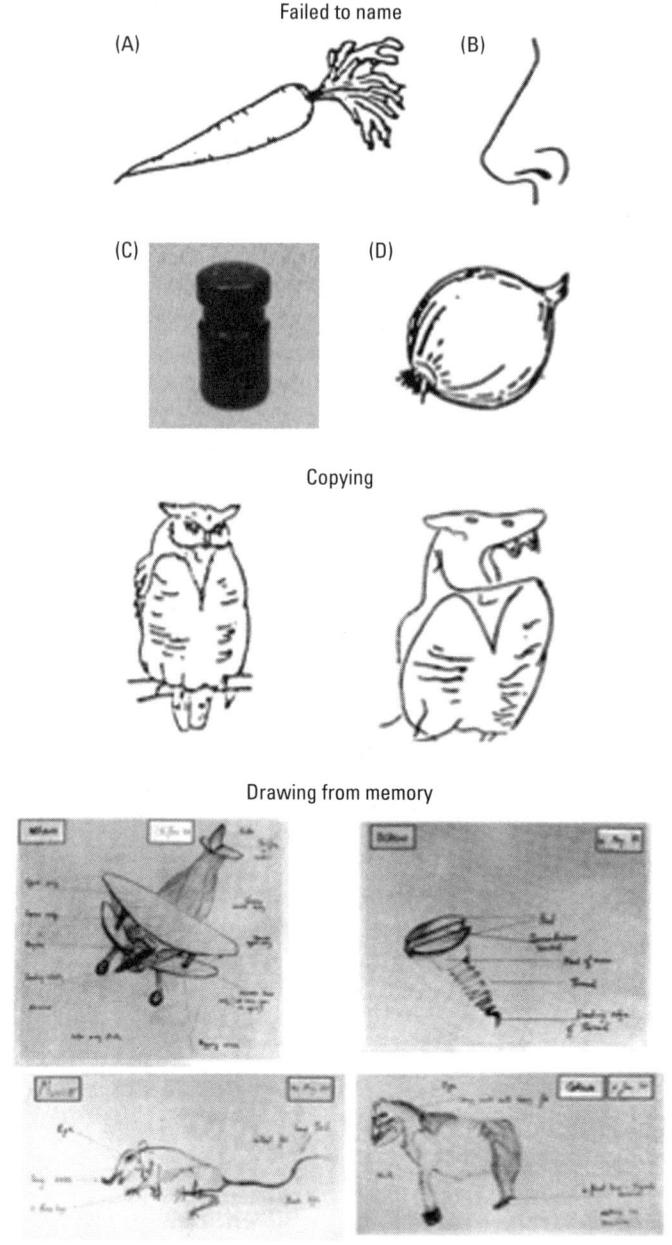

Figure 1.9 Integrative agnosia. The patient could not name objects in *A*. Copy (*B*) is focused on visually salient features that are misinterpreted with respect to the object. Drawing from memory (*C*) is excellent. The deficit lies in perceptual identification of visually presented objects.

believe there are separate "semantic memory" systems for visual and nonvisual features of objects (Paivio, 1986). Second, none of these features are part of the structural description of a car; they are all accessed through a structural description, according to the model presented. Third, any one of these features may or may not be part of a person's concept of cars. This last point leads to a discussion of what concepts are (note that the ideas of "concepts," "categories," and word "meanings" are highly related).

Thinking on the part of clinically oriented neurologists about concepts, and the related question of the meaning of words, has been heavily influenced by British empiricist philosophy, which emphasized the associations between information derived from different sensory modalities in forming a concept (Geschwind, 1965a, 1965b). Though there is no agreement about the answer to the questions "What are concepts?" and "What are word meanings?," the philosophical and psychological literature clearly shows that the view of concepts and word meanings as combinations of perceptual and motor features is too narrow, for two reasons.

First, concepts are not just combinations of features in instances of a concept that have been experienced, since we can classify new instances as falling under a concept. It may be the case that a person has only encountered tables made of wood, or tables that cost less than $3,000, but his or her concept of tables need not include the property "made of wood" or "costs less than $3,000"; these can be considered to be incidental properties of tables that he or she has experienced. Concepts are counterfactually supporting: If conditions x_1–x_n instantiate a concept, the concept would be instantiated if conditions x_1–x_n occurred, even if those conditions never *could* occur. If light rays could be manipulated to allow objects to come to a stable position on a surface parallel to the ground (and if something that allows objects to come to a stable position on a surface parallel to the ground is a table), a table could be made of light rays (the problem with making a table out of light rays is not that the concept of a table does not allow it to be made out of light rays, but that light rays cannot be manipulated in the required way).

Second, concepts are delineated in terms of intentions. Tables serve the function of allowing objects to rest on them, but an object is not a table simply because it allows objects to rest on it; it requires the intention on someone's part that it be used that way. A tree stump is not a table unless someone intends to use it as one; a table can be a desk (and vice versa) depending on intentions. Fodor (1998) noted in connection with the concept "to paint," that if you dip a paintbrush into a jar of paint and apply the paint to a wall with the intention of painting the wall, you have painted the wall but you have not painted the paintbrush.

Aristotle proposed that the set of properties that constitutes a concept (i.e., the "essential" properties of a concept) are those that are individually necessary and jointly sufficient to classify an item in a category (Aristotle, 1995). This formulation encounters a major problem in practice: The features that are necessary and sufficient for a concept are hard to determine. For natural categories, we can turn to experts in the relevant science, but science is always incomplete. For human-made items, it is even less clear what these features are. Thousands of years of study have failed to identify such features for almost any nonnatural concept (Wittgenstein [1921/1961] famously discussed the concept "game"). Many alternatives to the Aristotelian view have been proposed (see Margolis and Laurence [1991] for readings). One commonly invoked alternative is that concepts are determined by prototypes, whose features are not necessarily necessary and sufficient to determine a concept but are typical of items that fall under the concept. The idea that concepts are determined by a prototypical instance and a metric that determines the distance of any item from the prototype in a multidimensional space accounts for a great deal of psychological data regarding recognition and memory of items. It does, however, have significant limitations. The most important limitation is that prototypes of concepts do not combine to form other concepts. The prototypical fish for most Americans is perhaps a trout, perch, salmon, or some other medium-sized fish; the prototypical pet is a dog or a cat; but the prototypical pet fish is a goldfish or another small fish that survives in a glass bowl, not the combination of a trout and a dog. Fodor (1998) has argued that no existing theory answers the question of what a concept is; in his view, concepts are whatever the mind "locks" or "resonates" to when presented with prototypical instances. This view serves a number of philosophical purposes in his work, but it clearly leaves many basic questions unanswered.

Whatever they are, concepts are related to one another. The concept DOG is related to the concept ANIMAL by inclusion, to the concept TAIL by possession, and to the concept FRIEND by association. Tulving (1972) introduced the concept of "semantic memory" to describe a long-term memory system that contained "the organized knowledge a person possess[es] about words and other verbal symbols, their meaning and referents, about relations among them, and about rules, formulas, and algorithms for the manipulation of these symbols, concepts and relations" (p. 386). Concepts can be thought of as "nodes" in a network of associations and rule-related information in semantic memory.

One aspect of the network within which a concept is located that has received considerable attention is its hierarchical structure. Placing a concept within this hierarchy is one aspect of categorization. Concepts can be categorized at various levels of a hierarchy; for instance, Tibetan Terriers are dogs, which are mammals, which are animals. For many concepts, there is a "basic" level of categorization, characterized by items at this level inheriting relatively few features from the items above them, transmitting many features to the items below them, having considerable overlap in physical features with other items at the same level, being the most frequently referenced items in the hierarchy that includes them, and other properties. For example, most people consider "dog" to be the basic level in the hierarchy "Tibetan Terrier—dog—mammal—animal."

The basic level is relevant to perceptual identification: Most people recognize instances of dogs as dogs, not as species. However, expertise can change the basic level, with effects on perceptual identification and object recognition (Tanaka & Gauthier, 1997). The effect of expertise is to promote subordinate levels of the hierarchy to basic-level concepts. Since perceptual identification activates structural descriptions of basic-level categories, which differ as a function of expertise, what people with different levels of expertise "see" differs. Most people would "see" a Tibetan Terrier as a dog. My wife and I own Tibetan Terriers and are experts on what they look like, and, for us, "Tibetan Terrier" is the basic-level category in the hierarchy "Tibetan Terrier—dog—mammal—animal." My wife and I "see" Tibetan Terriers as Tibetan Terriers and can spot one at 100 paces.

A relatively simple cognitive "system" has been outlined in this section, showing several of its features. One is that, from the very first, the appearance of simplicity is deceiving; early aspects of object perception, such as color perception, are themselves complex processes. A second is that the process is shot through and through with effects of intentionality: We "see" (i.e., perceptually identify) objects that are visually presented instances of concepts, which require intention. Once we have perceptually identified an object, we activate the concept it is part of (what is here called "recognition") and often categorize it. The concept and its higher level categorization then can be used in other cognitive processes.

The way perceptual identification, recognition, and categorization of visually presented objects works is true of all primary cognitive processes. What differ across cognitive domains are the specific categories that are activated and the operations whereby this is achieved. Perception of spoken language, for instance, involves activation of categories such as the sound "/b/," the syntactic structure called "noun phrase," and the discourse-level structure called "topic"; none of these categories are activated when people identify objects on the basis of the their visual properties. As we have reviewed in visual object recognition, domain-specific categories are activated by specialized subroutines. In the case of language, such subroutines range from mapping acoustic waveforms onto linguistically relevant features of sounds through recognizing the form of a sentence and the content of a discourse. The extent to which the subroutines in different cognitive domains apply the same basic mechanisms to different categories is a topic of study (Anderson et al., 2004).

Control

Processes such as those described previously in the area of visual perception are subject to control. Control processes set goals, set criteria for success, deploy attention to input, choose operations to accomplish goals, plan sequences of operations and inhibit other sequences, and select responses. Control operations differ from the "basic" processes reviewed before inasmuch as they do not operate on a representation or a category themselves. Rather, they initiate, terminate, and enhance processes, such as those described previously, that do.

Basic processes do not operate normally or, in many cases, do not operate at all, without the involvement of control processes. This applies even to very early perceptual operations. For instance, perceptual identification and object recognition do not take place, or, at least, do not take place normally, if an object is not attended (see Wolfe & Bennett [1997], for evidence that unattended objects are perceived as "feature bundles," not as objects). Phenomena such as "change blindness" (failure to notice a difference between two images that are identical except for one change) provide evidence that items that are unattended are not registered in memory. Classic experiments using dichotic listening (playing different sounds to each ear) have shown that subjects cannot report the speech played to the unattended ear if they are required to understand speech played to the attended ear (Cherry, 1953; Treisman, 1964), indicating that unattended speech is processed only very "superficially." This is not to say that unattended items are not processed at all. Visual attention is attracted to unattended areas in the visual field that are visually dissimilar, or that change rapidly, indicating that unattended areas are processed to some degree (Wolfe, 1994); speech played to an unattended ear affects short-term memory for items played to the attended ear (Macken, Tremblay, Alford, & Jones, 1999), showing that it is not completely "blocked out." However, the level to which unattended items are processed is not sufficient to sustain the cognitive operations outlined previously.

Control processes are complex, as we have seen is the case with basic processes. For instance, attention has been divided along many lines. Different analyses have argued that it includes vigilance (being in a state that allows one to detect and respond to stimuli), selective attention (focusing on one of several stimuli), sustained attention (retaining attention on one item), divided attention (focusing on more than one item at a time, and/or switching from deploying attention to one item to deploying attention to another), and specialized attention processes such as visually directed attention. The processes of setting goals, setting criteria for success, choosing operations to accomplish goals, and other control processes have also been modeled in ways that include multiple subdivisions and subprocesses. As was the case for basic processes, it is impossible to review the entire range of control processes in this chapter. Instead, control processes will be illustrated through one simple example that builds on the discussion of visual object recognition. See Chapter 3 for additional discussion of control processes in the context of executive functions.

Imagine you are placed before a computer screen, as shown in Figure 1.10, and required to use a mouse to move a cursor from the resting spot (the rectangle) to the picture designated by a word you hear over headphones; when you finish one trial, you have to push a button to ask for the next. Performing this very simple task requires many steps. One possible set of steps is as follows: attending to the two pictures and processing them to the point of object recognition and concept activation; storing the representations that have been activated (e.g., the concepts evoked by the pictures) in memory for later use; attending to the spoken word and processing it to the point of activation of its meaning (for

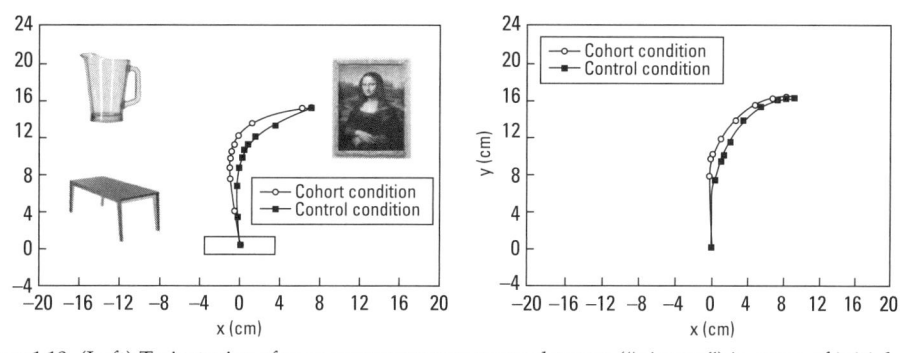

Figure 1.10 (Left) Trajectories of mouse movements toward target ("picture") in cases of initial phonological cohort competitor ("pitcher") and noncompetitor ("table"), showing continuous attraction of the phonological cohort competitor. (Right) Simulation based on interaction of phonological representation of target and foil interacting with perception of spoken word.

present purposes, its meaning can be considered to be the concept it evokes); comparing the concepts derived from object recognition with the meaning of the word; determining which concept-meaning pair is most similar; determining the location of the picture that corresponds to the concept that most closely matches the meaning of the word; planning a motor action that uses the mouse to move the cursor to that picture; and executing that program.

The task involves many control processes. The first "decision" is whether the set of steps outlined is going to be used. Here is another set of steps that would accomplish the task, which differs in the italicized steps: attending to the two pictures and processing them to the point of object recognition and concept activation; *activating the sound of the word that corresponds to the concepts activated by the pictures*; storing representations that have been activated (e.g., the *sounds* evoked by the pictures) in memory for later use; attending to the spoken word and *recognizing its sounds*; comparing the *sounds* derived from object recognition with the *sounds* of the word; determining which pair *of sounds* is most similar; determining the location of the picture that corresponds to the *sound* that most closely matches the *sound* of the word; planning a motor action that uses the mouse to move the cursor to that picture; and executing that program. A participant in the study would have to decide whether to use a semantic/conceptual basis for matching the word and the picture, a sound-based basis, or both. Whatever decision is made, the relevant operations have to be turned on. If a semantic/conceptual mechanism is used, the word has to be processed to the level of meaning; if a sound-based mechanism is used, the pictures have to be processed to the level of sounds. Even if one were to say that all these operations happen without control once a person attends to a picture or a word (which is doubtful; it is unlikely that we activate words for every object we perceive), control processes are required to compare the sounds or concepts that are the basis for the similarity judgment.

There is also the issue of the order to do things in. One could process one, or neither, of the pictures before one hears the word; one could process both pictures before processing the word and, if that made it impossible to process the word, one could stop processing the pictures or could try to store the sound of the word in memory and return to trying to understand it after one had finished processing both pictures. In fact, things could, and probably sometimes do, get much more complicated. If one were unsure about which concept-meaning pair or pair of sounds was most similar, it might be useful, or necessary, to reanalyze one or both pictures to see whether some other concept, which is closer to the meaning of the word and/or that has a different sound, could be evoked by a picture, and repeat the whole comparison-picture selection-motor planning process. The fact that timing of the processes in this task is flexible and might be changed depending on the results of the operations means that the operations listed previously have to be scheduled.

The choice of operations and their order is just one of many control problems that a participant in this simple task must deal with. Each of the operations listed in the decomposition of this task requires control, at the least in terms of shifting attention. And each of the operations listed in the decomposition of this task significantly understates the complexity of that "stage" of processing and has additional control operations embedded within it. Consider, for instance, the "response selection" process. In many models of this process (Ratcliff, 1978), the decision to make a response occurs when evidence in favor of that response reaches a threshold. At the onset of a trial, the evidence favoring both pictures is equal; as the trial progresses and the operations described previously are accomplished, evidence accrues favoring one picture over another. When evidence for a response reaches a threshold, that response is selected. The resting state of the evidence accumulator is a function of the probabilities of the set of choices, and the "drift rate" of evidence accrual is a function of the efficiency of the "basic" processes that analyze the input; the response threshold, however, is under participants' control. Older people, for instance, set higher thresholds (are more conservative) than younger people (Ratcliff, Thapar, & McKoon, 2011).

The discussion has focused so far on control processes that are internal to a task: scheduling and initiating operations, and setting certain parameters such as response selection thresholds. It is worth returning to the original outline of control processes and to note that these are the last items on that list: deploying attention to input, choosing operations to accomplish goals, planning sequences of operations and inhibiting other sequences, and selecting responses.[4] The first two items on the list should not be forgotten: setting goals and setting criteria for success. During all the activity described previously, the goal of the task must be maintained, and, at the end of each trial, the fact that the goal of the task has been satisfied must be established. The total extent of the control needed in this very simple task is hard to estimate; computer-based models that actually do tasks such as this routinely require much more control than experimental psychologists expect (Meyer & Keiras, 1997a, 1997b).

Interactions of Different Cognitive Domains

Examples of basic and control cognitive functions have been drawn from specific domains such as object recognition and word recognition. These domains interact; as with domain-specific operations themselves, this interaction occurs over very short time intervals (centiseconds). It is possible to name a familiar picture in less than 250 milliseconds, showing that the result of visual object recognition and categorization can be forwarded to word activation in a very short period of time. A dramatic example of the interaction of one domain (object recognition) with another (planning movement) is catching an object. When a person catches an object, she not only moves her body, arm, and hand in a way such that the trajectory of the movement intersects the trajectory of the object at a point where the object can be grasped. In addition, the person must program the force of the grasp in a way that is related to the nature of the object: Less force is exerted on an egg than on a baseball. This means that, if the object is not seen until after it is released, the object recognition system interacts with the system that computes the trajectory of the object and the motor planning system in the brief period during which the object is perceived and the action planned and executed.

One might expect that domains such as object recognition, trajectory estimation, and motor planning would be integrated, but integration of domains seems to be the general case. The experiment described, in which a person must move a curser to one of two pictures upon hearing a word, documents a case in which the output of one domain affects ongoing processing in another. If the distracter picture is named by a word that begins with the same sound as the target, the trajectory of the curser movement is bowed toward the distracter, compared to a situation in which the distracter and target start with different sounds (Fig. 1.10) (Spivey, Grosjean, & Knoblich, 2005). This shows that the concepts activated by the pictures activate words, that matching of the spoken word to the pictures is based not only on conceptual properties but also on phonological features of these words, and that this match interacts either with the perception of the word or the planning of motor movements. Computer simulations indicate that it can interact with the perception of the word (Fig. 1.10), which would indicate that there is a very rapid interaction of processes that can arise in association with picture identification (activation of the sound of the word that corresponds to the concept depicted in the picture) with those that recognize sounds from acoustic waveforms.

Closing Comments on Cognition

The presentation to this point begins to illustrate the nature and the extent of the operations that we can call "cognitive" under some definition of this term. They range from early vision through motor planning and include memory, language, higher level thought, and numerous control processes. The presentation begins to illustrate the truly daunting complexity of the basic operations, interactions, and control processes that occur in fractions of a second to produce behavior.

Before moving on to neurological issues, it is worth returning to the point that started this section: that cognition affects behavior by creating the content of propositional attitudes and connecting the propositions in these states to one another. The discussion so far does not deal with this but rather focuses on "lower level" aspects of cognition (though concepts and language would hardly be considered "lower level" compared to many neurological functions). There are three points about this that deserve additional brief discussion.

The first is that processes called cognitive (applying the criteria at the beginning of the chapter) affect behavior in more than one way. Object perception and language comprehension can affect behavior without running through fixation of belief. If you respond to the request "please pass the salt" by understanding it, looking for the salt, recognizing it, and getting and passing it over, you have behaved in response to cognitive operations that have nothing to do with fixation of belief. Fixation of belief, and its relation to desires, is one way—perhaps the most important way, but who knows?—that cognition affects behavior. With an expanded vision of how cognition affects behavior, we appreciate the pervasiveness of cognitive functions in human life even more.

Second, the output of modular processes is used to fixate beliefs. Relating the meanings of words to one another in propositions is probably the major source of information in semantic memory, and it requires word recognition, comprehension, sentence analysis and comprehension, and many other basic operations.

Third, little is known about how beliefs are fixated. This is what some consider to be one of the two highest areas of cognition at the frontiers of scientific understanding (the other being consciousness). From a mechanistic point of view, however, the basic types of operations outlined previously—lawful transformation of semantically evaluable symbols—have been argued to be the types of operation that apply in these processes (Fodor, 1998). There is some reason to be hopeful that, if we can understand cognitive operations at lower, domain-specific, levels, both psychologically and neurologically, the features we discover about them will be relevant to these higher levels as well.

Neural Mechanisms

Overview

Operations of the sort described previously have been related to neural activity in a variety of ways. Studies in animals have shown that long-term changes in synaptic numbers and activity, associated with gene expression, accompany the acquisition of stable long-term behaviors, such as habituation (Bailey, Bartsch, & Kandel, 1996). These types of neural events are thought to underlie long-term memories. Episodic changes in stimulus conditions and behavioral responses are associated with short-term stimulus- and response-related changes in spike trains, synaptic function, and other cellular physiologic markers of plasticity. Electrophysiological, metabolic, and neurovascular imaging in humans shows systematic relations to stimuli and behaviors. These studies provide the basis for models of the neural substrates for operations of the sort described previously. Along with studies of the effects of lesions, these data have clearly documented regional functional specialization of the brain. Evidence for a more widely distributed basis for cognitive functions also exists. Before turning to examples of localized and distributed functions, two general issues will be briefly discussed: the determinants of neural involvement in a function, and the nature of neural "networks."

The function of an area of the brain is in part determined by intrinsic properties of the neurons it contains, and in part by their connectivity (itself partly intrinsically determined). The role of intrinsic factors is easy to see at the sensory periphery, where receptor cells (e.g., cones, hair cells) contain elements that allow for the transduction of particular forms of energy. The features of cells in more central areas of the brain that allow them to accomplish the operations they do is less clear, but the finding of cells with specific morphology exclusively (Purkinje cells) or predominantly (Betz cells) in certain areas suggests that their intrinsic properties are highly connected or essential to the functions of those areas. The operations that particular cell layers play in particular functional domains have begun to be understood by the combination of theoretical modeling and experimental studies (Olson & Grossberg, 1998). These operations are not completely determined by the input to these layers, pointing to intrinsic features of cells in particular cortical layers in different brain regions contributing to the computational functions of the neuron. At a larger scale level, cytoarchitectonic, receptotonic, and other features of cortical organization are among the intrinsic properties of cell organization that contribute to, or determine, their functions (Zilles & Amunts, 2010).

The second factor that determines the function of an area is its input, both in the obvious sense that cells can only respond to the type of information they receive and in the less obvious sense that cell responses are in part caused by the patterns of their input (Mesulam, 1998). The effect of input (and input-output pairings) is to trigger molecular and genetic events that shape or determine features of cells such as synaptic elements that in turn affect future responses of the neuron (Bailey et al., 1996). The effect of input is greater in younger animals and can be quite dramatic: In neonatal ferrets whose visual cortex has been ablated, when connections are experimentally established from retinal receptor to medial geniculate cells (rather than the normal retinal to lateral geniculate pathway), responses to visual stimuli can be detected in auditory cortex (which receives medial geniculate afferents) that are very similar to those normally detected in primary visual cortex (Angelucci et al., 1998).[5]

Turning to the notion of "neural networks," this aspect of neural organization is directly related to the "systems"-level analyses presented here. Although the focus here will be on the scientific challenge of characterizing the functions of the parts of a "network," it is worth noting that there is also a challenge in delineating "networks." All behaviors involve coordinated activity of multiple brain areas, but one hesitates to say that the set of brain structures that support a person's responding to the request "pass the salt," which include areas that process language, those responsible for the perceptual identification of the salt, and those that plan and execute the motor response, are all one "network." Intuitions suggest there are three systems involved in this behavior, but the boundaries of systems/networks are hard to draw. The relation between words and concepts and the influence of concepts on perceptual identification raise the question of whether aspects of language and visual object recognition constitute a "network," and the integrated nature of object recognition and motor planning (illustrated in the example of catching an egg) raises questions about whether perceptual identification and motor planning do so. There is empirical evidence regarding these large-scale sets of areas. Functional connectivity patterns in resting-state functional magnetic resonance imaging (fMRI) have identified sets of structures that correspond to what has traditionally been considered the motor network, a network underlying attention, and other systems, including a previously unimagined "default network" that appears to play a role in non-stimulus-directed cognitive activity and which appears to be particularly vulnerable to degeneration in Alzheimer's disease (Buckner et al., 2005; De Luca, Beckmann, De Stefano, Matthews, & Smith, 2006). Such evidence helps define networks.

As is the case regarding cognition itself, the literature on the neural correlates of cognitive functions is vast, even excluding work at the molecular and genetic levels, and cannot be covered in any depth and breadth in this chapter. Once again, results will be reviewed in one area that are representative of more general features of the neural organization that supports cognition. In keeping with the systems-level discussion in this chapter, data will be reviewed from physiological, imaging, and lesion studies. For continuity with the first part of this chapter, the example employed will review the neural correlates of aspects of visual object recognition.

Neurological Correlates of Aspects of Visual Object Recognition

As discussed in the section on "Perceptual Identification, Recognition, and Categorization of Visually Presented Objects," the processes of visual object perceptual identification and object recognition reconstructs three-dimensional representations that contain many visual features (shape, color, texture) from a two-dimensional retinal image in which these features are segregated and associates other properties with this representation. In this section, four of the many processes that apply in this transformation will be discussed: construction of three-dimensional object-centered shapes from luminance, aspects of binding different visual features, identification of one special class of objects (faces), and activation of concepts. The discussion is largely based on Connor et al. (2009), Goebel and de Weerd (2009), and McKone et al. (2009).

Reconstruction of Three-Dimensional Object-Centered Representations

The construction of three-dimensional representations from two-dimensional input is an extremely difficult and computationally expensive process, so much so that many operational systems that "recognize" and manipulate objects avoid it and instead rely instead on object-centered two-dimensional reconstructions (Fei-Fei, Fergus, & Perona, 2006). The computational problem is that the retina contains approximately 10^6 channels of information in a two-dimensional array, which must be compressed into a single piece of information representing a three-dimensional object. Despite the obvious challenge this compression poses, there are a number of proposals regarding how three-dimensional object-centered representations might be constructed by the nervous system that have received empirical support. One such proposal will be reviewed here, based on progressively higher order geometric derivatives of luminance.

Visual stimuli yield a nonrandom pattern of retinal luminance that can be summarized in terms of progressively higher order contrast derivatives. Areas with little change have small first-order derivatives, while areas with larger changes have larger first-order derivatives (Fig. 1.11A); the former are guides to surfaces and the latter to boundaries between surfaces. Higher order derivatives (Fig. 1.11B) can be used to describe curves. The continuity and smoothness of most object boundaries can be summarized as combinations of first- and second-order derivatives.

Neurophysiological correlates of these transformations have been discovered in the tuning curves of neurons. Some neurons in V1 interblobs (areas of V1 that stain less intensely for cytochrome oxidase) and V2 interstripe regions (one of two areas of V2 that V1 interblobs project to) with small receptive fields can be modeled as being sensitive to first-order derivatives of luminance that are oriented in particular directions; that is, their tuning curves are sensitive to orientation and spatial frequency (Hubel & Weisel, 1959, 1962). These neurons respond to both chromatic and achromatic stimuli. Local increases in activity of these orientation-frequency sensitive neurons can be thought of as representing short oriented lines, which are parts of object boundaries. V4 neurons have larger receptive fields in which object boundaries can no longer be expressed as a single first-order derivative of luminance. However, some V4 neurons have tuning functions in the curvature/orientation domain that can be expressed as a combination of first- and second-order derivatives (Pasupathy & Connor, 1999). For instance, the cells depicted in Figure 1.12 respond to sharp convex curvature oriented to the left. Other V4 neurons respond to combinations of boundary fragments in fixed relations to one another, regardless of the overall shape of the object (Brincat & Connor, 2004). Studies of cell populations have shown how these sets of boundary fragments could be assembled into complete shape representations (Pasupathy & Connor, 2002). Some neurons in posterior inferior temporal lobe (PIT) and higher levels of the ventral visual pathway are tuned for spatial configurations of boundary configurations, independent of retinal position (Ito, Tamura, Fujita, & Tanaka, 1995). Figure 1.13 shows the response profile of a PIT neuron that responds to an ellipse in the top left and a rectangle in the bottom right of its receptive field. The fact that these

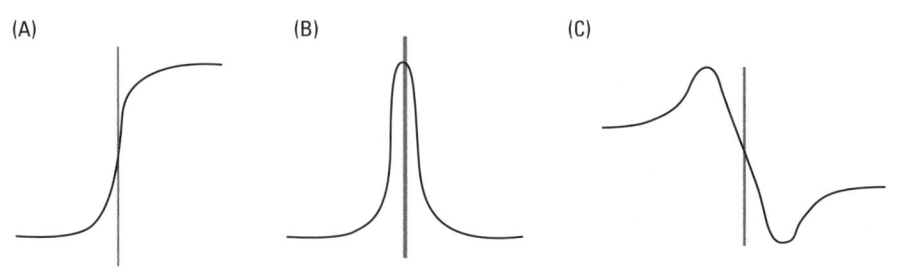

Figure 1.11 (A) Base curve. (B) First-order derivative of A at point of vertical line. (C) Second-order derivative of A at point of vertical line.

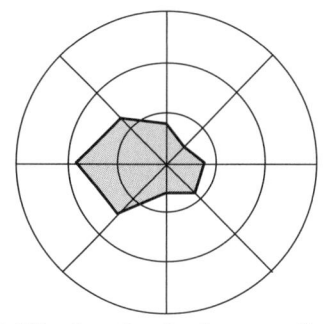

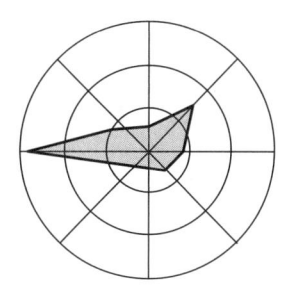

Figure 1.12 Effective stimulus for two cells in V4 (sharp convex curvature oriented to the left).

responses are independent of retinal position and scale with object size moves them from a retinotopic to an object-centered reference frame. The further step from these two-dimensional object-centered representations to three-dimensional object-centered representations may in part take place in more anterior portions of the inferior temporal gyrus, where some cells respond to three-dimensional spatial configurations of surface fragments characterized by their three-dimensional orientations and joint principal curvatures (Fig. 1.14) (Yamane, Carlson, Bowman, Wang, & Connor, 2008).

A related process consists of reconstructing object surfaces. The reconstruction of the surfaces of viewed objects has been modeled in at least three ways. Active interpolation models maintain that surface reconstruction involves interpolation of surface features from edges. Multiscale spatial frequency models create surface representations from low-frequency information. Both these models maintain that surfaces are created in retinotopic visual areas; they differ inasmuch as multiscale spatial frequency models rely only on low-frequency information. These two models contrast with a symbol-encoding model in which surfaces are encoded implicitly as

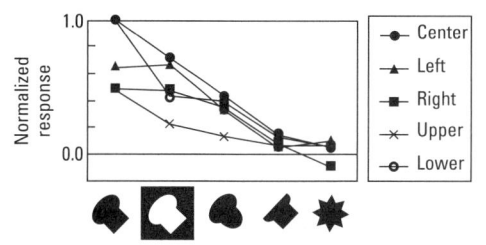

Figure 1.13 Effective stimulus for a cell in the posterior inferior temporal lobe (an ellipse in the top left and a rectangle in the bottom right of its receptive field).

a lack of discontinuity between boundaries (i.e., not retinotopically). The neural mechanisms that are consistent with interpolation will be outlined next.

Interpolation involves filling-in of surfaces from features near boundaries. Local discontinuities in features such as luminance are used to create boundaries, as discussed. Boundaries (edges) both initiate and constrain the spread of surface features (Grossberg, 2003). Points adjacent to boundaries serve as seeds for the spread of features, and inhibitory signals from the boundary constrain the spreading activation to within-boundary areas. This can be seen psychologically in the Craik O'Brien Cornsweet (COC) figure (Fig. 1.15A), in which alternate panels are perceived as differing in brightness. This is an illusion due to features near the boundaries, as Figure 1.15B shows, where the boundaries are blocked and the surfaces appear equally bright. Filling-in of brightness occurs within several hundred milliseconds of images that are artificially stabilized on the retina (Riggs & Ratliff, 1952) and can take several seconds when an image is stabilized by fixation. These findings have suggested that filling-in occurs within a few hundred milliseconds of determination of contours, which can take seconds to develop when images are not stably projected to the retina.

Physiologically, the role of edges in brightness control has been documented using optical imaging by Roe et al. (2005), who found differences in responses of cells in V2 to the Cornsweet figure and a baseline without the boundary (the Cornsweet figure and the baseline were therefore equivalent in total luminance). The time course of filling-in has been studied using the Troxler fading paradigm (Fig. 1.16). When a monkey fixates away from

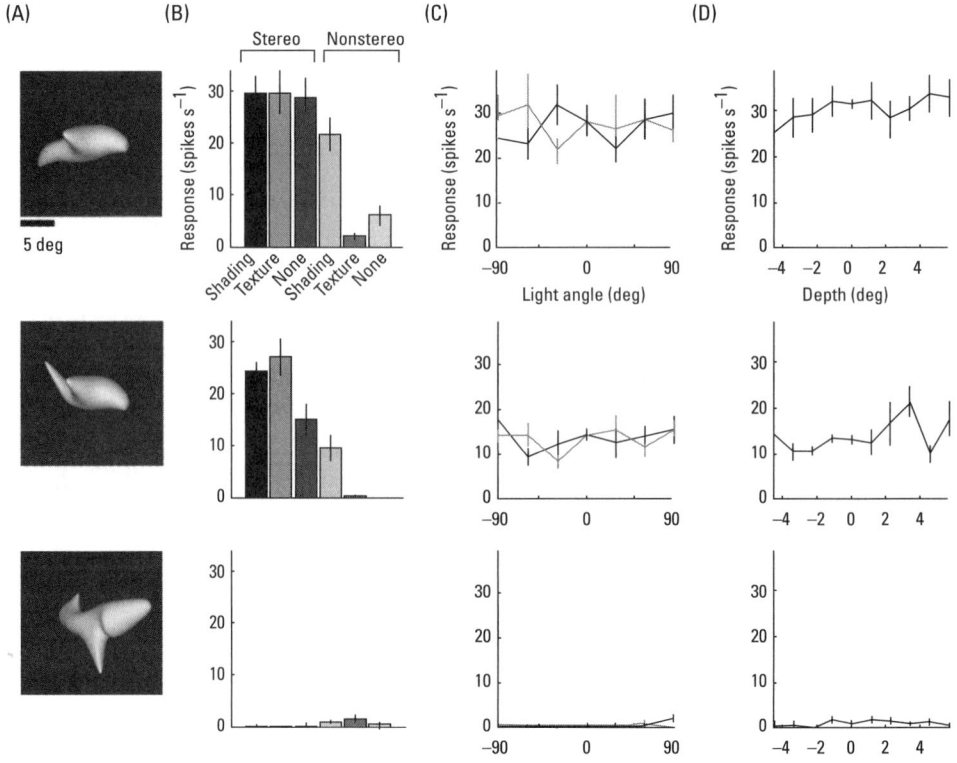

Figure 1.14 (*A*) Responses to highly effective (top), moderately effective (middle), and ineffective (bottom) example stimuli as a function of depth cues. Responses remained strong as long as disparity (black, green, and blue) or shading (gray) cues were present. The cell did not respond to stimuli with only texture cues (pale green) or silhouettes with no depth cues (pale blue). (*B*) Response consistency across lighting direction. The implicit direction of a point source at infinity was varied across 180° in the horizontal (left to right, black curve) and vertical (below to above, green curve) directions, creating very different two-dimensional shading patterns. (*C*) Response consistency across stereoscopic depth. (*D*) Response consistency across xy position.

the square, responses in neurons in V2 and V3 whose receptive fields include the square increase over several seconds to the level seen when the square is filled with the background. Humans report filling-in of the square at the same time point at which neural responses reach this level (Fig. 1.17) (de Weerd, 2006). The process of filling-in surface features has been related to V1 blobs (areas of V1 that stain more intensely for cytochrome oxidase) and

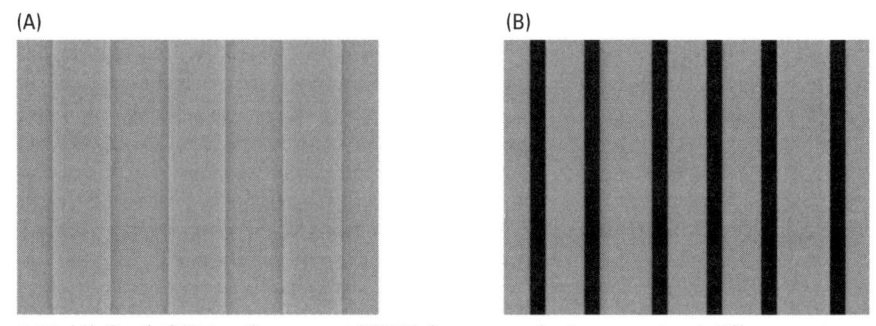

Figure 1.15 (*A*) Craik O'Brien Cornsweet (COC) figure, producing perceived differences in brightness in alternating panels. (*B*) COC figure with boundaries obscured, in which the perception in *A* is lost.

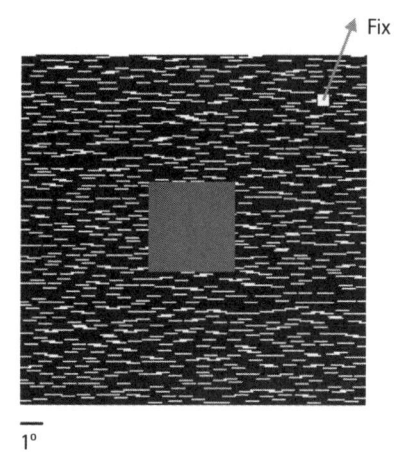

Figure 1.16 Troxler stimulus. With fixation as marked, the central patch fills in with the texture of the background.

V2 thin stripe regions (one of two areas of V2 that V1 blobs project to), which contain neurons that respond strongly to homogenous chromatic and achromatic stimuli in their receptive fields (Roe, Lu, & Hung, 2005; Roe & Ts'o, 1995).

Binding

Turning from individual visual features to their integration, the segregation of different types of visual features that begins in the retina is maintained throughout retinotopically projected visual areas. These features must be "bound" to form object representations. The notion of "binding" is complex and refers to functions as diverse as "perceptual grouping" of features of the same type under conditions

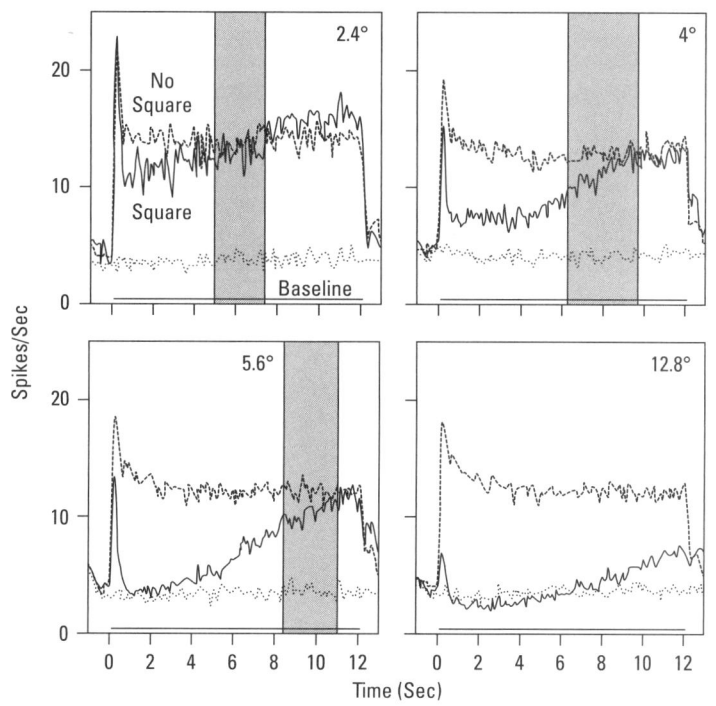

Figure 1.17 Correlation between increased neural activity in V2/V3 and perceptual filling-in. Average activity in stimulus conditions with a gray square over or inside the receptive field (solid line) and in conditions in which the square, and thus the RF, were physically filled in with texture (heavy dotted line) in subsets of V2 and V3 neurons with significant activity increases. Fine dots show baseline activity recorded without any stimulus. Square size is given at the top of the panels. The horizontal line on top of each abscissa indicates the 12-second stimulus presentation time, preceded and followed by a 1-second period in which activity was recorded in the absence of a stimulus. Human observers reported filling-in for the same stimuli as used during physiological recordings in the monkey in a time range indicated by the shaded zones.

where there are ambiguities in possible boundaries (e.g., "cluttered" scenes; scenes with several moving items whose trajectories overlap), through attributing different features (e.g., color, shape) to an individual object, to matching responses to percepts. Some of these "binding" processes, such as aspects of perceptual grouping, appear to be largely, if not entirely, preattentive, and others require attention. A sense of the role of attention in the "binding problem" can be gained by considering Treisman's influential feature integration theory (FIT) (Treisman & Gelade, 1980). The theory maintains that features are coded by position and bound when attention is directed toward a position. The theory explains several empirical findings: (1) that greater attention is required when binding is necessary to distinguish targets from nontargets ("conjunction search"—Fig. 1.18); (2) that when attention is directed elsewhere, illusory conjunctions wrongly recombining features of different objects are frequently seen; (3) that cueing the location of a target helps more when a conjunction must be reported than when the targets are defined as a disjunction of separate features; and (4) that grouping by single features occurs in parallel across the field, whereas grouping by conjunctions is much less salient and also seems to require active attention.

There are two major views regarding the neural basis for binding: feedforward hierarchical convergence ("directed line") models (Barlow, 1972, 1995, presented a classical statement of this type of model; for a more recent review, see Riesenhuber & Poggio, 1999) and oscillatory synchrony models (Singer, 1999). These theories are not incompatible, and it is possible that binding operations—or perhaps different types of binding operations—are supported by different neural processes.

Feedforward hierarchical convergence models are the type of model described previously regarding reconstruction of three-dimensional representations. They claim that "earlier," "lower order" cells send information to "later," "higher order" cells that respond to ever-more-complex aspects of a stimulus. The discussion of these models was simplified in several ways. One is that it relied on single-cell tuning curves. These models do not, however, require that higher level representations be correlated with single-cell responses; they can be related to local cell assemblies, in particular if information is coarse coded. Second, the presentation ignored the existence of local feedback, but the inclusion of such feedback does not change the essence of the process. Applying this approach to binding of different features encounters a number of problems, however. For instance, the number of possible combinations of features found in objects has suggested to many researchers that this approach would lead to a computational explosion and is beyond the capacity of the brain. Answers to some of these issues have been proposed (Reynolds & Desimone, 1999). Evidence that "later," "higher order" neurons respond to complex features of stimuli (see discussion of face recognition below) supports this class of models.

Oscillatory synchrony models maintain that binding of features involves interactions among cells and brain areas. Considerable work has pointed to synchrony of electroencephalographic (EEG) activity in the gamma frequency range (30–60 Hz), and, in some studies, the beta range up to 110–120 Hz, as the basis for aspects of binding. Oscillations that have been related to psychological functions have been described for both neocortex and allocortex (the olfactory bulb and hippocampus; see Gray [1994] for review). Singer (1999) reviews the advantages of synchronous oscillatory coding and possible physiological mechanisms that could produce it (largely related to lateral inhibitory circuits). Oscillations in the beta range or their synchronization could themselves be the neural "code" that represents psychologically relevant features and categories, and they have been argued to augment firing rates of individual neurons, thus enhancing spike train frequency coding (Fries, 2009). Gamma oscillations are related to oscillations at lower frequencies (in the theta and alpha ranges), which have been interpreted as resetting gamma cycles in psychologically relevant ways such as alternating attention (see Fries, 2009, for review). Synchronous oscillatory patterns have been associated with a wide range of cognitive processes, ranging from early aspects of perception (Gray & Singer, 1989), through effects of attention on perception (Landau & Fries, 2012) to motor planning (Salenius & Hari, 2003). Different forms of

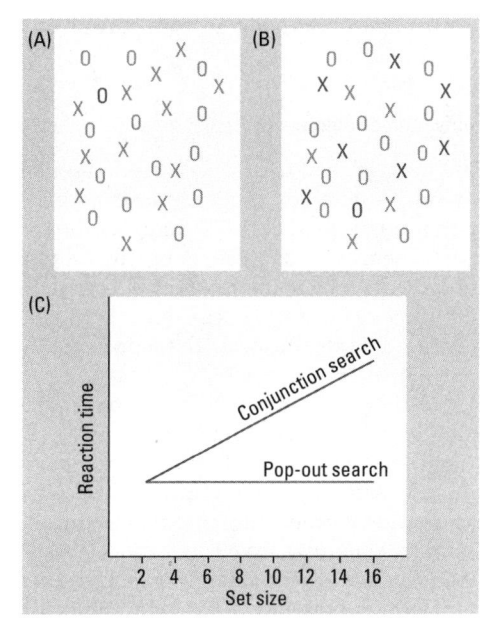

Figure 1.18 Conjunction and pop-out search. In both A and B, the task is to determine whether a red circle is present. In A, the target is defined as the feature in red; in B, the target is defined by the conjunction of red and circle. In C reaction time is shown for correct detections of present stimuli as a function of set size, consistent with parallel search not requiring serial deployment of attention in A and requiring serial deployment of attention in B. (See color plate section)

synchrony (e.g., onset synchrony, induced synchrony) need to be identified and may be related to different cognitive operations (Tallon-Baudry & Bertrand, 1999).[6]

With respect to visual object identification, one result pertains to the Gestalt principles that affect perceptual grouping. Gray (1994) reviewed evidence that proximity, similarity, common motion, continuity, closure, and segmentation all lead to increases in synchrony of firing of cells in striate cortex whose visual receptive fields do not overlap. He argued that these results are evidence for a role for synchrony in preattentive binding processes in vision. He cited results of Fries (1997) connecting synchronous activity in visual areas to control of motor responses as evidence of the biological relevance of these response patterns. Fries (1997) showed that synchronous activity in areas 17 and 18 was greater for cells that drove optikokinetic responses to the movement of the one of two gratings that drifted in opposite directions in strabismic cats in which cortical columns were responsive to only one eye.

In summary, "binding" of various types is a ubiquitous operation whose neural basis appears to involve both localized and distributed processes.

Face Recognition

The third aspect of high-level visual object processing whose neural basis will be briefly reviewed is identification of a specialized set of objects: faces.

There is strong psychological evidence that face recognition is a specialized perceptual process. McKone et al. (2009) review evidence that face identification depends more on configurational aspects of a face—the exact spacing between features—than on individual features. This appears as the "composite effect"—the finding that identification of one half of a combination face (in which the top half of the image contains the top half of one person's face and the bottom half contains the bottom half of another person's face) is much harder when the top and bottom images are aligned to form a face than when they are offset; as the "part-whole" effect, in which recognition of a face part is better if the part had previously been presented in the context of a face; as sensitivity to spatial changes, in which spatial distance between parts greatly affects face identification; and in a perceptual bias to upright face identification, in which subjects identify the upright face when an upright and inverted face are superimposed. All these effects are stronger for faces than for other classes of objects (McKone et al., 2009).

The neural basis for face recognition involves a specialized area of inferior temporal gyrus (ITG) in macaque and human. In macaque, face-selective cells have been identified in parts of ITG (Foldiak, Xiao, Keysers, Edwards, & Perrett, 2004), whose location corresponds to BOLD signal increases during viewing of faces (Tsao, Freiwald, Tootell, & Livingstone, 2006). Hasselmo et al. (1989) have shown that some of these neurons are projection and movement insensitive, indicating they respond to object-centered representations of faces. In humans, a right-lateralized area in the fusiform gyrus (called the "fusiform face area [FFA]") has been identified using fMRI. This area shows greater BOLD signal response to faces than to other classes of objects that have been presented (letter strings, flowers, houses, hands, everyday objects, and others) (Kanwisher, McDermott, & Chun, 1997). The FFA is sensitive to face identity (Rotshtein, Henson, Treves, Driver, & Dolan, 2005), but not facial expression (Winston, Vuilleumier, & Dolan, 2003). It shows a face inversion effect that correlates with the behavioral inversion effect (Yovel & Kanwisher, 2005) and a composite effect (Schiltz & Rossion, 2006).

Face recognition is a naturally developing process that resembles general object recognition in a variety of ways: Its input is three dimensional, mobile, presented from multiple angles, and often occluded. On the other hand, it is atypical of object recognition in many ways. All faces have characteristic features (overall shape, location relative to other objects such as parts of the body, parts, the geometrical layout of parts, and the range of relative spacing between parts). Faces convey biologically critical information about identity and therefore are highly salient, especially in precocial species in which survival and social adaptation are contingent on visually recognizing a mother and a small number of family members. Faces convey information that is useful in predicting behavioral responses (e.g., mood, whether a person is lying; Ekman, Friesen, & O'Sullivan, 1988). Evolutionary psychologists (Duchaine, Cosmides, & Tooby, 2001) and others (Caramazza & Shelton, 1998) have argued that these features of faces may have fostered the evolution of neural specializations for face recognition that do not apply to recognition of more "standard" classes of objects. People and members of many other species attend to faces a great deal, arguably more than to any other class of objects. This presumably encourages neutrally specialized mechanisms for their perceptual identification and memory. It is therefore not clear whether perceptual identification of the wide range of objects that we encounter relies on specialization of parts of high-level visual cortex that operate in the way that the FFA does. However, single cells have been found that respond selectively to other classes of objects (Grill-Spector, Kourtzi, & Kanwisher, 2001; Hasselmo, Rolls, Baylis, & Nalwa, 1989), pointing to a similar neural mechanism underlying at least part of their perceptual identification.

Activation of Concepts

The two views of neural organization—feedforward, direct line models, in which information coalesces in individual neurons or small neural assemblies, and distributed models, in which information is carried in distributed sets of neurons—have both been advanced as the basis for the representation and activation of concepts.

The first view is found in the paper that inaugurated the modern era of behavioral neurology—Geschwind's (1965a, 1965b) paper on "disconnection syndromes." Geschwind argued that the meanings of words—which he did not distinguish from concepts—consisted of the integration of modality-specific features of objects (themselves activated in unimodal association cortex adjacent to koniocortex) in inferior parietal lobe. The absence of strong direct connections from unimodal association cortex to inferior parietal multimodal association cortex in nonhuman species accounted for the absence of words with meaning in nonhumans. This theoretical account based on neuroanatomy has received mixed empirical support. Lesions in inferior parietal lobule do not cause word comprehension deficits or loss of nominal concepts (for selective review, see Binder, Desai, Graves, & Conant, 2009), but the inferior parietal lobule is one of many areas that are activated by tasks that require conceptual processing (for reviews, see Binder et al., 2009; Binder & Desai, 2011). The strongest evidence regarding the possible site of neural assemblies that might support the integration of various types of features into a concept in humans comes from semantic dementia, a degenerative disease that progressively affects the anterior temporal lobes, usually more so in the dominant left hemisphere (Hodges, Graham, & Patterson, 1995; Hodges, Patterson, Oxbury, & Funnell 1995; Jefferies & Lambon Ralph, 2006; Mummery et al., 2000; Snowden, Goulding, & Neary, 1989). Patients with semantic dementia show progressive loss of nominal concepts, evident no matter what the mode of access (verbal, pictorial, conceptual). This area is rarely activated by semantic tasks, however (but see Rogers et al., 2006, for an account of these apparently discrepant findings).

Evidence for distributed activity that constitutes the neural code for concepts comes primarily from neurovascular and neurophysiological activation studies. A number of studies have shown regional activation in sensory and/or motor areas that support processing of the perceptual features of objects or their use. Martin (2007) summarized this model as follows:

> Evidence from functional neuroimaging of the human brain indicates that information about salient properties of an object, such as what it looks like, how it moves, and how it is used, is stored in sensory and motor systems active when that information was acquired. As a result, object concepts belonging to different categories like animals and tools are represented in partially distinct, sensory- and motor property-based neural networks. This suggests that object concepts are not explicitly represented, but rather emerge from weighted activity within property-based brain regions. However, some property-based regions seem to show a categorical organization, thus providing evidence consistent with category-based, domain-specific formulations as well. (p. 25)

In addition to well-known results of this sort was the finding that reading words denoting specific actions involving the tongue (*lick*), finger (*pick*), and leg (*kick*) activated regions in premotor cortex that were also active when subjects made tongue, finger, and leg movements, respectively (Hauk, Johnsrude, & Pulvermuller, 2004). Damasio (1989) argued that objects were represented as patterns of activity in modality-specific regions of the brain.

A significant limitation of this literature is that, as the discussion of concepts in the section on "Perceptual Identification, Recognition, and Categorization of Visually Presented Objects" indicates, concepts are more than just the amalgamation of physical features and functional operations but have features that allow them to be counterfactually supporting and are delineated in intentional terms. Therefore, the way sensory and motor features of concepts are bound together only captures a part of the neural basis for concepts. Because of their relation to intentionality, human concepts differ fundamentally from those in other species, which cannot develop the range of intentions that we can; therefore, important aspects of the neural basis for human concepts will require human studies.

Overview of Perceptual Identification and Object Recognition

This brief review of physiological studies of aspects of visual object perception is highly selective, leaving out the great majority of mechanisms used in this process (e.g., use of color, texture, motion, and other features), discussion of alternate models, and even integration of the topics that were discussed (e.g., the role of surfaces in producing three-dimensional object-centered shapes). It is only intended to provide a glimpse of some of the features of cortical function and organization that underlie this domain-specific function. This section will be concluded by reviewing some of these mechanisms.

One feature of cortical organization that these results demonstrate is localization of function. Cells in particular brain areas can be thought of as performing particular operations on their input. Returning to the issues raised in the outset of this section, the operations of these cells are determined by their intrinsic features (e.g., the ability of cells in V4 to respond to the features they do is an intrinsic capacity, not one that can be understood by considering their input alone, even if the development of this computational capacity requires particular input at a critical time in development). Although the studies reported tended to rely on single-cell recording, as noted several times, there is evidence that many operations correspond to responses in considerably larger cell assemblies, which are localized in small areas of the brain (Georgopoulos, Kalaska, Caminiti, & Massey, 1982). Localization of function is a well-established feature of the cortical organization that supports all levels of psychological functions, from "line" detection through face recognition and activation of concepts.

Narrow localization is, however, only part of the basis for cortical support of cognitive functions. The other aspect of cortical organization is a more widespread basis for supporting cognitive operations. Some models of cortical organization (e.g., Mesulam, 1990, 1998) have argued that areas as large as the entire perisylvian association cortex (in the case of human language) support particular cognitive functions, in some cases with "gradients" of involvement toward "poles" of these large areas. These models use terms such as "distributed functions" or "neural nets" to describe cortical organization, and they draw upon mathematical models as the basis for distributed representations and processes (McClelland & Rumelhart, 1986; Rumelhart & McClelland, 1986).

From the point of view of relating cognitive operations to the brain, two different notions of "distributed," "neural net" cortical organization need to be distinguished. One is that individual cognitive operations are related to the activity of "distributed neural nets." The second is that sets of related cognitive operations are related to the activity of contiguous and directly connected areas of the brain.

To the best of my knowledge, although mathematical models have demonstrated that distributed representations are important candidates as neural mechanisms and that these systems can develop gradients of weights in hidden unit layers as they engage in what are considered individual processes over time (e.g., Plaut, McClelland, Seidenberg, & Patterson, 1996, in the case of reading), there is no evidence for distributed systems or for a gradient of activity in areas of the brain as large as those envisaged by Mesulam (1998) that supports individual cognitive operations. The evidence reviewed indicates that synchronous oscillations appear to "unite" areas of the brain in the service of what may be individual operations such as the Gestalt perceptual grouping processes, but the synchronous oscillations that apply in these "single operation" cases are quite spatially restricted. More widespread synchronous oscillations are observed in cases where different modalities or operations are involved, but this is an example of the second type of "distributed neural nets."

On the other hand, there is little doubt that the second of these modes of organization—that sets of related individual cognitive operations are related to the activity of contiguous and directly connected areas of the brain—applies in the cortex. We have seen that related operations apply in spatially contiguous and directly connected occipito-temporal cortex in the process of object recognition; the same is true of other sensory modalities, language, motor planning, control functions, and different aspects of memory and attention. These areas are integrated in a number of ways. This chapter has reviewed "direct line" feedforward hierarchical processing and synchronous oscillations, and mentioned local feedback, as aspects of their integration. Modern models add notions of "hubs" and "small world" organization to the ways these sets of areas interact to support related functions (Bassett & Bullmore, 2009).

Localized cell groups and larger areas are grouped together into "neural systems" that involve not only the cortex but also cortical-subcortical sets of neurons (see Chapter 2). For instance, the motor system includes premotor cortex, motor cortex, basal ganglia and other hemispheric subcortical areas, and the cerebellum and connected brain stem nuclei. At the highest level of organization, these systems interact: Voluntary motor function is determined by control operations, is dependent upon input from proprioceptive and vestibular systems, and in many cases initiated and modified by teleoceptive perceptual processing, especially vision.

Overall, the basic principles of the cortical organization that appears to support cognitive functions are (a) a high degree of specialization of cellular computational capacity (which develops in part based on input and shows a high, but presumably bounded, degree of plasticity); (b) localized cell groups that accomplish particular operations; (c) feedforward, correlated, and hub/small world organization of contiguous and densely interconnected areas to support related cognitive operations; (d) interaction of spatially disparate areas into "systems"; and (e) interaction of "systems" to accomplish tasks. As far as is known, these basic features of neural function and organization apply to all aspects of cognition—both "primary" and "control" operations.

Regional Functional Specialization for Cognitive Functions

This chapter will be concluded with a very brief overview of the regional functional specialization of the cortex at the third level of organization: organization of cortical areas to support related cognitive operations.

Large contiguous areas of the cortex tend to be devoted to operations of the same sort. A picture of the functions associated with different cortical regions is presented in Figure 1.19. This cartoon, or similar ones, is highly familiar to most clinicians, and details of some of the functions depicted in it are presented in other chapters. It will not be described further here, but rather a few comments will be made on how these localizations arise, as well as some caveats about this image.

The localization of these large cognitive domains is in part attributable to the operation of direct-line feedforward processing in cell groups with particular patterns of connectivity (Geschwind, 1965a, 1965b; Mesulam, 1990, 1998). On the sensory side, simpler representations are formed in koniocortex, whose efferents synapse exclusively in unimodal sensory association cortex, and cell groups in unimodal sensory association cortex have many reciprocal connections with one another. In conjunction with feedforward computations, this creates large areas of cortex devoted to higher level visual, auditory, and somasthetic processing. On the motor side, a similar phenomenon occurs in reverse: Primary motor cortex receives many afferents from adjacent unimodal motor association cortex, where aspects of movement are planned.

These factors do not account for all aspects of regional cortical functional specialization, however. On the surface of things, it does not appear that different types of control operations could be functionally related by the same types of feedforward mechanisms that apply to perceptual analysis and motor planning, making the localization of many control operations in prefrontal lobe unlikely to be due to these factors. The same is true of the different aspects of language (phonology, syntax, discourse structure). The location of the "default system" (see Chapters 3 and 4) close to a large number of primary systems and the location of episodic memory encoding in mesial temporal structures are also not easily attributable to these factors.

A final comment is that, although these gross functional localizations are quite well documented, ongoing work has consistently complicated the picture. The evidence for semantic processing in inferior

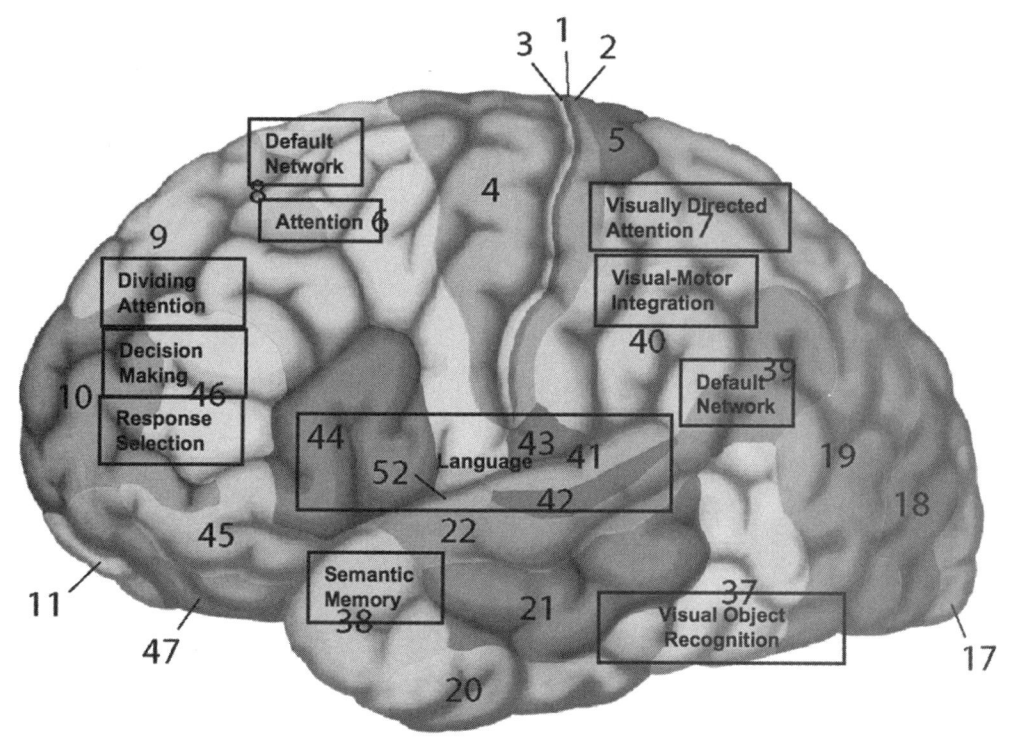

Figure 1.19 Cartoon of location of the major cognitive systems in the lateral human cortex. (See color plate section)

anterior temporal lobe, for instance, was unexpected; the existence of a default network was unsuspected. Traditional models of language processing localized spoken language comprehension in posterior superior temporal gyrus (Wernicke's area) and adjacent cortex and speech planning in posterior inferior frontal gyrus (Broca's area), but both deficit-lesion correlations (Caramazza & Zurif, 1976) and functional neuroimaging (Stromswold, Caplan, Alpert, & Rauch, 1986) have shown that aspects of comprehension related to the assignment of sentence syntactic structure are supported by Broca's area in at least some individuals. Though clinicians can reasonably rely on the picture in Figure 1.19 and can reasonably expect to be able to rely on that picture in the future, exceptions, additions, and modifications of these localizations are very likely to be documented as we learn more about cognitive functions themselves and their neural bases.

Notes

1. A category can sometimes be described in terms drawn from "lower" levels of science (e.g., "lightning" can be described in terms drawn from the theory of electromagnetism). The partial success of reductionism does not entail that something is not a category: "Lightning," and not its electromagnetic reformulation, plays a role in theories of climate (all "special sciences" have this structure).
2. The stimuli that provoke these neural responses are not circles, but the output of the cells can be considered to correspond to circles, subject to noise, which is sufficient for it to be used as a circle in subsequent computations in visual perception. (It is doubtful that either circles actually exist in either nature or serious models of perception; they are being used here simply as familiar descriptors.)
3. On the negative side, these descriptions at least risk circularity, as noted in the text. Operations that preserve the information in a representation cannot be non–circularly defined as cognitive operations if what makes something a representation is that it is subject to information-preserving operations and what makes something cognitive is that it operates on representations. This problem may be avoided if we say that the operations that preserve information are not themselves cognitive; it is the application of an operation to a semantically evaluable item that makes it cognitive. It bears repeating after considering these descriptions that, even if circularity can be avoided, it is not clear that these accounts will identify a set of psychological operations that cohere scientifically. But they are a start. And folk psychology and intuitions do not do better: The set of processes that are called "cognitive" in practice is highly heterogeneous on its face.
4. Setting response criteria thresholds might be considered setting criteria for success, applied within a task, not to the task itself.
5. There is a logical relation between plasticity due to altered input and the intrinsic properties of cells and their organization that determine their functional roles. These intrinsic features must be sufficiently generally present in cells to allow cells to perform new functions when presented with new inputs at certain points of development. The extent to which plasticity applies (e.g., whether non-koniocortical cells in the auditory system (or in the visual system, for that matter) would develop the response sensitivity of normally wired V1 or rewired A1 cells if they were presented with thalamic efferents) must reflect the nature of the experience-mutable, shared cellular properties that give a cell its computational potential.
6. The evidence for the relevance of synchronous oscillations to these processes is strong but remains controversial. Controversy arises for technical reasons (higher level oscillations may be harmonics of lower frequency, or they may be confounded with spike train frequencies; Dong, Mihalas, Qiu, von der Heydt, & Niebur, 2008) and because some phenomena that would seem to be supported by this process have not been associated with synchronous oscillations (cf. Dong et al., 2008, who found no evidence for synchrony associated with object stimuli).

References

Anderson, J. R., Bothell, D., Byrne, M. D., Douglass, S., Lebiere, C., & Qin, Y. (2004). An integrated theory of the mind. *Psychological Review, 111*, 1036–1060.

Angelucci, A., Clasca, F., & Sur, M. (1998). Brainstem inputs into the ferret medial geniculate nucleus and the effect of early deafferentation on novel retinal projections to the auditory thalamus. *Journal of Comparative Neurology, 400*, 417–439.

Aristotle. (1995). Categories. In *The complete works of Aristotle, 2 vols* (J. Barnes, Ed., & J. L. Ackrill, Trans., pp. 3–24). Princeton, NJ: Princeton University Press.

Bailey, C. H., Bartsch, D., & Kandel, E. R. (1996). Toward a molecular definition of long-term memory storage. *Proceedings of the National Academy of Sciences USA, 93*(24), 1344–1345.

Barlow, H. B. (1972). Single units and sensation: A neuron doctrine for perceptual psychology. *Perception, 1*, 371–394.

Barlow, H. B. (1995). The neuron in perception. In M. S. Gazzaniga (Ed.), *The cognitive neurosciences* (pp. 415–34). Cambridge, MA: MIT Press.

Bassett, D. S., & Bullmore, E. T. (2009). Human brain networks in health and disease. *Current Opinion in Neurology, 22*(4), 340–347.

Binder, J. R., & Desai, R. H. (2011). The neurobiology of semantic memory. *Trends in Cognitive Sciences, 15*(11), 527–536.

Binder, J. R., Desai, R. H., Graves, W. W., & Conant, L. L. (2009). Where is the semantic system? A critical review and meta-analysis of 120 functional neuroimaging studies. *Cerebral Cortex, 19*(12), 2767–2796.

Brincat, S. L., & Connor, C. E. (2004). Underlying principles of visual shape selectivity in posterior inferotemporal cortex. *Nature Neuroscience, 7*, 880–886.

Buckner, R. L., Snyder, A. Z., Shannon, B. J., LaRossa, G., Sachs, R., Fotenos, A. F.,…Mintun, M. A. (2005). Molecular, structural, and functional characterization of Alzheimer's disease: Evidence for a relationship between default activity, amyloid, and memory. *Journal of Neuroscience, 25*, 7709–7717.

Caramazza, A., & Zurif, E. (1976). Dissociations of algorithmic and heuristic processes in sentence comprehension: Evidence from aphasia. *Brain and Language, 3*, 572–582.

Cherry, E. C. (1953). Some experiments on the recognition of speech, with one and with two ears. *Journal of the Acoustical Society of America, 25*(5), 975–979.

Connor, C. E., Pasupathy, A., Brincat, S., & Yamane, Y. (2009). Neural transformation of object information by ventral pathway visual cortex. In M. S. Gazzaniga (Ed.), *The cognitive neurosciences* (4th ed., pp. 455–467). Cambridge, MA: MIT Press.

Damasio, A. R. (1989). Time-locked multiregional retroactivation: A systems-level proposal for the neural substrates of recall and recognition. *Cognition, 33*, 25–62.

De Luca, M., Beckmann, C. F., De Stefano, N., Matthews, P. M., & Smith, S. M. (2006). fMRI resting state networks define distinct modes of long-distance interactions in the human brain. *Neuroimage, 29*, 1359–1367.

De Weerd, P. (2006). Perceptual filling-in: More than the eye can see. *Progress in Brain Research, 154*, 227–245.

Dong, Y., Mihalas, S., Qiu, F., von der Heydt, R., & Niebur, E. (2008). Synchrony and the binding problem in macaque visual cortex. *Journal of Vision, 8*, 1–16.

Duchaine, B., Cosmides, L., & Tooby, J. (2001). Evolutionary psychology and the brain. *Current Opinion in Neurobiology, 11*, 225–230.

Ekman, P., Friesen, W. V., & O'Sullivan, M. (1988). Smiles when lying. *Journal of Personality and Social Psychology, 54*, 414–420.

Fei-Fei, L., Fergus, R., & Perona, P. (2006). One-shot learning of object categories. *IEEE Transactions, Pattern Analysis and Machine Intelligence, 28*(4), 594–611.

Fodor, J. (1998). *Concepts: Where cognitive science went wrong. The 1996 John Locke Lectures.* Oxford, UK: Oxford University Press.

Foldiak, P., Xiao, D., Keysers, C., Edwards, R., & Perrett, D. I. (2004). Rapid serial visual presentation for the determination of neural selectivity in area STSa. *Progress in Brain Research, 144*, 107–116.

Fries, P., Roelfsema, P. R., Engel, A. K., König, P., & Singer, W. (1997). Synchronization of oscillatory responses in visual cortex correlates with perception in interocular rivalry. *Proceedings of the National Academy of Sciences, 94*(23), 12699–12704.

Fries, P. (2009). Neuronal gamma-band synchronization as a fundamental process in cortical computation. *Annual Review of Neuroscience, 32*, 209–224.

Georgopoulos, A. P., Kalaska, J. F., Caminiti, R., & Massey, J. T. (1982). On the relations between the direction of twodimensional arm movements and cell discharge in primate motor cortex. *Journal of Neuroscience, 2*(11), 1527–1537.

Geschwind, N. (1965a). Disconnexion syndromes in animals and man. I. *Brain, 88*, 237–294.

Geschwind, N. (1965b). Disconnexion syndromes in animals and man. II. *Brain, 88*, 585–644.

Goebel, R., & De Weerd, P. (2009). Perceptual filling-in from experimental data to neural network modeling. In M. S. Gazzaniga (Ed.), *The cognitive neurosciences* (4th ed., pp. 435–454). Cambridge, MA: MIT Press.

Gray, C. M. (1994). Synchronous oscillations in neuronal systems: Mechanisms and functions. *Journal of Computational Neuroscience, 1*, 11–38.

Gray, C. M., & Singer, W. (1989). Stimulus-specific neuronal oscillations in orientation columns of cat visual cortex. *Proceedings of the National Academy of Sciences USA, 86*, 1698–1702.

Grill-Spector, K., Kourtzi, N., & Kanwisher, N. (2001). The lateral occipital complex and its role in object recognition. *Vision Research, 41*, 1409–1422.

Grossberg, S. (2003). Filling-in the forms: Surface and boundary interactions in visual cortex. In L. Pessoa & P. de Weerd (Eds.), *Filling-in: From perceptual completion to skill learning* (pp. 13–37). New York, NY: Oxford University Press.

Hasselmo, M. E., Rolls, E. T, Baylis, G. C., & Nalwa V. (1989). Object-centered encoding by face-selective neurons in the cortex in the superior temporal sulcus of the monkey. *Experimental Brain Research, 75,* 417–429.

Hauk, O., Johnsrude, I., & Pulvermuller, F. (2004). Somatotopic representation of action words in human motor and premotor cortex. *Neuron, 41,* 301–307.

Hodges, J. R., Graham, N., & Patterson, K. (1995). Charting the progression in semantic dementia: Implications for the organisation of semantic memory. *Memory, 3,* 463–495.

Hodges, J. R., Patterson, K., Oxbury, S., & Funnell, E. (1992) Semantic dementia: progressive fluent aphasia with temporal lobe atrophy. *Brain, 115,* 1783–1806.

Hubel, D. H., & Wiesel, T. N. (1959). Receptive fields of single neurones in the cat's striate cortex. *Journal of Physiology, 148,* 574–591.

Hubel, D. H., & Wiesel, T. N. (1962). Receptive fields, binocular interaction and functional architecture in the cat's visual cortex. *Journal of Physiology, 160,* 106–154.

Humphreys, G. W., & Riddoch, M. J. (Eds.). (1987). *Visual object processing: A cognitiveneuropsychological approach.* Hillsdale, NJ: Erlbaum.

Ito, M., Tamura, H., Fujita, I., & Tanaka, K. (1995). Size and position invariance of neuronal responses in monkey inferotemporal cortex. *Journal of Neurophysiology, 73,* 218–226.

Jefferies, E., & Lambon Ralph, M. A. (2006). Semantic impairment in stroke aphasia versus semantic dementia: A case-series comparison. *Brain, 129,* 2132–2147.

Kanwisher, N. G., McDermott, J., & Chun, M. M. (1997). The fusiform face area: A module in human extrastriate cortex specialized for face perception. *Journal of Neuroscience, 17*(11), 4302–4311.

Land, E. (1974). The retinex theory of colour vision. *Proceedings of the Royal Institute of Great Britain, 47,* 23–58.

Landau, A. N., & Fries, P. (2012). Attention samples stimuli rhythmically. *Current Biology, 22*(11), 1000–1004.

Macken, W. J., Tremblay, S., Alford, D., & Jones, D. M. (1999). Attentional selectivity in short-term memory: Similarity of process, not similarity of content, determines disruption. *International Journal of Psychology, 34,* 322–327.

Margolis, E., & Laurence, S. (Eds.). (1991). *Concepts: Core readings.* Cambridge, MA: MIT Press.

Martin, A. (2007). The representation of object concepts in the brain. *Annual Review of Psychology, 58,* 25–45.

McClelland, J. L., Rumelhart, D. E., & PDP Research Group. (1986). *Parallel distributed processing: Explorations in the microstructure of cognition, Vol. 2. Psychological and biological models.* Cambridge, MA: MIT Press.

McKone, E., Crookes, K., & Kanwisher, N. (2009). The cognitive and neural development of face recognition in humans. In M. S. Gazzaniga (Ed.), *The cognitive neurosciences* (4th ed., pp. 467–482). Cambridge, MA: MIT Press.

Meyer, D. E., & Kieras, D. E. (1997a). A computational theory of executive control processes and human multiple-task performance: Part 1. Basic mechanisms. *Psychological Review, 104,* 3–65.

Meyer, D. E., & Kieras, D. E. (1997b). A computational theory of executive control processes and human multiple-task performance: Part 2. Accounts of psychological refractory-period phenomena. *Psychological Review, 104,* 749–791.

Mesulam, M. M. (1990). Large-scale neurocognitive networks and distributed processing for attention, language, and memory. *Annals of Neurology, 28,* 597–613.

Mesulam, M. M. (1998). From sensation to cognition. *Brain, 121,* 1013–1052.

Mummery, C. J., Patterson, K., Price, C. J., Ashburner, J., Frackowiak, R. S., & Hodges, J. R. (2000). A voxel-based morphometry study of semantic dementia: Relationship between temporal lobe atrophy and semantic memory. *Annals of Neurology, 47,* 36–45.

Olson, S., & Grossberg, S. (1998). A neural network model for the development of simple and complex cell receptive fields within cortical maps of orientation and ocular dominance. *Neural Networks, 11,* 189–208.

Paivio, A. (1986). *Mental representations: A dual coding approach.* Oxford, UK: Oxford University Press.

Pasupathy, A., & Connor, C. E. (1999). Responses to contour features in macaque area V4. *Journal of Neurophysiology, 82,* 2490–2502.

Pasupathy, A., & Connor, C. E. (2002). Population coding of shape in area V4. *Nature Neuroscience, 5,* 1332–1338.

Plaut, D. C., McClelland, J. L., Seidenberg, M. S., & Patterson, K. (1996). Understanding normal and impaired word reading: Computational principles in quasi-regular domains. *Psychological Review, 103,* 56–115.

Ratcliff, R. (1978). A theory of memory retrieval. *Psychological Review, 85,* 59–108.

Ratcliff, R., Thapar, A., & McKoon, G. (2011). Effects of aging and IQ on item and associative memory. *Journal of Experimental Psychology: General, 140,* 464–487.

Reynolds, J. H., & Desimone, R. (1999). The role of neural mechanisms of attention in solving the binding problem. *Neuron, 24,* 19–29.

Riesenhuber, M., & Poggio, T. (1999). Are cortical models really bound by the "binding problem"? *Neuron, 24,* 87–93.

Riggs, L. A., & Ratliff, F. (1952). The effects of counteracting the normal movements of the eye. *Journal of the Optical Society of America, 42,* 872–873.

Roe, A. W., Lu, H. D., & Hung, C. P. (2005). Cortical processing of a brightness illusion. *Proceedings of the National Academy of Sciences USA, 102*(10), 3869–3874.

Roe, A. W., & Ts'o, D. Y. (1995). Visual topography in primate V2: Multiple representation across functional stripes. *Journal of Neuroscience, 15,* 3689–3715.

Rogers, T. T., Hocking, J., Noppeney, U., Mechelli, A., Gorno-Tempini, M., Patterson, K., & Price, C. (2006). The anterior temporal cortex and semantic memory: Reconciling findings from neuropsychology and functional imaging. *Cognitive, Affective and Behavioral Neuroscience, 6,* 201–213.

Rotshtein, P., Henson, R. N., Treves, A., Driver, J., & Dolan, R. J. (2005). Morphing Marilyn into Maggie dissociates physical and identity face representations in the brain. *Nature Neuroscience, 8*(1), 107–113.

Rumelhart, D. E., McClelland, J. L., & PDP Research Group. (1986). *Parallel distributed processing: Explorations in the microstructure of cognition, Vol. 1. Foundations.* Cambridge, MA: MIT Press.

Salenius, S., & Hari, R. (2003). Synchronous cortical oscillatory activity during motor action. *Current Opinion in Neurobiology, 13,* 678–684.

Schiltz, C., & Rossion, B. (2006). Faces are represented holistically in the human occipito-temporal cortex. *NeuroImage, 32,* 1385–1394.

Singer, W. (1999). Neuronal synchrony: A versatile code for the definition of relations? *Neuron, 24,* 49–65.

Snowden, J. S., Goulding, P. J., & Neary, D. (1989). Semantic dementia: A form of circumscribed temporal atrophy. *Behavioural Neurology, 2,* 167–182.

Spivey, M. J., Grosjean, M., & Knoblich, G. (2005). Continuous attraction toward phonological competitors. *Proceedings of the National Academy of Sciences USA, 102,* 10393–10398.

Stromswold, K., Caplan, D., Alpert, N., & Rauch, S. (1996). Localiza ion of syntactic comprehension by positron emission tomography. *Brain and Language, 52,* 452–473.

Tallon-Baudry, C., & Bertrand, O. (1999). Oscillatory gamma activity in humans and its role in object representation. *Trends in Cognitive Sciences, 3,* 151–162.

Tanaka, J. W., & Gauthier, I. (1997). Expertise in object and face recognition. In R. L. Goldstone, P. G. Schyns, & D. L. Medin (Eds.), *Psychology of learning and motivation, Vol. 36. Perceptual mechanisms of learning* (pp. 83–125). San Diego, CA: Academic Press.

Treisman, A. (1964). Monitoring and storage of irrelevant messages in selective attention. *Journal of Verbal Learning and Behavior, 3,* 449–459.

Treisman, A., & Gelade, G. (1980). A feature-integration theory of attention. *Cognitive Psychology, 12*(1), 97–136.

Tsao, D. Y., Freiwald, W. A., Tootell, R. B., & Livingstone, M. S. (2006). A cortical region consisting entirely of face-selective cells. *Science, 311,* 670–674.

Tulving, E. (1972). Episodic and semantic memory. In E. Tulving & W. Donaldson (Eds.), *Organization of memory* (pp. 381–403). New York, NY: Academic Press.

Turing, A. M. (1936). On computable numbers, with an application to the Entscheidungs problem. *Proceedings of the London Mathematical Society, 2*(42), 230–265.

Winston, J. S., Vuilleumier, P., & Dolan, R. J. (2003). Effects of low-spatial frequency components of fearful faces on fusiform cortex activity. *Current Biology, 13*(20), 1824–1829.

Wittgenstein, L. (1961). *Tractatus logico-philosophicus* (D. F. Pears & B. F. McGuinness, Trans.). New York, NY: Humanities Press. (original work published 1921)

Wolfe, J. M. (1994). Guided search 2.0: A revised model of visual search. *Psychonomic Bulletin and Review, 1*(2), 202–238.

Wolfe, J. M., & Bennett, S. C. (1997). Preattentive object files: Shapeless bundles of basic features. *Vision Research, 37*(1), 25–44.

Yamane, Y., Carlson, E. T., Bowman, K. C., Wang, Z., & Connor, C. E. (2008). A neural code for three-dimensional object shape in macaque inferotemporal cortex. *Nature Neuroscience, 11,* 1352–1360.

Yovel, G., & Kanwisher, N. (2005). The neural basis of the behavioral faceinversion effect. *Current Biology, 15*(24), 2256–2262.

Zilles, K., & Amunts, K. (2010). Centenary of Brodmann's map—Conception and fate. *Nature Reviews Neuroscience, 11*(2), 139–145.

2

Neuroanatomy and Behavioral Neurology of Subcortical Systems

Jeremy D. Schmahmann and Deepak N. Pandya

All behaviors are subserved by distributed neural systems that comprise anatomic regions, or nodes, each displaying unique architectural properties, distributed geographically throughout the nervous system, and linked anatomically and functionally in a precise and unique manner (Geschwind 1965a, 1965b; Goldman-Rakic, 1988; Jones & Powell, 1970a; Luria, 1966; Mesulam, 1981, 1990; Nauta, 1964; Pandya & Kuypers, 1969; Ungerleider & Mishkin, 1982). Subcortical structures are incorporated into the distributed neural circuits subserving cognition, a realization supported by the recognition of neurobehavioral syndromes following lesions of cerebral white matter and subcortical regions, and imaging studies in psychiatric patients demonstrating abnormalities in subcortical areas. This chapter presents an overview of the anatomical organization in monkey of the white matter tracts linking different cerebral cortical areas with each other, the connections between the cerebral cortex and subcortical areas, and a consideration of the clinical manifestations in patients of lesions in white matter tracts, the basal ganglia, thalamus, and cerebellum. We regard these as disconnection syndromes: focal disruptions of the distributed cortical and subcortical neural circuits that subserve neurologic function. Understanding the neurobiology of subcortical cognition and its clinical manifestations is essential to the evaluation and care of patients with dementia and the neurobehavioral consequences of many debilitating neurological diseases, including neurodegenerative diseases associated with dementia.

White Matter Tracts of the Cerebral Hemispheres

Anatomical Organization

The white matter tracts in the cerebral hemispheres are composed of axons coursing between cortico-cortical and cortico-subcortical territories. Neurons within any cortical area give rise to three distinct categories of efferent fibers that can be identified within the white matter immediately beneath the gyrus (Schmahmann & Pandya, 2006). These are association fibers, striatal fibers, and a confluence of fibers (the "cord") that carries commissural and subcortical (projection) fibers (Fig. 2.1).

Association fibers comprise local, neighborhood, and long association fibers. Local,

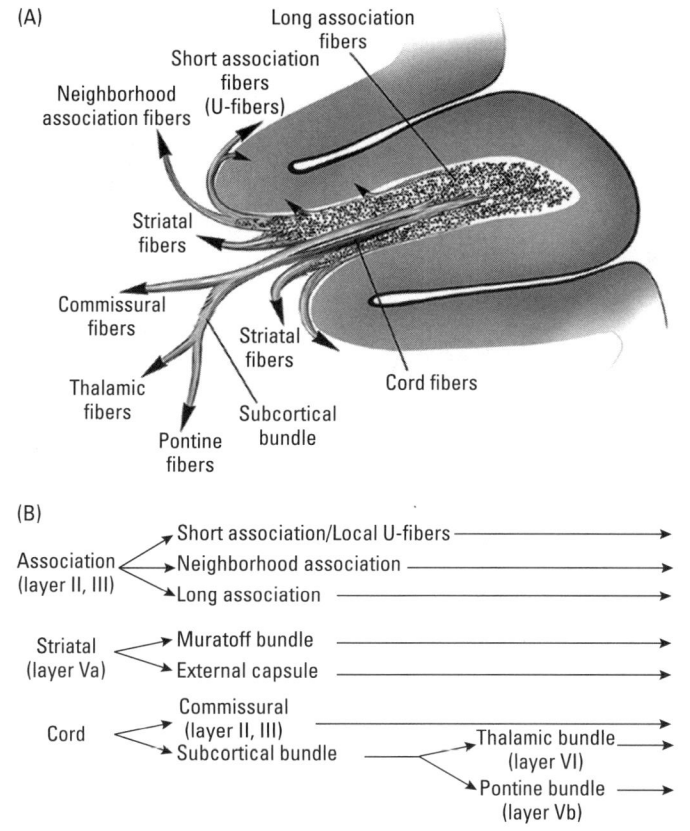

Figure 2.1 Diagram (A) and schema (B) of the principles of organization of white matter fiber pathways emanating from the cerebral cortex. Long association fibers are seen end-on as the stippled area within the white matter of the gyrus. In their course, these fibers either remain confined to the white matter of the gyrus, or they travel deeper in the white matter of the hemisphere. Short association fibers, or U-fibers, link adjacent gyri. Neighborhood association fibers link nearby regions usually within the same lobe. Striatal fibers intermingle with the association fibers early in their course, before coursing in the subcallosal fascicle of Muratoff or in the external capsule. Cord fibers segregate into commissural fibers that arise in cortical layers II and III, and the subcortical bundle, which further divides into fibers destined for thalamus arising from cortical layer VI, and those to brainstem and spinal cord in the pontine bundle arising from cortical layer V. (From Schmahmann & Pandya, 2006)

or U-fibers, are closely apposed to the undersurface of the sixth layer and are directed to cortical regions in the same or adjacent gyri. Neighborhood association fibers are distinct from local U-fibers and are directed to nearby cortical regions; for example, the fibers that connect the inferior parietal lobule to the medial parietal cortex. Long association fibers are the named fiber tracts that travel within the central part of the white matter of the core of the gyrus and link distant cortical areas within the same hemisphere.

Corticostriatal fibers course initially with the long association fibers before separating from them, then travel within one of two major fiber bundles. Fibers in the subcallosal fasciculus of Muratoff lead mainly to the caudate nucleus and putamen. Fibers in the external capsule target the ventral part of the caudate nucleus, the putamen and claustrum (Fig. 2.2).

The cord of fibers comprises a dense aggregation of fibers occupying the central core of the white matter of the gyrus and contains commissural fibers and the subcortical projection bundle. The commissural bundle travels to the opposite hemisphere via the corpus callosum or the anterior commissure

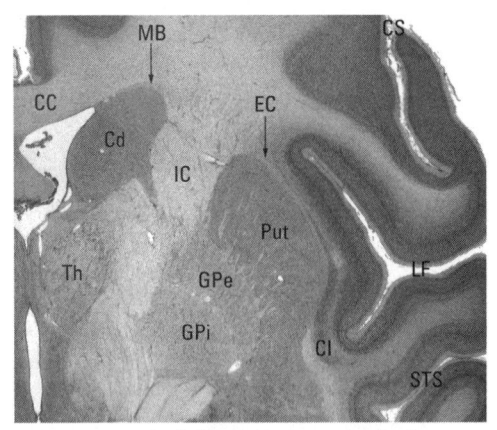

Figure 2.2 Light field photomicrograph of a coronal hemisphere of a monkey brain stained for Nissl substance, to show the locations of the Muratoff bundle (MB) coursing above the body of the caudate nucleus and below the corpus callosum, and the external capsule (EC) situated between the claustrum laterally and the putamen medially. CC = corpus callosum, Cd = caudate nucleus, Cl = claustrum, CS = central sulcus, GPe = globus pallidus external, GPi = globus pallidus internal, IC = internal capsule, LF = lateral fissure, Put = putamen, STS = superior temporal sulcus, Th = thalamus

(Fig. 2.3). The subcortical bundle (SB) travels within the internal capsule (anterior or posterior limb) or the sagittal stratum, and segregates into thalamic fibers that travel via thalamic peduncles to the thalamus, and a pontine fiber bundle that courses via the cerebral peduncle to the pons. The SB also gives rise to fibers to other diencephalic and brainstem structures.

Knowledge of these tracts and their putative functional properties is useful when considering the clinical consequence of white matter diseases, and in understanding the neurobehavioral consequence of subcortical lesions that affect white matter tracts. The following is a brief anatomical overview of the fiber tracts of the brain of Rhesus monkey (from Schmahmann & Pandya, 2006). These observations in monkey are supported by magnetic resonance imaging (MRI) findings in monkey (Schmahmann, Pandya, et al., 2007), and they closely match those in the human brain as determined using diffusion tensor imaging (DTI; e.g., Catani, Howard, Pajevic, & Jones, 2002; Makris et al., 2005; Thiebaut de Schotten, Dell'Acqua, Valabregue, & Catani, 2012; Wedeen et al., 2008), probabilistic

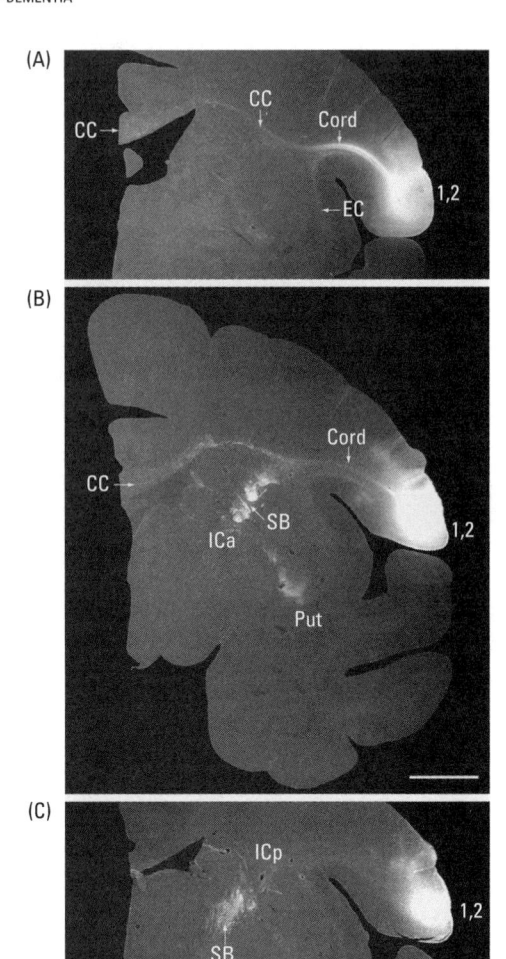

Figure 2.3 Photomicrographs of selected coronal sections of a Rhesus monkey following injection of radioisotope into the frontal operculum in the precentral aspects of areas 1 and 2. (A) The cord of fibers is seen emanating from the injection site, with some commissural fibers (Comm) continuing medially towards the opposite hemisphere through the corpus callosum. (B) The cord segregates into the commissural fibers and the subcortical bundle (SB) that descends into the anterior limb of the internal capsule. (C) Caudal to the injection site the subcortical bundle continues its course in the posterior limb of the internal capsule. Note terminations in the putamen. Magnification = 0.5×, bar = 5 mm. (Adapted from Schmahmann & Pandya, 2006; figure reproduced from Schmahman & Pandya, 2008). CC = corpus callosum, EC = external caspule, ICa = internal capsule, anterior limb, ICp = internal capsule, posterior limb, Put = putamen.

tractography (e.g., Johansen-Berg et al., 2005; Lehericy et al., 2004), and resting-state functional connectivity mapping (Greicius, Supekar, Menon, & Dougherty, 2009; Raichle et al., 2001). There are a few notable exceptions, however, exemplified by the finding of an apparent inferior fronto-occipital fascicle in humans (Forkel et al., 2012) that has not been identified in nonhuman primate tract tracing studies (Schmahmann & Pandya, 2006, 2007).

Association Fiber Tracts

The long association fiber tracts are the essential anatomic substrates for the interdomain communication between cortical areas that subserve different behaviors, and they deserve particular emphasis.

The superior longitudinal fasciculus (SLF) has three subcomponents:

SLF I (Fig. 2.4A) lies medially situated in the white matter of the superior parietal lobule and the superior frontal gyrus. It links the superior parietal region and adjacent medial parietal cortex in a reciprocal manner with the frontal lobe supplementary and premotor areas. It is thought to play a role in the regulation of higher aspects of motor behavior that require information about body part location, and it may contribute to the initiation of motor activity.

SLF II (Fig. 2.4B) is more laterally situated and occupies a position in the central core of the hemisphere white matter, lateral to the corona radiata and above the Sylvian fissure. It links the caudal inferior parietal lobule (equivalent in human to the angular gyrus) and the parieto-occipital areas, with the posterior part of the dorsolateral and mid-dorsolateral prefrontal cortex. It

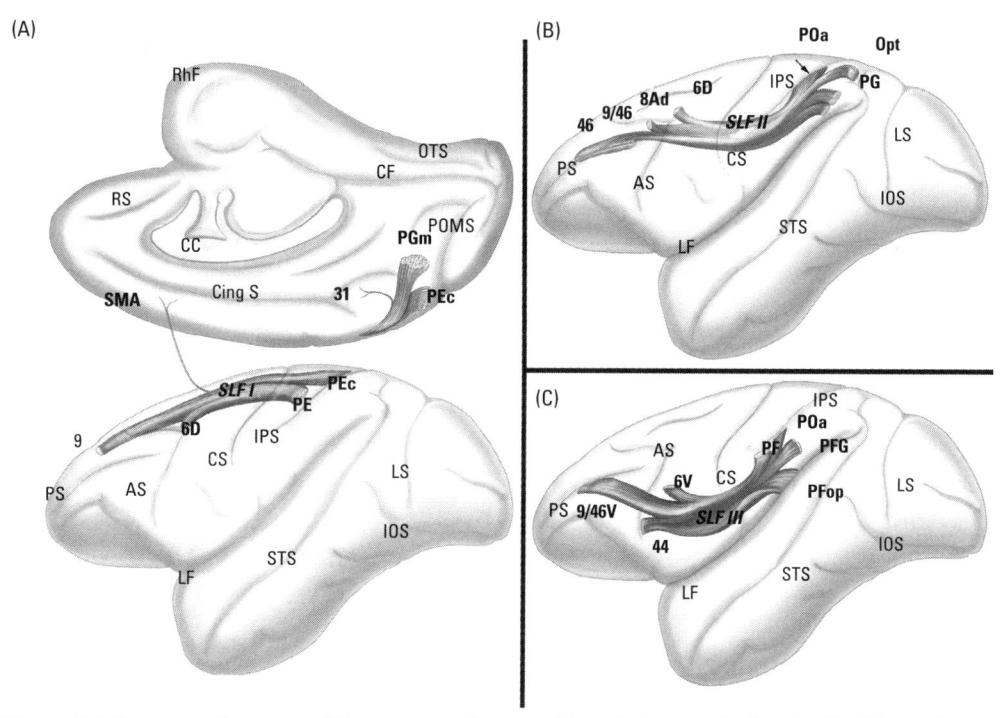

Figure 2.4 Summary diagrams of the course and composition of the superior longitudinal fasciculus (SLF) in the Rhesus monkey. (A) SLF I; (B) SLF II; and (C) SLF III. The lateral and medial views of the cerebral hemispheres show the trajectory of the three components of the SLF and the cortical areas that contribute axons to these fiber pathways. (Adapted from Schmahmann & Pandya, 2006). AS = arcuate sulcus, CC = corpus callosum, CF = calcarine fissure, Cing S = cingulate sulcus, CS = central sulcus, IOS = inferior occipital sulcus, IPS = intraparietal sulcus, LF = lateral fissure, LS = lunate sulcus, OTS = occipitotemporal sulcus, POMS = parieto-occipital medial sulcus, PS = principal sulcus, RhF = rhinal fissure, RS = rostral sulcus, SMA = supplementary motor area, STS = superior temporal sulcus

is thought to serve as the conduit for the neural system subserving visual awareness, the maintenance of attention, and engagement in the environment. It provides a means whereby the prefrontal cortex can regulate the focusing of attention within different parts of space.

SLF III (Fig. 2.4C) is further lateral and ventral, and it is located in the white matter of the parietal and frontal operculum. It provides the ventral premotor region and pars opercularis with higher order somatosensory input, it may be crucial for monitoring orofacial and hand actions, and in the human it may be engaged in articulatory aspects of language.

The arcuate fasciculus (AF) (Fig. 2.5A) runs in the white matter of the superior temporal gyrus and deep to the upper shoulder of the Sylvian fissure. By linking the caudal temporal lobe with the dorsolateral prefrontal cortex, it may be viewed as an auditory spatial bundle, important for the spatial attributes of acoustic stimuli and auditory-related processing. The AF has historically been regarded as linking the posterior (Wernicke) and anterior (Broca) language areas in the human brain, and to be involved in conduction aphasia. The connectional studies in monkey are consistent with the evolving notion that the AF subserves a dorsal stream of linguistic processing (Saur et al., 2008; Petrides & Pandya, 2009). Together with the SLF III, it appears that the AF is engaged in the phonemic aspects of language (sound appreciation and production).

The extreme capsule (EmC) (Fig. 2.5B) is situated between the claustrum and the insular cortex caudally, and between the claustrum and the orbital frontal cortex rostrally. In monkey, the extreme capsule is the principal association pathway linking the middle superior temporal region with the caudal parts of the orbital cortex and the ventral-lateral prefrontal cortex, including area 45. These areas are homologous to the Wernicke and Broca language cortices in human. The EmC, together with the MdLF (see Fig. 2.5), is thought to be implicated in a ventral stream processing of language, concerned with the semantic aspects of communication, namely, the meanings of words (Weiller, Bormann, Saur, Musso, & Rijntjes, 2011).

The middle longitudinal fasciculus (MdLF) (Fig. 2.5C) is situated within the white matter of the caudal inferior parietal lobule and extends into the white matter of the superior temporal gyrus. It links a number of high-level association and paralimbic cortical areas, including the inferior parietal lobule, caudal cingulate gyrus, parahippocampal gyrus, and prefrontal cortex. In the human the MdLF may play a role in language, possibly imbuing linguistic processing with information dealing with spatial organization, memory, and motivational valence.

The fronto-occipital fasciculus (FOF) (Fig. 2.6A) travels above the body and head of the caudate nucleus and the subcallosal fasciculus of Muratoff (Muratoff bundle; see Fig. 2.6), lateral to the corpus callosum, and medial to the corona radiata. It links the parieto-occipital region with dorsal premotor and prefrontal cortices. The FOF is the long association system of the dorsomedial aspects of the dorsal visual stream, and it appears to be an important component of the anatomical substrates involved in peripheral vision and the processing of visual spatial information.

The inferior longitudinal fasciculus (ILF) (Fig. 2.6B) is in the white matter between the sagittal stratum medially and the parieto-occipital and temporal cortices laterally. It has a vertical limb in the parietal and occipital lobes, and a horizontal component contained within the temporal lobe. The ILF is the long association system of the ventral visual pathways in the occipitotemporal cortices. Visual agnosia and prosopagnosia are two clinical syndromes that may arise from ILF damage.

The uncinate fasciculus (UF) (Fig. 2.7A) is a ventral limbic bundle that occupies the white matter of the rostral part of the temporal lobe, the limen insula, and the white matter of the orbital and medial frontal cortex. By connecting these temporal and prefrontal areas, the uncinate fasciculus may be a crucial component of the system that regulates emotional responses to auditory stimuli. It may also be involved in attaching emotional valence to visual information, is likely to be an important component of the circuit underlying recognition memory, and is implicated in cognitive tasks that are inextricably linked with emotional associations (Ghashghaei & Barbas, 2002). The UF has been shown to be clinically relevant in disorders of social and moral cognition, such as psychopathy

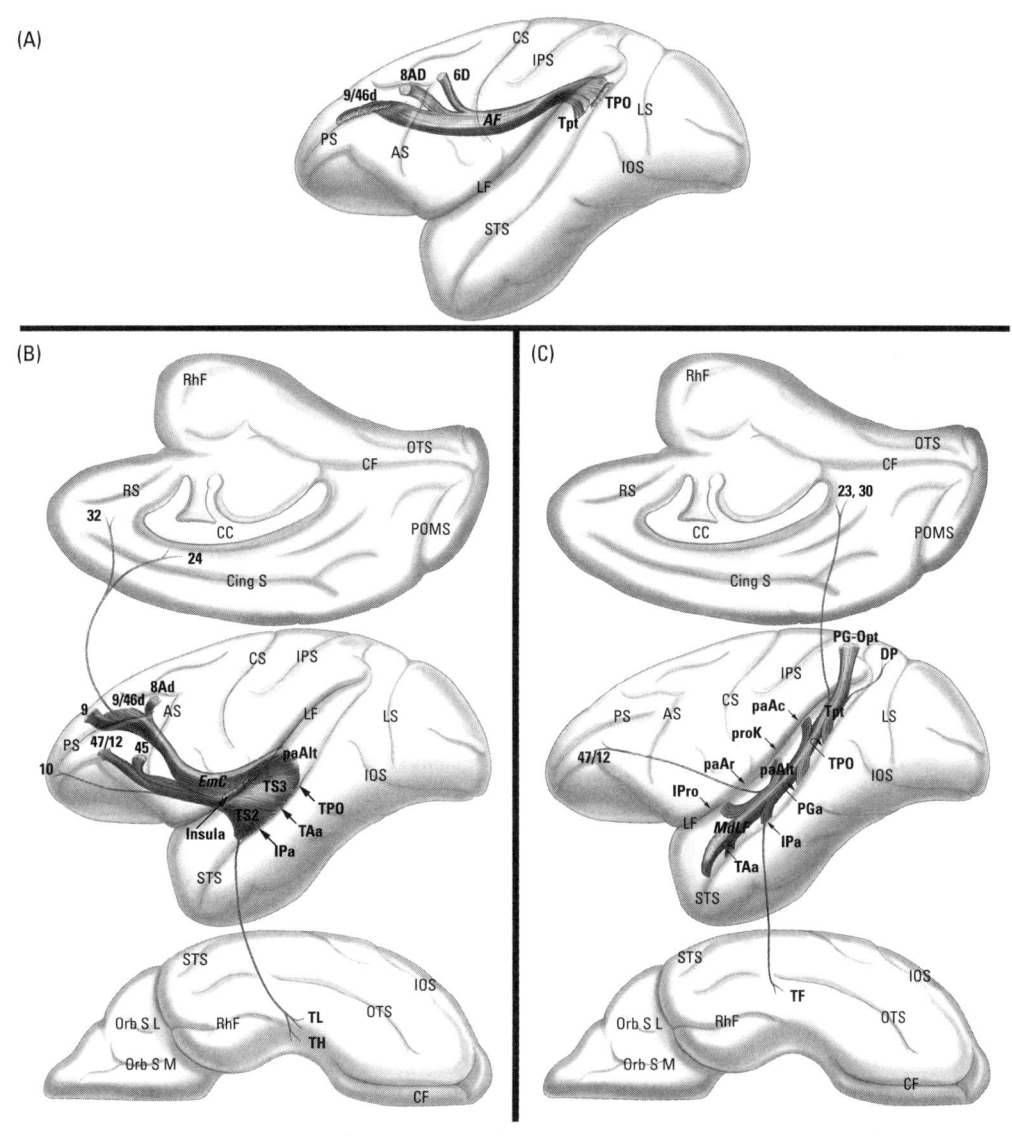

Figure 2.5 Summary diagrams of the course and composition in the Rhesus monkey of the (A) arcuate fasciculus (AF); (B) extreme capsule (EmC); and (C) middle longitudinal fasciculus (MdLF). The lateral and medial views of the cerebral hemispheres show the trajectory of the three components of the SLF and the cortical areas that contribute axons to these fiber pathways. (Adapted from Schmahmann & Pandya, 2006). AS = arcuate sulcus, CC = corpus callosum, CF = calcarine fissure, Cing S = cingulate sulcus, CS = central sulcus, IOS = inferior occipital sulcus, IPS = intraparietal sulcus, LF = lateral fissure, LS = lunate sulcus, Orb S L = lateral orbital sulcus, Orb S M = medial orbital sulcus, OTS = occipitotemporal sulcus, POMS = parieto-occipital medial sulcus, PS = principal sulcus, RhF = rhinal fissure, RS = rostral sulcus, STS = superior temporal sulcus

and sociopathy (Motzkin, Newman, Kiehl, & Koenigs, 2011; Sarkar et al., 2013), and in psychiatric illness including schizophrenia (Kawashima et al., 2009; Kubicki et al., 2002).

The cingulum bundle (CB) (Fig. 2.7B) nestles in the white matter of the cingulate gyrus. This dorsal limbic bundle links the rostral and caudal sectors of the cingulate gyrus with each other; with the dorsolateral, orbital, and medial prefrontal cortices; and with the parietal, retrosplenial, and ventral temporal cortices (including the parahippocampal

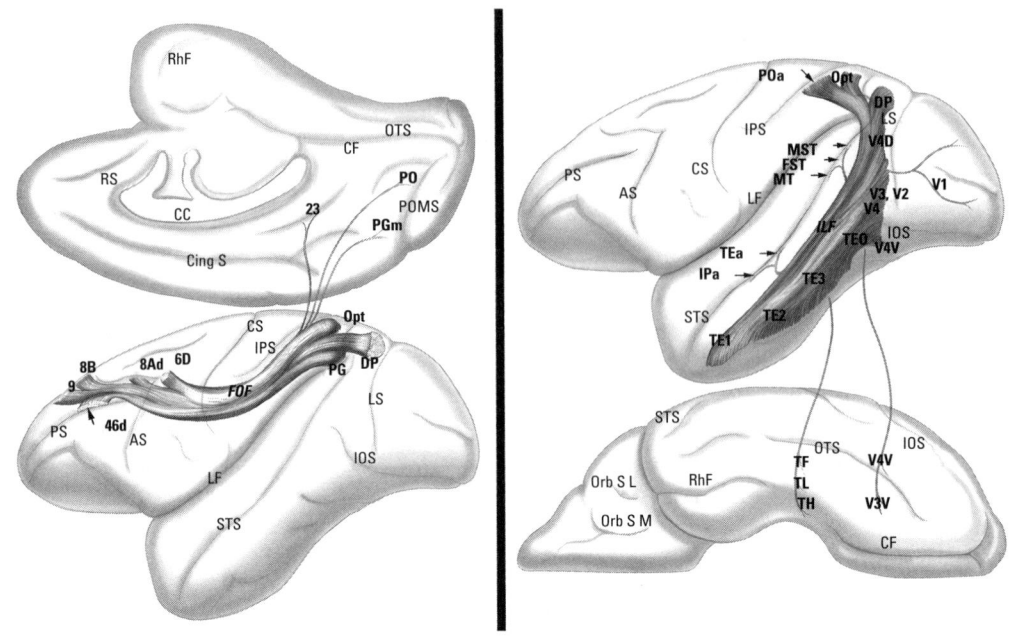

Figure 2.6 Summary diagrams of the course and composition in the Rhesus monkey of the (A) fronto-occipital fasciculus (FOF); and (B) inferior longitudinal fasciculus (ILF). The lateral, medial, and basal views of the hemisphere show the trajectory of these fiber pathways and the cortical areas that contribute axons to them. (Adapted from Schmahmann & Pandya, 2006). AS = arcuate sulcus, CC = corpus callosum, CF = calcarine fissure, Cing S = cingulate sulcus, CS = central sulcus, IOS = inferior occipital sulcus, IPS = intraparietal sulcus, LF = lateral fissure, LS = lunate sulcus, Orb S L = lateral orbital sulcus, Orb S M = medial orbital sulcus, OTS = occipitotemporal sulcus, POMS = parieto-occipital medial sulcus, PS = principal sulcus, RhF = rhinal fissure, RS = rostral sulcus, STS = superior temporal sulcus

gyrus and entorhinal cortex). By virtue of these connections, the CB may facilitate the emotional valence inherent in somatic sensation, nociception, attention, motivation, and memory (references in Schmahmann & Pandya, 2006). Cingulectomy, and subsequently bilateral stereotaxic cingulotomy, have achieved the status of established management for certain forms of neuropsychiatric illness, such as obsessive-compulsive disorder, and for intractable pain (Ballantine, Bouckoms, Thomas, & Giriunas, 1987; Ballantine, Cassidy, Flanagan, & Marino, 1967, 1987; Cosgrove & Rauch, 2003; Foltz & White, 1962; Jenike et al., 1991; Price et al., 2001; Spangler et al., 1996). The CB also links areas implicated in the default mode network—the retrosplenial cortex, medial prefrontal cortex, and medial temporal lobe, and thus likely plays a role in inner thought and creativity (autobiographical memory retrieval, envisioning the future, and conceiving the perspectives of others; Buckner, Andrews-Hanna, & Schacter, 2008).

Striatal Fibers

Corticostriatal fibers to the caudate nucleus, putamen, and claustrum are conveyed mainly by the subcallosal fasciculus of Muratoff and the external capsule.

Muratoff Bundle (Subcallosal Fasciculus of Muratoff)

The Muratoff bundle (MB) is a semilunar condensed fiber system situated immediately above the head and body of the caudate nucleus. It conveys axons to the striatum principally from association and limbic areas, with some fibers also from the dorsal part of the motor cortex.

External Capsule

The external capsule lies between the putamen medially and the claustrum laterally. It conveys fibers from the ventral and medial prefrontal cortex, ventral premotor cortex, precentral gyrus, the rostral superior

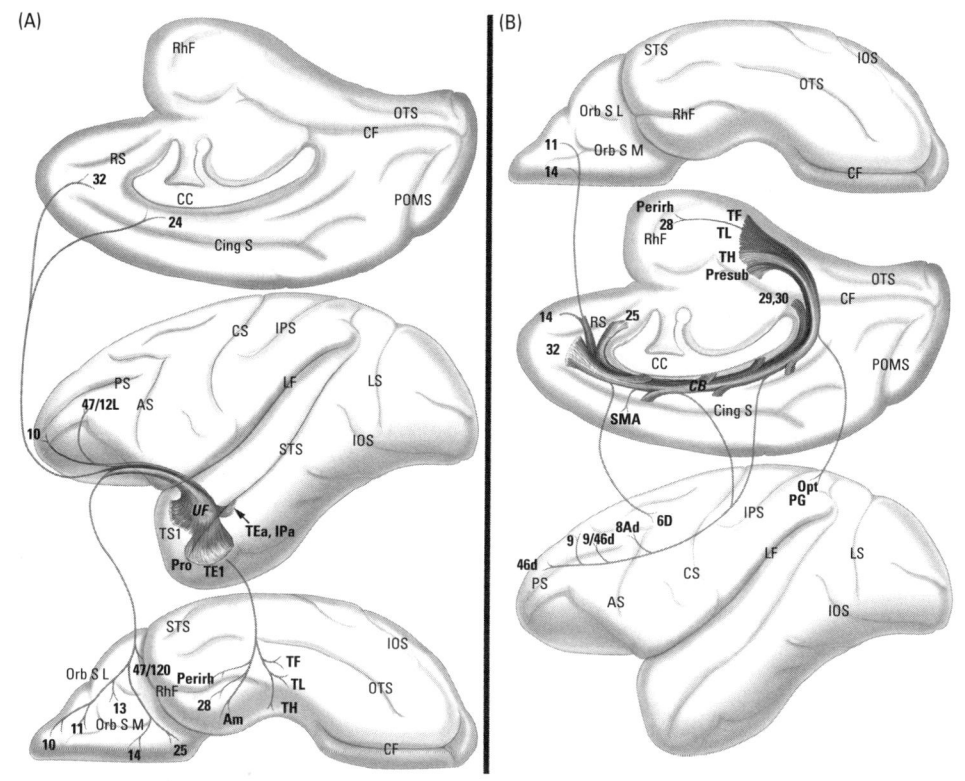

Figure 2.7 Summary diagrams of the course and composition in the Rhesus monkey of the (A) uncinate fasciculus (UF) and (B) cingulum bundle (CB). The lateral and medial views of the cerebral hemisphere show the trajectory of these fiber pathways and the cortical areas that contribute axons to them. (Adapted from Schmahmann & Pandya, 2006). Am = amygdala, AS = arcuate sulcus, CC = corpus callosum, CF = calcarine fissure, Cing S = cingulate sulcus, CS = central sulcus, IOS = inferior occipital sulcus, IPS = intraparietal sulcus, LF = lateral fissure, LS = lunate sulcus, Orb S L = lateral orbital sulcus, Orb S M = medial orbital sulcus, OTS = occipitotemporal sulcus, Perirh = perirhinal area, POMS = parieto-occipital medial sulcus, Pro = proisocortex, PS = principal sulcus, RhF = rhinal fissure, RS = rostral sulcus, STS = superior temporal sulcus

temporal region, and the inferotemporal and preoccipital regions. Projections from primary sensorimotor cortices are directed to the putamen; those from the supplementary motor area and association cortices terminate also in the caudate nucleus.

The MB and external capsule thus convey fibers from sensorimotor, cognitive, and limbic regions of the cerebral cortex to areas within the striatum in a topographically arranged manner. These corticostriatal pathways provide the critical links that enable different regions with the basal ganglia to contribute to motor control, cognition, and emotion.

Cord Fiber System

In addition to association and corticostriatal systems, every cortical region gives rise to a dense aggregation of fibers, termed "the cord," which occupies the central core of the white matter of the gyrus. The fibers in the cord separate into two distinct segments: commissural fibers and projection fibers in the subcortical bundle.

Commissural Fibers

Anterior Commissure
The anterior commissure (AC) traverses the midline in front of the anterior columns of the fornix, above the basal forebrain and beneath the medial and ventral aspect of the anterior limb of the internal capsule. Its fibers link the caudal part of the orbital frontal cortex, the temporal pole, the rostral superior temporal region, the major part of the inferotemporal area, and the parahippocampal

gyrus with their counterparts in the opposite hemisphere. In the nonhuman primate the AC is concerned with functional coordination across the hemispheres of highly processed information in the auditory and visual domains, particularly when imbued with mnemonic and limbic valence.

Corpus Callosum
The corpus callosum (CC) is divisible into five equal sectors conveying fibers across the hemispheres from the following locations: 1, the rostrum and genu contain fibers from the prefrontal cortex, rostral cingulate region, and supplementary motor area; 2, premotor cortex; 3, ventral premotor region and the motor cortex (face representation most rostral, followed by the hand and the leg, and postcentral gyrus fibers behind the motor fibers); 4, posterior parietal cortex; 5, the splenium contains superior temporal fibers rostrally, and inferotemporal and preoccipital fibers caudally. These comments regarding CC topography apply to the midsagittal plane.

Studies of the CC have led to novel understanding of the anatomic underpinnings of perception, attention, memory, language, and reasoning and have provided insights into consciousness, self-awareness, and creativity (Bogen & Bogen, 1988; Gazzaniga, 1967, 2000; Sperry, 1964, 1984). Knowledge of the CC topography is relevant in the clinical context of callosal section for control of seizures.

Hippocampal Commissures
Three fiber systems link the ventral limbic and paralimbic regions across the hemispheres.

Anterior (uncal and genual) hippocampal fibers are conveyed in the ventral hippocampal commissure, and those from the presubiculum, entorhinal cortex, and posterior parahippocampal gyrus are conveyed in the dorsal hippocampal commissure. The hippocampal decussation conveys fibers from the body of the hippocampal formation to the contralateral septum (Demeter, Rosene, & Van Hoesen, 1985). Damage to the hippocampal commissures in patients with lesions of the splenium of the corpus callosum may be responsible in part for the amnesia that occurs in this setting along with damage to the fornix that links the frontal and temporal lobes (Rudge & Warrington, 1991; Schmahmann, unpublished observations; Valenstein et al., 1987).

Projection Fibers

Projection (cortico-subcortical) fibers in the subcortical bundle are conveyed to their destinations via the internal capsule (anterior and posterior limbs) and the sagittal stratum. Each fiber system differentiates further as it progresses in the white matter into two principal systems: one destined for thalamus, and the other destined for brainstem and/or spinal cord.

Internal Capsule
The anterior limb of the internal capsule (ICa) conveys fibers from the prefrontal cortex, rostral cingulate region, and supplementary motor area (coursing through the genu of the capsule), principally to the thalamus, hypothalamus, and basis pontis.

The posterior limb of the internal capsule (ICp) conveys descending fibers from the premotor and motor cortices. Face, hand, arm, and leg fibers are arranged in a progressively caudal position. The ICp also conveys descending fibers from the parietal, temporal, and occipital lobes, and the caudal cingulate gyrus. These are topographically arranged within the capsule, in the rostral-caudal and superior-inferior dimensions.

Focal motor and sensory deficits follow infarction of the ICp, and complex behavioral syndromes result from lesions of the genu of the ICa and genu (Chukwudelunzu, Meschia, Graff-Radford, & Lucas, 2001; Schmahmann, 1984; Tatemichi et al., 1992). Deficits include fluctuating alertness, inattention, memory loss, apathy, abulia, and psychomotor retardation, with neglect of contralateral space and visual-spatial impairment from lesions of the genu in the right hemisphere, and severe verbal memory loss following genu lesions on the left. Deep brain stimulation has been successfully applied to the ICa in some patients with obsessive-compulsive disorder (Anderson & Ahmed, 2003) and intractable pain (Kumar, Toth, & Nath, 1997).

Sagittal Stratum
The sagittal stratum (SS) is a major cortico-subcortical white matter bundle that conveys fibers from the parietal, occipital, cingulate, and temporal regions to thalamus, basis pontis, and other

brainstem structures. It also conveys afferents principally from thalamus to cortex. The SS comprises an internal segment conveying corticofugal fibers efferent from the cortex and an external segment that contains incoming corticopetal fibers. The rostral sector of the SS corresponds to the anteriorly reflected fibers of the Flechsig-Meyer loop, while the ventral parts of the midsection of the SS contain the optic radiations and thalamic fibers of the caudal inferior temporal and occipitotemporal areas.

The SS is the equivalent of the internal capsule of the posterior part of the hemispheres. The functional implications are also analogous to those of the ICa and ICp. Whereas damage to the optic radiations in the ventral sector of the SS can lead to hemianopsia, damage to the dorsal part of the SS may result in distortion of high-level visual information.

Thalamic Peduncles

Cortico-subcortical fibers enter the thalamus in locations determined by their site of origin. The afferent and efferent fibers between thalamus and cerebral cortex are arrayed around the thalamus, and they are collectively termed "the thalamic peduncles" (details in Schmahmann & Pandya, 2006). The mammillothalamic tract that links the mammillary bodies with the anterior thalamic nuclei is particularly pertinent to the memory system; when damaged by lesions of thalamus, it can produce a profound amnestic syndrome.

Clinical Features of White Matter Lesions

Lesions of white matter fiber pathways themselves produce clinical consequences. Neuropsychiatric disturbances or dementia occurs in the setting of disseminated white matter damage from a large number of diseases, including small vessel cerebrovascular disease and multiple sclerosis (Filley, 2001, 2012; Schmahmann, Smith, Eichler, & Filley, 2007). Some neurodegenerative diseases, particularly tauopathy forms of frontotemporal lobar degeneration, are associated with primary neurodegenerative pathology within the frontotemporal white matter subjacent to frontotemporal cortex.

Poststroke language recovery depends on involvement of the subcallosal fasciculus of Muratoff (Naeser, Palumbo, Helm-Estabrooks, Stiassny-Eder, & Albert, 1989), parietal pseudothalamic pain results from white matter lesions that disconnect second somatosensory (SII) cortex from thalamus (Schmahmann & Leifer, 1992), and deficits in executive dysfunction and episodic memory are associated with white matter hyperintensities in aging (Smith et al., 2011). Focal white matter lesions result in aphasia, apraxia, and agnosia (Filley, 2001, 2012; Geschwind, 1965a,b), hemispatial neglect occurs with lesions in the anterior limb and genu of the internal capsule (Schmahmann, 1984; Schmahmann & Pandya, 2006; Tatemichi et al., 1992), frontal behavioral disturbances are noted in Marchiafava-Bignami disease of the corpus callosum (Leventhal, Baringer, Arnason, & Fisher, 1965), fornix lesions impair memory (D'Esposito, Verfaellie, Alexander, & Katz, 1995; Heilman & Sypert, 1977), and alexia without agraphia is seen with dual lesions in the splenium of the corpus callosum and the left occipital pole (Dejerine, 1892) as well as from a single subcortical lesion undercutting Wernicke's area (Schmahmann & Pandya, 2006).

The clinical deficits from loss of the white matter tracts linking different nodes may differ from those following lesions of the cortex or subcortical nodes for a number of reasons. White matter lesions may disrupt information destined for more than one node; they may involve association, projection, and striatal fibers; and they may affect more than one functional domain. Involvement of afferent versus efferent fibers may have clinical significance—striatal fibers are unidirectional from cortex to caudate-putamen; the middle cerebellar peduncle is essentially exclusively afferent from pons to cerebellum, whereas the superior cerebellar peduncle is predominantly efferent from cerebellum to the cerebral hemispheres; and the thalamic peduncles are bidirectional. Fiber tract disruptions are often incomplete by virtue of the anatomical arrangement of the pathways and the pathologic conditions that affect white matter, and the effects of partial versus complete disconnection are likely to be pertinent.

Basal Ganglia

Connectional Neuroanatomy of the Basal Ganglia

There are multiple parallel loops, or circuits, in the corticostriatal system, each of which comprises a parent cerebral cortical area (motor, association, or limbic cortex) that projects in a topographically arranged manner to nuclei of the basal ganglia, which in turn project via thalamus back to the cortical region of origin (Alexander, DeLong, & Strick, 1986; Mega & Cummings, 1994; Nauta & Domesick, 1984; Selemon & Goldman-Rakic, 1990). Each of these loops supports distinct domains of behavior. Sensorimotor and parietal intramodality sensory association cortices project predominantly to the dorsal and midsectors of the putamen. Association areas in prefrontal, posterior parietal, and superior temporal polymodal cortices project preferentially to the caudate nucleus. Orbital and medial prefrontal cortices and the cingulate gyrus project to the ventral striatum, and the rostral and inferior temporal and parahippocampal cortices project to the ventral striatum and ventral part of the putamen (Schmahmann & Pandya, 2006; Yeterian & Pandya, 1993, 1994, 1998). All these projections are arranged with a high degree of topographic specificity (Fig. 2.8).

Clinical Features of Basal Ganglia Lesions

Subcortical dementia as a clinical entity was first recognized in progressive supranuclear palsy and Huntington's disease (Albert, Feldman, & Willis, 1974), characterized by slowness of mental processing, forgetfulness, apathy, and depression. This notion was later expanded when it became apparent that focal subcortical lesions play a role in arousal, attention, mood, motivation, language, memory, abstraction, and visuospatial skills (Cummings & Benson, 1984). Patients with Parkinson's disease experience apathy with diminished emotional responsiveness (Dujardin et al., 2007) and cognitive decline, including impairment of concentration (bradyphrenia; Naville, 1922), loss of mental and behavioral flexibility with impaired strategic planning, sequential organization, constructional praxis, verbal fluency, working memory, attentional set shifting, initial encoding of information, procedural learning and spontaneous recall, and aspects of language that rely on procedural memory (Cronin-Golomb, Corkin, & Growdon, 1994; Growdon & Corkin, 1987; Muslimovic, Post, Speelman, & Schmand, 2007; Owen et al., 1992; Smith & McDowall, 2006; Williams-Gray, Foltynie, Brayne, Robbins, & Barker, 2007). These deficits are thought to reflect damage to fronto-striatal interactions, and interference with the role of basal ganglia in the cognitive processes that lead to habit formation (Graybiel, 1998; Barnes, Kubota, Hu, Jin, & Graybiel, 2005) and goal-directed behaviors (Delgado, 2007).

The major behavioral-cognitive syndromes that arise following basal ganglia lesions reflect the anatomic connections with the cerebral cortex. Three broad categories of behavioral-cognitive syndromes are recognized.

1. Lesions of the dorsal and midregions of the putamen that receive afferents from motor cortices lead to extrapyramidal motor syndromes and akinesia, and apathy and unconcern can follow damage to the dorsolateral striatum (Levy & Dubois, 2006). Hypophonic dysarthria is common in Parkinson's disease, reflecting involvement of the putamen.

2. Deficits in executive function and spatial cognition from lesions of the rostral head of the caudate nucleus reflect the connections with the dorsolateral prefrontal cortex concerned with attention and executive functions, and the posterior parietal cortex concerned with personal and extrapersonal space. Caudate head lesions can result in impaired working memory, strategy formation, and cognitive flexibility. Focal lesions are associated with impairments true to hemisphere—hemineglect and visual-spatial disorientation following right caudate lesions, aphasia after left caudate stroke (Caplan et al., 1990; Kumral, Evyapan, & Balkir, 1999). The precisely arranged topography of the associative projections to the striatum is likely to account for the observation that different regions of striatum engage in different aspects of cognition.

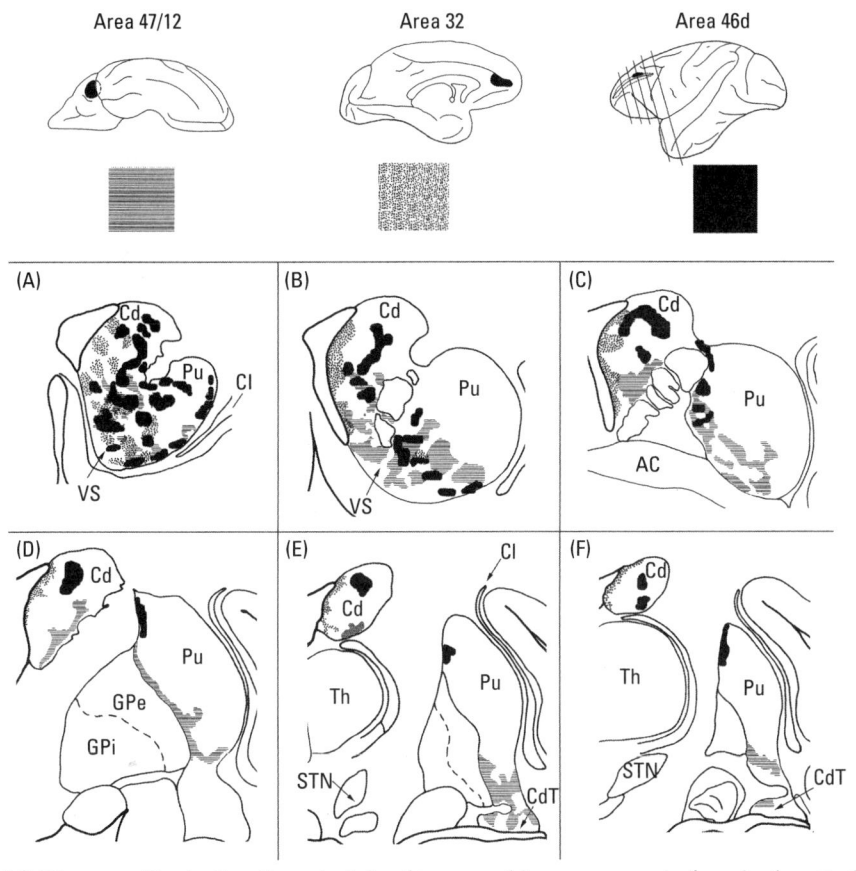

Figure 2.8 Diagrams illustrating the principle of topographic arrangement of cerebral cortical projections to the caudate nucleus (Cd) and putamen (Pu) from prefrontal cortex in the Rhesus monkey. Injections of anterogradely transported isotope tracer were placed in the prefrontal cortex. From left to right—orbital prefrontal cortex area 47/12 encroaching posteriorly on the insular proisocortex; medial prefrontal convexity area 32; and area 46d above the midportion of the principal sulcus. Coronal images through the striatum are shown in the columns below, from rostral above to caudal at the bottom. Black dots represent terminations in the striatum. (Adapted from Schmahmann & Pandya, 2006). AC = anterior commissure, CdT = tail of caudate nucleus, Cl = claustrum, GPe = globus pallidus external, GPi = globus pallidus internal, STN = subthalamic nucleus, Th = thalamus, VS = ventral striatum

3. Lesions of the ventral striatum produce disinhibited, irritable, and labile behaviors, and they are implicated in the neurobiology of addiction (Peoples, Kravitz, & Guillem, 2007) and obsessive-compulsive disorder (Remijnse et al., 2006). These disturbances of social and emotional function (behaviors with limbic valence) reflect the ventral striatal connections with the orbital and medial prefrontal cortices concerned with drive, motivation, emotional aspects of performance, inhibition of inappropriate responses, and reward-guided behaviors. Apathy most likely reflects involvement of the limbic ventral striato-pallidal system, but it can also occur following damage to dorsolateral striatum and may reflect connections with the medial prefrontal and anterior cingulate regions.

Motor and behavioral consequences of pallidotomy are also determined by lesion location. Posterior and ventrolateral regions (linked to motor cortical areas) have a beneficial impact on bradykinesia but no influence on cognitive performance (Lombardi et al., 2000). Rostral and dorsomedial GPi lesions (linked to prefrontal cortical areas 9 and 46) produce impaired semantic fluency, mathematical ability, and memory under conditions of proactive interference. Left-sided lesions produce deficits in verbal fluency and verbal encoding (Trépanier, Saint-Cyr, Lozano, & Lang, 1998). And bilateral pallidotomy, while generally effective at reducing the disabling features of Parkinson's disease (Scott, Gregory, & Hines, 1998), can result in prominent behavioral changes, disinhibition, reckless and socially inappropriate behaviors, apathy, poor judgment, and lack of insight (Ghika et al., 1999).

Thalamus

The neurobehavioral syndromes resulting from thalamic lesions may be understood by considering the functional properties of the thalamic nuclei as determined by tract-tracing investigations in monkeys, and physiological and clinical studies in patients. Thalamic nuclei have been grouped into five functional classes: reticular and intralaminar that subserve arousal and nociception; limbic nuclei concerned with mood and motivation; specific sensory nuclei; effector nuclei concerned with movement and aspects of language; and associative nuclei participating in high-level cognition (Schmahmann, 2003; Fig. 2.9; Table 2.1).

Anatomical Features and Connections

Reticular Thalamic Nucleus

This nuclear shell surrounds thalamus and conveys afferents from cerebral cortex. It contributes to synchrony and rhythms of thalamic neuronal activity and is relevant in the pathophysiology of epilepsy (Huguenard & Prince, 1997) and neural substrates of consciousness (Llinas & Ribary, 2001).

Intralaminar Thalamic Nuclei

The paracentral (Pcn), central lateral (CL), centromedian (CM), parafascicular (Pf), and midline nuclei such as paraventricular, rhomboid, and reunions play a role in autonomic drive. They receive afferents from brainstem, spinal cord, and cerebellum and have reciprocal connections with cerebral hemispheres.

The CM/Pf nuclei are linked with the basal ganglia in tightly connected functional circuits. A sensorimotor circuit links putamen with CM through the ventrolateral part of the internal segment of the globus pallidus (GPi). Cognitive circuits link the caudate with Pf through the dorsal GPi and through the substantia nigra pars reticulata (Sidibe, Pare, & Smith, 2002). A limbic circuit links the ventral striatum with the Pf through the rostromedial GPi, and midline nuclei receiving input from the periaqueductal gray and spinothalamic tract are involved in processing the motivational-affective components of pain (Bentivoglio, Kultas-Ilinsky, & Ilinsky, 1993; Lenz & Dougherty, 1997; Willis, 1997).

Limbic Thalamic Nuclei

The functions of the anterior nuclear group— ventral, medial, and dorsal (AV, AM, and AD nuclei), and the lateral dorsal (LD) nucleus are determined by their reciprocal anatomic connections with limbic structures in the cingulate gyrus, hippocampus, parahippocampal formation, entorhinal cortex, retrosplenial cortex, orbitofrontal and medial prefrontal cortices, and with subcortical structures, including the mamillary bodies and amygdala (Locke, Angevine, & Yakovlev, 1961; Yakovlev & Locke, 1961; Yakovlev, Locke, Koskoff, & Patton, 1960; Yeterian & Pandya, 1988). The magnocellular part of the medial dorsal nucleus (MDmc), parts of the medial pulvinar, and parts of the VA nucleus are also reciprocally interconnected with the cingulate gyrus and other components of the limbic system and thus may also be considered limbic. Like their cortical and subcortical counterparts (Devinsky & Luciano, 1997; Mesulam, 1988), limbic thalamic nuclei are likely to be essential for learning and memory, emotional experience and expression, drive, and motivation. The tuberothalamic artery irrigates these nuclei as well as the mamillothalamic and ventral amygdalofugal tracts that link the anterior thalamic nuclei with the limbic regions, accounting for the profound amnestic and limbic deficits resulting from tuberothalamic stroke.

Specific Sensory Thalamic Nuclei

The specific sensory nuclei include the medial geniculate nucleus (MGN), lateral geniculate

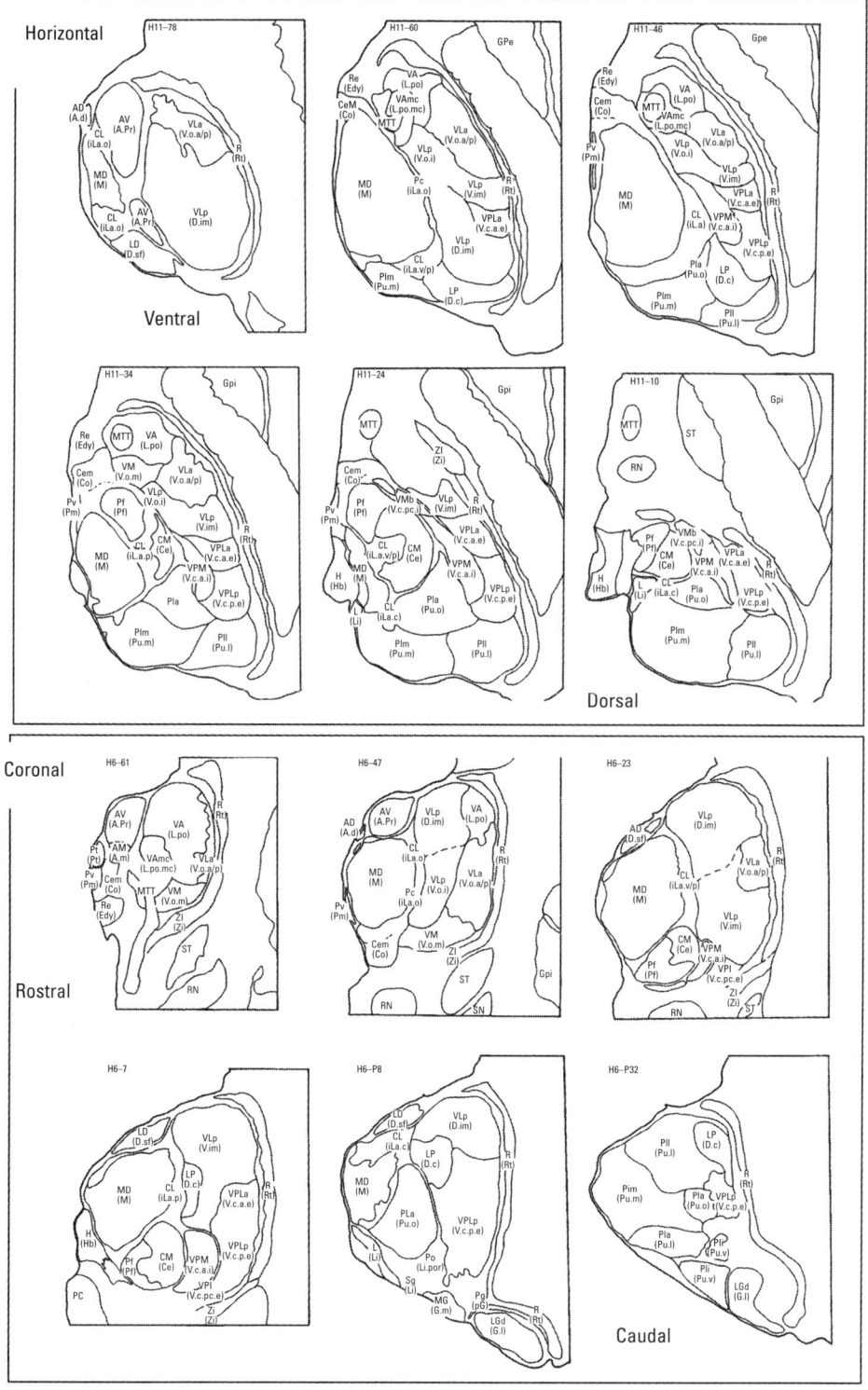

Figure 2.9 Diagram illustrating the nuclei of the human thalamus. Horizontal sections are seen above, from ventral to dorsal. Coronal sections below proceed from rostral to caudal. The revised nomenclature correlates with terminology used in the monkey. An earlier nomenclature is shown in parentheses. (Adapted from Jones, 1997; figure reproduced from Schmahmann & Pandya, 2008)

TABLE 2.1 Behavioral Roles of Thalamic Nuclei (From Schmahmann, 2003)

Major Functional Grouping	Thalamic Nuclei	Putative Functional Attributes
Reticular	Reticular	Arousal, rhythmicity, role in epileptogenesis
Intralaminar	CM, Pf, CL, Pcn, midline (reunions, paraventricular, rhomboid)	Arousal, attention, motivation, affective components of pain
Limbic	Anterior nuclear group (AD, AM, AV), Lateral dorsal nucleus Other—MDmc, medial pulvinar, ventral anterior.	Learning, memory, emotional experience and expression, drive, motivation
Specific Sensory	Medial geniculate	Auditory
	Lateral geniculate	Visual
	Ventroposterior—lateral (VPL)	Somatosensory body and limbs
	—medial (VPM)	Somatosensory head and neck
	—medial, parvicellular (VPMpc)	Gustatory
	—inferior (VPI)	Vestibular
Effector	Ventral anterior—reticulata recipient	Complex behaviors
	—pallidal recipient	Motor programming
	Ventral medial	Motor
	Ventral lateral—ventral part	Motor
	—dorsal part	Language (dominant hemisphere)
Associative	Lateral posterior	High-order somatosensory and visuospatial integration—spatial cognition
	Medial dorsal—medial, magnocellular (MDmc)	Drive, motivation, inhibition, emotion
	—intermediate, parvicellular (MDpc)	Executive functions, working memory
	—lateral, multiform (MDmf)	Attention, horizontal gaze
	Pulvinar—medial	Supramodal, high-level association region across multiple domains
	—Lateral	Somatosensory, visual association
	—Inferior	Visual association
	—Anterior (pulvinar oralis)	Intramodality somatosensory association, pain appreciation

AD = anterodorsal thalamic nucleus, AM = anteromedian thalamic nucleus, AV = anteroventral thalamic nucleus, CL = central lateral thalamic nucleus, CM = centromedian thalamic nucleus, Pcn = paracentral thalamic nucleus, Pf = parafascicular thalamic nucleus

nucleus (LGN), and ventroposterior nuclei (lateral, medial, and inferior—VPL, VPM, and VPI).

Medial geniculate nucleus connections with primary and association auditory cortices infer a role in higher level auditory processing as well as in elementary audition (Hackett, Stepniewska, & Kaas, 1998; Mesulam & Pandya, 1973; Pandya, Rosene, & Doolittle, 1994). The lateral geniculate projects to primary and secondary visual cortices (Kennedy & Bullier, 1985). It also receives projections back from visual areas (Shatz & Rakic, 1981), indicating that higher order processing can influence visual perception at an early stage.

The VPL and VPM nuclei are reciprocally interconnected with primary somatosensory cortices; VPL serves body and limbs, and VPM serves head and neck (Jones & Powell, 1970b). Gustatory function is subserved by the parvicellular division of VPM (Pritchard, Hamilton, Morse, & Norgren, 1986). The somatotopy of these nuclei is precise, and lacunar infarcts of the inferolateral artery produce focal sensory deficits. The VPI nucleus is linked with the rostral inferior parietal lobule and the second somatosensory area in the parietal operculum (SII; Schmahmann & Pandya, 1990; Yeterian & Pandya, 1985) and with the frontal operculum engaged in vestibular functions (Deecke, Schwarz, & Fredrickson, 1977).

Spinothalamic and trigeminothalamic inputs, and topographically organized wide dynamic neurons and nociceptive specific neurons in the ventroposterior nuclei facilitate their role in the specific component of the pain system (Willis, 1997). Disruption of SII cortex connections with these nuclei has been postulated to cause the parietal pseudothalamic pain syndrome (Schmahmann & Leifer, 1992).

Effector Thalamic Nuclei

Motor nuclei include the ventral anterior (VA), ventromedial (VM), and ventral lateral (VL) nuclei. Subregions within VA receive afferents from the internal globus pallidus (Ilinsky & Kultas-Ilinsky, 1987), are linked with premotor cortices (Jones, 1997), and may be responsible for dystonia in rostral thalamic lesions. Neurons in VA receive afferents from the substantia nigra pars reticulata (Francois, Tande, Yelnik, & Hirsch, 2002; Jones, 1985); are linked with premotor, supplementary motor (Schell & Strick, 1984), prefrontal (Goldman-Rakic & Porrino, 1985), caudal parts of the posterior parietal (Schmahmann & Pandya, 1990) and rostral cingulate cortices (Vogt, Pandya, & Rosene, 1987); and may account for complex behavioral syndromes following lesions of the ventral anterior thalamus.

The ventral sector of the posterior part of VL is linked with the motor cortex (Strick, 1976) and causes ataxia and mild motor weakness following thalamic stroke (Gutrecht, Zamani, & Pandya, 1992; Murthy, 1988; Solomon, Barohn, Bazan, & Grissom, 1994). The dorsal part is linked with the posterior parietal (Schmahmann & Pandya, 1990), prefrontal (Kievit & Kuypers, 1977; Künzle & Akert, 1977; Middleton & Strick, 1994), and superior temporal cortices (Yeterian & Pandya, 1989) and has a role in articulation and language (perseveration results from electrical stimulation of left medial VL; misnaming and omissions with stimulation of left posterior VL), as well as in the encoding and retrieval of verbal (left) and nonverbal information (right) (Hugdahl & Wester, 2000; Johnson & Ojemann, 2000; Ojemann, Fedio, & Van Buren, 1968; Ojemann & Ward, 1971).

Associative Thalamic Nuclei

The lateral posterior, medial dorsal, and pulvinar nuclei are interconnected with cerebral association areas and have no peripheral afferents or links with primary sensorimotor cortices.

The lateral posterior (LP) nucleus is reciprocally linked with the posterior parietal (Schmahmann & Pandya, 1990; Weber & Yin, 1984; Yeterian & Pandya, 1985), medial and dorsolateral extrastriate (Yeterian & Pandya, 1997), and posterior cingulate and medial parahippocampal cortices (Yeterian & Pandya, 1988). It is able to integrate intramodal and multimodal associative somatosensory and visual information, and it is likely engaged in spatial functions, goal-directed reaching (Acuña, Cudeiro, Gonzalez, Alonso, & Perez, 1990), and possibly in conceptual and analytical thinking.

The medial dorsal (MD) nucleus has reciprocal connections with the prefrontal cortex (Barbas, Henion, & Dermon, 1991; Giguere & Goldman-Rakic, 1988; Goldman-Rakic & Porrino, 1985; Siwek & Pandya, 1991; Tobias, 1975). The laterally placed multiformis part (MDmf) is linked with the area 8 in the arcuate concavity, and lesions produce impairments of horizontal gaze and attention. The intermediate part of MD (the parvicellular MDpc) is linked with dorsolateral and dorsomedial prefrontal cortices, areas 9 and 46, possibly accounting for poor working memory and perseveration resulting from MD lesions. The medial part (magnocellular MDmc) is linked with paralimbic regions—medial and orbital prefrontal cortices, amygdala, basal forebrain, and olfactory and entorhinal cortices (Graff-Radford, Tranel, Van Hoesen, & Brandt, 1990; Russchen, Amaral, & Price, 1987). Apathy, abulia, disinhibition, and failure to inhibit inappropriate behaviors are likely to result from MDmc lesions, along with memory (Victor, Adams, & Collins, 1971) and language deficits (Bogousslavsky, Regli, & Uske, 1988).

Different subregions within medial pulvinar (PM) are topographically linked with prefrontal (Asanuma, Andersen, & Cowan, 1985; Romanski, Giguere, Bates, & Goldman-Rakic, 1997; Yeterian & Pandya, 1988), posterior parietal (Asanuma, Andersen, & Cowan, 1985; Schmahmann & Pandya, 1990; Yeterian & Pandya, 1985), and auditory-related

(Pandya, Rosene, & Doolittle, 1994) and multimodal superior temporal cortices (Yeterian & Pandya, 1991), and with the cingulate, parahippocampal (Yeterian & Pandya, 1988), and insula cortices (Mufson & Mesulam, 1984). Aphasia (Ojemann, Fedio, & Van Buren, 1968), spatial neglect (Karnath, Himmelbach, & Rorden, 2002), and psychosis (Guard et al., 1986) may result from PM lesions. The lateral pulvinar (PL) is linked with posterior parietal (Asanuma, Andersen, & Cowan, 1985; Schmahmann & Pandya, 1990), superior temporal (Yeterian & Pandya, 1991), and medial and dorsolateral extrastriate cortices (Yeterian & Pandya, 1997), and the superior colliculus (Robinson & Cowie, 1997). It is engaged in the integration of somatosensory and visual information. Inferior pulvinar (PI) is linked with temporal lobe areas concerned with visual feature discrimination, and with ventrolateral and ventromedial extrastriate areas concerned with visual motion (Cusick, Scripter, Darensbourg, & Weber, 1993; Yeterian & Pandya, 1997). It also receives input from retinal ganglion cells (Cowey, Stoerig, & Bannister, 1994) and visual neurons of the superior colliculus (Robinson & Cowie, 1997). The anterior pulvinar (pulvinar oralis, PO) is interconnected with intramodality somatosensory association cortices in the rostral part of the inferior parietal region, and with the second somatosensory area (SII; Acuna, Cudeiro, Gonzalez, Alonso, & Perez, 1990; Asanuma, Andersen, & Cowan, 1985; Schmahmann & Pandya, 1990; Yeterian & Pandya, 1985). The PO nucleus may be important in the appreciation of pain, as are the suprageniculate, limitans, and posterior nuclei (Jones, 1985).

Sensorimotor, effector, limbic, and associative regions of cerebral cortex are therefore linked with distinctly different sets of thalamic nuclei. Thalamic projections to the posterior parietal lobe exemplify this concept (Schmahmann & Pandya, 1990). Connections become progressively elaborated as one moves from rostral to caudal within both the superior and the inferior parietal lobules. Rostral areas concerned with intramodality somatosensory processing are related to modality-specific thalamic nuclei, whereas caudal regions, concerned with complex functions, derive their input from multimodal and limbic nuclei (Fig. 2.10). This rostral-caudal cortical topography is represented within the LP and PO nuclei that project to both superior and inferior parietal lobules. Rostral parietal subdivisions receive projections from ventral regions within these thalamic nuclei, caudal parietal afferents arise from the dorsal parts of these nuclei, and the intervening cortical levels receive projections from intermediate positions within the nuclei. A similar topographic arrangement is present also in the medial pulvinar projections to the inferior parietal lobule (Fig. 2.11).

Clinical Features of Thalamic Lesions

C. Miller Fisher (1913–2012) first described neglect ("modified anosognosia and hemisomatognosia"), global "dysphasia," confusion, and visual hallucinations in patients with thalamic hemorrhage (Fisher, 1959). Accounts followed of thalamic dementia from prion diseases (Martin, 1997) and behavioral changes in patients with thalamic tumors (Nass et al., 2000; Ziegler, Kaufman, & Marshall, 1977), but these lesions are seldom confined to thalamus. Focal lesions in thalamus occur in the setting of ischemic infarction. There are four main vascular syndromes of the thalamus. A review of these vascular syndromes illustrates the behavioral roles of the different thalamic nuclei and highlights the clinical relevance of the thalamic afferent and efferent connections (Schmahmann, 2003; Fig. 2.12; Table 2.2).

Tuberothalamic Artery Infarction

These patients demonstrate fluctuating levels of consciousness, disorientation in time and place, and personality changes, including euphoria, lack of insight, apathy, lack of spontaneity, and emotional unconcern (Bogousslavsky, Regli, & Assal, 1986; Bogousslavsky, Regli, & Uske, 1988; Graff-Radford, Damasio, Yamada, Eslinger, & Damasio, 1985; Graff-Radford, Eslinger, Damasio, & Yamada, 1984; Lisovoski et al., 1993) (Fig. 2.13A and B). New learning and verbal and visual memory are impaired. Amnesia is greater following left thalamic lesions, along with anomia, impaired comprehension, fluent and meaningless discourse with semantic and phonemic paraphasic errors, neologisms, and perseveration. In contrast, repetition and reading aloud are preserved. Acalculia, buccofacial

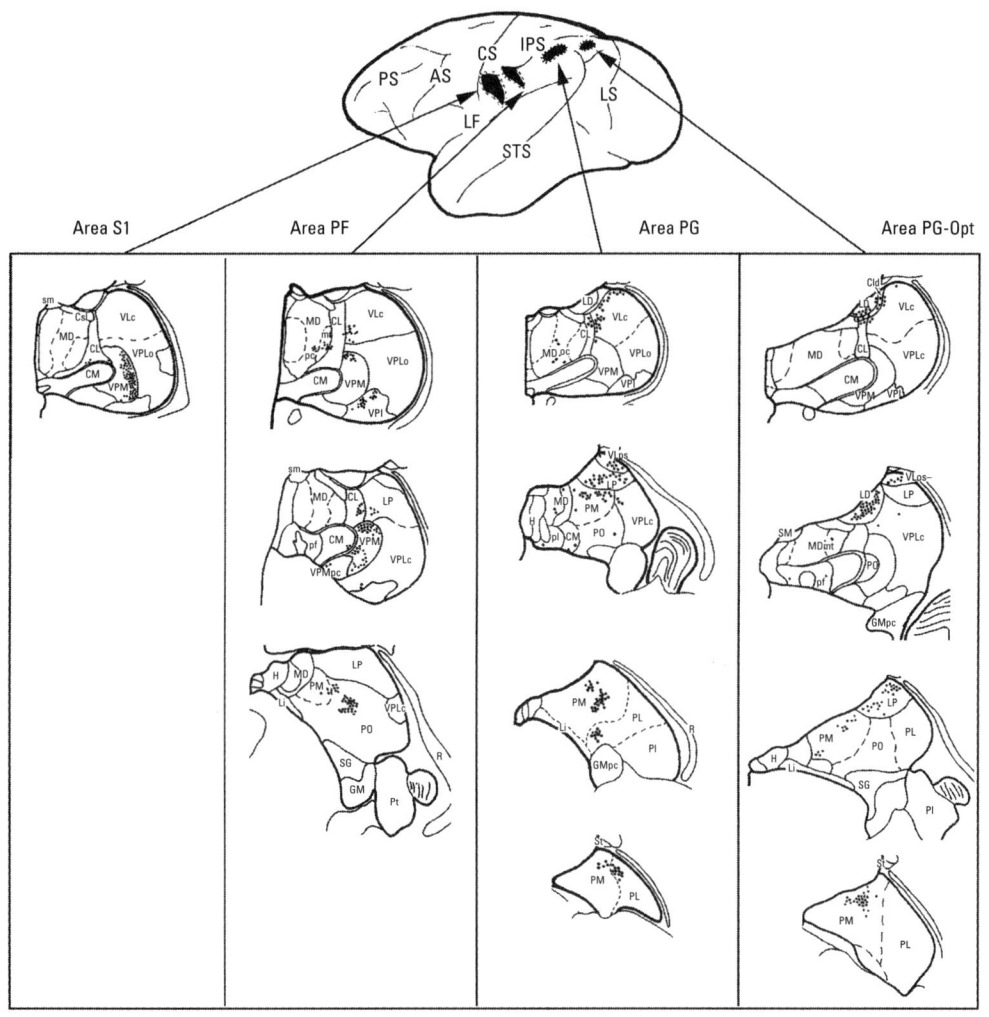

PARIETAL CORTICAL REGION	S1	Area PF	Area PG	Area PG-Opt
PRINCIPAL THALAMIC NUCLEAR AFFERENTS	Sensory Ventral posterior medial (VPM)	Sensory Ventral posterior medial (VPM) Ventral posterior inferior (VPI) Associative Pulvinar oralis (PO) Lateral posterior (LP) Pulvinar medialis (PM)	Associative Pulvinar medialis (PM) Lateral posterior (LP) Effector Ventral lateral (caudal (VLc) and pars postrema (VLps))	Associative Pulvinar medialis (PM) Lateral posterior (LP) Effector Ventral lateral (pars postrema) (VLps) Intralaminar Paracentralis (Pcn) Limbic Lateral dorsal (LD) Anterior nuclei
PUTATIVE FUNCTIONAL PROPERTIES	Primary unimodal somatosensory	Intramodality association within somatosensory domain: for graphesthesia, stereognosis	Multimodal somatosensory and visual: for integration of visual and cutaneo-kinesthetic spatial information	Multimodal associative and paralimbic: visual spatial and somesthetic stimuli invested with emotional and motivational valence

Figure 2.10 Diagrammatic representation of projections from thalamus (black dots) to primary somatosensory cortex S1, area PF, area PG, and area PG-Opt of the parietal lobe in Rhesus monkey following cortical injections (blackened areas) of wheat germ agglutinated horseradish peroxidase. Representative rostral to caudal levels of thalamus are shown. (Thalamic nomenclature according to Olszewski, 1952. Parietal lobe nomenclature according to Pandya & Seltzer, 1982.) The table summarizes the areas injected with tracer, the principal thalamic nuclei demonstrating retrogradely labeled neurons, and the putative functional attributes of the cortical areas studied. (Derived from Schmahmann & Pandya, 1990; figure reproduced from Schmahmann & Pandya, 2008)

temporally unrelated information (*palipsychism*). Apathy, inattention, disorientation, impaired sequencing, and perseveration are prominent. Dysarthria, hypophonia, anomia, and decreased verbal fluency are noted, but comprehension, writing, reading, and repetition are preserved (Clarke et al., 1994; Ghika-Schmid & Bogousslavsky, 2000).

Paramedian Artery Infarction

Disturbances of arousal and memory, confusion, agitation, aggression, apathy, and perseveration are common (Bogousslavsky, Regli, & Uske, 1988; Castaigne et al., 1981; Graff-Radford et al., 1984, 1985) (Fig. 2.13C). Left thalamic strokes produce a number of language impairments (Nadeau & Crosson, 1997) including adynamic aphasia (Guberman & Stuss, 1983) with reduced verbal fluency, preserved syntax, occasional paraphasias, and normal repetition. Right paramedian strokes impair visual-spatial functions. Bilateral infarction produces disorientation, confusion, hypersomnolence, and akinetic mutism (awake unresponsiveness) (Castaigne et al., 1981; Graff-Radford et al., 1984, 1985; Reilly, Connolly, Stack, Martin, & Hutchinson, 1992) as well as severe anterograde and retrograde memory deficits, apathy, inappropriate social behaviors, and a reported absence of spontaneous thoughts or mental activities (see Bogousslavsky et al., 1991; Engelborghs, Marien, Pickut, Verstraeten, & De Deyn, 2000; Guberman & Stuss, 1983). Distortion of personally relevant autobiographical memory with relative sparing of knowledge of famous people and public events has been observed—a thematic retrieval memory disorder (Hodges & McCarthy, 1993). Disorientation in time (*chronotaraxis*; Spiegel, Wycis, Orchinik, & Freed, 1956), apraxia, and dysgraphia are also reported (Castaigne et al., 1981; Graff-Radford, Tranel, Van Hoesen, & Brandt, 1990).

Inferolateral Artery Infarction

The thalamic syndrome of Dejerine and Roussy (1906) includes sensory loss, hemiparesis, and postlesion pain, particularly following right-sided lesions (Fig. 2.13D) (Bogousslavsky, Regli, & Uske, 1988; Caplan, DeWitt, Pessin, Gorelick, & Adelman, 1988; Fisher, 1978; Garcin & Lapresle, 1954; Lapresle & Haguenau, 1973;

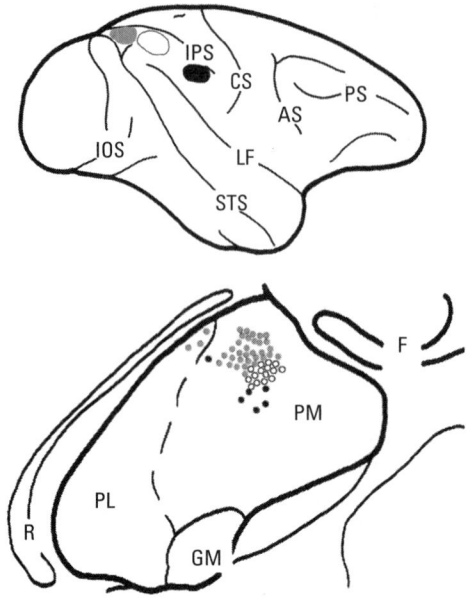

Figure 2.11 Diagrammatic representation of the projections from the medial pulvinar nucleus of thalamus (PM) to the inferior parietal lobule in Rhesus monkey. Fluorescent retrograde tracers were placed in area PF (shaded black), area PG (open circle), and area PG-Opt (shaded gray) in a Rhesus monkey, and the resulting retrogradely labeled neurons were identified in the PM nucleus. Shading of labeled neurons was according to the injection site in each case. (Adapted from Schmahmann & Pandya, 1990). AS = arcuate sulcus, CS = central sulcus, F = fornix, GM = medial geniculate, IOS = inferior occipital sulcus, IPS = intraparietal sulcus, LF = lateral fissure, PL = lateral pulvinar, PS = principal sulcus, R = reticular nucleus, STS = superior temporal sulcus.

apraxia, and limb apraxia may occur (Warren, Thompson, & Thompson, 2000). Right thalamic lesions produce the amnestic syndrome along with impairments in visual processing and visual memory, and hemispatial neglect. Lesions on either side produce emotional central facial paralysis (good facial movement with volition, but facial asymmetry during emotional display) and constructional apraxia. Motor findings are mild, and sensory disturbances are rare.

Stroke confined to the anterior/polar branch of the tuberothalamic artery affects memory and personality. Autobiographic memory and newly acquired information are disorganized with respect to temporal order, with patients displaying superimposition of

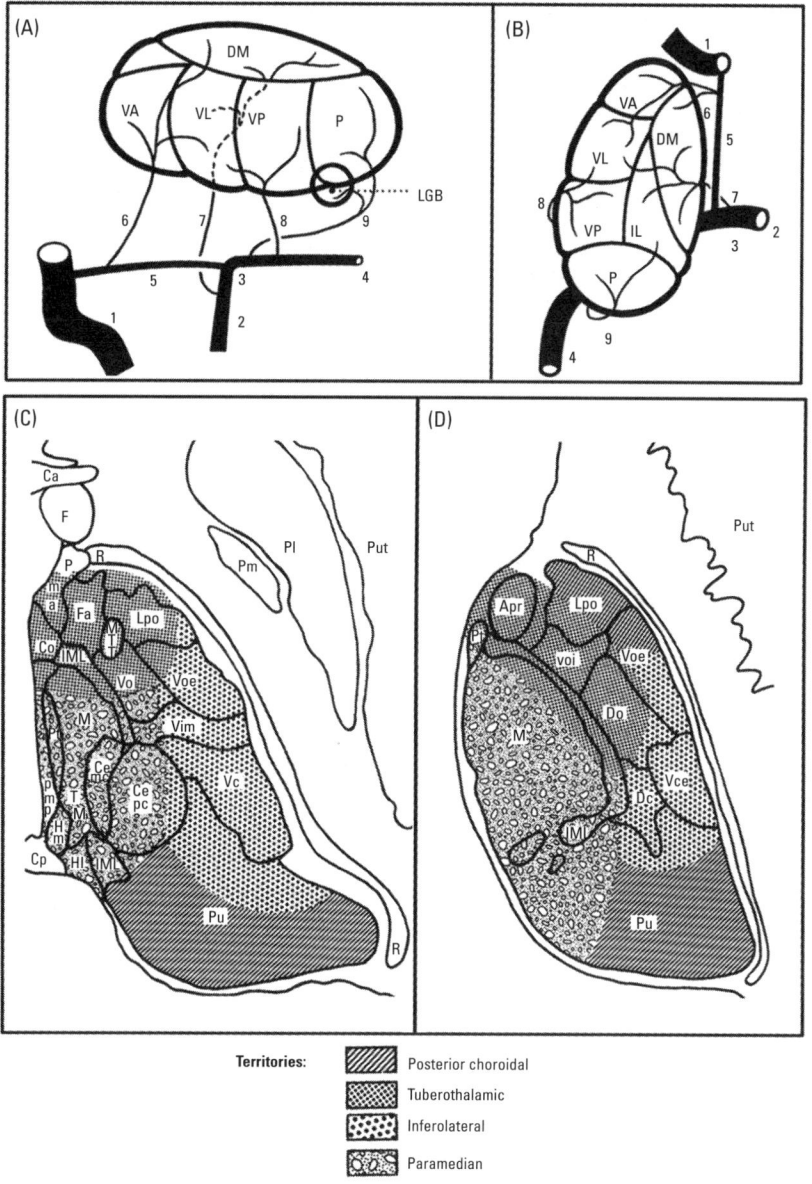

Figure 2.12 Thalamic vascular supply. Schematic diagram of the lateral (A) and dorsal (B) views of the four major thalamic arteries, and the nuclei they irrigate, according to Bogousslavsky, Regli, and Uske (1988). 1 = carotid artery, 2 = basilar artery, 3 = P1 region of the posterior cerebral artery (mesencephalic artery), 4 = posterior cerebral artery, 5 = posterior communicating artery, 6 = tuberothalamic artery, 7 = paramedian artery, 8 = inferolateral artery, 9 = posterior choroidal artery. DM, dorsomedial nucleus; IL, intralaminar nuclear complex; P, pulvinar; VA, Ventral anterior; VL, Ventral lateral; VP, ventral posterior complex. The illustrations in C and D from De Freitas and Bogousslavsky (2002) are an adapted version of the conclusions of von Cramon, Hebel, and Schuri (1985) regarding the patterns of irrigation by the thalamic arterial supply to the thalamic nuclei. (Composite image from Schmahmann, 2003)

Nasreddine & Saver, 1997). Sensory loss may be the sole clinical manifestation, involve all modalities, or impair spinothalamic sensation (temperature, pinprick) without loss of posterior column sense (position, vibration). These strokes produce a flexed and pronated "thalamic hand" (Foix & Hillemand, 1925) with the thumb buried beneath the other

TABLE 2.2 Thalamic Arterial Supply and Principal Clinical Features of Focal Infarction (From Schmahmann, 2003)

Thalmic Blood Vessel	Nuclei Irrigated	Clinical Features Reported
Tuberothalamic artery 22 (arises from middle third of P.Comm)	Reticular, intralaminar, VA, rostral VL, ventral pole of MD, anterior nuclei—AD, AM, AV, ventral internal medullary lamina, ventral amygdalofugal pathway, mamillothalamic tract	*Confusion, memory, emotion, behavior* Fluctuating arousal and orientation Impaired learning, memory, autobiographical memory Superimposition of temporally unrelated information Personality changes, apathy, abulia Executive failure, perseveration True to hemisphere—language if VL involved on left; hemispatial neglect if right sided Emotional facial, acalculia, apraxia
Paramedian artery 22 (arises from P1)	MD, intralaminar—CM, Pf, CL, posteromedial VL, ventromedial pulvinar, paraventricular, LD, dorsal internal medullary lamina	*Confusion, memory, language, behavior* Decreased arousal (coma vigil if bilateral) Impaired learning and memory, confabulation, temporal disorientation, poor autobiographical memory Aphasia if left sided, spatial deficits if right sided Altered social skills and personality, including apathy, aggression, agitation
Inferolateral artery 22 (arises from P2) Principal inferolateral branch	Ventroposterior complex—VPM, VPL, VPI Ventral lateral nucleus, ventral (motor) part	*Variable elements of a triad—hemisensory loss, hemiataxia, and hemiparesis* Sensory loss (variable extent, all modalities) Hemiataxia Hemiparesis Post-lesion pain syndrome (Dejerine-Roussy)—right hemisphere predominant
Medial branch	Medial geniculate	auditory consequences
Inferolateral pulvinar branches	Rostral and lateral pulvinar, LD nucleus	behavioral
Posterior choroidal artery (arises from P2) Lateral branches	LGN, LD, LP, inferolateral parts of pulvinar	Visual field loss (hemianopsia, quadrantanopsia) Variable sensory loss, weakness, aphasia, memory impairment, dystonia, hand tremor
Medial branches	MGN, posterior parts of CM and CL, pulvinar	

AD = anterodorsal thalamic nucleus, AM = anteromedian thalamic nucleus, AV = anteroventral thalamic nucleus, CL = central lateral thalamic nucleus, CM = centromedian thalamic nucleus, LD = lateral dorsal thalamic nucleus, LGN = lateral geniculate nucleus, LP = lateral posterior thalamic nucleus, MD = medial dorsal thalamic nucleus, VA = ventral exterior thalamic nucleus, VL = ventral lateral thalamic nucleus, VPI = ventral posterior inferior thalamic nucleus, VPL = ventral posterior lateral thalamic nucleus, VPM = ventral posterior medial thalamic nucleus.

fingers; and ataxia and hemiparesis in the same extremities (Caplan, DeWitt, Pessin, Gorelick, & Adelman, 1988; Dejerine & Roussy, 1906; Foix & Hillemand, 1925; Garcin, 1955; Gutrecht, Zamani, & Pandya, 1992). Cognitive and psychiatric presentations are notably absent.

Posterior Choroidal Artery Infarction

These strokes produce complex visual field deficits reflecting involvement of the lateral geniculate nucleus, hemisensory loss, transcortical aphasia, and memory deficits (Bogousslavsky, Regli, & Uske, 1988) as well as a delayed complex hyperkinetic motor syndrome with

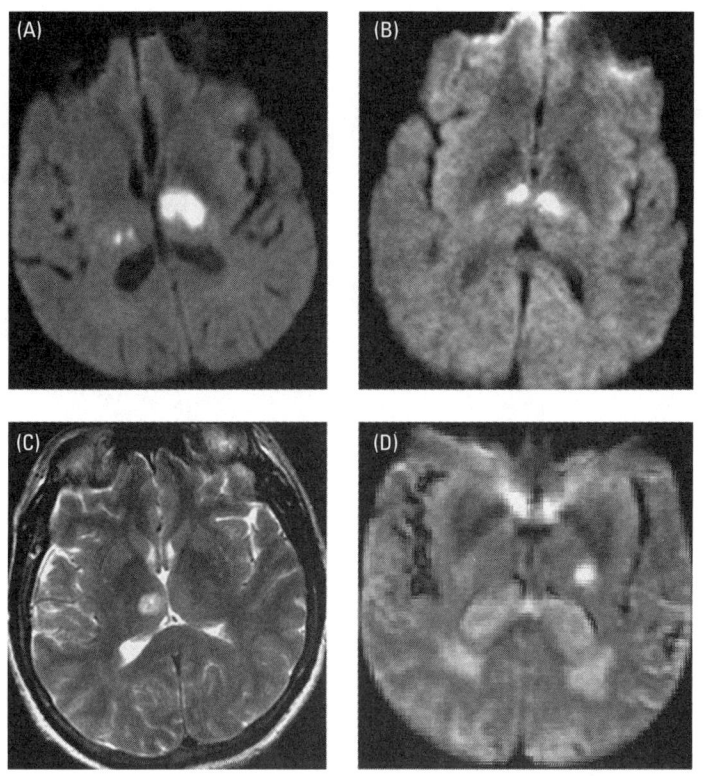

Figure 2.13 (A) Diffusion weighted image (DWI) of left tuberothalamic artery territory infarction (right of diagram). (B) DWI showing infarction bilaterally in the territory of the polar branch of the tuberothalamic artery, likely representing an example of the paramedian artery irrigating both the paramedian and tuberothalamic "territories." (C) Right paramedian artery territory infarction, seen on T2-weighted magnetic resonance imaging. (D) Acute infarction in the left inferolateral artery territory on DWI. (From Schmahmann & Pandya, 2008)

ataxia, rubral tremor, dystonia, myoclonus, and chorea (Neau & Bogousslavsky, 1996). Spatial neglect has been reported (Karnath, Himmelbach, & Rorden, 2002).

Damage to thalamic fiber pathways may have clinical consequences. The mamillothalamic tract (MMT) connects the anterior thalamic nuclei with the mamillary body, which is linked with hippocampus and entorhinal cortex. The MMT and fornix bind the anterior thalamic nuclei into the neural system for learning and memory. The ventral amygdalofugal pathway links the amygdala with the medial part of MD, and damage contributes to amnesia and emotional dysregulation (Graff-Radford, Tranel, Van Hoesen, & Brandt, 1990). Lesions of the superior, medial and inferior, and lateral thalamic peduncles and of the anterior limb of the internal capsule (conveying prefrontal and anterior cingulate interactions; Schmahmann & Pandya, 2006) can produce corticothalamic disconnection and complex behavioral syndromes (Chukwudelunzu, Meschia, Graff-Radford, & Lucas, 2001; Schmahmann, 1984; Tatemichi et al., 1992). Disorders of eye movement result from medial thalamic lesions destroying descending tracts from motor and premotor cortices to the midbrain nuclei of Darkschewitz and the interstitial nucleus of Cajal (upgaze and downgaze), and the rostral nucleus of the medial longitudinal fasciculus in the tectum (downgaze) (Bogousslavsky, Regli, & Uske, 1988; Fisher, 1959; Guberman & Stuss, 1983; Leigh & Zee, 1983).

Cerebellum

The cerebellum is subcortical only in the sense that it is distinct from cerebral cortex (Fig. 2.14). The traditional view that

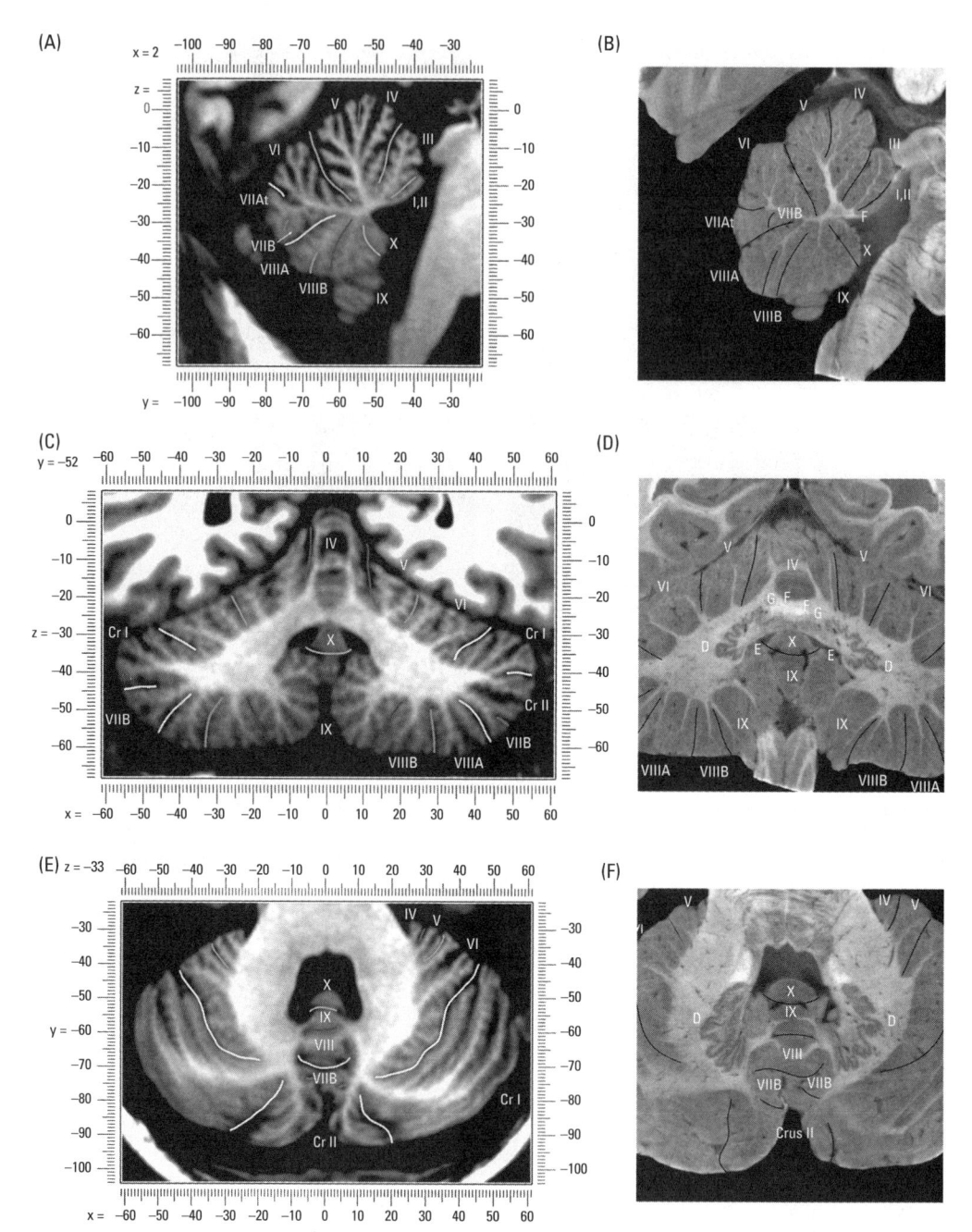

Figure 2.14 Images of the human cerebellum on magnetic resonance imaging (left) and postmortem cryosection (right). The cerebellum is sectioned in the sagittal plane 2 mm to the right of midline in *A* and *B*; in the coronal plane 52 mm behind the anterior commissure—posterior commissure (AC-PC) line in *C* and *D*; and in the transverse plane 33 mm below the AC-PC line in *E* and *F*. Cerebellar fissures are demarcated and the lobules are designated. Deep cerebellar nuclei are identified in the cryosection brain: D, dentate nucleus; E, emboliform nucleus; F, fastigial nucleus; G, globose nucleus. (From Schmahmann et al., 1999; Schmahmann et al., 2000)

cerebellar function is confined to the coordination of voluntary motor activity has evolved (Schmahmann, 1991, 1997). Evidence from patients has made it plain that cerebellar pathology is related to intellectual and emotional deficits in addition to motor incoordination. The wider role of the cerebellum in nervous system function has far-ranging implications for understanding the neural substrates of higher order behavior and neuropsychiatric disorders. There appears to be a double dissociation in the organization of motor and nonmotor functions in the cerebellum, a conclusion derived from clinical neurology as well as anatomy, physiology, and functional imaging studies.

Connectional Neuroanatomy of the Cerebellum

It is now known that cerebellar connections with the cerebral cortex are not confined to motor-related cortices projecting through basis pontis nuclei to cerebellum, and dentate nucleus of cerebellum sending efferents back through VL thalamus to motor cortex. Rather, the association and paralimbic regions of the cerebral cortex have topographically organized feedforward projections through the nuclei in the basis pontis into the cerebellum, as well as feedback projections from the cerebellum. Association cortex projections arise from the prefrontal, posterior parietal, superior temporal polymodal regions, and dorsal parastriate cortices. Paralimbic projections arise from the posterior parahippocampal cortex, limbic regions of the cingulate gyrus, and the anterior insular cortex involved in autonomic and pain modulation systems (Schmahmann, 1996; Schmahmann & Pandya, 1997a, 1997b). These corticopontine pathways are funneled through the cerebrocerebellar circuit within multiple parallel but partially overlapping loops converging with topographic ordering throughout the pons, whereas the motor corticopontine projections are mostly in the caudal half of the pons (Brodal, 1978; Schmahmann & Pandya, 1997b; Schmahmann, Rosene, & Pandya, 2004) (Fig. 2.15).

A precise pattern of organization is probably present also in the pontine projections to the cerebellar cortex, although this still remains to be demonstrated. The cerebellar anterior lobe and part of lobule VI receive afferents from motor and premotor cortices, whereas the association areas in the prefrontal and posterior parietal cortices are linked predominantly with crus I and crus II of the posterior lobe (Allen & Tsukahara, 1974; Kelly & Strick, 2003) (Fig. 2.16). Once conveyed to the cerebellar cortex, these streams of information are acted upon by the cerebellar corticonuclear microcomplexes (Ito, 1984), and then transmitted via the deep cerebellar nuclei to thalamus, on their way back to the cerebral cortex.

Cerebellar projections to thalamus arise from fastigial and interpositus nuclei as well as from the dentate nucleus, and they are directed not only to the cerebellar recipient VL but also to CL, Pcn, the CM-Pf complex, and MD that have efferent projections to association cortices. The cerebellar dentate nucleus sends projections through thalamus to different areas of the frontal lobe in the monkey (Middleton & Strick, 1997). The dorsomedial part of the dentate nucleus sends its projections to the motor cortex, whereas the ventrolateral and ventromedial parts of the dentate nucleus are connected with the prefrontal cortex, including area 9/46 (Kelly & Strick, 2003). Further anatomical details of the cerebrocerebellar linkage and of the olivary inputs to cerebellum may be found elsewhere (Schmahmann, 1996, 2006, 2013; Schmahmann & Pandya, 1997b; Voogd & Glickstein, 1998).

Resting state functional connectivity magnetic resonance imaging (rs-fcMRI) extends these anatomical investigations to humans by using the physiological feature of fluctuating blood oxygen level–dependent (BOLD) signal to infer anatomical connectivity. These studies show that activity in the cerebellar anterior lobe (most notably in lobules III through V), the adjacent part of lobules VI, and lobule VIII correlates with sensorimotor regions of the cerebral cortex. In contrast, activity in the cerebellar posterior lobe (mostly Crus I and II of lobule VII) correlates with prefrontal, parietal, and temporal association areas and the cingulate gyrus (Habas et al., 2009; Krienen & Buckner, 2009; O'Reilly, Beckmann, Tomassini, Ramnani, & Johansen-Berg, 2010). Further, cerebellar correlations with intrinsic functional connectivity networks in the cerebral hemispheres reveal a pattern such that lobules VI,

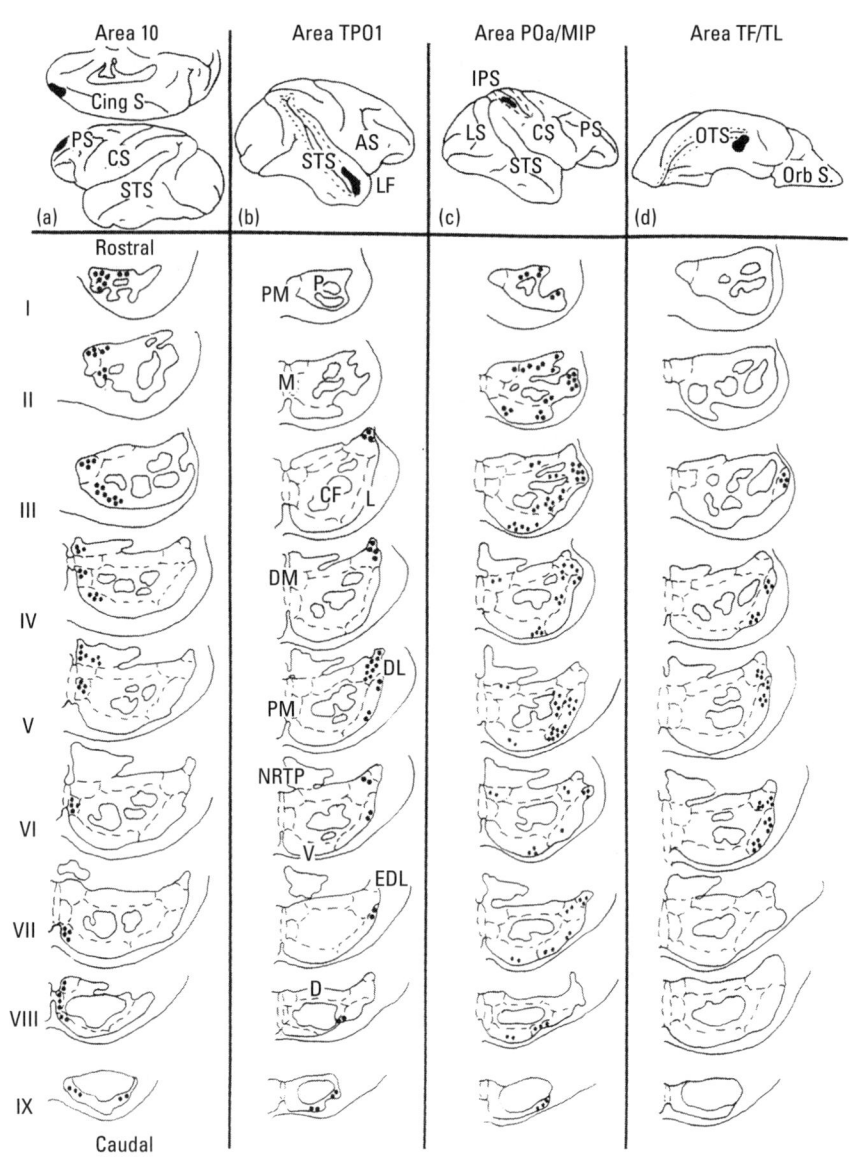

Figure 2.15 Diagram of the projections to the basis pontis from selected regions within the cerebral association areas. The pons is the obligatory synaptic step in the feedforward limb of the cerebrocerebellar circuit. Radiolabeled amino acids (shaded black area in the cerebral hemispheres) were placed in the medial and lateral parts of the rostral prefrontal cortex (area 10) in *A*; in the cortex buried within the rostral upper bank of the superior temporal sulcus (area TPO$_1$) in *B*; in cortex buried within the lower bank of the intraparietal sulcus (area POa, or MIP) in *C*; and in the parahippocampal gyrus (areas TF/TL) in *D*. The label was transported in an anterograde fashion and terminated (black dotes) in the ipsilateral half of the basis pontis from rostral level I to caudal level IX. Each cerebral area is connected with a unique and distributed subset of pontine neurons. The projections appear to be arranged in an interdigitating, but not overlapping manner. (From Schmahmann, 1996). AS = arcuate sulcus, Cing S = cingulate sulcus, CF = calcarine fissure, CS = central sulcus, D = dorsal nucleus, DL = dorsolateral nucleus, DM = dorsomedial nucleus, EDL = extreme dorsolateral nucleus, IPS = intraparietal sulcus, L = lateral nucleus, LF = lateral fissure, LS = lunate sulcus, M = medial nucleus, NRTP = nucleus reticularis tegmenti pontis, Orb S = orbital sulcus, OTS = occipitotemporal sulcus, P = peduncular nucleus, PM = paramedian nucleus, PS = principal sulcus, STS = superior temporal sulcus, V = ventral nucleus.

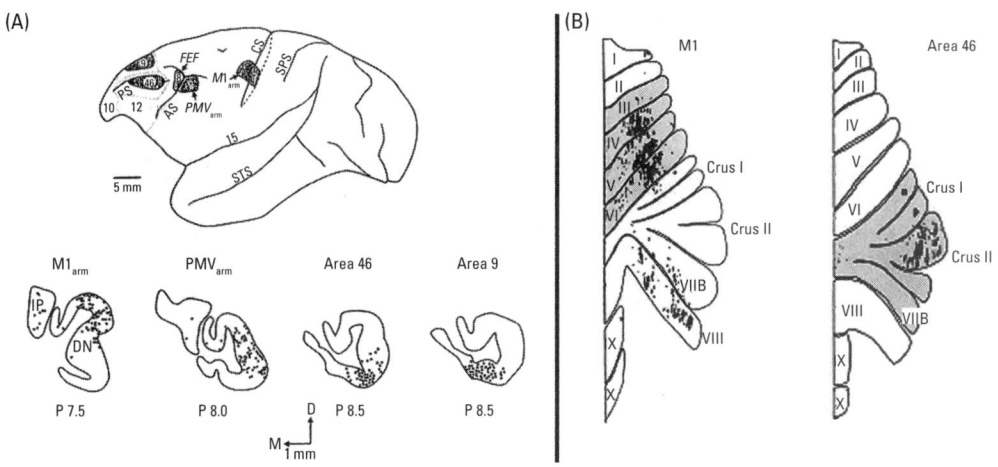

Figure 2.16 (A) Lateral view of a cebus monkey brain (top) to show the location of injections of McIntyre-B strain of Herpes simplex virus type 1 in the primary motor cortex, ventral premotor cortex, and areas 9 and 46. The resulting retrogradely labeled neurons in the cerebellar dentate nucleus (below) are indicated by solid dots. (From Middleton and Strick, 1997) (B) Flattened views of cerebellar cortex of monkey showing areas labeled in anterograde and retrograde fashion following injection of neurotropic virus tracers in the primary motor cortex at left, and prefrontal cortex area 46 at right. (Adapted from Kelly & Strick, 2003)

Crus I and Crus II, and lobule IX correlate with the executive control network; lobule VI with the salience network; and lobule IX with the default network (Buckner, Krienen, Castellanos, Diaz, & Yeo, 2011). Task-based functional MRI studies indicate that the cerebellar anterior lobe, adjacent parts of lobule VI, and lobule VIII are activated in sensorimotor tasks; lobules VI and VII in the posterior lobe are active during language, spatial, and executive function tasks; and affective processing engages the posterior lobes, including the vermis (Stoodley & Schmahmann, 2009; Stoodley, Valera, & Schmahmann, 2012) (Fig. 2.17). Working memory and executive functions engage lobules VI and VII, language recruits posterolateral cerebellum on the right, and spatial tasks recruit it on the left. Affective/emotional processing and pain and autonomic functions involve lobules VI and VII in the vermis more than the hemispheres (Moulton et al., 2011).

The anterior lobe is not engaged in cognitive tasks; the posterior lobe is not involved in motor tasks with the exception of parts of lobule VI and the second sensorimotor representation in lobule VIII (Stoodley & Schmahmann, 2009, 2010; Stoodley, Valera, & Schmahmann, 2010, 2012). This recognition that sensorimotor control is topographically separate and distinct from cognitive and emotional regulation in the cerebellum represents a major departure from earlier conventional wisdom. In sum, the cerebellar anterior lobe and parts of medial lobule VI, together with lobule VIII of the posterior lobe and the globose and emboliform nuclei (or, more accurately the interpositus nucleus in the experimental animal), constitute the sensorimotor cerebellum. Lobule VII (that includes Crus I and Crus II of lobule VIIA, and lobule VIIB), parts of lobule VI, and the ventral part of the dentate nucleus constitute the anatomical substrate of the cognitive cerebellum. The limbic cerebellum appears to have an anatomical signature in the fastigial nucleus and the cerebellar vermis, particularly the posterior vermis. Lobule IX is likely part of the default mode network, and lobule X is an essential node in the vestibular system.

There are few published details regarding the anatomical organization of cerebellar white matter at the systems level, that is, which parts of the cerebellar white matter convey afferent and efferent fibers to which specific cerebellar lobules. Nuclei in the rostral part of the basis pontis project via the middle cerebellar peduncle (MCP) to the posterior lobe of the cerebellum, and those in the caudal basis pontis project to the anterior cerebellum (Bechterew, 1885; Takahashi, Song, Folkerth, Grant, & Schmahmann,

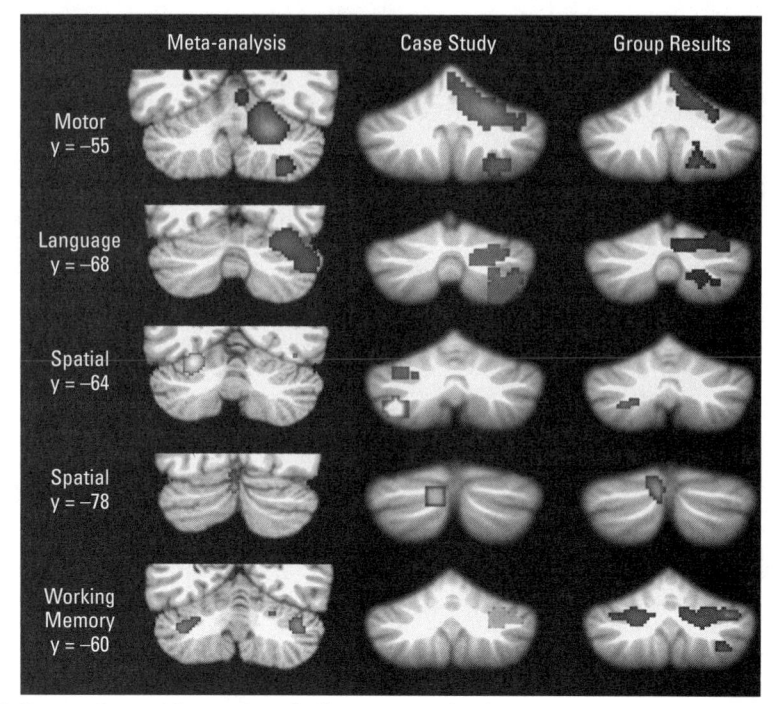

Figure 2.17 Converging evidence of cerebellar topography from a meta-analysis of published imaging data (Stoodley & Schmahmann, 2009), functional magnetic resonance imaging (fMRI) investigation in a single case study (Stoodley, Valera, & Schmahmann, 2010), and an fMRI evaluation of nine subjects (Stoodley, Valera, & Schmahmann, 2012). Consistently active clusters during motor (finger tapping), language tasks, spatial cognition, and working memory paradigms are shown on coronal cerebellar slices. Left is shown on the left. (From Stoodley, Valera, & Schmahmann, 2012)

2013), but more precise information concerning MCP organization remains to be elucidated. Similarly, the degree to which there is anatomical and functional differentiation within the superior cerebellar peduncle efferents to thalamus is not presently known. The topographical organization of motor, cognitive, and affective domains in cerebellum (Schmahmann, 1991, 2004) suggests that defining the arrangement of the cerebellar white matter pathways that connect with extracerebellar structures will be of great interest.

Clinical Features of Cerebellar Lesions

The cerebellar motor syndrome of gait ataxia, appendicular dysmetria, dysarthric speech, and oculomotor abnormalities results from lesions that affect the anterior lobe of the cerebellum, notably lobules I through V, with lobule VI (Fig. 2.18A) likely engaged in motor control in a manner possibly equivalent to premotor regions of the cerebral cortex (Schmahmann, MacMore, Gardner, & Vangel, 2009; Schmahmann, MacMore, & Vangel, 2009; Stoodley & Schmahmann, 2009; Stoodley, Valera, & Schmahmann, 2012). There is a second sensorimotor area identified by physiology and functional imaging, located in lobule VIII at the medial part of the posterior lobe (Grodd, Hülsmann, Lotze, Wildgruber, & Erb, 2001; Snider & Eldred, 1952). Oculomotor abnormalities along with prominent vestibular symptoms (vertigo, nausea, emesis) arise from lesions that involve lobules IX and X of the posterior and flocculonodular lobes (Duncan, Parker, & Fisher, 1975; Lee et al., 2006). Remarkably, large lesions in the major expansion of the cerebellar hemisphere (i.e., lobules Crus I and II and lobule VIIB in the posterior lobe; Fig. 2.18B) do not result in the cerebellar motor syndrome. Indeed, when these patients are examined a few days after

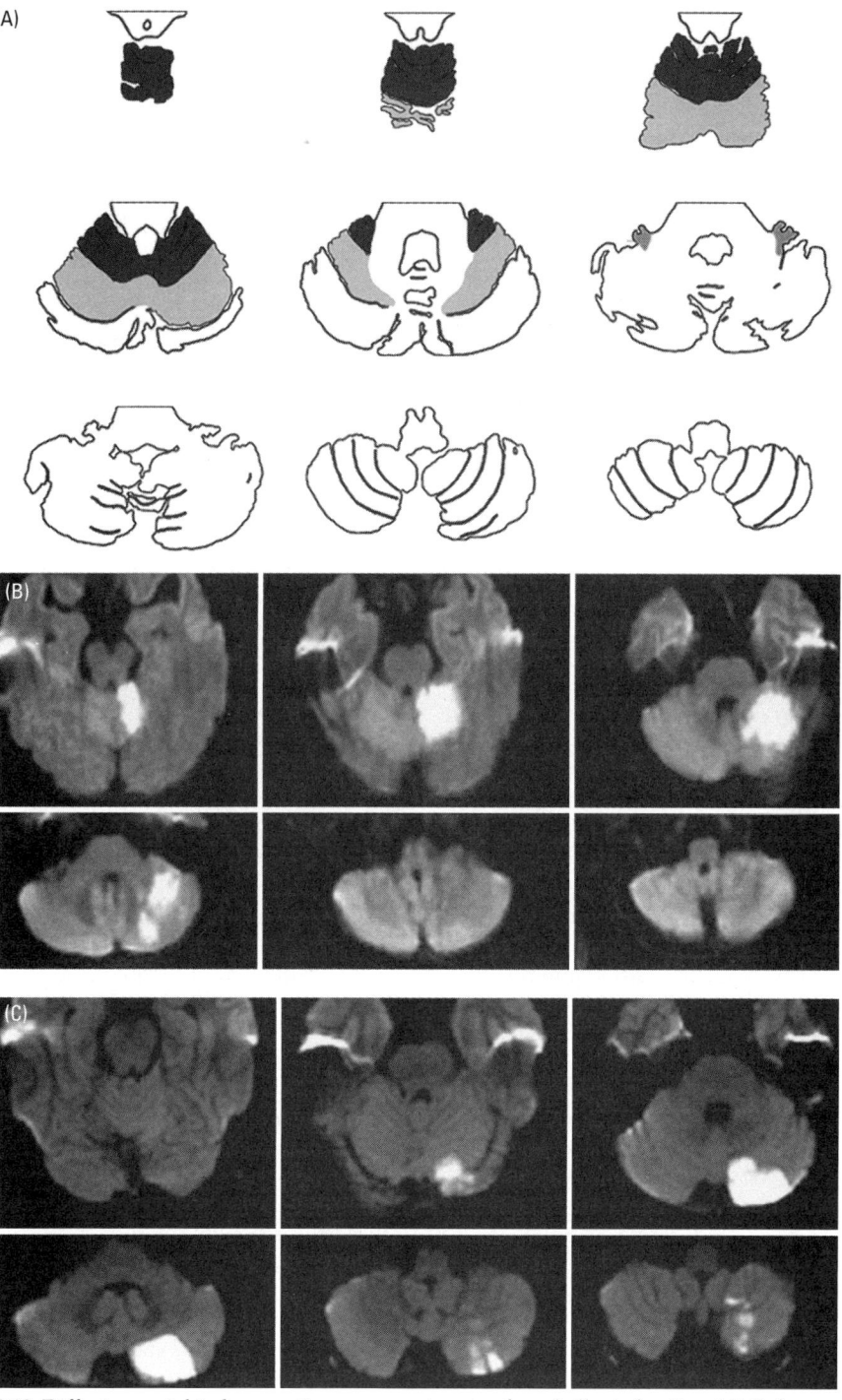

Figure 2.18 Diffusion weighted magnetic resonance image of cerebellar infarction. (*A*) Reference diagram in the horizontal plane of the major cerebellar lobular groupings (top left: superior, to bottom right: inferior). The anterior lobe (lobules I through V) is shaded black; lobule VI of the posterior lobe is shaded gray; lobules VII through IX of the posterior lobe, and lobule X (flocculonodular lobe) are not shaded. (*B*) Stroke in the territory of the superior cerebellar artery, involving the anterior lobe (cerebellar lobules I–V) and part of the posterior lobe. This patient had a cerebellar motor syndrome, scoring 20 of possible 120 points on the Modified International Cooperative Ataxia Rating Scale (MICARS; Schmahmann, Gardner, MacMore, & Vangel, 2009; Schmahmann, MacMore, & Vangel, 2009; Trouillas et al., 1997). (*C*) Stroke in the posterior inferior cerebellar artery territory, sparing the anterior lobe. The patient was motorically normal, with a MICARS score of 1. (Reproduced from Schmahmann & Pandya, 2008)

stroke, and the vestibular symptoms have subsided, it can be difficult to detect any sign of a motor disorder (Schmahmann, MacMore, & Vangel, 2009), a straightforward clinical finding that defies two centuries of dogma about the cerebellar role being confined exclusively to motor coordination.

The other side of the double dissociation is that the cerebellar cognitive affective syndrome (CCAS; Schmahmann & Sherman, 1998) occurs following lesions of the cerebellar posterior lobe, but not the anterior lobe (Exner, Weniger, & Irle, 2004; Schmahmann & Sherman, 1998). The CCAS is characterized by deficits in executive function, visual spatial performance, linguistic processing, and affective dysregulation. Executive impairments include deficits in working memory, motor or ideational set shifting, and perseveration. Verbal fluency is impaired to the point of telegraphic speech or mutism. Visuospatial disintegration impairs attempts to draw or copy a diagram, conceptualization of figures can be disorganized, and some patients display simultanagnosia. Anomia, agrammatic speech, and abnormal syntactic structure are observed, with abnormal prosody characterized by high-pitched, hypophonic whining. Abnormal modulation of behavior and personality is notable with posterior lobe lesions that involve the vermis and fastigial nucleus. This manifests as flattening of affect alternating or coexistent with disinhibited behaviors such as overfamiliarity, flamboyant and impulsive actions, and humorous but inappropriate and flippant comments. Regressive, childlike behaviors and obsessive-compulsive traits can be observed. Autonomic changes are noted following lesions of the fastigial nucleus and vermis, manifesting as bradycardia and syncope, or tachycardia in the setting of acquired panic disorder (Schmahmann & Sherman 1998; Schmahmann, Weilburg, & Sherman, 2007). The principal features and clinical relevance of the CCAS as defined by Schmahmann and Sherman (1998) have been replicated in adults with stroke (Malm et al., 1998; Neau, Arroyo-Anllo, Bonnaud, Ingrand, & Gil, 2000), in children who have undergone excision of cerebellar tumors (Levisohn, Cronin-Golomb, & Schmahmann, 2000; Riva & Giorgi, 2000; Scott et al., 2001), and in other acquired and developmental disorders of the cerebellum (Allin et al., 2001; Chheda, Sherman, & Schmahmann, 2002; van Harskamp, Rudge, & Cipolotti, 2005; Limperopoulos et al., 2006; Tavano et al., 2007; Tedesco et al., 2011). Deficits in emotional expression in patients with strokes and neurodegenerative lesions have also been linked to involvement of the cerebellar system (Parvizi, Anderson, Martin, Damasio, & Damasio, 2001; Parvizi, Joseph, Press, & Schmahmann, 2007).

The posterior fossa syndrome represents a particularly acute form of the CCAS (Levisohn, Cronin-Golomb, & Schmahmann, 2000; Pollack, 1997; Riva & Giorgi, 2000; Wisoff & Epstein, 1984). Within 48 hours following surgical resection of midline tumors of the cerebellum, children develop mutism, buccal and lingual apraxia, apathy, and poverty of spontaneous movement. Emotional lability is marked by rapid fluctuation between irritability and agitation to giggling and easy distractibility. The range of neuropsychiatric impairments in the setting of cerebellar lesions falls into five major behavioral domains: attentional control, emotional control, social skill set, autism spectrum disorders, and psychosis spectrum disorders (Schmahmann, Weilburg, & Sherman, 2007; Table 2.3).

The cerebrocerebellar system thus consists of discretely organized parallel anatomic subsystems that serve as the substrates for differentially organized functional subsystems (or loops) within the framework of distributed neural circuits. This anatomical organization is the substrate for dysmetria of thought theory (Schmahmann, 1991, 1996, 2000, 2004, 2010) and the notion of the universal cerebellar transform. This idea holds that the cerebellum plays an essential role in automatization and optimizing behavior around a homeostatic baseline according to context; that the cerebellum modulates cognition and emotion in the same way that it coordinates motor control; and that disruption of the neural circuitry linking the cerebellum with the association and paralimbic cerebral regions prevents the cerebellar modulation of functions subserved by the affected subsystems, thereby impairing the regulation of movement, cognition, and emotion. This loss of the "cerebellumizing" of behavior leads not only to gait and appendicular ataxia, dysarthria, and oculomotor abnormalities when the motor cerebellum is involved but also to the various aspects of the cerebellar cognitive affective syndrome (Schmahmann &

TABLE 2.3 Neuropsychiatric Manifestations in Cerebellar Disorders (From Schmahmann, Weilburg, & Sherman, 2007)

	Positive (Exaggerated) Symptoms	Negative (Diminished) Symptoms
Attentional control	Inattentiveness	Ruminativeness
	Distractibility	Perseveration
	Hyperactivity	Difficulty shifting focus of attention
	Compulsive and ritualistic behaviors	Obsessional thoughts
Emotional control	Impulsiveness, disinhibition	Anergy, anhedonia
	Lability, unpredictability	Sadness, hopelessness
	Incongruous feelings, pathological laughing/crying	Dysphoria
	Anxiety, agitation, panic	Depression
Autism spectrum	Stereotypical behaviors	Avoidant behaviors, tactile defensiveness
	Self-stimulation behaviors	Easy sensory overload
Psychosis spectrum	Illogical thought	Lack of empathy
	Paranoia	Muted affect, emotional blunting, apathy
Social skill set	Anger, aggression	Passivity, immaturity, childishness
	Irritability	Difficulty with social cues and interactions
	Overly territorial	Unawareness of social boundaries
	Oppositional behavior	Overly gullible and trusting

Sherman, 1998) when the cognitive and limbic cerebellar regions are damaged.

Conclusions

Two overarching principles govern the clinical manifestations resulting from lesions of the subcortical nodes of the distributed neural circuits discussed in this chapter. First, each node is engaged in multiple loops of information processing with anatomically and functionally distinct regions of the cerebral cortex and other subcortical nodes. The topography of the lesion within the node itself determines which behavioral domain is affected. Second, the histology of each node enables a computation, or transform, that is unique to that node. Loss of the nodal transform by a lesion therefore affects the motor/cognitive/affective outcome in a manner that is specific to the node. A more detailed discussion of the theoretical underpinnings of the behavioral neurology of these subcortical areas can be found in Schmahmann and Pandya (2008). It is worth restating, however, that a cortical area can be defined by its pattern of subcortical and cortical connections; that lesions of subcortical structures mimic deficits resulting from lesions of the cerebral cortex; and that there are qualitative differences between the clinical manifestations of lesions in functionally related areas of different cortical and subcortical nodes. Note that there is, by and large, no cross-modal communication within subcortical nodes (e.g., thalamic nuclei do not communicate with each other), although a possible exception has been reported in the striatonigrostriatal system (Haber, Fudge, & McFarland, 2000). Given that behavior is the result of complex interactions between different functional domains, at some point in the anatomy of cognition, mood must inform movement, strategy must rely on memory, and so on. The problem of segregated loops in cortical-subcortical interactions is resolved by the cerebral cortical association areas that, alone among the many nodes of the distributed neural system, facilitate the integration of information across multiple domains in a feedforward and feedback manner. This capability is made possible by the association fiber pathways, which are themselves exclusive to the cerebral cortex.

Acknowledgments

Supported in part by RO1 MH067980, MH64044, the Sidney R. Baer Jr. Foundation, the National Organization of Rare Disorders, the National Ataxia Foundation, and the MINDlink and Birmingham Foundations. The assistance of Jason MacMore, BA, is gratefully acknowledged.

References

Acuna, C., Cudeiro, J., Gonzalez, F., Alonso, J. M., & Perez, R. (1990). Lateral-posterior and pulvinar reaching cells--comparison with parietal area 5a: A study in behaving Macaca nemestrina monkeys. *Experimental Brain Research, 82*(1), 158–166.

Albert, M. L., Feldman, R. G., & Willis, A. L. (1974). The "subcortical dementia" of progressive supranuclear palsy. *Journal of Neurology Neurosurgery and Psychiatry, 37*(2), 121–130.

Alexander, G. E., DeLong, M. R., & Strick, P. L. (1986). Parallel organization of functionally segregated circuits linking basal ganglia and cortex. *Annual Review Neuroscience, 9*, 357–381.

Allen, G. I., & Tsukahara, N. (1974). Cerebrocerebellar communication systems. *Physiological Reviews, 54*(4), 957–1006.

Allin, M., Matsumoto, H., Santhouse, A. M., Nosarti, C., AlAsady, M. H., Stewart, A. L.,…Murray, R. M. (2001). Cognitive and motor function and the size of the cerebellum in adolescents born very pre-term. *Brain, 124*(Pt. 1), 60–66.

Anderson, D., & Ahmed, A. (2003). Treatment of patients with intractable obsessive-compulsive disorder with anterior capsular stimulation. Case report. *Journal of Neurosurgery, 98*(5), 1104–1108.

Asanuma, C., Andersen, R. A., & Cowan, W. M. (1985). The thalamic relations of the caudal inferior parietal lobule and the lateral prefrontal cortex in monkeys: Divergent cortical projections from cell clusters in the medial pulvinar nucleus. *Journal of Comparative Neurology, 241*(3), 357–381.

Ballantine, H. T., Jr., Bouckoms, A. J., Thomas, E. K., & Giriunas, I. E. (1987). Treatment of psychiatric illness by stereotactic cingulotomy. *Biological Psychiatry, 22*(7), 807–819.

Ballantine, H. T., Jr., Cassidy, W. L., Flanagan, N. B., & Marino, R., Jr. (1967). Stereotaxic anterior cingulotomy for neuropsychiatric illness and intractable pain. *Journal of Neurosurgery, 26*(5), 488–495.

Barbas, H., Henion, T. H., & Dermon, C. R. (1991). Diverse thalamic projections to the prefrontal cortex in the Rhesus monkey. *Journal of Comparative Neurology, 313*(1), 65–94.

Barnes, T. D., Kubota, Y., Hu, D., Jin, D. Z., & Graybiel, A. M. (2005). Activity of striatal neurons reflects dynamic encoding and recoding of procedural memories. *Nature, 437*(7062), 1158–1161.

Bechterew, W. (1885). Zur Anatomie der Schenkel des Kleinhirns, insbesondere der Brückenarme. *Neurologisches Centralblatt, 4*, 121–125.

Bentivoglio, M., Kultas-Ilinsky, K., & Ilinsky, I. (1993). Limbic thalamus: Structure, intrinsic organization, and connections. In B. A. Vogt & M. Gabriel (Eds.), *Neurobiology of cingulate cortex and limbic thalamus* (pp. 71–122). Boston, MA: Birkhäuser.

Bogen, J. E., & Bogen, G. M. (1988). Creativity and the corpus callosum. *Psychiatric Clinics of North America, 11*(3), 293–301.

Bogousslavsky, J., Regli, F., & Assal, G. (1986). The syndrome of unilateral tuberothalamic artery territory infarction. *Stroke, 17*(3), 434–441.

Bogousslavsky, J., Regli, F., Delaloye, B., Delaloye-Bischof, A., Assal, G., & Uske, A. (1991). Loss of psychic self-activation with bithalamic infarction. Neurobehavioural, CT, MRI and SPECT correlates. *Acta Neurologica Scandinavica, 83*(5), 309–316.

Bogousslavsky, J., Regli, F., & Uske, A. (1988). Thalamic infarcts: Clinical syndromes, etiology, and prognosis. *Neurology, 38*(6), 837–848.

Brodal, P. (1978). The corticopontine projection in the Rhesus monkey. Origin and principles of organization. *Brain, 101*(2), 251–283.

Buckner, R. L., Andrews-Hanna, J. R., & Schacter, D. L. (2008). The brain's default network: Anatomy, function, and relevance to disease. *Annals of the New York Academy of Sciences, 1124*, 1–38.

Buckner, R. L., Krienen, F. M., Castellanos, A., Diaz, J. C., & Yeo, B. T. (2011). The organization of the human cerebellum estimated by intrinsic functional connectivity. *Journal of Neurophysiology, 106*(5), 2322–2345.

Caplan, L. R., DeWitt, L. D., Pessin, M. S., Gorelick, P. B., & Adelman, L. S. (1988). Lateral thalamic infarcts. *Archives of Neurology, 45*(9), 959–964.

Caplan, L. R., Schmahmann, J. D., Kase, C. S., Feldmann, E., Baquis, G., Greenberg, J. P.,…Hier, D. B. (1990). Caudate infarcts. *Archives of Neurology, 47*(2), 133–143.

Castaigne, P., Lhermitte, F., Buge, A., Escourolle, R., Hauw, J. J., & Lyon–Caen, O. (1981). Paramedian thalamic and midbrain infarct: Clinical and neuropathological study. *Annals of Neurology, 10*(2), 127–148.

Catani, M., Howard, R. J., Pajevic, S., & Jones, D. K. (2002). Virtual in vivo interactive dissection of white matter fasciculi in the human brain. *Neuroimage, 17*(1), 77–94.

Chheda, M., Sherman, J., & Schmahmann, J. D. (2002). Neurologic, psychiatric and cognitive manifestations in cerebellar agenesis. *Neurology, 58*(Suppl. 3), 356.

Chukwudelunzu, F. E., Meschia, J. F., Graff-Radford, N. R., & Lucas, J. A. (2001). Extensive metabolic and neuropsychological abnormalities associated with discrete infarction of the genu of the internal capsule. *Journal of Neurology Neurosurgery and Psychiatry, 71*(5), 658–662.

Clarke, S., Assal, G., Bogousslavsky, J., Regli, F., Townsend, D. W., Leenders, K. L., & Blecic, S. (1994). Pure amnesia after unilateral left polar thalamic infarct: Topographic and sequential neuropsychological and metabolic (PET) correlations. *Journal of Neurology Neurosurgery and Psychiatry, 57*(1), 27–34.

Cosgrove, G. R., & Rauch, S. L. (2003). Stereotactic cingulotomy. *Neurosurgery Clinics of North America, 14*(2), 225–235.

Cowey, A., Stoerig, P., & Bannister, M. (1994). Retinal ganglion cells labelled from the pulvinar nucleus in macaque monkeys. *Neuroscience, 61*(3), 691–705.

Cronin-Golomb, A., Corkin, S., & Growdon, J. H. (1994). Impaired problem solving in Parkinson's disease: Impact of a set-shifting deficit. *Neuropsychologia, 32*(5), 579–593.

Cummings, J. L., & Benson, D. F. (1984). Subcortical dementia. Review of an emerging concept. *Archives of Neurology, 41*(8), 874–879.

Cusick, C. G., Scripter, J. L., Darensbourg, J. G., & Weber, J. T. (1993). Chemoarchitectonic subdivisions of the visual pulvinar in monkeys and their connectional relations with the middle temporal and rostral dorsolateral visual areas, MT and DLr. *Journal of Comparative Neurology, 336*(1), 1–30.

D'Esposito, M., Verfaellie, M., Alexander, M. P., & Katz, D. I. (1995). Amnesia following traumatic bilateral fornix transection. *Neurology, 45*(8), 1546–1550.

Deecke, L., Schwarz, D. W., & Fredrickson, J. M. (1977). Vestibular responses in the Rhesus monkey ventroposterior thalamus. II. Vestibulo-proprioceptive convergence at thalamic neurons. *Experimental Brain Research, 30*(2–3), 219–232.

DeFreitas, G., & Bogousslavsky, J. (2002). Thalamic infarcts. In G. Donnan, B. Norving, J. Bamford, & J. Bogousslavsky (Eds.), *Subcortical stroke* (pp. 255–285). New York, NY: Oxford University Press.

Déjerine, J. (1892). Contribution à l'étude anatomo-pathologique et clinique des differentes variétés de cécité verbale. *Mémoires de la Société de Biologie, 4*, 61–90.

Déjerine, J., & Roussy, G. (1906). Le syndrome thalamique. *Revue Neurologique (Paris), 14*, 521–532.

Delgado, M. R. (2007). Reward-related responses in the human striatum. *Annals of the New York Academy of Sciences, 1104*, 70–88.

Demeter, S., Rosene, D. L., & Van Hoesen, G. W. (1985). Interhemispheric pathways of the hippocampal formation, presubiculum, and entorhinal and posterior parahippocampal cortices in the Rhesus monkey: The structure and organization of the hippocampal commissures. *Journal of Comparative Neurology, 233*(1), 30–47.

Devinsky, O., & Luciano, D. (1997). The contributions of cingulate cortex to human behavior. In B. Vogt & M. Gabriel (Eds.), *Neurobiology of cingulate cortex and limbic thalamus* (pp. 527–556). Boston, MA: Birkhäuser.

Dujardin, K., Sockeel, P., Devos, D., Delliaux, M., Krystkowiak, P., Destee, A., & Defebvre, L. (2007). Characteristics of apathy in Parkinson's disease. *Movement Disorders, 22*(6), 778–784.

Duncan, G. W., Parker, S. W., & Fisher, C. M. (1975). Acute cerebellar infarction in the PICA territory. *Archives of Neurology, 32*(6), 364–368.

Engelborghs, S., Marien, P., Pickut, B. A., Verstraeten, S., & De Deyn, P. P. (2000). Loss of psychic self-activation after paramedian bithalamic infarction. *Stroke, 31*(7), 1762–1765.

Exner, C., Weniger, G., & Irle, E. (2004). Cerebellar lesions in the PICA but not SCA territory impair cognition. *Neurology, 63*(11), 2132–2135.

Filley, C. M. (2001). *The behavioral neurology of white matter*. New York, NY: Oxford University Press.

Filley, C. M. (2012). *Behavioral neurology of white matter* (2nd ed.). New York, NY: Oxford University Press.

Fisher, C. M. (1959). The pathologic and clinical aspects of thalamic hemorrhage. *Transactions of the American Neurological Association, 84*, 56–59.

Fisher, C. M. (1978). Thalamic pure sensory stroke: A pathologic study. *Neurology, 28*(11), 1141–1144.

Foix, C., & Hillemand, P. (1925). Les arte`res de l'axe ence´phalique jusqu'au dience ´phale inclusivement. *Revue Neurologique (Paris), 2*, 705–739.

Foltz, E. L., & White, L. E., Jr. (1962). Pain "relief" by frontal cingulumotomy. *Journal of Neurosurgery, 19*, 89–100.

Forkel, S. J., Thiebaut de Schotten, M., Kawadler, J. M., Dell'acqua, F., Danek, A., & Catani, M. (2012). The anatomy of fronto-occipital connections from early blunt dissections to contemporary tractography. *Cortex*, doi:10.1016/j.cortex.2012.09.005. Epub ahead of print.

Francois, C., Tande, D., Yelnik, J., & Hirsch, E. C. (2002). Distribution and morphology of nigral axons projecting to the thalamus in primates. *Journal of Comparative Neurology, 447*(3), 249–260.

Garcin, R. (1955). [Cerebello-thalamic syndrome caused by localized lesion of the thalamus; sign of so-called main creuse and its symptomatologic value]. *Revue Neurologique (Paris), 93*(1), 143–149.

Garcin, R., & Lapresle, J. (1954). [Sensory syndrome of the thalamic type and with hand-mouth topography due to localized lesions of the thalamus]. *Revue Neurologique (Paris), 90*(2), 124–129.

Gazzaniga, M. S. (1967). The human brain is actually two brains, each capable of advanced mental functions. When the cerebrum is divided surgically, it is as if the cranium contained two separate spheres of consciousness. *Scientific American, 217*(2), 24–29.

Gazzaniga, M. S. (2000). Cerebral specialization and interhemispheric communication: Does the corpus callosum enable the human condition? *Brain, 123*(Pt. 7), 1293–1326.

Geschwind, N. (1965a). Disconnexion syndromes in animals and man. I. *Brain, 88*(2), 237–294.

Geschwind, N. (1965b). Disconnexion syndromes in animals and man. II. *Brain, 88*(3), 585–644.

Ghashghaei, H. T., & Barbas, H. (2002). Pathways for emotion: Interactions of prefrontal and anterior temporal pathways in the amygdala of the Rhesus monkey. *Neuroscience, 115*(4), 1261–1279.

Ghika, J., Ghika-Schmid, F., Fankhauser, H., Assal, G., Vingerhoets, F., Albanese, A., ... Favre, J. (1999). Bilateral contemporaneous posteroventral pallidotomy for the treatment of Parkinson's disease: Neuropsychological and neurological side effects. Report of four cases and review of the literature. *Journal of Neurosurgery, 91*(2), 313–321.

Ghika-Schmid, F., & Bogousslavsky, J. (2000). The acute behavioral syndrome of anterior thalamic infarction: A prospective study of 12 cases. *Annals of Neurology, 48*(2), 220–227.

Giguere, M., & Goldman-Rakic, P. S. (1988). Mediodorsal nucleus: Areal, laminar, and tangential distribution of afferents and efferents in the frontal lobe of Rhesus monkeys. *Journal of Comparative Neurology, 277*(2), 195–213.

Goldman-Rakic, P. S. (1988). Topography of cognition: Parallel distributed networks in primate association cortex. *Annual Review Neuroscience, 11*, 137–156.

Goldman-Rakic, P. S., & Porrino, L. J. (1985). The primate mediodorsal (MD) nucleus and its projection to the frontal lobe. *Journal of Comparative Neurology, 242*(4), 535–560.

Graff-Radford, N. R., Damasio, H., Yamada, T., Eslinger, P. J., & Damasio, A. R. (1985). Nonhaemorrhagic thalamic infarction. Clinical, neuropsychological and electrophysiological findings in four anatomical groups defined by computerized tomography. *Brain, 108*(Pt. 2), 485–516.

Graff-Radford, N. R., Eslinger, P. J., Damasio, A. R., & Yamada, T. (1984). Nonhemorrhagic infarction of the thalamus: Behavioral, anatomic, and physiologic correlates. *Neurology, 34*(1), 14–23.

Graff-Radford, N. R., Tranel, D., Van Hoesen, G. W., & Brandt, J. P. (1990). Diencephalic amnesia. *Brain, 113*(Pt. 1), 1–25.

Graybiel, A. M. (1998). The basal ganglia and chunking of action repertoires. *Neurobiology of Learning and Memory, 70*(1–2), 119–136.

Greicius, M. D., Supekar, K., Menon, V., & Dougherty, R. F. (2009). Resting-state functional connectivity reflects structural connectivity in the default mode network. *Cerebral Cortex, 19*(1), 72–78.

Grodd, W., Hulsmann, E., Lotze, M., Wildgruber, D., & Erb, M. (2001). Sensorimotor mapping of the human cerebellum: fMRI evidence of somatotopic organization. *Human Brain Mapping, 13*(2), 55–73.

Growdon, J. H., & Corkin, S. (1987). Cognitive impairments in Parkinson's disease. *Advances in Neurology, 45*, 383–392.

Guard, O., Bellis, F., Mabille, J. P., Dumas, R., Boisson, D., & Devic, M. (1986). [Thalamic dementia after a unilateral hemorrhagic lesion of the right pulvinar]. *Revue Neurologique (Paris), 142*(10), 759–765.

Guberman, A., & Stuss, D. (1983). The syndrome of bilateral paramedian thalamic infarction. *Neurology, 33*(5), 540–546.

Gutrecht, J. A., Zamani, A. A., & Pandya, D. N. (1992). Lacunar thalamic stroke with pure cerebellar and proprioceptive deficits. *Journal of Neurology Neurosurgery and Psychiatry, 55*(9), 854–856.

Habas, C., Kamdar, N., Nguyen, D., Prater, K., Beckmann, C. F., Menon, V., & Greicius, M. D. (2009). Distinct cerebellar contributions to intrinsic connectivity networks. *Journal of Neuroscience, 29*(26), 8586–8594.

Haber, S. N., Fudge, J. L., & McFarland, N. R. (2000). Striatonigrostriatal pathways in primates form an ascending spiral from the shell to the dorsolateral striatum. *Journal of Neuroscience, 20*(6), 2369–2382.

Hackett, T. A., Stepniewska, I., & Kaas, J. H. (1998). Thalamocortical connections of the parabelt auditory cortex in macaque monkeys. *Journal of Comparative Neurology, 400*(2), 271–286.

Heilman, K. M., & Sypert, G. W. (1977). Korsakoff's syndrome resulting from bilateral fornix lesions. *Neurology, 27*(5), 490–493.

Hodges, J. R., & McCarthy, R. A. (1993). Autobiographical amnesia resulting from bilateral paramedian thalamic infarction. A case study in cognitive neurobiology. *Brain, 116*(Pt. 4), 921–940.

Hugdahl, K., & Wester, K. (2000). Neurocognitive correlates of stereotactic thalamotomy and thalamic stimulation in Parkinsonian patients. *Brain and Cognition, 42*(2), 231–252.

Huguenard, J., & Prince, D. (1997). Basic mechanisms of epileptic discharges in the thalamus. In M. Steriade, E. G. Jones, & D. A. McCormick (Eds.), *Thalamus, Vol. 2. Experimental and clinical aspects* (pp. 295–330). New York, NY: Elsevier.

Ilinsky, I. A., & Kultas-Ilinsky, K. (1987). Sagittal cytoarchitectonic maps of the Macaca mulatta thalamus with a revised nomenclature of the motor-related nuclei validated by observations on their connectivity. *Journal of Comparative Neurology, 262*(3), 331–364.

Ito, M. (1984). *The cerebellum and neural control.* New York, NY: Raven Press.

Jenike, M. A., Baer, L., Ballantine, T., Martuza, R. L., Tynes, S., Giriunas, I., . . . Cassem, N. H. (1991). Cingulotomy for refractory obsessive-compulsive disorder. A long-term follow-up of 33 patients. *Archives of General Psychiatry, 48*(6), 548–555.

Johansen-Berg, H., Behrens, T. E., Sillery, E., Ciccarelli, O., Thompson, A. J., Smith, S. M., & Matthews, P. M. (2005). Functional-anatomical validation and individual variation of diffusion tractography-based segmentation of the human thalamus. *Cerebral Cortex, 15*(1), 31–39.

Johnson, M. D., & Ojemann, G. A. (2000). The role of the human thalamus in language and memory: Evidence from electrophysiological studies. *Brain and Cognition, 42*(2), 218–230.

Jones, E. (1985). *The thalamus.* New York, NY: Plenum Press.

Jones, E. (1997). A description of the human thalamus. In M. Steriade, E. G. Jones, & D. A. McCormick (Eds.), *Thalamus, Vol. 2. Experimental and clinical aspects* (pp. 425–499). New York, NY: Elsevier.

Jones, E. G., & Powell, T. P. (1970a). An anatomical study of converging sensory pathways within the cerebral cortex of the monkey. *Brain, 93*(4), 793–820.

Jones, E. G., & Powell, T. P. (1970b). Connexions of the somatic sensory cortex of the Rhesus monkey. 3. Thalamic connexions. *Brain, 93*(1), 37–56.

Karnath, H. O., Himmelbach, M., & Rorden, C. (2002). The subcortical anatomy of human spatial neglect: Putamen, caudate nucleus and pulvinar. *Brain, 125*(Pt. 2), 350–360.

Kawashima, T., Nakamura, M., Bouix, S., Kubicki, M., Salisbury, D. F., Westin, C. F., . . . Shenton, M. E. (2009). Uncinate fasciculus abnormalities in recent onset schizophrenia and affective psychosis: A diffusion tensor imaging study. *Schizophrenia Research, 110*(1–3), 119–126.

Kelly, R. M., & Strick, P. L. (2003). Cerebellar loops with motor cortex and prefrontal cortex of a nonhuman primate. *Journal of Neuroscience, 23*(23), 8432–8444.

Kennedy, H., & Bullier, J. (1985). A double-labeling investigation of the afferent connectivity to cortical areas V1 and V2 of the macaque monkey. *Journal of Neuroscience, 5*(10), 2815–2830.

Kievit, J., & Kuypers, H. G. (1977). Organization of the thalamo-cortical connexions to the frontal lobe in the Rhesus monkey. *Experimental Brain Research, 29*(3–4), 299–322.

Krienen, F. M., & Buckner, R. L. (2009). Segregated fronto-cerebellar circuits revealed by intrinsic functional connectivity. *Cerebral Cortex, 19*(10), 2485–2497.

Kubicki, M., Westin, C. F., Maier, S. E., Frumin, M., Nestor, P. G., Salisbury, D. F., . . . Shenton, M. E. (2002). Uncinate fasciculus findings in schizophrenia: A magnetic resonance diffusion tensor imaging study. *American Journal of Psychiatry, 159*(5), 813–820.

Kumar, K., Toth, C., & Nath, R. K. (1997). Deep brain stimulation for intractable pain: A 15-year experience. *Neurosurgery, 40*(4), 736–746; discussion 746–737.

Kumral, E., Evyapan, D., & Balkir, K. (1999). Acute caudate vascular lesions. *Stroke, 30*(1), 100–108.

Kunzle, H., & Akert, K. (1977). Efferent connections of cortical, area 8 (frontal eye field) in Macaca fascicularis. A reinvestigation using the autoradiographic technique. *Journal of Comparative Neurology, 173*(1), 147–164.

Lapresle, J., & Haguenau, M. (1973). Anatomico-chemical correlation in focal thalamic lesions. *Zeitschrift für Neurologie, 205*(1), 29–46.

Lee, H., Sohn, S. I., Cho, Y. W., Lee, S. R., Ahn, B. H., Park, B. R., & Baloh, R. W. (2006). Cerebellar infarction presenting isolated vertigo: Frequency and vascular topographical patterns. *Neurology, 67*(7), 1178–1183.

Lehericy, S., Ducros, M., Krainik, A., Francois, C., Van de Moortele, P. F., Ugurbil, K., & Kim, D. S. (2004). 3-D diffusion tensor axonal tracking shows distinct SMA and pre-SMA projections to the human striatum. *Cerebral Cortex, 14*(12), 1302–1309.

Leigh, R., & Zee, D. (1983). *The neurology of eye movements.* Philadelphia, PA: FA Davis.

Lenz, F., & Dougherty, P. (1997). Pain processing in the human thalamus. In M. Steriade, E. G. Jones, & D. A. McCormick (Eds.), *Thalamus, Vol. 2. Experimental and clinical aspects* (pp. 617–651). New York, NY: Elsevier.

Leventhal, C. M., Baringer, J. R., Arnason, B. G., & Fisher, C. M. (1965). A case of Marchiafava-Bignami disease with clinical recovery. *Transactions of the American Neurological Association, 90,* 87–91.

Levisohn, L., Cronin-Golomb, A., & Schmahmann, J. D. (2000). Neuropsychological consequences of cerebellar tumour resection in children: Cerebellar cognitive affective syndrome in a paediatric population. *Brain, 123*(Pt. 5), 1041–1050.

Levy, R., & Dubois, B. (2006). Apathy and the functional anatomy of the prefrontal cortex-basal ganglia circuits. *Cerebral Cortex, 16*(7), 916–928.

Limperopoulos, C., Robertson, R. L., Estroff, J. A., Barnewolt, C., Levine, D., Bassan, H., &

du Plessis, A. J. (2006). Diagnosis of inferior vermian hypoplasia by fetal magnetic resonance imaging: Potential pitfalls and neurodevelopmental outcome. *American Journal of Obstetrics and Gynecology*, 194(4), 1070–1076.

Lisovoski, F., Koskas, P., Dubard, T., Dessarts, I., Dehen, H., & Cambier, J. (1993). Left tuberothalamic artery territory infarction: Neuropsychological and MRI features. *European Neurology*, 33(2), 181–184.

Llinas, R., & Ribary, U. (2001). Consciousness and the brain. The thalamocortical dialogue in health and disease. *Annals of the New York Academy of Sciences*, 929, 166–175.

Locke, S., Angevine, J. B., Jr., & Yakovlev, P. I. (1961). Limbic nuclei of thalamus and connections of limbic cortex. II. Thalamocortical projection of the lateral dorsal nucleus in man. *Archives of Neurology*, 4, 355–364.

Lombardi, W. J., Gross, R. E., Trepanier, L. L., Lang, A. E., Lozano, A. M., & Saint-Cyr, J. A. (2000). Relationship of lesion location to cognitive outcome following microelectrode-guided pallidotomy for Parkinson's disease: Support for the existence of cognitive circuits in the human pallidum. *Brain*, 123(Pt. 4), 746–758.

Luria, A. (1966). *Higher cortical functions in man*. (B. Haigh, Trans.). New York, NY: Basic Books.

Makris, N., Schlerf, J. E., Hodge, S. M., Haselgrove, C., Albaugh, M. D., Seidman, L. J.,...Schmahmann, J. D. (2005). MRI-based surface-assisted parcellation of human cerebellar cortex: An anatomically specified method with estimate of reliability. *Neuroimage*, 25(4), 1146–1160.

Malm, J., Kristensen, B., Karlsson, T., Carlberg, B., Fagerlund, M., & Olsson, T. (1998). Cognitive impairment in young adults with infratentorial infarcts. *Neurology*, 51(2), 433–440.

Martin, J. (1997). Degenerative diseases of the human thalamus. In M. Steriade, E. G. Jones, & D. A. McCormick (Eds.), *Thalamus, Vol. 2. Experimental and clinical aspects* (pp. 653–687). New York, NY: Elsevier.

Mega, M. S., & Cummings, J. L. (1994). Frontal-subcortical circuits and neuropsychiatric disorders. *Journal of Neuropsychiatry and Clinical Neurosciences*, 6(4), 358–370.

Mesulam, M. (1988). Patterns in behavioral neuroanatomy: Association areas, the limbic system, and hemispheric specialization. In M. Mesulam (Ed.), *Principles of behavioral neurology* (pp. 1–70). Philadelphia, PA: F. A. Davis.

Mesulam, M. M. (1981). A cortical network for directed attention and unilateral neglect. *Annals of Neurology*, 10(4), 309–325.

Mesulam, M. M. (1990). Large-scale neurocognitive networks and distributed processing for attention, language, and memory. *Annals of Neurology*, 28(5), 597–613.

Mesulam, M. M., & Pandya, D. N. (1973). The projections of the medial geniculate complex within the sylvian fissure of the Rhesus monkey. *Brain Research*, 60(2), 315–333.

Middleton, F. A., & Strick, P. L. (1994). Anatomical evidence for cerebellar and basal ganglia involvement in higher cognitive function. *Science*, 266(5184), 458–461.

Middleton, F. A., & Strick, P. L. (1997). Cerebellar output channels. *International Review of Neurobiology*, 41, 61–82.

Motzkin, J. C., Newman, J. P., Kiehl, K. A., & Koenigs, M. (2011). Reduced prefrontal connectivity in psychopathy. *Journal of Neuroscience*, 31(48), 17348–17357.

Moulton, E., Elman, I., Pendse, G., Schmahmann, J., Becerra, L., & Borsook, D. (2011). Aversion-related circuity in the cerebellum: Responses to noxious heat and unpleasant images. *Journal of Neuroscience*, 31(10), 3795–3804.

Mufson, E. J., & Mesulam, M. M. (1984). Thalamic connections of the insula in the Rhesus monkey and comments on the paralimbic connectivity of the medial pulvinar nucleus. *Journal of Comparative Neurology*, 227(1), 109–120.

Murthy, J. M. (1988). Ataxic hemiparesis--ventrolateral nucleus of the thalamus: yet another site of lesion. *Stroke*, 19(1), 122.

Muslimovic, D., Post, B., Speelman, J. D., & Schmand, B. (2007). Motor procedural learning in Parkinson's disease. *Brain*, 130(Pt. 11), 2887–2897.

Nadeau, S. E., & Crosson, B. (1997). Subcortical aphasia. *Brain and Language*, 58(3), 355–402; discussion 418–423.

Naeser, M. A., Palumbo, C. L., Helm-Estabrooks, N., Stiassny-Eder, D., & Albert, M. L. (1989). Severe nonfluency in aphasia. Role of the medial subcallosal fasciculus and other white matter pathways in recovery of spontaneous speech. *Brain*, 112(Pt. 1), 1–38.

Nasreddine, Z. S., & Saver, J. L. (1997). Pain after thalamic stroke: Right diencephalic predominance and clinical features in 180 patients. *Neurology*, 48(5), 1196–1199.

Nass, R., Boyce, L., Leventhal, F., Levine, B., Allen, J., Maxfield, C.,...George, A. (2000). Acquired aphasia in children after surgical resection of left-thalamic tumors. *Developmental Medicine and Child Neurology*, 42(9), 580–590.

Nauta, W. (1964). Some efferent connections of the prefrontal cortex in the monkey. In J. M. Warren & K. Akert (Eds.), *The frontal granular cortex and behavior* (pp. 397–409). New York, NY: McGraw-Hill.

Nauta, W. J., & Domesick, V. B. (1984). Afferent and efferent relationships of the basal ganglia. *Ciba Foundation Symposium*, 107, 3–29.

Naville, F. (1922). Etudes sur les complications et les sequelles mentales de l'encephalite epidemique. La bradyphrenie. *Encephale, 17*, 369–375, 423–336.

Neau, J. P., Arroyo-Anllo, E., Bonnaud, V., Ingrand, P., & Gil, R. (2000). Neuropsychological disturbances in cerebellar infarcts. *Acta Neurologica Scandinavica, 102*(6), 363–370.

Neau, J. P., & Bogousslavsky, J. (1996). The syndrome of posterior choroidal artery territory infarction. *Annals of Neurology, 39*(6), 779–788.

O'Reilly, J. X., Beckmann, C. F., Tomassini, V., Ramnani, N., & Johansen-Berg, H. (2010). Distinct and overlapping functional zones in the cerebellum defined by resting state functional connectivity. *Cerebral Cortex, 20*(4), 953–965.

Ojemann, G. A., Fedio, P., & Van Buren, J. M. (1968). Anomia from pulvinar and subcortical parietal stimulation. *Brain, 91*(1), 99–116.

Ojemann, G. A., & Ward, A. A., Jr. (1971). Speech representation in ventrolateral thalamus. *Brain, 94*(4), 669–680.

Olszewski, J. (1952). *The thalamus of the Macaca mulatta: An atlas for use with the stereotaxic instrument*. Basel, Switzerland and New York, NY: S. Karger.

Owen, A. M., James, M., Leigh, P. N., Summers, B. A., Marsden, C. D., Quinn, N. P.,...Robbins, T. W. (1992). Fronto-striatal cognitive deficits at different stages of Parkinson's disease. *Brain, 115*(Pt. 6), 1727–1751.

Pandya, D. N., & Kuypers, H. G. (1969). Cortico-cortical connections in the Rhesus monkey. *Brain Research, 13*(1), 13–36.

Pandya, D. N., Rosene, D. L., & Doolittle, A. M. (1994). Corticothalamic connections of auditory-related areas of the temporal lobe in the Rhesus monkey. *Journal of Comparative Neurology, 345*(3), 447–471.

Pandya, D. N., & Seltzer, B. (1982). Intrinsic connections and architectonics of posterior parietal cortex in the Rhesus monkey. *Journal of Comparative Neurology, 204*(2), 196–210.

Parvizi, J., Anderson, S. W., Martin, C. O., Damasio, H., & Damasio, A. R. (2001). Pathological laughter and crying: A link to the cerebellum. *Brain, 124*(Pt. 9), 1708–1719.

Parvizi, J., Joseph, J., Press, D. Z., & Schmahmann, J. D. (2007). Pathological laughter and crying in patients with multiple system atrophy-cerebellar type. *Movement Disorders, 22*(6), 798–803.

Peoples, L. L., Kravitz, A. V., & Guillem, K. (2007). The role of accumbal hypoactivity in cocaine addiction. *ScientificWorldJournal, 7*, 22–45.

Petrides, M., & Pandya, D. N. (2009). Distinct parietal and temporal pathways to the homologues of Broca's area in the monkey. *PLoS Biololgy, 7*(8), e1000170.

Pollack, I. F. (1997). Posterior fossa syndrome. *International Review of Neurobiology, 41*, 411–432.

Price, B. H., Baral, I., Cosgrove, G. R., Rauch, S. L., Nierenberg, A. A., Jenike, M. A., & Cassem, E. H. (2001). Improvement in severe self-mutilation following limbic leucotomy: A series of 5 consecutive cases. *Journal of Clinical Psychiatry, 62*(12), 925–932.

Pritchard, T. C., Hamilton, R. B., Morse, J. R., & Norgren, R. (1986). Projections of thalamic gustatory and lingual areas in the monkey, Macaca fascicularis. *Journal of Comparative Neurology, 244*(2), 213–228.

Raichle, M. E., MacLeod, A. M., Snyder, A. Z., Powers, W. J., Gusnard, D. A., & Shulman, G. L. (2001). A default mode of brain function. *Proceedings of the National Academy of Science USA, 98*(2), 676–682.

Reilly, M., Connolly, S., Stack, J., Martin, E. A., & Hutchinson, M. (1992). Bilateral paramedian thalamic infarction: A distinct but poorly recognized stroke syndrome. *Quarterly Journal of Medicine, 82*(297), 63–70.

Remijnse, P. L., Nielen, M. M., van Balkom, A. J., Cath, D. C., van Oppen, P., Uylings, H. B., & Veltman, D. J. (2006). Reduced orbitofrontal-striatal activity on a reversal learning task in obsessive-compulsive disorder. *Archives of General Psychiatry, 63*(11), 1225–1236.

Riva, D., & Giorgi, C. (2000). The cerebellum contributes to higher functions during development: Evidence from a series of children surgically treated for posterior fossa tumours. *Brain, 123*(Pt. 5), 1051–1061.

Robinson, D., & Cowie, R. (1997). The primate pulvinar: Structural, functional and behavioral components of visual salience. In M. Steriade, E. G. Jones, & D. A. McCormick (Eds.), *Thalamus, Vol. 2. Experimental and clinical aspects* (pp. 53–92). New York, NY: Elsevier.

Romanski, L. M., Giguere, M., Bates, J. F., & Goldman-Rakic, P. S. (1997). Topographic organization of medial pulvinar connections with the prefrontal cortex in the Rhesus monkey. *Journal of Comparative Neurology, 379*(3), 313–332.

Rudge, P., & Warrington, E. K. (1991). Selective impairment of memory and visual perception in splenial tumours. *Brain, 114*(Pt. 1B), 349–360.

Russchen, F. T., Amaral, D. G., & Price, J. L. (1987). The afferent input to the magnocellular division of the mediodorsal thalamic nucleus in the monkey, Macaca fascicularis. *Journal of Comparative Neurology, 256*(2), 175–210.

Sarkar, S., Craig, M. C., Catani, M., Dell'acqua, F., Fahy, T., Deeley, Q., & Murphy, D. G.

(2013). Frontotemporal white-matter microstructural abnormalities in adolescents with conduct disorder: A diffusion tensor imaging study. *Psychological Medicine, 43*(2), 401–411.

Saur, D., Kreher, B. W., Schnell, S., Kummerer, D., Kellmeyer, P., Vry, M. S.,...Weiller, C. (2008). Ventral and dorsal pathways for language. *Proceedings of the National Academy of Science USA, 105*(46), 18035–18040.

Schell, G. R., & Strick, P. L. (1984). The origin of thalamic inputs to the arcuate premotor and supplementary motor areas. *Journal of Neuroscience, 4*(2), 539–560.

Schmahmann, J. D. (1984). *Hemi-inattention from right hemisphere subcortical infarction*. Boston, MA: Society of Neurology and Psychiatry.

Schmahmann, J. D. (1991). An emerging concept. The cerebellar contribution to higher function. *Archives of Neurology, 48*(11), 1178–1187.

Schmahmann, J. D. (1996). From movement to thought: Anatomic substrates of the cerebellar contribution to cognitive processing. *Human Brain Mapping, 4*, 174–198.

Schmahmann, J. D. (Ed.). (1997). *The cerebellum and cognition. International review of neurobiology* (Vol. 47). San Diego, CA: Academic Press.

Schmahmann, J. D. (2000). The role of the cerebellum in affect and psychosis. *Journal of Neurolinguistics, 13*, 189–214.

Schmahmann, J. D. (2003). Vascular syndromes of the thalamus. *Stroke, 34*(9), 2264–2278.

Schmahmann, J. D. (2004). Disorders of the cerebellum: Ataxia, dysmetria of thought, and the cerebellar cognitive affective syndrome. *Journal of Neuropsychiatry and Clinical Neurosciences, 16*(3), 367–378.

Schmahmann, J. D. (2006). Cerebellum and spinal cord - principles of development, anatomical organization, and functional relevance. In A. Brice & S. Pulst (Eds.), *Spinocerebellar degenerations: The ataxias and spastic paraplegias* (pp. 1–60). New York, NY: Elsevier.

Schmahmann, J. D. (2010). The role of the cerebellum in cognition and emotion: Personal reflections since 1982 on the dysmetria of thought hypothesis, and its historical evolution from theory to therapy. *Neuropsychology Review, 20*(3), 236–260.

Schmahmann, J. D. (2013). Cerebellum and ataxia. In H. R. Jones, T. M. Burns, M. J. Aminoff, & S. L. Pomeroy (Eds.), *The Netter Collection of medical illustrations, Frank H. Netter, MD, Vol. 7. Nervous system Part 1, Brain* (2nd ed., pp. 177–197). Philadelphia, PA: Elsevier/Saunders.

Schmahmann, J. D., Doyon, J., McDonald, D., Holmes, C., Lavoie, K., Hurwitz, A. S.,...Petrides, M. (1999). Three-dimensional MRI atlas of the human cerebellum in proportional stereotaxic space. *Neuroimage, 10*(3 Pt. 1), 233–260.

Schmahmann, J. D., Doyon, J., Toga, A., Evans, A., & Petrides, M. (2000). *MRI atlas of the human cerebellum*. San Diego, CA: Academic Press.

Schmahmann, J. D., Gardner, R., MacMore, J., & Vangel, M. G. (2009). Development of a brief ataxia rating scale (BARS) based on a modified form of the ICARS. *Movement Disorders, 24*(12), 1820–1828.

Schmahmann, J. D., & Leifer, D. (1992). Parietal pseudothalamic pain syndrome. Clinical features and anatomic correlates. *Archives of Neurology, 49*(10), 1032–1037.

Schmahmann, J. D., MacMore, J., & Vangel, M. (2009). Cerebellar stroke without motor deficit: Clinical evidence for motor and non-motor domains within the human cerebellum. *Neuroscience, 162*(3), 852–861.

Schmahmann, J. D., & Pandya, D. N. (1990). Anatomical investigation of projections from thalamus to posterior parietal cortex in the Rhesus monkey: A WGA-HRP and fluorescent tracer study. *Journal of Comparative Neurology, 295*(2), 299–326.

Schmahmann, J. D., & Pandya, D. N. (1997a). Anatomic organization of the basilar pontine projections from prefrontal cortices in Rhesus monkey. *Journal of Neuroscience, 17*(1), 438–458.

Schmahmann, J. D., & Pandya, D. N. (1997b). The cerebrocerebellar system. *International Review of Neurobiology, 41*, 31–60.

Schmahmann, J. D., & Pandya, D. N. (2006). *Fiber pathways of the brain*. New York, NY: Oxford University Press.

Schmahmann, J. D., & Pandya, D. N. (2007). The complex history of the fronto-occipital fasciculus. *Journal of the History of the Neurosciences, 16*(4), 362–377.

Schmahmann, J. D., & Pandya, D. N. (2008). Disconnection syndromes of basal ganglia, thalamus, and cerebrocerebellar systems. *Cortex, 44*(8), 1037–1066.

Schmahmann, J. D., Pandya, D. N., Wang, R., Dai, G., D'Arceuil, H. E., de Crespigny, A. J., & Wedeen, V. J. (2007). Association fibre pathways of the brain: Parallel observations from diffusion spectrum imaging and autoradiography. *Brain, 130*(Pt. 3), 630–653.

Schmahmann, J. D., Rosene, D. L., & Pandya, D. N. (2004). Motor projections to the basis pontis in Rhesus monkey. *Journal of Comparative Neurology, 478*(3), 248–268.

Schmahmann, J. D., & Sherman, J. C. (1998). The cerebellar cognitive affective syndrome. *Brain, 121*(Pt. 4), 561–579.

Schmahmann, J. D., Smith, E. E., Eichler, F. S., & Filley, C. M. (2008). Cerebral white matter: Neuroanatomy, clinical neurology, and neurobehavioral correlates. *Annals of the New York Academy of Sciences, 1142*, 266–309.

Schmahmann, J. D., Weilburg, J. B., & Sherman, J. C. (2007). The neuropsychiatry of the cerebellum - insights from the clinic. *Cerebellum*, 6(3), 254–267.

Scott, R., Gregory, R., Hines, N., Carroll, C., Hyman, N., Papanasstasiou, V.,...Aziz, T. (1998). Neuropsychological, neurological and functional outcome following pallidotomy for Parkinson's disease. A consecutive series of eight simultaneous bilateral and twelve unilateral procedures. *Brain*, 121(Pt. 4), 659–675.

Scott, R. B., Stoodley, C. J., Anslow, P., Paul, C., Stein, J. F., Sugden, E. M., & Mitchell, C. D. (2001). Lateralized cognitive deficits in children following cerebellar lesions. *Developmental Medicine and Child Neurology*, 43(10), 685–691.

Selemon, L. D., & Goldman-Rakic, P. S. (1990). Topographic intermingling of striatonigral and striatopallidal neurons in the Rhesus monkey. *Journal of Comparative Neurology*, 297(3), 359–376.

Shatz, C. J., & Rakic, P. (1981). The genesis of efferent connections from the visual cortex of the fetal Rhesus monkey. *Journal of Comparative Neurology*, 196(2), 287–307.

Sidibe, M., Pare, J. F., & Smith, Y. (2002). Nigral and pallidal inputs to functionally segregated thalamostriatal neurons in the centromedian/parafascicular intralaminar nuclear complex in monkey. *Journal of Comparative Neurology*, 447(3), 286–299.

Siwek, D. F., & Pandya, D. N. (1991). Prefrontal projections to the mediodorsal nucleus of the thalamus in the Rhesus monkey. *Journal of Comparative Neurology*, 312(4), 509–524.

Smith, E. E., Salat, D. H., Jeng, J., McCreary, C. R., Fischl, B., Schmahmann, J. D.,...Greenberg, S. M. (2011). Correlations between MRI white matter lesion location and executive function and episodic memory. *Neurology*, 76(17), 1492–1499.

Smith, J. G., & McDowall, J. (2006). When artificial grammar acquisition in Parkinson's disease is impaired: The case of learning via trial-by-trial feedback. *Brain Research*, 1067(1), 216–228.

Snider, R. S., & Eldred, E. (1952). Cerebrocerebellar relationships in the monkey. *Journal of Neurophysiology*, 15(1), 27–40.

Solomon, D. H., Barohn, R. J., Bazan, C., & Grissom, J. (1994). The thalamic ataxia syndrome. *Neurology*, 44(5), 810–814.

Spangler, W. J., Cosgrove, G. R., Ballantine, H. T., Jr., Cassem, E. H., Rauch, S. L., Nierenberg, A., & Price, B. H. (1996). Magnetic resonance image-guided stereotactic cingulotomy for intractable psychiatric disease. *Neurosurgery*, 38(6), 1071–1076; discussion 1076–1078.

Sperry, R. (1984). Consciousness, personal identity and the divided brain. *Neuropsychologia*, 22(6), 661–673.

Sperry, R. W. (1964). The great cerebral commissure. *Scientific American, 210*, 42–52.

Spiegel, E. A., Wycis, H. T., Orchinik, C., & Freed, H. (1956). Thalamic chronotaxis. *American Journal of Psychiatry*, 113(2), 97–105.

Stoodley, C. J., & Schmahmann, J. D. (2009). Functional topography in the human cerebellum: A meta-analysis of neuroimaging studies. *Neuroimage*, 44(2), 489–501.

Stoodley, C. J., & Schmahmann, J. D. (2010). Evidence for topographic organization in the cerebellum of motor control versus cognitive and affective processing. *Cortex*, 46(7), 831–844.

Stoodley, C. J., Valera, E. M., & Schmahmann, J. D. (2010). An fMRI study of intra–individual functional topography in the human cerebellum. *Behavioural Neurology*, 23(1–2), 65–79.

Stoodley, C. J., Valera, E. M., & Schmahmann, J. D. (2012). Functional topography of the cerebellum for motor and cognitive tasks: An fMRI study. *Neuroimage*, 59(2), 1560–1570.

Strick, P. L. (1976). Anatomical analysis of ventrolateral thalamic input to primate motor cortex. *Journal of Neurophysiology*, 39(5), 1020–1031.

Takahashi, E., Song, J. W., Folkerth, R. D., Grant, P. E. & Schmahmann, J. D. (2013). Detection of postmortem human cerebellar cortex and white matter pathways using high angular resolution diffusion tractography: A feasibility study. *Neuroimage, 68*, 105–111.

Tatemichi, T. K., Desmond, D. W., Prohovnik, I., Cross, D. T., Gropen, T. I., Mohr, J. P., & Stern, Y. (1992). Confusion and memory loss from capsular genu infarction: A thalamocortical disconnection syndrome? *Neurology*, 42(10), 1966–1979.

Tavano, A., Grasso, R., Gagliardi, C., Triulzi, F., Bresolin, N., Fabbro, F., & Borgatti, R. (2007). Disorders of cognitive and affective development in cerebellar malformations. *Brain*, 130(Pt. 10), 2646–2660.

Tedesco, A. M., Chiricozzi, F. R., Clausi, S., Lupo, M., Molinari, M., & Leggio, M. G. (2011). The cerebellar cognitive profile. *Brain*, 134(Pt. 12), 3672–3686.

Thiebaut de Schotten, M., Dell'Acqua, F., Valabregue, R., & Catani, M. (2012). Monkey to human comparative anatomy of the frontal lobe association tracts. *Cortex*, 48(1), 82–96.

Tobias, T. J. (1975). Afferents to prefrontal cortex from the thalamic mediodorsal nucleus in the Rhesus monkey. *Brain Research*, 83(2), 191–212.

Trepanier, L. L., Saint-Cyr, J. A., Lozano, A. M., & Lang, A. E. (1998). Neuropsychological consequences of posteroventral pallidotomy for the treatment of Parkinson's disease. *Neurology*, 51(1), 207–215.

Trouillas, P., Takayanagi, T., Hallett, M., Currier, R. D., Subramony, S. H., Wessel, K.,...Manyam, B. (1997). International

Cooperative Ataxia Rating Scale for pharmacological assessment of the cerebellar syndrome. The Ataxia Neuropharmacology Committee of the World Federation of Neurology. *Journal of the Neurological Sciences*, *145*(2), 205–211.

Ungerleider, L., & Mishkin, M. (1982). Two cortical visual systems. In D. Ingle, M. A. Goodale, & R. J. W. Mansfield (Eds.), *Analysis of visual behavior* (pp. 549–586). Cambridge, MA: MIT Press.

Valenstein, E., Bowers, D., Verfaellie, M., Heilman, K. M., Day, A., & Watson, R. T. (1987). Retrosplenial amnesia. *Brain*, *110*(Pt. 6), 1631–1646.

van Harskamp, N. J., Rudge, P., & Cipolotti, L. (2005). Cognitive and social impairments in patients with superficial siderosis. *Brain*, *128*(Pt. 5), 1082–1092.

Victor, M., Adams, R. D., & Collins, G. H. (1971). The Wernicke-Korsakoff syndrome. A clinical and pathological study of 245 patients, 82 with post-mortem examinations. *Contemporary Neurology Series*, *7*, 1–206.

Vogt, B. A., Pandya, D. N., & Rosene, D. L. (1987). Cingulate cortex of the Rhesus monkey: I. Cytoarchitecture and thalamic afferents. *Journal of Comparative Neurology*, *262*(2), 256–270.

von Cramon, D. Y., Hebel, N., & Schuri, U. (1985). A contribution to the anatomical basis of thalamic amnesia. *Brain*, *108*(Pt. 4), 993–1008.

Voogd, J., & Glickstein, M. (1998). The anatomy of the cerebellum. *Trends in Neuroscience*, *21*(9), 370–375.

Warren, J. D., & Thompson, P. D. (2000). Diencephalic amnesia and apraxia after left thalamic infarction. *Journal of Neurology Neurosurgery and Psychiatry*, *68*(2), 248.

Weber, J. T., & Yin, T. C. (1984). Subcortical projections of the inferior parietal cortex (area 7) in the stump-tailed monkey. *Journal of Comparative Neurology*, *224*(2), 206–230.

Wedeen, V. J., Wang, R. P., Schmahmann, J. D., Benner, T., Tseng, W. Y., Dai, G., … de Crespigny, A. J. (2008). Diffusion spectrum magnetic resonance imaging (DSI) tractography of crossing fibers. *Neuroimage*, *41*(4), 1267–1277.

Weiller, C., Bormann, T., Saur, D., Musso, M., & Rijntjes, M. (2011). How the ventral pathway got lost: And what its recovery might mean. *Brain and Language*, *118*(1–2), 29–39.

Williams-Gray, C. H., Foltynie, T., Brayne, C. E., Robbins, T. W., & Barker, R. A. (2007). Evolution of cognitive dysfunction in an incident Parkinson's disease cohort. *Brain*, *130*(Pt. 7), 1787–1798.

Willis, W. J. (1997). Nociceptive functions of thalamic neurons. In M. Steriade, E. G. Jones, & D. A. McCormick (Eds.), *Thalamus, Vol. 2. Experimental and clinical aspects* (pp. 373–424). New York, NY: Elsevier.

Wisoff, J. H., & Epstein, F. J. (1984). Pseudobulbar palsy after posterior fossa operation in children. *Neurosurgery*, *15*(5), 707–709.

Yakovlev, P. I., & Locke, S. (1961). Limbic nuclei of thalamus and connections of limbic cortex. III. Corticocortical connections of the anterior cingulate gyrus, the cingulum, and the subcallosal bundle in monkey. *Archives of Neurology*, *5*, 364–400.

Yakovlev, P. I., Locke, S., Koskoff, D. Y., & Patton, R. A. (1960). Limbic nuclei of thalamus and connections of limbic cortex. *Archives of Neurology*, *3*, 620–641.

Yeterian, E. H., & Pandya, D. N. (1985). Corticothalamic connections of the posterior parietal cortex in the Rhesus monkey. *Journal of Comparative Neurology*, *237*(3), 408–426.

Yeterian, E. H., & Pandya, D. N. (1988). Corticothalamic connections of paralimbic regions in the Rhesus monkey. *Journal of Comparative Neurology*, *269*(1), 130–146.

Yeterian, E. H., & Pandya, D. N. (1989). Thalamic connections of the cortex of the superior temporal sulcus in the Rhesus monkey. *Journal of Comparative Neurology*, *282*(1), 80–97.

Yeterian, E. H., & Pandya, D. N. (1991). Corticothalamic connections of the superior temporal sulcus in Rhesus monkeys. *Experimental Brain Research*, *83*(2), 268–284.

Yeterian, E. H., & Pandya, D. N. (1993). Striatal connections of the parietal association cortices in Rhesus monkeys. *Journal of Comparative Neurology*, *332*(2), 175–197.

Yeterian, E. H., & Pandya, D. N. (1994). Laminar origin of striatal and thalamic projections of the prefrontal cortex in Rhesus monkeys. *Experimental Brain Research*, *99*(3), 383–398.

Yeterian, E. H., & Pandya, D. N. (1997). Corticothalamic connections of extrastriate visual areas in Rhesus monkeys. *Journal of Comparative Neurology*, *378*(4), 562–585.

Yeterian, E. H., & Pandya, D. N. (1998). Corticostriatal connections of the superior temporal region in Rhesus monkeys. *Journal of Comparative Neurology*, *399*(3), 384–402.

Ziegler, D. K., Kaufman, A., & Marshall, H. E. (1977). Abrupt memory loss associated with thalamic tumor. *Archives of Neurology*, *34*(9), 545–548.

3

Executive Control, the Regulation of Goal-Directed Behaviors, and the Impact of Dementing Illness

Kirk R. Daffner and Kim C. Willment

The executive control functions encompass a wide range of high-level cognitive and behavioral capacities that allow an individual to pursue goal-directed and context-appropriate behavior. Some of the most disturbing neurological disorders include those in which executive functions have been compromised, perhaps because those affected have lost capacities that we associated most with being human. While the research literature on the executive control is vast and spans decades and many different experimental modalities, there are still many questions regarding the discrete component functions implicated in executive control, how these component functions are organized, and what underlying neural structures support them. However, there is little disagreement that the executive control functions mediate vital human capacities, such as long-term planning, execution of goals, and perspective taking. This chapter will focus on elucidating principles and concepts associated with executive control functions and their neuroanatomic substrates. We will then briefly illustrate several representative patterns of executive dysfunction in the dementias, with a particular emphasis on distinguishing the profiles associated with the behavioral variant of frontotemporal lobar degeneration (bvFTD) and Alzheimer's disease (AD).

Historical Perspective

The classic work on executive control functions initially emerged from observations of patients with neurological illness or brain injury. In his work in the late 19th and early 20th centuries, John Hughlings Jackson inferred that some abnormalities in behavior resulted from the effects of pathology at the "higher centers" of the nervous systems, which led to a loss of influence over the "lower centers" (Jackson, 1932; Wozniak & Jackson, 1999). He proposed that when lower centers of the nervous system were "liberated" and no longer under control of the higher centers, due to disease, injury, or disruption from some other reason, this led to a "reduction to a more automatic condition," or what would later be termed "loss of inhibition." Leonardo Bianchi (1922) also observed that ablating areas in the frontal cortex in monkeys and other animals caused a constellation of symptoms, including a reduction in purposeful behavior, impaired ability to coordinate actions in order to achieve a higher goal, and problems in socially appropriate behavior, which he called the "frontal lobe syndrome." Early in the 20th century, Kurt Goldstein coined the term "abstract attitude," which he believed was lost in many individuals with brain injuries, as suggested by the display of a more "concrete attitude," or a tendency to focus on the physical and not the conceptual properties of their environments (Goldstein & Scheerer, 1941). His discussion of abstract versus concrete attitudes laid the foundation for ongoing study of abstraction and how it plays an important role in *internally guided versus automatic behavior*. Among many other important contributions, he provided an insightful case study of the loss of abstract attitude in bvFTD, at the time referred to as Pick's disease (Goldstein & Katz, 1937).

The introduction of the concept of working memory by Baddeley and Hitch (1974) played an important role in the conceptual evolution of executive functioning. Their model posits that working memory is a system of temporary storage and manipulation of information that links perception and controlled action. An attentional control system (the central executive) actively regulates the distribution of limited attentional resources and coordinates information within three subsidiary "slave systems" (the visuospatial sketchpad, phonological loop, and the more recently characterized episodic memory buffer). Shallice (1982) later proposed the notion of the supervisory attentional system (SAS), which he described as the highest level of a larger model of cognitive function that serves to handle *nonroutine goal achievement in a slow but flexible manner*. He suggested that the SAS operates when the selection of known behavioral programs fails, or when there is no clear or obvious solution to a problem. Around the same time, Posner proposed a link between attention and "cognitive control" (Posner & Snyder, 1975) and suggested that there is a separate "executive" branch of the attention system that is responsible for focusing attention (Posner & Petersen, 1990).

Over the past 25 years, others have expanded these ideas to identify individual, lower level executive control components that enable higher order goal-directed behaviors, such as inhibition, resolving interference, updating working memory, and mental set shifting (e.g., Friedman & Miyake, 2004; Logie, Cocchini, Delia, & Baddeley, 2004; Miyake et al., 2000; Salthouse, Atkinson, & Berish, 2003). Muriel Lezak (1995, 2004) proposed a framework of four broad domains that interact to produce goal-directed behavior that include volition, planning, purposive action, and effective performance. This model has widespread appeal because of its simplicity; however, it has been criticized for lacking a strong theoretical basis and research support (Anderson, 2008). One of the major difficulties that have surfaced as a result of defining distinct constructs of executive control is the relative interrelatedness of various component functions and the variability in the patterns of impairments that can be seen in patient populations with similar pathology or lesion focus. Patients described as exhibiting executive dysfunction can present with one or a number of cognitive and affective difficulties, such as impulsivity, disinhibition, inattention, reduced working memory, difficulty with task monitoring, planning and organizing problems, poor reasoning ability, and difficulty switching between tasks, among others. Problems with the regulation of emotions can lead to apathy, affective lability, socially inappropriate behavior, and reduced motivation and energy. In addition, disturbances in executive functions can lead to impairment in performance in many other cognitive domains, such as memory, language, and visuospatial functioning, that rely on executive control. The widespread influence of executive functions on other cognitive domains has led researchers to question whether different component functions actually represent a common underlying executive process (Duncan, Emslie, Williams, Johnson, & Freer, 1996; Duncan, Johnson, Swales, & Freer, 1997; Engle, Kane, & Tuholski, 1999; Kimberg & Farah, 1993). Miyake et al.'s (2000) work on individual differences in executive functioning has been quite influential to this line of research. Using confirmatory factor analysis, they demonstrated that three aspects of executive functioning—updating, inhibition, and shifting—are interrelated and moderately correlated constructs. However, they also found that each component function also contributed its own independent power to separate task functions. They theorized that the overlap of executive constructs may relate to a common task requirement that is inherent in all executive control tasks, even those that are chosen specifically to tap a particular executive function: the maintenance of goal and context information in working memory.

Barkley's self-regulatory model (1997) addresses another important aspect that has not been emphasized in many modern frameworks of executive control: the involvement of emotion and affect in goal-directed behavior. This model, which is primarily derived from work examining behavioral inhibition, is composed of four main constructs, including (1) working memory, which allows for individuals to resist interfering information; (2) management of emotional responses; (3) internalized self-directed speech, which is used to control and sustain rule-based behavior and facilitate planning and problem solving; and (4) the analysis and synthesis of information into new behavioral responses to meet a goal. This model emphasizes that the goal-directed behavior cannot be met without emotional regulation and the integration of factors related to an individual's self, such as prior knowledge and experience.

Executive Control and the Frontal Networks

Executive control processes are strongly associated with involvement of the frontal lobes, particularly the prefrontal cortex (PFC). The frontal lobes consist of motor, premotor, and "prefrontal" cortices. The PFC, whose damage leads to the classic "frontal lobe syndromes," is made up of paralimbic and heteromodal components (Mesulam, 1986). The paralimbic component of the frontal lobes includes the anterior cingulate (Brodmann areas [BA] 24, 32, 33), paraolfactory (BA 25), and caudal orbitofrontal regions (BA 11, 13, 14, 47/12) and the frontoinsular cortex (BA 13, 14). The largest part of the PFC consists of the granular, heteromodal (higher order) association cortex, and it is located in the lateral and anterior parts of the frontal lobes (BA 9, 10, 11, 45, 46, 47) (Fig. 3.1).

While the PFC is critically involved in executive control processes, dysfunction may not necessarily be the direct result of prefrontal pathology and instead may be related to network disruptions at the level of white matter damage or dysfunction of

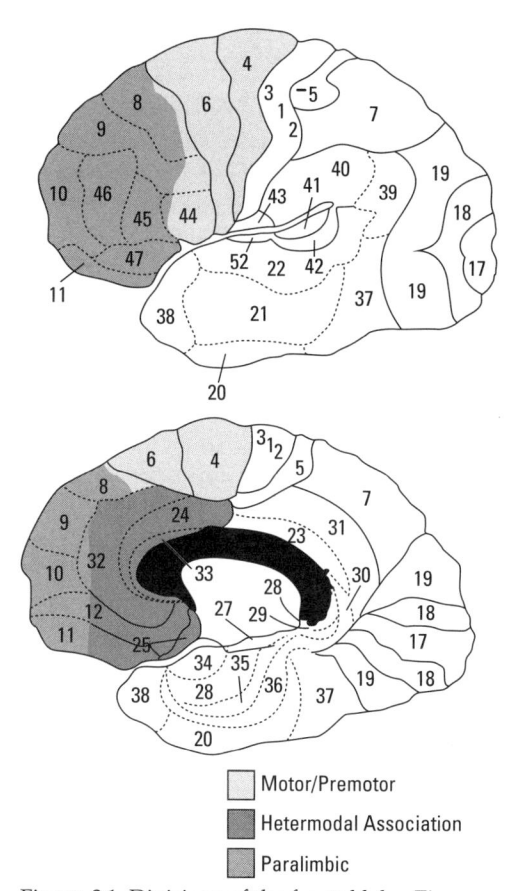

Figure 3.1 Divisions of the frontal lobe. Figure adapted from Mesulam (1986). (See color plate section)

critical "nodes" within a distributed system (Alexander & Stuss, 2000; Andres, 2003; Stuss & Knight, 2002). Alexander et al. (1986) initially reported on the multiple connections that run between sites of the frontal cortex, basal ganglia, and thalamus. They described five major circuits: (1) dorsolateral prefrontal, (2) lateral orbitofrontal, (3) anterior cingulate, (4) motor, and (5) oculomotor. On the basis of advanced multisynaptic circuit tracing techniques, Middleton and Strick (2002) proposed that two additional "circuits" be included: the medial orbitofrontal and inferotemporal/posterior parietal. All follow the same general pattern of connectivity, and lesions at any point along the frontal-subcortical circuits can lead to dysexecutive symptoms (Fig. 3.2).

The major cortical inputs to the dorsolateral prefrontal circuit within the heteromodal association cortex come from (1) modality-specific association areas

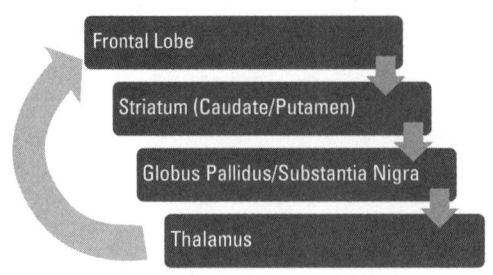

[Frontal Lobe → Striatum (Caudate/Putamen) → Globus Pallidus/Substantia Nigra → Thalamus → (back to Frontal Lobe)]

Figure 3.2 Schema of the frontal-striatal-thalamic circuits first proposed by Alexander et al. (1986).

(dedicated to the processing of information in only one sensory modality); (2) other heteromodal, high-order association cortical areas in the posterior parietal and superior temporal lobes; and (3) paralimbic regions, including the orbitofrontal, cingulate cortices, and the frontoinsular cortex (Barbas & Mesulam, 1985; Chavis & Pandya, 1976). Regions within the paralimbic prefrontal cortex receive extensive, direct input from limbic areas, including the amygdala and other nonfrontal paralimbic regions, as well as the frontal heteromodal association cortex to which they also send extensive projections.

The exact neurophysiologic features that distinguish the prefrontal heteromodal association cortex from other multisensory integration regions and allow it to perform the high-level functions associated with executive control have not been fully delineated, although several characteristics have been proposed. First, compared to other heteromodal cortices in the lateral temporal and posterior parietal lobes, the heteromodal association regions of the PFC appear to have more pronounced paralimbic connections, which may underlie its unique role in regulation or integration of complex cognitive and affective processes (Mesulam, 1986). Second, in terms of synaptic connections, neurons of the PFC are several steps removed from direct sensory processing, and therefore the sensory data it receives about the external environment are more highly processed (Mesulam, 2000). This implies that cognitive resources typically recruited to process sensory input or facilitate motor output are available in the prefrontal heteromodal association cortices, allowing these regions to devote more resources to higher level processing and integration. Finally, similar to other heteromodal regions, the PFC contains a special class of neurons that fire during delay periods of a delay response task (Goldman-Rakic, 1987; Miller, Erickson, & Desimone, 1996; Rainer, Asaad, & Miller, 1998). Such activity may provide the physiological underpinnings of the ability to hold information online. However, what seems unique to the PFC is that these cells can maintain their delay-period activity in the presence of distracters (i.e., persist in firing across memory delays even when distracting events occur before a behavioral response is permitted), which differs from memory-sensitive neurons outside of the PFC (Kane & Engle, 2002). This capacity may be a critical to the role of the PFC in maintaining representations of goals in the face of competing, task-irrelevant stimuli.

Neuroimaging research utilizing intrinsic network connectivity mapping has expanded our understanding of the functional connectivity of the PFC and its involvement in large-scale networks (Bressler & Menon, 2010). Both paralimbic prefrontal regions within medial frontal cortex (MFC) and heteromodal association regions within lateral prefrontal regions are consistently coactivated by cognitively demanding tasks (Curtis & D'Esposito, 2003; Kerns et al., 2004; Menon, Adleman, White, Glover, & Reiss, 2001; Ridderinkhof, Ullsperger, Crone, & Nieuwenhuis, 2004) and have been frequently interpreted as constituting a unitary network (Vincent, Kahn, Snyder, Raichle, & Buckner, 2008). However, regions of the MFC, including the dorsal anterior cingulate cortex (dACC) and orbital frontoinsula (FI), also activate in response to pain, uncertainty, and other threats to homeostasis (Craig, 2002; Grinband, Hirsch, & Ferrera, 2006; Peyron, Laurent, & Garcia-Larrea, 2000). Therefore, it has been suggested that the MFC is perhaps responding to homeostatic significance and signaling whether a change in cognitive or emotional "tone" is required (Critchley, 2005; Critchley, Wiens, Rotshtein, Ohman, & Dolan, 2004). While the number of distinct intrinsic brain networks and the complexity of their interactions have not been fully delineated (Vincent et al., 2008; Yeo et al., 2011), a fundamental network model of cognitive control that accounts for both paralimbic and prefrontal heteromodal cortex contributions has been proposed by Seeley and colleagues (2007). In this model, paralimbic regions, including the dorsal anterior cingulate (dACC) and anterior insular (AI) cortices comprise the "salience network," while regions of the prefrontal heteromodal cortex, including dorsolateral frontal and superior parietal cortices, constitute an "executive control" network (Seeley et al., 2007) (Fig. 3.3). The salience network can be thought of as providing ongoing surveillance of internal (and external) events or activity that is homeostatically relevant. In doing so, the salience network helps to allocate, and may even compete for, resources with the executive control network, in order to account for emotional factors that influence goal-directed processes (Seeley et al., 2007). In addition to the salience and executive control networks, intrinsic networks responsible for attentional control (Corbetta & Shulman, 2002) and internally focused operations, such as re-experiencing one's past and imagining one's future (Buckner, Andrews-Hanna, & Schacter, 2008; Gusnard, Raichle, & Raichle, 2001; Schacter, Addis, & Buckner, 2007), also play important roles in goal-directed behavior. These networks will be discussed in more detail in the following sections.

Executive Control and Goal-Directed Behavior

As a heuristic, we have found it helpful to break down the complex processes involved in goal-directed behavior into different classes of functions. At the center of this heuristic model is the concept of a "goal." A goal can be defined as a cognitive representation of an objective that one is committed or motivated to accomplish via directed behavioral or mental activity. The complexity of goals can vary along many dimensions. For example, a goal can range from committing to follow a concrete motor command (i.e., "open your eyes") to such complex and abstract notions as devoting oneself to the eradication of homelessness. Goals can also be conceptualized as varying across several other facets, including temporal proximity (immediate to long term), how planful they are (proactive vs. reactive), and their level of abstractness or meaningfulness.

Execution of Goals

The ability to flexibly adapt one's behavior in pursuit of a goal could not be accomplished

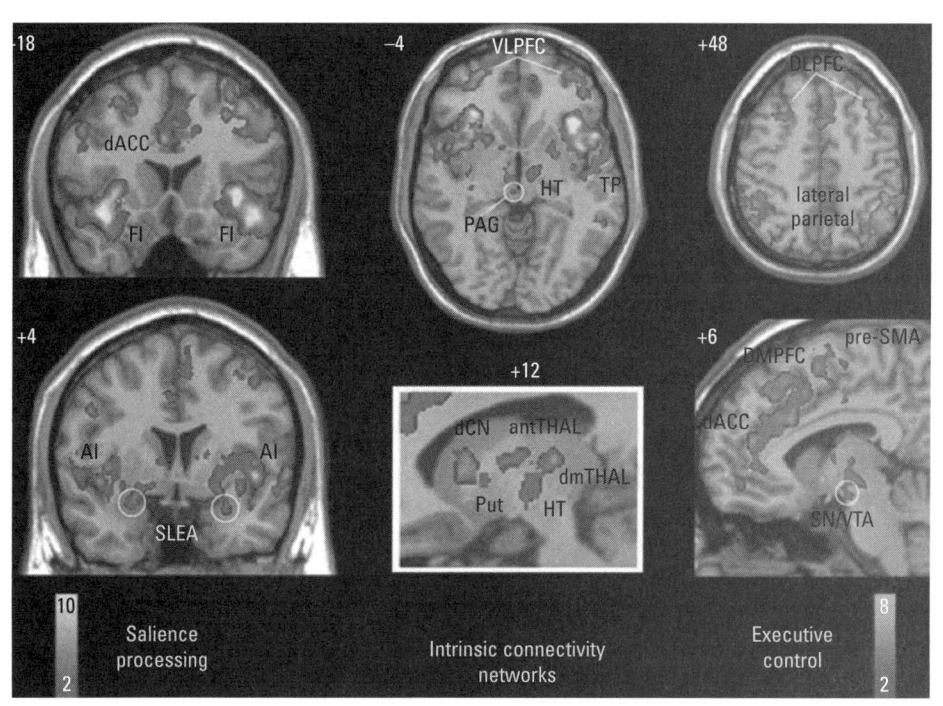

Figure 3.3 Salience and executive control networks revealed through intrinsic connectivity mapping. Image adapted from Seeley et al., 2007. (See color plate section)

without executive control. Executive control is not a unitary construct but instead refers to a complex set of processes that allow for an organism to carry out goal-directed behavior. We divide the process of executive control into three classes of operations: working memory, outcome/reward anticipation and monitoring, and response/behavioral selection.

Working Memory

Working memory is a theoretical construct that describes a system of limited capacity where information is temporarily stored (or maintained) and manipulated, which is critical for successful cognition (Baddeley, 2003). Therefore, working memory subsumes several executive control functions itself (referred to as the central executive by Baddeley), including attentional control, reasoning, planning, and ordering/organizing, which facilitate goal-directed behavior. Information represented in working memory is subject to evaluation and manipulation and serves as the basis for decisions and the planning of complex behaviors (Genovesio, Brasted, & Wise, 2006; Yoshida & Ishii, 2006).

Neuroanatomically, the lateral PFC has long been considered one of the most important brain regions involved in working memory processes. Imaging studies, using delayed match-to-sample tasks, have consistently documented prefrontal activation (see D'Esposito et al., 1998; Fletcher & Henson, 2001 for reviews). However, the functional anatomic distinctions within the lateral PFC remain an area of controversy. There is some evidence to support the lateralization of function in the PFC, with the right PFC more engaged by spatial working memory tasks and the left PFC more engaged by verbal working memory tasks (D'Esposito et al., 1998; Schumacher et al., 1996; Smith, Jonides, & Koeppe, 1996). Some studies support the specialization of function in the PFC that parallels the dorsal ("where") versus the ventral ("what") pathways for visual processing in the posterior cortex, such that dorsolateral PFC subserves spatial working memory and ventrolateral PFC may preferentially subserve object working memory (Courtney, Ungerleider, Keil, & Haxby, 1996; Wilson & O'Scalaidhe, 1993). Other studies support a dissociation of PFC according to processing demands, with the ventral PFC supporting the maintenance aspects of working memory and the dorsal lateral PFC facilitating the manipulation of information (D'Esposito, Postle, Ballard, & Lease, 1999; Petrides, 2000; Wagner, Maril, Bjork, & Schacter, 2001). Still other work has suggested that the dorsal lateral PFC is more likely to be activated as the task demands increase, to provide the needed support and scaffolding offered by executive control functions (D'Esposito et al., 1999; Petrides, 2000; Rypma, Prabhakaran, Desmond, Glover, & Gabrieli, 1999; Wagner et al., 2001). Clinical reports in humans and lesion studies in monkeys generally confirm a central role of the PFC in working memory (for a review see Miller & Cohen, 2001). However, several lesion studies suggest that working memory can be left relatively unimpaired following unilateral PFC damage (D'Esposito & Postle, 1999), perhaps by means of compensatory activity in the intact hemisphere (Corbetta, Kincade, Lewis, Snyder, & Sapir, 2005; Voytek et al., 2010).

In addition to the PFC, data from functional imaging studies have also consistently revealed activity within the posterior parietal cortex (PPC; BA 7) during working memory tasks (Curtis & D'Esposito, 2006; Owen et al., 2004; Wager & Smith, 2003). Supporting their functional interactions, lateral PFC and PPC tract-tracing studies have confirmed reciprocal interconnections (Schwartz & Goldman-Rakic, 1984). More recent neuroimaging research focused on identifying large-scale intrinsic brain networks has also revealed that lateral PFC interacts in a functionally cohesive manner with lateral superior parietal regions (Seeley et al., 2007) to support working memory and attention control. As introduced previously, this network has been termed the executive control network (Seeley et al., 2007). Others have reported on an intrinsic network that also includes lateral prefrontal and parietal regions, often called the fronto-parietal network (Niendam et al., 2012; Vincent et al., 2008). However, this network is more extensive and includes regions that overlap with the medial PFC and fronto-insular cortex, which Seeley and colleagues (2007) separate into the salience network.

Task Setting

Task setting refers to the high-level coordination of several types of working memory and executive control functions in order to establish a goal-directed plan upon which motor or mental activity is enacted. At its simplest level, task setting describes the process of creating mappings of a stimulus to a designated response (Stuss & Alexander, 2007) or coding an action with a goal. As goals become more complex, they require sequencing of multiple responses or actions. Therefore, task setting may occur several times during the execution of a single goal, and/or multiple tasks may be set simultaneously to facilitate a goal. *Planning* plays a critical role in the process of task setting and subsumes several executive control functions, each with heavy working memory demands. Planning occurs when a goal or "planned" event, held in working memory, triggers the generation of a new order of mental representations. These mental representations may consist of one or more intermediate steps or tasks upon which the goal is predicated. For example, if one visualizes going on vacation, the anticipated event (vacation) will not occur unless a series of intermediate steps or tasks (e.g., choosing a date, a place, a method of transportation) is first generated. *Organization* involves the ordering or manipulation of tasks or responses, such that the individual tasks are eventually arranged in a manner that, when viewed as a whole, conforms to some type of higher order logic or scheme. Organization also has a heavy working memory demand, as the higher order scheme must be held in mind so that the individual parts can be manipulated according to the scheme. For example, it is impossible to organize a bookshelf without holding in mind a chosen organizational scheme (e.g., arranging books alphabetically, by size, by color, etc.).

Several groups have proposed that tasks or actions are organized in a gradient that extends from posterior to anterior lateral PFC. That is, the more immediate/less abstract tasks or actions are processed in posterior regions of the lateral PFC, closer to premotor cortex, where they are more immediately accessible by motor cortex. The more abstract, less temporally immediate tasks or actions that do not require motor responses are organized more anteriorly toward the frontal pole (Badre, 2008; Badre & D'Esposito, 2007, 2009; Barbalat, Chambon, Franck, Koechlin, & Farrer, 2009; Kouneiher, Charron, & Koechlin, 2009).

To elicit the process of task setting, researchers often employ paradigms that ask participants to act contrary to an overlearned tendency or prepotent response, as in the Stroop Interference (Egner & Hirsch, 2005), Simon (Peterson et al., 2002), and stop-signal tasks (Aron & Poldrack, 2006). Other common paradigms require participants to learn and implement experimenter-provided rules for mapping stimuli to responses, often under conditions that require flexible switching between task rules or response strategies (Bunge, 2004). These tasks tend to emphasize experimental control of behavior, requiring participants to pursue artificial goals or respond according to rules dictated by the experimenter.

Attentional Control and Processing Priorities

Top-down attentional control, also referred to as goal-driven or endogenous attention, is responsible for selecting the information that gains access to working memory (Knudsen, 2007). Given the amount of information and stimuli that confront humans, the process of selecting which information has access to working memory is highly competitive (Desimone & Duncan, 1995). This is generally thought to occur through one of two mechanisms: (1) by directing resources (sensory or motor) toward a target in the environment (Andersen et al., 2004), and (2) by means of attentional biasing in order to improve the signal-to-noise in all information processing domains (sensory, motor, internal state, and memory) (Knudsen, 2007). The process of directing resources to goal-appropriate stimuli or events via the top-down control of spatial attention and eye movement has been linked to the dorsal attention network, which includes regions in the dorsolateral PFC, frontal eye fields, and superior parietal cortex (Corbetta & Shulman, 2002; Fox et al., 2005; Vincent et al., 2008) (Fig. 3.4a).

Regions of this system overlap partially with the executive control network, although there is evidence that they are two distinct networks (Vincent et al., 2008). However, the functional properties and organization of the posterior parietal cortex (PPC; which encompasses the superior parietal cortex) indicate that it is likely to be more involved in top-down modulation of spatial attention as opposed to working memory (Colby & Goldberg, 1999).

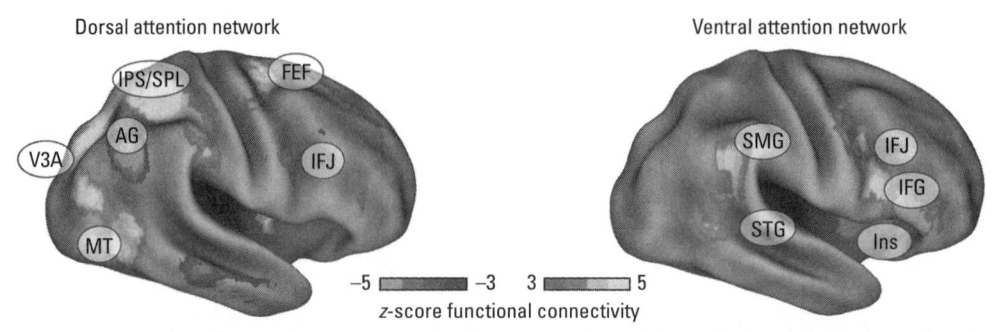

Figure 3.4 Dorsal and ventral attention networks. Image adapted from Corbetta & Shulman (2011). (See color plate section)

For example, the PPC appears to be more susceptible to interruption by distracting stimuli (Powell & Goldberg, 2000), which results in a pattern of functional activity that is less persistent than the PFC (Fuster, 1995; Miller et al., 1996). Instead, activity in the PPC may represent the integration of sensorimotor information in order to visually guide movements (Buneo & Andersen, 2006).

The second mechanism of top-down attentional control, attentional biasing, is thought to be facilitated by *top-down modulation*, which refers to neuronal enhancement or excitation, inhibition, or possibly both. The role of top-down modulation in cognitive control and goal-directed behavior is explained in more detail in Box 3.1.

Although attention and working memory are generally thought of as two distinct cognitive constructs, this notion has been challenged in favor of a model in which attention and working memory mutually influence each other (Gazzaley & Nobre, 2012; Kiyonaga, Egner, & Soto, 2012). First, the contents of working memory have been conceptualized as active internal representations maintained within the focus of attention (Zanto & Gazzaley, 2009). Second, while attentional control can determine what has access to working memory, it is perhaps also true that representations held within working memory can affect the allocation of attentional resources. As such, working memory may allow for the active maintenance of current processing priorities (Lavie, Hirst, de Fockert, & Viding, 2004). Processing priorities refer to important contextual information, such as rules, instructions, and intentions that are associated with a goal representation (Cohen, Braver, & O'Reilly, 1996; Cohen & Servan-Schreiber, 1992).

Outcome/Reward Anticipation and Monitoring

Selecting the best course of action in goal-directed behavior describes a very active mental state in which the brain is dynamically making predictions and generating expectations based on reinforcement values of previous actions and experiences (O'Doherty, Kringelbach, Rolls, Hornak, & Andrews, 2001; Ullsperger & von Cramon, 2004). Much of the work on decision-making and reward-maximizing behavior comes from models of reinforcement learning (Sutton & Barto, 1998), which suggest that the flexibility of this process relies on one's ability to rapidly monitor and update prediction values based on actual outcomes and experience. Outcome and reward anticipation and monitoring are essential motivators of goal-directed behavior. Regions within the medial PFC, particularly the orbitofrontal cortex (OFC) and anterior cingulate cortex (ACC), play complementary and reciprocal roles in this process (Berns, McClure, Pagnoni, & Montague, 2001; Elliott, Friston, & Dolan, 2000).

Anticipating Consequences/Outcomes

The ability to anticipate consequences is a critical factor in making controlled decisions among competing tasks or strategies. It may be the case that consequences and reward values associated with context-relevant information, such as sensory signals, as well as knowledge of similar events and their associated consequences, are gathered to inform us of our options. This process of anticipating consequences can be thought of as a type of internal *monitoring*, which involves keeping track of a designated set of external or internal stimuli or responses and associated

BOX 3.1 Executive Control via Top-Down Modulation

Miller and Cohen (2001) proposed that the primary function of the prefrontal cortex is to support cognitive control by actively maintaining rules or goals online in order to evaluate incoming information and internal states to guide response or task selection toward a current goal. They suggest that this control is implemented by bias signals throughout much of the rest of the brain, which increase or decrease the gain of sensory or motor neurons that are engaged in goal-oriented behavior. According to Miller and Cohen, this biasing mechanism is a special case of cognitive control within the sensory domain and the term "cognitive control" is applied to any situation where a biasing signal is used to promote task-appropriate responding.

Extending on the work of Miller and Cohen, Gazzaley and D'Esposito (2007) proposed that cognitive control can be thought of as applying to not only sensory input but different kinds of processing as well, including thought/cognition, emotion, and motor output. Within the Gazzaley and D'Esposito (2007) framework, the control of *sensory input* involves the selective focus of limited cognitive resources on features of the external environment that are relevant, ignoring those elements that are irrelevant. Such control is particularly pertinent during processes such as selective attention, working memory encoding, and long-term memory (LTM) encoding. Control of our *internal state* involves influence over both emotive and cognitive features of the internal milieu, such as affect and emotion, as well as generating and maintaining representations in the absence of external stimuli (cognition). Emotional control includes regulating internal feeling states and emotion-related cognitions, physiologic states, and behaviors, while cognitive control includes working memory maintenance and manipulation, mental imagery, introspection, organization, and planning. Gazzaley and D'Esposito (2007) suggest that it is the extensive interaction between control of emotional and cognitive internal states that leads to complex processes such as social conduct and decision making. Control of *motor output* entails regulation of all body movements, with eye movements and reaching behavior being the most extensively studied. Gazzaley and D'Esposito (2007) propose a framework that is biologically plausible based on extensive animal research on neuronal excitation and inhibition (Alexander, Newman, & Symmes, 1976; Funahashi, Bruce, & Goldman-Rakic, 1993; Fuster, 1985; Skinner & Yingling, 1977). Abnormalities within each of these domains of processing (sensory input, cognition, emotion, and motor output) can be understood in terms of impairments in *top-down modulation*, reflecting disorders of enhancement (activation), inhibition (suppression), or both. The clinical features of enhancement and inhibition deficits across domains of executive control are discussed in more detail in Box 3.2), including the the two executive control functions discussed thus far, task setting and attentional control.

reward values linked to distinct tasks or strategies. This process then sets the necessary means for performance monitoring, in which discrepancies register in the mind of the person monitoring or trigger a particular reaction. Individuals who have difficulty modulating the process of anticipating consequences may be poorly motivated to perform goal-directed behavior or may have trouble making a decision regarding competing tasks and strategies because of difficulty disengaging from the process of gathering information and generating possible outcomes (Table 3.1).

As mentioned previously, both the OFC and ACC interact as critical nodes in the process of anticipating consequences and outcomes. In primates, the OFC (BA 11, 13, 14, 47/12) appears to contain neural processors that help to store or code the reinforcement value of sensory signals (learning stimulus-reward associations). OFC is seen as binding events with consequences or learning how stimuli will impact an individual emotionally and physically. This is facilitated, in part, by the OFC's reciprocal interactions between the amygdala (Schoenbaum, Chiba, & Gallagher, 1998, 1999). The organization of function within the OFC has been described as a series of gradients. First, medial OFC has been associated with activity in response to

TABLE 3.1 Top-Down Modulation Clinical Features of Enhancement (Activation) and Inhibition (Suppression) Deficits

	Sensory Input	Thought/Cognition	Emotion	Motor Output
Executive control functions	Attentional control	Task setting Working memory Maintenance Anticipation Performance Monitoring Planning	Regulation of affective and motivational states Reward-related decision making/motivation	Eye movements (saccades) Motor preparation Motor control (initation/inhibition) Response maintenance
Enhancement deficits (cannot turn it on)	Reduced ability to focus attention	Inability to set about coordinating goal-directed behavior Inability to hold information or task priorities online Fewer "cognitive degrees of freedom" and limited behavioral repertoire Reduced ability to anticipate consequences necessary to carry out goal-directed behavior Reduced ability to flexibly modify behavior Poor planning and organization	Emotional blunting Apathy—motivational inability to carry out goal-directed behavior Inability to update the reward value of actions	Reduced ability to initiate movements Impairments in motor sequencing Inability to sustain a response over time
Inhibition deficits (cannot turn it off)	Increased distractibility by task-irrelevant sensory input	Difficulty disengaging or switching between tasks Difficulty with decision making Increased distractibility by task-irrelevant cognitive input	Disinhibited behavior Context-inappropriate behavior Emotional lability	Impulsivity Perseveration Utilization behavior Impairments in motor sequencing Inability for delayed gratification

Note. Extrapolation of schema presented in Gazzaley and D'Esposito (2007).

reward value of a stimulus, while lateral OFC has been shown to encode stimuli in terms of potential for punishment. In addition, an anterior-posterior gradient has also been proposed, and it suggests that posterior OFC encodes reward value for concrete primary reinforcers like taste and touch, while anterior OFC encodes the value of more abstract, symbolic complex secondary reinforcing factors like money (Kringelbach & Rolls, 2004; Rankin et al., 2006).

The ability of the OFC to alter contingencies between stimuli and their expected reinforcement value is critical for flexible behavior (Schoenbaum & Roesch, 2005). In fact, a particular class of neurons, called "reversal" neurons (Thorpe, Rolls, & Maddison, 1983), has been identified within the OFC that are associated with flexibly coding representations between predictive cues and outcomes during discrimination learning (Rolls, Critchley, Mason, & Wakeman, 1996; Schoenbaum et al., 1999; Schoenbaum, Setlow, Nugent, Saddoris, & Gallagher, 2003). Normal aging is associated with a decline in cognitive flexibility, and work from the animal literature has shown that aged animals often have difficulty modifying responses when contingencies change. Specifically, activity recorded in OFC "reversal" neurons of aged rats fails to show the same level of sensitivity or ability to flexibly encode stimulus-outcome associations relative to young control rats (Schoenbaum, Setlow, Saddoris, & Gallagher, 2006).

The ACC also plays a critical role in anticipating outcomes and consequences of actions. The ACC is located in the neural "cross-road" of motor, cognitive, and affective/arousal systems. It receives afferents from amygdala, fronto-insular cortex, OFC, midline thalamus, and monoaminergic centers of the brainstem. While OFC cells have been shown to encode the expected value of stimuli (Schoenbaum et al., 2006), cells within the ACC appear to encode the expected value of actions (Matsumoto, Matsumoto, Abe, & Tanaka, 2007; Walton, Devlin, & Rushworth, 2004) and are perhaps more closely tied to the action-selection process (Rushworth & Behrens, 2008).

In addition, ACC activity in neuroimaging studies has also been associated with coding conflict between competing responses (Botvinick, Braver, Barch, Carter, & Cohen, 2001; Holroyd & Coles, 2002). The conflict monitoring theory (Botvinick et al., 2001; Carter & van Veen, 2007) proposes that the ACC and more broadly regions within the medial prefrontal cortex (MPFC) monitor the level of conflict arising across potential responses, including situations that require the overriding of prepotent responses, situations requiring selection among a set of equally permissible responses, and situations involving errors. For example, in one version of the Stroop Interference Task, the word "red" is printed in the color blue, and the task is to name the color. Two divergent responses compete to determine behavioral output. The automatic tendency to read the word "red" must be countered in order to correctly execute the task of naming the color, which is blue. The ACC is recruited during this task. A signal from the ACC regarding the detection of conflict seems to call upon other brain regions to exercise cognitive control. As discussed later, the ACC is also integrally involved in performance monitoring and detecting prediction errors.

Based on the information presented thus far on anticipating consequences and outcomes, one might assume that action is therefore chosen simply based on the highest anticipated or most rewarded outcome. However, this would significantly constrain an individual's behavioral repertoire, as a limited number of actions or behaviors would likely be repeated over and over (Rushworth & Behrens, 2008). Therefore, there likely needs to be an incentive to explore other available options, as well as a level of flexibility or breadth (i.e., additional degrees of freedom) within working memory to support the range of strategic possibilities that exist to achieve a goal. In statistics, "degrees of freedom" refers to a number of values in an equation that are free to vary. The term "degrees of freedom," when applied metaphorically to cognition, captures an important property of goal-directed behavior (Daffner & Searl, 2008). *Task or plan management* refers to the process of holding multiple tasks or strategies (determined by the complexity of the goal), their expected or anticipated outcomes, and the relative value of these outcomes in working memory. The efficiency or quality of task management is influenced by an individual's ability to inhibit prepotent responses and the capacity of working memory to maintain and manipulate a range of task/strategy options. Individuals with dysexecutive syndromes typically follow the "path of least resistance" because their limited capacity for working memory, monitoring, inhibition, and initiation cannot provide the cognitive support necessary for the enactment of alternative responses. Fewer "cognitive degrees of freedom" usually results in the generation of behavioral responses that are most directly tied to their sources of input, with few modulating influences.

Performance/Reward Monitoring

Performance monitoring refers to the ability to track actions and their expected outcomes and utilize information signaling success or failure in performance. In general, successful monitoring necessitates intact working memory because the expected outcome must be kept "in mind" to serve as a comparison point to the actual outcome. This information is then utilized to update reinforcement associations of stimuli and actions. Without performance monitoring, an individual would have difficulty modifying behavior to achieve a goal (Table 3.1). Of note, the process of performance/reward monitoring is inextricably linked to the process of anticipating consequences/outcomes and is subserved by similar neuroanatomical networks with nodes within the ACC and OFC.

The ACC has been associated with holding a central role in tracking one's performance, particularly when it deviates from expectations or from what is known to result in reward. The ACC may index conflict at the level of divergence from expectation, response errors (Falkenstein, Hohnsbein, Hoormann, & Blanke, 1991; Niki & Watanabe, 1979), and task difficulty/mental effort (Botvinick et al., 2001; Botvinick, Cohen, & Carter, 2004). According to the performance monitoring theory (Holroyd & Coles, 2008), medial PFC monitors actual performances and detects both negative and positive prediction errors that subsequently engage cognitive control processes to enact behavioral adjustments (Holroyd & Coles, 2002; Holroyd, Yeung, Coles, & Cohen, 2005). While ACC activation is most often present in neuroimaging studies during tasks where subjects have to evaluate the outcome of their chosen action and use this information to guide future behavior (Bush et al., 2002; Knutson, Adams, Fong, & Hommer, 2001; Ullsperger & von Cramon, 2003), the OFC is also likely involved in updating related stimulus-outcome associations (Schoenbaum et al., 2006).

Response/Behavioral Selection

Response or behavioral selection involves the parallel processes of initiating/sustaining a task response and/or inhibiting responses or activity in the service of carrying out goal-directed behavior.

Initiating and Sustaining Motor and Mental Activity

Initiation is the purposeful, self-generated commencement of an overt behavior or mental activity. The process of initiating and sustaining any response is sometimes referred to as "energization" (Stuss & Alexander, 2007). Without guidance from working memory and the process of task setting, initiation cannot occur and behaviors may be limited to reflexive and automatic responses to environmental stimuli (Table 3.1).

Response maintenance, or sustaining a response over time, is thought to reflect the accumulation of activation sufficient to produce and sustain a response over time (Alexander, Stuss, Shallice, Picton, & Gillingham, 2005). Stuss and Alexander (2007) argue that the response maintenance aspect of energization is responsible for countering the neurophysiological tendency for any neural activity to become inactive in the absence of input. They suggest that to optimize responding, particularly when activation becomes low (e.g., detecting occasional stimuli or performing occasional motor acts), lower level perceptual or motor representations require energization or re-energization. Without such a process, performance over a prolonged period will inevitably waiver (Table 3.1).

Medial frontal structures, including the anterior cingulate cortex (BA 24, 25, 32), the supplementary motor area (BA 6), and pre-supplementary motor area (BA 6), are thought to play an important role in the initiation and maintenance of behavior (Passingham, 1995; Paus, 2001; Ridderinkhof et al., 2004). As noted in the preceding sections, the ACC is critical to the process of anticipating the potential reward value of various actions, which serves as a basis of motivating/energizing behavior. Paus (2001) has reviewed how components of the ACC send efferents to skeletal muscle, oculomotor, and vocalization systems. The ACC also has major connections with the lateral PFC, giving it access to the extensive cognitive processing of this area. Patients with medial frontal damage often demonstrate impairments in the initiation of speech and motor movements or deficits in inhibiting reflexive motor responses (Paus, 2001) (e.g., grasp reflex) or control of the contralateral limb (e.g., alien hand syndrome) (Banks, 1989; Hashimoto, 1998). Bilateral lesions of the anterior cingulate can cause akinetic mutism, a condition characterized by a failure to speak (mutism) or to begin volitional movements (akinesis) (Barris & Schuman, 1953; Nemeth, Hegedus, & Molnar, 1988).

Inhibiting or Stopping Motor and Mental Activity

Inhibition involves the suppression of specific behavioral output, mental activity, or an emotional response (usually an automatic or prepotent/overlearned response). Inhibition is an important component of self-regulation, which requires both inhibition of automatic responses (suppression) and execution of different, consciously chosen responses in their place. Behavioral inhibition also includes the ability to cease a particular behavior at the appropriate time and is the basis of delayed gratification, which involves denying oneself something satisfying, presumably in order to achieve a more important goal (Table 3.1).

There is growing evidence that the lateral PFC, especially in the right hemisphere, is activated during the inhibition of behavioral responses, for example, in motor go-no go tasks, when a response must be withheld (Liddle, Kiehl, & Smith, 2001). Functional imaging studies have indicated that the inferior lateral PFC (BA 44/45) is recruited when a person's cognitive set needs to be shifted—for example, during the Wisconsin Card Sorting Task (Konishi et al., 1999) or inhibiting memory processing of word associates (Anderson et al., 2004). Anderson and colleagues (2004) provide evidence that the lateral PFC (BA 45/46) is activated during a task in which subjects are asked to control (inhibit) memory processing of word associates. The increase in lateral prefrontal activity is linked to a reduction in hippocampal activation and an increased probability of not recalling a test item. As mentioned previously, the lateral PFC is also involved in top-down control of selective attention.

Inhibitory activity also plays an important role in *emotion regulation* and social interactions (Box 3.2), and it is associated with activity in the orbitofrontal cortex. Specifically, the OFC has been shown to mediate top-down regulation of the amygdala, critical for affective processing by PFC (Davidson, 2000). OFC (and lateral PFC) show increased neural activity when participants are actively regulating their emotions and activity within the OFC, and lateral PFC has been shown to be inversely correlated with activity of amygdala (Ochsner, Bunge, Gross, & Gabrieli, 2002). Patients with damage to OFC or difficulty modulating OFC function often exhibit poor emotional regulation and strikingly disinhibited, inappropriate behavior (Box 3.2). In patients with neurodegenerative diseases, emotional control has even been predicted primarily by right OFC thickness, while cognitive control was predicted by DLPFC structures (Krueger et al., 2011).

How Are Goals Selected?

In order for individuals to pursue goal-directed behaviors, they need to be sufficiently motivated. According to the classic psychological theory of motivation proposed by Hull (1943), motivation describes a global modulation or regulation factor that is based on the expected possible gains (rewards/meaningfulness/punishment) of a range of behavioral options. The expected gains of pursuing actions that lead to a particular goal are coded or controlled by several factors, including, but likely not limited to, representations of

---

BOX 3.2 Inhibitory Control and Emotion Regulation

Affect or emotion regulation involves modulating one's external expression of emotions in accordance with perceived social expectations by using top-down processes to modulate internal emotional states. It is what we do to influence the emotions we have, when we have them, and how we experience and express them (Gross, 1998). At times, it may be necessary to inhibit the influence of emotional information in order to successfully facilitate goal-directed behavior. Emotion regulation can be initiated intrinsically (by the individual) or extrinsically (by someone else), or it can be motivated by hedonic (feeling less negative or more positive) or instrumental (to achieve one's long-term goals) factors (Tamir, 2009). In addition, the emotion regulatory goal may be explicit (deliberate and conscious) or implicit (activated outside of an individual's awareness) (Bargh & Williams, 2006; Mauss, Bunge, & Gross, 2007).

There may be times in social situations when inherent conflict arises between what is enjoyable for an individual and what is best for a group. To maintain harmonious social relationships at these times, it may be necessary to inhibit one's own desires and immediate needs (Heatherton, 2011). For example, individuals may have to put aside sadness in service of performing their job responsibilities or refrain from voicing anger to someone in authority. The emotion regulatory goal in these circumstances is influenced or motivated by one's desire to maintain social harmony, and top-down control mechanisms are recruited to inhibit emotion generation.

the self (information regarding personal values and beliefs that are carried across time), representations of the past and the future (information about past experiences and expectation or the anticipation of a specific outcome), and representations of external and internal importance (how critical the behavior is to an individual's external and internal homeostasis or survival). Input from systems that generate homeostatic/survival value, representations of the self, and representations of the past/future provide higher order or top-down mechanisms that determine long-term and immediate goals. A prerequisite for these systems to function is that the brain be in an active state, which is facilitated by the first system discussed here.

Ascending Arousal System

The ascending arousal system or the ascending reticular activating system (ARAS) is a bottom-up process that can be thought of as acting as the brain's "furnace." It is responsible for producing the "heat" or a global activating influence that provides the scaffolding for wakefulness and alertness. The ARAS is composed of two major pathways: (1) the reticulothamalocortical pathway that promotes cortical arousal, and (2) the extrathalamic pathway, which originates in the brainstem and basal forebrain and sends direct projections to the cortex (Kinomura, Larsson, Gulyas, & Roland, 1996). The Yerkes-Dodson law has provided the classic framework for understanding the relationship between arousal and task performance, and it suggests that there is an optimal level of arousal that follows an inverted u-shaped curve. Either end of the spectrum (too little or too much arousal) can adversely affect task performance (Yerkes & Dodson, 1908). While the "heat" or activating influence produced by this system is necessary for goal-directed behavior, it is not sufficient. The "heat" then needs to be channeled where it can be used to fuel executive control functions. Mesulam (2000) has referred to the paralimbic PFC as the "bridge" that channels raw motivational energy toward context-appropriate objects.

Representations of the Self

The self-concept describes a uniquely human ability to consciously represent personal attributes, such as abilities/skills, social roles, psychological characteristics, and preferences (D'Argembeau & Salmon, 2012). Humans also hold multiple representations of their self-concept, including views about themselves across different contexts or relationships (Chen, Boucher, & Tapias, 2006) and how they are seen by others. Aside from personal traits, the self-concept is also thought to include knowledge about personal goals, which plays a critical role in guiding and motivating behavior (Higgins, 1997; Markus & Nurius, 1986).

Imaging studies of the self-concept or self-knowledge most frequently ask participants to represent or reflect on their own psychological traits. Participants are asked to judge whether different trait adjectives (e.g., funny, loud, hard-working) describe their own psychological traits or those of another person, such as a famous person (Kelley et al., 2002) or a personally familiar person (e.g., a best friend) (Heatherton et al., 2006). These studies have strongly implicated the MPFC as being most active when thinking about the self versus another. Other work has shown that the MPFC may also play an important role in thinking about how we are seen by others. That is, the pattern of increased MPFC activation is consistent when self-judgments are made from one's own perspective and when judgments are made while taking the perspective of a personally familiar other (D'Argembeau et al., 2007). These findings suggest that perhaps the neural architecture that supports self-cognition is similar to that which supports social cognition (Amodio & Frith, 2006).

Studies investigating the neural correlates of reflecting on personal goals have also implicated several regions in the MPFC, in addition to regions of the posterior cingulate/precuneus (Johnson et al., 2006; Johnson, Nolen-Hoeksema, Mitchell, & Levin, 2009; Mitchell et al., 2009). More specifically, Johnson and colleagues (2006) found that regions within the MPFC showed greater activation when thinking about hopes and aspirations, while non-PFC medial regions showed greater activation when thinking of duties and obligations. The MPFC may also play a role in processing the self-relatedness or self-relevance of information, such that representations that elicit high activity in the MPFC may be those that constitute the mental model of the self that is held in mind at a given moment (D'Argembeau & Salmon, 2012).

Representation of the Future and Past

The human ability to revisit or re-experience one's past and imagine one's future provides an individual with a sense of personal continuity over time (Klein, Loftus, & Kihlstrom, 2002; Schacter et al., 2007; Tulving, 2005). In these instances, the individual creates or re-creates an experience outside of his or her personal present moment (Buckner & Carroll, 2007). This ability to represent the future and the past is also thought to influence our self-concept or self-knowledge (Conway, 2005), an important function of which may be to provide episodic forms of self-knowledge, or representations of specific personal experiences that support or perhaps even constrain representations of the self (D'Argembeau & Salmon, 2012). Together, the self-concept and the ability to represent episodic forms of self-knowledge have been referred to as *self-referential processing*. As mentioned previously, self-referential processing is thought to play a critical role in goal-directed behavior by helping to determine self-relevance, which may vary across time and context (Markus & Wurf, 1987). The self-relevance of information plays a critical role in motivating goal-directed behavior.

The default-mode network is proposed to play an integral role in representing one's future and past by adaptively integrating "information about relationships and associations from past experiences, in order to construct mental simulations about possible future events" (Schacter et al., 2007, p. 660). The default-mode network comprises a set of interconnected brain regions, including MPFC, posterior cingulate cortex (PCC)/precuneus, lateral and medial temporal lobes, and posterior inferior parietal lobule (pIPL) that are suppressed during tasks that demand externalized attention (Buckner et al., 2008; Gusnard, Akbudak, Shulman, & Raichle, 2001; Laird et al., 2009; Shulman et al., 1997) (Fig. 3.5). These regions, particularly the medial frontal and posteromedial regions, overlap with the structures involved in representations of the self-concept discussed in the previous section and likely support a mechanism for interaction to support

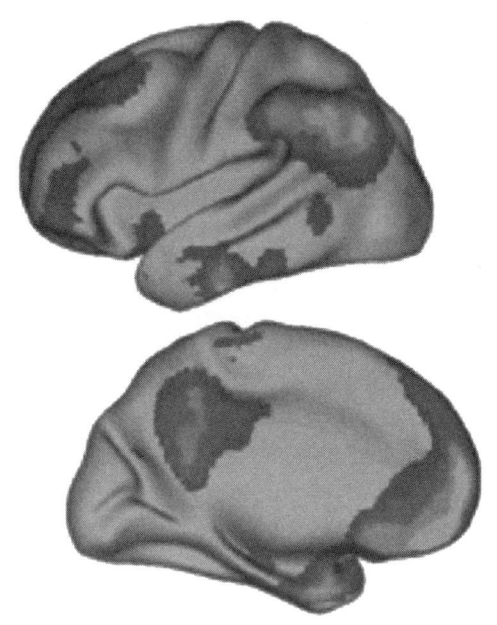

Figure 3.5 Default-mode network—The displayed positron emission tomography (PET) data include nine studies (132 participants) from Shulman et al. (1997, reanalyzed in Buckner et al., 2005). Image from Buckner et al. (2012).

self-referential processing. The default-mode network has been shown to be involved in cognitive processes that are internally focused, such as mind wandering (Christoff, Gordon, Smallwood, Smith, & Schooler, 2009; Mason et al., 2007), self-reference (D'Argembeau et al., 2005; Gusnard, Akbudak, et al., 2001), and recollecting one's past or imagining one's personal future (Schacter et al., 2007; Spreng, Mar, & Kim, 2009). The brain's default-mode network is most frequently engaged during tasks where participants are asked to remember specific past events, imagine specific future events, or imagine specific events that involve a familiar other, in response to event cues (Addis, Wong, & Schacter, 2007; Buckner & Carroll, 2007; Okuda et al., 2003; Szpunar, Watson, & McDermott, 2007).

How Changes in Salience Influence Goal-Directed Behavior

An individual's internal and external environment is continuously flooded by stimuli, some of which are more important to act on than others. Two systems, the salience network and the ventral attention network (which are partially overlapping), play critical roles in deciding what information or stimuli are most urgent or task relevant (Corbetta & Shulman, 2002; Seeley et al., 2007). They also facilitate an individual's ability to disengage from one's way of thinking, current activity, or present circumstances and re-engage in a different way of thinking or responding when the context or environment demands it. This ability, often referred to as set shifting, allows a person to manage transitions, cope with unexpected changes in plans, shift perspectives as relevant information becomes available, and think flexibly and creatively when solving problems. *Perseveration* is the continued engagement in a previous behavior despite the presence of cues in the environment that signal the need to shift or reorient (Table 3.1).

The Salience Network

The salience network likely plays two important roles in goal-directed behavior. First, it is uniquely positioned to identify the most homeostatically relevant stimuli through the rapid integration of sensory, visceral, autonomic, and hedonic signals (Seeley et al., 2007). In this way, it is well positioned to participate in the selection of an individual's current goal. However, the salience network is also thought to continuously survey the internal (and external) terrain to signal the occurrence of a salient event that may require the rapid modification of current processing priorities to ensure survival or homeostatic balance. Thus, the salience network can disrupt executive control processing underlying goal-directed behavior when a more immediately relevant event requires attention/action.

Within the salience network, the anterior cingulate cortex (ACC), orbitofrontal cortex (OFC), and the frontoinsular cortex (FI) have been identified as specialized nodes for sympathetic efference and interoceptive feedback (Craig, 2002; Critchley, 2005; Critchley, Elliott, Mathias, & Dolan, 2000; Critchley et al., 2004; Saper, 2002) (Fig. 3.3). Specifically, the FI is uniquely situated at the interface of the cognitive, homeostatic, and affective systems of the human brain, providing a link between stimulus-driven processing and brain regions involved in monitoring the internal milieu (Craig, 2009). A recent model suggests that the integration of information by the FI serves to motivate goal-directed behavior to utilize attention and working memory resources (Menon & Uddin, 2010). The right FI has been referred to as a convergence zone that may represent a "global emotional moment," built from the integration of interoceptive inputs, with goals, hedonic conditions, and contextual information (Craig, 2009).

The ACC is also a critical node within the salience network and is also positioned where motor, cognitive, and affective/arousal systems converge, similar to the FI. As such, the ACC is capable of integrating changes in motivational and arousal states, with expected outcomes and potential reinforcements to motivate behavior (Kerns et al., 2004; Menon et al., 2001; Ridderinkhof et al., 2004).

The Ventral Attention Network

Similar to the salience network, the ventral attention network plays a critical role in keeping track of external events that may impact our safety or survival. The ventral attention network includes temporal-parietal junction (TPJ) and regions of the ventral frontal cortex (VFC) (inferior frontal gyrus, frontal opercular cortex, and anterior insula) and is lateralized to the right hemisphere (Corbetta & Shulman, 2002) (Fig. 3.4b). This system shows activity increases upon detection of salient targets, especially when they appear in unexpected locations (Astafiev et al., 2003; Astafiev, Stanley, Shulman, & Corbetta, 2004; Corbetta, Kincade, Ollinger, McAvoy, & Shulman, 2000; Kincade, Abrams, Astafiev, Shulman, & Corbetta, 2005).

The ventral attention network mediates *bottom-up*, stimulus-driven reorienting of attention (Shulman et al., 2009) and acts as a "circuit breaker" in response to novel, salient, or potentially significant stimuli (Corbetta & Shulman, 2002). A stimulus may be salient based on hard-wired (e.g., looming stimuli) or learned (e.g., voice of a parent) biological importance (Knudsen, 2007). The nervous system responds automatically to such salient stimuli with unusually strong responses. Unexpected or highly salient stimuli can trigger the orienting response that calls upon top-down control mechanisms to evaluate whether the salient stimuli is of greater importance than the current contents of working memory (Miller & Cohen, 2001; Miller & D'Esposito, 2005).

Behaviorally, the function of the ventral attention system manifests as the orienting response, or the reorienting of attention toward a salient stimuli. A functional interaction between the dorsal and ventral attention networks has been proposed such that task-relevant signals from the dorsal system "filter" stimulus-driven signals in the ventral system, whereas stimulus-driven "circuit-braking" signals from the ventral system provide an interrupt to the dorsal system, reorienting it toward salient stimuli (Corbetta & Shulman, 2002; Shulman et al., 2003). Pavlov's (1960) classic descriptions of the orienting response illustrate the importance of the ventral attention network in supporting higher level cognitive functioning:

> The biological significance [of the orienting reflex] is obvious. If the animal were not provided with such a reflex its life would hang at every moment by a thread.... In man this reflex has been greatly developed in its highest form by inquisitiveness—the parent of that scientific method through which we hope one day to come to a true orientation in knowledge of the world around us. (p. 12)

Contributions of Neurotransmitter Function to Executive Control

Dopamine is probably the best characterized neurotransmitter associated with the executive functions (Cohen & Servan-Schreiber, 1992). It contributes to the adequate function of working memory (Goldman-Rakic, 1996; Williams & Goldman-Rakic, 1995) and helps to regulate motivational states and reward systems (Horvitz, Stewart, & Jacobs, 1997; Schultz, Dayan, & Montague, 1997; Wickelgren, 1997). Evidence in the animal literature points to an "optimal" amount of dopamine, which follows an inverted "u-shaped" curve. Too much or too little dopamine is detrimental to working memory performance (Arnsten, 1997; Arnsten & Rubia, 2012). Dopamine originates from structures in the midbrain, including the ventral tegmental area (VTA), that project to frontal cortex. In rats, lesions to either midbrain VTA cell bodies or frontal cortical areas result in very similar behavioral effects (hyperactivity) (Pycock, Kerwin, & Carter, 1980). In monkeys, destruction of dopamine terminals leads to impaired performance on the delayed alternation task in a manner similar to that seen after destruction of the frontal cortex itself (Brozoski, Brown, Rosvold, & Goldman, 1979).

Dopamine also plays an important role in anticipating outcomes and reward monitoring. It appears to do this by coding a prediction error, such that a reward that is better than predicted elicits an activation (positive prediction error), a predicted reward that matches its outcome elicits no response, and a reward that is worse than predicted induces a reduction in neural response (negative error) (Bayer & Glimcher, 2005; Morris, Arkadir, Nevet, Vaadia, & Bergman, 2004; Nakahara, Itoh, Kawagoe, Takikawa, & Hikosaka, 2004; Tobler, Fiorillo, & Schultz, 2005; Zaghloul et al., 2009). This reward-predicting signal specifies the value of future rewards, including information regarding the probability of encountering a stimulus or performing an action that will lead to a particular reward. This probability distribution of reward values would ideally be normally distributed, such that extreme rewards occur less frequently than intermediate rewards (Schultz, 2010).

Norepinephrine, released from neurons originating in the brainstem's locus coeruleus, serves as a central neurotransmitter mediating arousal and vigilance, and helps to improve the ratio of signal-to-noise (Arnsten & Li, 2005; Mesulam, 2000; Nieuwenhuis, Aston-Jones, & Cohen, 2005; Petersen & Posner, 2012; Usher, Cohen, Servan-Schreiber, Rajkowski, & Aston-Jones, 1999). Specifically, norepinephrine stimulation of postsynaptic, alpha-2A adrenoceptors on PFC pyramidal cell spines is critical for strengthening appropriate PFC network connections (increasing or enchancing "signals") (Arnsten & Li, 2005), whereas dopamine D1 stimulation on a separate set of spines is important for reducing inappropriate network connections (decreasing or inhibiting "noise") (Arnsten & Rubia, 2012). Alpha-2a noradrenergic receptors in the PFC are important in the modulation of focused attention (Wang et al., 2011). Disruption of these receptors can lead to increased distractibility. Alpha-2a autoreceptors on neurons in the locus coeruleus also many modulate its discharge rates, leading to improved attention (Taylor & Russo, 2001).

Acetylcholine is released by neurons projecting from basal forebrain to frontal cortex and hippocampus in response to behaviorally significant or novel events (Acquas, Wilson, & Fibiger, 1996; Davidson & Marrocco, 2000). This neurotransmitter has been strongly implicated in the modulation of selective attention (Petersen & Posner, 2012). Positron emission tomography (PET) studies in healthy volunteers have suggested that inhibition of cholinesterase activity (thus increasing cholinergic tone) is associated with more efficient working memory (faster reaction times and more circumscribed activation of the right PFC) (Freo et al., 2005; Furey et al., 1997).

Depletion of *serotonin* from OFC (but not DLPFC) has been shown to markedly impair OFC regulation of emotion and inhibition (Clarke, Walker, Dalley, Robbins, & Roberts, 2007; Rubia et al., 2005). Less is known about the role of serotonin in other aspects of executive control. Similar to dopamine, serotonin has been shown to affect working memory function (Goldman-Rakic, 1999); however, serotonin may play a unique role in reversal learning (Clarke, 2006; Clarke, Dalley, Crofts, Robbins, & Roberts, 2004; Clarke et al., 2005). Deficits in reversal learning tend to result in marked perseveration to above rewarded stimuli. Disruption of a number of mechanisms may explain the pattern of perseverative, inflexible behavior associated with serotonin depletion in PFC, including altered responsiveness to punishment, loss of reward, or deficits in inhibitory control (Robbins & Roberts, 2007).

Orexin has key arousing effects needed for the brain to enter a wakeful state (Saper, Chou, & Scammell, 2001). Orexin-rich neurons directly project to the PFC and thalamus (Moore, Abrahamson, & Van Den, 2001) but also to NE cell bodies in the locus coeruleus (Horvath, Diano, & van den Pol, 1999). Orexins excite the same synapses in the PFC as nicotine and have been show to improve attentional function (Lambe, Olausson, Horst, Taylor, & Aghajanian, 2005). In fact, the antinarcolepsy medication, modafinil, is thought to work via the orexin system (Turner et al., 2003) to enhance excitatory projections to the cortex (Lin, Hou, & Jouvet, 1996; Scammell et al., 2000). Orexins also activate a group of DA neurons in the ventral tegmental area that project to the PFC (Vittoz, Schmeichel, & Berridge, 2008). NE and DA tend to be low during periods of drowsiness, moderate during conditions of alert interest, and high during uncontrollable stress (Vijayraghavan, Wang, Birnbaum, Williams, & Arnsten, 2007). Under optimal conditions, NE and DA neurons tend to produce relatively low levels of tonic firing, but they fire to stimuli that are relevant and/or predict reward (Aston-Jones, Rajkowski, & Cohen, 2000; Berridge & Waterhouse, 2003; Schultz, 2002).

Consistent with these observations, pharmacological interventions that have been employed to improve arousal, motivation, attention, and executive control functions include stimulant medications, catecholamine "boosters," alpha-2 agonists, dopaminergic agents, modafinil, and cholinergic agents. Stimulant medications increase the availability of catecholamines (dopamine and norepinephrine). They may improve arousal level, motivational tone, and attentional focus (Chiarello & Cole, 1987; Greenhill & Osman, 2000; Marin, Fogel, Hawkins, Duffy, & Krupp, 1995; Taylor & Russo, 2001; Wilens, Biederman, Spencer, & Prince, 1995). Stimulants have been studied most extensively in patients with attention-deficit/hyperactivity disorders (ADHD) but also have been used with variable success for other disorders that lead to dysexecutive syndromes (Challman & Lipsky, 2000; Rahman et al., 2005; Siddall, 2005; Whyte et al., 2004). Nonstimulant medications boost norepinephrine (atomoxetine) or norepinephrine and dopamine (e.g., buprorion). As mentioned previously, modafinil promotes wakefulness and can treat narcolepsy and other sleep-related disorders. It seems to be an effective treatment for attention and executive dysfunction (Muller, Steffenhagen, Regenthal, & Bublak, 2004; Taylor & Russo, 2000; Turner, Clark, Dowson, Robbins, & Sahakian, 2004), but it does not tend to improve motivation.

Dopaminergic agents (e.g., pramipexole, bromocriptine, selegiline, L-dopa) are most often prescribed in the context of treating Parkinson's disease. However, these medications have also been used to help improve motivation, diminish apathy, and to augment working memory and other executive functions (Luciana & Collins, 1997; Luciana,

Depue, Arbisi, & Leon, 1992; Marin et al., 1995; McDowell, Whyte, & D'Esposito, 1998; Muller, von Cramon, & Pollman, 1998; Muller & von Cramon, 1994). In particular, activation of D1 receptors may be more important than activating D2 receptors when attempting to improve working memory performance in neurologically healthy individuals with low working memory capacity (Kimber, Watson, & Mathias, 1997; Muller et al., 1998). However, the use of dopaminergic agents must be monitored closely because they may increase behavioral and neuropsychiatric symptoms, including impulse control difficulties, repetitive/stereotyped behaviors, agitation, and psychosis.

Cholinesterase inhibitors (e.g., donepezil, rivastigimine, galantamine), which increase the availability of acetylcholine, were developed for the symptomatic treatment of probable AD. However, this class of medications also appears to have a modest effect on aspects of executive functions, attention, and neuropsychiatric well-being associated with aging and other neurologic disorders (Furey et al., 1997; Furey, Pietrini, & Haxby, 2000; Khateb, Ammann, Annoni, & Diserens, 2005; Yesavage et al., 2008; Zhang, Plotkin, Wang, Sandel, & Lee, 2004). Cholinesterase inhibitors have been found to be effective in boosting cognition in patients with AD, Parkinson's disease, dementia with Lewy bodies, and mixed dementia, but not in patients with bvFTLD.

Executive Control and Cognitive Aging

The gradual decline in cognitive abilities, particularly memory and executive function, of many older adults is well documented (Craik & Salthouse, 2000; Greenwood, 2000). Several major theories of cognitive aging suggest a salient role for changes in the functioning of frontal networks, including (1) *the executive deficit (frontal aging) hypothesis*, which proposes that executive abilities dependent on frontal lobe integrity are affected earlier and to a greater magnitude than other processes (West, 1996); (2) *the inhibitory deficit hypothesis*, which suggests a reduction in the efficiency of inhibitory mechanisms (Hasher & Zacks, 1988); and (3) *the processing speed hypothesis*, in which performance deficits are attributed to generalized slowing of processing speed (Salthouse, 1996). Aging-related volume reductions, or atrophy, have been associated with lower synaptic densities in older adults, as opposed to cell death (Terry, 2000). The PFC and medial temporal structures have been shown to be particularly affected by normal aging, as well as so-called pathological aging (Raz et al., 2003, 2004; Resnick, Pham, Kraut, Zonderman, & Davatzikos, 2003; West, 1996). In addition, to aging-related structural changes, evidence for white matter abnormalities (Decarli & Scheltens, 2002; Pantoni & Garcia, 1997; Pugh & Lipsitz, 2002), neurophysiological changes (Almaguer, Estupinan, Uwe, & Bergado, 2002; Chao & Knight, 1997; Pelosi & Blumhardt, 1999; Shankar, Teyler, & Robbins, 1998), and changes in neurotransmitters levels (Gazzaley, Thakker, Hof, & Morrison, 1997; Volkow et al., 1996) have also been reported.

The functional imaging literature commonly reports that older adults often exhibit "overrecruitment" of neural activity relative to their younger counterparts to carry out episodic memory tasks (Cabeza, 2002), working memory tasks (Grady et al., 1998; Reuter-Lorenz et al., 2000), and novelty processing tasks (Daffner, Sun, et al., 2011; Riis et al., 2008). The functional significance of this increased activation likely varies depending on the perceptual, memory, verbal, spatial, or executive functioning task; however, there is evidence to suggest that age-related increases in neural activity when carrying out executive tasks may be compensatory. Several hypotheses have been proposed to explain these activation pattern changes and their relationship to cognitive performance. The compensation-related utilization of neural circuits hypothesis (CRUNCH) (Reuter-Lorenz & Cappell, 2008) is based on imaging work in verbal and spatial working memory tasks that shows a discrepant pattern of prefrontal activation between younger and older adults. Specifically, while younger adults tend to show lateralized prefrontal activation that is domain dependent, older adults demonstrate pattern bilateral prefrontal activation that is not domain dependent (Reuter-Lorenz et al., 2000). CRUNCH is in the tradition of cognitive resource theory, which suggests that while bilateral activation may be compensatory, it comes at a computational cost (Reuter-Lorenz & Cappell, 2008) and that the differences in PFC activity patterns of old and young adults may be a function of age-associated differences in processing capacity. As such, while recruiting more resources for tasks with relatively low demands may help the older adult maintain task performance, at levels of higher demand older adults may be limited by a resource ceiling (Daffner, Chong, et al., 2011).

The posterior-anterior shift in aging (PASA) hypothesis (Davis, Dennis, Daselaar, Fleck, & Cabeza, 2008) explains the pattern of increased frontal activation in aging by proposing that there is a simultaneous reduction in occipital activity coupled with an increase in frontal activity. The link between declines in occipital function and sensory-perceptual deficits is consistent with abundant evidence that perceptual processing declines as a function of aging (for a review, see Schneider & Pichora-Fuller, 2000) and studies that show age-related dedifferentiation in early sensory processing (Gazzaley, Cooney, Rissman, & D'Esposito, 2005; Park et al., 2004). For example, Park and colleagues (2004) demonstrated an aging-related reduction in category-specific activation within ventral visual cortex, including the fusiform face area. Therefore, PASA is thought to indicate that the recruitment of higher order cognitive processes is in response to deficits in posterior brain regions, although the exact function of the compensatory frontal activity has yet to be identified (Davis et al., 2008).

An alternative theory regarding increased recruitment of frontal regions is that it reflects the process of dedifferentiation or loss of specialized neural circuits. Age-related dedifferentiation of function refers to decreases in signal-to-noise ratio in cortical processing that correlate with age and result in reduced regional process specificity and increases in nonspecific cortical activation (Li, Lindenberger, & Sikstrom, 2001). Within this framework, age-related activity increases in frontal regions are thought to reflect generalized spreading of activity due to reduced specialization of function.

Executive Control and the Dementias

Behavioral Variant Frontotemporal Dementia and Alzheimer's Disease

Frontotemporal lobar degeneration (FTLD) describes a group of clinically, pathologically, and genetically heterogenous diseases (Mackenzie et al., 2009) that are associated with atrophy in the frontal and temporal lobes. The most common clinical syndrome associated with FTLD is behavioral variant frontotemporal dementia (bvFTD), which is characterized by a progressive deterioration of personality, social comportment, and cognition (Rascovsky et al., 2011). In bvFTD, degeneration often begins in the paralimbic prefrontal regions, including the pregenual anterior cingulate cortex (pACC) and frontoinsular cortex (Boccardi et al., 2005; Broe et al., 2003; Schroeter, Raczka, Neumann, & von Cramon, 2008; Seeley et al., 2008). As a result of the prominent impact that the disease has on paralimbic prefrontal regions, initial symptoms of bvFTD include changes in personality, impaired social interaction, disinhibition, deficits in impulse control, and loss of insight (Hodges & Miller, 2001). Disease progression often spreads to adjacent orbital and dorsolateral frontal regions (Seeley, Zhou, & Kim, 2012). Right-hemisphere structures often show more pronounced involvement than the left, although the pattern can be symmetrical. Intrigued by this atrophy pattern that preferentially affects paralimic prefrontal structures, Seeley, Menon, and colleagues (2007) studied healthy young adults in an attempt to clarify regions functionally correlated with the right fronto-insular cortex. The resulting map revealed that the bilateral ACC, left FI, and subcortical, limbic, and brainstem sites with known connections from primate and rodent axonal tracer studies (Mesulam & Mufson, 1982; Ongur & Price, 2000; Saper, 2002) all shared functional connectivity with the right FI. In addition, these network findings overlapped with the bvFTD atrophy pattern. As described earlier, this circuit was referred to as the "salience network" in light of observations that ACC and FI coactivate in response to emotionally significant ambient stimuli and events, from pain, thirst, and hunger to social rejection, embarrassment, collaboration, and adoration (Craig, 2002; Critchley, 2005). Deficits in executive control and social cognition are core features of bvFTD (Kipps & Hodges, 2006; Rascovsky et al., 2007). Specifically, the neuropsychological profile specified by the international consensus criteria (Rascovsky et al., 2011) includes executive function deficits with relative sparing of memory and visuospatial functions. Early in the course of bvFTD, performance on formal neuropsychological tests of executive functioning may be spared; however, reports of day-to-day difficulties with decision making, context-appropriate behavior, and impulse control highlight the importance of executive dysfunction early in the course of bvFTD, even if we are not yet able to measure these deficits psychometrically.

The presentation and profile of bvFTD is antithetical to that of Alzheimer's disease (AD), whose pathology preferentially impacts medial temporal lobe structures, before progressing to lateral temporal, parietal, and frontal regions (Arnold, Hyman, Flory, Damasio, & Van Hoesen, 1991; Braak & Braak, 1991). The classic pattern of cognitive decline typically associated with AD is characterized by early impairment of episodic memory functioning, in addition to changes in visuospatial functioning and semantic processing (Aggarwal, Wilson, Beck, Bienias, & Bennett, 2005). Social graces and conduct are generally well preserved into the middle stages of the disease. However, AD patients often exhibit declines in aspects of executive functioning, including divided attention and attentional control, which are over and above that which is typically associated with normal aging. When focused specifically on executive functioning, research has had difficulty disentangling the patterns of compromised executive function seen in AD from other disorders that primarily affect frontal lobe functioning (Baddeley, Baddeley, Bucks, & Wilcock, 2001; Baddeley, Cocchini, Sala, Logie, & Spinnler, 1999); however, the classic pattern of episodic, visuospatial, and language deficits clearly distinguishes AD from disorders such as bvFTD.

Additional Profiles

Although a large percentage of patients with dementia have mixed underlying etiologies that often include AD or cerebrovascular pathology, the cognitive profiles of these separate processes are associated with distinct clinical features. What we present can be described as "pure" syndromic types associated with each condition.

Vascular Cognitive Impairment

Vascular cognitive impairment (VCI) refers to all forms of cognitive dysfunction caused by vascular disease, ranging from mild cognitive dysfunction to dementia (Bowler, 2003; Hachinski & Bowler, 1993; Snowdon et al., 1997). The characteristic neuropsychological profile of VCI, particularly subcortical ischemic vascular disease, includes early impairment of attention and executive functioning, with slowing of information processing and motor performance (Desmond, 2004; Garrett et al., 2004). In contrast to bvFTLD, patients with VCI typically do not tend to present with severe behavior and personality changes. In terms of relative patterns of executive functioning deficits, VCI patients tend to be more impaired than AD patients on measures of initiation, freedom from perseveration (Kertesz, Hudson, Mackenzie, & Munoz, 1994; Kramer, Reed, Mungas, Weiner, & Chui, 2002; Libon et al., 1997; Starkstein et al., 1996), planning, and self-regulation (Villardita, 1993).

Dementia With Lewy Bodies

Dementia with Lewy bodies (DLB) is characterized by prominent deficits in visuospatial ability, attention, executive functioning, and relatively spared memory (McKeith et al., 2005). Within the realm of attention and executive functioning, fluctuations in attention are the cardinal sign in DLB. In general, basic span tests have not proven to be sensitive, but instead, measures of attention that combine the components of selection, vigilance, and executive control of attention have resulted in more consistent findings (Calderon et al., 2001; Crowell, Luis, Cox, & Mullan, 2007; Forstl et al., 1993; Guidi, Paciaroni, Paolini, De Padova, & Scarpino, 2006). Computerized attention-based reaction time variability has been shown to be correlated with questionnaires of fluctuating cognition and electroencephalogram-measured fluctuations (Walker et al., 2000), suggesting that attentional variability may be a useful measure of fluctuating cognition in DLB.

Parkinson's Disease

Parkinson's disease, which causes disruption of the fronto-striatal-thalamic circuit, particularly within the substantia nigra, can present with working memory deficits, difficulties with initiation, perseveration, trouble with mental flexibility, and apathy. The literature on cognitive impairment in PD is extensive and there are several comprehensive reviews (Caballol, Marti, & Tolosa, 2007; Levin & Katzen, 2005; Owen, 2004; Pillon, Boller, Levy, & Dubois, 2001; Zgaljardic, Borod, Foldi, & Mattis, 2003). Kudlicka et al. (2011) conducted a meta-analysis of the studies focusing on executive impairment in PD. In particular, they searched for studies of PD patients without dementia or depression and a Hoehn and Yahr score of I to III. Significant difficulties were found in PD patients compared with controls across measures of executive functioning, including verbal fluency, digit span backward, Wisconsin Card Sorting Test, Stroop Test, and Trail Making Test B. Impairments in some areas of functioning, particularly executive functions, are evident even at the early stages of the disease and may predict the onset of dementia (Muslimovic, Post, Speelman, & Schmand, 2005; Woods & Troster, 2003). Of particular interest was the finding that PD patients do not show deficits in all subcomponents of executive functioning; instead, there is evidence for variable performance, with the strongest differences between PD and controls groups found in working memory, problem solving, verbal fluency, and inhibition (Marinus et al., 2003; Muslimovic et al., 2005; Uekermann et al., 2004; Weintraub & Stern, 2005).

Clinical Assessment of Executive Functions

History

Patients with significant executive and behavioral dysfunction rarely initiate clinical evaluation. Obtaining a careful history from reliable informants regarding changes in the patient's personality and behavior is essential. Given the lack of insight that often accompanies frontal systems dysfunction, it can be helpful to obtain ratings of behavior by family members, caregivers, or other individuals who know the patient well. Several questionnaires have been specifically designed to elicit information about a patient's degree of executive dysfunction (Table 3.2).

Qualitative Observation

Often a clinician's qualitative observations of a patient's behavior during the examination can provide a wealth of information with regard to executive dysfunction. Symptoms that are likely to be detectable by behavioral observation include disinhibition, impaired context-appropriate behavior, disorganization, poor initiation, affect dysregulation, and poor self-monitoring. Features of a patient's presentation likely to reveal dysexecutive symptoms include dress and hygiene (diminished ability to organize or monitor oneself or to adhere to social expectations), spontaneous speech (poor organization of thought processes, inappropriate content, failure to engage in reciprocal conversation), nonverbal communication (lack of appreciation of personal space, failure to perceive social cues, poor eye contact), and inappropriate behavior.

Formal Neuropsychological Testing

In a previous chapter (Daffner & Searl, 2008), we described several neuropsychological batteries specifically developed to measure symptoms of frontal systems and

TABLE 3.2 Executive Function Questionnaires

The Behavior Rating Inventory of Executive Function (BRIEF-A) (Gioia, Isquith, Guy, & Kenworthy, 2000)
    Designed to assess the frequency and severity of dysexecutive symptoms (problems in inhibition, shifting, emotional control, initiation, working memory, planning and organization, organization of materials, and monitoring)

The Frontal Systems Behavior Scale (FrSBE) (Grace & Malloy, 2001)
    A rating scale for adults age 18–95 designed to measure changes in apathy, disinhibition, and dysexecutive symptoms often associated with damage to frontal networks.

The Frontal Behavioral Inventory (FBI) (Blair et al., 2007; Kertesz, Davidson, & Fox, 1997)
    Developed to track the evolution of symptoms, as well as record and monitor behavioral changes over time, as it assesses both the presence of certain symptoms but also severity of disrupted behaviors.

executive dysfunction, including the Frontal Assessment Battery (FAB; Dubois, Slachevsky, Litvan, & Pillon, 2000), the Delis-Kaplan Executive Function System (DKEFS; Delis & Kaplan, 2001), the Behavioral Assessment of Dysexecutive Syndromes (BADS; Wilson, Alderman, Burgess, Emsile, & Evans, 1996), and the Executive Control Battery (ECB; Goldberg, Podel, Bilder, & Jaeger, 2000). However, classic tests of executive function can fail to detect the dysexecutive changes in early frontally mediated neurodegenerative processes, such as bvFTD (Gregory et al., 2002). Here we have chosen to focus on alternative measures that can be added to traditional assessment batteries, including ecologically valid neuropsychological tests and tests of social cognition, which show promise in improving our ability to detect change in the earlier stages of frontal dysfunction.

Ecologically Valid Neuropsychological Tests

A growing number of studies are showing that impairment in ecologically valid, or "real life," tests of complex decision making and planning have the potential to be more sensitive to the earliest stages of frontally mediated processes (Gregory et al., 2002; Torralva, Roca, Gleichgerrcht, Bekinschtein, & Manes, 2007). Examples of these tasks include the Multiple Errands Test (Knight, Alderman, & Burgess, 2002) and the Hotel Test (Manly, Hawkins, Evans, Woldt, & Robertson, 2002). Shallice and Burgess (1991) have shown that patients with frontal lobe damage, who demonstrate normal performance on standard neuropsychological measures, tend to make more errors in everyday situations that require planning and multitasking. The MET and the abbreviated hospital version, MET-HV, require individuals to perform a number of everyday tasks within four different sets of categories: (1) attain specific goals, such as purchasing items, collecting an envelope from a reception area, using the phone, and sending a letter; (2) obtain and write down pieces of information; (3) call a number 20 minutes after the test has begun (prospective memory); and (4) inform the examiner when every task has been completed. Errors are coded over five categories (inefficiencies, rule breaks, interpretation failures, task failures, and total fails). Patients are typically followed at a distance to code these errors where needed.

The Hotel Test (Manly et al., 2002) is made up of six activities that would be completed in order to run a hotel. A patient is provided with a list of tasks to be attempted over a 15-minute period, with the goal that at the end of the time period the patient will make an informed estimate of how long each task would take to complete. Each task on its own may take longer than 15 minutes to complete, and patients are informed that they will not complete each task. The Hotel Test is made up of six tasks, including compiling individual bills, sorting a collection of charity coins, looking up telephone numbers, proofreading the hotel leaflet, sorting conference labels, and a prospective task requiring the patient to remember to open and close the delivery doors at specific times. The patient is provided with the materials needed to complete the tasks and a clock. Scoring is based on several categories, including (1) number of tasks attempted; (2) number of tasks attempted correctly; (3) time allocation; and (4) prospective memory performance. Similar to the MET, the patient is typically observed from a distance. A version of the Hotel Test is available commercially (with normative data) as part of the Behavioural Assessment of the Dysexecutive Syndrome (Wilson et al., 1996).

While there is evidence for these tests to be quite sensitive to early changes in PFC function, they can be quite time intensive; in the case of the MET, it requires clinicians and their patients to leave the safety of the examination room. Although normative data do exist for these tests (Alderman, Burgess, Knight, & Henman, 2003; Dawson et al., 2009; Knight et al., 2002; Manly et al., 2002), standardization of the procedures (particularly on the MET) is difficult because no two assessments will be exactly alike.

Tests of Social Cognition

Although tests of social cognition do not strictly tap executive functions, they have shown promise in improving diagnostic accuracy of early frontally mediated neurodegenerative processes. Theory of mind tests have been proposed to assess social and emotional cognition, especially when classic executive tests show few abnormalities or normal performance (Adenzato,

Cavallo, & Enrici, 2010; Funkiewiez, Bertoux, de Souza, Levy, & Dubois, 2012; Lough et al., 2006; Rahman, Sahakian, Hodges, Rogers, & Robbins, 1999; Torralva et al., 2007; Torralva, Roca, Gleichgerrcht, Bekinschtein, & Manes, 2009). One proposed battery, the Social cognition and Emotional Assessment (SEA) (Funkiewiez et al., 2012), provides six weighted composite scores based on performance on four tests and a questionnaire: (1) a facial emotional recognition test (from 35 Ekman pictures) (Ekman & Friesen, 1975) in which patients must identify which emotion (fear, sadness, disgust, surprise, happiness, or neutral) is being expressed; (2) a shortened version of the Faux Pas recognition test (Stone, Baron-Cohen, & Knight, 1998) that evaluates theory of mind on the basis of patients' answers to questions about 10 stories, five of which feature social faux pas (Gregory et al., 2002; Stone et al., 1998); (3) a behavioral control test in which patients must learn to apply a strategy of choice and to modify their choice based on a monetary reward; (4) a reversal learning and extinction test (adapted from Hornak et al., 2004) in which patients must reverse a pattern of reinforced choice after contingencies are unexpectedly reversed; and (5) completion of the Starkstein Apathy Scale, a questionnaire/structured interview (Starkstein et al., 1992). The social cognition tests from the SEA most accurately discriminated bvFTD patients from controls or patients with AD (Funkiewiez et al., 2012). As a result of these findings, the mini-SEA was developed, which is comprised of the sum of the facial emotion recognition and the Faux Pas test scores. The estimated completion time for the mini-SEA is 30 minutes.

The Reading the Mind in the Eyes Test (RMET) (Baron-Cohen, Wheelwright, Hill, Raste, & Plumb, 2001) is another widely used theory of mind test consisting of 36 photographs of eyes expressing a complex mental state. Patients are directed to choose one of four words describing the mental states. Recent data suggest that the RMET is sensitive to early prefrontal dysfunction associated with bvFTD (Pardini et al., 2012).

Conclusion

The past several decades of research have greatly extended our understanding of the neuroanatomy, physiology, and cognitive processing that underlies executive functions, and they have informed our understanding of the different clinical syndromes resulting from various neurodegenerative processes and conditions associated with aging. When executive functions fail, the negative impact on individuals affected and those who care for them can be extraordinary. We anticipate that future research will lead to increasingly effective diagnostic tools for executive dysfunction and hopefully treatments that will improve the quality of life of our patients these disorders.

Acknowledgments

Work on this chapter was made possible by the support of the Wimberly family, Muss family, and Mortimer/Grubman family. The authors would also like to thank Marissa Keppley for her excellent administrative assistance.

References

Acquas, E., Wilson, C., & Fibiger, H. C. (1996). Conditioned and unconditioned stimuli increase frontal cortical and hippocampal acetylcholine release: Effects of novelty, habituation, and fear. *Journal of Neuroscience, 16,* 3089–3096.

Addis, D. R., Wong, A. T., & Schacter, D. L. (2007). Remembering the past and imagining the future: Common and distinct neural substrates during event construction and elaboration. *Neuropsychologia, 45,* 1363–1377.

Adenzato, M., Cavallo, M., & Enrici, I. (2010). Theory of mind ability in the behavioural variant of frontotemporal dementia: An analysis of the neural, cognitive, and social levels. *Neuropsychologia, 48,* 2–12.

Aggarwal, N. T., Wilson, R. S., Beck, T. L., Bienias, J. L., & Bennett, D. A. (2005). Mild cognitive impairment in different functional domains and incident Alzheimer's disease. *Journal of Neurology, Neurosurgery and Psychiatry, 76,* 1479–1484.

Alderman, N., Burgess, P. W., Knight, C., & Henman, C. (2003). Ecological validity of a simplified version of the multiple errands shopping test. *Journal of the International Neuropsychology Society, 9,* 31–44.

Alexander, G. E., DeLong, M. R., & Strick, P. L. (1986). Parallel organization of functionally segregated circuits linking basal ganglia and cortex. *Annual Review of Neuroscience, 9,* 381.

Alexander, G. E., Newman, J. D., & Symmes, D. (1976). Convergence of prefrontal and acoustic inputs upon neurons in the superior temporal gyrus of the awake squirrel monkey. *Brain Research, 116,* 334–338.

Alexander, M. P., & Stuss, D. T. (2000). Disorders of frontal lobe functioning. *Seminars in Neurology, 20,* 427–437.

Alexander, M. P., Stuss, D. T., Shallice, T., Picton, T. W., & Gillingham, S. (2005). Impaired concentration due to frontal lobe damage from two distinct lesion sites. *Neurology, 65,* 572–579.

Almaguer, W., Estupinan, B., Uwe, F. J., & Bergado, J. A. (2002). Aging impairs amygdala-hippocampus interactions involved in hippocampal LTP. *Neurobiology of Aging, 23,* 319–324.

Amodio, D. M., & Frith, C. D. (2006). Meeting of minds: The medial frontal cortex and social cognition. *Nature Reviews Neuroscience, 7,* 268–277.

Andersen, R., Meeker, D., Pesaran, B., Brezen, B., Buneo, C., & Scherberger, H. (2004). Sensorimotor transformations in the posterior parietal portex. In M. S. Gazzaniga (Ed.), *The cognitive neurosciences III* (pp. 463–478). Cambridge, MA: MIT Press.

Anderson, M. C., Ochsner, K. N., Kuhl, B., Cooper, J., Robertson, E., Gabrieli, S. W.,...Gabrieli, J. D. (2004). Neural systems underlying the suppression of unwanted memories. *Science, 303,* 232–235.

Anderson, P. J. (2008). Models of executive function. In V. Anderson, R. Jacobs, & P. J. Anderson (Eds.), *Executive functions and the frontal lobes: A lifespan perspective* (pp. 3–21). New York, NY: Taylor & Francis.

Andres, P. (2003). Frontal cortex as the central executive of working memory: Time to revise our view. *Cortex, 39,* 871–895.

Arnold, S. F., Hyman, B. T., Flory, J., Damasio, A. R., & Van Hoesen, G. W. (1991). The topographical and neuroanatomical distribution of neurofibrillary tangles and neuritic plaques in the cerebral cortex of patients with Alzheimer's disease. *Cerebral Cortex, 1,* 103–116.

Arnsten, A. F. (1997). Catecholamine regulation of the prefrontal cortex. *Journal of Psychopharmacology, 11,* 151–162.

Arnsten, A. F., & Li, B. M. (2005). Neurobiology of executive functions: Catecholamine influences on prefrontal cortical functions. *Biological Psychiatry, 57,* 1377–1384.

Arnsten, A. F., & Rubia, K. (2012). Neurobiological circuits regulating attention, cognitive control, motivation, and emotion: Disruptions in neurodevelopmental psychiatric disorders. *Journal of the American Academy of Child and Adolescent Psychiatry, 51,* 356–367.

Aron, A. R., & Poldrack, R. A. (2006). Cortical and subcortical contributions to stop signal response inhibition: Role of the subthalamic nucleus. *Journal of Neuroscience, 26,* 2424–2433.

Astafiev, S. V., Shulman, G. L., Stanley, C. M., Snyder, A. Z., Van Essen, D. C., & Corbetta, M. (2003). Functional organization of human intraparietal and frontal cortex for attending, looking, and pointing. *Journal of Neuroscience, 23,* 4689–4699.

Astafiev, S. V., Stanley, C. M., Shulman, G. L., & Corbetta, M. (2004). Extrastriate body area in human occipital cortex responds to the performance of motor actions. *Nature Neuroscience, 7,* 542–548.

Aston-Jones, G., Rajkowski, J., & Cohen, J. (2000). Locus coeruleus and regulation of behavioral flexibility and attention. *Progress in Brain Research, 126,* 165–182.

Baddeley, A. (2003). Working memory: Looking back and looking forward. *Nature Reviews Neuroscience, 4,* 829–839.

Baddeley, A., Baddeley, H. A., Bucks, R. S., & Wilcock, G. K. (2001). Attentional control in Alzheimer's disease. *Brain, 124,* 1492–1508.

Baddeley, A., Cocchini, G., Sala, S. D., Logie, R. H., & Spinnler, H. (1999). Working memory and vigilance: Evidence from normal aging and Alzheimer's disease. *Brain and Cognition, 41,* 87–108.

Baddeley, A. D., & Hitch, G. J. (1974). Working memory. In G. Bower (Ed.), *The psychology of learning and motivation* (pp. 47–89). New York, NY: Academic Press.

Badre, D. (2008). Cognitive control, hierarchy, and the rostro-caudal organization of the frontal lobes. *Trends in Cognitive Science, 12,* 193–200.

Badre, D., & D'Esposito, M. (2007). Functional magnetic resonance imaging evidence for a hierarchical organization of the prefrontal cortex. *Journal of Cognitive Neuroscience, 19,* 2082–2099.

Badre, D., & D'Esposito, M. (2009). Is the rostro-caudal axis of the frontal lobe hierarchical? *Nature Reviews Neuroscience, 10,* 659–669.

Barbalat, G., Chambon, V., Franck, N., Koechlin, E., & Farrer, C. (2009). Organization of cognitive control within the lateral prefrontal cortex in schizophrenia. *Archives of General Psychiatry, 66,* 377–386.

Barbas, H., & Mesulam, M. M. (1985). Cortical afferent input to the principalis region of the rhesus monkey. *Neuroscience, 15,* 619–637.

Bargh, J. A., & Williams, E. L. (2006). The automaticity of social life. *Current Directions in Psychological Science, 15,* 1–4.

Barkley, R. A. (1997). Behavioral inhibition, sustained attention, and executive functions: Constructing a unifying theory of ADHD. *Psychological Bulletin, 121*, 65–94.

Baron-Cohen, S., Wheelwright, S., Hill, J., Raste, Y., & Plumb, I. (2001). The "reading the mind in the eyes" test revised version: A study with normal adults, and adults with Asperger syndrome or high-functioning autism. *Journal of Child Psychology and Psychiatry, 42*, 241–251.

Barris, R. W., & Schuman, H. R. (1953). [Bilateral anterior cingulate gyrus lesions; Syndrome of the anterior cingulate gyri.]. *Neurology, 3*, 44–52.

Bayer, H. M., & Glimcher, P. W. (2005). Midbrain dopamine neurons encode a quantitative reward prediction error signal. *Neuron, 47*, 129–141.

Berns, G. S., McClure, S. M., Pagnoni, G., & Montague, P. R. (2001). Predictability modulates human brain response to reward. *Journal of Neuroscience, 21*, 2793–2798.

Berridge, C. W., & Waterhouse, B. D. (2003). The locus coeruleus-noradrenergic system: Modulation of behavioral state and state-dependent cognitive processes. *Brain Research and Brain Research Reviews, 42*, 33–84.

Bianchi, L (1922). *The mechanism of the brain and the function of the frontal lobes.* Edinburgh, UK: E & S Livingstone.

Blair, M., Kertesz, A., Davis-Faroque, N., Hsiung, G. Y., Black, S. E., Bouchard, R. W., ... Feldman, H. (2007). Behavioural measures in frontotemporal lobar dementia and other dementias: The utility of the frontal behavioural inventory and the neuropsychiatric inventory in a national cohort study. *Dementia and Geriatric Cognitive Disorders, 23*, 406–415.

Boccardi, M., Sabattoli, F., Laakso, M. P., Testa, C., Rossi, R., Beltramello, A., ... Frisoni, G. B. (2005). Frontotemporal dementia as a neural system disease. *Neurobiology of Aging, 26*, 37–44.

Botvinick, M. M., Braver, T. S., Barch, D. M., Carter, C. S., & Cohen, J. D. (2001). Conflict monitoring and cognitive control. *Psychological Review, 108*, 624–652.

Botvinick, M. M., Cohen, J. D., & Carter, C. S. (2004). Conflict monitoring and anterior cingulate cortex: An update. *Trends in Cognitive Sciences, 8*, 539–546.

Bowler, J. (2003). Epidemiology: Identifying vascular cognitive impairment. *International Psychogeriatrics, 15*(Suppl 1), 115–122.

Braak, H., & Braak, E. (1991). Neuropathological stageing of Alzheimer-related changes. *Acta Neuropathologica, 82*, 239–259.

Bressler, S. L., & Menon, V. (2010). Large-scale brain networks in cognition: Emerging methods and principles. *Trends in Cognitive Sciences, 14*, 277–290.

Broe, M., Hodges, J. R., Schofield, E., Shepherd, C. E., Kril, J. J., & Halliday, G. M. (2003). Staging disease severity in pathologically confirmed cases of frontotemporal dementia. *Neurology, 60*, 1005–1011.

Brozoski, T. J., Brown, R. M., Rosvold, H. E., & Goldman, P. S. (1979). Cognitive deficit caused by regional depletion of dopamine in prefrontal cortex of rhesus monkey. *Science, 205*, 929–932.

Buckner, R. L. (2012). The serendipitous discovery of the brain's default network. *Neuroimage, 62*, 1137–1145.

Buckner, R. L., Andrews-Hanna, J. R., & Schacter, D. L. (2008). The brain's default network: Anatomy, function, and relevance to disease. *Annals of the New York Academy of Sciences, 1124*, 1–38.

Buckner, R. L., & Carroll, D. C. (2007). Self-projection and the brain. *Trends in Cognitive Sciences, 11*, 49–57.

Buneo, C. A. & Andersen, R. A. (2006). The posterior parietal cortex: Sensorimotor interface for the planning and online control of visually guided movements. *Neuropsychologia, 44*, 2594–2606.

Bunge, S. A. (2004). How we use rules to select actions: A review of evidence from cognitive neuroscience. *Cognitive, Affective, and Behavioral Neuroscience, 4*, 564–579.

Bush, G., Vogt, B. A., Holmes, J., Dale, A. M., Greve, D., Jenike, M. A., & Rosen, B. R. (2002). Dorsal anterior cingulate cortex: A role in reward-based decision making. *Proceedings of the National Academy of Science USA, 99*, 523–528.

Caballol, N., Marti, M. J., & Tolosa, E. (2007). Cognitive dysfunction and dementia in Parkinson disease. *Movement Disorders, 22*(Suppl 17), S358–S366.

Cabeza, R. (2002). Hemispheric asymmetry reduction in older adults: The HAROLD model. *Psychology of Aging, 17*, 85–100.

Calderon, J., Perry, R. J., Erzincioglu, S. W., Berrios, G. E., Dening, T. R., & Hodges, J. R. (2001). Perception, attention, and working memory are disproportionately impaired in dementia with Lewy bodies compared with Alzheimer's disease. *Journal of Neurology, Neurosurgery and Psychiatry, 70*, 157–164.

Carter, C. S., & van Veen, V. (2007). Anterior cingulate cortex and conflict detection: An update of theory and data. *Cognitive, Affective, and Behavioral Neuroscience, 7*, 367–379.

Challman, T. D., & Lipsky, J. J. (2000). Methylphenidate: Its pharmacology and uses. *Mayo Clinic Proceedings, 75*, 711–721.

Chao, L. L., & Knight, R. T. (1997). Prefrontal deficits in attention and inhibitory control with aging. *Cerebral Cortex, 7*, 63–69.

Chavis, D. A., & Pandya, D. N. (1976). Further observations on corticofrontal connections in the rhesus monkey. *Brain Research, 117,* 369–386.

Chen, S., Boucher, H. C., & Tapias, M. P. (2006). The relational self revealed: Integrative conceptualization and implications for interpersonal life. *Psychological Bulletin, 132,* 151–179.

Chiarello, R. J., & Cole, J. O. (1987). The use of psychostimulants in general psychiatry. A reconsideration. *Archives of General Psychiatry, 44,* 286–295.

Christoff, K., Gordon, A. M., Smallwood, J., Smith, R., & Schooler, J. W. (2009). Experience sampling during fMRI reveals default network and executive system contributions to mind wandering. *Proceedings of the National Academy of Science USA, 106,* 8719–8724.

Clarke, H. F., Dalley, J. W., Crofts, H. S., Robbins, T. W., & Roberts, A. C. (2004). Cognitive inflexibility after prefrontal serotonin depletion. *Science, 304,* 878–880.

Clarke, H. F., Walker, S. C., Crofts, H. S., Dalley, J. W., Robbins, T. W., & Roberts, A. C. (2005). Prefrontal serotonin depletion affects reversal learning but not attentional set shifting. *Journal of Neuroscience, 25,* 532–538.

Clarke, H. F., Walker, S. C., Dalley, J. W., Robbins, T. W., & Roberts, A. C. (2007). Cognitive inflexibility after prefrontal serotonin depletion is behaviorally and neurochemically specific. *Cerebral Cortex, 17,* 18–27.

Clarke, R. (2006). Vitamin B12, folic acid, and the prevention of dementia. *New England Journal of Medicine, 354,* 2817–2819.

Cohen, J. D., Braver, T. S., & O'Reilly, R. C. (1996). A computational approach to prefrontal cortex, cognitive control and schizophrenia: Recent developments and current challenges. *Philosophical Transactions of the Royal Society of Londong B: Biological Sciences, 351,* 1515–1527.

Cohen, J. D., & Servan-Schreiber, D. (1992). Context, cortex, and dopamine: A connectionist approach to behavior and biology in schizophrenia. *Psychological Review, 99,* 45–77.

Colby, C. L., & Goldberg, M. E. (1999). Space and attention in parietal cortex. *Annual Review of Neuroscience, 22,* 319–349.

Conway, M. A. (2005). Memory and the self. *Journal of Memory and Language, 53,* 594–628.

Corbetta, M., Kincade, J. M., Ollinger, J. M., McAvoy, M. P., & Shulman, G. L. (2000). Voluntary orienting is dissociated from target detection in human posterior parietal cortex. *Nature Neuroscience, 3,* 292–297.

Corbetta, M., Kincade, M. J., Lewis, C., Snyder, A. Z., & Sapir, A. (2005). Neural basis and recovery of spatial attention deficits in spatial neglect. *Nature Neuroscience, 8,* 1603–1610.

Corbetta, M., & Shulman, G. L. (2002). Control of goal-directed and stimulus-driven attention in the brain. *Nature Reviews Neuroscience, 3,* 201–215.

Corbetta, M., & Shulman, G. L. (2011). Spatial neglect and attention networks. *Annual Review of Neuroscience, 34,* 569–599.

Courtney, S. M., Ungerleider, L. G., Keil, K., & Haxby, J. V. (1996). Object and spatial visual working memory activate separate neural systems in human cortex. *Cerebral Cortex, 6,* 39–49.

Craig, A. D. (2002). How do you feel? Interoception: The sense of the physiological condition of the body. *Nature Reviews Neuroscience, 3,* 655–666.

Craig, A. D. (2009). How do you feel—now? The anterior insula and human awareness. *Nature Reviews Neuroscience, 10,* 59–70.

Craik, F. I. M., & Salthouse, T. A. (2000). *The handbook of aging and cognition.* Mahwah, NJ: Erlbaum.

Critchley, H. D. (2005). Neural mechanisms of autonomic, affective, and cognitive integration. *Journal of Comparative Neurology, 493,* 154–166.

Critchley, H. D., Elliott, R., Mathias, C. J., & Dolan, R. J. (2000). Neural activity relating to generation and representation of galvanic skin conductance responses: A functional magnetic resonance imaging study. *Journal of Neuroscience, 20,* 3033–3040.

Critchley, H. D., Wiens, S., Rotshtein, P., Ohman, A., & Dolan, R. J. (2004). Neural systems supporting interoceptive awareness. *Nature Neuroscience, 7,* 189–195.

Crowell, T. A., Luis, C. A., Cox, D. E., & Mullan, M. (2007). Neuropsychological comparison of Alzheimer's disease and dementia with lewy bodies. *Dement Geriatr Cogn Disord, 23,* 120–125.

Curtis, C. E., & D'Esposito, M. (2003). Persistent activity in the prefrontal cortex during working memory. *Trends in Cognitive Sciences, 7,* 415–423.

D'Argembeau, A., Collette, F., Van der, L. M., Laureys, S., Del Fiore, G., Degueldre, C.,…Salmon, E. (2005). Self-referential reflective activity and its relationship with rest: A PET study. *Neuroimage, 25,* 616–624.

D'Argembeau, A., Ruby, P., Collette, F., Degueldre, C., Balteau, E., Luxen, A.,…Salmon, E. (2007). Distinct regions of the medial prefrontal cortex are associated with self-referential processing and perspective taking. *Journal of Cognitive Neuroscience, 19,* 935–944.

D'Argembeau, A., & Salmon, E. (2012). The neural basis of semantic and episodic forms of self-knowledge: Insights from functional neuroimaging. *Advances in Experimental Medicine and Biology, 739,* 276–290.

D'Esposito, M., Aguirre, G. K., Zarahn, E. K., Ballard, D., Shin, R. K., & Lease, J. (1998). Functional MRI studies of spatial and non-spatial working memory. *Brain Research Cognitive Brain Research, 7,* 1–13.

D'Esposito, M., & Postle, B. R. (1999). The dependence of span and delayed-response performance on prefrontal cortex. *Neuropsychologia, 37,* 1303–1315.

D'Esposito, M., Postle, B. R., Ballard, D., & Lease, J. (1999). Maintenance versus manipulation of information held in working memory: An event-related fMRI study. *Brain and Cognition, 41,* 66–86.

Daffner, K. R., & Searl, M. M. (2008). The dysexecutive syndromes. In G. Goldenberg & B. Miller (Eds.), *Handbook of clinical neurology: Neuropsychology and behavioral neurology* (pp. 249–267). New York, NY: Elsevier Press.

Daffner, K. R., Chong, H., Sun, X., Tarbi, E. C., Riis, J. L., McGinnis, S. M., & Holcomb, P. J. (2011). Mechanisms underlying age- and performance-related differences in working memory. *Journal of Cognitive Neuroscience, 23,* 1298–1314.

Daffner, K. R., Sun, X., Tarbi, E., Rentz, D. M., Holcomb, P. J., & Riis, J. L. (2011). Does compensatory neural activity survive old-old age? *NeuroImage, 54,* 427–438.

Davidson R. J. (2000). Affective style, psychopathology, and resilience: Brain mechanisms and plasticity. *American Psychologist, 55,* 1196–1214.

Davidson, M. C., & Marrocco, R. T. (2000). Local infusion of scopolamine into intraparietal cortex slows covert orienting in rhesus monkeys. *Journal of Neurophysiology, 83,* 1536–1549.

Davis, S. W., Dennis, N. A., Daselaar, S. M., Fleck, M. S., & Cabeza, R. (2008). Que PASA? The posterior anterior shift in aging. *Cerebral Cortex, 18,* 1201–1209.

Dawson, D. R., Anderson, N. D., Burgess, P., Cooper, E., Krpan, K. M., & Stuss, D. T. (2009). Further development of the Multiple Errands Test: Standardized scoring, reliability, and ecological validity for the Baycrest version. *Archives of Physical Medicine and Rehabilitation, 90,* S41–S51.

Decarli, C., & Scheltens, P. (2002). Structural brain imaging. In T. Erkinjuntti & S. Gauthier (Eds.), *Vascular cognitive impairment* (pp. 433–457). London, UK: Martin Dunitz.

Delis, D., & Kaplan, E. (2001). *Delis-Kaplan Executive Function System (DKEFS).* San Antonio, TX: Psychological Corporation.

Desimone, R., & Duncan, J. (1995). Neural mechanisms of selective visual attention. *Annual Review of Neuroscience, 18,* 193–222.

Desmond, D. W. (2004). The neuropsychology of vascular cognitive impairment: Is there a specific cognitive deficit? *Journal of the Neurological Sciences, 226,* 3–7.

Dubois, B., Slachevsky, A., Litvan, I., & Pillon, B. (2000). The FAB: A frontal assessment battery at bedside. *Neurology, 55,* 1621–1626.

Duncan, J., Emslie, H., Williams, P., Johnson, R., & Freer, C. (1996). Intelligence and the frontal lobe: The organization of goal-directed behavior. *Cognitive Psychology, 30,* 257–303.

Duncan, J., Johnson, R., Swales, M., & Freer, C. (1997). Frontal lobe deficit after head injury: Unity and diversity of function. *Cognitive Neuropsychology, 14,* 713–741.

Egner, T., & Hirsch, J. (2005). Cognitive control mechanisms resolve conflict through cortical amplification of task-relevant information. *Nature Neuroscience, 8,* 1784–1790.

Ekman, P., & Friesen, W. V. (1975). *Unmasking the face.* Englewood Cliffs, NJ: Prentice-Hall.

Elliott, R., Friston, K. J., & Dolan, R. J. (2000). Dissociable neural responses in human reward systems. *Journal of Neuroscience, 20,* 6159–6165.

Engle, R. W., Kane, M. J., & Tuholski, S. W. (1999). Individual differences inworking memory capacity and what they tell us about controlled attention, general fluid intelligence and functions of the prefrontal cortex. In A. Miyake & P. Shah (Eds.), *Models of working memory* (pp. 102–134). Cambridge, UK: Cambridge University Press.

Falkenstein, M., Hohnsbein, J., Hoormann, J., & Blanke, L. (1991). Effects of crossmodal divided attention on late ERP components. II. Error processing in choice reaction tasks. *Electroencephalography and Clinical Neurophysiology, 78,* 447–455.

Fletcher, P. C., & Henson, R. N. (2001). Frontal lobes and human memory: Insights from functional neuroimaging. *Brain, 124,* 849–881.

Forstl, H., Burns, A., Levy, R., Cairns, N., Luthert, P., & Lantos, P. (1993). Neuropathological correlates of behavioural disturbance in confirmed Alzheimer's disease. *British Journal of Psychiatry, 163,* 364–368.

Fox, M. D., Snyder, A. Z., Vincent, J. L., Corbetta, M., Van Essen, D. C., & Raichle, M. E. (2005). The human brain is intrinsically organized into dynamic, anticorrelated functional networks. *Proceedings of the National Academy of Science USA, 102,* 9673–9678.

Freo, U., Ricciardi, E., Pietrini, P., Schapiro, M. B., Rapoport, S. I., & Furey, M. L. (2005). Pharmacological modulation of prefrontal cortical activity during a working memory task in young and older humans: A PET study with physostigmine. *American Journal of Psychiatry, 162,* 2061–2070.

Friedman, N. P., & Miyake, A. (2004). The relations among inhibition and interference control functions: A latent-variable analysis. *Journal of Experimental Psychology: General, 133,* 101–135.

Funahashi, S., Bruce, C. J., & Goldman-Rakic, P. S. (1993). Dorsolateral prefrontal lesions and oculomotor delayed-response performance: Evidence for mnemonic "scotomas." *Journal of Neuroscience, 13,* 1479–1497.

Funkiewiez, A., Bertoux, M., de Souza, L. C., Levy, R., & Dubois, B. (2012). The SEA (Social cognition and Emotional Assessment): A clinical neuropsychological tool for early diagnosis of frontal variant of frontotemporal lobar degeneration. *Neuropsychology, 26,* 81–90.

Furey, M. L., Pietrini, P., & Haxby, J. V. (2000). Cholinergic enhancement and increased selectivity of perceptual processing during working memory. *Science, 290,* 2315–2319.

Furey, M. L., Pietrini, P., Haxby, J. V., Alexander, G. E., Lee, H. C., VanMeter, J.,…Freo, U. (1997). Cholinergic stimulation alters performance and task-specific regional cerebral blood flow during working memory. *Proceedings of the National Academy of Science USA, 94,* 6512–6516.

Fuster, J. M. (1985). The prefrontal cortex, mediator of cross-temporal contingencies. *Human Neurobiology, 4,* 169–179.

Fuster, J. M. (1995). *Memory in the cerebral cortex: An empirical approach to neural networks in the human brain and nonhuman primate.* Cambridge, MA: Dorsey Press.

Garrett, K. D., Browndyke, J. N., Whelihan, W., Paul, R. H., DiCarlo, M., Moser, D. J.,…Ott, B. R. (2004). The neuropsychological profile of vascular cognitive impairment—no dementia: Comparisons to patients at risk for cerebrovascular disease and vascular dementia. *Archives of Clinical Neuropsychology, 19,* 745–757.

Gazzaley, A., Cooney, J. W., Rissman, J., & D'Esposito, M. (2005). Top-down suppression deficit underlies working memory impairment in normal aging. *Nature Neuroscience, 8,* 1298–1300.

Gazzaley, A., & D'Esposito, M. (2007). Unifying prefrontal cortex function: Executive control, neural networks, and top-down modulation. In B. Miller & J. Cummings (Eds.), *The human frontal lobes* (pp. 187–206). New York, NY: Guildford Press.

Gazzaley, A., & Nobre, A. C. (2012). Top-down modulation: Bridging selective attention and working memory. *Trends in Cognitive Sciences, 16,* 129–135.

Gazzaley, A. H., Thakker, M. M., Hof, P. R., & Morrison, J. H. (1997). Preserved number of entorhinal cortex layer II neurons in aged macaque monkeys. *Neurobiology of Aging, 18,* 549–553.

Genovesio, A., Brasted, P. J., & Wise, S. P. (2006). Representation of future and previous spatial goals by separate neural populations in prefrontal cortex. *Journal of Neuroscience, 26,* 7305–7316.

Gioia, G., Isquith, P., Guy, S., & Kenworthy, L. (2000). *Behavior rating inventory of executive function.* Odessa, FL: Psychological Assessment Resources.

Goldberg, E., Podel, K., Bilder, R., & Jaeger, J (2000). *The executive control battery.* Melbourne, Australia: PsychPress.

Goldman-Rakic, P. S. (1987). Circuitry of primate prefrontal cortex and regulation of behavior by representational memory. In F. Plum, V. B. Mountcastle, & S. T. Geiger (Eds.), *The handbook of physiology, Section 1. The nervous system, Vol. 5. Higher functions of the brain part 1* (pp. 373–417). Bethesda, MD: American Physiological Society.

Goldman-Rakic, P. S. (1996). Regional and cellular fractionation of working memory. *Proceedings of the National Academy of Science USA, 93,* 13473–13480.

Goldman-Rakic, P. S. (1999). The "psychic" neuron of the cerebral cortex. *Annals of the New York Academy of Sciences, 868,* 13–26.

Goldstein, K., & Katz, E. (1937). The psychopathology of Pick's Disease. *Archives of Neurology and Psychiatry, 38*(3), 473–490.

Goldstein, K., & Scheerer, M. (1941). Abstract concrete behavior. *Psychological Monographs, 53,* 110–130.

Grace, J., & Malloy, P. (2001). *Frontal systems behavior scale (FrSBe).* Odessa, FL: Psychological Assessment Resources.

Grady, C. L., McIntosh, A. R., Bookstein, F., Horwitz, B., Rapoport, S. I., & Haxby, J. V. (1998). Age-related changes in regional cerebral blood flow during working memory for faces. *NeuroImage, 8,* 409–425.

Greenhill, L. L., & Osman, B. B. (2000). *Ritalin: Theory and practice.* New York, NY: Mary Ann Liebert.

Greenwood, P. M. (2000). The frontal aging hypothesis evaluated. *Journal of the International Neuropsychological Society, 6,* 705–726.

Gregory, C., Lough, S., Stone, V., Erzinclioglu, S., Martin, L., Baron-Cohen, S., & Hodges, J. R. (2002). Theory of mind in patients with frontal variant frontotemporal dementia and Alzheimer's disease: Theoretical and practical implications. *Brain, 125,* 752–764.

Grinband, J., Hirsch, J., & Ferrera, V. P. (2006). A neural representation of categorization uncertainty in the human brain. *Neuron, 49,* 757–763.

Gross, J. J. (1998). The emerging field of emotion regulation: An integrative review. *Review of General Psychology, 2,* 271–299.

Guidi, M., Paciaroni, L., Paolini, S., De Padova, S., & Scarpino, O. (2006). Differences and similarities in the neuropsychological profile of dementia with Lewy bodies and Alzheimer's disease in the early stage. *Journal of the Neurological Sciences, 248,* 120–123.

Gusnard, D. A., Akbudak, E., Shulman, G. L., & Raichle, M. E. (2001). Medial prefrontal cortex and self-referential mental activity: Relation to a default mode of brain function. *Proceedings of the National Academy of Sciences USA, 98,* 4259–4264.

Gusnard, D. A., Raichle, M. E., & Raichle, M. E. (2001). Searching for a baseline: Functional imaging and the resting human brain. *Nature Reviews Neuroscience, 2,* 685–694.

Hachinski, V. C., & Bowler, J. V. (1993). Vascular dementia. *Neurology, 43,* 2159–2160.

Hasher, L., & Zacks, R. T. (1988). Working memory, comprehension, and aging: A review and a new view. *Psychology of Learning and Motivation, 22,* 193–225.

Heatherton, T. F. (2011). Neuroscience of self and self-regulation. *Annual Review of Psychology, 62,* 363–390.

Heatherton, T. F., Wyland, C. L., Macrae, C. N., Demos, K. E., Denny, B. T., & Kelley, W. M. (2006). Medial prefrontal activity differentiates self from close others. *Social Cognitve and Affective Neuroscience, 1,* 18–25.

Higgins, E. T. (1997). Beyond pleasure and pain. *American Psychologist, 52,* 1280–1300.

Hodges, J. R., & Miller, B. (2001). The classification, genetics and neuropathology of frontotemporal dementia. Introduction to the special topic papers: Part I. *Neurocase, 7,* 31–35.

Holroyd, C. B., & Coles, M. G. (2002). The neural basis of human error processing: Reinforcement learning, dopamine, and the error-related negativity. *Psychological Review, 109,* 679–709.

Holroyd, C. B., & Coles, M. G. (2008). Dorsal anterior cingulate cortex integrates reinforcement history to guide voluntary behavior. *Cortex, 44,* 548–559.

Holroyd, C. B., Yeung, N., Coles, M. G., & Cohen, J. D. (2005). A mechanism for error detection in speeded response time tasks. *Journal of Experimental Psychology: General, 134,* 163–191.

Hornak, J., O'Doherty, J., Bramham, J., Rolls, E. T., Morris, R. G., Bullock, P. R., & Polkey, C. E. (2004). Reward-related reversal learning after surgical excisions in orbito-frontal or dorsolateral prefrontal cortex in humans. *Journal of Cognitive Neuroscience, 16,* 463–478.

Horvath, T. L., Diano, S., & van den Pol, A. N. (1999). Synaptic interaction between hypocretin (orexin) and neuropeptide Y cells in the rodent and primate hypothalamus: A novel circuit implicated in metabolic and endocrine regulations. *Journal of Neuroscience, 19,* 1072–1087.

Horvitz, J. C., Stewart, T., & Jacobs, B. L. (1997). Burst activity of ventral tegmental dopamine neurons is elicited by sensory stimuli in the awake cat. *Brain Research, 759,* 251–258.

Hull, C. L. (1943). *Principles of behavior.* New York, NY: Appleton-Century.

Jackson, J. H. (1932). *Selected writings of John Hughlings Jackson.* London, UK: Hodder and Stoughton.

Johnson, M. K., Nolen-Hoeksema, S., Mitchell, K. J., & Levin, Y. (2009). Medial cortex activity, self-reflection and depression. *Social Cognitive and Affective Neuroscience, 4,* 313–327.

Johnson, M. K., Raye, C. L., Mitchell, K. J., Touryan, S. R., Greene, E. J., & Nolen-Hoeksema, S. (2006). Dissociating medial frontal and posterior cingulate activity during self-reflection. *Social Cognitive and Affective Neuroscience, 1,* 56–64.

Kane, M. J., & Engle, R. W. (2002). The role of prefrontal cortex in working-memory capacity, executive attention, and general fluid intelligence: An individual-differences perspective. *Psychonomic Bulletin Review, 9,* 637–671.

Kelley, W. M., Macrae, C. N., Wyland, C. L., Caglar, S., Inati, S., & Heatherton, T. F. (2002). Finding the self? An event-related fMRI study. *Journal of Cognitive Neuroscience, 14,* 785–794.

Kerns, J. G., Cohen, J. D., MacDonald, A. W., III, Cho, R. Y., Stenger, V. A., & Carter, C. S. (2004). Anterior cingulate conflict monitoring and adjustments in control. *Science, 303,* 1023–1026.

Kertesz, A., Davidson, W., & Fox, H. (1997). Frontal behavioral inventory: Diagnostic criteria for frontal lobe dementia. *Canadian Journal of the Neurological Sciences, 24,* 29–36.

Kertesz, A., Hudson, L., Mackenzie, I. R. A., & Munoz, D. G. (1994). The pathology and nosology of primary progressive aphasia. *Neurology, 44,* 2065–2072.

Khateb, A., Ammann, J., Annoni, J. M., & Diserens, K. (2005). Cognition-enhancing effects of donepezil in traumatic brain injury. *European Neurology, 54,* 39–45.

Kimber, J. R., Watson, L., & Mathias, C. J. (1997). Distinction of idiopathic Parkinson's disease from multiple-system atrophy by stimulation of growth-hormone release with clonidine. *Lancet, 349,* 1877–1881.

Kimberg, D. Y., & Farah, M. J. (1993). A unified account of cognitive impairments following frontal damage: The role of working memory in complex organized behavior. *Journal of Experimental Psychology: General, 122,* 411–428.

Kincade, J. M., Abrams, R. A., Astafiev, S. V., Shulman, G. L., & Corbetta, M. (2005). An event-related functional magnetic resonance imaging study of voluntary and stimulus-driven orienting of attention. *Journal of Neuroscience, 25,* 4593–4604.

Kinomura, S., Larsson, J., Gulyas, B., & Roland, P. E. (1996). Activation by attention of the human reticular formation and thalamic intralaminar nuclei. *Science, 271,* 512–515.

Kipps, C. M., & Hodges, J. R. (2006). Theory of mind in frontotemporal dementia. *Society for Neuroscience, 1,* 235–244.

Kiyonaga, A., Egner, T., & Soto, D. (2012). Cognitive control over working memory biases of selection. *Psychonomic Bulletin Review, 19,* 639–646.

Klein, S. B., Loftus, J., & Kihlstrom, J. F. (2002). Memory and temporal experience: The effects of episodic memory loss on an amnesic patient's ability to remember the past and imagine the future. *Social Cognition, 20,* 353–379.

Knight, C., Alderman, N., & Burgess, P. W. (2002). Development of a simplified version of the multiple errands test for use in hospital settings. *Neuropsychological Rehabiltation, 12,* 231–255.

Knudsen, E. I. (2007). Fundamental components of attention. *Annual Review of Neuroscience, 30,* 57–78.

Knutson, B., Adams, C. M., Fong, G. W., & Hommer, D. (2001). Anticipation of increasing monetary reward selectively recruits nucleus accumbens. *Journal of Neuroscience, 21,* RC159.

Konishi, S., Nakajima, K., Uchida, I., Kikyo, H., Kameyama, M., & Miyashita, Y. (1999). Common inhibitory mechanism in human inferior prefrontal cortex revealed by event-related functional MRI. *Brain, 122,* 981–991.

Kouneiher, F., Charron, S., & Koechlin, E. (2009). Motivation and cognitive control in the human prefrontal cortex. *Nature Neuroscience, 12,* 939–945.

Kramer, J. H., Reed, B. R., Mungas, D., Weiner, M. W., & Chui, H. C. (2002). Executive dysfunction in subcortical ischaemic vascular disease. *Journal of Neurology, Neurosurgery and Psychiatry, 72,* 217–220.

Kringelbach, M. L., & Rolls, E. T. (2004). The functional neuroanatomy of the human orbitofrontal cortex: Evidence from neuroimaging and neuropsychology. *Progress in Neurobiology, 72,* 341–372.

Krueger, C. E., Laluz, V., Rosen, H. J., Neuhaus, J. M., Miller, B. L., & Kramer, J. H. (2011). Double dissociation in the anatomy of socioemotional disinhibition and executive functioning in dementia. *Neuropsychology, 25,* 249–259.

Kudlicka, A., Clare, L., & Hindle, J. V. (2011). Executive functions in Parkinson's disease: Systematic review and meta-analysis. *Movement Disorders, 26,* 2305–2315.

Laird, A. R., Eickhoff, S. B., Li, K., Robin, D. A., Glahn, D. C., & Fox, P. T. (2009). Investigating the functional heterogeneity of the default mode network using coordinate-based meta-analytic modeling. *Journal of Neuroscience, 29,* 14496–14505.

Lambe, E. K., Olausson, P., Horst, N. K., Taylor, J. R., & Aghajanian, G. K. (2005). Hypocretin and nicotine excite the same thalamocortical synapses in prefrontal cortex: Correlation with improved attention in rat. *Journal of Neuroscience, 25,* 5225–5229.

Lavie, N., Hirst, A., de Fockert, J. W., & Viding, E. (2004). Load theory of selective attention and cognitive control. *Journal of Experimental Psychology: General, i,* 339–354.

Levin, B. E., & Katzen, H. L. (2005). Early cognitive changes and nondementing behavioral abnormalities in Parkinson's disease. *Advances in Neurology, 96,* 84–94.

Lezak, M. D. (1995). *Neuropsychological assessment.* New York, NY: Oxford University Press.

Lezak, M. D., Howieson, D., Loring, D. W., Hannay, H., & Fischer, J. (2004). *Neuropsychological assessment.* New York, NY: Oxford University Press.

Li, S. C., Lindenberger, U., & Sikstrom, S. (2001). Aging cognition: From neuromodulation to representation. *Trends in Cognitive Sciences, 5,* 479–486.

Libon, D. J., Bogdanoff, B., Bonavita, J., Skalina, S., Cloud, B. S., Resh, R., ... Ball, S. K. (1997). Dementia associated with periventricular and deep white matter alterations: A subtype of subcortical dementia. *Archives of Clinical Neuropsychology, 12,* 239–250.

Liddle, P. F., Kiehl, K. A., & Smith, A. M. (2001). Event-related fMRI study of response inhibition. *Human Brain Mapping, i,* 100–109.

Lin, J. S., Hou, Y., & Jouvet, M. (1996). Potential brain neuronal targets for amphetamine-, methylphenidate-, and modafinil-induced wakefulness, evidenced by c-fos immunocytochemistry in the cat. *Proceedings of the National Academy of Science USA, 93,* 14128–14133.

Logie, R. H., Cocchini, G., Delia, S. S., & Baddeley, A. D. (2004). Is there a specific executive capacity for dual task coordination? Evidence from Alzheimer's disease. *Neuropsychology, 18,* 504–513.

Lough, S., Kipps, C. M., Treise, C., Watson, P., Blair, J. R., & Hodges, J. R. (2006). Social reasoning, emotion and empathy in frontotemporal dementia. *Neuropsychologia, 44,* 950–958.

Luciana, M., & Collins, P. F. (1997). Dopaminergic modulation of working memory for spatial but not object cues in normal humans. *Journal of Cognitive Neuroscience, 9,* 330–347.

Luciana, M., Depue, R. A., Arbisi, P., & Leon, A. (1992). Facilitation of working memory in humans by a D2 dopamine receptor agonist. *Journal of Cognitive Neuroscience, 4,* 58–68.

Mackenzie, I. R., Neumann, M., Bigio, E. H., Cairns, N. J., Alafuzoff, I., Kril, J.,...Mann, D. M. (2009). Nomenclature for neuropathologic subtypes of frontotemporal lobar degeneration: Consensus recommendations. *Acta Neuropathologica, 117,* 15–18.

Manly, T., Hawkins, K., Evans, J., Woldt, K., & Robertson, I. H. (2002). Rehabilitation of executive function: Facilitation of effective goal management on complex tasks using periodic auditory alerts. *Neuropsychologia, 40,* 271–281.

Marin, R. S., Fogel, B. S., Hawkins, J., Duffy, J., & Krupp, B. (1995). Apathy: A treatable syndrome. *Journal of Neuropsychiatry and Clinical Neuroscience, 7,* 23–30.

Marinus, J., Visser, M., Verwey, N. A., Verhey, F. R., Middelkoop, H. A., Stiggelbout, A. M., & van Hilten, J. J. (2003). Assessment of cognition in Parkinson's disease. *Neurology, 61,* 1222–1228.

Markus, H., & Nurius, P. (1986). Possible selves. *American Psychologist, 41,* 954–969.

Markus, H., & Wurf, E. (1987). The dynamic self-concept: A social psychological perspective. In Rosenweig, M.R. & Porter, L.W. (Eds.) *Annual Review of Psychology* (pp. 299–337). Palo Alto, Ca: Annual Reviews.

Mason, M. F., Norton, M. I., Van Horn, J. D., Wegner, D. M., Grafton, S. T., & Macrae, C. N. (2007). Wandering minds: The default network and stimulus-independent thought. *Science, 315,* 393–395.

Matsumoto, M., Matsumoto, K., Abe, H., & Tanaka, K. (2007). Medial prefrontal cell activity signaling prediction errors of action values. *Nature Neuroscience, 10,* 647–656.

Mauss, I. B., Bunge, S. A., & Gross, J. J. (2007). Automatic emotion regulation. *Social and Personality Psychology Compass, 1,* 146–167.

McDowell, S., Whyte, J., & D'Esposito, M. (1998). Differential effect of a dopaminergic agonist on prefrontal function in traumatic brain injury patients. *Brain, 121,* 1155–1164.

McKeith, I. G., Dickson, D. W., Lowe, J., Emre, M., O'Brien, J. T., Feldman, H.,...Yamada, M. (2005). Diagnosis and management of dementia with Lewy bodies: Third report of the DLB Consortium. *Neurology, 65,* 1863–1872.

Menon, V., Adleman, N. E., White, C. D., Glover, G. H., & Reiss, A. L. (2001). Error-related brain activation during a Go/NoGo response inhibition task. *Human Brain Mapping, 12,* 131–143.

Menon, V., & Uddin, L. Q. (2010). Saliency, switching, attention and control: A network model of insula function. *Brain Structure and Function, 214,* 655–667.

Mesulam, M. M. (1986). Frontal cortex and behavior. *Annals of Neurology, 19,* 320–325.

Mesulam, M. M. (2000). *Principles of behavioral and cognitive neurology.* Oxford, UK: Oxford University Press.

Mesulam, M. M., & Mufson, E. J. (1982). Insula of the old world monkey. I. Architectonics in the insulo-orbito-temporal component of the paralimbic brain. *Journal of Comparative Neurology, 212,* 1–22.

Middleton, F. A., & Strick, P. L. (2002). Basal-ganglia "projections" to the prefrontal cortex of the primate. *Cerebral Cortex, 12,* 926–935.

Miller, B. T., & D'Esposito, M. (2005). Searching for "the top" in top-down control. *Neuron, 48,* 535–538.

Miller, E. K., & Cohen, J. D. (2001). An integrative theory of prefrontal cortex function. *Annual Review of Neuroscience, 24,* 167–202.

Miller, E. K., Erickson, C. A., & Desimone, R. (1996). Neural mechanisms of visual working memory in prefrontal cortex of the macaque. *Journal of Neuroscience, 16,* 5154–5167.

Mitchell, K. J., Raye, C. L., Ebner, N. C., Tubridy, S. M., Frankel, H., & Johnson, M. K. (2009). Age-group differences in medial cortex activity associated with thinking about self-relevant agendas. *Psychology of Aging, 24,* 438–449.

Miyake, A., Friedman, N. P., Emerson, M. J., Witzki, A. H., Howerter, A., & Wager, T. D. (2000). The unity and diversity of executive functions and their contributions to complex "frontal lobe" tasks: A latent variable analysis. *Cognitive Psychology, 41,* 49–100.

Moore, R. Y., Abrahamson, E. A., & Van Den, P. A. (2001). [The hypocretin neuron system: An arousal system in the human brain]. *Archives Italiennes de Biologie, 139,* 195–205.

Morris, G., Arkadir, D., Nevet, A., Vaadia, E., & Bergman, H. (2004). Coincident but distinct messages of midbrain dopamine and striatal tonically active neurons. *Neuron, 43,* 133–143.

Muller, U., Steffenhagen, N., Regenthal, R., & Bublak, P. (2004). Effects of modafinil on working memory processes in humans. *Psychopharmacology (Berlin), 177,* 161–169.

Muller, U., & von Cramon, D. Y. (1994). The therapeutic potential of bromocriptine in neuropsychological rehabilitation of patients with acquired brain damage. *Progress in Neuropsychopharmacology and Biological Psychiatry, 18,* 1103–1120.

Muller, U., von Cramon, D. Y., & Pollman, S. (1998). D1- versus D2-receptor modulation of visuospatial working memory in humans. *Journal of Neuroscience, 18,* 2720–2728.

Muslimovic, D., Post, B., Speelman, J. D., & Schmand, B. (2005). Cognitive profile of patients with newly diagnosed Parkinson disease. *Neurology, 65,* 1239–1245.

Nakahara, H., Itoh, H., Kawagoe, R., Takikawa, Y., & Hikosaka, O. (2004). Dopamine neurons can represent context-dependent prediction error. *Neuron, 41,* 269–280.

Nemeth, G., Hegedus, K., & Molnar, L. (1988). Akinetic mutism associated with bicingular lesions: Clinicopathological and functional anatomical correlates. *European Archives of Psychiatry and Neurological Science, 237,* 218–222.

Niendam, T. A., Laird, A. R., Ray, K. L., Dean, Y. M., Glahn, D. C., & Carter, C. S. (2012). Meta-analytic evidence for a superordinate cognitive control network subserving diverse executive functions. *Cognitive, Affective, and Behavioral Neuroscience, 12,* 241–268.

Nieuwenhuis, S., Aston-Jones, G., & Cohen, J. D. (2005). Decision making, the P3, and the locus coeruleus-norepinephrine system. *Psychological Bulletin, 131,* 510–532.

Niki, H., & Watanabe, M. (1979). Prefrontal and cingulate unit activity during timing behavior in the monkey. *Brain Research, 171,* 213–224.

O'Doherty, J., Kringelbach, M. L., Rolls, E. T., Hornak, J., & Andrews, C. (2001). Abstract reward and punishment representations in the human orbitofrontal cortex. *Nature Neuroscience, 4,* 95–102.

Ochsner, K. N., Bunge, S. A., Gross, J. J., & Gabrieli, J. D. (2002). Rethinking feelings: An FMRI study of the cognitive regulation of emotion. *Journal of Cognitive Neuroscience, 14,* 1215–1229.

Okuda, J., Fujii, T., Ohtake, H., Tsukiura, T., Tanji, K., Suzuki, K.,...Yamadori A. (2003). Thinking of the future and past: The roles of the frontal pole and the medial temporal lobes. *Neuroimage, 19,* 1369–1380.

Ongur, D., & Price, J. L. (2000). The organization of networks within the orbital and medial prefrontal cortex of rats, monkeys and humans. *Cerebral Cortex, 10,* 206–219.

Owen, A. M. (2004). Cognitive dysfunction in Parkinson's disease: The role of frontostriatal circuitry. *Neuroscientist, 10,* 525–537.

Pantoni, L., & Garcia, J. H. (1997). Cognitive impairment and cellular/vascular changes in the cerebral white matter. *Annals of the New York Academy of Sciences, 826,* 92–102.

Pardini, M., Emberti, G. L., Mascolo, M., Benassi, F., Abate, L., Guida, S.,...Cocito L. (2012). Isolated theory of mind deficits and risk for frontotemporal dementia: A longitudinal pilot study. *Journal of Neurology, Neurosurgery and Psychiatry, 84*(7), 818–821.

Park, D. C., Polk, T. A., Park, R., Minear, M., Savage, A., & Smith, M. R. (2004). Aging reduces neural specialization in ventral visual cortex. *Proceedings of the National Academy of Sciences USA, 101,* 13091.

Passingham, D (1995). *The frontal lobes and voluntary action.* Oxford, UK: Oxford University Press.

Paus, T. (2001). Primate anterior cingulate cortex: Where motor control, drive and cognition interface. *Nature Reviews Neuroscience, 2,* 417–424.

Pavlov, I. P. (1960). *Conditioned Reflexes. An investigation of the physiological activity of the cerebral cortex.* New York, NY: Dover Publications, Inc.

Pelosi, L., & Blumhardt, L. D. (1999). Effects of age on working memory: An event-related potential study. *Brain Research Cognitive Brain Research, 7,* 321–334.

Petersen, S. E., & Posner, M. I. (2012). The attention system of the human brain: 20 years after. *Annual Review of Neuroscience, 35,* 73–89.

Peterson, B. S., Kane, M. J., Alexander, G. M., Lacadie, C., Skudlarski, P., Leung, H. C.,...Gore JC. (2002). An event-related functional MRI study comparing interference effects in the Simon and Stroop tasks. *Brain Research Cognitive Brain Research, 13,* 427–440.

Petrides, M. (2000). Dissociable roles of mid-dorsolateral prefrontal and anterior inferotemporal cortex in visual working memory. *Journal of Neuroscience, 20,* 7496–7503.

Peyron, R., Laurent, B., & Garcia-Larrea, L. (2000). Functional imaging of brain responses to pain. A review and meta-analysis (2000). *Neurophysiologie Clinique, 30,* 263–288.

Pillon, B., Boller, F., Levy, R., & Dubois, B. (2001). Cognitive deficits and dementia in Parkinson's disease. In F. Boller & S. F. Cappa (Eds.), *Handbook of neuropsychology* (pp. 311–371). Elsevier, Amsterdam.

Posner, M. I., & Petersen, S. E. (1990). The attention system of the human brain. *Annual Review of Neuroscience, 13,* 25–42.

Posner, M. I., & Snyder, C. R. R. (1975). Attention and cognitive control. In R. L. Solso (Ed.), *Information processing and cognition, the Loyola Symposium* (pp. 55–85). Hillsdale, NJ: Erlbaum.

Powell, K. D., & Goldberg, M. E. (2000). Response of neurons in the lateral intraparietal area to a distractor flashed during the delay period of a memory-guided saccade. *Journal of Neurophysiology, 84,* 301–310.

Pugh, K. G., & Lipsitz, L. A. (2002). The microvascular frontal-subcortical syndrome of aging. *Neurobiology of Aging, 23,* 421–431.

Pycock, C. J., Kerwin, R. W., & Carter, C. J. (1980). Effect of lesion of cortical dopamine terminals on subcortical dopamine receptors in rats. *Nature, 286,* 74–76.

Rahman, S., Robbins, T. W., Hodges, J. R., Mehta, M. A., Nestor, P. J., Clark, L., & Sahakian, B. J. (2005). Methylphenidate ("Ritalin") can ameliorate abnormal risk-taking behavior in the frontal variant of frontotemporal dementia. *Neuropsychopharmacology, 31*(3), 651–658.

Rahman, S., Sahakian, B. J., Hodges, J. R., Rogers, R. D., & Robbins, T. W. (1999). Specific cognitive deficits in mild frontal variant frontotemporal dementia. *Brain, 122*(Pt 8), 1469–1493.

Rainer, G., Asaad, W. F., & Miller, E. K. (1998). Selective representation of relevant information by neurons in the primate prefrontal cortex. *Nature, 393,* 577–579.

Rankin, K. P., Gorno-Tempini, M. L., Allison, S. C., Stanley, C. M., Glenn, S., Weiner, M. W., & Miller, B. L. (2006). Structural anatomy of empathy in neurodegenerative disease. *Brain, 129,* 2945–2956.

Rascovsky, K., Hodges, J. R., Kipps, C. M., Johnson, J. K., Seeley, W. W., Mendez, M. F.,…Miller, B. M. (2007). Diagnostic criteria for the behavioral variant of frontotemporal dementia (bvFTD): Current limitations and future directions. *Alzheimer Disease and Associative Disorders, 21,* S14–S18.

Rascovsky, K., Hodges, J. R., Knopman, D., Mendez, M. F., Kramer, J. H., Neuhaus, J.,…Miller, B. L. (2011). Sensitivity of revised diagnostic criteria for the behavioural variant of frontotemporal dementia. *Brain, 134,* 2456–2477.

Raz, N., Gunning-Dixon, F., Head, D., Rodrigue, K. M., Williamson, A., & Acker, J. D. (2004). Aging, sexual dimorphism, and hemispheric asymmetry of the cerebral cortex: Replicability of regional differences in volume. *Neurobiology of Aging, 25,* 377–396.

Raz, N., Rodrigue, K. M., Kennedy, K. M., Head, D., Gunning-Dixon, F., & Acker, J. D. (2003). Differential aging of the human striatum: Longitudinal evidence. *American Journal of Neuroradiology, 24,* 1849–1856.

Resnick, S. M., Pham, D. L., Kraut, M. A., Zonderman, A. B., & Davatzikos, C. (2003). Longitudinal magnetic resonance imaging studies of older adults: A shrinking brain. *Journal of Neuroscience, 23,* 3295–3301.

Reuter-Lorenz, P. A., & Cappell, K. A. (2008). Neurocognitive aging and the compensation hypothesis. *Current Directions in Psychological Science, 17,* 177–182.

Reuter-Lorenz, P. A., Jonides, J., Smith, E. E., Hartley, A., Miller, A., Marshuetz, C., & Koeppe, R. A. (2000). Age differences in the frontal lateralization of verbal and spatial working memory revealed by PET. *Journal of Cognitive Neuroscience, 12,* 174–187.

Ridderinkhof, K. R., Ullsperger, M., Crone, E. A., & Nieuwenhuis, S. (2004). The role of the medial frontal cortex in cognitive control. *Science, 306,* 443–447.

Riis, J. L., Chong, H., Ryan, K. K., Wolk, D. A., Rentz, D. M., Holcomb, P. J., & Daffner, K. R. (2008). Compensatory neural activity distinguishes different patterns of normal cognitive aging. *NeuroImage, 39,* 441–454.

Robbins, T. W., & Roberts, A. C. (2007), "Differential regulation of fronto-executive function by the monoamines and acetylcholine." *Cerebral Cortex, 17*(1), 151–160.

Rolls, E. T., Critchley, H. D., Mason, R., & Wakeman, E. A. (1996). Orbitofrontal cortex neurons: Role in olfactory and visual association learning. *Journal of Neurophysiology, 75,* 1970–1981.

Rubia, K., Lee, F., Cleare, A. J., Tunstall, N., Fu, C. H., Brammer, M., & McGuire, P. (2005). Tryptophan depletion reduces right inferior prefrontal activation during response inhibition in fast, event-related fMRI. *Psychopharmacology (Berlin), 179,* 791–803.

Rushworth, M. F., & Behrens, T. E. (2008). Choice, uncertainty and value in prefrontal and cingulate cortex. *Nature Neuroscience, 11,* 389–397.

Rypma, B., Prabhakaran, V., Desmond, J. E., Glover, G. H., & Gabrieli, J. D. (1999). Load-dependent roles of frontal brain regions in the maintenance of working memory. *Neuroimage, 9,* 216–226.

Salthouse, T. A. (1996). The processing-speed theory of adult age differences in cognition. *Psychological Review, 103,* 403–428.

Salthouse, T. A., Atkinson, T. M., & Berish, D. E. (2003). Executive functioning as a potential mediator of age-related cognitive decline in normal adults. *Journal of Experimental Psychology: General, 132,* 566–594.

Saper, C. B. (2002). The central autonomic nervous system: Conscious visceral perception and autonomic pattern generation. *Annual Review of Neuroscience, 25,* 433–469.

Saper, C. B., Chou, T. C., & Scammell, T. E. (2001). The sleep switch: Hypothalamic control of sleep and wakefulness. *Trends in Neuroscience, 24,* 726–731.

Scammell, T. E., Estabrooke, I. V., McCarthy, M. T., Chemelli, R. M., Yanagisawa, M., Miller, M. S., & Saper, C. B. (2000). Hypothalamic arousal regions are activated during modafinil-induced wakefulness. *Journal of Neuroscience, 20,* 8620–8628.

Schacter, D. L., Addis, D. R., & Buckner, R. L. (2007). Remembering the past to imagine the future: The prospective brain. *Nature Reviews Neuroscience, 8,* 657–661.

Schneider, B. A., & Pichora-Fuller, M. K. (2000). Age-related changes in temporal processing: Implications for listening comprehension. *Seminars in Hearing, 22,* 227–239.

Schoenbaum, G., Chiba, A. A., & Gallagher, M. (1998). Orbitofrontal cortex and basolateral amygdala encode expected outcomes during learning. *Nature Neuroscience, 1,* 155–159.

Schoenbaum, G., Chiba, A. A., & Gallagher, M. (1999). Neural encoding in orbitofrontal cortex and basolateral amygdala during olfactory discrimination learning. *Journal of Neuroscience, 19,* 1876–1884.

Schoenbaum, G., & Roesch, M. (2005). Orbitofrontal cortex, associative learning, and expectancies. *Neuron, 47,* 633–636.

Schoenbaum, G., Setlow, B., Nugent, S. L., Saddoris, M. P., & Gallagher, M. (2003). Lesions of orbitofrontal cortex and basolateral amygdala complex disrupt acquisition of odor-guided discriminations and reversals. *Learning and Memory, 10,* 129–140.

Schoenbaum, G., Setlow, B., Saddoris, M. P., & Gallagher, M. (2006). Encoding changes in orbitofrontal cortex in reversal-impaired aged rats. *Journal of Neurophysiology, 95,* 1509–1517.

Schroeter, M. L., Raczka, K., Neumann, J., & von Cramon, D. Y. (2008). Neural networks in frontotemporal dementia—a meta-analysis. *Neurobiology of Aging, 29,* 418–426.

Schultz, W. (2002). Getting formal with dopamine and reward. *Neuron, 36,* 241–263.

Schultz, W. (2010). Dopamine signals for reward value and risk: Basic and recent data. *Behavior and Brain Function, 6,* 24.

Schultz, W., Dayan, P., & Montague, P. (1997). A neural substrate of prediction and reward. *Science, 275,* 1593–1599.

Schumacher, E. H., Lauber, E., Awh, E., Jonides, J., Smith, E. E., & Koeppe, R. A. (1996). PET evidence for an amodal verbal working memory system. *Neuroimage, 3,* 79–88.

Schwartz, M. L., & Goldman-Rakic, P. S. (1984). Callosal and intrahemispheric connectivity of the prefrontal association cortex in rhesus monkey: Relation between intraparietal and principal sulcal cortex. *Journal of Comparative Neurology, 226,* 403–420.

Seeley, W. W., Crawford, R., Rascovsky, K., Kramer, J. H., Weiner, M., Miller, B. L., & Gorno-Tempini, M. L. (2008). Frontal paralimbic network atrophy in very mild behavioral variant frontotemporal dementia. *Archives of Neurology, 65,* 249–255.

Seeley, W. W., Menon, V., Schatzberg, A. F., Keller, J., Glover, G. H., Kenna, H., . . . Greicius, M. D. (2007). Dissociable intrinsic connectivity networks for salience processing and executive control. *Journal of Neuroscience, 27,* 2349–2356.

Seeley, W. W., Zhou, J., & Kim, E. J. (2012). Frontotemporal dementia: What can the behavioral variant teach us about human brain organization? *Neuroscientist, 18,* 373–385.

Shallice, T. (1982). Specific impairments of planning. *Philosophical Transactions of the Royral Society of London B: Biological Sciences, 298,* 199–209.

Shallice, T., & Burgess, P. W. (1991). Deficits in strategy application following frontal lobe damage in man. *Brain, 114,* 727–741.

Shankar, S., Teyler, T. J., & Robbins, N. (1998). Aging differentially alters forms of long-term potentiation in rat hippocampal area CA1. *Journal of Neurophysiology, 79,* 334–341.

Shulman, G. L., Astafiev, S. V., Franke, D., Pope, D. L., Snyder, A. Z., McAvoy, M. P., & Corbetta, M. (2009). Interaction of stimulus-driven reorienting and expectation in ventral and dorsal frontoparietal and basal ganglia-cortical networks. *Journal of Neuroscience, 29,* 4392–4407.

Shulman, G. L., Fiez, J. A., Corbetta, M., Buckner, R. L., Miezin, F. M., Raichle, M. E., & Petersen, S. E. (1997). Common blood flow changes across visual tasks: II Decreases in cerebral cortex. *Journal of Cognitive Neuroscience, 9,* 648–663.

Shulman, G. L., McAvoy, M. P., Cowan, M. C., Astafiev, S. V., Tansy, A. P., d'Avossa, G., & Corbetta, M. (2003). Quantitative analysis of attention and detection signals during visual search. *Journal of Neurophysiology, 90,* 3384–3397.

Siddall, O. M. (2005). Use of methylphenidate in traumatic brain injury. *Annals of Pharmacotherapy, 39,* 1309–1313.

Skinner, J. E., & Yingling, C. D. (1977). Central gating mechanisms that regulate event-related potentials and behavior. *Progress in Clinical Neurophysiology, 1,* 30–69.

Smith, E. E., Jonides, J., & Koeppe, R. A. (1996). Dissociating verbal and spatial working memory using PET. *Cerebral Cortex, 6,* 11–20.

Snowdon, D. A., Greiner, L. H., Mortimer, J. A., Riley, K. P., Greiner, P. A., & Markesbery, W. R. (1997). Brain infarction and the clinical expression of Alzheimer disease. The Nun Study. *Journal of the American Medical Association, 277,* 813–817.

Spreng, R. N., Mar, R. A., & Kim, A. S. (2009). The common neural basis of autobiographical memory, prospection, navigation, theory of mind, and the default mode: A quantitative meta-analysis. *Journal of Cognitive Neuroscience, 21,* 489–510.

Starkstein, S. E., Mayberg, H. S., Preziosi, T. J., Andrezejewski, P., Leiguarda, R., & Robinson,

R. G. (1992). Reliability, validity, and clinical correlates of apathy in Parkinson's disease. *Journal of Neuropsychiatry and Clinical Neuroscience*, *4*, 134–139.

Starkstein, S. E., Sabe, L., Vazquez, S., Teson, A., Petracca, G., Chemerinski, E.,...Leiguarda, R. (1996). Neuropsychological, psychiatric, and cerebral blood flow findings in vascular dementia and Alzheimer's disease. *Stroke*, *27*, 408–414.

Stone, V. E., Baron-Cohen, S., & Knight, R. T. (1998). Frontal lobe contributions to theory of mind. *Journal of Cognitive Neuroscience*, *10*, 640–656.

Stuss, D. T., & Alexander, M. P. (2007). Is there a dysexecutive syndrome? *Philosophical Transactions of the Royal Society of London B: Biological Sciences*, *362*, 901–915.

Stuss, D. T., & Knight, R. T. (2002). *Principles of frontal lobe function*. New York, NY: Oxford University Press.

Sutton, R. S., & Barto, A. G. (1998). *Reinforcement learning: An introduction*. Cambridge, MA: MIT Press.

Szpunar, K. K., Watson, J. M., & McDermott, K. B. (2007). Neural substrates of envisioning the future. *Proceedings of the National Academy of Science USA*, *104*, 642–647.

Tamir, M. (2009). Differential preferences for happiness: Extraversion and trait-consistent emotion regulation. *Journal of Personality*, *77*, 447–470.

Taylor, F. B., & Russo, J. (2000). Efficacy of modafinil compared to dextroamphetamine for the treatment of attention deficit hyperactivity disorder in adults. *Journal of Child and Adolescent Psychopharmacology*, *10*, 311–320.

Taylor, F. B., & Russo, J. (2001). Comparing guanfacine and dextroamphetamine for the treatment of adult attention-deficit/hyperactivity disorder. *Journal of Clinical Psychopharmacology*, *21*, 223–228.

Terry, R. D. (2000). Cell death or synaptic loss in Alzheimer disease. *Journal of Neuropathology and Experimental Neurology*, *59*, 1118–1119.

Thorpe, S. J., Rolls, E. T., & Maddison, S. (1983). The orbitofrontal cortex: Neuronal activity in the behaving monkey. *Experimental Brain Research*, *49*, 93–115.

Tobler, P. N., Fiorillo, C. D., & Schultz, W. (2005). Adaptive coding of reward value by dopamine neurons. *Science*, *307*, 1642–1645.

Torralva, T., Kipps, C. M., Hodges, J. R., Clark, L., Bekinschtein, T., Roca, M.,...Manes F. (2007). The relationship between affective decision-making and theory of mind in the frontal variant of fronto-temporal dementia. *Neuropsychologia*, *45*, 342–349.

Torralva, T., Roca, M., Gleichgerrcht, E., Bekinschtein, T., & Manes, F. (2009). A neuropsychological battery to detect specific executive and social cognitive impairments in early frontotemporal dementia. *Brain*, *132*, 1299–1309.

Tulving, E. (2005). Episodic memory and autonoesis: Uniquely human? In H. S. Terrace & J. Metcalfe (Eds.), *The missing link in cognition* (pp. 4–56). New York, NY: Oxford University Press.

Turner, D. C., Clark, L., Dowson, J., Robbins, T. W., & Sahakian, B. J. (2004). Modafinil improves cognition and response inhibition in adult attention-deficit/hyperactivity disorder. *Biological Psychiatry*, *55*, 1031–1040.

Turner, D. C., Robbins, T. W., Clark, L., Aron, A. R., Dowson, J., & Sahakian, B. J. (2003). Cognitive enhancing effects of modafinil in healthy volunteers. *Psychopharmacology (Berlin)*, *165*, 260–269.

Uekermann, J., Daum, I., Bielawski, M., Muhlack, S., Peters, S., Przuntek, H., & Mueller, T. (2004). Differential executive control impairments in early Parkinson's disease. *Journal of Neural Transmission Supplementa*, 39–51.

Ullsperger, M., & von Cramon, D. Y. (2003). Error monitoring using external feedback: Specific roles of the habenular complex, the reward system, and the cingulate motor area revealed by functional magnetic resonance imaging. *Journal of Neuroscience*, *23*, 4308–4314.

Ullsperger, M., & von Cramon, D. Y. (2004). Neuroimaging of performance monitoring: Error detection and beyond. *Cortex*, *40*, 593–604.

Usher, M., Cohen, J. D., Servan-Schreiber, D., Rajkowski, J., & Aston-Jones, G. (1999). The role of locus coeruleus in the regulation of cognitive performance. *Science*, *283*, 549–554.

Vijayraghavan, S., Wang, M., Birnbaum, S. G., Williams, G. V., & Arnsten, A. F. (2007). Inverted-U dopamine D1 receptor actions on prefrontal neurons engaged in working memory. *Nature Neuroscience*, *10*, 376–384.

Villardita, C. (1993). Alzheimer's disease compared with cerebrovascular dementia. Neuropsychological similarities and differences. *Acta Neurologica Scandinavica*, *87*, 299–308.

Vincent, J. L., Kahn, I., Snyder, A. Z., Raichle, M. E., & Buckner, R. L. (2008). Evidence for a frontoparietal control system revealed by intrinsic functional connectivity. *Journal of Neurophysiology*, *100*, 3328–3342.

Vittoz, N. M., Schmeichel, B., & Berridge, C. W. (2008). Hypocretin/orexin preferentially activates caudomedial ventral tegmental area dopamine neurons. *European Journal of Neuroscience*, *28*, 1629–1640.

Volkow, N. D., Ding, Y. S., Fowler, J. S., Wang, G. J., Logan, J., Gatley, S. J.,...Gur R. (1996).

Dopamine transporters decrease with age. *Journal of Nuclear Medicine, 37*, 554–559.

Voytek, B., Davis, M., Yago, E., Barcelo, F., Vogel, E. K., & Knight, R. T. (2010). Dynamic neuroplasticity after human prefrontal cortex damage. *Neuron, 68*, 401–408.

Wager, T. D. & Smith, E. E. (2003). Neuroimaging and working memory: A metaanalysis. *Cognitive, Affective, and Behavioral Neuroscience, 3*, 255–274.

Wagner, A. D., Maril, A., Bjork, R. A., & Schacter, D. L. (2001). Prefrontal contributions to executive control: fMRI evidence for functional distinctions within lateral Prefrontal cortex. *NeuroImage, 14*, 1337–1347.

Walker, M. P., Ayre, G. A., Cummings, J. L., Wesnes, K., McKeith, I. G., O'Brien, J. T., & Ballard, C. G. (2000). Quantifying fluctuation in dementia with Lewy bodies, Alzheimer's disease, and vascular dementia. *Neurology, 54*, 1616–1625.

Walton, M. E., Devlin, J. T., & Rushworth, M. F. (2004). Interactions between decision making and performance monitoring within prefrontal cortex. *Nature neuroscience, 7*(11), 1259–1265.

Wang, M., Gamo, N. J., Yang, Y., Jin, L. E., Wang, X. J., Laubach, M.,...Arnsten, A. F. (2011). Neuronal basis of age-related working memory decline. *Nature, 476*, 210–213.

Weintraub, D., & Stern, M. B. (2005). Psychiatric complications in Parkinson disease. *American Journal of Geriatric Psychiatry, 13*, 844–851.

West, R. L. (1996). An application of prefrontal cortex function theory to cognitive aging. *Psychological Bulletin, 120*, 272–292.

Whyte, J., Hart, T., Vaccaro, M., Grieb-Neff, P., Risser, A., Polansky, M., & Coslett, H. B. (2004). Effects of methylphenidate on attention deficits after traumatic brain injury: A multidimensional, randomized, controlled trial. *American Journal of Physical Medicine and Rehabilitation, 83*, 401–420.

Wickelgren, I. (1997). Getting the brain's attention. *Science, 278*, 35–37.

Wilens, T. E., Biederman, J., Spencer, T. J., & Prince, J. (1995). Pharmacotherapy of adult attention deficit/hyperactivity disorder: A review. *Journal of Clinical Psychopharmacology, 15*, 270–279.

Williams, G. V., & Goldman-Rakic, P. S. (1995). Modulation of memory fields by dopamine D1 receptors in prefrontal cortex. *Nature, 376*, 572–575.

Wilson, B., Alderman, N., Burgess, P., Emsile, H., & Evans, J. (1996). *Behavioral assessment of the dysexecutive syndrome*. Suffolk, UK: Thames Valley Test Company.

Wilson, F. A. W., & O'Scalaidhe, S. P. (1993). Dissociation of object and spatial processing domains in primate prefrontal cortex. *Science, 260*, 1955–1958.

Woods, S. P., & Troster, A. I. (2003). Prodromal frontal/executive dysfunction predicts incident dementia in Parkinson's disease. *Journal of the International Neuropsychology Society, 9*, 17–24.

Wozniak, R. H., & Jackson, J. H. (1999). *Evolution and dissolution of the nervous system. Classics in psychology, 1855-1941: Historical essays*. London, UK: Thoemes Continuum.

Yeo, B. T., Krienen, F. M., Sepulcre, J., Sabuncu, M. R., Lashkari, D., Hollinshead, M.,...Buckner, R. L. (2011). The organization of the human cerebral cortex estimated by intrinsic functional connectivity. *Journal of Neurophysiology, 106*, 1125–1165.

Yerkes, R. M., & Dodson, J. D. (1908). The relation of strength of stimulus to rapidly of habit-formation. *Journal of Comparative Neurology and Psychology, 18*, 459–482.

Yesavage, J. A., Friedman, L., Ashford, J. W., Kraemer, H. C., Mumenthaler, M. S., Noda, A., & Hoblyn, J. (2008). Acetylcholinesterase inhibitor in combination with cognitive training in older adults. *Journal of Gerontology B: Psychological Sciences and Social Sciences, 63*, 288–294.

Yoshida, W., & Ishii, S. (2006). Resolution of uncertainty in prefrontal cortex. *Neuron, 50*, 781–789.

Zaghloul, K. A., Blanco, J. A., Weidemann, C. T., McGill, K., Jaggi, J. L., Baltuch, G. H., & Kahana, M. J. (2009). Human substantia nigra neurons encode unexpected financial rewards. *Science, 323*, 1496–1499.

Zanto, T. P., & Gazzaley, A. (2009). Neural suppression of irrelevant information underlies optimal working memory performance. *Journal of Neuroscience, 29*, 3059–3066.

Zgaljardic, D. J., Borod, J. C., Foldi, N. S., & Mattis, P. (2003). A review of the cognitive and behavioral sequelae of Parkinson's disease: Relationship to frontostriatal circuitry. *Cognitive and Behavioral Neurology, 16*, 193–210.

Zhang, L., Plotkin, R. C., Wang, G., Sandel, M. E., & Lee, S. (2004). Cholinergic augmentation with donepezil enhances recovery in short-term memory and sustained attention after traumatic brain injury. *Archives of Physical Medicine and Rehabilitation, 85*, 1050–1055.

4

Memory Systems in Dementia

Andrew E. Budson

Memory problems are the most common issue that patients and families mention when coming to see a clinician for what turns out to be dementia. Memory dysfunction can be due to almost any type of neurodegenerative disease, as well as by a diverse group of disorders, including strokes, tumors, head trauma, hypoxia, cardiac surgery, malnutrition, attention-deficit/hyperactivity disorder, depression, anxiety, and medication effects (Budson & Solomon, 2011; Mesulam, 2000; Newman, Carpenter, Varma, & Just, 2003). Memory function can also be altered by normal aging. Although once thought to be a simple concept, we now consider memory to be a collection of cognitive processes that are subserved by several major neural systems. Memory research, which began with neuropsychological studies of patients with focal brain lesions using pencil and paper and now relies on sophisticated neuroscientific methods such as positron emission tomography, functional magnetic resonance imaging, and event-related potentials, has provided the rationale for a more refined and improved classification system (Schacter, Wagner, & Buckner, 2000). In this chapter a number of different types of memory will be reviewed, including the important anatomical structures for each and the major neurological disorders that disrupt them (Tables 4.1 and 4.2).

A greater understanding of these memory systems will aid clinicians in their diagnosis and treatment of the memory disorders of their patients. Accurate diagnosis will become more important as new therapeutic interventions for underlying causes of memory impairment or dementia are developed.

A memory system can be thought of as a mechanism by which the brain processes information so that it is available for use at a later time (Schacter & Tulving, 1994). Some systems are associated with conscious awareness (explicit) and can be recalled verbally (declarative), whereas others are typically unconscious (implicit) and are instead expressed by a change in behavior (nondeclarative; Squire, 1992). Memory can also be categorized in other ways, such as whether the material to be remembered is verbal (Wagner et al., 1998) or visual (Ally, 2012; Brewer, Zhao, Desmond, Glover, & Gabrieli, 1998).

Episodic Memory

Episodic memory is the explicit and declarative memory system used to remember a particular episode of life, such as sharing a meal with a friend on a specific date. This memory system is dependent upon the medial

TABLE 4.1 Selected Memory Systems

Memory System	Examples	Awareness	Length of Storage	Major Anatomical Structures
Episodic memory	Remembering a short story, what you had for dinner last night, and what you did on your last birthday	Explicit Declarative	Minutes to years	Medial temporal lobe, anterior thalamic nucleus, mamillary body, fornix, prefrontal cortex
Semantic memory	Knowing who was the first President of the United States, the color of a lion, and how a fork and comb are different	Explicit Declarative	Minutes to years	Inferior lateral temporal lobes
Autonomic simple classical conditioning	Pavlov's dog; a fear response	Implicit Nondeclarative	Minutes to years	Amygdala and basolateral limbic system
Motoric simple classical conditioning	Eye-blink conditioning	Implicit Nondeclarative	Minutes to months	Cerebellum
Procedural memory	Driving a standard transmission car, and learning the sequence of numbers on a touch-tone phone without trying	Implicit Nondeclarative	Minutes to years	Basal ganglia, cerebellum, supplementary motor area
Perceptual priming	Word-stem completion: octopus→oct___	Implicit Nondeclarative	Minutes to days	Cortical sensory association areas (e.g., extrastriate visual cortex for visual perceptual priming)
Conceptual priming	Word-stem completion: sea creatures→oct___	Implicit Nondeclarative	Minutes to days	Inferior prefrontal cortex
Working memory	Phonological: keeping a phone number "in your head" before dialing Spatial: mentally following a route, or rotating an object in your mind	Explicit Declarative	Seconds to minutes; information actively rehearsed or manipulated	Phonological: prefrontal cortex, Broca's area, Wernike's area. Spatial: Prefrontal cortex, visual association areas

TABLE 4.2 Selective Memory System Disruptions in Common Clinical Disorders

Disease	Episodic Memory	Semantic Memory	Simple Classical Conditioning	Procedural Memory	Priming	Working Memory
Alzheimer's disease	+++	++	+	−	−perceptual +conceptual	++
Frontotemporal dementia	++	++	?	−	?	+++
Semantic dementia	+	+++	?	?	?	−
Lewy body dementia	++	?	?	?	?	++
Stroke and vascular dementia	+	+	±	+	±	++
Parkinson's disease	+	+	−	+++	−	++
Huntington's disease	+	+	−	+++	−	+++
Progressive supranuclear palsy	+	+	?	−++	?	+++
Korsakoff syndrome	+++	−	+	−	±	±
Multiple sclerosis	+	±	±	?	−	++
Transient global amnesia	+++	±	?	−	−	−
Hypoxic-ischaemic injury	++	−	−	−	±	±
Head trauma	+	+	±	±	?	++
Tumors	±	±	±	±	±	±
Depression	+	±	?	++	?	±
Anxiety	+	−	±	−	±	±
Obsessive-compulsive disorder	+	−	±	++	±	++
Attention-deficit/ hyperactivity disorder	−	−	−	?	±	+

+++, Early and severe impairment; ++, moderate impairment; +, mild impairment; ±, occasional impairment or impairment in some studies but not others; −, no significant impairment; ?, unknown.

temporal lobes (including the hippocampus); episodic memory has been largely defined by what patients with medial temporal lobe lesions cannot remember relative to healthy individuals. Other critical structures in the episodic memory system (some of which are associated with a circuit described by Papez in 1937) include the basal forebrain with the medial septum and diagonal band of Broca's area, the retrosplenial cortex, the presubiculum, the fornix, mammillary bodies, the mammillothalamic tract, and the anterior nucleus of the thalamus (Fig. 4.1) (Mesulam, 2000). A lesion in any one of these structures may cause dysfunction of the episodic memory system.

Memory loss due to dysfunction of the episodic memory system generally follows a pattern known as Ribot's law. Starting with the onset of the injury to the brain, there is greatest disruption in the ability to learn new information (anterograde amnesia), moderate disruption in the ability to recall recently learned information (retrograde amnesia), and the ability to recall remotely learned information is generally intact (Fig. 4.2; Ribot, 1881).

The core of the episodic memory system is the hippocampus and other regions of the medial temporal lobe. It is worth examining these structures more closely. The medial temporal lobes are neuroanatomically complex structures with multiple regions and subregions. Figure 4.3 shows the medial temporal lobe structures, including the parahippocampal gyrus, presubiculum, subiculum,

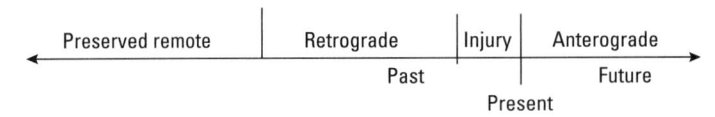

Figure 4.2 Ribot's law.

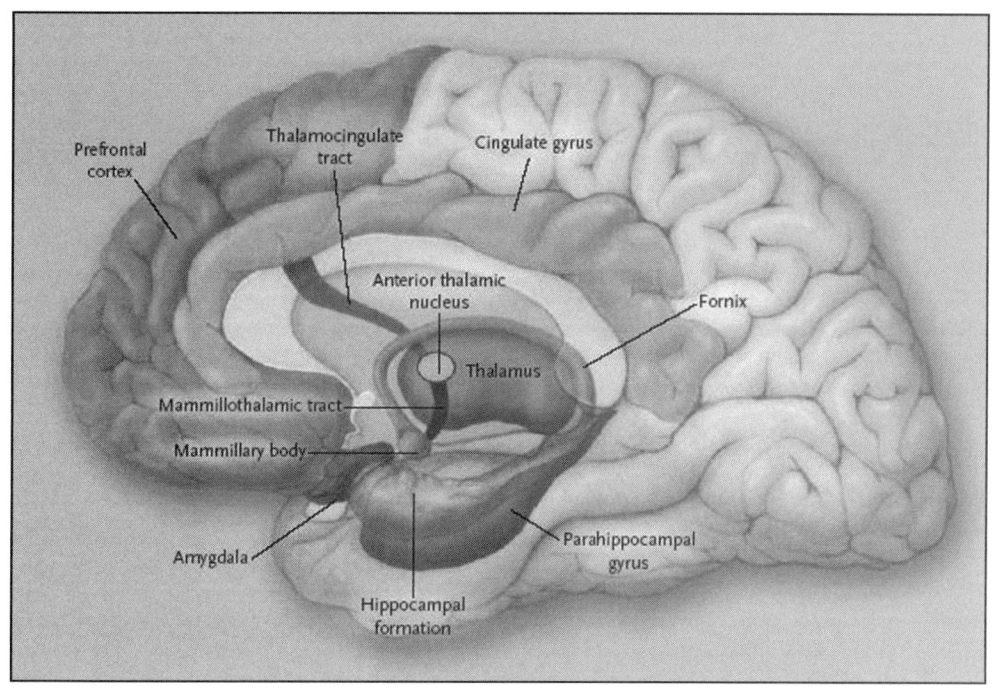

Figure 4.1 Episodic memory. The medial temporal lobes, including the hippocampus and parahippocampus, form the core of the episodic memory system. Other brain regions are also necessary for episodic memory to function correctly. In addition to being involved in episodic memory, the amygdala is also important for the autonomic conditioning. (From Budson and Price, 2005; permission granted by the *New England Journal of Medicine*)

and hippocampus proper, including its subregions.

Although exactly how the medial temporal lobes store and retrieve memories is still an active area of research, our current understanding from cognitive neuroscience is as follows. An individual experiences an episode of her life, such as having lunch that day. The cortically distributed patterns of neural activity representing the sights, sounds, smells, tastes, emotions, and thoughts during that episode are transferred first to the parahippocampal region (including perirhinal and parahippocampal cortex), then to the entorhinal cortex, and then to the hippocampus proper, specifically the dentate gyrus, where the disparate threads of experience are bound together as a single memory (Fig. 4.4) (Wolosin, Zeithamova, & Preston, 2012). This bound information is then transferred to the CA3 region, where it is further processed (Fig. 4.5). It is in this CA3 region where the critically important hippocampal index is assigned, allowing the memory to be stored in a unique way so that it can later be recalled.

Typically memories are retrieved when a cue from the environment matches a part of the stored memory. Continuing our breakfast example, years later the individual might now bite into a little cookie that tastes remarkably like the one that she had previously at lunch. This sensory cue is transferred from the cortex to the parahippocampal region and to the hippocampus (Fig. 4.4). After the cue is transferred from the entorhinal cortex, it goes directly to the CA3 region, where the original hippocampal index is retrieved (Fig. 4.6). The hippocampal index may be used to retrieve much of the original pattern of the neural activity representing the original episode stored in memory. This retrieved pattern of activity may then be transferred to the CA1 region, the subiculum, the entorhinal cortex, and then back out to the cortex—actively re-creating all of sights, sounds, smells, tastes, emotions, and thoughts of the original memory episode (Fig. 4.4).

The hippocampus remains critical for memory retrieval until a process known as *consolidation* occurs. Much research still

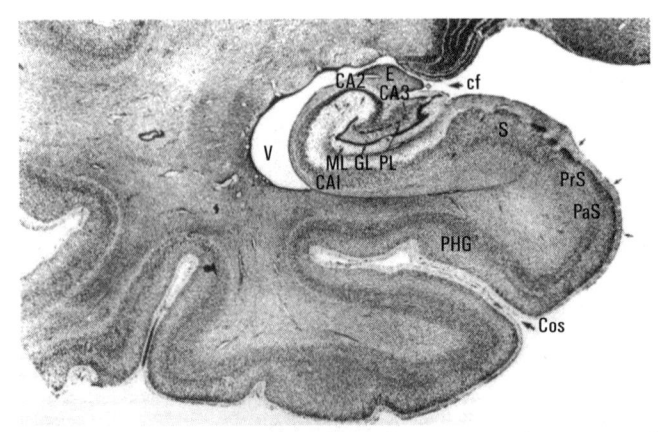

Figure 4.3 Detailed anatomy of the medial temporal lobe. PHG, parahippocampal gyrus; Pr, presubiculum; v, ventricle; S, subiculum. CA1, CA2, and CA3 are subregions of the hippocampus, and ML, GL, and PL are different regions of the dentate gyrus of the hippocampus. (From Martin JH. *Neuroanatomy: Text and Atlas*. New York, NY.: Elsevier, 1989, p. 391; permission granted by *Elsevier*)

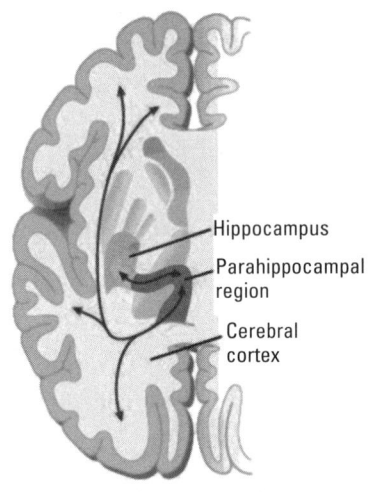

Figure 4.4 Areas of the cerebral cortex, including sensory areas, are connected bidirectionally to the parahippocampal region, which is in turn bidirectionally connected to the hippocampus. (From Eichenbaum, 1997; permission granted by *Science* Magazine)

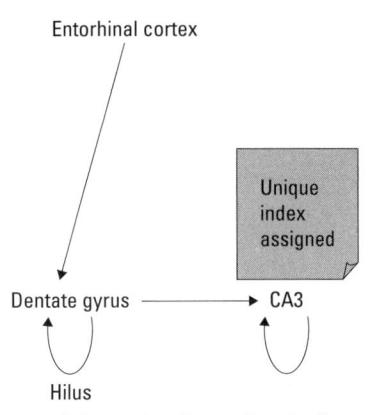

Figure 4.5 Schematic of encoding in the medial temporal lobe.

needs to be done to better understand consolidation, but one thought is that once a memory is consolidated the distributed pattern of cortical neural activity is directly linked together, such that when a cue is encountered, the memory may be retrieved directly from cortical-cortical connections, without the need for the hippocampus. And although there are many details that need to be learned, there are significant data to suggest that sleep is critical for consolidation to occur (Aly & Moscovitch, 2010; Potkin & Bunney, 2012; Ruch et al., 2012; Stickgold, 2005, 2006; Wamsley & Stickgold, 2011).

The CA3 region of the hippocampus, the region in which the hippocampal index is formed and where pattern matching of cues and memories occurs, is one of the most critical regions. Although it is not known exactly how the CA3 region is involved in these activities, a number of models using neural networks have been proposed. A simplified example of such a model will show how an individual can find his car when he parks in a parking garage over three successive days—and also why it is sometimes difficult for an individual to find his car. In

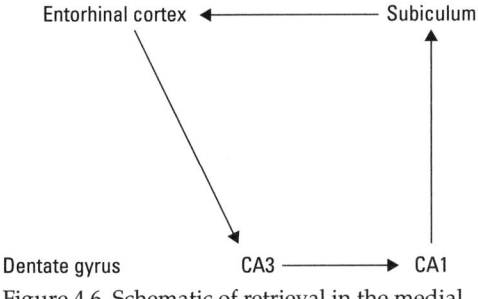

Figure 4.6 Schematic of retrieval in the medial temporal lobe.

this imaginary parking garage there are two areas, green and yellow, and two levels, first and second. Two affective states, happy and sad, are also shown to represent not only emotions but other contextual details that may differ between days. On the first day the car is parked in the green area, on the first floor, and it was a happy day. From this distributed pattern of neural activity a hippocampal index can be formed that helps one remember that the car was parked in the green area, on the first floor, and halfway down the aisle on the left (Fig. 4.7A). On the second day the car is parked in the yellow area, on the second floor, and it was a sad day. Nonetheless, this distinct pattern of neural activity allows a unique hippocampal index to form that enables one to remember that the car was parked in the yellow area, on the second floor, and halfway down the aisle on the right (Fig. 4.7B). On the third day the car is also parked in the yellow area, on the second floor, and it again was a sad day (Fig. 4.7C). Although one might wish that a hippocampal index will form to enable one to remember that the car was parked in the in the yellow area, on the second floor,

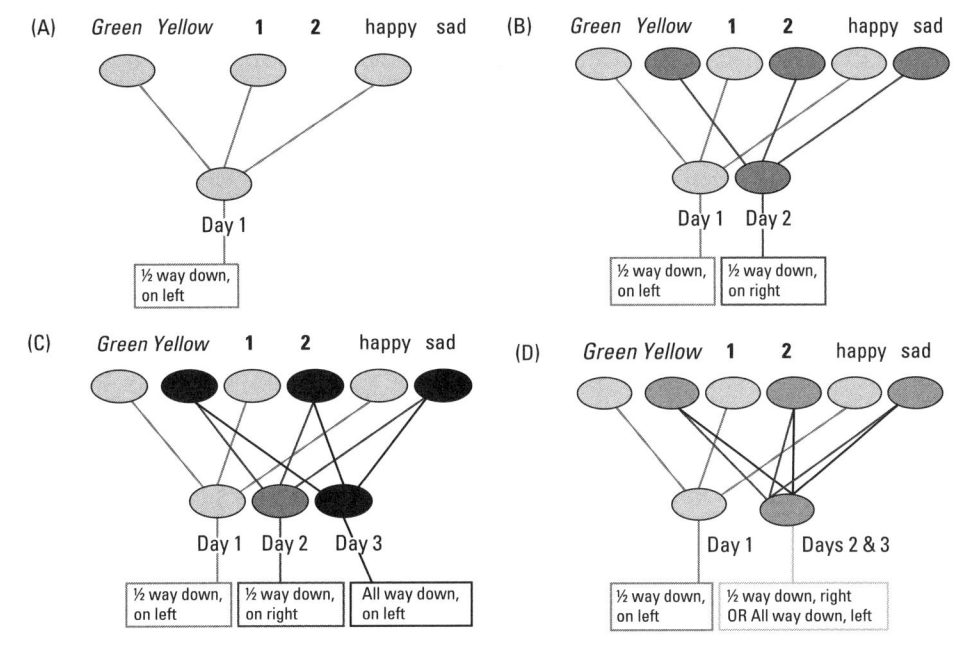

Figure 4.7 A neural network model of episodic memory. (A) On the first day, a hippocampal index helps one remember that the car is parked in the Green area, on the 1st floor, and it was a happy day. (B) On the second day, a unique hippocampal index indicates that the car is parked in the Yellow area, on the 2nd floor, and it was a sad day. (C) On the third day, the car is also parked in the Yellow area, on the 2nd floor, and it again was a sad day. (D) There is a single hippocampal index that forms for both days two and three. This hippocampal index is strengthened for the common aspects of the two memories: parking in the Yellow area, on the 2nd floor. But this index also contains divergent aspects of the memory: half-way down the aisle on the right and all the way down the aisle on the left. Thus, on day three it is easy to remember that the car is parked in the Yellow area on the 2nd floor, but it is difficult to remember if it is parked half-way down the aisle on the right or all the way down the aisle on the left.

and all the way down the aisle on the left, there is a problem. When there are completely overlapping patterns of neural activity, a separate hippocampal index cannot form. Instead, there is a single hippocampal index that forms for both days two and three (Fig. 4.7D). This hippocampal index is strengthened for the common aspects of the two memories: parking in the yellow area, on the second floor. But this index also contains divergent aspects of the memory: halfway down the aisle on the right and all the way down the aisle on the left. Thus, on day three it is easy to remember that the car is parked in the yellow area on the second floor, but it is difficult to remember whether it is parked halfway down the aisle on the right or all the way down the aisle on the left.

In addition to the medial temporal lobes and Papez's circuit, the frontal lobes are also important for episodic memory (Ally, McKeever, Waring, & Budson, 2009; Fletcher & Henson, 2001; Simons & Spiers, 2003). Whereas the medial temporal lobes are critical for the retention of information, the frontal lobes are important for the acquisition, registration, or encoding of information (Wagner et al., 1998); the retrieval of information without contextual and other cues (Petrides, 2002); the recollection of the source of information (Johnson, Kounios, & Nolde, 1997); and the assessment of the temporal sequence and recency of events (Kopelman, Stanhope, & Kingsley, 1997). It is also notable that the left medial temporal and left frontal lobes are most active when a person is learning words (Wagner et al., 1998), and that the right medial temporal and right frontal lobes are most active when learning visual scenes (Brewer et al., 1998).

In episodic memory the frontal lobes enable the individual to focus attention on the information to be remembered and to engage the medial temporal lobes. Dysfunction of the frontal lobes may cause a number of memory problems, including distortions of episodic memory and false memories, such as when information becomes associated with the wrong context (Johnson, O'Connor, & Cantor, 1997) or incorrect specific details (Budson et al., 2002). Extreme memory distortions are often synonymous with confabulations: "Memories" are created to be consistent with current information (Johnson, O'Connor, & Cantor, 1997), such as

TABLE 4.3 A Filing Analogy of Episodic Memory

Brain Structure	Analogy
Frontal lobes	File clerk
Medial temporal lobes	Recent memory files
Other cortical regions	Remote memory files

"remembering" that someone broke into the house and rearranged household items.

A useful analogy can help conceptualize the dysfunction in episodic memory that occurs due to damage to the medial temporal lobes (and Papez's circuit) versus damage to the frontal lobes (Budson & Price, 2002, 2005) (Table 4.3). The frontal lobes are the "file clerk" of the episodic memory system, the medial temporal lobes are the "recent memory file cabinet," and other cortical regions are the "remote memory file cabinet" (Fig. 4.8). Thus, if the frontal lobes are impaired, it is difficult—but not impossible—to get information in and out of storage. Placing new information into storage may require stronger encoding, and retrieving information from storage may require stronger cues from the environment. When the frontal lobes are impaired, the information stored in memory may also be distorted due to "improper filing" that leads to an inaccurate source, context, or sequence. If the medial temporal lobes are impaired, on the other hand, it may be impossible for recent information to be stored. This will often lead to the patient asking for the same information again and again—perhaps a dozen times in an hour. Older information that has been consolidated over months to years is likely stored in other cortical regions and will therefore be available for retrieval even when the medial temporal lobes or Papez's circuit are damaged. To illustrate this analogy, we can compare the episodic memory dysfunction attributable to depression versus Alzheimer's disease. Patients with depression have a dysfunctional "file clerk," whereas patients with Alzheimer's disease have a dysfunctional "recent memory file cabinet."

Recent evidence has suggested that the parietal lobes also play an important role in episodic memory (Dulas & Duarte, 2013). In fact, in functional imaging studies the parietal lobes are more frequently associated

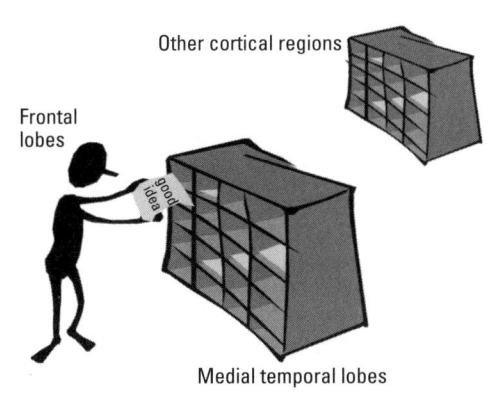

Figure 4.8 Semantic, procedural, and working memory. The inferolateral temporal lobes are important in the naming and categorization tasks by which semantic memory is typically assessed. However, in the broadest sense, semantic memory may reside in multiple and diverse cortical areas that are related to various types of knowledge. The basal ganglia, cerebellum, and supplementary motor area are critical for procedural memory. The prefrontal cortex is active in virtually all working memory tasks; other cortical and subcortical brain regions will also be active, depending on the type and complexity of the working memory task. In addition to being involved in procedural memory, the cerebellum is also important for the motoric conditioning. (From Budson and Price; permission granted by the *New England Journal of Medicine*)

with successful memory retrieval than either the frontal or medial temporal lobes (Simons et al., 2008). Despite this ubiquitous activation, the precise role of the parietal lobes in memory is not clear. Theories include attention to memory in both top-down and bottom-up roles (Cabeza, 2008), working memory's contribution to episodic memory (Berryhill & Olson, 2008), its role in retrieval and recollection (Davidson et al., 2008; Vilberg & Rugg, 2008, 2009), and the subjective memorial experience (Ally et al., 2008a; Simons, Peers, Mazuz, Berryhill, & Olson, 2010).

Because the hippocampus and other medial temporal lobe structures are the earliest and most severely affected brain regions in Alzheimer's disease, episodic memory—and in particular the file cabinet component of episodic memory—is the earliest and most impaired cognitive function. Common symptoms include asking the same questions repeatedly, repeating the same stories, forgetting appointments, and leaving the stove on. Following Ribot's law, patients with Alzheimer's disease show *anterograde amnesia* or difficulty learning new information. They also show *retrograde amnesia* or difficulty retrieving previously learned information. However, the patients typically demonstrate preserved memory for remote information. Thus, a patient may report, "I've got short-term memory problems—I cannot remember what I did yesterday but I can still remember things from 30 years ago." Not understanding that this pattern is suggestive of the memory impairment common in Alzheimer's disease, family members may report that they feel confident that whatever the patient's problem is, that "it isn't Alzheimer's disease," because the patient can still remember what happened many years ago.

Another hallmark of the episodic memory impairment in Alzheimer's disease is that memory is impaired even when the learning or encoding of information is maximized by multiple rehearsals, and after retrieval demands have been minimized with the use of a multiple-choice recognition test. In other words, even when patients appear to have successfully learned new information by repeating it back over several learning trials, they are often unable to recognize this information on a multiple-choice test. This type of memory loss is often referred to as a "rapid rate of forgetting," although whether the information has been truly learned or not in the first place has been a matter of debate (e.g., Budson et al., 2007).

In addition to rapid forgetting, patients with Alzheimer's disease also experience distortions of memory and false memories. These distortions may include falsely remembering that they have already turned off the stove or taken their medications, leading patients to neglect performing these tasks. More dramatic distortions of memory may occur when patients substitute one person in a memory for another, combine two memories together, or think that an event that happened long ago occurred recently. Sometimes a false memory can be confused with a psychotic delusion or hallucination. For example, a patient may claim to have recently seen and spoken with a long-deceased family member. This patient is much more likely to be suffering from a memory distortion or a false memory than a true hallucination. The same is true for the patient who claims that people are breaking into the house and moving around things. That these symptoms likely represent memory distortions rather than true hallucinations or delusions has implications when it comes time for treatment; that is, memory distortions are best treated with memory-enhancing medications (such as cholinesterase inhibitors) rather than antipsychotic medications.

Although not as impaired as medial temporal lobes, the frontal lobes are involved in both Alzheimer's disease and mild cognitive impairment (Dickerson et al., 2009; Koivunen et al., 2012). Frontal lobe dysfunction may be one reason that patients with Alzheimer's disease experience memory distortions and false memories. That they show frontal lobe dysfunction also means that, in addition to a major impairment with their "file cabinet," patients with Alzheimer's disease also show milder but definite impairment with their "file clerk" as well. Additionally, patients with Alzheimer's disease have major pathology in parietal cortex, and this pathology may occur quite early in the disease (McKee et al., 2006). Thus, although the medial temporal lobe pathology is most relevant in the majority, patients with Alzheimer's disease have multiple components impaired in their episodic memory system.

As vascular dementia is dementia due to multiple strokes, whether a patient experiences episodic memory dysfunction and of what quality depends upon the size, number, and location of the cerebrovascular disease. However, the most common type of vascular dementia is that due to small vessel ischemic disease. Because small vessel ischemic disease has a predilection for the subcortical white matter, and because most of the white matter in the brain is carrying neural signals going to or from the frontal lobes, patients with vascular dementia experience a "frontal" memory disorder. In other words, because their frontal lobes are not working (or are not properly connected to the rest of the brain), they show impairment in the "file clerk" component of episodic memory. Consequently encoding is often impaired, as is free recall, whereas relative preservation is typically seen when tasks that assist in retrieval, such as cued recall and recognition, are used.

Patients with frontotemporal dementia often show no impairment in episodic memory until late in the disease. If they do demonstrate early episodic memory impairment, it is generally that of a frontal memory disorder, similar to that of a patient with vascular dementia. Many other dementias also affect the frontal lobes and thus may also lead to a frontal episodic memory disorder. These dementias include progressive supranuclear palsy, corticobasal degeneration, multiple system atrophy, and normal pressure hydrocephalus.

Semantic Memory

Semantic memory refers to our store of conceptual and factual knowledge that is not related to any specific memory, such as the color of broccoli or what a fork is used for. Like episodic memory, semantic memory is an explicit and declarative memory. Evidence that semantic memory and episodic memory are separate memory systems has come from both neuroimaging studies (Schacter et al., 2000) and the fact that previously acquired semantic memory is spared in patients who have severe impairment of the episodic memory system, such as with disruption of Papez's circuit or surgical removal of the medial temporal lobes (Corkin, 1984).

In its broadest sense, semantic memory includes all our knowledge of the world not related to any specific episodic memory. It could therefore be argued that semantic memory resides in multiple cortical areas throughout the brain. For example, there is evidence that visual images are stored in nearby visual association areas (Vaidya, Zhao, Desmond, & Gabrieli, 2002). A more restrictive view of semantic memory justified in light of the naming and categorization tasks by which it is usually tested, however, localizes semantic memory to the inferolateral temporal lobes (Fig. 4.9; Damasio, Grabowski, Tranel, Hichwa, & Damasio, 1996; Perani et al., 1999).

The most common clinical disorder disrupting semantic memory is Alzheimer's disease (Gardini et al., 2013). This disruption may be due to pathology in the inferolateral temporal lobes (Price & Morris, 1999) or to pathology

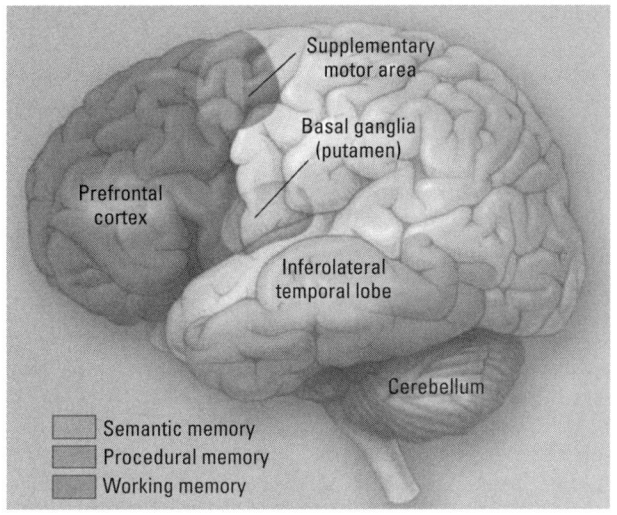

Figure 4.9 Semantic, Procedural, and Working Memory. The inferolateral temporal lobes are important in the naming and categorization tasks by which semantic memory is typically assessed. However, in the broadest sense, semantic memory may reside in multiple and diverse cortical areas that are related to various types of knowledge. The basal ganglia, cerebellum, and supplementary motor area are critical for procedural memory. The prefrontal cortex is active in virtually all working memory tasks; other cortical and subcortical brain regions will also be active, depending on the type and complexity of the working memory task. In addition to being involved in procedural memory, the cerebellum is also important for the motoric conditioning. (From Budson and Price, 2005; permission granted by the *New England Journal of Medicine*.) (See color plate section)

in frontal cortex (Lidstrom et al., 1998), leading to poor activation and retrieval of semantic information (Balota, Watson, Duchek, & Ferraro, 1999). Supporting the idea that two separate memory systems are impaired in Alzheimer's disease, episodic and semantic memory decline independently of each other in this disorder (Green & Hodges, 1996).

Almost any disorder that can disrupt the inferolateral temporal lobes may cause impairment of semantic memory, including traumatic brain injury, stroke, surgical lesions, encephalitis, and tumors (Table 4.2). Patients with semantic dementia (the temporal variant of frontotemporal dementia) exhibit deficits in all functions of semantic memory, such as naming, single-word comprehension, and impaired general knowledge (such as the color of common items) (Hoffman, Meteyard, & Patterson, 2012). Other aspects of cognition, however, are relatively preserved, including components of speech, perceptual and nonverbal problem-solving skills, and episodic memory (Hodges, 2001).

Although naming difficulties (particularly with proper nouns) are common in healthy older adults, naming difficulties may also be a sign of a disorder of semantic memory. When a disorder of semantic memory is suspected, the evaluation should include the same components as the workup for episodic memory disorders. One of the first aspects of the history and cognitive examination that should be ascertained is whether the problem is solely one of difficulty in recalling people's names and other proper nouns (common in healthy older adults) or to a true loss of semantic information. Patients with mild dysfunction of semantic memory may show only reduced generation of words in a semantic category (e.g., the number of grocery items that can be generated in 1 minute), whereas patients with a more severe impairment of semantic memory usually show a two-way naming deficit: They are unable to name an item when it is described, and they are also unable to describe an item when it is named. General knowledge is also impoverished in these more severely affected patients. Treatment will depend upon the specific disorder identified.

Simple Classical Conditioning

Simple classical conditioning involves the pairing of two stimuli: an unconditioned stimulus and a conditioned stimulus. When paired together repeatedly, the response can then be elicited by the conditioned stimulus alone (Table 4.1). Think of the famous case of Pavlov's dog: the meat (the unconditioned stimulus) is paired with the bell (the conditioned stimulus). After a number of pairings, the response—salivation—is elicited by the bell (the conditioned stimulus) alone (Pavlov, 1927). This form of memory is nondeclarative and implicit, because conscious awareness (although often present) is not necessary for the learning to take place. Two types of conditioning are that of an *autonomic conditioned response* (such as a fear response) and a *motoric conditioned response* (such as an eyeblink). The amygdala, related structures, and connections in the basolateral limbic system (including the dorsomedial thalamic nuclei, subcallosal area, and the stria terminalis) are important for autonomic conditioning (Fig. 4.1; Markowitsch, 1995). In motoric conditioning, the cerebellum appears to play the most important role (Fig. 4.9; Dimitrova et al., 2002; Solomon, Stowe, & Pendlbeury, 1989).

Although disruption of this form of memory rarely comes to clinical attention, patients have been described with selective impairment of simple classical conditioning. In one study, three patients are reported. The first, who had selective bilateral amygdala damage, had no difficulty with episodic memory (remembering a new list of items) but could not acquire a classical conditioning autonomic response. The second, who had selective bilateral hippocampal damage, showed episodic memory dysfunction (being unable to remember the list of items) but did acquire the classical conditioning. The third, who had bilateral damage to both amygdala and hippocampi, showed both impairment in episodic memory and did not acquire the classical conditioning (Bechara et al., 1995). Other patients who have disruption of the amygdala, thalamus, or cerebellum may also show impairments of one or more types of simple classical conditioning, including those with Alzheimer's disease (impaired autonomic conditioning due primarily to pathology in amygdala), frontotemporal dementia (Hoefer et al., 2008), and those with damage to the cerebellum or its connections (impaired motor conditioning; Heindel, Salmon, Shults, Walicke, & Butters, 1989).

Procedural Memory

Procedural memory refers to the ability to learn cognitive and behavioral skills and algorithms that operate at an automatic, unconscious level. Procedural memory is nondeclarative and implicit. Examples include learning to ride a bike or play the piano (Table 4.1). Because procedural memory is spared in patients who have severe deficits of the episodic memory system (such as those who have undergone surgical removal of the medial temporal lobes), it is clear that the procedural memory system is separate and distinct from the episodic memory system (Corkin, 1984; Heindel et al., 1989).

Functional imaging research has shown that a number of brain regions involved in procedural memory become active as a new task is learned, including the supplementary motor area, basal ganglia, and cerebellum (Fig. 4.9; Daselaar, Rombouts, Veltman, Raaijmakers, & Jonker, 2003). Convergent evidence comes from studies of patients with damage to the basal ganglia or cerebellum who show impairment in learning procedural skills (Exner, 2002). Because the basal ganglia and cerebellum are relatively spared in early Alzheimer's disease, despite their episodic memory deficit these patients show normal acquisition and maintenance of their procedural memory skills (Beaunieux et al., 2012). As in episodic memory, sleep is critical for consolidation of procedural memory (Holz et al., 2012).

Parkinson's disease is the most common disorder disrupting procedural memory. Patients in the early stages of Huntington's disease and olivopontocerebellar degeneration also show impaired procedural memory while performing nearly normally on episodic memory tests (Holl, Wilkinson, Tabrizi, Painold, & Jahanshahi, 2012; Heindel et al., 1989; Salmon, Lineweaver, & Heindel, 1998). Other causes of damage to the basal ganglia or cerebellum, including tumors, strokes, and hemorrhages, may also disrupt procedural memory. Patients with major depression also show impairment in procedural memory tasks, perhaps because depression involves dysfunction of the basal ganglia (Sabe Jason, Juejati, Leiguarda, & Starkstein, 1995).

Disruption of procedural memory should be suspected when patients show evidence of either substantial difficulties in learning new skills (compared to their baseline) or the loss of previously learned skills. For example, patients may lose the ability to perform automatic, skilled movements, such as writing, swinging a tennis racket, or playing a musical instrument. Although these patients may be able to relearn the fundamentals of these skills, explicit thinking becomes required for their performance. As a result, patients with damage to the procedural memory system lose the automatic, effortlessness of simple motor tasks that healthy individuals take for granted. The evaluation of disorders of procedural memory is similar to that of disorders of episodic memory; treatment depends upon the specific disease process. Lastly, it is worth noting that patients whose episodic memory has been devastated by a static disorder, such as encephalitis, have had successful rehabilitation by using procedural memory (and other nondeclarative forms of memory) to learn new skills (Glisky & Schacter, 1989).

Priming

Priming occurs when a prior encounter with a particular item changes the response to the current item (Table 4.1). Because this phenomenon occurs even if the individual does not consciously remember encountering the prior item, priming is another example of an implicit and nondeclarative form of memory. Priming is often divided into *perceptual priming*, which is modality specific (e.g., auditory, visual) and does not benefit from elaborate encoding at study, versus *conceptual priming*, which is not modality specific and shows enhancement with increased encoding.

Perceptual priming depends upon a perceptual representation system, involved in processing information regarding the form and structure of items but not their meanings (Tulving & Schacter, 1990). Converging evidence suggests that posterior cortical regions involved in processing of sensory information are important for perceptual priming. A patient with bilateral occipital lobe lesions demonstrated normal episodic memory and conceptual priming while failing to show perceptual priming (Keane, Gabrieli, Mapstone, Johnson, & Corkin, 1995). Neuroimaging studies of visual perceptual priming using positron emission tomography and functional magnetic resonance imaging show changes in activation of visual peristriate cortex (Schacter & Buckner, 1998). By contrast, neuroimaging studies of conceptual priming typically show changes in left prefrontal regions (Schacter & Buckner, 1998). Most studies have shown that patients with early degenerative diseases that do not affect the sensory association cortices, such as Alzheimer's, Parkinson's, and Huntington's diseases, demonstrate normal perceptual priming (Koivisto, Portin, & Rinne, 1996). For conceptual priming, however, many (but not all) studies have found these groups to be impaired (Heindel et al., 1989; Millet, Le Goff, Bouisson, Dartigues, & Amieva, 2010).

Working Memory

Bringing together the traditional fields of attention, concentration, and short-term memory, working memory refers to the ability to temporarily maintain and manipulate information that one needs to keep in mind. Requiring active and conscious participation, working memory is an explicit and declarative memory system. Working memory has traditionally been divided into three components: one that processes phonologic information (e.g., keeping a phone number "in your head"), one that processes spatial information (e.g., mentally following a route), and an executive system that allocates attentional resources (Baddeley, 1998).

Studies have demonstrated that working memory involves a network of cortical and subcortical areas, which differ depending on the particular task (Borst & Anderson, 2013; Rowe, Toni, Josephs, Frackowiak, & Passingham, 2000). Participation of the prefrontal cortex, however, is involved in virtually all working memory tasks (Fig. 4.9;

Fletcher & Henson, 2001). The network of cortical and subcortical areas typically includes posterior brain regions (e.g., visual association areas) that are linked with prefrontal regions to form a circuit. Research suggests that spatial working memory tends to involve more regions on the right side, and phonologic working memory tends to involve more regions on the left side of the brain. Bilateral brain activation is observed, however, in more difficult working memory tasks, regardless of the nature of the material being processed (Newman et al., 2003). Additionally, an increase in the number of brain regions activated in prefrontal cortex is observed as the complexity of the task increases (Jaeggi et al., 2003).

Because working memory depends upon networks which include frontal and parietal cortical regions as well as subcortical structures, most neurodegenerative diseases impair working memory. Studies have demonstrated that working memory may be impaired in patients with Alzheimer's disease, Parkinson's disease, Huntington's disease, and dementia with Lewy bodies (Schneider et al., 2012), as well as less common disorders such as progressive supranuclear palsy (Table 4.2; Calderon et al., 2001; Gotham, Brown, & Marsden, 1988). In fact, even prior to the onset of clinical symptoms, Alzheimer's disease and vascular pathology can lead to impairment in working memory (Bennett, Wilson, Boyle, Buchman, & Schneider, 2012). In addition to these neurodegenerative diseases, almost any disease process that disrupts the frontal lobes or their connections to posterior cortical regions and subcortical structures can interfere with working memory. Such processes include tumors, strokes, multiple sclerosis, head injury, and others (Kubat-Silman, Dagenbach, & Absher, 2002; Sfagos et al., 2003). Because it involves the silent rehearsal of verbal information, almost any type of aphasia may impair phonologic working memory. Disorders that diminish attentional resources, including attention-deficit/hyperactivity disorder, obsessive-compulsive disorder, depression, and schizophrenia, can also impair working memory (Egeland et al., 2003; Klingberg, Forssberg, & Westerberg, 2002; Purcell, Maruff, Kyrios, & Pantelis, 1998).

Disorders of working memory may present in several different ways. Often the patient will exhibit an inability to concentrate or pay attention. Impairment in performing a new task with multistep instructions is frequently seen. Interestingly, a disorder of working memory may also present as a problem with episodic memory because information must first be "kept in mind" by working memory in order for episodic memory to encode it (Fletcher & Henson, 2001). Such cases will therefore show a primary impairment in encoding.

The evaluation of disorders of working memory is similar to that of disorders of episodic memory. Treatment depends upon the underlying cause. Stimulants, approved by the FDA for the treatment of attention-deficit/hyperactivity disorder (Mehta, Goodyer, & Sahakian, 2004), are often helpful in disorders of working memory.

Improving Memory in Dementia

Nonpharmacological treatments are invaluable and can often help improve and/or preserve daily function as much as medications. Almost all of us use some type of external system or device to enhance memory. Lists, calendars, date and address books, smart phones, and iPads can help patients with mild to moderate Alzheimer's disease in addition to healthy individuals. Participating in social activities has been shown to reduce apathy and improve mood, memory, and overall cognitive function. Other strategies that have been shown to improve memory include using habits, pictures, strategies, and participating in aerobic exercise.

Habit can compensate for poor memory. Although patients with Alzheimer's disease have great difficulty in remembering verbal instructions such as "Please remember to put your keys on the hall table," they can learn to place them there through habit as well as anyone. Learning through habit, sometimes called "muscle memory" and formally classified as procedural memory, is learning through doing. Because the brain regions involved in procedural memory, basal ganglia and cerebellum, are relatively spared by Alzheimer's disease, patients can learn to do tasks such as put their keys on the hall table by doing the action or activity repetitively.

It is said that a picture is worth a thousand words. Some of our research has shown that, although memory is enhanced by pictures relative to words for young adults, this effect of pictures is even greater for healthy older adults, greater still for patients with mild cognitive impairment, and is the greatest for patients with Alzheimer's disease (Embree et al., 2012). This enhancement of memory for pictures versus words in Alzheimer's disease is likely attributable to increased attention to pictures (over words), as well as the distinctiveness of pictures that makes them easier to remember. We also may process a picture once as an image and once as its meaning. Bottom line: Let the family know that instead of simply telling the patient that his granddaughter will be visiting today, show him her picture, and he will be more likely to remember.

Another study we conducted explored patients' memory for statements that they were told were true versus statements that they were told were false. We found that patients with Alzheimer's disease correctly remembered that the true statements were true 69% of the time, but they also incorrectly remembered that the false statements were true 59% of the time—more than half (Mitchell, Sullivan, Schacter, & Budson, 2006). This result means that if you tell a patient with Alzheimer's disease what not to do, the patient will be more likely to think that he should do it than if you never said anything at all. We therefore caution all of our families to only tell their loved ones what they should do, not what they should not do. It is one strategy that has been proven to work.

Conclusion

When patients come to the clinic because of cognitive impairment, the complaint from patients and families is typically that of memory loss. Understanding exactly which memory system is impaired will lead to a more accurate diagnosis of the patient's disorder. As more specific therapeutic strategies are developed for the treatment of diseases that cause memory dysfunction, this knowledge will become increasingly important (Budson & Solomon, 2011).

Acknowledgments

This work was supported by National Institute on Aging grant P30 AG13846. This material is also the result of work supported with resources and the use of facilities at the Veterans Affairs Boston Healthcare System, Boston, MA.

References

Ally, B. A. (2012). Using pictures and words to understand recognition memory deterioration in amnestic mild cognitive impairment and Alzheimer's disease: A review. *Current Neurology and Neuroscience Reports, 12*(6), 687–694.

Ally, B. A., McKeever, J. D., Waring, J. D., & Budson, A. E. (2009). Preserved frontal memorial processing for pictures in patients with mild cognitive impairment. *Neuropsychologia, 47*(10), 2044–2055.

Ally, B. A., Simons, J. S., McKeever, J. D., Peers, P. V., & Budson, A. E. (2008a). Parietal contributions to recollection: Electrophysiological evidence from aging and patients with parietal lesions. *Neuropsychologia, 46*(7), 1800–1812.

Aly, M., & Moscovitch, M. (2010). The effects of sleep on episodic memory in older and younger adults. *Memory, 18*(3), 327–334.

Baddeley, A. D. (1998). Recent developments in working memory. *Current Opinion in Neurobiology, 8*:234–238.

Balota, D. A., Watson, J. M., Duchek, J. M., & Ferraro, F. R. (1999). Cross-modal semantic and homographic priming in healthy young, healthy old, and in Alzheimer's disease individuals. *Journal of the International Neuropsychological Society, 5*, 626–640.

Beaunieux, H., Eustache, F., Busson, P., de la Sayette, V., Viader, F., & Desgranges, B. (2012). Cognitive procedural learning in early Alzheimer's disease: Impaired processes and compensatory mechanisms. *Journal of Neurophysiology, 6*(1), 31–42.

Bechara, A., Tranel, D., Damasio, H., Adolphs, R., Rockland, C., & Damasio, A. R. (1995). Double dissociation of conditioning and declarative knowledge relative to the amygdala and hippocampus in humans. *Science, 269*, 115–118.

Bennett, D. A., Wilson, R. S., Boyle, P. A., Buchman, A. S., & Schneider, J. A. (2012). Relation of neuropathology to cognition in persons without cognitive impairment. *Annals of Neurology*, 72(4), 599–609.

Berryhill, M. E., & Olson, I. R. (2008). Is the posterior parietal lobe involved in working memory retrieval? Evidence from patients with bilateral parietal lobe damage. *Neuropsychologia*, 46(7), 1775–1786.

Borst, J. P., & Anderson, J. R. (2013). Using model-based functional MRI to locate working memory updates and declarative memory retrievals in the fronto-parietal network. *Proceedings of the National Academy of Science USA*, 110(5), 1628–1633

Brewer, J. B., Zhao, Z., Desmond, J. E., Glover, G. H., & Gabrieli, J. D. (1998). Making memories: Brain activity that predicts how well visual experience will be remembered. *Science*, 281, 1185–1187.

Budson, A. E., & Price, B. H. (2002). Memory: Clinical disorders. In: *Encyclopedia of life sciences*. Vol. 11. London: Nature Publishing Group, 529–536.

Budson, A. E., & Price, B. H. (2005). Memory dysfunction. *New England Journal Medicine*, 352, 692–699.

Budson, A. E., Simons, J. S., Waring, J. D., Sullivan, A. L., Hussoin, T., & Schacter, D. L. (2007). Memory for the September 11, 2001, terrorist attacks one year later in patients with Alzheimer's disease, patients with mild cognitive impairment, and healthy older adults. *Cortex*, 43(7), 875–888.

Budson, A. E., & Solomon, P. R. (2011). *Memory loss: A practical guide for clinicians*. Philadelphia, PA: Elsevier.

Budson, A. E., Sullivan, A. L., Mayer, E., Daffner, K. R., Black, P. M., & Schacter. D. L. (2002). Suppression of false recognition in Alzheimer's disease and in patients with frontal lobe lesions. *Brain*, 125, 2750–2765.

Cabeza, R. (2008). Role of parietal regions in episodic memory retrieval: The dual attentional processes hypothesis. *Neuropsychologia*, 46(7), 1813–1827.

Calderon, J., Perry, R. J., Erzinclioglu, S. W., Berrios, G. E., Dening, T. R., & Hodges, J. R. (2001). Perception, attention, and working memory are disproportionately impaired in dementia with Lewy bodies compared with Alzheimer's disease. *Journal of Neurology, Neurosurgery and Psychiatry*, 70, 157–164.

Corkin, S. (1984). Lasting consequences of bilateral medial temporal lobectomy: Clinical course and experimental findings in H. M. *Seminars in Neurology*, 4, 249–259.

Damasio, H., Grabowski, T. J., Tranel, D., Hichwa, R. D., & Damasio, A. R. (1996). A neural basis for lexical retrieval. *Nature*, 380, 499–505.

Daselaar, S. M., Rombouts, S. A., Veltman, D. J., Raaijmakers, J. G., & Jonker, C. (2003). Similar network activated by young and old adults during the acquisition of a motor sequence. *Neurobiology of Aging*, 24, 1013–1019.

Davidson, P. S., Anaki, D., Ciaramelli, E., Cohn, M., Kim, A. S., Murphy, K. J., ...Levine, B. (2008). Does lateral parietal cortex support episodic memory? Evidence from focal lesion patients. *Neuropsychologia*, 46(7), 1743–1755.

Dickerson, B. C., Bakkour, A., Salat, D. H., Feczko, E., Pacheco, J., Greve, D. N., ...Buckner, R. L. (2009). The cortical signature of Alzheimer's disease: Regionally specific cortical thinning relates to symptom severity in very mild to mild AD dementia and is detectable in asymptomatic amyloid-positive individuals. *Cerebral Cortex*, 19(3), 497–510.

Dimitrova, A., Weber, J., Maschke, M., Elles, H. G., Kolb, F. P., Forsting, M., ...Timmann, D. (2002). Eyeblink-related areas in human cerebellum as shown by fMRI. *Human Brain Mapping*, 17, 100–115.

Dulas, M. R., & Duarte, A. (2013). The influence of directed attention at encoding on source memory retrieval in the young and old: An ERP study. *Brain Research*, 1500, 55–71.

Egeland, J., Sundet, K., Rund, B. R., Asbjørnsen, A., Hugdahl, K., Landrø, N. I., ...Stordal, K. I. (2003). Sensitivity and specificity of memory dysfunction in schizophrenia: A comparison with major depression. *Journal of Clinical and Experimental Neuropsychology*, 25, 79–93.

Eichenbaum, H. (1997). How does the brain organize memories? *Science*, 277(5324), 330–332.

Embree, L. M., Budson, A. E., & Ally, B. A. (2012). Memorial familiarity remains intact for pictures but not for words in patients with amnestic mild cognitive impairment. *Neuropsychologia*, 50(9), 2333–2340.

Fletcher, P. C., & Henson, R. N. A. (2001). Frontal lobes and human memory: Insights from functional neuroimaging. *Brain*, 124, 849–881.

Gardini, S., Cuetos, F., Fasano, F., Pellegrini, F. F., Marchi, M., Venneri, A., & Caffarra, P. (2013). Brain structural substrates of semantic memory decline in mild cognitive impairment. *Current Alzheimer Research*, 10(4), 373–389.

Glisky, E. L., & Schacter, D. L. (1989). Extending the limits of complex learning in organic amnesia: Computer training in a vocation domain. *Neuropsychologia*, 27, 173–178.

Gotham, A. M., Brown, R. G., & Marsden, C. D. (1988). "Frontal" cognitive functions in patients with Parkinson's disease "on" and "off" levodopa. *Brain*, 111, 299–321.

Green, J. D., & Hodges, J. R. (1996). Identification of famous faces and famous names in early Alzheimer's disease. Relationship to anterograde episodic and general semantic memory. *Brain, 119,* 111–128.

Heindel, W. C., Salmon, D. P., Shults, C. W., Walicke, P. A., & Butters, N. (1989). Neuropsychological evidence for multiple implicit memory systems: A comparison of Alzheimer's, Huntington's, and Parkinson's disease patients. *Journal of Neuroscience, 9,* 582–587.

Hodges, J. R. (2001). Frontotemporal dementia (Pick's disease): Clinical features and assessment. *Neurology, 56,* S6-S10

Hoefer, M., Allison, S. C., Schauer, G. F., Neuhaus, J. M., Hall, J., Dang, J. N.,...Rosen, H. J. (2008). Fear conditioning in frontotemporal lobar degeneration and Alzheimer's disease. *Brain, 131*(Pt 6), 1646–1657.

Hoffman, P., Meteyard, L., & Patterson, K. (2012). Broadly speaking: Vocabulary in semantic dementia shifts towards general, semantically diverse words. *Cortex,* doi: 10.1016/j.cortex.2012.11.004. Epub ahead of print.

Holl, A. K., Wilkinson, L., Tabrizi, S. J., Painold, A., & Jahanshahi, M. (2012). Probabilistic classification learning with corrective feedback is selectively impaired in early Huntington's disease—evidence for the role of the striatum in learning with feedback. *Neuropsychologia, 50*(9), 2176–2186.

Holz, J., Piosczyk, H., Landmann, N., Feige, B., Spiegelhalder, K., Riemann, D.,...Voderholzer, U. (2012). The timing of learning before night-time sleep differentially affects declarative and procedural long-term memory consolidation in adolescents. *PLoS One, 7*(7), e40963.

Jaeggi, S. M., Seewer, R., Nirkko, A. C., Eckstein, D., Schroth, G., Groner, R., & Gutbrod, K. (2003). Does excessive memory load attenuate activation in the prefrontal cortex? Load-dependent processing in single and dual tasks: Functional magnetic resonance imaging study. *Neuroimage, 19,* 210–225.

Johnson, M. K., Kounios, J., & Nolde, S. F. (1997). Electrophysiological brain activity and memory source monitoring. *NeuroReport, 8,* 1317–1320.

Johnson, M. K., O'Connor, M., & Cantor, J. (1997). Confabulation, memory deficits, and frontal dysfunction. *Brain and Cognition, 34,* 189–206.

Keane, M. M., Gabrieli, J. D., Mapstone, H. C., Johnson, K. A., & Corkin, S. (1995). Double dissociation of memory capacities after bilateral occipital-lobe or medial temporal-lobe lesions. *Brain, 118*(Pt 5), 1129–1148.

Klingberg, T., Forssberg, H., & Westerberg, H. (2002). Training of working memory in children with ADHD. *Journal of Clinical and Experimental Neuropsychology, 24,* 781–791.

Koivisto, M., Portin, R., & Rinne, J. O. (1996). Perceptual priming in Alzheimer's and Parkinson's diseases. *Neuropsychologia, 34,* 449–457.

Koivunen, J., Karrasch, M., Scheinin, N. M., Aalto, S., Vahlberg, T., Någren, K.,...Rinne, J. O. (2012). Cognitive decline and amyloid accumulation in patients with mild cognitive impairment. *Dementia and Geriatric Cognitive Disorders, 34*(1), 31–37.

Kopelman, M. D., Stanhope, N., & Kingsley, D. (1997). Temporal and spatial contex memory in patients with focal frontal, temporal lobe, and diencephalic lesions. *Neuropsychologia, 35,* 1533–1545.

Kubat-Silman, A. K., Dagenbach, D., & Absher, J. R. (2002). Patterns of impaired verbal, spatial, and object working memory after thalamic lesions. *Brain and Cognition, 50,* 178–193.

Lidstrom, A. M., Bogdanovic, N., Hesse, C., Volkman, I., Davidsson, P., & Blennow, K. (1998). Clusterin (apolipoprotein J) protein levels are increased in hippocampus and in frontal cortex in Alzheimer's disease. *Experimental Neurology, 154,* 511–521.

Markowitsch, H. J. (1995). Anatomical basis of memory disorders. In M. S. Gazzaniga (Ed.). *The cognitive neurosciences* (pp. 765–779). Cambridge, MA: MIT Press.

McKee, A. C., Au, R., Cabral, H. J., Kowall, N. W., Seshadri, S., Kubilus, C. A.,...Wolf, P. A. (2006). Visual association pathology in preclinical Alzheimer disease. *Journal of Neuropathology and Experimental Neurology, 65*(6), 621–630.

Mehta, M. A., Goodyer, I. M., & Sahakian, B. J. (2004). Methylphenidate improves working memory and set-shifting in AD/HD: Relationships to baseline memory capacity. *Journal of Child Psychology and Psychiatry, 45,* 293–305.

Mesulam, M-M. (2000). *Principles of behavioral and cognitive neurology* (2nd ed). New York, NY: Oxford University Press.

Millet, X., Le Goff, M., Bouisson, J., Dartigues, J. F., & Amieva, H. (2010). Encoding processes influence word-stem completion priming in Alzheimer's disease: A meta-analysis. *Journal of Clinical and Experimental Neuropsychology, 32*(5), 494–504.

Mitchell, J. P., Sullivan, A. L., Schacter, D. L., & Budson, A. E. (2006). Mis-attribution errors in Alzheimer's disease: The illusory truth effect. *Neuropsychology, 20*(2), 185–192.

Newman, S. D., Carpenter, P. A., Varma, S., & Just, M. A. (2003). Frontal and parietal participation in problem solving in the Tower of London: fMRI and computational modeling of planning and high-level perception. *Neuropsychologia, 41*, 1668–1682.

Papez, J. W. (1937). A proposed mechanism of emotion. *Archives of Neurology and Psychiatry, 38*, 725–743.

Pavlov, I. P. (1927). *Conditioned reflexes: An investigation of the physiological activity of the cerebral cortex.* London, UK: Oxford University Press.

Perani, D., Cappa, S. F., Schnur, T., Tettamanti, M., Collina, S., Rosa, M. M., & Fazio, F. (1999). The neural correlates of verb and noun processing. A PET study. *Brain 122*(Pt 12), 2337–2344.

Petrides, M. (2002). The mid-ventrolateral prefrontal cortex and active mnemonic retrieval. *Neurobiology of Learning and Memory, 78*, 528–538.

Potkin, K. T., & Bunney, W. E., Jr. (2012). Sleep improves memory: The effect of sleep on long term memory in early adolescence. *PLoS One, 7*(8), e42191.

Price, J. L., & Morris, J. C. (1999). Tangles and plaques in nondemented aging and "preclinical" Alzheimer's disease. *Annals of Neurology, 45*, 358–368.

Purcell, R., Maruff, P., Kyrios, M., & Pantelis, C. (1998). Cognitive deficits in obsessive-compulsive disorder on tests of frontal-striatal function. *Biological Psychiatry 43*, 348–357.

Ribot, T. (1881). *Les maladies de la mémoire.* Paris, France: Félix Alcan.

Rowe, J. B., Toni, I., Josephs, O., Frackowiak, R. S., & Passingham, R. E. (2000). The prefrontal cortex: Response selection or maintenance within working memory? *Science 2000*;288:1656–1660.

Ruch, S., Markes, O., Duss, S. B., Oppliger, D., Reber, T. P., Koenig, T.,...Henke, K. (2012). Sleep stage II contributes to the consolidation of declarative memories. *Neuropsychologia, 50*(10), 2389–2396.

Sabe, L., Jason, L., Juejati, M., Leiguarda, R., & Starkstein, S. E. (1995). Dissociation between declarative and procedural learning in dementia and depression. *Journal of Clinical and Experimental Neuropsychology, 17*, 841–848.

Salmon, D. P., Lineweaver, T. T., & Heindel, W. C. (1998). Nondeclarative memory in neurodegenerative disease. In A. I. Troster (Ed.), *Memory in neurodegenerative disease: Biological, cognitive, and clinical perspectives* (pp. 210–225). Cambridge, UK: Cambridge University Press.

Schacter, D. L., & Buckner, R. L. (1998). Priming and the brain. *Neuron, 20*, 185–195.

Schacter, D. L., & Tulving, E. (1994). What are the memory systems of 1994? In D. L. Schacter & E. Tulving (Eds.), *Memory systems 1994* (pp. 1–38). Cambridge, MA: MIT Press.

Schacter, D. L., Wagner, A. D., & Buckner, R. L. (2000). Memory systems of 1999. In E. Tulving & F. I. M. Craik (Eds.), *The Oxford handbook of memory* (pp. 627–643). New York, NY: Oxford University Press.

Schneider, J. A., Arvanitakis, Z., Yu, L., Boyle, P. A., Leurgans, S. E., & Bennett, D. A. (2012). Cognitive impairment, decline and fluctuations in older community-dwelling subjects with Lewy bodies. *Brain, 135*(Pt 10), 3005–3014.

Sfagos, C., Papageorgiou, C. C., Kosma, K. K., Kodopadelis, E., Uzunoglu, N. K., Vassilopoulos, D., & Rabavilas, A. D. (2003). Working memory deficits in multiple sclerosis: A controlled study with auditory P600 correlates. *Journal of Neurology, Neurosurgery and Psychiatry, 74*, 1231–1235.

Simons, J. S., Peers, P. V., Hwang, D. Y., Ally, B. A., Fletcher, P. C., & Budson, A. E. (2008). Is the parietal lobe necessary for recollection in humans? *Neuropsychologia, 46*(4), 1185–1191.

Simons, J. S., Peers, P. V., Mazuz, Y. S., Berryhill, M. E., & Olson, I. R. (2010). Dissociation between memory accuracy and memory confidence following bilateral parietal lesions. *Cereb Cortex.* 2010 Feb;20(2), 479–485.

Simons, J. S., & Spiers, H. J. (2003). Prefrontal and medial temporal lobe interactions in long-term memory. *Nature Reviews Neuroscience, 4*, 637–648.

Solomon, P. R., Stowe, G. T., & Pendlbeury, W. W. (1989). Disrupted eyelid conditioning in a patient with damage to cerebellar afferents. *Behavioral Neuroscience, 103*, 898–902.

Squire, L. R. (1992). Memory and the hippocampus: A synthesis from findings with rats, monkeys, and humans. *Psychological Review, 99*, 195–231.

Stickgold, R. (2005). Sleep-dependent memory consolidation. *Nature, 437*, 1272–1278.

Stickgold, R. (2006). Neuroscience: A memory boost while you sleep. *Nature, 444*, 559–560.

Tulving, E., & Schacter, D. L. (1990). Priming and human memory systems. *Science, 247*, 301–306.

Vaidya, C. J., Zhao, M., Desmond, J. E., & Gabrieli, J. D. (2002). Evidence for cortical encoding specificity in episodic memory: Memory-induced re-activation of picture processing areas. *Neuropsychologia, 40*, 2136–2143.

Vilberg, K. L., & Rugg, M. D. (2008). Memory retrieval and the parietal cortex: A review of evidence from a dual-process perspective. *Neuropsychologia, 46*(7), 1787–1799.

Vilberg, K. L., & Rugg, M. D. (2009). Functional significance of retrieval-related activity in lateral parietal cortex: Evidence from fMRI and ERPs. *Human Brain Mapping, 30*(5), 1490–1501.

Wagner, A. D., Schacter, D. L., Rotte, M., Koutstaal, W., Maril, A., Dale, A. M., ... Buckner, R. L. (1998). Building memories: Remembering and forgetting of verbal experiences as predicted by brain activity. *Science*, *281*, 1188–1191.

Wamsley, E. J., & Stickgold, R. (2011). Memory, sleep and dreaming: Experiencing consolidation. *Sleep Medicine Clinics*, *6*(1), 97–108.

Wolosin, S. M., Zeithamova, D., & Preston, A. R. (2012). Reward modulation of hippocampal subfield activation during successful associative encoding and retrieval. *Journal of Cognitive Neuroscience*, *24*(7), 1532–1547.

5

Motor Programming Disorders in Dementia

Kenneth M. Heilman

Dementia is pragmatically defined as a decrement in cognitive abilities such that people affected can no longer successfully care for themselves and their family nor successfully interact with their environment. Except for verbal communication, it is our upper limbs that primarily allow us to perform these interactions. Thus, this chapter will focus on the effects of dementing diseases on action programming of the upper limbs.

The neural innervation, muscles, and joints of our upper limbs (forelimbs), which include the arm, forearm, hand, and fingers, allow us to perform almost an infinite number of movements. To perform successful interactions, the nerves and muscles that implement movements of the forelimbs must be guided by instructions from the brain. In general, there are two major forms of instructions. One type deals with "when" decisions and the other with "how" instructions. Whereas the major goal of this chapter is to discuss disorders of the "how" system or apraxic disorders, "when" or action-intentional disorders can be a major source of disability in patient with diseases of the brain and thus will be briefly discussed.

Action-Intentional Disorders

There are at least four "when" action decisions that people must make and these include the following: (1) when to initiate a movement or action; (2) when to persist at an action; (3) when the task is complete and actions should be terminated or when an action is not accomplishing the goal and much be changed; and (4) when not to initiate an action.

A deficit in initiating an action is called *akinesia*, and a delay in initiating an action is called *hypokinesia*. Patients who have trouble sustaining an action or actions until a task is complete have what is called *impersistence*. If a person continues performing an action or actions after a task has been completed, or this action is not accomplishing the person's goal and should be altered but is not, this disorder is called *motor perseveration*. There appears to be at least two main forms of perseveration: repeatedly continuing the same action, which is called *continuous perseveration*, or after altering an action returning to a previous action pattern, which is called *recurrent perseveration*. Performing an action when no action is required is called *defective response inhibition*. Often when patients act and there is no action needed, their inappropriate action is initiated by a stimulus. For example, Lhermitte (1983) noted that some patients, when in the presence of objects (e.g., a pen and paper), will utilize these objects (e.g., write or draw) without an apparent goal. He called this "utilization behavior" and subsequently "the environmental dependency syndrome." Luria (1962) had previously described an echopraxia task that may also examine for "environmental dependency." In this echopraxia task the examiner asks the patient to put up two fingers when the examiner puts up one finger and vice versa. Patients perform abnormally when they put the same number of fingers as does the examiner. Crucian et al. (2007) reported that some patients who are tested with the crossed response task, in which they are instructed to close their eyes and move the hand opposite that touched, will have a propensity to move the hand that has been stimulated.

These "when" disorders, also called "action intentional disorders" (Heilman, 2004), are most often observed in patients who suffer with frontal-subcortical-basal ganglia dysfunction. The presence of these action-intentional disorders can be a major cause of a decrement in a person's ability to successfully care for oneself or one's family, and to successfully interact with one's environment. Thus, while not commonly assessed by clinicians who evaluate patients for dementia, these disorders are a major cause of disability. Some of the most common dementing diseases that may induce these disorders are forms of vascular dementia, multiple sclerosis, head trauma, Parkinson's disease, and other degenerative movement disorders, such as progressive supranuclear palsy, corticobasal degeneration, and multiple systems atrophy.

Apraxic Disorders

Relevance

To successfully care for ourselves and our family as well as successfully interact with our environment, people need to know "how" to move or act. For example, a person has to know how to posture one's forelimb to hold a tool or implement to work with an object, how to move one's joints to correctly accomplish the required action, how to direct one's hand and fingers to the object with which one wants to act upon, how fast to move portions of one's forelimb, and how much force to use. A person also needs to know the mechanical advantage that tools and implement may afford, how to use these tools, and how to sequence one's action to successfully complete one's goal-directed behavior. The diagnosis of *apraxia* may be important for several reasons. First, it may help the clinician understand the form of dementia from which a patient is suffering. Second, all the limb-apraxic disorders discussed here can cause a disability, and detecting the form of apraxia may help patients and caregivers to understand the types of activities in which these patients should not engage because they may hurt themselves or other people. Third, knowledge of the disability may allow patients and caregivers (ideally with the assistance of an occupational therapist) to develop strategies that may limit the disabilities caused by these disorders.

Whereas disorders of the brain that impair the "how" networks that program purposeful actions of the forelimb are called apraxia, this term in Greek literally means "without action." As mentioned previously, we now call an absence of action, when an action is required, akinesia; however, this term "apraxia" was a term originally used by Steinthal (1871) to describe impairment of patients' abilities to correctly carry out "how" motor programs.

Task Specific Versus General Forms of Limb Apraxia

In regard to the forelimbs, there are two major forms of apraxia. One form is task specific and the other form is general. Task-specific apraxia includes disorders limited primarily to one activity. For example, dressing apraxia and constructional apraxia are examples of task-specific apraxia. In these two forms of specific apraxia there are impairments of the "how" to dress or "how" to draw, but these how deficits can be caused by disorders such as inattention or neglect so that the person with dressing apraxia does not dress one's left side, or deficits in one's body image-schema, and most commonly visuospatial deficits. Therefore, while disorders such as constructional apraxia are commonly associated with dementia and are often assessed in neuropsychological batteries such as the Mini-Mental Status Examination and the Montreal Cognitive Assessment, these task-specific disorders will not be discussed in this chapter.

Exclusionary Criteria

In addition to apraxia, there are many disorders that might impair a person's ability to perform purposeful skilled movements. Therefore, in part, as noted by Geschwind (1965), the diagnosis of apraxia is partly dependent on the exclusion of other disorders that may interfere with the performance of goal-oriented actions. For example, if a patient is impaired in performing purposeful movements because the patient has deficits such as weakness, abnormal movements such as tremor, chorea, ballismus, myoclonus, severe sensory-perceptual deficits, attentional deficits such as neglect, or cognitive impairments such as an impaired comprehension, then the patient's inability to perform purposeful goal-oriented actions is not considered a form or apraxia. If a patient with dementia has one or more of these disorders and this disorder prevents the examiner from fully investigating this patient, then it may not be possible to learn whether this patient has apraxia; however, if in the presence of some of these disorders some patients can be tested, the interpretation of these tests must be considered in light of these patients' other disabilities.

Forms of Upper Limb Apraxia

The term "apraxia" was a term originally used by Steinthal (1871) to describe impairment of the human to correctly carry out "how" motor programs. Although the term "apraxia" was first used by Steinthal (1871), it was primarily Hugo Liepmann who made some of the first important contributions to the understanding of these "how" disorders. Liepmann (1920) described three major forms of apraxia: (1) limb-kinetic apraxia; (2) ideomotor apraxia; and (3) ideational apraxia. All three of these forms of apraxia can be seen with patients who have dementia. We described a fourth type that we called conceptual apraxia (Heilman, Maher, Greenwald, & Rothi, 1997; Ochipa, Rothi, & Heilman, 1992) and that may also be associated with dementia. The diagnosis of these specific types of apraxia is dependent upon the types of motor programming errors made by the patient. In this section we will describe these four different forms of general forelimb apraxia, including (1) the mean by which patients may be tested for each of these forms of apraxia, (2) the types of errors made by patients who exhibit these forms of apraxia, and (3) the pathophysiology that might account for these "how" program deficits. We will also briefly discuss the diseases that can induce dementia and also may cause each of these types of apraxia.

Conceptual Apraxia

Clinical

Although there are animals that use tools, and even some animals that fashion tools such as ravens, crows, and apes, it is primarily humans who use tools to aid them in altering their environment. Humans have mechanical knowledge, and when the proper tool is not available, they are able to use alternative tools or even develop new tools. Although often not assessed, there are patients who, when presented with a problem that requires an action, sometimes cannot recognize the tool they need to fulfill the required action. There are also patients who might not recall the type of actions associated with specific tools, utensils, or objects (tool-object action associative knowledge). Unlike patients with ideomotor apraxia who make spatial and temporal errors, patients with conceptual apraxia make content errors (Ochipa, Rothi, & Heilman, 1989). For example, when shown a picture of a screwdriver and asked to demonstrate by pantomiming the use of this tool, the patients with ideomotor apraxia may move the incorrect joints, such as twisting their wrist in circles; however, the patient with conceptual apraxia might pantomime a hammering motion by making pounding movements.

Patients with conceptual apraxia may have another problem where they are unable to recall which specific tool (e.g., hammer) is associated with a specific object (e.g., nail) (tool-object associative knowledge); however, the sign that appears to be sensitive for the presence of this disorder is a loss of mechanical knowledge. There are two major means by which mechanical knowledge can be tested. One is an alternative tool task. For example, when attempting to drive a nail into a piece of wood and there is no hammer, the patient with conceptual apraxia might select a screwdriver rather than a wrench in an attempt to pound in the nail (Ochipa et al., 1992). The second is tool development, such as bending a wire to make a hook to retrieve an item in the bottom of a tube (Heilman et al., 1997; Ochipa et al., 1992).

Pathophysiology

Right-handed patients with a callosal disconnection can demonstrate conceptual apraxia of the nonpreferred nondominant left hand (Watson & Heilman, 1983). Heilman et al. (1997) also studied right-handed patients who had either right or left hemispheric cerebral infarctions for conceptual apraxia. We found that conceptual apraxia was more commonly associated with left than right hemisphere injury, suggesting that in people who are right handed it is their left hemisphere that stores this mechanical knowledge. In this study (Heilman et al., 1997) we also want to learn the locus of injury that induced conceptual apraxia within the left hemisphere, but no specific anatomic region appeared to be critical, and most patients had injury to their parietal and/or frontal cortex. The failure to find a specific locus may have been caused by a lack of power, and with more subjects we may have found the loci of lesions that induce this disorder. It is also possible that tool-object, tool movement, and mechanical knowledge are stored in different areas of the brain. In addition, it is possible that the representations that store mechanical knowledge are widely distributed in the left hemisphere. This latter hypothesis has been supported by a functional imaging study which revealed that when the conceptual tasks were compared with the control tasks, there was overlapping activation in left parietal temporal occipital junction, prefrontal, dorsal premotor, cuneus, and inferior temporal areas (Ebisch et al., 2007).

Diseases That Can Cause Conceptual Apraxia and May Be Associated With Cognitive Disorders

As mentioned, conceptual apraxia can be associated with diseases that cause focal brain damage, such as stroke, but it is commonly seen in patients suffering with Alzheimer's disease (Ochipa et al., 1992), and this disorder may be one of the early cognitive signs in this disease. There is also some evidence that patients with the semantic dementia form of frontotemporal lobar degeneration may also have conceptual apraxia (Silveri & Ciccarelli, 2009).

Ideomotor Apraxia

Clinical

When performing transitive acts, especially those that involve tools, such as scissors, and implements, such as knives, patients with ideomotor apraxia (IMA) primarily make spatial errors. Whereas these spatial errors can also be observed during the performance of intransitive acts (such as saluting), patients with IMA are more likely to make errors with transitive than intransitive acts. These apraxic patients can also make temporal errors; however, with bedside clinic testing these temporal errors are often more difficult to detect than are the spatial errors. There are three major types of spatial errors that can be observed in patients who have IMA and these included (1) postural errors, (2) egocentric spatial movement errors, and (3) allocentric spatial movement errors. Each of these forms of errors is described subsequently.

Postural errors, which are also called internal configuration errors, are most likely seen when patients are asked to pantomime a transitive act such as making believe they are holding a pair of scissors in their hand and are using these scissors to cut a piece of paper in half. Typically when patients with IMA are requested to pantomime a transitive movement, they will fail to correctly place their fingers, hand, forearm, and arm in the position that would enable them to correctly hold a tool or implement. Goodglass and Kaplan (1963) reported that when patients are asked to pantomime the use of a tool or implement, such as scissors, these patients often use their hand and fingers as the tool. For example, when the patients with IMA are asked to demonstrate how they would use a pair of scissors to cut a piece of paper in half, they will often extend their forefinger as well as their middle finger and then abduct and adduct these fingers as if these fingers were the blades of the scissors. When making this posture, these patients are not correctly demonstrating the posture used for holding a pair of scissors but rather are making the emblem of scissors. Goodglass and Kaplan (1963) called these types of errors "body-part as object errors," but when using the fingers as the blades of scissor, these patients are using their body part as the tool rather than the object upon which the tool works. Hence, we termed these errors "body-part as tool errors (BPTEs)."

BPTEs are, however, not always indicator of the presence of IMA. When asked to pantomime the use of a tool, such as a pair of scissors, even normal people will often make BPTEs. This failure to correctly carry out this request may be related to the rarity of occasions that people use transitive pantomimes versus emblems and using the finger as blades is an emblem of scissors rather than pantomime. However, when normal people are asked to not use their hand and fingers or other body parts as the tools and instead to show the examiner how they would use the actual tool, most normal people will stop making BPTEs. In contrast, many patients with IMA, unlike normal people, continue to make BPTEs even when the examiner repeatedly attempts to correct this abnormal behavior (Raymer, Maher, Foundas, Heilman, & Rothi, 1997).

Sometimes when patients with IMA do stop making BPTEs and attempt to pantomime, they will incorrectly posture their fingers, hand, forearm, and arm. For example, when attempting to hold a pair of scissors, they may place their thumb below their forefinger.

In addition to positioning one's upper limb in the correct posture, when correctly pantomiming a transitive act a person needs to correctly move the joints in one's upper limb in order that the tool will be able to correctly move through space and be able to perform its proper function. Independent of the position of the object on which this tool will act, patients with IMA often either move the incorrect joints or move these joins in an incorrect fashion. For example, if asked to pantomime using a hammer to hit a nail in a board that is placed horizontally, below eye level, patients with IMA may flex and extend their arm at the elbow, but not flex and extend (or ulnar and radial deviate) their hand at their wrist. Thus, if they were holding an actual hammer, the head of this hammer would not decent to hit the head of the nail.

Whereas hammering can be performed with just movements of the wrist, some actions with tools require the coordination of two or more joints. For example, if a person is asked to carve a slice of turkey with a knife, normal people may fix their wrist and as they bring their arm at the shoulder forward they extend their arm at the elbow. After they have made this forward movement they have to reverse these movements, and as they move their arm backward at their shoulder they have to flex their arm at the elbow; however, with each stroke the elbow flexion is reduced to allow the knife to move downward. In contrast to normal people, patients with IMA will often just move one joint, either at the shoulder or elbow and thus rather than making a slicing movement, they will make stabbing or chopping movements (Poizner, Mack, Verfaellie, Rothi, & Heilman, 1990; Rothi, Mack, Verfaellie, Brown, & Heilman, 1988).

In addition to these egocentric postural and movement errors, patients with IMA can also make allocentric or target-oriented movement errors. If a person is going to use a tool properly, the person must direct this tool to the object upon which the tool works. For example, when using a hammer to pound a nail, the hammer has to be directed to the head of the nail. In addition to making egocentric postural and movement errors, patients with IMA make allocentric errors by failing to direct their real or pretended actions toward the real or imaginary target of these actions (Poizner et al., 1990; Rothi et al., 1988).

Assessment for Ideomotor Apraxia

Some patients or their families-caregivers may be able to give a history of an impairment using tools and implements; however, the construct of apraxia is not well known to the general public, and thus it is uncommon that patients or family members-caregivers will complain about the presence of this disorder.

There are three means for testing for the presence of IMA: observing patients work with actual tools and the objects upon which these tools act, by having patients imitate the examiner pantomiming transitive acts, and having the patient pantomime to command. When using actual tools or imitating the examiner, the patient is provided with cues and thus the most sensitive test for IMA is asking patients to pantomime transitive acts to verbal command. As mentioned, patients with IMA often perform more poorly with transitive ("Show me how you would scramble eggs with a fork") than intransitive acts ("Wave bye-bye") (Haaland, Harrington, & Knight, 2000; Rothi et al., 1988), and thus patients should be assessed by having them pantomime transitive actions.

Although patients with IMA typically improve when imitating the examiner pantomime a transitive act, their performance often remains impaired. In addition, when using actual tools or implements, their performance might improve even further, but often they may continue to make errors (Poizner et al., 1990). For example, after being reminded not to use their body part as the tool, patients with IMA will continue to make these BPTEs or other postural errors, but when provided with scissors, which have two circular or oval holes for forefinger and thumb placement, it would be unlikely that a patient will make a BPTE by extending the forefinger and middle finger.

In addition to the postural, egocentric, and allocentric movement errors discussed previously, patients with IMA may also make movement speed errors; however, these may be difficult to recognize. For example, when using a knife to slice turkey, normally the arm moves most slowly as the knife approaches the turn (from extension of the arm to flexion and vice versa); however, patients with IMA often do not follow this speed-temporal pattern (Poizner et al., 1990).

As we will discuss, some patients will have ideomotor apraxia primarily of one forelimb, and thus both upper limbs should be tested. In addition, patients with IMA often have an impairment of comprehending other people's meaningful pantomimes and may also be impaired at discriminating correct form incorrect postures (Mozaz, Rothi, Anderson, Crucian, & Heilman, 2002), as well as pantomimed actions (Heilman, Rothi, & Valenstein, 1982). Thus, tests of comprehension of well-performed pantomimes and discrimination between correctly and incorrectly performed pantomimes should also be tested.

Pathophysiology

The diseases that can cause IMA will be discussed in the subsequent section; however, in this section we will discuss the areas of the brain that when injured may cause IMA. Studies of patients with stroke have revealed that IMA is associated with injury to several structures, including the inferior parietal lobe, the premotor cortex (supplementary motor area and convexity premotor cortex), and the corpus callosum. Subcortical lesions that involve the basal ganglia, the thalamus, and the white matter connecting these areas with the cerebral cortex can be associated with IMA.

One of the first people to perform systematic research on the pathology accounting for IMA was Hugo Liepmann. In an early study, Liepmann & Maas (1907) investigated a population of right-handed patients who had damage confined to either their left or right hemisphere. Liepmann found that none of the patients with right hemisphere injury had an IMA; however, about 50% of those with left hemispheric strokes had IMA.

Paul Broca (1861) was the first to report that aphasia in right-handed patients is almost always associated with left hemisphere damage. Thus, based on both Broca's and Liepmann's reports, it is not surprising that most patients with IMA are also aphasic. The frequent coexistence of aphasia and IMA, where patients can neither speak nor gesture correctly, has led to the hypothesis that both aphasia and apraxia are symptoms of an inability to use symbols and signs, a deficit that has been termed "asymbolia" (Finkelburg, 1873); however, as noted by Liepmann (1907), some patients with IMA are not aphasic and some aphasic patients are not apraxic. This dissociation suggests that while there may be overlap, there are parts of the brain that mediate speech-language that are not important in the control of purposeful skilled movement and vice versa. The frequent co-occurrence of these two disorders is therefore probably related to two factors. One factor is the cause of the cerebral dysfunction. For example, strokes in the middle cerebral artery distribution damage multiple cortical areas including those that mediate speech and those subserving purposeful skilled movements. It is also possible that certain portions of the cerebral cortex have neuronal networks that perform more than one function; when these areas are damaged, there may be a loss of more than one function.

Parietal Lobe

Liepmann (1920) noted that when a person with a left hemisphere injury demonstrated signs of IMA, the person often had an injury to the inferior parietal lobe. Geschwind (1965) posited that lesions in this region caused apraxia because they disconnected Wernicke area (posterior portion of the left superior temporal lobe), which is critical for comprehension of speech, from the premotor cortex, which is important in programming the primary motor cortex. This disconnection hypothesis is similar to that proposed by Wernicke (1874) and Lichtheim (1885) to account for conduction aphasia and that conduction aphasia often accompanies IMA. According to Geschwind's hypothesis, the incoming verbal message that provides the patient with the knowledge of the pantomime that the examiner requested is decoded in Wernicke's area, but this message must then be transmitted to the premotor cortex in the left frontal lobe. When the pantomime is to be carried out with the right hand, then the premotor cortex activates the corticospinal neurons in the motor cortex, which activate the appropriate motor neurons and then muscles. When the left hand is used, the left premotor cortex transfers this information to the right premotor cortex, and the information activates the motor neurons in the right hemisphere. Thus, according to Geschwind's hypothesis, a lesion of the left supramarginal gyrus could injure the white matter pathway (arcuate fasciculus) that connects Wernicke's area, located in the posterior-superior temporal lobe, with the left hemisphere's convexity premotor cortex. This could, in turn, produce an IMA because the area of the brain important in comprehension is disconnected from the area of the frontal lobe important in providing the motor cortex with the movement program.

This verbal-motor disconnection hypothesis, however, cannot entirely explain why patients with IMA from a left parietal lesion are also impaired when imitating. Geschwind posited that to perform imitation the connections between the visual association area, on the left side, and premotor cortex, which is in the white matter under the inferior parietal cortex, is also interrupted; Geschwind suggested that this left hemispheric white matter pathway from the occipital cortex to the premotor cortex was dominant for carrying this information, but he did not explain why it was dominant. When patients with IMA are given a tool to hold in the hand (right or left) and attempt to use this tool, they also make errors (Poizner et al., 1990) and Geschwind's left parietal white matter disconnection hypotheses cannot also explain this observation. As we will discuss in a subsequent section, patients with degenerative diseases such as Alzheimer's disease may also demonstrate IMA, and many of these patient have degeneration of their parietal lobe cortex; thus, white matter disconnection could not explain the IMA observed in these patients.

About three decades ago we put forth an alternative "movement representation" hypothesis (Heilman et al., 1982; Rothi, Heilman, & Watson, 1985) that may account for the IMA associated with left inferior parietal lesions. We suggested that in right-handed people these movement formula or movement representations, which we also have called "praxicons," contain the spatial and temporal parameters of purposeful actions. The inferior parietal lobe of the left hemisphere receives visual information from both the ventral "what" system important in recognizing tool, implements, and the objects upon which these tool interact and the dorsal "where" visual association system that provides information about the relationship of the arm with an object in peripersonal space. In addition, the inferior parietal lobe also receives input from the superior parietal association areas that contain kinesthetic representations of upper limb movements. Based on this visuo-kinesthetic input, the left inferior parietal lobe develops visuospatial kinesthetic representations of skilled movement. Thus, if there is an injury to these movement representations or praxicons, the patients with this injury should demonstrate deficits of pantomiming to command, imitating both meaningful and meaningless gestures and even using actual tools. In addition, if these representations are degraded, patients should not be able to comprehend other people's pantomimes and these patients should not be able to discriminate between correctly and incorrectly performed transitive pantomimes performed by the examiner.

In contrast, if these praxicons are intact, but patients have injury to the premotor cortex or the pathways that connect these movement representations to premotor cortex, these patients would also be expected to have performance deficits characteristic of IMA. In contrast to patients with parietal lesions, the patients with a premotor injury should be able to discriminate between incorrect and correct pantomimes performed by the examiner. We (Heilman et al., 1982; Rothi et al., 1985) tested patients with anterior and posterior left hemisphere cerebral cortical lesions by assessing for IMA by having these patients produce transitive pantomimes as well as assessing their pantomime discrimination. We found that some patients with both left hemispheric anterior and posterior lesions had the production deficits typical of IMA. In contrast, we found that it was primarily the patients with posterior damage who had both production and discrimination disturbances. More recently, Halsband and coworkers (2001) replicated Heilman et al. (1982) and Rothi et al.'s (1985) results. These results provided evidence against Geschwind's disconnection hypothesis of IMA from parietal lesions and instead support the postulate that injury of the left inferior parietal lobe induces IMA because injury to this area degrades the movement representations that are stored in this area.

Haaland and her coinvestigators (2000) were interested in attempting to more precisely localize the left hemispheric lesions that induce and do not induce IMA and found that patients with IMA had injury to the cortical regions adjacent to the intraparietal sulcus, which is in part at the top of the supramarginal gyrus. Functional imaging has provided convergent evidence that the left inferior parietal lobe stores movement representations in right-handed subjects (Moll et al., 2000).

Pramstaller and Marsden (1996) noted that subcortical lesions, which injure the superior longitudinal fasciculus, are associated with IMA and thus this form of apraxia can be induced by a disconnection syndrome. However, this disconnection is not between the areas important for language comprehension and the motor cortex, but rather between the movement representations stored in the inferior parietal cortex and the premotor cortex.

Supplementary Motor Area

As mentioned previously, the movement representations or praxicons that are stored in the left parietal lobe are probably stored in a three-dimensional visual and kinesthetic spatial-temporal code. In order for the motor cortex to correctly activate the motor nerves and the muscles to which these nerves are connected, and move a person's joints in the correct fashion, these visual-kinesthetic spatial-temporal representations have to be translated into a motor program that selectively activates specific portions of the motor cortex in a specific temporal pattern.

The medial portion of the premotor cortex (Brodmann's area 6), called the supplementary motor area (SMA), receives projections from parietal neurons. The SMA projects to the convexity premotor cortex as well as to primary motor cortex and also has direct projections to the neurons of the spinal cord that control upper limb movement. When the primary motor cortex in the hand area is stimulated, one or more fingers may twitch and if during functional imaging a person moves just one finger in a repetitive motion, the hand area in Brodmann's area 4, the primary motor cortex on the contralateral side, will demonstrate activation. In contrast, if the SMA is stimulated, the person will perform complex arm, forearm, hand, and finger movements; and during functional imaging when normal people perform transitive pantomimes, there is activation of the SMA, as well as primary motor cortex (Lauritzen, Henriksen, & Lassen, 1981; Rao et al., 1993). Based on these reports, it appears that premotor cortex and especially SMA is the area or areas of the brain that convert the polymodal (visual-kinesthetic) temporo-spatial movement representation into a motor program, and it is this portion of the premotor cortex that directs the activation of the motor neurons in primary motor cortex. Watson et al. (1986) reported several patients who sustained left-sided medial frontal lesions that included the supplementary motor area, and these patients demonstrated an impairment in performing transitive purposeful movements and these errors were consistent with IMA; however, in contrast to the patients with left parietal lesions, these patients were able to discriminate between correctly and incorrectly performed pantomimes, and the reason for this dichotomy may be related to these patients' preservation of their praxicons (visuo-kinesthetic spatial temporal movement representations).

Convexity Premotor Cortex

The role of injury-degeneration of the convexity premotor cortex in the development of IMA is not well known. For example, Faglioni and Basso (1985) wrote that they had difficulty finding any well-documented cases where patients had IMA as a result of injury to convexity premotor region. Subsequently, Barrett et al. (1998) and Haaland et al. (2000) did report patients with frontal premotor injury who appeared to have an IMA. Barrett et al's (1998) report described a study of one patient who could properly make a movement if it only required the movement of one joint of the upper limb, but it was impaired when she was required to make movements that required the coordination between two or more joints.

Haaland et al. (2000) studied a population of patients with stroke who had ideomotor apraxia, using the lesion overlap method for localization; in addition to finding parietal injury was associated with IMA, they found that injury of a portion of the convexity premotor cortex, the middle frontal gyrus, also appeared to be a critical area. In contrast, however, Freund and Hummelsheim (1985) studied a population of patients with convexity premotor lesions and also found that these patients were apraxic but instead of having IMA they had limb-kinetic apraxia, a disorder that will be discussed later.

Basal Ganglia and Thalamus

In the prior sections the relationships between IMA and cortical dysfunction was discussed; however, subcortical structures have a great influence on cortical functions, and there have been several reports that subcortical lesions can also induce IMA (Agostoni, Coletti, Orlando, & Tredici, 1983; Basso & Della Sala, 1986; Della Sala, Basso, Laiacona, & Papagno, 1992; DeRenzi, Faglioni, Scarpa, & Crisi, 1986; Kertesz & Ferro, 1984; Kleist, 1907; von Monakov, 1914). To learn the subcortical structures that may cause IMA when damaged, Pramstaller and Marsden (1996) performed a meta-analysis. In this analysis they reviewed the case reports of 82 patients who had an IMA caused by a subcortical lesion. They concluded that lesions confined to the basal ganglia, including the putamen, caudate, and the globus pallidus, rarely, if ever, cause an IMA. Unfortunately, in most of the studies reviewed by these investigators the patients were only tested with imitation. In addition, these patients' performance was only scored as either correct or incorrect. The most sensitive test for IMA is having patients pantomime to command, and Pramstaller and Marsden's (1996) results may have been related to the insensitivity of the testing procedure used to assess these patients.

Subsequently, Hanna-Pladdy et al. (2001) studied patients for IMA and compared patients with cortical and subcortical strokes. These investigators studied these patients using transitive and intransitive gestures, both to command and with imitation. They found that both the group of patients with cortical and subcortical lesions made the spatial and temporal error associated with IMA; however, they also found some differences. Whereas the patients with cortical lesions were impaired in the production of transitive and intransitive gestures-to-verbal command and imitation, as well as impaired gesture discrimination, the participants who had subcortical lesions only demonstrated mild production-execution deficits for transitive pantomimes to verbal command; consistent with Pramstaller and Marsden's (1996) report, the patients with subcortical lesions had normal imitation. In addition, unlike the patients with cortical lesions, the group of patients with the subcortical lesions were unimpaired on a gesture (correct versus incorrect) discrimination task. The subcortical group, however, made more postural errors than the cortical group. Unlike the Pramsteller and Marsden study, this study by Hanna-Pladdy et al. does suggest that the subcortical structures make an independent contribution to the praxis processing system. Unfortunately, we have not learned the role of these subcortical structures in controlling the performance of purposeful skilled upper limb movement.

Subcortical injury can also damage the thalamus, and there have been several case reports of patients who developed apraxia from lesions of the left thalamus in the region of the pulvinar nucleus (Nadeau, Roeltgen, Sevush, Ballinger, & Watson, 1994; Shuren, Maher, & Heilman, 1994). This thalamic nucleus has strong connections with the inferior parietal lobes, which, as discussed, play a critical role in storing movement representations; thus, damage to this nucleus might impair the activation of these movement representations.

Diseases That May Be Associated With Cognitive Disorders and Ideomotor Apraxia

Vascular

In the previous discussion of the pathophysiology of IMA, most of the patients studied had vascular disease, and thus patients with vascular dementia may reveal an IMA. The most common vascular lesion to cause IMA is a thrombosis in the distribution of the left middle cerebral artery, which infarcts the parietal cortex; however, injury to the left hemisphere premotor cortex either medially with a left anterior cerebral artery distribution infarction or laterally with an infarction in distribution of the anterior branches of the middle cerebral artery can also cause IMA.

Studies of disability have revealed that the presence of apraxia is one of the major reasons patients with strokes cannot perform independently (Hanna-Pladdy et al., 2003) and often cannot return to work (Saeki & Hachisuka, 2004).

Alzheimer's Disease

Along with impairments of episodic memory, language (e.g., anomia), visuospatial skills and elements of the Gerstmann's syndrome, ideomotor apraxia is one of the most common deficits observed in patients with Alzheimer's disease. In addition to making postural, spatial, and temporal errors when performing (pantomiming, imitating, or using actual tools and implements) purposeful movements that are typical of ideomotor apraxia, patients with Alzheimer's disease also are impaired at pantomime recognition and discrimination (Rousseaux, Rénier, Anicet, Pasquier, & Mackowiak-Cordoliani, 2012). Mozaz et al. (2006), using a posture recognition test, also demonstrated that patients with Alzheimer's disease are impaired. These comprehension discrimination studies suggest that patients with Alzheimer's disease have a decrement in the movement representations.

An unusual form of dementia called "posterior cortical atrophy" that often starts with visuospatial disabilities and visual agnosic disorders can also be associated with ideomotor apraxia (Goethals & Santens, 2001)

Parkinson's Disease

There have been several studies that have revealed that patients with Parkinson's disease can have an ideomotor apraxia (Goldenberg, Wimmer, Auff, & Schnaberth, 1986; Leiguarda et al., 1997). Goldenberg et al. (1986) found that the severity of apraxia was not directly related to the severity of these patients' Parkinsonian motor signs but instead appeared to be related to their visuospatial and visuoperceptual skills. Leiguarda et al. (1997) found that there were no differences when patients with Parkinson's disease were "on" versus "off" their medication, suggesting that this apraxic disorder was not related to a dopamine deficit. The patients with Parkinson's disease who had ideomotor apraxia had normal pantomime comprehension and were able to discriminate well-performed from improperly performed pantomimes, suggesting that their impairment was not related to degradation of their movement representation, but rather an inability to translate these representation into motor programs. In addition, the apraxia appeared to be related to their performance on tests of frontal-executive functions, such as the Tower of Hanoi, Trailmaking, and verbal fluency tests.

Parkinson Plus Syndromes: Corticobasal Degeneration, Progressive Supranuclear Palsy, Multiple System Atrophy

One of the earliest and most prominent signs associated with corticobasal degeneration is ideomotor apraxia. Most commonly, patients with corticobasal degeneration have a more severe apraxia of one upper (right or left) limb than the opposite upper limb. We have noted that many patients with corticobasal degeneration who demonstrate severe ideomotor apraxia on tests of pantomime, imitation, and object use can still discriminate correct from incorrect gestures performed by the examiner, suggesting that that their movement representations are still intact (Leiguarda et al., 1994) and that their ideomotor apraxia may be related to degeneration of the supplementary motor area.

Leiguarda et al. (1997) found that about 75% of patients with progressive supranuclear palsy did demonstrate an ideomotor apraxia. Leiguarda et al. did find that in those patients with Parkinson plus syndrome with ideomotor apraxia their Mini-Mental Status Examination (MMSE) scores correlated with the severity of their apraxia. In most of these patients their apraxia was characterized by spatial errors, including postural errors as well as ego and allocentric movement errors. Sometimes corticobasal degeneration and supranuclear palsy are difficult to clinically differentiate; however, Pharr et al. (2001) did note that patients with supranuclear palsy had less severe apraxia than those with corticobasal degeneration and also have impaired vertical ocular saccades and gait impairments.

Leiguarda et al. (1997) also reported that patients with multisystem atrophy did not exhibit ideomotor apraxia, but in contrast, Uluduz et al. (2010) reported that patients with multisystem atrophy did exhibit ideomotor apraxia and found that the patients with multisystem atrophy were more impaired than those with Parkinson's disease. Monza et al. (1998) also found that patients with multisystem atrophy can have an ideomotor apraxia and that the patients with multisystem atrophy who have an ideomotor apraxia often also have executive dysfunction.

Huntington's Disease

Since patients with Huntington's disease do have chorea, it may be difficult to determine when making purposeful movement if the errors observed in patients with Huntington's disease are related to their chorea or the presence of an ideomotor apraxia. Holl and coworkers (2011), however, attempted to learn whether patients with Huntington's disease did have an ideomotor apraxia and found that when these patients developed dementia they often demonstrated ideomotor apraxia.

Limb-Kinetic Apraxia (Melokinetic Apraxia, Innervatory Apraxia)

Clinical

Patients with limb-kinetic apraxia (Liepmann, 1920) have a loss of hand-finger deftness and thus are impaired in making precise movements of the upper limbic as well as being impaired in making independent but coordinated finger movements. Activities of daily living such as buttoning a shirt or blouse or tying shoelaces require dexterity or movement deftness. In addition, there are many instrumental activities that also require precise independent finger and arm movements.

There are many tests of deftness or dexterity. Patients can be assessed by having them button shirts, but this requires the use of both hands and is difficult to quantitate. To assess patients for the presence of limb-kinetic apraxia, we use the coin rotation task. When performing this test, the patient is asked to rotate a nickel between the thumb, index, and middle fingers, as rapidly as possible for 20 revolutions (Hanna-Pladdy, Mendoza, Apostolos, & Heilman, 2002). This test is easy to perform, gives quantitative results, and appears to be sensitive. Another test is to have patients pick up dimes from a flat surface. Normal adults will pick up these dimes using their thumb and forefinger using a pincher grasp. Patients with limb-kinetic apraxia will use a palmer grasp or slide the dime off the table, and as it drops, they grab it. Another test that can be used to assess for limb-kinetic apraxia is the pegboard. Both lifting the peg from a well and placing these pegs into small holes requires deftness, but patients may perform poorly on this test for many other reasons.

Typically, patients with hemispheric damage have a contralesional loss of deftness.

Heilman, Meador, and Loring (2000), as well as Hanna-Pladdy and colleagues (2002), have found that people with right-hand preference are more likely to have an additional ipsilateral loss of deftness (limb-kinetic apraxia) with left than right hemispheric injury.

Pathophysiology

Liepmann (1920) thought that the injury of the primary sensorimotor cortex caused limb-kinetic apraxia, and subsequently, Lawrence and Kuypers (1968) demonstrated a loss of a precision pincher grasp in monkeys with lesions of the pyramid that interrupted the corticospinal tract. Freund and Hummelsheim (1985) as well as Fogassi and colleagues (2001) reported that damage to the premotor cortex (Brodmann's area 6) can also induce limb-kinetic apraxia. Converging evidence for the role of premotor cortex in programming deft finger movements comes from the work of Nirkko and coworkers (2001), who performed functional magnetic resonance imaging while participants were performing unilateral deft finger movements and found that performance of these movements were associated with activation of the convexity premotor cortex.

There also appears to be hemispheric asymmetries in the development of limb-kinetic apraxia in people who are right handed, such that left hemisphere dysfunction, such as stroke, can induce ipsilateral (as well as contralesional) limb-kinetic apraxia (Heilman, Meador, & Loring, 2000; Hanna-Pladdy and colleagues, 2002); however, when right-handed patients have a right hemisphere stroke they may develop limb-kinetic apraxia of their contralesional left hand, but their right hand will often perform normally. This lesion-induced hemispheric asymmetry suggests than in right-handed people the left hemisphere has stronger ipsilateral control of spinal motor neurons than does the right hemisphere, and physiological studies in normal participants appear to support this postulate (Ghacibeh et al., 2007); however, it is not known whether this ipsilateral control is mediated by ipsilateral corticospinal pathways or by means of the corpus callosum.

Diseases That Can Cause Limb-Kinetic Apraxia and May Be Associated With Cognitive Disorders

Limb-kinetic apraxia can often be associated with cerebrovascular disease. In addition, we have reported that many patients with Parkinson's disease have this disorder, and their loss of deftness does not appear to be related to their bradykinesia (Quencer et al., 2007). Limb-kinetic apraxia can also be seen with the Parkinson's plus syndromes such as progressive supranuclear palsy (Leiguarda et al., 1997) and corticobasal degeneration, and, like the ideomotor apraxia, it may be asymmetrical. Gebhardt and coworkers (2008) studied finger tapping, as a measure of bradykinesia, and coin rotation, as a measure of limb-kinetic apraxia, while both on and off dopaminergic treatment and found that this treatment primarily improved bradykinesia (finger tapping) and did not have a substantial influence on coin rotation, suggesting that in these patients it is not the dopaminergic deficit that is causing this disorder.

Ideational Apraxia

Clinical

Unfortunately the diagnostic term "ideational apraxia" has been used to label many different disorders. This term has been used for patients with what we now call conceptual apraxia. De Renzi & Lucchelli (1968) used this term for patients who had severe ideomotor apraxia and were impaired when they attempted to use actual tools. I also used this term for patients who could not produce the correct transitive pantomime to verbal command but could perform normally when seeing the tool or the object upon which the tool normally works (Heilman, 1973). We now call this disorder "dissociation apraxia" because it appears that in these patients there is a dissociation of the systems important in comprehending speech and those important in programming movements (Heilman & Watson, 2008). Liepmann (1920) initially used this term for a disorder first described by Marcuse (1904) and Pick (1905), where patients have an inability to correctly sequence a series of acts, an ideational plan, that are required to successfully complete a goal. Poeck (1983) noted that while some patients may have perseveration, this disorder is not solely caused by perseveration but rather a disturbance in the conceptual organization of actions. Some investigators now call this disorder the "action disorganization syndrome" (Forde & Humphreys, 2002). Thus, the most important test for making the diagnosis of ideational apraxia is having the patient perform a task that requires several sequential motor acts, such as making a sandwich. Some clinicians test patients for ideational apraxia by having them verbally describe the means by which they would make something such as a sandwich. To assess for ideational apraxia, Qureshi et al. (2011) assessed participants with sets of pictures that showed the steps in completing a task, but the steps were shown out of order. The participants were required to point to the pictures in the correct sequence to complete each task. In another test, the Natural Action Test (NAT), subjects are presented with real objects and are required to perform multistep tasks that lead to a completed goal (Schwartz et al., 2002).

Pathophysiology

Although some of the diseases that cause this disorder are reviewed later in the chapter, the pathophysiology is not well understood. Liepmann (1920) thought that the lesion that induced this disorder was located in the left occipital parietal region. A functional imaging study performed with normal subjects performing a sequential action task appeared to activate the parietal lobe, as suggested by Liepmann (1920); however, the critical anatomic focus of dysfunction in ideational apraxia remains unknown (Humphreys & Forde, 1998). The frontal lobes are thought to be important in sequencing and Niki et al. (2009) reported several patients with frontal lobe tumors who had evidence of the "action disorganization syndrome" or ideational apraxia.

Diseases Associated With Ideational Apraxia

Most often the patients with ideational apraxia have some form of dementia such as Alzheimer's disease (Chainay, Louarn, & Humphreys, 2006). Giovannetti et al. (2006) demonstrated that patients with vascular dementia are more likely to have ideational apraxia (deficits on the NAT) than patients with Alzheimer's disease. We assessed patients for Parkinson's disease for ideational apraxia and found that ideational apraxia is associated with this condition. These patients' errors were predominantly in sequencing rather than repetition or omission, indicating that the poor performance was not caused by perseveration (Qureshi, Williamson, & Heilman, 2011). Leiguarda et al. (1997) reported that some patients with Parkinsons plus syndromes such as progressive supranuclear palsy also have problems with tasks involving multiple steps.

Summary

This chapter describes the clinical characteristics that define the various forms of upper limb apraxia, including conceptual, ideomotor, limb-kinetic, and ideational apraxia.

When a person determines that something needs to be altered, he or she must make some conceptual decisions, including whether a tool is needed and, if so, what tool can best accomplish this goal. The person must also know the action that this tool performs and the movements needed to operate this tool. If the correct tool is not available or a new tool is needed, the person also has to have the ability to understand the mechanical advantage this tools affords and how this could be accomplished by an alternative tool or the development of a new tool. A loss of this mechanical knowledge is called conceptual apraxia. In right-handed people this knowledge is stored in the left hemisphere, but the exact locations of these representations are unknown.

After a person selects a tool to work on an object, he or she also needs to have knowledge of the posture required to hold this tool as well as the egocentric and allocentric movements that permit this tool to be properly moved through space. In people who are right handed, these movement (temporo-spatial) representations appeared to be stored in the left parietal lobe, and degradation of these movement representations or damage to the premotor cortex that translates these spatial-temporal representations into motor programs induces ideomotor apraxia.

The motor program formulated by the premotor cortex must be implemented by the motor cortex that activates the motor neurons in the spinal cord. Injury to the premotor cortex or corticospinal system induces a loss of deftness and a disability when performing independent but coordinated finger movement, which is called limb-kinetic apraxia. Finally, many goal-oriented behaviors require a series of independent actions and often these actions must be performed in a specific temporal sequence. The inability to correctly sequence a series of acts, to achieve a goal, is called ideational apraxia, and this disorder may be a sign of frontal-executive dysfunction.

These limb-apraxic disorders can be a major cause of disability, both when performing instrumental activities and in activities of day living. Thus, testing for these forms of apraxia may not only aid in diagnosis but also help patients and caregivers manage their disabilities.

References

Agostoni, E., Coletti, A., Orlando, G., & Tredici, G. (1983). Apraxia in deep cerebral lesions. *Journal of Neurology, Neurosurgery and Psychiatry, 46*, 804–808.

Barrett, A. M., Schwartz, R. L., Raymer, A. L., Crucian, G. P., Rothi, L. J. G., & Heilman, K. M. (1998). Dyssynchronous apraxia: Failure to combine simultaneous preprogrammed movements. *Cognitive Neuropsychology, 15*, 685–703.

Basso, A., & Della Sala, S. (1986). Ideomotor apraxia arising from a purely deep lesion [letter]. *Journal of Neurology, Neurosurgery and Psychiatry, 49*(4), 437–454.

Broca, P. (1861). Remarques sur le siege de la faculte du language articule, suivies d'une observation d'aphemie. *Bulletin Société Anatomique (Paris), 2*, 330–357.

Chainay, H., Louarn, C., & Humphreys, G. W. (2006). Ideational action impairments in Alzheimer's disease. *Brain and Cognition, 62*(3), 198–205.

Crucian, G. P., Heilman, K., Junco, E., Maraist, M., Owens, W. E., Foote, K. D., & Okun, M. S. (2007). The crossed response inhibition task in Parkinson's disease: Disinhibition hyperkinesia. *Neurocase, 13*(3), 158–164

Della Sala, S., Basso, A., Laiacona, M., & Papagno, C. (1992). Subcortical localization of ideomotor apraxia: A review and an experimental study. In G. Vallar, S. F. Cappa, & C-W. Wellesch (Eds.), *Neuropsychological disorders associated with subcortical lesions* (pp. 357–380). Oxford, UK: Oxford University Press.

DeRenzi, E., & Lucchelli, F. (1968). Ideational apraxia. *Brain, 113*, 1173–1188.

DeRenzi, E., Faglioni, P., Scarpa, M., & Crisi, G. (1986). Limb apraxia in patients with damage confined to the left basal ganglia and thalamus. *Journal of Neurology, Neurosurgery and Psychiatry, 49*, 1030–1038.

Ebisch, S. J., Babiloni, C., Del Gratta, C., Ferretti, A., Perrucci, M. G., Caulo, M.,...Romani, G. L.(2007). Human neural systems for conceptual knowledge of proper object use: A functional magnetic resonance imaging study. *Cerebral Cortex, 17*(11), 2744–2751.

Faglioni, P., & Basso, A. (1985). Historical perspective on apraxia. In E. A. Roy (Ed.), *Neuropsychological studies of apraxia and related disorders* (pp. 2–44). New York, NY: North Holland Press.

Finkelburg, F. (1873). Uber Aphasie und Aysombolie Nebst Versuch Elmer Theorie der Sprachbildung. *Archiv fur Psychiatrie, 6*.

Fogassi, L., Gallese, V., Buccino, G., Craighero, L., Fadiga, L., & Rizzolatti, G. (2001). Cortical mechanism for the visual guidance of hand grasping movements in the monkey: A reversible inactivation study. *Brain, 124*(Pt 3), 571–586.

Forde, E. M., & Humphreys, G. W. (2002). Dissociations in routine behaviour across patients and everyday tasks. *Neurocase, 8*(1-2), 151–167.

Freund, H. J., & Hummelsheim, H. (1985). Lesions of premotor cortex in man. *Brain, 108*, 697–733.

Gebhardt, A., Vanbellingen, T., Baronti, F., Kersten, B., & Bohlhalter, S. (2008). Poor dopaminergic response of impaired dexterity in Parkinson's disease: Bradykinesia or limb kinetic apraxia? *Movement Disorders, 23*(12), 1701–1706.

Geschwind, N. (1965). Disconnection syndromes in animals and man. *Brain, 88*, 237–294, 585–644.

Ghacibeh, G. A., Mirpuri, R., Drago, V., Jeong, Y., Heilman, K. M., & Triggs, W. J. (2007). Ipsilateral motor activation during unimanual and bimanual motor tasks. *Clinical Neurophysiology, 118*(2), 325–332.

Giovannetti, T., Schmidt, K. S., Gallo, J. L., Sestito, N., & Libon, D. J. (2006). Everyday action in dementia: Evidence for differential deficits in Alzheimer's disease versus subcortical vascular dementia. *Journal of the International Neuropsychology Society, 12*(1), 45–53.

Goethals, M., & Santens, P. (2001). Posterior cortical atrophy. Two case reports and a review of the literature. *Clinical Neurology and Neurosurgery, 103*(2), 115–119.

Goldenberg, G., Wimmer, A., Auff, E., & Schnaberth, G. (1986). Impairment of motor planning in patients with Parkinson's disease: Evidence from ideomotor apraxia testing. *Journal of Neurology, Neurosurgery and Psychiatry, 49*(11), 1266–1272.

Goodglass, H., & Kaplan, E. (1963). Disturbance of gesture and pantomime in aphasia. *Brain, 86*, 703–720.

Haaland, K. Y., Harrington, D. L., & Knight, R. T. (2000). Neural representations of skilled movement. *Brain, 123*(Pt 11), 2306–2313.

Halsband, U., Schmitt, J., Weyers, M., Binkofski, F., Grutzner, G., & Freund, H. J. (2001). Recognition and imitation of pantomimed motor acts after unilateral parietal and premotor lesions: A perspective on apraxia. *Neuropsychologia, 39*(2), 200–216.

Hanna-Pladdy, B., Heilman, K. M., & Foundas, A. L. (2001). Cortical and subcortical contributions to ideomotor apraxia: Analysis of task demands and error types. *Brain, 124*, 2513–2527.

Hanna-Pladdy, B., Mendoza, J. E., Apostolos, G. T., & Heilman, K. M. (2002). Lateralised motor control: Hemispheric damage and the loss of deftness. *Journal of Neurology, Neurosurgery and Psychiatry, 73*, 574–577.

Hanna-Pladdy, B., Heilman, K. M., & Foundas, A. L. (2003). Ecological implications of ideomotor apraxia: Evidence from physical activities of daily living. *Neurology, 60*(3), 487–490.

Heilman, K. M. (1973). Ideational apraxia—a re-definition. *Brain, 96*, 861–864.

Heilman, K. M. (2004). Intentional neglect. *Frontiers in Bioscience, 9*, 694–705.

Heilman, K. M., Maher, L. M., Greenwald, M. L., & Rothi, L. J. R. (1997). Conceptual apraxia from lateralized lesions. *Neurology, 49*, 457–464.

Heilman, K. M., Meador, K. J., & Loring, D. W. (2000). Hemispheric asymmetries of limb-kinetic apraxia: A loss of deftness. *Neurology, 55*, 523–526.

Heilman, K. M., Rothi, L. J. G., & Valenstein, E. (1982). Two forms of ideomotor apraxia. *Neurology, 32*, 415–426.

Heilman, K. M., & Watson, R. T. (2008). The disconnection apraxias. *Cortex, 44*(8), 975–982.

Holl, A. K., Ille, R., Wilkinson, L., Otti, D. V., Hödl, E., Herranhof, B.,...Bonelli, R. M. (2011). Impaired ideomotor limb apraxia in cortical and subcortical dementia: A comparison of Alzheimer's and Huntington's disease. *Neurodegenerative Disorders, 8*(4), 208–215.

Humphreys, G. W., & Forde, E. M. E. (1998). Disordered action schema and action disorganization syndrome. *Cognitive Neuropsychology, 15*, 771–811.

Kertesz, A., & Ferro, J. M. (1984). Lesion size and location in ideomotor apraxia. *Brain, 107*, 921–933.

Kleist, K. (1907). Kortikale (innervatorische) Apraxie. *Jahrbuch fur Psychiatrie und Neurologie, 28*, 46–112.

Lauritzen, M., Henriksen, L., & Lassen, N. A. (1981). Regional cerebral blood flow during rest and skilled hand movements by Xenon-133 inhalation and emission computerized tomography. *Journal of Cerebral Blood Flow and Metabolism, 1*, 385–389.

Lawrence, D. G., & Kuypers, H. G. (1968). The functional organization of the motor system in the monkey. II. The effects of lesions of the descending brain-stem pathways. *Brain, 91*(1), 15–36.

Leiguarda, R., Lees, A. J., Merello, M., Starkstein, S., & Marsden, C. D. (1994). The nature of apraxia in corticobasal degeneration. *Journal of Neurology, Neurosurgery and Psychiatry, 57*(4), 455–459.

Leiguarda, R. C., Pramstaller, P. P., Merello, M., Starkstein, S., Lees, A. J., & Marsden, C. D. (1997). Apraxia in Parkinson's disease, progressive supranuclear palsy, multiple system atrophy and neuroleptic-induced parkinsonism. *Brain, 120*(Pt 1), 75–90.

Lhermitte, F. (1983). "Utilization behaviour" and its relation to lesions of the frontal lobes. *Brain, 106*(Pt 2), 237–255.

Lichtheim, L. (1885). On aphasia. *Brain, 7*, 433–484.

Liepmann, H. (1920). Apraxia. *Erbgn der ges Med, 1*, 516–543.

Liepmann, H., & Maas, O. (1907). Fall von linksseitiger Agraphie und Apraxie bei rechsseitiger Lahmung. *Zeitschrift fur Psychologie und Neurologie, 10*, 214–227.

Luria, A. R. (1962). *Higher cortical functions in man*. Moscow, Russia: Moscow University Press.

Marcuse, H. (1904). Apraktische Symptome bei einen Falle von seniler Demenz. *Zentrlball fur Neurologie, 15*, 737–751.

Moll, J., de Oliveira-Souza, R., Passman, L. J., Cunha, F. C., Souza-Lima, F., & Andreiuolo, P. A. (2000). Functional MRI correlates of real and imagined tool-use pantomimes. *Neurology, 54*, 1331–1336.

Monza, D., Soliveri, P., Radice, D., Fetoni, V., Testa, D., Caffarra, P.,...Girotti, F. (1998). Cognitive dysfunction and impaired organization of complex motility in degenerative Parkinsonian syndromes. *Archives of Neurology, 55*(3), 372–378.

Mozaz, M., Rothi, L. J., Anderson, J. M., Crucian, G. P., & Heilman, K. M. (2002). Postural knowledge of transitive pantomimes and intransitive gestures. *Journal of the International Neuropsychology Society, 8*(7), 958–962.

Mozaz, M., Garaigordobil, M., Gonzalez, Rothi, L. J., Anderson, J., Crucian, G. P., & Heilman, K. M. (2006). Posture recognition in Alzheimer's disease. *Brain and Cognition*, *62*(3), 241–245.

Nadeau, S. E., Roeltgen, D. P., Sevush, S., Ballinger, W. E., & Watson, R. T. (1994). Apraxia due to a pathologically documented thalamic infarction. *Neurology*, *44*(11), 2133–2137.

Niki, C., Maruyama, T., Muragaki, Y., & Kumada, T. (2009). Disinhibition of sequential actions following right frontal lobe damage. *Cognitive Neuropsychology*, *26*(3), 266–285.

Nirkko, A. C., Ozdoba, C., Redmond, S. M., Bürki, M., Schroth, G., Hess, C. W., & Wiesendanger, M. (2001). Different ipsilateral representations for distal and proximal movements in the sensorimotor cortex: activation and deactivation patterns. *Neuroimage*. *13*(5), 825–835.

Ochipa, C., Rothi, L. J. G., & Heilman, K. M. (1989). Ideational apraxia: A deficit in tool selection and use. *Annals of Neurology*, *25*, 190–193.

Ochipa, C., Rothi, L. J. G., & Heilman, K. M. (1992). Conceptual apraxia in Alzheimers disease. *Brain*, *114*, 2593–2603.

Pharr, V., Uttl, B., Stark, M., Litvan, I., Fantie, B., & Grafman, J. (2001). Comparison of apraxia in corticobasal degeneration and progressive supranuclear palsy. *Neurology*, *56*(7), 957–963.

Pick, A. (1905). *Sudien uber Motorische Apraxia und ihre Mahestenhende Erscheinungen*. Leipzig, Germany: Deuticke.

Poeck, K. (1983). Ideational apraxia. *Journal of Neurology*, *230*(1), 1–5.

Poizner, H., Mack, L., Verfaellie, M., Rothi, L. J. G., & Heilman, K. M. (1990). Three dimensional computer graphic analysis of apraxia. *Brain*, *113*, 85–101.

Pramstaller, P. P., & Marsden, C. D. (1996). The basal ganglia and apraxia. *Brain*, *119*(Pt 1), 319–340.

Quencer, K., Okun, M. S., Crucian, G., Fernandez, H. H., Skidmore, F., & Heilman, K. M. (2007). Limb-kinetic apraxia in Parkinson disease. *Neurology*, *68*(2), 150–151.

Qureshi, M., Williamson, J. B., & Heilman, K. M. (2011). Ideational apraxia in Parkinson disease. *Cognitive and Behavioral Neurology*, *24*(3), 122–127.

Rao, S. M., Binder, J. R., Bandettini, P. A., Hammeke, T. A., Yetkin, F. Z., Jesmanowicz, A., . . . Estkowski, L. D. (1993). Functional magnetic resonance imaging of complex human movements. *Neurology*, *43*(11), 2311–2318.

Raymer, A. M., Maher, L. M., Foundas, A. L., Heilman, K. M., & Rothi, L. J. G. (1997). The significance of body part as tool errors in limb apraxia. *Brain and Cognition*, *34*, 287–292.

Rousseaux, M., Rénier, J., Anicet, L., Pasquier, F., & Mackowiak-Cordoliani, M. A. (2012). Gesture comprehension, knowledge and production in Alzheimer's disease. *European Journal of Neurology*, *19*(7), 1037–1044.

Rothi, L. J. G., Heilman, K. M., & Watson, R. T. (1985). Pantomime comprehension and ideomotor apraxia. *Journal of Neurology, Neurosurgery and Psychiatry*, *48*, 207–210.

Rothi, L. J. G., Mack, L., Verfaellie, M., Brown, P., & Heilman, K. M. (1988). Ideomotor apraxia: Error pattern analysis. *Aphasiology*, *2*, 381–387.

Saeki, S., & Hachisuka, K. (2004). The association between stroke location and return to work after first stroke. *Journal of Stroke and Cerebrovascular Disease*, *13*(4), 160–163.

Schwartz, M. F., Buxbaum, L. J., Ferraro, M., Veramonti, T., & Segal, M. (2002). *Naturalistic action test*. Suffolk, England: Thames Valley Test Company.

Shuren, J. E., Maher, L. M., & Heilman, K. M. (1994). Role of the pulvinar in ideomotor praxis. *Journal of Neurology, Neurosurgery and Psychiatry*, *57*(10), 1282–1283.

Silveri, M. C., & Ciccarelli, N. (2009). Semantic memory in object use. *Neuropsychologia*, *47*(12), 2634–2641.

Steinthal, P. (1871). *Abriss der Sprach wissenschaft*. Berlin.

Uluduz, D., Ertürk, O., Kenangil, G., Ozekmekçi, S., Ertan, S., Apaydin, H., & Erginöz, E. (2010). Apraxia in Parkinson's disease and multiple system atrophy. *European Journal of Neurology*, *17*(3), 413–418.

Von Monakov, C. (1914). *Die Lokalisation im Grosshirn und der Abbau der Function durch Kortikale Herde*. Wiesbaden, Germany: Bergmann.

Watson, R. T., & Heilman, K. M. (1983). Callosal apraxia. *Brain*, *106*, 391–403.

Wernicke, C. (1874). *Das Aphasiche Symptomenkomplex*. Breslau, Poland: Cohn and Weigart.

Part II

The Dementias: The Major Diseases and Clinical Syndromes

6

The Neuropathology of Neurodegenerative Dementias

Etty P. Cortes Ramirez and Jean-Paul G. Vonsattel

In all neurodegenerative diseases, it is thought that the degenerative pathologic process is well under way many years before symptom onset. A tremendous amount of our knowledge of these diseases has been learned through careful neuropathological examination of brain tissue from patients whose symptoms have been well characterized during life. Nevertheless, despite this progress and the ability of experts to predict pathology with a reasonable degree of sensitivity and specificity, many specific aspects of the relationships between pathological measures of neurodegenerative pathology and clinical symptoms prior to death remain poorly understood. Perhaps the biggest conceptual issue relates to the question of what is disease and what is aging. Some longitudinal prospective studies have demonstrated convincingly that individuals who are cognitively, emotionally, and physically intact within 1 year prior to their death may have a substantial burden of clinically silent neuropathology.

Some of the changes seen by pathologists in the brains of healthy elderly individuals can be seen macroscopically and some can be seen microscopically. Some of these changes appear to be present in most older individuals regardless of neuropsychiatric clinical status, while others are thought to be specific for a neurodegenerative disease.

This chapter employs the basic approach of clinicopathological correlations as it was fostered by Drs. E. P. Richardson, R. D. Adams, C. M. Fisher, and E. T. Hedley-Whyte at the Massachusetts General Hospital. Thus, the emphasis is placed on the relationships between the types of macroscopic and microscopic pathology, their localization in different brain regions, and the symptoms that may ensue. First, however, we describe the neurodegenerative changes that can be commonly seen in the aging brain. We then focus on representative neurodegenerative diseases, highlighting the outstanding pathologic hallmarks associated with each clinical condition.

Neurodegenerative Neuropathology in Cognitively Normal Individuals

The aging central nervous system undergoes changes that are gradual and relentless, which at some point cause physical deficits or cognitive dysfunction attributed to "normal aging." The initial phase of this process most likely consists of a subtle decline of physical and mental performance without definite physical changes detectable in the brain, probably as a result of physiologic changes in neurotransmitter and electrophysiologic function. It has long been known, however, that many cognitively intact older adults exhibit neuropathologic changes identical to those of Alzheimer's disease (AD) dementia, but to a lesser extent (Knopman et al., 2003; Lace et al., 2009; Polvikoski et al., 2001; Price et al., 2009; Tomlinson, Blessed, & Roth, 1968). Some authors have suggested that a possible pathologic continuum exists between "aging" and AD. For example, as early as 1924, Simchowicz concluded that "senile dementia consists of both acceleration and increased intensity of the age-related physiological involution of the brain" (Simchowicz, 1924). Drachman formulated Simchowicz's hypothesis 70 years later as follows: "If we live long enough, will we all become demented? With our present lack of means to prevent the most common dementia, AD, more and more of us will decline cognitively, as life expectancy increases, evidently with an age-related acceleration of incidence" (Drachman, 1994; p. 1563).

While the brain changes associated with "normal age-related cognitive changes" continue to be studied, many contemporary theorists view the occurrence of AD neuropathology in cognitively intact individuals as evidence that the neuropathological disease process of AD gradually takes place for many years prior to the manifestation of symptoms. Many such investigators view this as an opportunity for intervention (see Chapter 18).

Briefly, on postmortem examination, the outstanding changes found in the brains of cognitively normal elderly individuals include the following (Fig. 6.1). Macroscopically, atrophy is often present, which is evidenced by weight loss (up to 200 grams [normal: women 1,260 g; men 1,360 g]), narrowing of gyri and widening of sulci, and ventricular dilatation. Microscopically, some neuronal loss is often seen but with less decrease of the neuronal density than expected because of the shrinkage of the neuropil; occurrence of neurofibrillary tangles of Alzheimer; immature and diffuse type plaques, and neuritic plaques; granulovacuolar degeneration, and Hirano bodies especially within the hippocampus; Marinesco bodies (pars compacta of the substantia nigra); and vasculopathies (e.g., atherosclerosis, arteriolosclerosis, hypertensive angiopathy, amyloid angiopathy, or cerebral amyloid angiopathy [CAA]), and ferro-calcic angiopathy, especially involving the lenticular nucleus (globus pallidus > putamen). Microhemorrhages, criblures, lacunes, glial scars, or infarcts result from the vasculopathies, which cause frequently mixed pathological changes (Schneider, Arvanitakis,

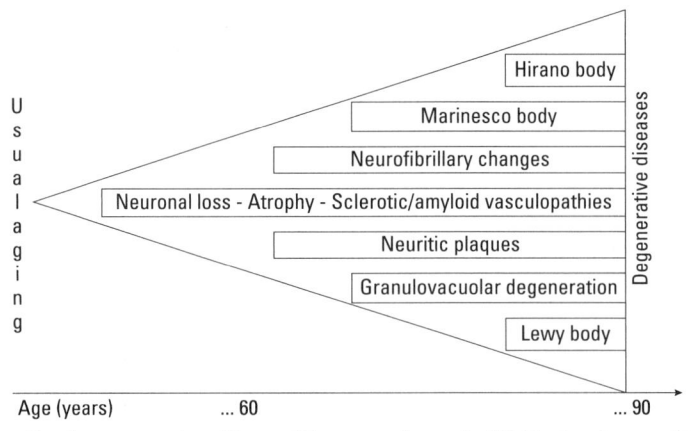

Figure 6.1 "If we live long enough, will we all become demented?" During "normal" aging, the brains of most individuals show changes similar to those occurring in Alzheimer's disease, albeit to a much lesser extent. Thus, a quantitative continuum might exist between "normal" age-related changes and the neuropathology of some neurodegenerative diseases. It is also possible that these pathological changes mark the preclinical stages of neurodegenerative diseases, which would ultimately manifest as symptomatic illnesses.

Bang, & Bennett, 2007). Lewy body–containing neurons and Lewy neurites are found in 10%–15% of brains from allegedly asymptomatic elderly individuals (Frigerio et al., 2009; Jellinger, 2009; Ross et al., 2004). The association of degenerative pathological changes and the occurrence of dementia is stronger in younger old persons than in older old persons (Savva et al., 2009).

Selective Regional Vulnerability of the Aging Brain

The neuropathologist must attempt to infer the localization of the origin of the neurodegenerative process. Gross atrophy results from the loss of neurons, including their synapses and their myelinated or bare axons, which constitute the brunt of the white matter. The constellation of the loss of neurons and neuropil along with the occurrence of reactive gliosis gradually blurs normal neuronal and glial cytoarchitecture. Perhaps because the clearance of the cellular debris is overwhelmed or hypofunctional, there is accumulation of proteinaceous aggregates such as amyloid-β. Usually proteinaceous aggregates develop without acute or chronic inflammatory infiltrates, although, as mentioned, the microgliocytes participate in the process.

By the time the patient dies, the severity of the degenerative process is usually widespread but often uneven. Putatively the most involved sites might have been the starting injury points or primary centers of degeneration (Grünthal, 1930). The hypothesis of the occurrence of initial primary centers of degeneration is supported by the variable severity of the degenerative process, especially evidenced on postmortem examination. Thus, one can assume that degeneration spread from these primary sites within one or more especially vulnerable systems while simultaneously contaminating the adjacent parenchyma whether or not being part of the main system involved (Spatz, 1938). At some point during the degenerative process, the waning function of the network involved results in distinctive symptoms localizable to that system. As we have begun to learn about the pathologic features that appear to be specifically associated with a particular neurodegenerative disease process, we have begun to think of the processes as having a potentially long presymptomatic or prodromal period (see Chapters 17 and 18).

The development of dementia with or without motor deficit results from the degeneration of structures, including the cerebral cortex, as in AD; the cerebral white matter, as in multiples sclerosis or cerebrovascular disease; the hippocampal formation, entorhinal region, amygdala, nucleus basalis of Meynert, as in AD; the striatum, as in Huntington's disease (HD); the mesencephalon, especially the pars compacta of substantia nigra, as in Parkinson's disease (PD), or in Lewy body diseases; or the brainstem, subthalamic nucleus, striatum, and cerebellum as in progressive supranuclear palsy (PSP). A key clinicopathologic lesson learned over the past decades is the tenet that it is the localization—rather than the molecular composition—of neuropathology that determines the clinical phenotype. That is, many reports have described multiple neuropathologies underlying a given clinical phenotype and conversely a singular molecular neuropathology (in some cases associated with a single genetic mutation) in association with multiple clinical phenotypes (see Chapters 8, 9, 10).

Cerebral Cortex

Despite this variability, the localization and apparent progression of some neurodegenerative pathological processes occurs with a remarkable reproducibility (Morrison, Hof, & Morrison, 1998). Phylogenetically the cerebral cortex is composed of the allocortex, and the more recent, neocortex, both with their respective subdivisions and their selective vulnerability characteristically associated with the neurodegenerative dementias. The allocortex includes archicortex (hippocampal formation [cornu ammonis, dentate fascia]) and paleocortex (piriform cortex [entorhinal area, olfactory cortex]). The neocortex includes both homotypical cortex (six distinct layers, such as in posterior parietal cortex) and heterotypical cortex, including both agranular (motor) cortex and granular (visual) cortex. The allocortical regions are particularly prone to degeneration in AD and frontotemporal lobar degeneration (FTLD; Kemper, 1994). The large pyramidal neurons, notably those of the Sommer sector of the hippocampus, are susceptible to neurofibrillary tangle formation, granulovacuolar degeneration, and Hirano body formation (Lace et al., 2009). The stellate neurons of layer 2 of the entorhinal cortex are highly susceptible to neurofibrillary tangle formation, most conspicuously in AD. The large and small pyramidal neurons of the hippocampus, and the granule neurons of the fascia dentata, are susceptible to Pick bodies (Ball, 1979; Binetti, Growdon, & Vonsattel, 1998).

Within the neocortex (Fig. 6.2), the homotypical cortex is usually more vulnerable than the heterotypical cortex (motor cortex, where the pyramidal neurons including Betz cells predominate, or visual cortex, where the granular neurons prevail) (Kemper, 1994). Neocortical neurons can be categorized as pyramidal and nonpyramidal cells. The pyramidal neurons have extensive intracortical and extracortical connections; it is these neurons that are most affected in neurodegenerative diseases associated with dementia. The unipolar pyramidal projection neurons of the anterior insula and cingulate cortex known as Von Economo neurons are particularly vulnerable to FTLD (Seeley, et al., 2006).

Cerebral White Matter

The cerebral white matter harbors myelinated and bare axons, fibrillary astrocytes, oligodendrocytes, and blood vessels. Extensive loss of the white matter with subsequent dementia may be caused by vasculopathies. Indeed, hypertensive vascular changes (fibrosis of the walls of the vessels; i.e., arteriolosclerosis) cause hypoperfusion of central white matter. A gradual loss of oligodendrocytes, myelin, and neuronal processes occurs with a reactive gliosis and widening of the perivascular spaces (criblures). Especially involved is the subcortical white matter, as in Binswanger disease. Nearly 30% of cohort of individuals with cerebral autosomal dominant arteriopathy with subcortical infarcts and leukoencephalopathy (CADASIL) developed dementia and a pathological phenotype similar to that of Binswanger disease (Davous & Bequet, 1995; Dichgans et al., 1998; Tournier-Lasserve et al., 1993). Dementing illnesses with a predominantly myelinoclastic or demyelinating process include progressive multifocal leukoencephalopathy (PML), the encephalopathy of the acquired immune deficiency syndrome (AIDS), and multiple sclerosis (Brew, Rosenblum, Cronin, & Price, 1995; Fontaine et al., 1994).

Subcortical Nuclei

The amygdala is often severely involved in neurodegenerative dementing diseases. In AD, the amygdala often shows neuronal loss,

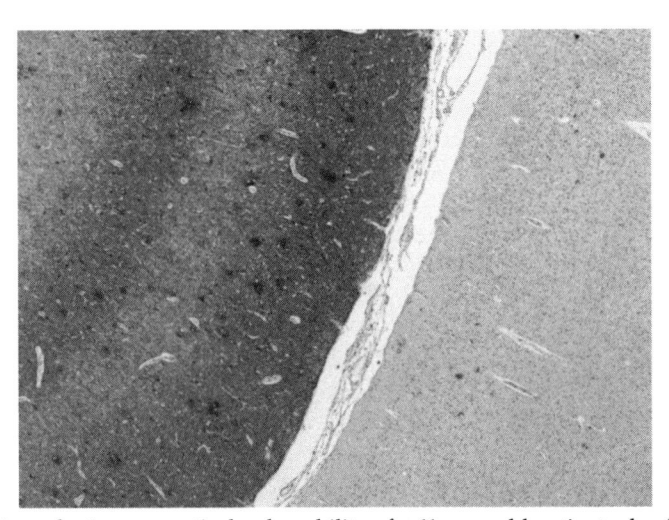

Figure 6.2 Relative selective neocortical vulnerability of a 61-year-old patient who died of cardiac arrest and who carried the clinical diagnosis of possible Alzheimer's disease: The cuneus (left, homotypic cortex) contains many neuropil threads that are labeled with AT8 antibodies directed against phosphorylated tau, and scattered neuritic plaques. In contrast, the calcarine cortex (right, heterotypic cortex) is relatively spared. (AT8 immunohistochemistry; original magnification, 25×)

neurofibrillary tangles, neuritic plaques, and gliosis. In up to 60% of AD brains, the amygdala exhibits Lewy body–containing neurons and Lewy neurites (Hamilton, 2000; Wakisaka et al., 2003). In DLB, the amygdala exhibits neuronal loss, neurons with Lewy body or Lewy body–containing neurons, and spongiform changes (small, round or oval vacuoles), neuronal tangles, and neuritic plaques. In the classic Pick's disease form of FTLD, the amygdala exhibits severe neuronal loss, gliosis, ballooned neurons, status spongiosus (large, irregular vacuoles with coarse glial margins), and Pick bodies.

The cholinergic neurons of the nucleus basalis of Meynert, or substantia innominata, undergo either primary or retrograde degeneration in AD, DLB, PD, and PSP. The large cholinergic neurons of the neostriatum (caudate nucleus, putamen, nucleus accumbens) undergo neurofibrillary degeneration in AD and in PSP. The striatum (neostriatum plus globus pallidus) bears the brunt of the cerebral atrophy in HD. The dorsomedian and the anterior nuclei of the thalamus, which are the limbic nuclei, are prone to neuronal loss with the occurrence of neurofibrillary tangles in AD. The rostral half of the thalamus may be atrophic (usually medial > lateral) in Pick's disease. These thalamic changes are frequently encountered in the context of dementia (Schmahmann, 2003).

Brainstem

The brainstem often shows degenerative changes in dementing illnesses with or without symptoms of movement disorders (Parvizi, Van Hoesen, & Damasio, 2001). Neuronal loss involves the substantia nigra pars compacta (mainly dopaminergic) in DLB, up to 70% of cases of classic Pick's disease, PD, PSP, and to a lesser extent AD. The nucleus coeruleus (norepinephrine—catecholamine) is especially involved in AD, DLB, and PD. The neuronal loss of the nucleus coeruleus is usually less severe in PSP than in PD. The neurons of the dorsal and median raphe nuclei (serotoninergic) are vulnerable in AD, DLB, PD, and PSP. The dorsal nucleus of vagus (cholinergic) shows neuronal loss in DLB and PD. In addition, neurofibrillary tangles or Lewy body–containing neurons can occur in the reticular formation.

In summary, neurodegenerative dementias share at least partly in common their involvement of vulnerable cortical and subcortical regions, including allocortex (entorhinal and pyriform cortices, hippocampus), neocortex (homotypical > heterotypical), amygdala, mammillary bodies, anterior and dorsomedian nuclei of thalamus, neostriatum, nucleus coeruleus, and raphe nuclei.

Pathological Hallmarks of the Major Neurodegenerative Dementias

Cerebral Atrophy

The hallmarks of cerebral atrophy on gross examination of the brains are the narrowing of the gyri and widening of the sulci, including up to 20%–30% weight loss (Fig. 6.3).

A surprising degree of cerebral atrophy may occur in cognitively normal elderly individuals (Ezekiel et al., 2004; Hulette et al., 1998). Likewise, atrophy may be absent or subtle early during any neurodegenerative process. Brain atrophy becomes conspicuous in about 90% of brains of patients with advanced dementia without or with movement disorders (Fig. 6.3). However, severe dementia may occur in patients whose brains show little or no atrophy. Brains of patients with DLB, or of a few patients with AD, especially those who are older then 80 at the time of death, may appear normal on external gross examination (Polvikoski et al., 2001). Likewise, the brains of patients with "dementia lacking distinctive histology" or Creutzfeldt Jakob disease or other prion diseases may be unremarkable on gross examination. Some patients with frontotemporal dementia may exhibit prominent circumscribed atrophy.

Ventricular Enlargement

The volume of each lateral ventricle is about 7.0–10.0 cc in individuals without neurological or psychiatric diseases. The ventricular volume may reach up to 50 cc or more in demented people (Fig. 6.3 B). The widening of the ventricles in conjunction with parenchymal loss is referred to as hydrocephalus ex vacuo. The severity and topography of ventricular enlargement tend to match that of the atrophy of the encompassing parenchyma.

(A) (B)

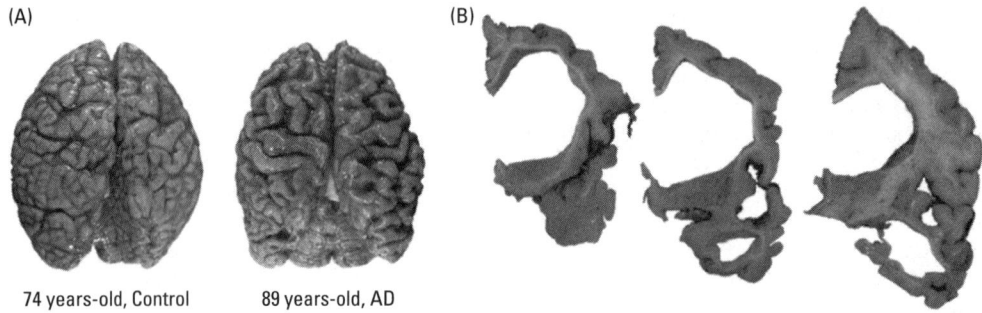

74 years-old, Control   89 years-old, AD

Figure 6.3 (*A*) Dorsal aspect of a normal fresh brain (left) of a 74-year-old cognitively intact individual and of an atrophic fresh brain (right) of a demented, 89-year-old patient with end-stage Alzheimer's disease (AD). Note the widening of the sulci and the narrowing of the gyri in the brain of the person with AD (*B*) compared to the individual who was cognitively intact (*A*). (*B*) Fixed coronal slices of the right cerebral hemisphere of a 78-year-old patient with end-stage AD. There is severe atrophy of the gray (cortex, hippocampus, amygdaloid nucleus, striatum, and thalamus) and white matter (left, rostral; right, caudal). The lateral ventricle is severely widened. At the end stage, brain atrophy tends to become diffuse, thus making it difficult to identify brain regions selectively vulnerable early in the course of the disease.

Neuritic Plaques

Neuritic plaques (or senile plaques, amyloid argyrophilic plaques) are extracellular deposits that are abundant in AD and can also be seen in many intellectually normal older subjects. Neuritic plaques develop in the cerebral cortex, amygdala, hippocampal formation, and in the striatum, especially in the nucleus accumbens. They may occur in the thalamus, particularly within the dorsomedian and anterior nuclei, and occasionally within the cerebellar cortex.

The "classical" or "neuritic plaques" are spherical lesions with a 50–180 μm diameter (Fig. 6.4B). They are composed of a centrally located Congo red–positive amyloid core, which can be labeled with antibodies directed against amyloid-β (Aβ). This core of Aβ is surrounded by a halo of distorted neurites containing argyrophilic, paired helical filaments (PHF [dystrophic neurites]). Microglial cells and macrophages can be seen within the plaques. Reactive astrocytes tend to be at the periphery of the plaques or in the parenchyma surrounding the plaques.

Neurofibrillary Changes

Neurofibrillary changes are due to the cytoplasmic or intracellular accumulation of distorted, paired helical filaments caused by the hyperphosphorylation of tau. The hyperphosphorylation prevents the fulfillment of the normal function of tau, which is a microtubule-associated protein that promotes tubulin assembly and stabilizes microtubules.

Neurofibrillary changes consist of thin, fragmented, tortuous, and argyrophilic fibrils, which are labeled with AT8 antibodies directed against phosphorylated tau (Fig. 6.4B). Depending of the underlying degenerative process, they occur within the halo of neuritic plaques (dystrophic neurites), within the cytoplasm of pyramidal neurons (flame shaped neurofibrillary tangles), within the cytoplasm of oval neurons (globose tangles), and within the cytoplasm of oligodendrocytes or astrocytes (glial cytoplasmic tangles). The so-called tauopathies include AD, FTLD (including classic Pick's disease), PSP, corticobasal degeneration, and chronic traumatic encephalopathy, as well as a host of relatively rare neurodegenerative diseases.

Hirano Bodies and Granulovacuolar Degeneration

Hirano bodies and granulovacuolar degeneration are more frequent in people with dementia than in intellectually normal subjects; apparently, their density increases with age. Hirano bodies are ovoid, or rod-shaped, 10–30 μm in length, eosinophilic, amorphous structures found among, usually adjacent

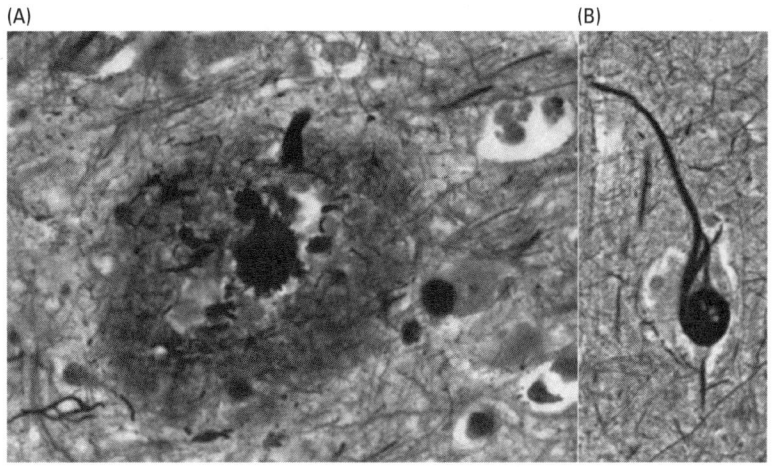

Figure 6.4 Hallmarks of Alzheimer's disease neuropathology: (A) neuritic plaques (about 180 μm in diameter; each one replaces an estimated 10^6 synapses and about 100 neurons). The centrally located core is made up of aggregates of amyloid-β, which results from incomplete degradation of a trans-membrane protein present in nerve terminals called amyloid-β precursor protein (APP). The gene for APP is located on chromosome 21. (B) Neurofibrillary tangles of Alzheimer and neuropil threads (argyrophilic neurons and threads) consist of intracellular accumulation of paired helical filaments caused by the hyperphosphorylation of tau. Tau protein is a phosphoprotein that binds to and promotes polymerization and stability of microtubules. The tau gene is located on chromosome 17. (Bielschowsky silver stain; original magnification, 630×) (See color plate section)

to, or within the cytoplasm of hippocampal pyramidal neurons, especially involved is the Sommer sector (CA-1) (Hirano, 1994). They may appear as a result of age-related alterations of the microfilamentous system.

Granulovacuolar degeneration consists of the presence of one or more cytoplasmic granules, 1–2 μm across, surrounded by an optically empty rim, or vacuole measuring 3–5 μm in diameter. Especially involved are the pyramidal neurons of the Sommer sector (CA1) and subiculum of the hippocampus. Tomlinson et al. reported severe involvement of the pyramidal cells of the Sommer sector in every demented patient and that "some degree" of this change was found in 70% of their control brains (Tomlinson et al., 1968). Both Hirano bodies and granulovacuolar degenerations are ubiquitinated and not labeled with AT8 antibodies directed against phosphorylated tau.

Pick Bodies

Pick bodies are neuronal, cytoplasmic, argyrophilic, well outlined, and round, or oval bodies measuring 10–15 μm across (Fig. 6.5). They are labeled with AT8 antibodies directed against phosphorylated tau, antibodies directed against ubiquitinated proteins, but not with antibodies directed against α-synuclein aggregates. They are found in cortical and hippocampal, pyramidal neurons; in neurons of the stratum granulosum of the dentate gyrus; and in the amygdala, and occasionally within the striatum and brainstem.

Ballooned Neurons (Pick Cells)

Ballooned neurons, also referred to as "Pick cells" are swollen neurons with convex contours, homogeneous glassy, pale, eosinophilic cytoplasm, and eccentric nuclei (Clark et al., 1986). The cytoplasm is diffusely argyrophilic with variable intensity. Ballooned neurons are found in a variety of neurodegenerative diseases including classic Pick's disease, PSP, corticobasal degeneration, and AD.

Status Spongiosus Versus Spongiform Changes

Status spongiosus consists of irregular cavitation of the neuropil in the presence of a dense

(A)   (B)

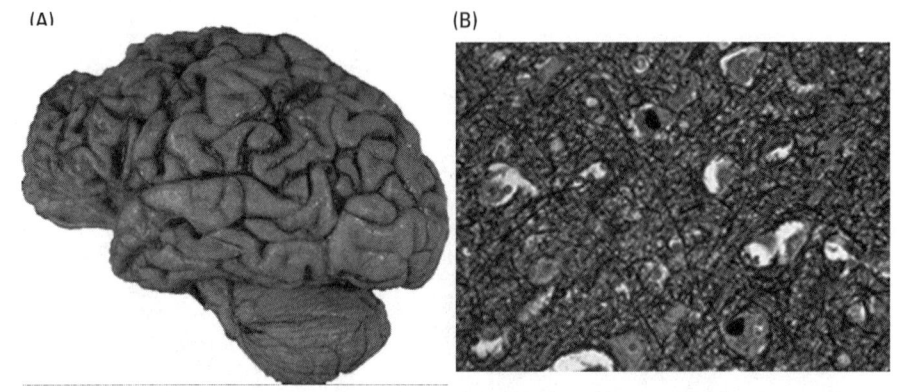

Figure 6.5 (A) Formalin fixed, lateral aspect of the left half brain of a 53-year-old patient with frontotemporal lobar degeneration (classical Pick's disease). Note the prominent circumscribed atrophy involving the frontal lobe, rostral temporal lobe, and the inferior parietal lobule. Although atrophic, the pre- and postcentral gyri, the caudal two thirds of the superior temporal gyrus, and occipital lobe are relatively preserved. (B) Microphotographs of Pick bodies. Pick bodies are argyrophilic (bottom left, Bielschowsky, 200×), are labeled with AT8 antibodies directed against phosphorylated tau (bottom right, AT8, 630×), or with antibodies directed against ubiquitinated proteins. They are not labeled with antibodies directed against α-synuclein aggregates, which is in contrast to Lewy bodies. (Bielschowsky silver stain; original magnification, 400×) (See color plate section)

glial meshwork (Masters & Richardson, 1978). It is nonspecific and characteristically is the manifestation of end-stage gliosis.

Spongiform changes consist of the presence of small, round, or ovoid, optically empty vacuoles within the neuropil. Transcortical or deep cortical spongiform changes associated with gliosis are hallmarks of the spongiform encephalopathies, including Creutzfeldt-Jakob disease (CJD). However, to some extent, spongiform changes (with mild, or without reactive astrocytosis) are observed in the Lewy body spectrum diseases, the FTD spectrum diseases, and occasionally in AD (Smith et al., 1987). In these instances, spongiform changes are usually confined to the superficial, cortical layers; but, at times, they are indistinguishable from those observed in spongiform encephalopathies, which must then be ruled out using Western blots.

Alzheimer's Disease

By the time a patient with AD typically dies, the gross appearance of the brain is diffusely atrophic with a predilection for the prefrontal, parietal, and temporal lobes. In 10% of cases, however, the atrophy may be circumscribed or minimal. On examination of the cut sections, the brunt of the atrophy involves the cerebral cortex and adjacent white matter in the areas mentioned previously, often particularly prominently in the medial temporal cortical regions, hippocampal formation, amygdaloid nucleus, and the anterior thalamus (Fig. 6.3). The ventricular system is widened proportionally to the volume loss of the parenchyma. In most instances, the nucleus coeruleus is paler than normally expected, which is in contrast to the usually well-pigmented pars compacta of the substantia nigra.

Microscopically, the characteristic lesions of AD are often widespread throughout the brain, although their severity varies regionally (Braak, Alafuzoff, Arzberger, Kretzschmar, & Del Tredici, 2006; K. A. Jellinger & Bancher 1998; Parvizi et al., 2001). Microscopic AD neuropathology is usually most prominent in the entorhinal/perirhinal cortex, hippocampal formation (Fig. 6.6), amygdaloid nucleus, basal forebrain including the substantia innominata (nucleus of Meynert), hypothalamus, thalamus, and the following regions of the cerebral cortex: temporal, prefrontal, and parietal. The motor and visual cortices are relatively preserved, although not spared. The characteristic lesions of AD include neuritic and diffuse amyloid plaques, neurofibrillary tangles of Alzheimer, with accompanying neuronal loss.

Neuritic plaques tend to predominate in cortical layers II and III (Fig. 6.4A).

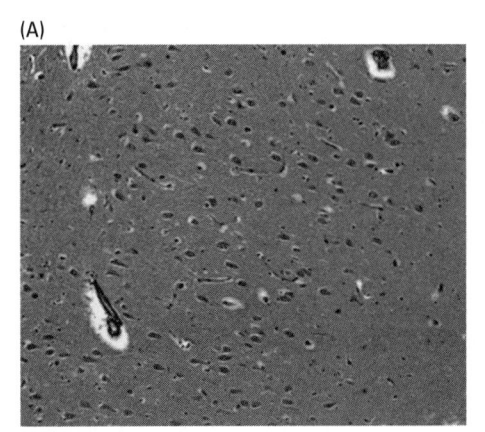

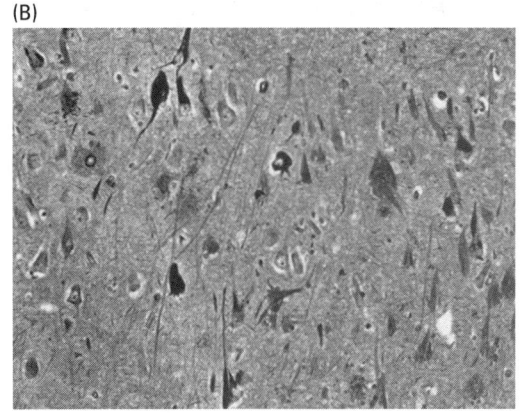

Figure 6.6 (A) The hippocampus (CA1 subfield, Sommer's sector) of a 100-year-old individual with mild cognitive impairment and apparently normal neuronal density. Rare argyrophilic neurons can be seen, (Original magnification, 100×). (B) The hippocampus of a 90-year-old patient with Alzheimer's disease. Compared to A, the neuronal density is severely decreased. Among the residual neurons, many are argyrophilic (Bielschowsky silver stain; original magnification, 200×)

Neurofibrillary tangles of Alzheimer usually predominate in layers III and V of the neocortex (Fig. 6.4B). Furthermore, neuronal tangles are scattered within the mesencephalic colliculi, raphe nuclei, periaqueductal gray, nucleus coeruleus, and reticular formation.

In addition to the neuropathology features of AD discussed previously, amyloid-β may also gradually accumulate within the walls of medium-sized leptomeningeal or cortical vessels (Attems, Jellinger, Thal, & Van Nostrand, 2011). This accumulation causes compression atrophy of the smooth muscle of the media with subsequent loss of the flexibility and contractibility of the vessel, which predisposes to blood leakage. The frequency of this vasculopathy increases with age and occurs often in elderly people, including those without cognitive impairment. The frequency and severity of CAA are enhanced in individuals with AD. Severe CAA may cause recurrent, lobar cerebral hemorrhages. See Chapter 14 for more information on CAA.

Frontotemporal Lobar Degeneration

In FTLD, grossly apparent atrophy usually predominates within the frontal, fronto-temporal, or fronto-temporal-parietal regions (Fig. 6.5). The anterior insula and anterior cingulate cortex are often devastated neuropathologically in FTLD and are thought by some investigators to be where the disease begins (Seeley et al., 2008). Other particularly vulnerable regions are the frontal cortex rostral to the motor strip, the temporal cortex with relative preservation of the caudal third of the superior temporal gyrus, and to a lesser degree the parietal cortex.

At the microscopic level, concepts of the neuropathology of FTLD have been rapidly evolving. At present, several broad subdivisions of FTLD are recognized. One important neuropathologic subtype of FTLD is known as FTLD-tau, characterized by the presence of hyperphosphorylated tau inclusions within neurons and glia. This is the classic Pick's disease, although other non-Pick tauopathies can be associated with the clinical phenotype of FTD as well. Pick's disease neuropathology includes neurons containing Pick bodies, scattered ballooned neurons or Pick cells, and status spongiosus. Tau protein is a microtubule associated protein thought to be critical in stabilizing microtubules and supporting intracellular molecular transport.

The other important neuropathologic subtype of FTLD is associated with TAR DNA-binding protein (TDP43) inclusions within neurons and glia (Cairns et al., 2007b; Neumann et al., 2007). TDP43 was discovered in 2006 as a major protein aggregate in approximately 50% of FTLD and also in the vast majority of cases of amyotrophic lateral sclerosis (ALS; Neumann et al., 2006). TDP43 is largely found within the nucleus and is involved in RNA regulation and transport. There appear to be four distinct subtypes of FTLD-TDP pathology based on the morphology of the inclusions and their cellular localization (Mackenzie et al., 2011). Emerging evidence indicates that each subtype may be associated with characteristic clinical and genetic features. To date, a number of genetic mutations in FTD and ALS patients have been identified in conjunction with TDP43 pathology, including mutations in *GRN* (the progranulin gene), the TDP gene itself (*TARDBP*), *VCP* (the valosin containing protein gene), and the recently identified *C9ORF72* hexanucleotide repeat expansion.

Another much less common neuropathologic subtype of FTLD, discovered in 2009, is characterized by intranuclear inclusions of the RNA-binding protein FUS (fused in sarcoma). This protein is implicated in nuclear transcriptional activities. FUS inclusions are seen in associated with mutations in the *FUS* gene in a small proportion of familial ALS cases and are seen in sporadic FTLD, often with a young age of onset. This is another key finding that has generated tremendous excitement in bringing together the FTLD and ALS research communities.

See Chapter 8 for discussion of the clinical aspects of FTD.

Neuropathology of Dementias Associated With Lewy Bodies

On gross examination of the brain of a patient with PD dementia or DLB, the most outstanding changes noticeable are pallor of the pars compacta of the substantia nigra (mesencephalon) and of the nucleus coeruleus (metencephalon) (Fig. 6.7). Usually the DLB or PDD brain is not atrophic or is only mildly atrophic.

Microscopically, the hallmark of DLB/PDD is intraneuronal cytoplasmic inclusions referred to as the "Lewy body" (Fig. 6.8). Lewy bodies are labeled with antibodies directed against ubiquitinated proteins, and specifically against α-synuclein. In contrast to Pick bodies, Lewy bodies are not argyrophilic. Their morphology varies, so two types of Lewy body can be distinguished: the brainstem or classical type involving mainly the pigmented neurons of the brainstem (Fig. 6.8), and the cortical type, found mainly within cortical neurons.

In PD, the outstanding findings are the presence of Lewy body–containing neurons and Lewy neurites, and loss of neurons within both the peripheral and central nervous systems. Within the peripheral nervous system, the olfactory bulb, autonomic ganglion, and myenteric plexus of the intestines (Kupsky, Grimes, Sweeting, Bertsch, & Cote, 1987) are involved. In the brainstem, the following structures are commonly affected: the dorsal motor nucleus of the vagus (cholinergic) and the reticular formation; the nucleus coeruleus (noradrenergic) and neurons of the median raphé (serotoninergic); the pars compacta of the substantia nigra and tegmental scattered pigmented neurons (dopaminergic), the Edinger-Westphal nucleus (cholinergic, preganglionic parasympathetic motor

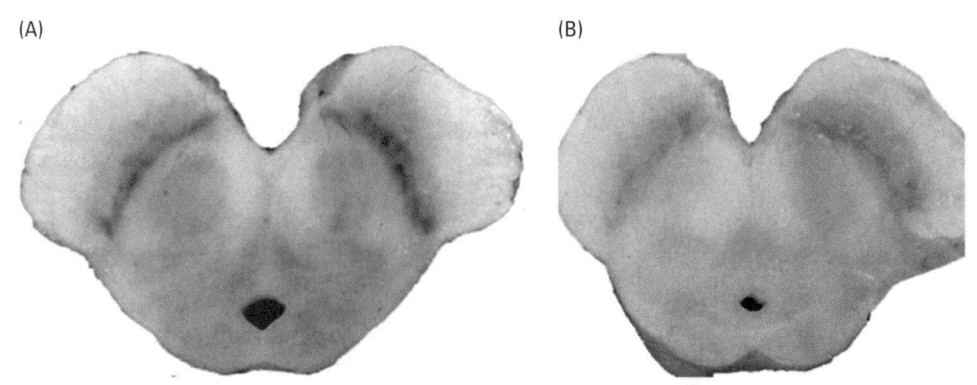

Figure 6.7 Transverse slices through the midbrain. (*A*) The normal adult pars compacta of the substantia nigra is well pigmented. (*B*) In contrast to *A*, in Parkinson disease (*B*), or in dementia with Lewy bodies, the normally expected pigment is decreased. This pigment, neuromelanin, is a by-product of neuronal function. The cytoplasmic density of neuromelanin gradually increases with age.

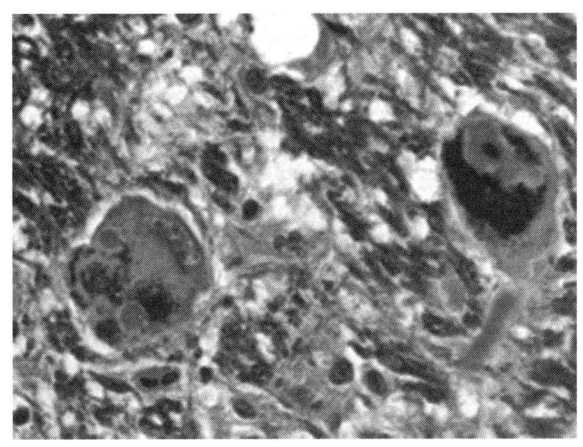

Figure 6.8 Lewy body (brainstem type) is usually round, 8–30 μm in diameter, and consists of a cytoplasmic, hyaline core with or without concentric lamellar bands, and with a peripheral, pale halo. These two Lewy body–containing neurons are from the nucleus coeruleus. One of them has two round Lewy bodies (lower left). The other has a somewhat bilobulated Lewy body with a visible, basophilic, and dark core (upper right). (LHE stain; original magnification, 630×) (See color plate section)

neurons that control lens accommodation and pupillary constriction, which lie near the midline, dorsal to the oculomotor nucleus [III cranial nerve nucleus]). In the diencephalon, the structures involved include the thalamus, hypothalamus, and substantia innominata, including nucleus of Meynert (cholinergic) (Braak et al., 2003; Halliday et al., 1990; Langston, 2006).

Neocortical neurons prone to contain Lewy bodies are those located mainly within layers V or VI with the following temporospatial pattern in the majority of patients with protracted disease: parahippocampal gyrus, occipitotemporalis gyrus, insular cortex, cingulate gyrus, homotypic neocortex, and then heterotypic neocortex (Braak et al., 2003; K. A. Jellinger, 2004, 2008). When Lewy body–containing neurons are widespread within the brain and brainstem, neuropathologists often refer to the condition as diffuse Lewy body disease. In DLB, Lewy body–containing neurons occur in the same areas as those involved in PD (see Fig. 6.8); in addition, they are widespread within the cerebral cortex and amygdaloid nucleus. Furthermore, in DLB, spongiform changes often occur and occasionally can mimic prion diseases. However, in contrast to CJD, the spongiform changes in DLBD tend to involve the superficial, cortical layers, and are either without or with mild reactive gliosis. In CJD, spongiform changes involve the deep cortical layers or are transcortical, especially in the late stage of the disease, and are associated with reactive gliosis.

Some patients exhibit the neuropathologic hallmarks of both AD and DLB. This diagnosis, sometimes referred to as the AD Lewy body variant (ADLBV), is made when the brain of a demented patient shows the changes of AD together with those of diffuse Lewy body disease. Perhaps patients with ADLV have both AD and PD given the shared clinical and pathological characteristics (Brown et al., 1998; Perl, Olanow, & Calne, 1998; Zaccai, Brayne, McKeith, Matthews, & Ince, 2008). In ADLBV, in addition to the widespread presence of the Lewy body–containing neurons, the density and distribution of neuritic plaques and neurofibrillary tangles are such that the patient meets AD neuropathologic criteria as well.

See Chapter 12 for discussion of the clinical aspects of DLB.

Huntington's Disease

HD is an autosomal dominant illness usually with midlife onset of psychiatric, cognitive, and motor symptoms. Death occurs 12–15 years from the time of symptomatic onset (Wexler et al., 2004). An unstable expansion of CAG (trinucleotide) repeats within the coding region of the gene "IT15" (for "Interesting Transcript. referred to as HD-IT15 CAG repeats) causes the disease. This gene, on chromosome 4 (4p16.3), encodes the 350-kDa-protein huntingtin whose function is only partially known (Huntington's Disease Collaborative Research Group, 1993). An expanded polyglutamine residue (polyQ) distinguishes the mutated huntingtin (with about 37 to 250 polyQ [mhtt]) from the wild type (with 8 to about 34–36 polyQ [whtt]). The disease manifests itself clinically when the critical threshold of about 37 polyQ is exceeded (Hendricks et al., 2008). This phenomenon is observed in a group of nine inherited, neurodegenerative diseases caused by polyQ extension, referred to as polyglutaminopathies.

The mhtt is expressed in all organs, yet the brunt of the changes of HD identified so far occurs in the brain. The degeneration initially involves the striatum (neuronal loss, gliosis), then the cerebral cortex, and eventually is fairly diffusely throughout the brain (Hadzi et al., 2012; Halliday et al., 1998; Rüb et al., 2013; Vonsattel & DiFiglia, 1998).

Examination of coronal slices reveals bilateral atrophy of the striatum in 95% of the HD brains. The striatal atrophy is prominent in 80%, mild in 15%, and subtle, if present at all, in 5% of the brains. Nonstriatal regions show atrophy of variable severity or have normal appearance. As a rule, the postmortem HD brain is diffusely smaller than normal in the late stage of the disease. The striatum is probably the only site where neuronal loss and "active" reactive, fibrillary astrocytosis coexist to be readily noticeable on postmortem examination using conventional methods of investigation.

The gradual atrophy of the striatum, which sequentially involves the neostriatum, external segment, then the internal segment of globus pallidus, typifies HD. In turn, the neostriatal loss has an ordered, topographic distribution. The tail of the caudate nucleus shows more degeneration than the body, which is more involved than the head. Similarly, the caudal portion of the putamen is more degenerated than the rostral portion.

Along the coronal (or dorsoventral) axis of the neostriatum, the dorsal, neostriatal regions are more involved than the ventral ones. Along the medio-lateral axis, the paraventricular half of the caudate nucleus is more involved than the paracapsular half.

In summary, the dorsal third of the rostral neostriatum is especially prone to degenerate in contrast to the relatively preserved ventral third, including the nucleus accumbens. Features that HD shares with the other eight, currently known polyglutaminopathies are ubiquitinated, neuronal, nuclear inclusions involving scattered neurons, and dystrophic neurites, and neuronal loss in regions more or less distinctive for each disease of this group. The observation of these ubiquitinated aggregates in HD human brains was made following the occurrence of widespread nuclear inclusions seen in neurons, glial, and ependymal cells of the first transgenic mice (R6/2) harboring exon 1 of the human gene. This genetic insertion encodes htt with expanded CAG-repeats, which translate into a series of consecutive glutamine residues or polyQ (Mangiarini et al., 1996).

Among the theories for the selective, cellular damage in HD, the most compelling involve impaired energy metabolism, excitotoxicity, and relative, selective endotoxicity.

The excitotoxicity theory proposes that subpopulations of striatal medium-sized spiny projection neurons are hypersensitive to corticostriatal and thalamostriatal glutamate, or excessive glutamate is released by these afferents, while striatal interneurons are less affected. Mutated *huntingtin* causes neuronal dysfunction long before cell death. Perhaps endotoxicity results from misfolding of mhtt. Wild-type *huntintin* is soluble. In contrast, *mhtt* is insoluble and forms aggregates. Despite the tremendous amount of recent important data obtained on *whtt*, or *mhtt*, the relatively selective loss of striatal neurons seen in HD continues to remain mysterious.

References

Attems, J., Jellinger, K., Thal, D. R., & Van Nostrand, W. (2011). Review: Sporadic cerebral amyloid angiopathy. *Neuropathology and Applied Neurobiology*, 37, 75–93.

Ball, M. J. (1979). Topography of Pick inclusion bodies in hippocampi of demented patients. A quantitative study. *Journal of Neuropathology and Experimental Neurology*, 38, 614–620.

Binetti, G., Growdon, J. H., & Vonsattel, J-P.G. (1998). Pick's disease. *Blue Books of Practical Neurology. The Dementias*, 19, 7–44.

Braak, H., Alafuzoff, I., Arzberger, T., Kretzschmar, H., & Del Tredici, K. (2006). Staging of Alzheimer disease-associated neurofibrillary pathology using paraffin sections and immunocytochemistry. *Acta Neuropathologica, 112*, 389–404.

Braak, H., Del Tredici, K., Rüb, U., de Vos, R. A., Jansen Steur, E. N., & Braak, E. (2003). Staging of brain pathology related to sporadic Parkinson's disease. *Neurobiology of Aging, 24*, 197–211.

Brew, B. J., Rosenblum, M., Cronin, K., & Price, R. W. (1995). AIDS dementia complex and HIV-1 brain infection: Clinical-virological correlations. *Annals of Neurology, 38*, 563–570.

Brown, D. F., Dababo, M. A., Bigio, E. H., Risser, R. C., Eagan, K. P., Hladik, C. L., & White, C. L., III. (1998). Neuropathologic evidence that the Lewy body variant of Alzheimer disease represents coexistence of Alzheimer disease and idiopathic Parkinson disease. *Journal of Neuropathology and Experimental Neurology, 57*, 39–46.

Cairns, N. J., Neumann, M., Bigio, E. H., Holm, I. E., Troost, D., Hatanpaa, K. J.,...Mackenzie, I. R. (2007b). TDP-43 in familial and sporadic frontotemporal lobar degeneration with ubiquitin inclusions. *American Journal of Pathology, 171*, 227–240.

Clark, A. W., Manz, H. J., White, C. L., III, Lehmann, J., Miller, D., & Coyle, J. T. (1986). Cortical degeneration with swollen chromatolytic neurons: Its relationship to Pick's disease. *Journal of Neuropathology and Experimental Neurology, 45*, 268–284.

Davous, P., & Bequet, D. (1995). CADASIL—un nouveau modèle de démence sous-corticale. *Revue Neurologique, 151*, 634–639.

Dichgans, M., Mayer, M., Uttner, I., Brüning, R., Müller-Höcker, J., Rungger, G.,...Gasser, T. (1998). The phenotypic spectrum of CADASIL: Clinical findings in 102 cases. *Annals of Neurology, 44*, 731–739.

Drachman, D. A. (1994). If we live long enough, will we all be demented?. *Neurology, 44*, 1563–1565.

Ezekiel, F., Chao, L., Kornak, J., Du, A. T., Cardenas, V., Truran, D.,...Weiner, M. (2004). Comparisons between global and focal brain atrophy rates in normal aging and Alzheimer disease. *Alzheimer Disease and Associated Disorders, 18*, 196–201.

Fontaine, B., Seilhean, D., Tourbah, A., Daumas-Duport, C., Duyckaerts, C., Benoit, N.,...Lyon-Caen, O. (1994). Dementia in two histologically confirmed cases of multiple sclerosis: One case with isolated dementia and one case associated with psychiatric symptoms. *Journal of Neurology, Neurosurgery, and Psychiatry, 57*, 353–359.

Frigerio, R., Fujishiro, H., Maraganore, D. M., Klos, K. J., DelleDonne, A., Heckman, M. G.,...Ahlskog, J. E. (2009). Comparison of risk factor profiles in incidental Lewy body disease and Parkinson disease. *Archives of Neurology, 66*(9), 1114–1119.

Huntington's Disease Collaborative Research Group. (1993). A novel gene containing a trinucleotide repeat that is expanded and unstable on Huntington's disease chromosomes. *Cell, 72*, 971–983.

Grünthal, E. (1930). Über ein Brüderpaar mit Pickscher Krankheit. Eine vergleichende Untersuchung, zugleich ein Beitrag zur Kenntnis der Verursachung und des Verlaufs der Erkrankung. *Zeitschrift für die gesamte Neurologie und Psychiatrie (Berlin), 129*, 350–375.

Hadzi, T. C., Hendricks, A. E., Latourelle, J. C., Lunetta, K. L., Cupples, L. A., Gillis, T.,...Vonsattel, J. P. (2012). Assessment of cortical and striatal involvement in 523 Huntington disease brains. *Neurology, 79*(16), 1708–1715.

Halliday, G. M., Li, Y. W., Blumbergs, P. C., Joh, T. H., Cotton, R. G., Howe, P. R.,...Geffen, L. B. (1990). Neuropathology of immunohistochemically identified brainstem neurons in Parkinson's disease. *Annals of Neurology, 27*, 373–385.

Halliday, G. M., McRitchie, D. A., Macdonald, V., Double, K. L., Trent, R. J., & McCusker, E. (1998). Regional specificity of brain atrophy in Huntington's disease. *Experimental Neurology, 154*, 663–672.

Hamilton, R. L. (2000). Lewy bodies in Alzheimer's disease: A neuropathological review of 145 cases. *Brain Pathology, 10*(3), 378–384.

Hendricks, A. E., Latourelle, J. C., Lunetta, K. L., Cupples, L. A., Wheeler, V., MacDonald, M. E.,...Myers, R. H. (2008). Estimating the probability of de novo HD cases from transmission of expanded penetrant CAG alleles in the Huntington disease gene from male carriers of hight normal alleles (27–35 CAG). *American Journal of Medical Genetics Part A, 149A*, 1375–1381.

Hirano, A. (1994). Hirano bodies and related neuronal inclusions. *Neuropathology and Applied Neurobiology, 20*, 3–11.

Hulette, C. M., Welsh-Bohmer, K. A., Murray, M. G., Saunders, A. M., Mash, D. C., & McIntyre, L. M. (1998). Neuropathological and neuropsychological changes in 'normal' aging: Evidence for preclinical Alzheimer disease in cognitively normal individuals. *Journal of Neuropathology and Experimental Neurology, 57*(12), 1168–1174.

Jellinger, K. (2009). A critical evaluation of current staging of α-synuclein pathology in

Lewy body disorders. *Biochimica et Biophysica Acta, 1792,* 730–740.

Jellinger, K. A. (2004). Lewy body-related α-synucleinopathy in the aged human brain. *Journal of Neural Transmission, 111,* 1219–1235.

Jellinger, K. A. (2008). A critical reappraisal of current staging of Lewy-related pathology in human brain. *Acta Neuropathologica, 116,* 1–16.

Jellinger, K. A., & Bancher, C. (1998). Neuropathology of Alzheimer's disease: A critical update. *Journal of Neural Transmission, 54,* 77–95.

Kemper, T. L. (1994). Neuroanatomical and meuropathological changes during aging and dementia. In M. L. Albert & J. E. Knoefel (Eds.), *Clinical neurology of aging* (2nd ed., pp. 3–67). New York, NY: Oxford University Press.

Knopman, D. S., Parisi, J. E., Salviati, A., Floriach-Robert, M., Boeve, B. F., Ivnik, R. J.,...Petersen, R. C. (2003). Neuropathology of cognitively normal elderly. *Journal of Neuropathology and Experimental Neurology, 62,* 1087–1095.

Kupsky, W. J., Grimes, M. M., Sweeting, J., Bertsch, R., & Cote, L. J. (1987). Parkinson's disease and megacolon: Concentric hyaline inclusions (Lewy bodies) in enteric ganglion cells. *Neurology, 37,* 1253–1255.

Lace, G., Savva, G. M., Forster, G., de Silva, R., Brayne, C., Matthews, F. E.,...Wharton, S. B. (2009). Hippocampal tau pathology is related to neuroanatomical connections: An ageing population-based study. *Brain, 132,* 1324–1334.

Langston, J. W. (2006). The Parkinsons's complex: Parkinsonism is just the tip of the iceberg. *Annals of Neurology, 59,* 591–596.

Mackenzie, I. R. A., Neumann, M., Bigio, E. H., Cairns, N. J., Alafuzoff, I., Kril, J.,...Mann, D. M. (2010). Nomenclature and nosology for neuropathologic subtypes of frontotemporal lobar degeneration: An update. *Acta Neuropathologica, 119,* 1–4.

Mangiarini, L., Sathasivam, K., Seller, M., Cozens, B., Harper, A., Hetherington, C.,...Bates, G. P. (1996). Exon 1 of the HD gene with an expanded CAG repeat is sufficient to cause a progressive neurological phenotype in transgenic mice. *Cell, 87,* 493–506.

Masters, C. L., & Richardson, E. P., Jr. (1978). Subacute spongiform encephalopathy (Creutzfeldt-Jakob disease). The nature and progression of spongiform change. *Brain, 101,* 333–344.

Neumann, M., Mackenzie, I. R., Cairns, N. J., Boyer, P. J., Markesbery, W. R., Smith, C. D.,...Forman, M. S. (2007). TDP-43 in the ubiquitin pathology of frontotemporal dementia with VCP gene mutations. *Journal of Neuropathology and Experimental Neurology, 66,* 152–157.

Neumann, M., Sampathu, D. M., Kwong, L. K., Truax, A. C., Micsenyi, M. C., Chou, T. T.,...Lee, V. M. (2006). Ubiquitinated TDP-43 in frontotemporal lobar degeneration and amyotrophic lateral sclerosis. *Science, 314,* 130–133.

Parvizi, J., Van Hoesen, G. W., & Damasio, A. (2001). The selective vulnerability of brainstem nuclei to Alzheimer's disease. *Annals of Neurology, 49,* 53–66.

Perl, D. P., Olanow, C. W., & Calne, D. (1998). Alzheimer's disease and Parkinson's disease: Dinstinct entities or extremes of a spectrum of neurodegeneration. *Annals of Neurology, 44*(Suppl 1), S19–S31.

Polvikoski, T., Sulkava, R., Myllykangas, L., Notkola, I. L., Niinistö, L., Verkkoniemi, A.,...Haltia, M. (2001). Prevalence of Alzheimer's disease in very elderly people. A prospective neuropathological study. *Neurology, 56,* 1690–1996.

Price, J. L., McKeel, D. W., Jr., Buckles, V. D., Roe, C. M., Xiong, C., Grundman, M.,...Morris, J. C. (2009). Neuropathology of nondemented aging: Presumptive evidence for preclinical Alzheimer disease. *Neurobiology of Aging, 30,* 1026–1036.

Ross, G. W., Petrovitch, H., Abbott, R. D., Nelson, J., Markesbery, W., Davis, D.,...White, L. R. (2004). Parkinsonian signs and substantia nigra neuron density in decendents elders without PD. *Annals of Neurology, 56,* 532–539.

Rüb, U., Hoche, F., Brunt, E. R., Heinsen, H., Seidel, K., Del Turco, D.,...den Dunnen, W. F. (2013). Degeneration of the cerebellum in Huntington's disease (HD): Possible relevance for the clinical picture and potential gateway to pathological mechanisms of the disease process. *Brain Pathology, 23,* 165–177.

Savva, G. M., Wharton, S. B., Ince, P. G., Forster, G., Matthews, F. E., & Brayne, C. (2009). Age, neuropathology, and dementia. *New England Journal of Medicine, 360*(22), 2302–2309.

Schmahmann, J. D. (2003). Vascular syndromes of the thalamus. *Stroke, 34,* 2264–2278.

Schneider, J. A., Arvanitakis, Z., Bang, W., & Bennett, D. A. (2007). Mixed brain pathologies account for most dementia cases in community-dwelling older persons. *Neurology, 69,* 2197–2204.

Seeley, W. W., Carlin, D. A., Allman, J. M., Macedo, M. N., Bush, C., Miller, B. L., & Dearmond, S. J. (2006). Early frontotemporal dementia targets neurons unique to apes and humans. *Annals of Neurology, 60*(6), 660–667.

Seeley, W. W., Crawford, R., Rascovsky, K., Kramer, J. H., Weiner, M., Miller, B. L.,

Gorno-Tempini, M. L. (2008). Frontal paralimbic network atrophy in very mild behavioral variant frontotemporal dementia. *Archives of Neurology.* 2008 Feb;*65*(2), 249–255.

Simchowicz, T. (1924). Sur la signification des plaques séniles et sur la formule sénile de l'écorce cérébrale. *Revue Neurologique, 1,* 221–227.

Smith, T. W., Anwer, U., DeGirolami, U., Drachman, D.A. (1987). Vacuolar change in Alzheimer's disease. *Archives of Neurology, 44,* 225–228.

Spatz, H. (1938). Die 'systematischen Atrophien'. Eine wohlgekenzeichnete Gruppe der Erbkrankheiten des Nervensystems. *Archiv für Psychiatrie und Nervenkrankheiten, 108,* 1–18.

Tomlinson, B. E., Blessed, G., & Roth, M. (1968). Observations on the brains of non-demented old people. *Journal of the Neurological Sciences, 7,* 331–356.

Tournier-Lasserve, E., Joutel, A., Melki, J., Weissenbach, J., Lathrop, G. M., Chabriat, H.,...Maciazek, J. (1993). Cerebral autosomal dominant arteriopathy with subcortical infarcts and leukoencephalopathy maps to chromosome 19q12. *Nature Genetics, 3,* 256–259.

Vonsattel, J-P.G., & DiFiglia, M. (1998). Huntington disease. *Journal of Neuropathology and Experimental Neurology, 57,* 369–384.

Wakisaka, Y., Furuta, A., Tanizaki, Y., Kiyohara, Y., Iida, M., & Iwaki, T. (2003). Age-associated prevalence and risk factors of Lewy body pathology in a general population: The Hisayama study. *Acta Neuropathologica, 106,* 374–382.

Wexler, N. S., Lorimer, J., Porter, J., Gomez, F., Moskowitz, C., Shackell, E.,... Landwehrmeyer, B. (2004). Venezuelan kindreds reveal that genetic and environmental factors modulate Huntington's disease age of onset. *Proceedings of the National Academy of Science USA, 101,* 3498–3503.

Zaccai, J., Brayne, C., McKeith, I., Matthews, F., & Ince, P. G. (2008). Patterns and stages of α-synucleinopathy. Relevance in a population-based cohort. *Neurology, 70,* 1042–1048.

7

Chronic Traumatic Encephalopathy

Ann C. McKee

Repetitive mild brain trauma is associated with the development of chronic traumatic encephalopathy (CTE), a progressive neurodegenerative tauopathy with distinctive clinical and pathological features. CTE is associated with the play of contact athletics, especially boxing and American football, but it has been linked to many other sports, including ice hockey, wrestling, rugby, and soccer, and to other traumatic exposures, including physical abuse, poorly controlled epilepsy, head-banging behaviors, and trauma experienced during military service (Corsellis, Bruton, & Freeman-Browne, 1973; Geddes, Vowles, Nicoll, & Revesz, 1999; Goldstein et al., 2012; Hof, Knabe, Bovier, & Bouras, 1991; McKee et al., 2009, 2010, 2013; Omalu et al., 2005, 2006). CTE is not restricted to professional athletes; early stages of CTE have been also found in high school and collegiate athletes and in military veterans after blast or concussive injury. Military service members are at risk for CTE due to heterogeneous traumatic exposures often involving a combination of athletic participation, recreational activities, training practices, as well as military combat (McKee et al., 2013).

Historically, the concept of a neurodegenerative disease developing after repeated minor trauma to the brain was first recognized in boxing. The first medical study of CTE, or "punch drunk" as it was originally known, was reported in 1928 by Harrison Martland, a New Jersey pathologist, who described the clinical symptom complex affecting boxers who "stayed in the ring long enough" (p. 1103). Millspaugh (1937) referred to the condition as "dementia pugilistica," while other terms such as the "psychopathic deterioration of pugilists" (Courville, 1962) and "traumatic encephalopathy" (Parker, 1934) were also used. Critchley introduced the term "chronic progressive traumatic encephalopathy" to highlight the progressive nature of the condition (1957) and noted that "Once established it not only does not permit of reversibility, but it ordinarily advances steadily…even though the boxer has retired from the ring. (p. 360)"

Acute Mild Traumatic Brain Injury: Subconcussion, Concussion, and Postconcussion

Although all cases of neuropathologically verified CTE have been associated with repetitive minor brain trauma, the pathophysiological mechanisms underlying how trauma triggers a progressive neurodegeneration and tauopathy remain inconclusive. Concussion and subconcussion are considered forms of mild traumatic brain injury (mTBI). Mild TBI is classified by a Glasgow Coma Score of 13 to 15 with transient neurologic deficits following an acute closed head injury. Although concussion and other forms of mTBI are usually self-limited and symptoms resolve over a period of several weeks, prolonged symptoms develop in 10%–30% of individuals, a condition referred to as postconcussive syndrome (PCS) if the symptoms do not resolve in 3 months (Dean & Sterr, 2013). Symptoms of concussion and postconcussion include headaches, dizziness, nausea, fatigue, anxiety, depression, irritability, sleep disturbances, sensitivity to noise and light, and changes in coordination, balance, appetite, vision, and hearing. In PCS, symptoms last for months to years following the injury and may produce permanent disability. Neuropsychological testing in PCS may reveal persistent, yet subtle, cognitive deficits, most often in the executive domain (Bohnen, Jolles, & Twijnstra, 1992). Percussive injuries less severe than concussion that do not produce overt neurological symptoms, yet are associated with slight neuropsychiatric deficits or changes in functional magnetic resonance imaging, are referred to as "subconcussion" (Talavage et al., 2010). Subconcussive injuries can be substantial in some sports; for instance, it has been reported that an offensive lineman can experience over 1,000 subconcussive hits over the level of 10 g in the course of a single season of college football (Crisco et al., 2012).

Acceleration and deceleration forces on the brain, either linear or rotational, produce concussion and subconcussion (Ommaya & Gennarelli, 1974). When the firmly gelatinous brain, which is suspended in cerebrospinal fluid inside a boney skull, is subjected to rapid acceleration, deceleration, and rotational forces, the brain elongates and deforms, stretching individual components such as neurons, glial cells, and blood vessels. These traumatic stretch injuries affect neuronal cell bodies, axons, dendrites, blood vessels, and glial cells; axons are especially vulnerable as they often extend long distances from the neuronal cell bodies and may be injured even without the death of the neuron of origin (Maxwell, Povlishock, & Graham, 1997; Medana & Esiri, 2003). Traumatic axonal injury (TAI) does not uniformly affect all axonal populations. Smaller unmyelinated axons are more damaged by concussive forces than larger myelinated axons; it remains unclear whether this is due to intrinsic susceptibility or because the myelin provides relative protection to axons (Reeves, Phillips, & Povlishock, 2005). The microscopic changes in the brain that are a consequence of concussive injury, such as TAI, are not detectable with conventional structural imaging studies, including computed tomography (CT) scan and magnetic resonance imaging (MRI). Diffusion tensor imaging (DTI), however, provides information about the white matter microstructure and fiber tract integrity that is useful in assessing the severity and predicting recovery in individuals with concussion and mTBI. The severity of symptoms after mTBI correlates with reduction of white matter integrity on DTI, providing evidence that persistent microstructural brain injury underlies the persistent symptoms of PCS (Johnson, Stewart, & Smith, 2012). Furthermore, DTI is emerging as a valuable tool in refining the diagnosis, prognosis, and management of mTBI (Bazarian, Zhu, Blyth, Borrino, & Zhong, 2012; Cubon, Putukian, Boyer, & Dettwiler, 2011).

In addition to the traumatic stretch injury of axons and other cellular compartments after mTBI, neurotransmitters, including glutamate, are abruptly released with massive increases in intracellular calcium, glucose hypermetabolism, kinase activation, and diminished cerebral blood flow (Giza & Hovda, 2001). These metabolical disturbances also improve with time and rest, but lasting changes may occur.

Functional MRI (fMRI) studies have detected significant alterations in brain activation patterns in individuals with persistent symptoms after mTBI (Chen, Johnston, Petrides, & Ptito, 2008; Chen et al., 2004; Gosselin et al., 2011; McAllister et al., 2001; Ptito, Chen, & Johnston, 2007). These abnormal brain activation patterns can remain for months after injury, despite normal neurocognitive task performance (Chen et al., 2004; Lovell et al., 2007; McAllister et al., 1999). The discrepancy between fMRI and neurocognitive testing may be the result of functional reallocation of neurocognitive resources as a compensatory mechanism, followed by a more prolonged period of microstructural recovery (Cubon et al., 2011). In a study of mTBI patients using fMRI to assess the neural correlate of working memory, patients with more severe postconcussive symptoms showed increased brain activity in the normal working memory network, as well as the recruitment of brain regions outside this network (Smits et al., 2009).

Pathological studies of acute concussion and PCS are rare and include subjects with more severe traumatic injuries as well, but both demonstrate the presence of multifocal TAI, microhemorrhage, and microglial activation (Blumbergs, 1944; Oppenheimer, 1968). Oppenheimer reported that acute TBI, including some cases of concussion, was associated with microscopic petechial hemorrhages and axonal injury associated with microglial clusters that were often perivascular. Blumbergs and colleagues examined five cases of human concussive head injury and reported multifocal axonal injury using beta-amyloid precursor (β-APP) immunohistochemistry in the fornices, a major hippocampal projection pathway thought to be important in memory (Blumbergs, 1944). The authors suggested that damage to the fornix might underlie some of the persisting memory deficits that occur in patients after concussion. In general, the amount and distribution of TAI is dependent on the severity of the TBI, with mild injury producing only microscopic axonal damage and moderate and severe TBI producing more severe axonal injury.

Axonal Injury in Mild Traumatic Brain Injury

Severe TAI is also referred to as diffuse axonal injury (DAI) and is characterized by hallmark lesions in the corpus callosum and dorsolateral quadrants of the brainstem, first described by Strich (Maxwell, McCreath, Graham, & Gennarelli, 1995). DAI is only present after the most severe TBIs. Patients who sustain DAI are usually unconscious from the moment of impact and remain unconscious, vegetative, or severely disabled until death. In DAI, axonal retraction balls and axonal swellings are found diffusely distributed in the corpus callosum, internal capsule, cerebral white matter, fornix, midbrain, pons, medulla, and cerebellum (Blumbergs, 1944).

It is now appreciated that axons are not physically transected or sheared at the time of injury, except in the most severe instances, but instead they undergo a series of changes that results in a secondary axotomy within 24 hours (Maxwell et al., 1995). The axolemma is one of the initial sites of injury; the increased permeability, uncontrolled influx of Ca^{2+}, swelling of mitochondria, disruption of microtubules, and alterations in axonal transport that follow mTBI produce axonal swelling and secondary axotomy (Giza & Hovda, 2001; Maxwell et al., 1995). In addition, even in the absence of additional traumatic or vascular injury, progressive axonal swelling and disconnection can continue for years after TBI (Blumbergs, 1944), which contribute to the development of progressively greater disability in some individuals (Johnson et al., 2012). Determining the pathogenetic mechanisms underlying continued axonal degeneration after TBI and the development of progressive late-life neurodegenerative disease is a critical focus of current research.

Chronic Traumatic Encephalopathy

The symptoms of CTE are insidious, often first manifested as disturbances in attention or concentration or depression that are occasionally associated with headaches. Short-term memory difficulties, aggressive tendencies, executive dysfunction, and explosivity are also frequent symptoms. Characteristically the first symptoms appear around ages 35–45 years, although the range is broad, from 26 years to 65 years (McKee et al., 2013). There is characteristically a long latent period (mean 8 years, range 0–37 years) between the last trauma and the development of symptoms (McKee et al., 2009). In young individuals, it is unclear whether the symptoms represent prolonged postconcussive symptoms or the early manifestations of CTE. Unlike other neurodegenerative disorders, headache is a persistent and early symptom in nearly half the individuals who develop CTE. The headache may be migrainous or a constant dull pain. Other personality and behavioral changes that are common in individuals with early (stage I or II) CTE are irritability, explosivity, and erratic behaviors (McKee et al., 2013). By stage III disease, most subjects are considered cognitively impaired and by stage IV CTE, executive dysfunction and memory loss are usually severe and most are demented. Other symptoms often include impulsivity, suicidality, language difficulties, paranoia, and visuospatial abnormalities;

approximately one third are suicidal at some point in their course. Gait disturbances, dysarthria, and parkinsonism are found in about 10% of individuals with CTE in association with late-stage disease.

In CTE, the severity of cognitive impairment is most likely associated with several pathologies, including neuroinflammation; axonal, neuronal, and synapse loss; and the accumulation of toxic aggregates of tau and TDP proteins. The severity of the tau pathology most likely contributes to cognitive decline and behavioral changes, as has been shown for Alzheimer's disease (AD; McKee, Kosik, & Kowall, 1991); however, there is also substantial axonal pathology in CTE, and axonal pathology likely accounts for some of the changes in personality and behavior, especially in early stages of disease when the accumulations of hyperphosphorylated-tau (p-tau) are minimal. Other contributors to clinical symptoms include toxic accumulations of TDP-43 and neuroinflammation. Although the clinical symptoms of CTE often begin with behavior and personality changes in a person's thirties or forties similar to those of frontotemporal dementia, the clinical course of CTE is considerably slower and might span three or four decades. When symptoms of CTE begin later in life, in persons in their fifties and sixties, memory loss similar to AD is often the outstanding symptom, usually associated with agitation, aggression, and combative behaviors.

Neuropathology of Chronic Traumatic Encephalopathy

In stage I CTE, there may be mild enlargement of the frontal horn of the lateral ventricle, but the brain is otherwise unremarkable. In stage II, the third ventricle may also be slightly enlarged. A small cavum septum and pallor of the locus coeruleus and substantia nigra are occasionally found in stage II. By stage III, mild cerebral atrophy with dilation of the lateral and third ventricles is characteristic. Septal abnormalities, either cavum septum or septal perforations; atrophy of the mammillary bodies, thalamus, and hypothalamus; and thinning of the mid-portion of the corpus callosum are found, and the locus coeruleus and substantia nigra are depigmented. By stage IV CTE, there is marked atrophy of the medial temporal lobe and, less so, of the cerebral cortex, white matter, thalamus, hypothalamus, and mammillary body. The brain weight is often significantly diminished and there is enlargement of the lateral and third ventricles, a sharply concave contour of the third ventricle, and septal abnormalities.

Microscopic Pathology

Criteria for the Pathological Diagnosis of Chronic Traumatic Encephalopathy

In stage I CTE, there are focal epicenters of perivascular p-tau neurofibrillary tangles (NFTs) and astrocytic tangles (ATs), most prominent in the sulcal depths and typically affecting superior and dorsolateral frontal cortices (Box 7.1 and Table 7.1; Figs. 7.1, 7.2, and 7.3). The cortex surrounding the epicenters is unremarkable except for rare isolated NFTs in superficial laminae of adjacent cortex. There are no NFTs in deep nuclei, including locus coeruleus and nucleus basalis of Meynert, hypothalamus, thalamus, brainstem, or spinal cord. In stage II CTE, p-tau pathology is found in multiple foci of the cerebral cortex,

---

BOX 7.1 Criteria for the Diagnosis of Chronic Traumatic Encephalopathy

1. Perivascular foci of p-tau immunoreactive astrocytic tangles (ATs) and neurofibrillary tangles (NFTs)
2. Irregular cortical distribution of p-tau immunoreactive NFTs and ATs with a predilection for the depth of cerebral sulci
3. Clusters of subpial and periventricular ATs in the cerebral cortex, diencephalon, and brainstem
4. NFTs in the cerebral cortex located preferentially in the superficial layers

Source: Adapted from McKee et al. (2013).

TABLE 7.1 Distinctions in Hyperphosphorylated Tau Pathology Between Alzheimer's Disease and Chronic Traumatic Encephalopathy

Pathological Features		Alzheimer's Disease	Chronic Traumatic Encephalopathy
Tau protein	Six isoforms 3 or 4 repeat tau	All six isoforms present 3 repeat and 4 repeat tau present	All six isoforms present[1] 3 repeat and 4 repeat tau present
Cell origin			
	Neuronal	NFTs and pretangles	NFTs and pretangles
	Astrocytic	Not present[2]	Prominent ATs
Neuronal domain			
	Cell body	Prominent	Prominent
	Dendrite	Prominent	Prominent
	Axon	Sparse	Prominent
Cell origin			
	Perivascular	Not present	Prominent NFTs and ATs
	Foci at depths of cerebral sulci	Not present	Prominent NFTs and ATs
	Irregular, patchy cortical distribution	Not present	Prominent
	Cortical laminae	Predominantly laminae III and V	Predominantly laminae I-III
	Subpial ATs	Not present	Prominent
	Periventricular ATs	Not present	Present
	Astrocytic plaques	May be present	Not present
Distribution			
	Mild pathology	Braak stages I–III: NFTs in entorhinal cortex, amygdala, and hippocampus	CTE stages I-II: NFTs in focal epicenters in cerebral cortex, usually frontal lobe
	Advanced pathology	Braak stages IV–VI: High density of NFTs in widespread cortical areas and medial temporal lobe, uniform distribution Low densities of NFTs in basal ganglia and brainstem; none in mammillary bodies White matter tracts relatively uninvolved.	CTE stages III-IV: High density of NFTs in widespread cortical areas and medial temporal lobe, patchy irregular distribution High densities of NFTs in thalamus, hypothalamus, mammillary bodies, brainstem. Moderate densities of NFTs in basal ganglia, especially nucleus accumbens. Prominent p-tau pathology in white matter tracts.

[1] Schmidt et al. (2001).
[2] Low densities of 4R immunoreactive "thorn-shaped astrocytes" are found in the temporal lobe of some older subjects and older subjects with Alzheimer's disease.
ATs, astrocytic tangles; NFTs, neurofibrillary tangles.
Source: Adapted from McKee et al. (2013).

most commonly in superior, dorsolateral, lateral, inferior, and subcallosal frontal; anterior, inferior, and lateral temporal; inferior parietal; insular and septal cortices. Scattered NFTs are also found in the superficial layers of cortex. NFTs are also found in the locus coeruleus, nucleus basalis of Meynert, and amygdala in stage II disease; rare NFTs and pretangles may be found in the hypothalamus, CA1 of hippocampus, entorhinal cortex, thalamus, substantia nigra, and dorsal and median raphe nuclei of the midbrain. In stage III CTE, there are patchy collections of subpial and perivascular in the sulcal depths, as well as superficial layers of superior frontal, dorsolateral frontal, inferior orbital, septal, insular, temporal pole, superior middle and inferior temporal, and inferior parietal cortices. There

Stage I

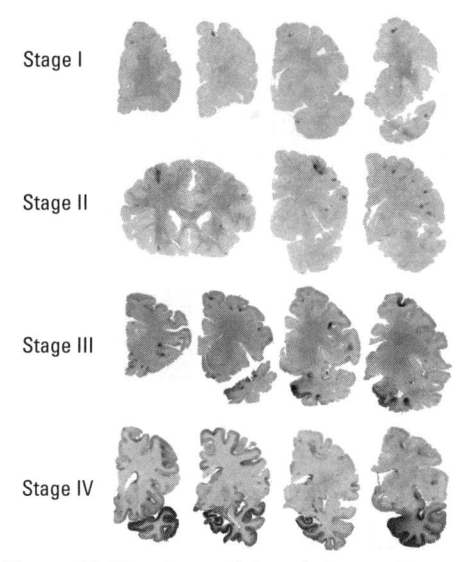

Stage II

Stage III

Stage IV

Figure 7.1 The stages of chronic traumatic encephalopathy (CTE). In stage I CTE, p-tau pathology is restricted to discrete foci in the cerebral cortex, most commonly in the superior, dorsolateral, or lateral frontal cortices, and typically around small vessels at the depths of sulci. In stage II CTE, there are multiple epicenters at the depths of the cerebral sulci and localized spread of neurofibrillary pathology from these epicenters to the superficial layers of adjacent cortex. The medial temporal lobe is spared neurofibrillary p-tau pathology in stage II CTE. In stage III, p-tau pathology is widespread; the frontal, insular, temporal, and parietal cortices show widespread neurofibrillary degeneration with greatest severity in the frontal and temporal lobe, concentrated at the depths of the sulci. Also in stage III CTE, the amygdala, hippocampus, and entorhinal cortex show neurofibrillary pathology. In stage IV CTE, there is widespread severe p-tau pathology affecting most regions of the cerebral cortex and the medial temporal lobe. (All images, CP-13 immunostained 50 μm tissue sections)

are high densities of NFTs in the hippocampus, entorhinal cortex, amygdala, nucleus basalis of Meynert, and locus coeruleus. NFTs are frequent in olfactory bulbs, hypothalamus, mammillary bodies, substantia nigra, and dorsal and median raphe nuclei. In stage III and IV, distinctive wall-to-wall NFTs may be present in medial temporal lobe regions and olfactory bulbs. In stage IV CTE, there are striking p-tau abnormalities widely distributed throughout the cerebrum, diencephalon, basal ganglia, brainstem, and spinal cord. Neuronal loss in the cortex and hippocampal sclerosis may be present. The primary visual cortex is generally spared. The p-tau NFTs at all stages are immunoreactive for both 3 repeat and 4 repeat tau, while ATs are predominantly immunoreactive for 4 repeat tau.

Hyperphosphorylated Tau Pathology in Deep Nuclei in Chronic Traumatic Encephalopathy

P-tau NFTs are found in locus coeruleus, nucleus basalis of Meynert, and amygdala even in young individuals with stage II disease. As the disease progresses to involve wider regions of the frontal, temporal, and parietal cortices in stage III disease, NFTs are found in the thalamus, hypothalamus, hippocampus, entorhinal cortex, substantia nigra, dorsal and median raphe nuclei, olfactory bulbs, mammillary bodies, nucleus accumbens, dorsal motor nucleus of the vagus, dentate nucleus of the cerebellum, and, more rarely, the spinal cord.

How Chronic Traumatic Encephalopathy Is Distinct From Alzheimer's Disease

In CTE, cortical sections show a distinctly irregular distribution of p-tau pathology with prominent subpial clusters of p-tau ATs, a prominent perivascular distribution, focal accentuation at depths of sulci, and NFTs distributed primarily in superficial cortical laminae, and the relative absence of beta-amyloid (Aβ) deposition (Table 7.1, Fig. 7.3). Periventricular regions show intense ependymal immunostaining for p-tau. Axonal varicosities and neuropil threads in the subcortical and deep white matter are also p-tau immunopositive. In AD, there is a diffuse cortical distribution of NFTs preferentially involving laminae III and V and without accentuation at depths of sulci. Small blood vessels at sulcal depths show no clustering of neurofibrillary pathology perivascularly. The subpial and periventricular regions show no p-tau positivity. Neuritic as well as diffuse Aβ plaques are a prominent feature of all cases of AD, whereas Aβ plaques are found in fewer than half of cases of CTE; when Aβ is found in CTE, the deposition tends to be less than

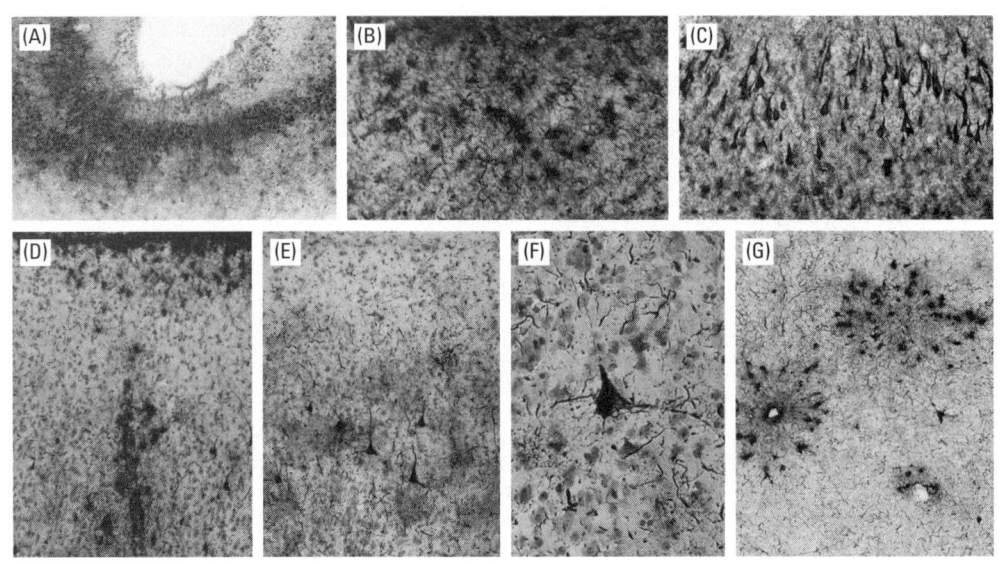

Figure 7.2 Distinctive pattern and morphology of tau immunoreactive neurofibrillary pathology in chronic traumatic encephalopathy. (*A*) Tau immunoreactive neurofibrillary degeneration is often most striking at depths of the sulci accompanied by focal thinning of the cortical ribbon (AT8 immunostain, original magnification, 60×). (*B*) Subpial tau immunoreactive tangles are found in both neurons and astrocytes (double immunostained section for GFAP [red] and AT8 [brown] showing colocalization of tau and GFAP [arrow]; original magnification, 350×). (*C*) Extremely dense NFTs and neuropil neurites are found in the medial temporal lobe structures, including CA1 of the hippocampus, shown here. Senile plaques are absent (AT8 immunostain, original magnification, 150×). (*D*) NFTs and astrocytic tangles tend to be centered around small blood vessels and in subpial patches (AT8 immunostain, original magnification, 150×). (*E*) NFTs characteristically involve cortical layers II and III in association with clusters of tau-positive astrocytic processes (AT8 immunostain, original magnification, 150×). (*F*) NFT in a Betz cell of primary motor cortex (AT8 immunostain, original magnification, 350×). (*G*) There is often a striking perivascular clustering of NFTs around small blood vessels (AT8, original magnification, 150×). (See color plate section)

ALZHEIMER'S DISEASE

CHRONIC TRAUMATIC ENCEPHALOPATHY

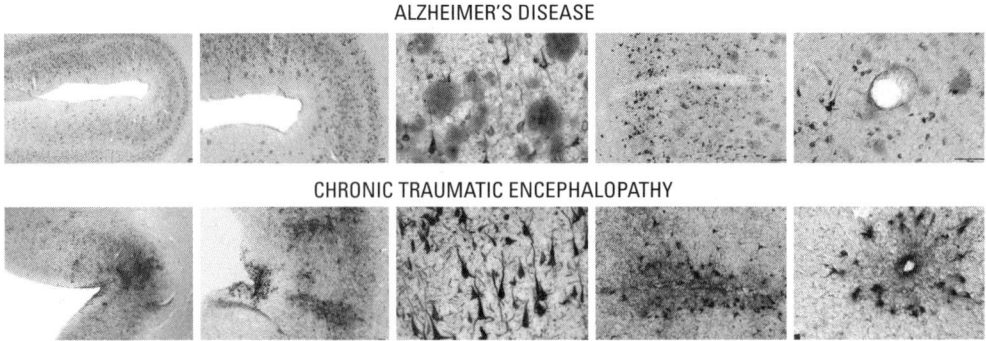

Figure 7.3 How the p-tau pathology of chronic traumatic encephalopathy is distinctive from Alzheimer's disease. (Top row) Alzheimer's disease: Double immunostained sections for Aß (red) and PHF-1 (brown) show diffuse, relatively uniform cortical distribution of NFTs preferentially involving laminae III and V, without accentuation at depths of sulci. Small blood vessels at sulcal depths show no clustering of neurofibrillary pathology perivascularly. There is also no clustering of neurofibrillary pathology in subpial or periventricular regions. (Bottom row) Chronic traumatic encephalopathy: Sections immunostained for AT8 showing irregular cortical distribution of p-tau pathology with prominent subpial clusters of p-tau astrocytic tangles, focal accentuation at depths of sulci, and distribution of NFTs in superficial cortical laminae I-III. Small blood vessels at bottom of cortical sulcus show prominent perivascular distribution of astrocytic tangles and NFTs (AT8). Double immunostained section for Aß (red) and PHF-1 (brown) (center panel) shows dense NFTs without Aß deposition. (See color plate section)

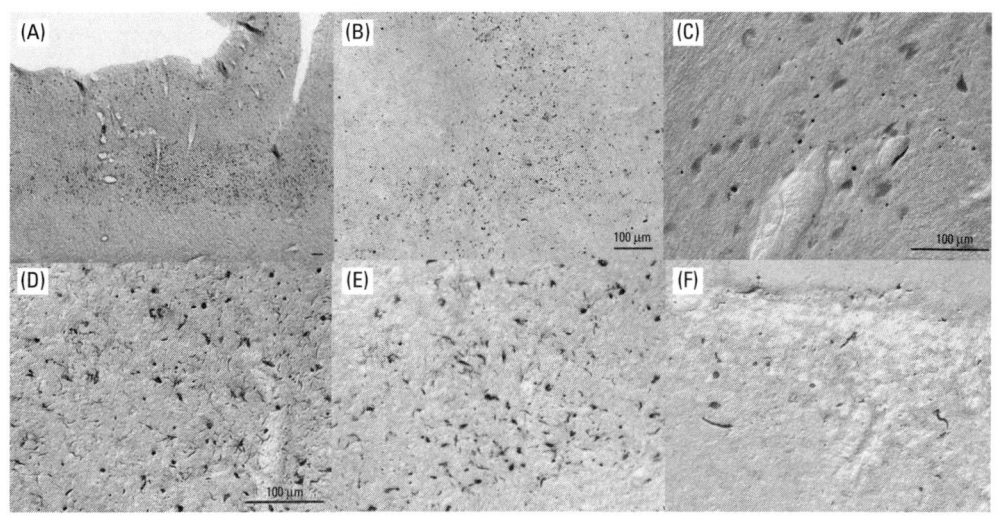

Figure 7.4 The phosphorylated TDP43 pathology of chronic traumatic encephalopathy (CTE). (A, B, D, and E) Dense pTDP-43 abnormalities are found in the cerebral cortex of stage IV CTE. (C) Dense pTDP-43 pathology in substantia nigra pars compacta. (F) Pronounced pTDP-43 immunopositive pathology in the periventricular region of the third ventricle. (All images: 50 μm tissue sections; all scale bars, 100 μm) (See color plate section)

AD and diffuse plaques predominate over neuritic plaques.

TDP-43 Pathology in Chronic Traumatic Encephalopathy

In stage I disease, TDP-43 immunopositive neurites are found in approximately 60% of cases in frontal subcortical white matter and fornix (Fig. 7.4). In stage II disease, 80% of CTE cases have TDP-43 immunopositivity, consisting of isolated neurites or inclusions in the cerebral subcortical white matter, brainstem, or medial temporal lobe, often in a subpial, periventricular, or perivascular distribution. By stage III CTE, TDP-43 immunoreactive neurites are found in the cerebral cortex, medial temporal lobe, or brainstem of most cases. TDP-43 immunoreactivity is found in all stage IV cases, as dense TDP-43-positive rounded and thread-like neurites, intraglial and intraneuronal inclusions in cerebral cortex, medial temporal lobe, diencephalon, basal ganglia, brainstem, and rarely, spinal cord. In cases with the most severe TDP-43 deposition, dense accumulations of TDP-43 inclusions and neurites are found in all layers of the neocortex, particularly layer II, as well as occasional TDP-43-positive inclusions in the dentate fascia of the hippocampus, a distribution pattern that overlaps with that found in the TDP pathologic subtype of frontotemporal lobar degeneration (FTLD).

Axonal Injury in Chronic Traumatic Encephalopathy

In CTE stages I and II, there are scattered axonal varicosities in the deep layers of the frontal and temporal cortices, subcortical white matter, and deep white matter tracts of the diencephalon. Some phosphorylated neurofilament axonal varicosities are also immunoreactive for p-tau. In more advanced disease, stages III and IV, axonal loss is usually severe with numerous distorted axonal profiles in frontal and temporal cortices and white matter (Fig. 7.5).

Chronic Traumatic Encephalopathy and Comorbidities

Chronic Traumatic Encephalopathy and Alzheimer's Disease

Deposition of Aß as diffuse plaques, neuritic plaques, or vascular amyloid is found in 30% of CTE cases; subjects who develop Aß are significantly older than those without Aß (McKee et al., 2013). Aß deposits are not present in CTE subjects younger than age 45 years. The

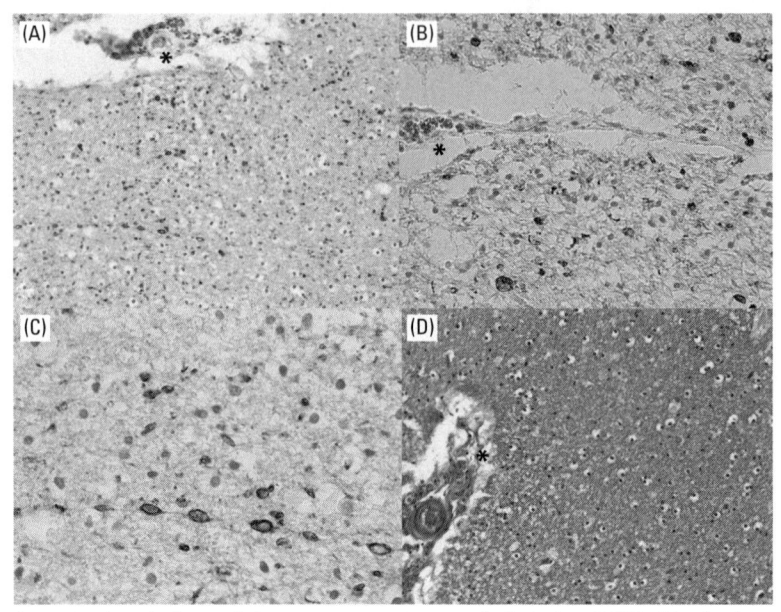

Figure 7.5 The axonal pathology of chronic traumatic encephalopathy (CTE). (*A–C*) Phosphorylated neurofilament staining (SMI-34) in cerebral white matter of stage III CTE shows marked reduction in axonal staining and numerous large, irregular axonal varicosities. A small arteriole shows marked infiltration with hemosiderin-laden macrophages (asterisks). (*D*) Luxol fast hematoxylin blue-stained section of white matter shows brisk astrocytosis, loss of myelinated fibers, and macrophages around vessel (asterisk). (10 μm tissue sections; scale bars: 100 μm) (See color plate section)

percentage of CTE subjects with Aß pathology is approximately the same that has been reported after severe acute TBI; diffuse cortical Aß plaques have been reported in 30% to 38% of cases after severe acute TBI as early as 2 hours after injury (Ikonomovic et al., 2004). In our recent series of 68 cases with CTE, approximately 11% were diagnosed with coexistent AD (McKee et al., 2013). In subjects with comorbid CTE and AD, significant memory loss generally begins in their forties or fifties, occasionally together with behavioral and personality changes, in the absence of a family history of early-onset AD. In subjects with CTE and AD, the p-tau pathology tends to be more florid than found with either disease alone; there is extreme involvement of most regions of cerebral cortex, diencephalon, basal ganglia, brainstem, and spinal cord as well as marked Aß deposition.

Chronic Traumatic Encephalopathy and Lewy Body Disease

Alpha-synuclein-positive Lewy bodies (LBs) are found in approximately 22% of CTE cases, in subjects who are significantly older than those without LBs (McKee et al., 2013). Approximately 16% of CTE cases meet criteria for the concomitant diagnosis of one of the Lewy body spectrum disorders, half as Parkinson's disease (PD) and half as dementia with Lewy bodies (DLB). When CTE is found in association with DLB-spectrum disorders, symptoms of CTE usually appear first with the development of slowness of movement, gait disturbance, tremor, and, if DLB is present, visual hallucinations late in the disease course.

Chronic Traumatic Encephalopathy and Frontotemporal Lobar Degeneration

Approximately 6% of subjects with CTE also develop FTLD either as FTLD-tau or FTLD-TDP (McKee et al., 2013). The most common FTLD, frontotemporal lobar degeneration with TDP-43-positive inclusions, FTLD-TDP, is defined by TDP-43-positive neuronal cytoplasmic and intranuclear inclusions, dystrophic neurites, and glial cytoplasmic inclusions in the superficial layers of cerebral cortex and dentate gyrus (Cairns et al., 2007; Dickson, 2009; Litvan et al., 1996). In advanced CTE, the distribution of TDP-43 is extremely widespread and in some areas overlaps with the pattern found in FTLD-TDP. It is probable that p-tau aggregates promote the aggregation and deposition of other pathological proteins such as TDP-43, Aß, and alpha-synuclein. Alternatively, repetitive trauma itself might trigger the deposition of multiple proteins (Uryu et al., 2002).

Chronic Traumatic Encephalopathy With Motor Neuron Disease

Approximately 10% of individuals with CTE develop a progressive motor neuron disease (CTE+MND), characterized by profound weakness, atrophy, spasticity, and fasciculations (McKee et al., 2010, 2013). Most individuals with CTE + MND present with symptoms of MND and develop mild cognitive and behavioral symptoms several years after the onset of motor weakness and fasciculations. One third of CTE + MND subjects present with depression and behavioral or cognitive changes prior to the development of symptoms of motor neuron disease. Individuals with motor neuron disease and CTE tend to die from respiratory failure at younger ages and in earlier stages of CTE (stage II-III) compared to subjects without MND. Independent of the stage of p-tau pathology, subjects with CTE+MND show severe TDP-43 pathology as neuronal, glial, and neuritic inclusions involving widespread regions of the central nervous system, including the cerebral hemispheres, basal ganglia, diencephalon, brainstem, anterior horn cells, and white matter tracts of the spinal cord (Fig. 7.5; Box 7.2). In CTE + MND there is also degeneration of lateral and ventral corticospinal tracts of the spinal cord and marked loss of anterior horn cells from the spinal cord. The accumulation of abnormal aggregates of p-tau and pTDP-43 is similar to Guam Parkinsonism-dementia complex, another example of an environmentally acquired tauopathy and TDP-43 proteinopathy (Hirano, 1992). The marked accumulation of pathological pTDP-43 aggregates in advanced stages of CTE, the partial immunohistochemical colocalization of ptau with pTDP-43, and the development of MND and FTLD in some individuals with CTE suggests that CTE and FTLD share similar pathogenic mechanisms (Costanza et al., 2011; King et al., 2010).

Pathogenetic Mechanisms of Chronic Traumatic Encephalopathy

As a result of the percussive stretch injury to neurons, the microtubule associated protein, tau, normally associated with microtubules in axons, becomes abnormally phosphorylated, misfolded, aggregated, and cleaved, all of which generate neurotoxicity (Amadoro et al., 2006; Chen, Wang, & Tseng, 2010; Khlistunova et al., 2006; McKee et al., 2013; Zilka et al., 2006). Although evidence suggests that tau phosphorylation and misfolding is a reversible process at least initially (Stieler et al., 2011; Van der Jeugd et al., 2012; Wolozin, 2012), repeated traumatic injuries and progressively greater accumulations of abnormal and toxic

---

BOX 7.2 Criteria for the Diagnosis of Chronic Traumatic Encephalopathy with Motor Neuron Disease

1. Clinical diagnosis of definite amyotrophic lateral sclerosis using the revised El Escorial criteria for the diagnosis of amyotrophic lateral sclerosis
2. The pathological diagnosis of chronic traumatic encephalopathy
3. Degeneration of lateral and ventral corticospinal tracts of the spinal cord
4. Marked loss of anterior horn cells from cervical, thoracic, and lumbar spinal cord with gliosis
5. TDP-43 or pTDP-43 positive neuronal, glial, neuritic, or intranuclear inclusions in anterior horn cells and white matter tracts of the spinal cord

Source: Adapted from McKee et al. (2013).

p-tau appear to become self-perpetuating at some point. Individuals who evolve from acute concussion and postconcussion states into a progressive tau-based neurodegeneration experience progressive clinical deterioration, even though they have retired from their sport or ceased the activities associated with brain trauma. How this progressive neurodegeneration develops after episodes of acute minor neurotrauma in all probability involves spreading of tau pathology intercellularly and extracellularly throughout the brain.

Direct and indirect evidence for interneuronal tau transmission in animal models suggests that the transfer of toxic tau species between neurons might be due to interneuronal spreading of tau mediated by a prion-like templated misfolding of tau (Clavaguera et al., 2009; de Calignon et al., 2012; Guo & Lee, 2011; Hall & Patuto, 2012; Kim et al., 2010; Liu et al., 2012). Other possible modes of transmission involve oligomeric or toxic N-terminal tau in the receiving neuron with dysregulation of intracellular calcium (Frost, Jacks, & Diamond, 2009; Park & Ferreira, 2005). Although spreading of tau pathology is thought to occur from one neuronal synapse to another, transmission involving astrocytes or microglia or cerebrospinal fluid (CSF) pathways is also possible. CSF fluid enters the brain parenchyma along the Virchow–Robin spaces surrounding penetrating arteries, and brain interstitial fluid is cleared along paravenous drainage pathways. Transfer of tau pathology to astrocytes and neurons surrounding this clearance pathway might be at least partially responsible for tau propagation, as has been shown recently for Aß (Iliff et al., 2012). Clearance through paravenous flow and the CSF might also regulate extracellular levels of p-tau and TDP-43 and explain the distinctive perivascular, subpial, and periventricular localization of both proteins (Hall & Patuto, 2012). The striking subpial and periventricular location of abnormal p-tau and p-TDP-43 deposits is a feature of CTE that is unique from other tauopathies such as AD and FTLD-tau, suggesting that CSF circulation of p-tau might be more severe in CTE compared to other tauopathies.

The patchy irregular location of the p-tau pathology suggests that the distribution is related to direct mechanical injury from blows to the top of the head; furthermore, the localization to the perivascular region and sulcal depths corresponds to focal stress points of the brain. In addition, the early and predominant involvement of the superior and dorsolateral frontal lobes in former football players parallels the high frequency of impacts to the top of the head compared to those to the front, back, and side of the head in football players (Guskiewicz et al., 2007; Mihalik, Bell, Marshall, & Guskiewicz, 2007), as well as fMRI data showing activation impairments in dorsolateral prefrontal cortex that was associated with significantly higher numbers of head collisions to the top-front of the head (Talavage et al., 2010).

One of the key features of CTE is that the disease continues to progress for decades after the activity that produced traumatic injury has stopped. It suggests that once the pathological cascades involved in CTE-related neurodegeneration are triggered, they continue to progress throughout the individual's lifetime. In our series of American football players, the number of years played ($p < .0001$), years since retirement ($p < .0001$), and age at death ($p < .0001$) significantly correlated with pathological stage of CTE (McKee et al., 2013). In addition, the degree of aggregated p-tau and TDP-43 protein deposition, neuronal and axonal loss, neuroinflammation, cerebral atrophy, and ventricular enlargement all increase with longer survival (McKee et al., 2013).

Clinical Diagnosis of Chronic Traumatic Encephalopathy

Presently, there are no available biomarkers for the diagnosis of CTE; however, many promising biomarkers appear to be on the horizon, including diffusion tensor imaging (DTI), functional connectivity (fMRI), or other advanced imaging measures of axonal integrity, magnetic resonance spectroscopy (MRS) to detect biochemical metabolites, CSF and plasma protein markers (including p-tau and total tau), and new p-tau ligands to identify p-tau deposition in the CSF and brain (Xia et al., 2013).

Genetic Risk for Chronic Traumatic Encephalopathy and the Role of the Apolipoprotein E Gene

In acute TBI, there is evidence that the cognitive and behavioral outcome of moderate and severe TBI is more severe in Apolipoprotein

E (ApoE) e4 positive individuals (Ariza et al., 2006; Chiang, Chang, & Hu, 2003; Friedman et al., 1999). In addition, in a study of professional boxers with high levels of traumatic exposure (more than 12 professional bouts), ApoE e4 carriers had more severe motor, cognitive, and psychiatric deficits than boxers without the ApoE e4 allele (Jordan et al., 1997). Preliminary analysis of ApoE genotyping in individuals with neuropathologically verified CTE indicates significantly more ApoE e4 homozygotes than would be predicted in an age-matched cohort without CTE ($p < .05$). While there are also more ApoE e3/ e4 heterozygotes in the CTE cohort than expected, the difference does not meet statistical significance.

Guidelines for Prevention and Treatment of Chronic Traumatic Encephalopathy

The most basic and effective way to decrease the incidence of CTE is to limit exposure to mTBI. In athletes, this is accomplished by restricting exposure to trauma and adhering to strict return to play guidelines. Proper care and management of mTBI in general and, in particular, in sports and military service will also reduce the incidence of CTE. Unfortunately, despite using the best preventative tools and proper management, mTBI will continue to occur as a result of accidental and unexpected injury. There are currently no reliable, specific measures of neurological dysfunction after mTBI, and most recommendations for concussion diagnosis center on the resolution of acute symptoms such as headache, confusion, and sensitivity to light (Harmon et al., 2013). However, studies using event-related potentials, transcranial magnetic stimulation, balance testing, rapid reading tasks, multitask effects on gait stability, positron emission tomography, and DTI MRI have all shown abnormalities after TBI that persist for weeks after symptoms have resolved, indicating that safe return to play guidelines based entirely on subjective symptoms might not be the best prognosticator. There is an urgent need to develop field-ready, user-friendly biomarkers to detect mTBI immediately at the time of injury and to guide management and therapeutic interventions in the postinjury period.

Conclusions

CTE develops after repetitive mTBI, including concussion and subconcussion. The exact pathogenetic relationship between acute mTBI and the development of CTE is not precisely clear but undoubtedly involves acute axonal injury, persistent axonal transport failure, microvascular injury, cytoskeletal disruption, and tau hyperphosphorylation and aggregation. The clinical symptoms of CTE usually develop many years after exposure to repetitive but minor brain trauma. The most common presenting symptoms of CTE are depression, headaches, attention and concentration difficulties, and short-term memory loss that typically appear in midlife. Neuropathologically, CTE is associated with significantly diminished brain weight; marked atrophy of the medial temporal lobe, cerebral cortex, subcortical white matter, thalamus, hypothalamus, and mammillary bodies; enlargement of the lateral and third ventricles; septal abnormalities; and depigmentation of the locus coeruleus and substantia nigra. The progression of p-tau pathology in CTE follows a predictable sequence that can be divided into four stages, stages I–IV. Stage I is characterized by focal, perivascular deposits of p-tau at the base of the cerebral sulci; later stages involve progressively more expansive regions of neocortex, medial temporal lobe, diencephalon, basal ganglia, brainstem, and spinal cord. The early, focal cortical p-tau pathology of CTE is distinctive from other tauopathies, and unlike the early limbic degeneration and later neocortical involvement typical of AD (Braak & Braak, 1991; Braak, Braak, & Bohl, 1993). TDP-43 abnormalities are also found in most CTE cases; in advanced CTE, TDP-43 pathology is often severe and widespread. As tau and TDP-43 deposition increases, there is a parallel increase in axonal pathology and loss. CTE may be associated with other neurodegenerative diseases, including AD, PD, DLB, FTLD, and MND. Most individuals with CTE and MND present with symptoms of motor neuron disease at young ages and develop subtle cognitive and behavioral symptoms a few years later. While the pathogenic mechanisms of CTE remain to be fully elucidated, progressive axonal degeneration, accumulation, and transneuronal propagation of toxic aggregated proteins appear to be essential components. CTE can only be diagnosed at autopsy at the present time; however, promising efforts to develop DTI, fMRI, MRS, CSF, and blood p-tau and neuroinflammatory markers, and p-tau PET ligands as biomarkers are under way to diagnose and monitor the course of disease in living subjects. Future therapeutic efforts in mTBI will need to address acute mTBI as well as the long-term progressive neurodegeneration that follows. Currently, the best therapies are prevention of the initial traumatic injuries and continued public education regarding proper detection and management of acute mTBI.

Dedication

This work is dedicated to Hyo Soon-Lee (August 24, 1961–November 13, 2012).

Acknowledgments

I gratefully acknowledge the use of resources and facilities at the Edith Nourse Rogers Memorial Veterans Hospital (Bedford, MA). I also gratefully acknowledge the help of all the codirectors and staff for the Center for the Study of Traumatic Encephalopathy at Boston University and the Boston VA, and the families whose participation made this work possible. This work was supported by The Department of Veterans Affairs; Veterans Affairs Biorepository (CSP 501); Translational Research Center for Traumatic Brain Injury and Stress Disorders (TRACTS); Veterans Affairs Rehabilitation Research and Development Traumatic Brain Injury Center of Excellence (B6796-C); National Institute of Aging Boston University Alzheimer's Disease Center (P30AG13846; supplement 0572063345-5); National Institute of Aging Boston University Framingham Heart Study R01 (AG1649); Sports Legacy Institute; and the National Operating Committee on Standards for Athletic Equipment. This work was also supported by an unrestricted gift from the National Football League and the Andlinger Foundation.

References

Amadoro, G., Ciotti, M. T., Costanzi, M., Cestari, V., Calissano, P., & Canu, N. (2006). NMDA receptor mediates tau-induced neurotoxicity by calpain and ERK/MAPK activation. *Proceedings of the National Academy of Science USA, 103*(8), 2892–2897.

Ariza, M., Pueyo, R., Matarin Mdel, M., Junque, C., Mataro, M., Clemente, I.,...Sahuquillo, J. (2006). Influence of APOE polymorphism on cognitive and behavioural outcome in moderate and severe traumatic brain injury. *Journal of Neurology, Neurosurgery and Psychiatry, 77*(10), 1191–1193.

Bazarian, J. J., Zhu, T., Blyth, B., Borrino, A., & Zhong, J. (2012). Subject-specific changes in brain white matter on diffusion tensor imaging after sports-related concussion. *Magnetic Resonance Imaging, 30*(2), 171–180.

Blumbergs, P. S. G. (1944). Staining of amyloid precursor protein to study axonal injury in mild head injury. *Lancet, 344*, 1055.

Bohnen, N., Jolles, J., & Twijnstra, A. (1992). Neuropsychological deficits in patients with persistent symptoms six months after mild head injury. *Neurosurgery, 30*(5), 692–695; discussion 5–6.

Braak, H., & Braak, E. (1991). Neuropathological stageing of Alzheimer-related changes. *Acta Neuropathologcia, 82*(4), 239–259.

Braak, H., Braak, E., & Bohl, J. (1993). Staging of Alzheimer-related cortical destruction. *European Neurology, 33*(6), 403–408.

Cairns, N. J., Bigio, E. H., Mackenzie, I. R., Neumann, M., Lee, V. M., Hatanpaa, K. J.,...Mann, D. M. (2007). Neuropathologic diagnostic and nosologic criteria for frontotemporal lobar degeneration: Consensus of the Consortium for Frontotemporal Lobar Degeneration. *Acta Neuropathologcia, 114*(1), 5–22.

Chen, J. K., Johnston, K. M., Frey, S., Petrides, M., Worsley, K., & Ptito, A. (2004). Functional abnormalities in symptomatic concussed athletes: An fMRI study. *Neuroimage, 22*(1), 68–82.

Chen, J. K., Johnston, K. M., Petrides, M., & Ptito, A. (2008). Recovery from mild head injury in sports: Evidence from serial functional magnetic resonance imaging studies in male athletes. *Clinical Journal of Sports Medicine, 18*(3), 241–247.

Chen, L. J., Wang, Y. J., & Tseng, G. F. (2010). Compression alters kinase and phosphatase activity and tau and MAP2 phosphorylation transiently while inducing the fast adaptive dendritic remodeling of underlying cortical neurons. *Journal of Neurotrama, 27*(9), 1657–1669.

Chiang, M. F., Chang, J. G., & Hu, C. J. (2003). Association between apolipoprotein E genotype and outcome of traumatic brain injury. *Acta Neurochirurgica (Wien), 145*(8), 649–653; discussion 53–4.

Clavaguera, F., Bolmont, T., Crowther, R. A., Abramowski, D., Frank, S., Probst, A.,...Tolnay, M. (2009). Transmission and spreading of tauopathy in transgenic mouse brain. *Nature Cell Biology*, *11*(7), 909–913.

Corsellis, J. A., Bruton, C. J., & Freeman-Browne, D. (1973). The aftermath of boxing. *Psychological Medicine*, *3*(3), 270–303.

Costanza, A., Weber, K., Gandy, S., Bouras, C., Hof, P. R., Giannakopoulos, P., & Canuto, A. (2011). Review: Contact sport-related chronic traumatic encephalopathy in the elderly: Clinical expression and structural substrates. *Neuropathology and Applied Neurobiology*, *37*(6), 570–584.

Courville, C. B. (1962). Punch drunk. Its pathogenesis and pathology on the basis of a verified case. *Bulletin of the Los Angeles Neurological Society*, *27*, 160–168.

Crisco, J. J., Wilcox, B. J., Machan, J. T., McAllister, T. W., Duhaime, A. C., Duma, S. M.,...Greenwald, R. M. (2012). Magnitude of head impact exposures in individual collegiate football players. *Journal of Applied Biomechanics*, *28*(2), 174–183.

Critchley, M. (1957). Medical aspects of boxing, particularly from a neurological standpoint. *British Medical Journal*, *1*(5015), 357–362.

Cubon, V. A., Putukian, M., Boyer, C., & Dettwiler, A. (2011). A diffusion tensor imaging study on the white matter skeleton in individuals with sports-related concussion. *Journal of Neurotrama*, *28*(2), 189–201.

Dean, P. J., & Sterr, A. (2013). Long-term effects of mild traumatic brain injury on cognitive performance. *Frontiers in Human Neuroscience*, *7*, 30.

de Calignon, A., Polydoro, M., Suarez-Calvet, M., William, C., Adamowicz, D. H., Kopeikina, K. J.,...Hyman, B. T. (2012). Propagation of tau pathology in a model of early Alzheimer's disease. *Neuron*, *73*(4), 685–697.

Dickson, D. W. (2009). Neuropathology of non-Alzheimer degenerative disorders. *International Journal of Clinical and Experimental Pathology*, *3*(1), 1–23.

Friedman, G., Froom, P., Sazbon, L., Grinblatt, I., Shochina, M., Tsenter, J.,...Groswasser, Z. (1999). Apolipoprotein E-epsilon4 genotype predicts a poor outcome in survivors of traumatic brain injury. *Neurology*, *52*(2), 244–248.

Frost, B., Jacks, R. L., & Diamond, M. I. (2009). Propagation of tau misfolding from the outside to the inside of a cell. *Journal of Biological Chemistry*, *284*(19), 12845–12852.

Geddes, J. F., Vowles, G. H., Nicoll, J. A., & Revesz, T. (1999). Neuronal cytoskeletal changes are an early consequence of repetitive head injury. *Acta Neuropathologcia*, *98*(2), 171–178.

Giza, C. C., & Hovda, D. A. (2001). The neurometabolic cascade of concussion. *Journal of Athletic Training*, *36*(3), 228–235.

Goldstein, L. E., Fisher, A. M., Tagge, C. A., Zhang, X. L., Velisek, L., Sullivan, J. A.,...McKee, A. C. (2012). Chronic traumatic encephalopathy in blast-exposed military veterans and a blast neurotrauma mouse model. *Science Translational Medicine*, *4*(134), 134ra60.

Gosselin, N., Bottari, C., Chen, J. K., Petrides, M., Tinawi, S., de Guise, E., & Ptito, A. (2011). Electrophysiology and functional MRI in post-acute mild traumatic brain injury. *Journal of Neurotrama*, *28*(3), 329–341.

Guo, J. L., & Lee, V. M. (2011). Seeding of normal Tau by pathological Tau conformers drives pathogenesis of Alzheimer-like tangles. *Journal of Biological Chemistry*, *286*(17), 15317–1531.

Guskiewicz, K. M., Mihalik, J. P., Shankar, V., Marshall, S. W., Crowell, D. H., Oliaro, S. M.,...Hooker, D. N. (2007). Measurement of head impacts in collegiate football players: Relationship between head impact biomechanics and acute clinical outcome after concussion. *Neurosurgery*, *61*(6), 1244–1252; discussion 52–3.

Hall, G. F., & Patuto, B. A. (2012). Is tau ready for admission to the prion club? *Prion*, *6*(3), 223–233.

Harmon, K. G., Drezner, J. A., Gammons, M., Guskiewicz, K. M., Halstead, M., Herring, S. A.,...Roberts, W. O. (2013). American Medical Society for Sports Medicine position statement: concussion in sport. *British Journal of Sports Medicine*, *47*(1), 15–26.

Hirano, A. (1992). Amyotrophic lateral sclerosis and parkinsonism-dementia complex on Guam: Immunohistochemical studies. *Keio Journal of Medicine*, *41*(1), 6–9.

Hof, P. R., Knabe, R., Bovier, P., & Bouras, C. (1991). Neuropathological observations in a case of autism presenting with self-injury behavior. *Acta Neuropathologcia*, *82*(4), 321–326.

Ikonomovic, M. D., Uryu, K., Abrahamson, E. E., Ciallella, J. R., Trojanowski, J. Q., Lee, V. M.,...DeKosky, S. T. (2004). Alzheimer's pathology in human temporal cortex surgically excised after severe brain injury. *Experimental Neurology*, *190*(1), 192–203.

Iliff, J. J., Wang, M., Liao, Y., Plogg, B. A., Peng, W., Gundersen, G. A.,...Nedergaard, M. (2012). A paravascular pathway facilitates CSF flow through the brain parenchyma and the clearance of interstitial solutes, including amyloid beta. *Science Translational Medicine*, *4*(147), 147ra11.

Johnson, V. E., Stewart, W., & Smith, D. H. (2012). Axonal pathology in traumatic brain injury. *Experimental Neurology*, *246*, 35–43.

Jordan, B. D., Relkin, N. R., Ravdin, L. D., Jacobs, A. R., Bennett, A., & Gandy, S. (1997). Apolipoprotein E epsilon4 associated with chronic traumatic brain injury in boxing. *Journal of the American Medical Association*, *278*(2), 136–140.

Khlistunova, I., Biernat, J., Wang, Y., Pickhardt, M., von Bergen, M., Gazova, Z.,...Mandelkow, E. M. (2006). Inducible expression of Tau repeat domain in cell models of tauopathy: aggregation is toxic to cells but can be reversed by inhibitor drugs. *Journal of Biological Chemistry*, *281*(2), 1205–1214.

Kim, W., Lee, S., Jung, C., Ahmed, A., Lee, G., & Hall, G. F. (2010). Interneuronal transfer of human tau between Lamprey central neurons in situ. *Journal of Alzheimers Disease*, *19*(2), 647–664.

King, A., Sweeney, F., Bodi, I., Troakes, C., Maekawa, S., & Al-Sarraj, S. (2010). Abnormal TDP-43 expression is identified in the neocortex in cases of dementia pugilistica, but is mainly confined to the limbic system when identified in high and moderate stages of Alzheimer's disease. *Neuropathology*, *30*(4), 408–419.

Litvan, I., Hauw, J. J., Bartko, J. J., Lantos, P. L., Daniel, S. E., Horoupian, D. S.,...Anderson, D. W. (1996). Validity and reliability of the preliminary NINDS neuropathologic criteria for progressive supranuclear palsy and related disorders. *Journal of Neuropathology and Experimental Neurology*, *55*(1), 97–105.

Liu, L., Drouet, V., Wu, J. W., Witter, M. P., Small, S. A., Clelland, C., & Duff, K. (2012). Trans-synaptic spread of tau pathology in vivo. *PLoS One*, *7*(2), e31302.

Lovell, M. R., Pardini, J. E., Welling, J., Collins, M. W., Bakal, J., Lazar, N.,...Becker, J. T. (2007). Functional brain abnormalities are related to clinical recovery and time to return-to-play in athletes. *Neurosurgery*, *61*(2), 352–359; discussion 9–60.

Martland, H. (1928). Punch drunk. *Journal of the American Medical Association*, *91*, 1103–1107.

Maxwell, W. L., McCreath, B. J., Graham, D. I., & Gennarelli, T. A. (1995). Cytochemical evidence for redistribution of membrane pump calcium-ATPase and ecto-Ca-ATPase activity, and calcium influx in myelinated nerve fibres of the optic nerve after stretch injury. *Journal of Neurocytology*, *24*(12), 925–942.

Maxwell, W. L., Povlishock, J. T., & Graham, D. L. (1997). A mechanical analysis of nondisruptive axonal injury: A review. *Journal of Neurotrama*, *14*(7), 419–440.

McAllister, T. W., Saykin, A. J., Flashman, L. A., Sparling, M. B., Johnson, S. C., Guerin, S. J.,...Yanofsky, N. (1999). Brain activation during working memory 1 month after mild traumatic brain injury: A functional MRI study. *Neurology*, *53*(6), 1300–1308.

McAllister, T. W., Sparling, M. B., Flashman, L. A., Guerin, S. J., Mamourian, A. C., & Saykin, A. J. (2001). Differential working memory load effects after mild traumatic brain injury. *Neuroimage*, *14*(5), 1004–1012.

McKee, A. C., Cantu, R. C., Nowinski, C. J., Hedley-Whyte, E. T., Gavett, B. E., Budson, A. E.,...Stern, R. A. (2009). Chronic traumatic encephalopathy in athletes: Progressive tauopathy after repetitive head injury. *Journal of Neuropathology and Experimental Neurology*, *68*(7), 709–735.

McKee, A. C., Gavett, B. E., Stern, R. A., Nowinski, C. J., Cantu, R. C., Kowall, N. W.,...Budson, A. E. (2010). TDP-43 proteinopathy and motor neuron disease in chronic traumatic encephalopathy. *Journal of Neuropathology and Experimental Neurology*, *69*(9), 918–929.

McKee, A. C., Kosik, K. S., & Kowall, N. W. (1991). Neuritic pathology and dementia in Alzheimer's disease. *Annals of Neurology*, *30*(2), 156–165.

McKee, A. C., Stein, T. D., Nowinski, C. J., Stern, R. A., Daneshvar, D. H., Alvarez, V. E.,...Cantu, R. C. (2013). The spectrum of disease in chronic traumatic encephalopathy. *Brain*, *136*(Pt 1), 43–64.

Medana, I. M., & Esiri, M. M. (2003). Axonal damage: A key predictor of outcome in human CNS diseases. *Brain*, *126*(Pt 3), 515–530.

Mihalik, J. P., Bell, D. R., Marshall, S. W., & Guskiewicz, K. M. (2007). Measurement of head impacts in collegiate football players: An investigation of positional and event-type differences. *Neurosurgery*, *61*(6), 1229–1235; discussion 35.

Millspaugh, J. (1937). Dementia pugilistica. *US Naval Medical Bulletin*, *35*, 297–261.

Omalu, B. I., DeKosky, S. T., Hamilton, R. L., Minster, R. L., Kamboh, M. I., Shakir, A. M., & Wecht, C. H. (2006). Chronic traumatic encephalopathy in a national football league player: Part II. *Neurosurgery*, *59*(5), 1086–1092; discussion 92–3.

Omalu, B. I., DeKosky, S. T., Minster, R. L., Kamboh, M. I., Hamilton, R. L., & Wecht, C. H. (2005). Chronic traumatic encephalopathy in a National Football League player. *Neurosurgery*, *57*(1), 128–134; discussion -34.

Ommaya, A. K., & Gennarelli, T. A. (1974). Cerebral concussion and traumatic unconsciousness. Correlation of experimental and clinical observations of blunt head injuries. *Brain*, *97*(4), 633–654.

Oppenheimer, D. R. (1968). Microscopic lesions in the brain following head injury. *Journal of Neurology, Neurosurgery and Psychiatry*, *31*(4), 299–306.

Park, S. Y., & Ferreira, A. (2005). The generation of a 17 kDa neurotoxic fragment: An alternative mechanism by which tau mediates beta-amyloid-induced neurodegeneration. *Journal of Neuroscience*, 25(22), 5365–5375.

Parker, H. L. (1934). Traumatic encephalopathy (`punch drunk') of professional pugilists. *Journal of Neurology and Psychopathology*, 15(57), 20–28.

Ptito, A., Chen, J. K., & Johnston, K. M. (2007). Contributions of functional magnetic resonance imaging (fMRI) to sport concussion evaluation. *NeuroRehabilitation*, 22(3), 217–227.

Reeves, T. M., Phillips, L. L., & Povlishock, J. T. (2005). Myelinated and unmyelinated axons of the corpus callosum differ in vulnerability and functional recovery following traumatic brain injury. *Experimental Neurology*, 196(1), 126–137.

Stieler, J. T., Bullmann, T., Kohl, F., Toien, O., Bruckner, M. K., Hartig, W.,...Arendt, T. (2011). The physiological link between metabolic rate depression and tau phosphorylation in mammalian hibernation. *PLoS One*, 6(1), e14530.

Smits, M., Dippel, D. W., Houston, G. C., Wielopolski, P. A., Koudstaal, P. J., Hunink, M. G., & van der Lugt, A. (2009). Postconcussion syndrome after minor head injury: Brain activation of working memory and attention. *Human Brain Mapping*, 30(9), 2789–803.

Talavage, T. M., Nauman, E., Breedlove, E. L., Yoruk, U., Dye, A. E., Morigaki, K.,...Leverenz, L. J. (2010). Functionally-detected cognitive impairment in high school football players without clinically-diagnosed concussion. *Journal of Neurotrauma*, 31(4), 327–328.

Uryu, K., Laurer, H., McIntosh, T., Pratico, D., Martinez, D., Leight, S.,...Trojanowski, J. Q. (2002). Repetitive mild brain trauma accelerates Abeta deposition, lipid peroxidation, and cognitive impairment in a transgenic mouse model of Alzheimer amyloidosis. *Journal of Neuroscience*, 22(2), 446–454.

Van der Jeugd, A., Hochgrafe, K., Ahmed, T., Decker, J. M., Sydow, A., Hofmann, A.,...Mandelkow, E. M. (2012). Cognitive defects are reversible in inducible mice expressing pro-aggregant full-length human Tau. *Acta Neuropathologcia*, 123(6), 787–805.

Wolozin, B. (2012). Regulated protein aggregation: Stress granules and neurodegeneration. *Molecular Neurodegeneration*, 7, 56.

Xia, C. F., Arteaga, J., Chen, G., Gangadharmath, U., Gomez, L. F., Kasi, D.,...Kolb, H. C. (2013). [(18)F]T807, a novel tau positron emission tomography imaging agent for Alzheimer's disease. *Alzheimers and Dementia*, 9(6), 666–676.

Zilka, N., Filipcik, P., Koson, P., Fialova, L., Skrabana, R., Zilkova, M.,...Novak, M. (2006). Truncated tau from sporadic Alzheimer's disease suffices to drive neurofibrillary degeneration in vivo. *FEBS Letters*, 580(15), 3582–3588.

8

Frontotemporal Dementia

Bradford C. Dickerson

The clinical and pathological investigation of frontotemporal dementia (FTD) has a complex history dating back over 100 years, and in the 21st century its clinical and pathological classification continues to evolve with groundbreaking new discoveries. This chapter will provide a comprehensive review of FTD with an emphasis on behavioral variant FTD; readers are referred to Chapter 9 for a detailed review of primary progressive aphasia, the major language variant of FTD.

In 1892, Arnold Pick described a 71-year-old patient with progressive cognitive decline, primarily manifesting as early loss of language (Pick, Girling, & Berrios, 1997). Pick noted the prominent anterior temporal lobe atrophy present in the brain of this patient, and he subsequently reported three further cases—including very clear descriptions of clinical and gross postmortem features. The associated histologic abnormalities identified microscopically were later described by Alois Alzheimer, and in the 1920s the term "Pick's disease" was coined by Onari and Spatz. As early as 1927, Schneider described the clinical course of the disease, highlighting the insidious early changes in behavior and personality and, contrasted with Alzheimer's disease (AD), the typical relative preservation of memory and orientation into the middle phases of the disease (Berrios & Girling, 1994). A few reports on these diseases were published through the middle of the 20th century, but it was not until the 1980s and 1990s that interest in these conditions was resurrected with advances in neuroimaging, neuropathology, genetics, and related fields. Although terminology continues to be confusing in this family of diseases, we now recognize patients with several major forms of the clinical entity "frontotemporal dementia (FTD)," including "behavioral variant FTD (bvFTD)," "semantic dementia (SD) or the semantic variant of PPA," the "nonfluent or agrammatic variant of PPA," and the "logopenic" variant of PPA. The neuropathological family of conditions is termed "frontotemporal lobar degeneration (FTLD)". FTLD is a loosely knit group of neurodegenerative diseases that preferentially affect the frontal and anterior temporal lobes, with relative sparing of other cortical regions in many cases, and often affects basal ganglia and in some cases basal forebrain and brainstem nuclei.

For most of the 20th century, patients with progressive dementias presenting with prominent early behavioral change were diagnosed with Pick's disease. In a series of studies starting in 1982, Mesulam reinvigorated the interest of the neurology and psychiatry communities in progressive degenerative aphasias, which he termed "primary progressive aphasia (PPA)" (Mesulam, 1982). In the 1980s, the Lund (Gustafson, 1987) and Manchester (Neary, Snowden, Northen, & Goulding, 1988) groups reported important early studies generating renewed interest in the behavioral phenotype of FTD, soon thereafter proposing clinical and pathological diagnostic criteria (Brun et al., 1994). In the late 1990s, formal international consensus research diagnostic criteria (Neary et al., 1998) were developed for three clinical subtypes of FTLD: frontotemporal dementia, progressive nonfluent aphasia, and semantic dementia. In 2001, McKhann and others proposed simpler criteria for the practicing clinician (McKhann et al., 2001), although some authors have criticized these criteria as being too vague. Important advances were formalized in 2011 when new consensus diagnostic criteria were published for PPA (Gorno-Tempini et al., 2011) and bvFTD (Rascovsky et al., 2011). These criteria were then largely incorporated with some simplification into the fifth edition of the American Psychiatric Association's *Diagnostic and Statistical Manual of Mental Disorders* in 2013.

Epidemiology

FTLD is thought to be the third most common degenerative dementia, after AD and dementia with Lewy bodies (DLB), accounting for 5%–15% of dementias. FTLD is often an early-onset dementia, typically manifesting itself in patients who are 45–65 years old. It is probably the second most common cause of dementia in people younger than 65. Yet it has been reported with pathological confirmation in patients as young as 21 (Snowden, Neary, & Mann, 2004) and as old as 85 (Gislason, Sjogren, Larsson, & Skoog, 2003). Some epidemiologic studies raise the question of whether it is being substantially underascertained (Ibach et al., 2003), suggesting that it may be more common than previously thought, including in the elderly (Borroni et al., 2010; Knopman, Petersen, Edland, Cha, & Rocca, 2004).

The incidence and prevalence rates of FTD have received little study with widely ranging results, from a prevalence of ~1.1 per 100,000 cases in a study from the Netherlands (Rosso et al., 2003) to 15–17 per 100,000 cases in two studies from the United Kingdom (Harvey Skelton-Robinson, & Rossor, 2003; Ratnavalli, Brayne, Dawson, & Hodges, 2002) and one from Northern Italy (Borroni et al., 2010) to 35 per 100,000 cases from a recent door-to-door investigation in Southern Italy (Bernardi et al., 2012). With regard to incidence, an American study revealed incidence rates in Rochester, Minnesota, of 2.2 per 100,000 between ages 40 and 49, 3.3 per 100,000 between ages 50 and 59, and 8.9 per 100,000 between ages 60 and 69 (Knopman et al., 2004).

One of the major challenges in this field is the large number of potential ways FTLD can be classified, yet this stems in part from many exciting new developments in the field. For instance, there is an the increasing number of ways these diseases overlap with other neurodegenerative diseases, including progressive supranuclear palsy (PSP), corticobasal degeneration (CBD), and amyotrophic lateral sclerosis (ALS).

Neuropathology of Frontotemporal Lobar Degeneration

The hallmark of the neuropathology of FTLD is its topographic distribution—which in some cases is strikingly focal—in the frontal and anterior temporal lobes, as well as a number of subcortical structures. Progress in this field in recent years has been rapid and has resulted in a number of reclassifications in the past decade based on new findings from immunohistochemistry, molecular biology, and genetics.

Dr. Arnold Pick first described the remarkably focal "knife-like" atrophy of frontal and anterior temporal cortex that can be seen in FTLD (Munoz, Morris, & Rosser, 2011; Pick, 1892). Using the new silver staining histopathologic techniques of the time, Dr. Alois Alzheimer first reported two microscopic lesions (Alzheimer, 1911): intraneuronal argyrophilic inclusion bodies, which later came to be known as the "Pick body," and achromatic neuronal balloon cells, which later were called "Pick cells" (Onari & Spatz, 1926). Multiple investigators throughout the 20th century reported detailed clinical and pathologic studies of such cases (Binns & Robertson, 1962; Neumann, 1949; Schenk, 1959), describing the major features of what was called "Pick's disease," which can be

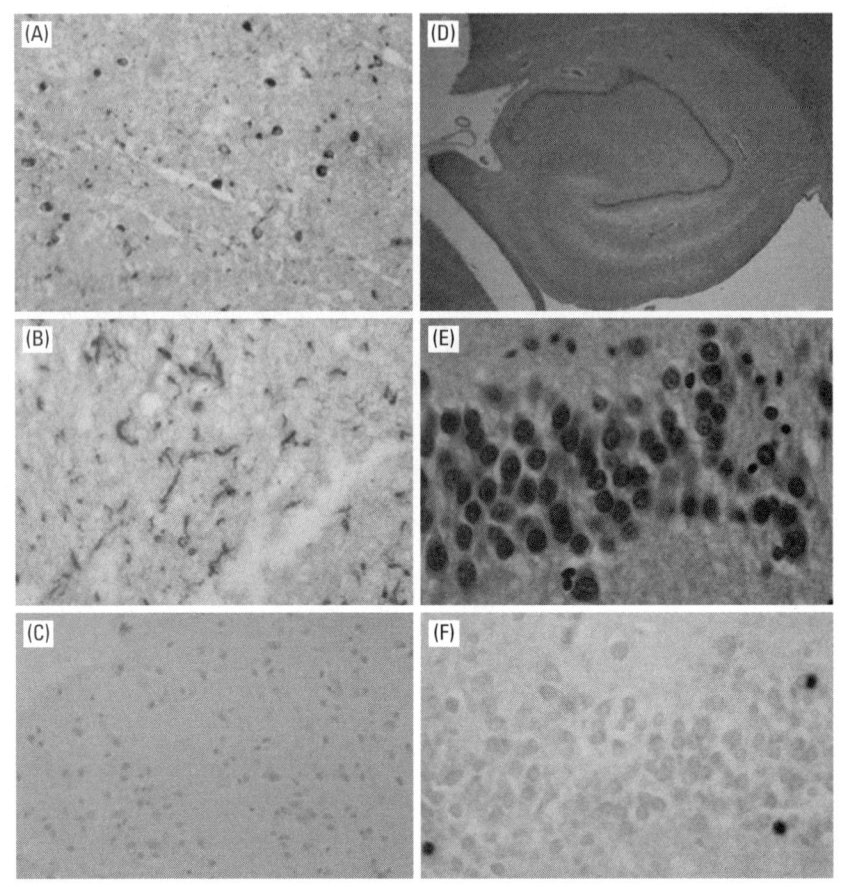

Figure 8.1 Tau pathology in a case of classical Pick's disease prominently affects neuronal and glial cells in gray matter (A, labeling with AT8 [phosphorylated tau] immunohistochemistry) and also usually demonstrates prominent abnormalities in white matter (B, labeling with AT8 immunohistochemistry) of frontal and temporal cortices, including the dentate gyrus of the hippocampus, with sparing of primary cortices particularly Heschl's and calcarine cortex (C, absent labeling with AT8 immunohistochemistry). The hippocampus (D, low-power hematoxylin and eosin stain) also classically shows dense, smooth-contoured rounded cytoplasmic inclusions in granule cells of the dentate gyrus (E, high-power hematoxylin and eosin stain), which are labeled with AT8 immunohistochemistry (F). (See color plate section)

summarized as atrophy and substantial tau pathology in prefrontal cortex, frontoinsula, anterior cingulate, and anterior temporal cortex with relative sparing of the superior temporal gyrus, especially its posterior third, as well as primary visual cortex (Hof, Bouras, Perl, & Morrison, 1994; Yoshimura, 1989) (see Fig. 8.1). Prominent white matter tau pathology is commonly present (Zhukareva et al., 2002). Some investigators have called attention to the heavy tau burden near the cortical gray matter–white matter junction, including deep cortical layers and immediately subjacent white matter (Dickson, 2001). The basal ganglia, basal forebrain, and brainstem structures are variably affected, with some patients showing minimal pathology and others exhibiting substantial pathology (Dickson, 2001). In recent years, Pick's disease has been conceptualized as part of a spectrum of tauopathies that can present as bvFTD, including progressive supranuclear palsy and corticobasal degeneration and other less common forms (Dickson, Kouri, Murray, & Josephs, 2011; Kertesz, Davidson, & Munoz, 1999).

Yet it eventually became clear that some patients with what otherwise appeared clinically to have a frontal lobe-type dementia did not exhibit classical Pick's disease.

Constantinidis developed a classification system that recognized three major types of so-called Pick's disease, the first of which is classical Pick's pathology, the second corticobasal degeneration, and the third lacked specific histological characteristics. Brun and Gustafson recognized a "frontal lobe degeneration of non-Alzheimer type" that was neither Alzheimer's nor classical Pick's disease, and this was similarly identified by other investigators (Clark et al., 1986; Neary et al., 1988) and referred to as "dementia lacking distinctive histology (DLDH)" (Knopman, Mastri, Frey, Sung, & Rustan, 1990).

In 2004–2006, it became clear that the majority of DLDH cases demonstrated immunoreactivity to ubiquitin (FTLD-U). In a major discovery in 2006, investigators demonstrated that the majority of these showed specific inclusions of TDP-43 (transactive DNA-binding protein, molecular weight 43 kDa) (Neumann et al., 2006) with a number of distinct subtypes based on the intracellular localization and morphology of the inclusions (Mackenzie, Rademakers, & Neumann, 2010). Furthermore, this protein has been found in most cases of ALS. In 2009, many of the remaining 10% of pathologically unclassified FTLD cases were shown to be immunoreactive to the fused in sarcoma (FUS) protein (Neumann et al., 2009). Thus, the current classification of FTLD neuropathology has emerged in the last 5 years as (1) FTLD-tau, (2) FTLD-TDP, (3) FTLD-FUS, and several other rare proteinopathies. There is still a small portion of cases unaccounted for using this schema.

It is unclear why particular brain regions are vulnerable to tau or TDP-43 pathology in FTLD. Selectively vulnerable cell types—the holy grail of most neurodegenerative disease research—were unknown until very recently. In 2006, Seeley et al. reported the selective loss of a specific cell type found in the anterior cingulate and frontoinsular cortex of great apes, whales, and humans (Seeley et al., 2006), although a primitive homologue was recently reported in the macaque insula (Evrard, Forro, & Logothetis, 2012). This spindle-shaped neuron, the Von Economo cell, was reported by Seeley et al. to be reduced by more than 60% in these brain regions in seven FTLD patients but not in five AD patients. Remaining VEN neurons showed pathologic features in FTLD but appeared morphologically normal in AD. Further research on this and potentially other selectively vulnerable cell types in FTLD may reveal new insights into the devastation of these cortical regions in FTLD syndromes.

Genetics of Frontotemporal Lobar Degeneration

Early reports of families in which Pick's disease was observed in multiple generations (Groen & Endtz, 1982; Heston, 1978; Schenk, 1959) prompted genetic investigations (Foster et al., 1997). It is now estimated that approximately 20%–40% of cases of FTLD exhibit a family history of a similar or related condition, with many families exhibiting an autosomal dominant pattern (Neary, Snowden, & Mann, 2005). Linkage studies have identified loci on chromosomes 3, 9, and 17.

In 1998, mutations of intronic regions of the microtubule associated protein tau (*MAPT*) gene on chromosome 17q21 were first reported in FTLD in families in which patients also exhibited parkinsonism (Hutton et al., 1998; Poorkaj et al., 1998). More than 44 *MAPT* mutations have been reported in over 100 families in the world (Rademakers, Cruts, & van Broeckhoven, 2004). Since many of the initial cases of FTLD linked to *MAPT* mutations also had a parkinsonian syndrome, they were initially designated as FTD-parkinsonism, or FTDP-17. Further study of the phenotypes of patients with *MAPT* mutations has revealed clinical syndromes of classic bvFTD, PSP, CBD, or rarely PPA. It was clear from the early years of investigation that patients within the same family with the same genetic mutation may present with distinct clinical phenotypes, such as CBD or bvFTD (Bugiani et al., 1999). An example pedigree from a family with autosomal dominant MAPT-related FTD is shown in Figure 8.2.

However, *MAPT* mutations account for only 5%–20% of familial FTLD. There were a number of cases of familial FTLD with linkage to chromosome 17q21 but without *MAPT* gene mutations—importantly, none of these cases had tau pathology, but instead demonstrated what was originally described as DLDH or FTLD-U.

A key discovery took place in 2006 when investigators identified mutations in the

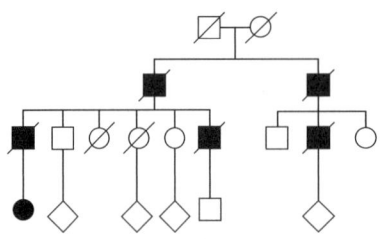

Figure 8.2 Pedigree of a family with autosomal dominant frontotemporal dementia (FTD) with all cases presenting with behavioral variant FTD with age of onset typically in the 60s. The genetic mutation identified in this family was *MAPT* P301L. The paternal progenitor presumably was a carrier but died in his 50s without symptoms.

progranulin (*GRN*) gene (Baker et al., 2006; Cruts et al., 2006), also on 17q21 and very close to the *MAPT* gene, as being associated with what is now known to be FTLD-TDP pathology (TDP-43 was discovered soon after the report of *GRN* mutations in FTLD). There are now more than 70 mutations known to occur, which are thought to result in a degraded protein whose function is lost ("loss of function"). The pathology associated with *GRN* mutations is TDP43-immunoreactive intranuclear inclusions with lentiform shape, localized primarily in cortex and striatum.

Together, *MAPT* and *GRN* mutations account for approximately 50%–60% of familial FTLD cases; mutations in other genes that have been discovered in association with FTLD, such as *CHMP2B* (Skibinski et al., 2005), are less common. In 2009, mutations in the *FUS* gene were discovered in amyotrophic lateral sclerosis (ALS; Kwiatkowski et al., 2009; Vance et al., 2009); nearly all FTLD-FUS cases examined to date do not appear to be associated with *FUS* mutations (Huey et al., 2011).

Another major discovery was made in the genetics of FTD in 2011. A number of families with members exhibiting FTD or ALS or both (FTD-ALS) had been reported with linkage to chromosome 9p, but the responsible gene remained mysterious until two groups reported an expanded GGGGCC hexanucleotide repeat in a noncoding region of the chromosome 9 open reading frame 72 gene (*C9ORF72*) (DeJesus-Hernandez et al., 2011; Renton et al., 2011). This important finding has catalyzed the FTD and ALS research communities, since the *C9ORF72* mutation appears to be the most common genetic cause of both conditions.

Detailed clinical and clinicopathologic studies have been undertaken of families in which FTLD is associated with particular genetic mutations. The key lessons learned to date underscore the fundamental heterogeneity of the FTLD umbrella. In two families with two different *GRN* mutations, similar underlying types of pathology were present but the topographic distribution of the pathology, and thereby the clinical phenotypes, were different (Snowden et al., 2006). In one family, the pathology was mostly in the left frontotemporal region, and the proband presented with progressive aphasia. In the other family, the pathology was distributed bilaterally and the phenotype was one of apathy and other behavioral disturbance, with less prominent language symptoms.

Yet even within the same family, the phenotype of FTLD associated with *GRN* mutations can be heterogeneous, as originally described by Bugiani et al. (1999) for a *MAPT* mutation. In one well-studied family (F337), the proband presented with aphasia and altered behavior with loss of insight. The proband's sister presented, however, with progressive aphasia with preserved comportment and insight. Other members of the family were reported to have prominent behavioral change without language symptoms. This family illustrates the spectrum of topographic distribution of pathology and behavioral phenotype within a family with the same genetic mutation associated with FTLD, suggestive of the influence of other contextual modifiers, possibly genetic or environmental.

The clinical phenotypes within families with *MAPT* mutations are also variable (Janssen et al., 2002; Rademakers et al., 2004). Patients differ in their degree of parkinsonism, and some have PSP or CBS signs. The presenting syndrome is often behavioral, commonly the overactive, disinhibited type. And families with the *C9ORF72* mutation are now the prototypical example of markedly different clinical phenotypes, with some patients exhibiting bvFTD, others with ALS, and others with FTD-ALS. The bvFTD phenotype associated with *C9ORF72* mutations is also different in that psychosis is much more prominent than in typical bvFTD; bizarre delusions are commonly a symptom very early in the course of the *C9ORF72* bvFTD phenotype (Boeve et al., 2012). PPA phenotypes appear to be uncommon in patients with this mutation. Thus, a growing research effort is being devoted to trying to understand genetic and other modifiers of these disease-associated mutations.

With regard to clinical practice of genetic testing in patients with FTD, we and other specialty groups follow an approach similar to that outlined in recent reviews (Fong, Karydas, & Goldman, 2012; Goldman et al., 2011; Quaid, 2011). First, we carefully obtain a family history ideally encompassing three generations, recording each blood relative's age of death, cause of death if known, and general cognitive/behavioral/neuropsychiatric status in later life. We acknowledge with the family that FTD and related conditions were often not diagnosed or may have been misdiagnosed in prior generations. Autopsy results from a family member provide critical information, but autopsies were not commonly obtained. If there is a potential family history of FTD or related disorders, we ask the family to try to obtain additional information or records about the affected relatives and to consider pursuing genetic testing after first meeting with our group's genetic counselor. If there is clearly not a family history of FTD or related disorders, and family members lived past typical age of onset, there is a low likelihood of the presence of a genetic mutation. If family history information is unavailable or blood relatives died at a younger age, we suggest that the patient/family work with our genetic counselor to discuss the issues involved. In a patient with an onset younger than 50, we and others often recommend that the patient/family consider genetic testing. A recent study presents a useful classification system for indicating the likelihood of a genetic mutation in a case of FTD (Wood et al., in press).

Clinical Characteristics of Frontotemporal Lobar Degeneration

The symptoms of these disorders are strongly related to the particular frontotemporal or frontostriatal brain regions that are affected. Symptoms referable to extrapyramidal, brainstem, and upper/lower motor neuron systems may be present because the pathology of any given case of FTLD may also involve these brain regions and systems. Nevertheless, although the clinical syndrome may include extrapyramidal symptoms, for example, the patient usually would not be mistaken for having Parkinson's disease because of the presence of prominent language and/or behavioral symptoms. Furthermore, the patient may not in fact have a phenotype best described as "parkinsonism" because the phenomenon is gait apraxia with axial rigidity, which would probably best be described more specifically as "PSP-like." These issues can be complicated, but it is important to recognize the wide range of clinical phenomena that can be caused by FTLD pathology.

For the purposes of diagnosis, it is essential to try to determine the earliest clinical symptoms that were initially present, which may or may not be the symptoms most troublesome to the patient and/or family at the time of presentation. Since many of the early symptoms are related to changes in affect or personality, it is not surprising that patients may first present to psychiatrists or other mental health professionals. In our initial visit with a new patient, we always interview and examine the patient independently from our interview of the informant(s). Although time consuming, this approach facilitates an open discussion of symptoms (informants may be uncomfortable discussing some issues in front of the patient) and enables the clinician to evaluate insight and concern in the patient separately from influence by informants. Lack of awareness or concern is often a core element of the clinical presentation in patients with bvFTD.

Behavioral Variant Frontotemporal Dementia

FTLD neuropathology is often associated with a clinical phenotype involving the insidious development of changes in interpersonal and emotional behavior, commonly accompanied by executive dysfunction. This clinical syndrome has traditionally been referred to as "Pick's disease," starting with descriptions by Arnold Pick followed by Onari and Spatz, Schneider, Goldstein, and a series of other early- to mid-20th-century investigators. Interest was resurrected by a number of groups later in the 20th century, but formal diagnostic criteria were not published until the

TABLE 8.1 Diagnostic Criteria for Behavioral Variant Frontotemporal Dementia

1. Evidence of Neurodegenerative Disease by Progressive Deterioration of Cognition or Behavior Based on Observation or History	
2. Possible Behavioral Variant Frontotemporal Dementia (bvFTD) (at least three of the following must be present early (<3 years) in the course)	
a. Behavioral disinhibition	Socially inappropriate behavior; loss of manners or decorum; impulsivity
b. Apathy or inertia	
c. Loss of sympathy or empathy	Diminished response to other people's needs and feelings; diminished social interest
d. Perseverative, stereotyped, or compulsive behavior	Simple repetitive movements; complex compulsive or ritualistic behavior; stereotypy of speech
e. Hyperorality and dietary changes	Altered food preferences; binge eating or increased consumption of alcohol or cigarettes; oral exploration of inedible objects
f. Neuropsychological profile of executive dysfunction with relative sparing of episodic memory and visuospatial skills	
3. Probable bvFTD	
a. Meets criteria for possible bvFTD	
b. Exhibits functional decline	
c. Imaging results consistent with bvFTD	Frontal and/or anterior temporal atrophy or hypometabolism or perfusion
4. bvFTD With Definite Frontotemporal Lobar Degeneration (FTLD) Pathology	
a. Meets criteria for possible or probable bvFTD	
b. Histopathological evidence of FTLD on biopsy or autopsy	
c. Presence of a known pathogenic mutation	
5. Exclusionary criteria for bvFTD	
a. Pattern of deficits is better accounted for by another neuromedical disorder	
b. Behavioral disturbance is better accounted for by a psychiatric disorder	
c. Biomarkers strongly indicative of Alzheimer's disease or another neurodegenerative process	

Source: Adapted with permission from Rascovsky et al., Brain 2011

Lund-Manchester criteria in 1994 (Brun et al., 1994), and then revised by an international consensus group in 1998 (Neary et al., 1998).

Based on a variety of concerns regarding prior criteria (Rascovsky et al., 2007), new international consensus diagnostic criteria were published in 2011 (Rascovsky et al., 2011) and are summarized in Table 8.1. BvFTD appears to be the most common variant of FTLD. The specific symptoms of this variant depend on the particular regions of frontotemporal cortical and frontostriatal brain systems that are involved and their laterality.

Disinhibition is a common early symptom, and it can manifest as socially inappropriate behavior such as overly familiar interactions with strangers; loss of manners or violations of social normative behavior such as public urination or changes in behavior during social meals; or impulsive actions such as unnecessary or excessive purchasing or shoplifting (Miller et al., 1991; Miller, Darby, Benson, Cummings, & Miller, 1997; Snowden et al., 2001). Sometimes patients who are very active, jocular, and make rash decisions or go on spending sprees can be mistakenly diagnosed with mania or hypomania. Disinhibition appears to be related particularly to orbitofrontal and cingulo-opercular abnormalities in FTD (O'Callaghan, Hodges, & Hornberger, 2013).

Another very common early symptom is apathy, including loss of interest in hobbies or leisure activities and social withdrawal (Chow et al., 2009; Massimo et al., 2009; Shinagawa, Ikeda, Fukuhara, & Tanabe, 2006); these behavioral changes are often mistaken for depression. Yet patients with bvFTD do not usually exhibit sadness or cry; do not talk about concerns, worries, or thoughts of worthlessness or hopelessness; and do not usually exhibit the loss of appetite or sleep disturbance often seen in depression. Some investigators have suggested that bvFTD may present as a "disinhibited" or "inert" (apathetic) subtype (Snowden et al., 2001), while many patients present with intermixed symptoms of both types (Le Ber et al., 2006). Atrophy in the anterior cingulate cortex, dorsolateral prefrontal cortex (Massimo et al., 2009), and striatum (Rosen et al., 2005) has been observed in association with apathy in bvFTD.

Loss of empathy or sympathy toward the spouse, other family members, and friends is very common and can be subtle in some cases, depending in part on premorbid personality traits (Lough et al., 2006; Mendez & Perryman, 2003; Rankin, Kramer, & Miller, 2005). These behavioral changes may concern family members for some time before it becomes obvious that something is wrong, which often occurs when the patient exhibits a highly unusual response to an event that almost universally provokes a vigorous, uniform emotion in most people, such as the death of a close friend or family member or the birth of a child. Even under these circumstances, the behavior is commonly attributed to depression or another psychiatric illness or to stress or a midlife crisis. Right anterior temporal cortex, anterior insula, and striatal abnormalities have been most consistently identified as related to loss of empathy (Perry et al., 2001; Rankin et al., 2006).

Compulsive, ritualistic, or repetitive behaviors are common in bvFTD, often early in the illness, and can be very distressing to family members (Ames, Cummings, Wirshing, Quinn, & Mahler, 1994; Nyatsanza et al., 2003). In some cases, they may be the presenting symptom (Mendez, Perryman, Miller, Swartz, & Cummings, 1997). Examples of these symptoms include repetitive "projects" (e.g., stereotyped writing of greeting cards), chores (e.g., repeated emptying of trash), or playing of card or computer games or repetitive watching of a particular television show (Bozeat, Gregory, Ralph, & Hodges, 2000). Speech patterns may be stereotyped (e.g., catch phrases, telling of stories as if by a script). Some of these symptoms appear similar to those of obsessive-compulsive disorder (OCD) but usually bvFTD patients do not describe obsessive thoughts or any relief of such thoughts by a compulsive activity, as is typically described in primary OCD. Some patients have very rigid routines that must be performed identically each day (often at a particular time, associated with "clock watching"); if these routines are disrupted, some patients become very upset. These symptoms may change as the disease progresses, in some cases becoming simpler. Simple repetitive behaviors include tapping or moving a limb, licking lips, picking skin, grunting, or moaning. These may appear similar to choreiform movements seen in dyskinetic movement disorders or tardive dyskinesia. Anatomic abnormalities associated with compulsive behaviors include striatal and anterior temporal atrophy (Josephs, Whitwell, & Jack, 2007; Perry et al., 2012; Rosso et al., 2001).

Changes in eating behavior are common and may include altered food preferences (such as an increased sweet tooth or a rigid stereotypy in the foods eaten from day to day) or gluttonous or binge-like eating (Bozeat et al., 2000; Miller, Darby, Swartz, Yener, & Mena, 1995). This may—but does not always—result in substantial weight gain. Normative social eating conventions are often violated, including rapid eating or stuffing food in the mouth, taking food from others' plates, or belching. Patients may exhibit changes in the consumption of alcohol or cigarettes, sometimes resulting in extreme intoxication or vomiting. Occasionally early, but more often later, in the course of the disease patients may explore inedible objects by placing them in their mouth, similar to the behavior seen in Kluver Bucy syndrome. The neurobiologic basis of changes in eating behavior in FTD has received little investigation, but it appears to involve right lateralized ventral anterior insula, striatum, and orbitofrontal cortex on structural magnetic resonance imaging (MRI) voxel-based morphometry (Whitwell et al., 2007; Woolley et al., 2007), as well as hypothalamus (Piguet, Petersen, et al., 2011).

Executive dysfunction (problems with organization, planning, sequencing, decision making, multitasking, or monitoring performance) is very common in bvFTD (Bozeat et al., 2000). Symptoms described by family members often include difficulty with financial management, poor decision making, inability to complete tasks (particularly novel tasks), or not recognizing or correcting mistakes. Despite the report of these symptoms in daily life, patients may still perform within normal limits on neuropsychological tests of executive function (Gregory & Hodges, 1996). Progressive loss of executive abilities may lead to job loss or disastrous mismanagement of money. In many cases, it can be difficult to determine which problems in daily life are caused by executive dysfunction as opposed to apathy. This is not surprising given that constructs of the executive functions usually include initiation or "energization" as a component process (see Chapter 3). Although executive dysfunction is typically thought of as being caused by dorsolateral prefrontal cortical involvement, as also discussed in Chapters 2 and 3, it can originate in anterior cingulate, insular, parietal, or subcortical nodes of large-scale executive systems.

Another important clinical feature of bvFTD is lack of insight. This symptom was considered a core element of the Neary et al. (1998) diagnostic criteria but was not included in the new international consensus diagnostic criteria because it was thought to be too difficult to ascertain consistently. Nevertheless, it is well established that many patients with bvFTD, and some patients with semantic dementia, have a striking lack of insight (Banks & Weintraub, 2008; Eslinger et al., 2005; Williamson et al., 2009) even when confronted with obvious impairments. Clinically, this can be particularly challenging when the patient refuses to make office follow-up visits because he or she is convinced there is not a problem. Lack of insight in FTD has been associated with right-lateralized ventromedial prefrontal atrophy (Rosen et al., 2010).

Another core feature of bvFTD is personality change. Alterations in personality can be prominent in bvFTD and also in semantic dementia (Rankin, Baldwin, Pace-Savitsky, Kramer, & Miller, 2005). Although questionnaire-based instruments to assess classical dimensional personality traits are readily available, changes in personality might be best understood clinically by considering more specific process-oriented functions contributing to personality traits. When faced with a family member who says, "My spouse is not the person I married, his/her personality is completely different," it is incumbent upon the clinician to probe further to ascertain the specific changes being described. Some symptoms may include changes in the expression or comprehension of emotion, social withdrawal or disinhibition, or loss of empathy. In some cases a previously gruff or aggressive individual becomes docile. The patient's insight into these changes is often poor. Other symptoms that may also be described as personality changes include obsessive-compulsive behaviors, such as hoarding, and those involving changes in appetitive drives, such as sexual, eating, or drinking behaviors.

Despite the inclusion in the new bvFTD diagnostic criteria of "the relative preservation of memory," memory impairment can be a prominent early feature in some cases of bvFTD (Hornberger, Piguet, Graham, Nestor, & Hodges, 2010; Pennington, Hodges, & Hornberger, 2011), including those that are pathologically proven (Graham et al., 2005). In some cases, memory symptoms are reported by the patient and/or family, but test performance is normal; this may reflect executive contributions to memory encoding or retrieval in daily life, which may be relatively controlled in the office setting (Pasquier, Grymonprez, Lebert, & Van der Linden, 2001). In other cases, day-to-day memory is preserved but psychometric test performance is impaired due to the magnitude of executive or semantic deficits, thereby resulting in an overestimation of memory impairment. In our clinical practice, we do not avoid the clinical diagnosis of bvFTD in a patient with well-documented amnesia if the remainder of the clinical presentation is consistent with bvFTD, especially if supported by neuroimaging test results.

Unlike the language-dominant types of FTLD, language may be relatively intact early in the course of bvFTD. This is particularly true on basic neuropsychological tests of language performance. Higher level language abilities at the level of discourse (Ash et al., 2006), as well as emotionally laden forms of communication, including prosody, irony, sarcasm, and humor, are often abnormal early in the course of bvFTD (Kipps, Nestor, Acosta-Cabronero, Arnold, & Hodges, 2009; Perry et al., 2001). As the disease progresses, semantic and other impairments often become prominent.

Psychosis has been thought unusual in bvFTD, but the discovery of the *C9ORF72* expansion has highlighted the common presence of psychosis in patients as well as nondemented family members with this genetic mutation (Boeve et al., 2012).

Progressive Aphasic Subtypes of Frontotemporal Lobar Degeneration

The other major clinical phenotype of FTLD involves a primary language disturbance. If a patient presents with an isolated, gradually progressive aphasia, he or she would be diagnosed by many specialists with primary progressive aphasia (PPA), as described in detail in Chapter 9. (Readers are referred to Chapter 9 for a detailed review of PPA; a few comments on points not made in that chapter will be made here.)

As originally suggested by Neary et al. (1998), such a patient would have been diagnosed as having a language-predominant form of FTD or FTLD, and further subtyped into progressive nonfluent aphasia (PNFA) or semantic dementia (SD). At present, the approach suggested by the recent international consensus diagnostic criteria for PPA (Gorno-Tempini et al., 2011) focuses on determining the precise clinical phenotype without reference to the presumed underlying pathology. Three clinical phenotypes are currently recognized: the agrammatic variant of PPA (PPA-g, which likely captures most of the patients formerly diagnosed with PNFA), the semantic variant of PPA (PPA-s, which likely captures most of the patients formerly diagnosed with SD), and the logopenic variant of PPA. The logopenic variant of PPA (PPA-l) is most frequently associated with biomarkers of underlying AD, and thus it would not be considered a major clinical subtype of FTLD. Nevertheless, a minority of PPA-l patients do not demonstrate biomarkers of AD pathobiology in vivo (Leyton et al., 2011) and in fact have FTLD neuropathology *postmortem* (usually FTLD-TDP) (Mesulam et al., 2008). Thus, while PPA-l is often considered nearly synonymous with an atypical language variant of AD, these recent observations support the inclusion of this clinical phenotype as a part—if small—of the FTLD spectrum.

Although patients with progressive aphasias may have personality, comportmental, and social symptoms, they are by definition less prominent than the language impairment early in the course of the disorder. The presence of prominent early neuropsychiatric or behavioral symptoms is generally considered exclusionary for PPA. Despite this distinction, which is particularly important for clinical research on these disorders, some patients whose diagnosis would be best considered as PPA have prominent early neuropsychiatric or behavioral symptoms (a point discussed briefly in the new diagnostic criteria). Many others have relatively mild but notable symptoms in these domains, particularly as PPA progresses to involve abilities beyond language (Modirrousta, Price, & Dickerson, 2013).

With regard to the PPA subtypes, the literature suggests that semantic variant PPA (PPA-s) patients commonly exhibit neuropsychiatric symptoms, often relatively early and in a fairly stereotypical fashion. Many of these symptoms are similar to those of bvFTD, including loss of empathy, changes in eating behavior, compulsive behavior, and disinhibition. Although these symptoms are highly consistent with FTD, depending on when they begin and how they are reported by informants, it may be difficult for the clinician to be confident in assigning a subtype diagnosis (i.e., bvFTD vs. PPA-s vs. SD). In fact, in the Neary et al. diagnostic criteria for FTD, features considered supportive of a diagnosis of SD included loss of sympathy or empathy and narrowed preoccupations (mental rigidity) (Neary et al., 1998). Aberrant motor behavior is also reported as common in some studies; in our experience this often includes elaborate kinds of movements related to repetitive or compulsive behaviors, although there has been little focused study of this topic. Depression is also reported as common in PPA-s in some studies; in our experience, however, at least some patients say certain phrases repetitively (i.e., "catch phrases") that appear to express negative emotion (e.g., "I feel so stupid," "I used to know that and now I just don't know anything"), but with minimal affective behavior consistent with depression, and a structured interview with some of these patients' caregivers reveals little behavior in daily life that appears consistent with a diagnosis of depression.

In PPA-g, neuropsychiatric symptoms are less frequent initially, but as the illness progresses it becomes increasingly common to see apathy, depression, or irritability. In some cases these symptoms are present early in the illness, which may lead to misdiagnosis as a primary psychiatric disorder (often depression).

In PPA-l, neuropsychiatric symptoms are relatively infrequent early but increase as the illness progresses and include agitation, anxiety, irritability, and apathy. In many cases we have seen, the clinical phenomenology of neuropsychiatric symptoms appears similar to that seen in AD.

Diagnostic Assessment of Suspected Frontotemporal Lobar Degeneration

As with all neurodegenerative diseases, a careful clinical history taken from the patient and a knowledgeable informant is usually the single most important element of assessment. Specific FTLD symptom inventories (Bozeat et al., 2000; Snowden et al., 2001), the Frontal Behavioral Inventory (Kertesz, Davidson, & Fox, 1997), and the Neuropsychiatric Inventory (NPI) (Cummings, 1997) are very useful in ascertaining symptoms of FTLD in a structured manner. Some of these instruments can be given to caregivers in advance as questionnaires or used to structure an office-based interview. We have developed structured interviews targeting social and language symptoms in FTLD (Bickart et al., 2014; Sapolsky et al., 2010). As mentioned previously, we believe it is essential to interview the patient separately from informants. The interview with the patient should include a psychiatric interview evaluating mood and affect, thought content (i.e., Is there evidence of psychosis?), and insight.

In the initial office assessment of a patient with suspected FTLD, a basic cognitive examination is essential. Most commonly used cognitive screening instruments, such as the Mini Mental State Examination, are insensitive to the cognitive and behavioral deficits of FTLD, as described in detail in Chapter 19. Office-based general cognitive testing instruments thought to be more sensitive to FTLD include the Montreal Cognitive Assessment (MOCA) and Addenbrooke's Cognitive Examination (ACE) (Mathuranath, Nestor, Berrios, Rakowicz, & Hodges, 2000). The Frontal Assessment Battery (Dubois, Slachevsky, Litvan, & Pillon, 2000) is a brief (~10 minutes) cognitive and psychomotor assessment that has demonstrated sensitivity to FTLD. Although these tests will often identify deficits in patients with FTD, some patients perform normally early in the course of the disease.

Finally, a neurologic examination is essential, working especially to determine whether there are abnormalities in eye movements or gait, limb or buccofacial apraxia, extrapyramidal signs, primitive reflexes, or evidence of motor neuron disease. Impersistence and distractibility can present challenges during the neurologic exam.

Neuropsychological assessment can be invaluable in patients suspected of having FTLD-spectrum disorders. Although some patients may perform adequately on brief office-based cognitive testing typically performed by a neurologist, psychiatrist, geriatrician, or other physician, the neuropsychologist may be able to detect abnormalities on extended testing. In at least some very mild cases, however, reasonably extensive neuropsychological assessment can be normal (Gregory, Serra-Mestres, & Hodges, 1999). Aiming to assemble a neuropsychological test battery tailored to bvFTD, Torralva, Manes, and colleagues compiled a set of previously developed tests emphasizing "real-life" elements of executive function as well as social cognition (Torralva, Roca, Gleichgerrcht, Bekinschtein, & Manes, 2009). This test battery demonstrated higher sensitivity to mild FTD than many standard tests included in typical dementia neuropsychological batteries. Another similar approach was taken by Funkiewiez, Dubois, and colleagues, who assembled the Social cognition and Emotion Assessment (SEA), and ultimately found that a subset (facial emotion recognition and faux pas) of the original tests were most sensitive to bvFTD, deriving the mini-SEA (Funkiewiez et al., 2012), as described in more detail in Chapter 3.

The combination of findings from the assessments described previously can be used to determine whether a patient fulfills current diagnostic criteria (Rascovsky et al., 2011) for "possible" bvFTD or one of the progressive aphasias. For bvFTD, the clinician's confidence can be formally elevated to "probable" bvFTD if neuroimaging findings are present as described next. A similar approach is taken by many clinicians in diagnosing PPA, although the criteria do not specify these levels of confidence formally (Gorno-Tempini et al., 2011).

Neuroimaging and Other Diagnostic Tests

Neuroimaging is an important part of the diagnostic workup of FTLD, and it has made valuable contributions to our understanding of the specific subtype disorders. Both structural (MRI) and functional (positron emission tomography [PET], single-photon emission computed tomography [SPECT]) neuroimaging may be valuable for the investigation of anatomic, metabolic, or perfusion abnormalities in FTLD. See Chapter 22 for more details about these techniques and data interpretation.

MRI is critical in the diagnostic workup of suspected FTLD for both the exclusion of other potential causes of slowly progressive frontal lobe syndromes, such as tumors, cerebrovascular disease, or the newly identified "sagging brain syndrome" (see Chapter 15) and for the identification of abnormalities consistent with FTLD neurodegenerative syndromes. Frontal and/or anterior temporal atrophy is the typical finding, and it is often more prominent in the right hemisphere in bvFTD and the left hemisphere in PPA (Fig. 8.3A). Metabolic or perfusion imaging can be useful in addition to MRI for the identification of abnormalities when anatomic changes are subtle or undetectable (Fig. 8.3B). In some cases, both structural and functional neuroimaging may be normal early in the course of what ultimately declares itself over time as FTD (Gregory et al., 1999). Electroencephalography is not commonly recommended in the diagnostic evaluation of suspected FTD, but it may demonstrate anterior or focal slowing consistent with frontal neurodegeneration.

Cerebrospinal fluid (CSF) biomarkers are being investigated in FTLD (Hu et al., 2011), but they are not yet mature enough for use in clinical practice. In some cases, the exclusion of an atypical form of AD can be helpful by analyzing CSF for amyloid-β and tau (see Chapter 22). General CSF investigation may be valuable to rule out other neurologic disorders if the patient has atypical features or a more rapid course (see Chapter 15).

If clinical evidence of motor neuron disease is present, especially if it is subtle, electromyography can provide valuable information regarding the presence of upper or lower

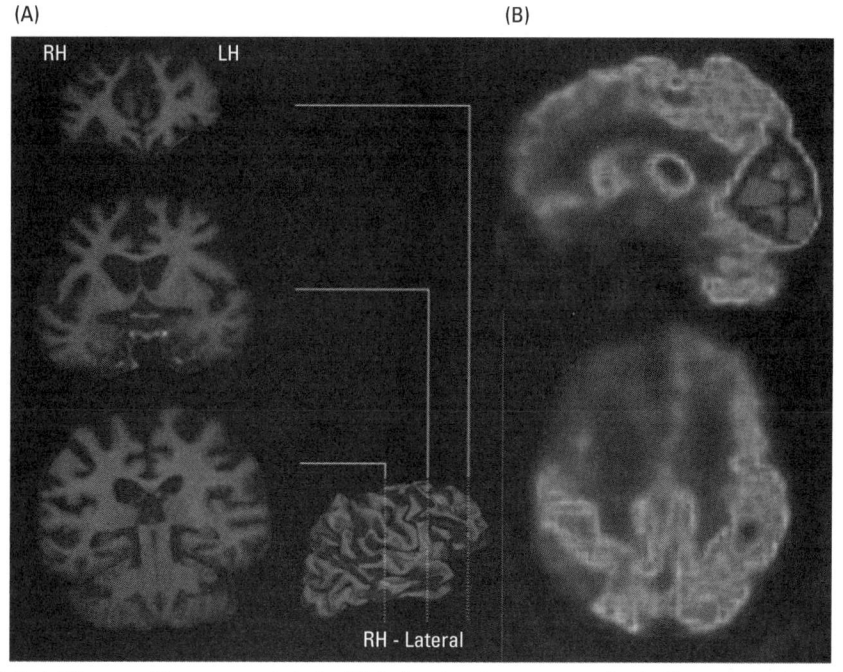

Figure 8.3 A 58-year-old man presented with behavioral symptoms (including apathy, impulsive eating) and executive dysfunction. (A) Magnetic resonance imaging (MRI) demonstrated bilateral (right greater than left) frontal, temporal, and parietal atrophy, quantified with a map of cortical thickness compared to controls. (B) Fludeoxyglucose positron emission tomography (FDG-PET) showed prominent bilateral (right greater than left) frontal and temporal hypometabolism. This man was found to have a Q300X (premature termination) mutation in *GRN*. He exhibited a 5-year clinical course from first symptoms to death. Postmortem examination revealed the expected TDP-43 pathology. (See color plate section)

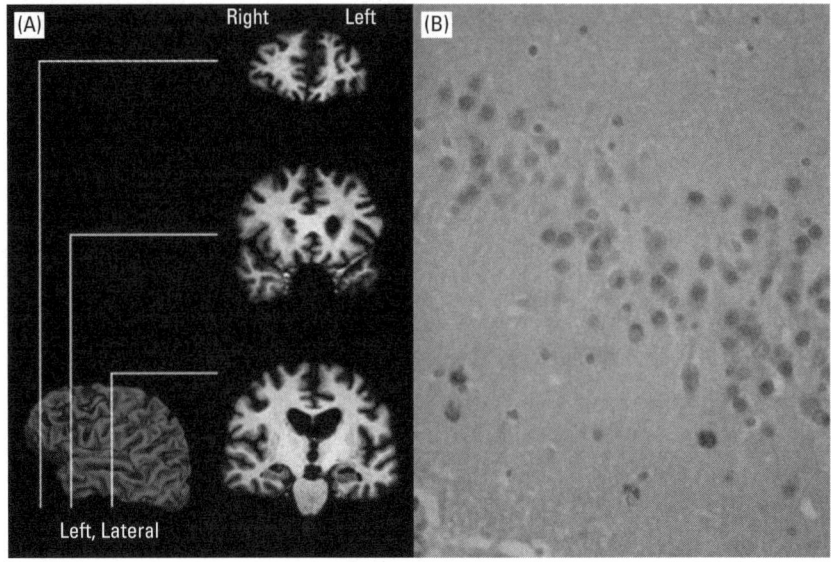

Figure 8.4 A 59-year-old man presented with behavioral symptoms (including loss of empathy, aggression, lack of insight), executive dysfunction, and word-finding difficulties. Shortly thereafter he developed dysarthria and dysphagia and was found to have clinical evidence of motor neuron disease with bulbar predominance (tongue weakness, fasciculations, lip weakness, as well as mild shoulder weakness and fasciculations with lower extremity hyperreflexia and extensor plantar responses). Electromyography showed sharp waves, fibrillation potentials, and fasciculation potentials in cervical, thoracic, and lumbar myotomes with long-duration, high-amplitude polyphasic potentials with reduced recruitment and rapid firing. (A) Magnetic resonance imaging (MRI) demonstrated bilateral (left greater than right) frontal atrophy, quantified with a map of cortical thickness compared to controls. He exhibited a 3.5-year clinical course from first symptoms to death. (B) Postmortem examination revealed the expected TDP-43 pathology (TDP-43 immunohistochemistry of dentate gyrus of hippocampus). (See color plate section)

motor neuron dysfunction, which may be critical for prognosis (Fig. 8.4).

In Vivo Neuroimaging of Neuropathologic Markers

With the advent of neuroimaging tracers that bind to specific pathologic molecules, such as Pittsburgh compound B (PiB) (Klunk et al., 2004) or the growing number of putative tau ligands (Chien et al., 2013; Fodero-Tavoletti et al., 2011; Maruyama et al., 2013; Small et al., 2006), it is possible to investigate clinicopathologic relationships in vivo. Extensive efforts are under way to develop tracers specific for additional pathologic markers. This will surely lead to a revolution in our understanding of the spectrum of frontotemporal dementias. In the first study of FTLD with PiB, a comparison was made between PiB tracer uptake in twelve FTLD cases, seven AD cases, and eight controls. The FTLD cases included five patients with behavioral FTD, two with FTD/ALS, four with semantic dementia, and one with progressive aphasia. The results indicated that all AD patients had "positive" PiB PET scans, seven out of eight controls had negative PiB scans, and eight of twelve FTLD cases had negative PiB PET scans.

Although this initially seemed to be a high number of amyloid-positive FTLD cases, it may not be particularly surprising in light of several autopsy studies showing the presence of AD pathology in 20%–30% of FTLD cases, with or without the presence of additional FTLD-type pathology (Davies et al., 2005; Forman et al., 2006; Kertesz, McMonagle, Blair, Davidson, & Munoz, 2005; Knibb, Xuereb, Patterson, & Hodges, 2006). The distribution of PiB tracer uptake in these four cases was similar to that typically seen in AD. Two of the cases carried clinical diagnoses of behavioral FTD, and the other two were clinically diagnosed with semantic dementia. Of note, however, some elements of the cognitive profiles and the fludeoxyglucose positron emission tomography (FDG-PET) metabolic deficits of these four cases showed features more often associated with AD than FTLD. Of the two FTLD patients who have come to autopsy in this series, one had a tauopathy and one had a ubiquitinopathy; both were PiB negative.

Subsequent to this initial study, Rabinovici and colleagues have performed further investigation of the utility of amyloid imaging in PPA and FTLD. A series of PPA patients produced results that were consistent with expectations from pathologic series, with elevated cortical PiB binding in one out of six cases of agrammatic/nonfluent PPA, one out of five cases of semantic PPA, and four out of four cases of logopenic PPA (Rabinovici et al., 2008). In a comparison of amyloid PET versus FDG-PET imaging in the differential diagnosis of AD versus FTLD, PiB and FDG showed similar overall accuracy in discriminating AD and FTLD, but PiB was more sensitive to AD when interpreted qualitatively or quantitatively. FDG was more specific, but only when scans were classified quantitatively. PiB slightly outperformed FDG in the small subset of patients with known histopathology (Rabinovici et al., 2012) (see Chapter 22 for further discussion).

Clinical Course of Frontotemporal Dementia

The early symptoms help determine the major subtypes of FTLD, but as the disease progresses, involvement of other frontotemporal and subcortical brain regions often result in the development of symptoms characteristic of the other subtypes of FTLD (Seeley et al., 2005). For example, patients with PPA-semantic variant may develop disinhibition, compulsivity, and other behavioral symptoms, while bvFTD patients may develop speech, language and/or semantic deficits.

Overall, survival after diagnosis is typically 6–10 years, with bvFTD patients having the shortest mean survival at 3.4 years, PPA survival at 4.5 years, and PPA-semantic variant patients having the longest survival (Grasbeck, Englund, Horstmann, Passant, & Gustafson, 2003). A more recent study suggests a slightly better prognosis for bvFTD patients, with a median survival of 4.2 years from diagnosis (Garcin et al., 2009). The development of early motor symptoms or signs is a poor prognostic feature in all forms of FTD (Hu et al., 2009), as is early language impairment in bvFTD (Garcin et al., 2009). Recent data suggest that semantic dementia patients may commonly have a very slow progression, with 50% of patients alive at 12.8 years after diagnosis in a large cohort of 100 patients (Hodges et al., 2010). The ultimate development of markers of the specific form of neuropathology may be important for prognostication, with one autopsy study of 71 patients indicating that tau pathology was associated with shorter (3 years) survival than non-tau forms of FTLD pathology (8 years) (Xie et al., 2008).

In our practice, we always discuss the value of autopsy with family members and with patients if possible. Despite continued improvements in the use of clinical and biomarker data for probabilistic prediction of FTLD or non-FTLD pathology, every specialized center continues to observe surprising cases (Figs. 8.5 and 8.6). Not only is this information important for providing family members with the greatest detail possible about the patient's disease, it also contributes in extremely valuable ways to ongoing research efforts.

Treatment of Frontotemporal Lobar Degeneration

Once a diagnosis of one of the forms of FTD is made, the clinician unfortunately needs to deliver the news that, at present, there are no disease-modifying therapies for FTD (as is the case for all other major neurodegenerative diseases). Nevertheless, despite the fact that we are not yet able to reverse or slow the progression of FTD and related disorders, these diseases are treatable, as discussed in detail in other chapters in this volume. Treatment includes empiric pharmacologic management of symptoms, nonpharmacologic management of symptoms, management of comorbid conditions that may exacerbate cognitive-behavioral impairment, psychosocial support, and education of the family and in some cases the patient as well

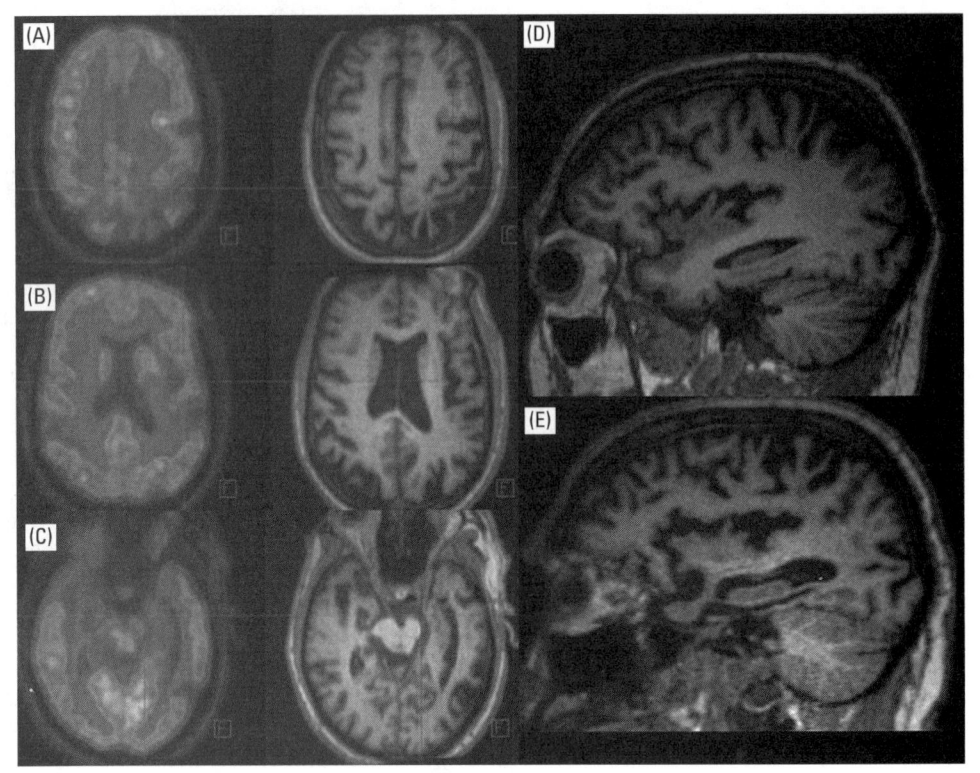

Figure 8.5 A 50-year-old man presented with unilateral dominant hand apraxia and depression without rigidity, alien hand syndrome, or eye movement abnormalities, followed shortly by executive dysfunction, word-finding difficulty, and memory loss. The initial neuroimaging examination revealed markedly asymmetric dominant hemisphere fludeoxyglucose positron emission tomography (FDG-PET) hypometabolism (A, B, C, left column) and atrophy (A, B, C, right column) extending from perirolandic and dorsal parietal cortex (A) into perisylvian cortex (B) and ventral temporal cortex (C) with relative preservation of frontal cortex and striatum. His symptoms progressed to include marked upper extremity apraxia with the eventual development of rigidity, aphasia, dysarthria, episodic and semantic memory impairment, compulsive behavior, impulsive eating, and agitation. Along with the progression of symptoms, atrophy progressed from (D) parietal and posterolateral temporal over a 4-year interval to include (E) ventral and anterior temporal, insular, and posterior frontal cortex. (See color plate section)

(Cardarelli, Kertesz, & Knebl, 2010). A multidisciplinary team of specialists is invaluable in caring for patients and families suffering from FTD (Wylie, Shnall, Onyike, & Huey, 2013). Pharmacologic and nonpharmacologic management depends on the identification and grading of severity of specific symptoms (including cognitive, behavioral, and motor symptoms), followed by their prioritization and monitoring over time. Once this is done, judicious empiric use of medications can be tackled. At present, no medications are approved for the symptomatic treatment of FTD, but many medications have demonstrated utility in small studies or case series (Jicha & Nelson, 2011; Manoochehri & Huey, 2012; Piguet, Hornberger, Mioshi, & Hodges, 2011). For example, selective serotonin reuptake inhibitors or other antidepressants can modulate disinhibition or compulsive behavior, stimulants or pro-dopaminergic agents can sometimes reduce apathy or attentional impairment, and anticonvulsants/mood stabilizers or antipsychotic compounds can ameliorate aggression or agitation. Yet side effects of these medications may in some cases outweigh benefits and always need close monitoring.

Nonpharmacologic symptom management strategies generally require the expertise of

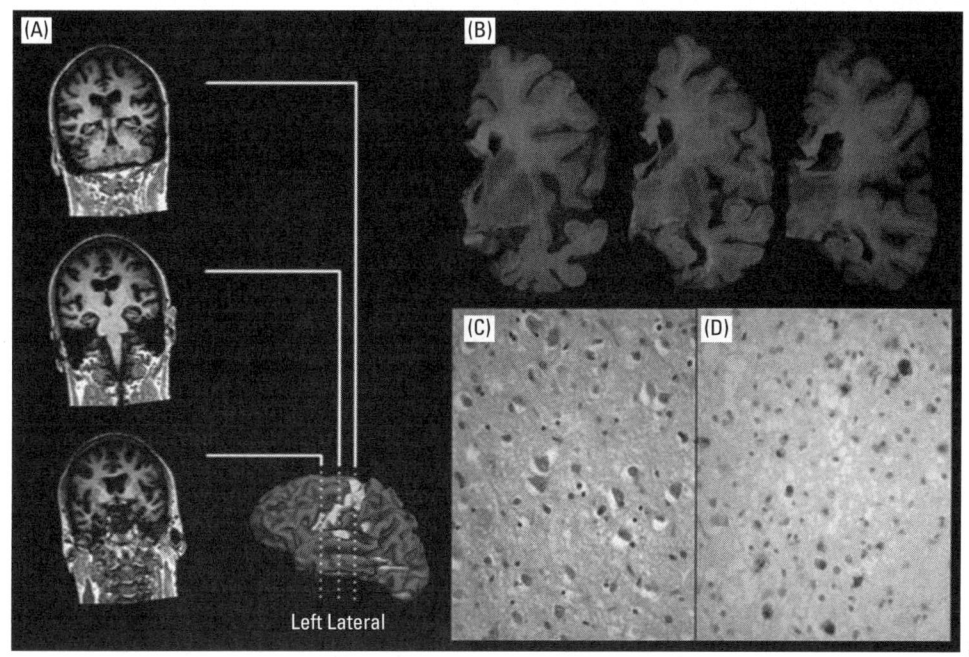

Figure 8.6 The 50-year-old man described in Figure 8.5 exhibited an 8-year clinical course from first symptoms to death. Despite (A) the clear magnetic resonance imaging (MRI) evidence of initial perirolandic and parietotemporal atrophy (left greater than right), quantified with a map of cortical thickness compared to controls with (B) postmortem support for these gross findings, histological examination revealed (C) Pick bodies and (D) tau immunoreactive pathology consistent with pathological Pick's disease. (See color plate section)

an experienced specialist clinician or team (Gitlin, Kales, & Lyketsos, 2012; Shnall et al., 2013). These include speech and language therapy for communication or swallowing issues, occupational therapy for problems with hand-eye coordination or planning that impacts instrumental or basic activities of daily living, physical therapy for gait disorders, and in some cases psychotherapy (for patient or family). A driving assessment is critical, as is determination of financial or health care competency. Social work assistance with facilitating disability compensation can be very helpful. Paid or volunteer companions or home health aides to help patients remain active yet safe can be invaluable. Day programs or respite residential programs may play important roles at some point in the course of the illness. Ultimately, because the myriad of resources that may be helpful to patients and family members can be difficult to identify, it is essential to dedicate time and effort toward specialized education for the patient/family through the clinician or multidisciplinary team or the Association for FTD (http://www.theaftd.org/) or Alzheimer's Association (http://www.alz.org). Psychosocial support resources can also be valuable for nearly all families and for some patients. The development of close links between the FTD specialty care team and the primary care physician is very important to assist in general management, including monitoring comorbid conditions and considering the role of standard prophylactic care in the context of FTD.

Finally, it is critical late in the course of the illness to assist patients and families with end-of-life care, facilitating access to palliative care resources and ideally obtaining nursing home and hospice care at the appropriate time. There continues to be a desperate need for residential or nursing facilities that have the capacity and skill to care for patients with FTD. And although research at present focuses largely on understanding the disease and offers little if any novel putative treatment options for patients with FTD, participation can provide some meaning in an otherwise entirely tragic situation.

Ultimately, the quality of the partnership between care providers experienced with FTD and patients/families with these diseases is a critical factor that influences the experience of living with FTD.

References

Alzheimer, A. (1911). Über eigenartige Krankheitsfälle der späteren Alters. *Zeitschrift für die gesamte Neurologie und Psychiatrie, 4*, 356–385.

Ames, D., Cummings, J. L., Wirshing, W. C., Quinn, B., & Mahler, M. (1994). Repetitive and compulsive behavior in frontal lobe degenerations. *Journal of Neuropsychiatry and Clinical Neuroscience, 6*, 100–113.

Ash, S., Moore, P., Antani, S., McCawley, G., Work, M., & Grossman, M. (2006). Trying to tell a tale: Discourse impairments in progressive aphasia and frontotemporal dementia. *Neurology, 66*, 1405–1413.

Baker, M., Mackenzie, I. R., Pickering-Brown, S. M., Gass, J., Rademakers, R., Lindholm, C.,...Hutton, M. (2006). Mutations in progranulin cause tau-negative frontotemporal dementia linked to chromosome 17. *Nature, 442*, 916–919.

Banks, S., & Weintraub, S. (2008). Self-awareness and self-monitoring of cognitive and behavioral deficits in behavioral variant frontotemporal dementia, primary progressive aphasia and probable Alzheimer's disease. *Brain and Cognition, 67*, 58–68.

Bernardi, L., Frangipane, F., Smirne, N., Colao, R., Puccio, G., Curcio, S. A.,...Bruni, A. C. (2012). Epidemiology and genetics of frontotemporal dementia: A door-to-door survey in southern Italy. *Neurobiology of Aging, 33*, 2948.e1–2948.e10.

Berrios, G. E., & Girling, D. M. (1994). Introduction: Pick's disease and the "frontal lobe" dementias. *History of Psychiatry, 5*, 539–547.

Bickart, K. C., Brickhouse, M., Negreira, A., Sapolsky, D., Feldman Barrett, L., & Dickerson, B. C. (2014) Atrophy in distinct corticolimbic networks predicts social impairments in frontotemporal dementia. *Journal of Neurology, Neurosurgery, and Psychiatry, 85*(4), 438–448.

Binns, J. K., & Robertson, E. E. (1962). Pick's disease in old age. *Journal of Mental Science, 108*, 804–810.

Boeve, B. F., Boylan, K. B., Graff-Radford, N. R., DeJesus-Hernandez, M., Knopman, D. S., Pedraza, O.,...Rademakers, R. (2012). Characterization of frontotemporal dementia and/or amyotrophic lateral sclerosis associated with the GGGGCC repeat expansion in C9ORF72. *Brain, 135*, 765–783.

Borroni, B., Alberici, A., Grassi, M., Turla, M., Zanetti, O., Bianchetti, A.,...Padovani, A. (2010). Is frontotemporal lobar degeneration a rare disorder? Evidence from a preliminary study in Brescia county, Italy. *Journal of Alzheimers Disease, 19*, 111–116.

Bozeat, S., Gregory, C. A., Ralph, M. A., & Hodges, J. R. (2000). Which neuropsychiatric and behavioural features distinguish frontal and temporal variants of frontotemporal dementia from Alzheimer's disease? *Journal of Neurology, Neurosurgery and Psychiatry, 69*, 178–186.

Brun, A., Englund, E., Gustafson, L., Passant, U., Mann, D., Neary, D., & Snowden, J. S. (1994). Clinical and neuropathological criteria for frontotemporal dementia. The Lund and Manchester Groups. *Journal of Neurology, Neurosurgery and Psychiatry, 57*, 416–418.

Bugiani, O., Murrell, J. R., Giaccone, G., Hasegawa, M., Ghigo, G., Tabaton, M.,...Ghetti, B. (1999). Frontotemporal dementia and corticobasal degeneration in a family with a P301S mutation in tau. *Journal of Neuropathology and Experimental Neurology, 58*, 667–677.

Cardarelli, R., Kertesz, A., & Knebl, J. A. (2010). Frontotemporal dementia: A review for primary care physicians. *American Family Physician, 82*, 1372–1377.

Chien, D. T., Bahri, S., Szardenings, A. K., Walsh, J. C., Mu, F., Su, M. Y.,...Kolb, H. C. (2013). Early clinical PET imaging results with the novel PHF-tau radioligand [F-18]-T807. *Journal of Alzheimers Disease, 34*, 457–468.

Chow, T. W., Binns, M. A., Cummings, J. L., Lam, I., Black, S. E., Miller, B. L.,...van Reekum, R. (2009). Apathy symptom profile and behavioral associations in frontotemporal dementia vs dementia of Alzheimer type. *Archives of Neurology, 66*, 888–893.

Clark, A. W., Manz, H. J., White, C. L., III, Lehmann, J., Miller, D., & Coyle, J. T. (1986). Cortical degeneration with swollen chromatolytic neurons: Its relationship to Pick's disease. *Journal of Neuropathology and Experimental Neurology, 45*, 268–284.

Cruts, M., Gijselinck, I., van der Zee, J., Engelborghs, S., Wils, H., Pirici, D.,...Van Broeckhoven, C. (2006). Null mutations in progranulin cause ubiquitin-positive frontotemporal dementia linked to chromosome 17q21. *Nature, 442*, 920–924.

Cummings, J. L. (1997). The Neuropsychiatric Inventory: Assessing psychopathology in dementia patients. *Neurology, 48*, S10–S16.

Davies, R. R., Hodges, J. R., Kril, J. J., Patterson, K., Halliday, G. M., & Xuereb, J. H. (2005).

The pathological basis of semantic dementia. *Brain, 128*, 1984–1995.

DeJesus-Hernandez, M., Mackenzie, I. R., Boeve, B. F., Boxer, A. L., Baker, M., Rutherford, N. J.,...Rademakers, R. (2011). Expanded GGGGCC hexanucleotide repeat in noncoding region of C9ORF72 causes chromosome 9p-linked FTD and ALS. *Neuron, 72*, 245–256.

Dickson, D. W. (2001). Neuropathology of Pick's disease. *Neurology, 56*, S16–S20.

Dickson, D. W., Kouri, N., Murray, M. E., & Josephs, K. A. (2011). Neuropathology of frontotemporal lobar degeneration-tau (FTLD-tau). *Journal of Molecular Neuroscience, 45*, 384–389.

Dubois, B., Slachevsky, A., Litvan, I., & Pillon, B. (2000). The FAB: A Frontal Assessment Battery at bedside. *Neurology 55*, 1621–1626.

Eslinger, P. J., Dennis, K., Moore, P., Antani, S., Hauck, R., & Grossman, M. (2005). Metacognitive deficits in frontotemporal dementia. *Journal of Neurology, Neurosurgery and Psychiatry, 76*, 1630–1635.

Evrard, H. C., Forro, T., & Logothetis, N. K. (2012). Von Economo neurons in the anterior insula of the macaque monkey. *Neuron, 74*, 482–489.

Fodero-Tavoletti, M. T., Okamura, N., Furumoto, S., Mulligan, R. S., Connor, A. R., McLean, C. A.,...Villemagne, V. L. (2011). 18F-THK523: A novel in vivo tau imaging ligand for Alzheimer's disease. *Brain, 134*, 1089–1100.

Fong, J. C., Karydas, A. M., & Goldman, J. S. (2012). Genetic counseling for FTD/ALS caused by the C9ORF72 hexanucleotide expansion. *Alzheimers Research Therapy, 4*, 27.

Forman, M. S., Farmer, J., Johnson, J. K., Clark, C. M., Arnold, S. E., Coslett, H. B.,...Grossman, M. (2006). Frontotemporal dementia: clinicopathological correlations. *Annals of Neurology, 59*, 952–962.

Foster, N. L., Wilhelmsen, K., Sima, A. A., Jones, M. Z., D'Amato, C. J., & Gilman, S. (1997). Frontotemporal dementia and parkinsonism linked to chromosome 17: A consensus conference. Conference Participants. *Annals of Neurology, 41*, 706–715.

Funkiewiez, A., Bertoux, M., de Souza, L. C., Lévy, R., & Dubois, B. (2012). The SEA (Social cognition and Emotional Assessment): a clinical neuropsychological tool for early diagnosis of frontal variant of frontotemporal lobar degeneration. *Neuropsychology, 26*(1):81–90.

Garcin, B., Lillo, P., Hornberger, M., Piguet, O., Dawson, K., Nestor, P. J., & Hodges, J. R. (2009). Determinants of survival in behavioral variant frontotemporal dementia. *Neurology, 73*, 1656–1661.

Gislason, T. B., Sjogren, M., Larsson, L., & Skoog, I. (2003). The prevalence of frontal variant frontotemporal dementia and the frontal lobe syndrome in a population based sample of 85 year olds. *Journal of Neurology, Neurosurgery and Psychiatry, 74*, 867–871.

Gitlin, L. N., Kales, H. C., & Lyketsos, C. G. (2012). Nonpharmacologic management of behavioral symptoms in dementia. *Journal of the American Medical Association, 308*, 2020–2029.

Goldman, J. S., Rademakers, R., Huey, E. D., Boxer, A. L., Mayeux, R., Miller, B. L., & Boeve, B. F. (2011). An algorithm for genetic testing of frontotemporal lobar degeneration. *Neurology, 76*, 475–483.

Gorno-Tempini, M. L., Hillis, A. E., Weintraub, S., Kertesz, A., Mendez, M., Cappa, S. F.,...Grossman, M. (2011). Classification of primary progressive aphasia and its variants. *Neurology, 76*, 1006–1014.

Graham, A., Davies, R., Xuereb, J., Halliday, G., Kril, J., Creasey, H.,...Hodges, J. (2005). Pathologically proven frontotemporal dementia presenting with severe amnesia. *Brain, 128*, 597–605.

Grasbeck, A., Englund, E., Horstmann, V., Passant, U., & Gustafson, L. (2003). Predictors of mortality in frontotemporal dementia: A retrospective study of the prognostic influence of pre-diagnostic features. *International Journal of Geriatric Psychiatry, 18*, 594–601.

Gregory, C. A., & Hodges, J. R. (1996). Clinical features of frontal lobe dementia in comparison to Alzheimer's disease. *Journal of Neural Transmission, Supplemntal 47*, 103–123.

Gregory, C. A., Serra-Mestres, J., & Hodges, J. R. (1999). Early diagnosis of the frontal variant of frontotemporal dementia: how sensitive are standard neuroimaging and neuropsychologic tests? *Neuropsychiatry Neuropsychol Behav Neurol 12*, 128–135.

Groen, J. J., & Endtz, L. J. (1982). Hereditary Pick's disease: Second re-examination of the large family and discussion of other hereditary cases, with particular reference to electroencephalography, a computerized tomography. *Brain, 105*(Pt 3), 443–459.

Gustafson, L. (1987). Frontal lobe degeneration of non-Alzheimer type. II. Clinical picture and differential diagnosis. *Archives of Gerontology and Geriatrics, 6*, 209–223.

Harvey, R. J., Skelton-Robinson, M., & Rossor, M. N. (2003). The prevalence and causes of dementia in people under the age of 65 years. *Journal of Neurology, Neurosurgery and Psychiatry, 74*, 1206–1209.

Heston, L. L. (1978). The clinical genetics of Pick's disease. *Acta Psychiatrica Scandinavica, 57*, 202–206.

Hodges, J. R., Mitchell, J., Dawson, K., Spillantini, M. G., Xuereb, J. H., McMonagle,

P.,...Patterson, K. (2010). Semantic dementia: Demography, familial factors and survival in a consecutive series of 100 cases. *Brain, 133,* 300–306.

Hof, P. R., Bouras, C., Perl, D. P., & Morrison, J. H. (1994). Quantitative neuropathologic analysis of Pick's disease cases: Cortical distribution of Pick bodies and coexistence with Alzheimer's disease. *Acta Neuropathologica, 87,* 115–124.

Hornberger, M., Piguet, O., Graham, A. J., Nestor, P. J., & Hodges, J. R. (2010). How preserved is episodic memory in behavioral variant frontotemporal dementia? *Neurology, 74,* 472–479.

Hu, W. T., Chen-Plotkin, A., Grossman, M., Arnold, S. E., Clark, C. M., Shaw, L. M.,...Trojanowski, J. Q. (2011). Novel CSF biomarkers for frontotemporal lobar degenerations. *Neurology, 75,* 2079–2086.

Hu, W. T., Seelaar, H., Josephs, K. A., Knopman, D. S., Boeve, B. F., Sorenson, E. J.,...Grossman, M. (2009). Survival profiles of patients with frontotemporal dementia and motor neuron disease. *Archives of Neurology, 66,* 1359–1364.

Huey, E. D., Ferrari, R., Moreno, J. H., Jensen, C., Morris, C. M., Potocnik, F.,...Momeni, P. (2011). FUS and TDP43 genetic variability in FTD and CBS. *Neurobiology of Aging, 33,* 1016 e1019–1017.

Hutton, M., Lendon, C. L., Rizzu, P., Baker, M., Froelich, S., Houlden, H.,...Heutink, P. (1998). Association of missense and 5'-splice-site mutations in tau with the inherited dementia FTDP-17. *Nature, 393,* 702–705.

Ibach, B., Koch, H., Koller, M., Wolfersdorf, M., Workgroup for Geriatric Psychiatry of the Psychiatric State Hospitals of G, & Workgroup for Clinical Research of the Psychiatric State Hospitals of G. (2003). Hospital admission circumstances and prevalence of frontotemporal lobar degeneration: A multicenter psychiatric state hospital study in Germany. *Dementia and Geriatric Cognitive Disorders, 16,* 253–264.

Janssen, J. C., Warrington, E. K., Morris, H. R., Lantos, P., Brown, J., Revesz, T.,...Rossor, M. N. (2002). Clinical features of frontotemporal dementia due to the intronic tau *10*(+16) mutation. *Neurology, 58,* 1161–1168.

Jicha, G. A., & Nelson, P. T. (2011). Management of frontotemporal dementia: Targeting symptom management in such a heterogeneous disease requires a wide range of therapeutic options. *Neurodegenerative Disease Management, 1,* 141–156.

Josephs, K. A., Whitwell, J. L., & Jack, C. R., Jr. (2007) Anatomic correlates of stereotypies in frontotemporal lobar degeneration. *Neurobiology of Aging.*

Kertesz, A., Davidson, W., & Fox, H. (1997). Frontal behavioral inventory: Diagnostic criteria for frontal lobe dementia. *Canadian Journal of Neurological Sciences, 24,* 29–36.

Kertesz, A., Davidson, W., & Munoz, D. G. (1999). Clinical and pathological overlap between frontotemporal dementia, primary progressive aphasia and corticobasal degeneration: the Pick complex. *Dementia and Geriatric Cognitive Disorders 10* Suppl 1, 46–49.

Kertesz, A., McMonagle, P., Blair, M., Davidson, W., & Munoz, D. G. (2005). The evolution and pathology of frontotemporal dementia. *Brain 128,* 1996–2005.

Kipps, C. M., Nestor, P. J., Acosta-Cabronero, J., Arnold, R., & Hodges, J. R. (2009) Understanding social dysfunction in the behavioural variant of frontotemporal dementia: the role of emotion and sarcasm processing. *Brain 132,* 592–603.

Klunk, W. E., Engler, H., Nordberg, A., Wang, Y., Blomqvist, G., Holt, D. P.,...Långström, B. (2004). Imaging brain amyloid in Alzheimer's disease with Pittsburgh Compound-B. *Annals of Neurology, 55,* 306–319.

Knibb, J. A., Xuereb, J. H., Patterson, K., & Hodges, J. R. (2006). Clinical and pathological characterization of progressive aphasia. *Annals of Neurology 59,* 156–165.

Knopman, D. S., Mastri, A. R., Frey, W. H., II, Sung, J. H., & Rustan, T. (1990). Dementia lacking distinctive histologic features: A common non-Alzheimer degenerative dementia. *Neurology, 40,* 251–256.

Knopman, D. S., Petersen, R. C., Edland, S. D., Cha, R. H., & Rocca, W. A. (2004). The incidence of frontotemporal lobar degeneration in Rochester, Minnesota, 1990 through 1994. *Neurology, 62,* 506–508.

Kwiatkowski, T. J., Jr., Bosco, D. A., Leclerc, A. L., Tamrazian, E., Vanderburg, C. R., Russ, C.,...Brown, R. H., Jr. (2009) Mutations in the FUS/TLS gene on chromosome 16 cause familial amyotrophic lateral sclerosis. *Science, 323,* 1205–1208.

Le Ber, I., Guedj, E., Gabelle, A., Verpillat, P., Volteau, M., Thomas-Anterion, C.,...Dubois, B. (2006). Demographic, neurological and behavioural characteristics and brain perfusion SPECT in frontal variant of frontotemporal dementia. *Brain, 129,* 3051–3065.

Leyton, C. E., Villemagne, V. L., Savage, S., Pike, K. E., Ballard, K. J., Piguet, O.,...Hodges, J. R. (2011). Subtypes of progressive aphasia: Application of the International Consensus Criteria and validation using beta-amyloid imaging. *Brain, 134,* 3030–3043.

Lough, S., Kipps, C. M., Treise, C., Watson, P., Blair, J. R., & Hodges, J. R. (2006). Social reasoning, emotion and empathy in frontotemporal dementia. *Neuropsychologia, 44,* 950–958.

Mackenzie, I. R., Rademakers, R., & Neumann, M. (2010). TDP-43 and FUS in amyotrophic lateral sclerosis and frontotemporal dementia. *Lancet Neurology, 9,* 995–1007.

Manoochehri, M., & Huey, E. D. (2012). Diagnosis and management of behavioral issues in frontotemporal dementia. *Current Neurology and Neuroscience Reports, 12,* 528–536.

Maruyama, M., Shimada, H., Suhara, T., Shinotoh, H., Ji, B., Maeda, J., ... Higuchi, M. (2013). Imaging of tau pathology in a tauopathy mouse model and in Alzheimer patients compared to normal controls. *Neuron, 79,* 1094–1108.

Massimo, L., Powers, C., Moore, P., Vesely, L., Avants, B., Gee, J., ... Grossman, M. (2009). Neuroanatomy of apathy and disinhibition in frontotemporal lobar degeneration. *Dementia and Geriatric Cognitive Disorders, 27,* 96–104.

Mathuranath, P. S., Nestor, P. J., Berrios, G. E., Rakowicz, W., & Hodges, J. R. (2000). A brief cognitive test battery to differentiate Alzheimer's disease and frontotemporal dementia. *Neurology, 55,* 1613–1620.

McKhann, G. M., Albert, M. S., Grossman, M., Miller, B., Dickson, D., & Trojanowski, J. Q. (2001). Clinical and pathological diagnosis of frontotemporal dementia: Report of the Work Group on Frontotemporal Dementia and Pick's Disease. *Archives of Neurology, 58,* 1803–1809.

Mendez, M. F., & Perryman, K. M. (2003). Disrupted facial empathy in drawings from artists with frontotemporal dementia. *Neurocase, 9,* 44–50.

Mendez, M. F., Perryman, K. M., Miller, B. L., Swartz, J. R., & Cummings, J. L. (1997). Compulsive behaviors as presenting symptoms of frontotemporal dementia. *Journal of Geriatric Psychiatry and Neurology, 10,* 154–157.

Mesulam, M., Wicklund, A., Johnson, N., Rogalski, E., Leger, G. C., Rademaker, A., ... Bigio, E. H. (2008). Alzheimer and frontotemporal pathology in subsets of primary progressive aphasia. *Annals of Neurology, 63,* 709–719.

Mesulam, M. M. (1982). Slowly progressive aphasia without generalized dementia. *Annals of Neurology, 11,* 592–598.

Miller, B. L., Darby, A. L., Swartz, J. R., Yener, G. G., & Mena, I. (1995). Dietary changes, compulsions and sexual behavior in frontotemporal degeneration. *Dementia, 6,* 195–199.

Miller, B. L., Darby, A., Benson, D. F., Cummings, J. L., & Miller, M. H. (1997). Aggressive, socially disruptive and antisocial behaviour associated with fronto-temporal dementia. *British Journal of Psychiatry, 170,* 150–154.

Miller, B. L., Cummings, J. L., Villanueva-Meyer, J., Boone, K., Mehringer, C. M., Lesser, I. M., & Mena, I. (1991). Frontal lobe degeneration: Clinical, neuropsychological, and SPECT characteristics. *Neurology, 41,* 1374–1382.

Modirrousta, M., Price, B. H., & Dickerson, B. C. (2013). Neuropsychiatric symptoms in primary progressive aphasia: Phenomenology, pathophysiology, and approach to assessment and treatment. *Neurodegenerative Disease Management, 3,* 133–146.

Munoz, D. G., Morris, H. R., & Rosser, M. (2011). Pick's disease. In D. W. Dickson & R. O. Weller (Eds.), *Neurodegeneration: The molecular pathology of dementia and movement disorders* (2nd ed., pp. xx–xx): Wiley-Blackwell.

Neary, D., Snowden, J., & Mann, D. (2005). Frontotemporal dementia. *Lancet Neurology 4,* 771–780.

Neary, D., Snowden, J. S., Northen, B., & Goulding, P. (1988). Dementia of frontal lobe type. *Journal of Neurology, Neurosurgery and Psychiatry, 51,* 353–361.

Neary, D., Snowden, J. S., Gustafson, L., Passant, U., Stuss, D., Black, S., ..., Benson, D. F. (1998). Frontotemporal lobar degeneration: A consensus on clinical diagnostic criteria. *Neurology, 51,* 1546–1554.

Neumann, M., Rademakers, R., Roeber, S., Baker, M., Kretzschmar, H. A., & Mackenzie, I. R. (2009). A new subtype of frontotemporal lobar degeneration with FUS pathology. *Brain, 132,* 2922–2931.

Neumann, M., Sampathu, D. M., Kwong, L. K., Truax, A. C., Micsenyi, M. C., Chou, T. T., ... Lee, V. M. (2006). Ubiquitinated TDP-43 in frontotemporal lobar degeneration and amyotrophic lateral sclerosis. *Science, 314,* 130–133.

Neumann, M. A. (1949). Pick's disease. *Journal of Neuropathology and Experimental Neurology, 8,* 255–282.

Nyatsanza, S., Shetty, T., Gregory, C., Lough, S., Dawson, K., & Hodges, J. R. (2003). A study of stereotypic behaviours in Alzheimer's disease and frontal and temporal variant frontotemporal dementia. *Journal of Neurology, Neurosurgery and Psychiatry, 74,* 1398–1402.

O'Callaghan, C., Hodges, J. R., & Hornberger, M. (2013). Inhibitory dysfunction in frontotemporal dementia: A review. *Alzheimer Disease and Associated Disorders, 27,* 102–108.

Onari, K., & Spatz, H. (1926). Anatomische Beiträge zur Lehre von der Pickschen umschriebenen Grosshirnrinden-Atrophie ("Picksche Krankheit"). *Z Neurol, 101,* 470–511.

Pasquier, F., Grymonprez, L., Lebert, F., & Van der Linden, M. (2001). Memory impairment differs in frontotemporal dementia and Alzheimer's disease. *Neurocase, 7,* 161–171.

Pennington, C., Hodges, J. R., & Hornberger, M. (2011). Neural correlates of episodic memory in behavioral variant frontotemporal dementia. *Journal of Alzheimers Disease*, 24, 261–268.

Perry, D. C., Whitwell, J. L., Boeve, B. F., Pankratz, V. S., Knopman, D. S., Petersen, R. C., ...Josephs, K. A. (2012). Voxel-based morphometry in patients with obsessive-compulsive behaviors in behavioral variant frontotemporal dementia. *European Journal of Neurology*, 19, 911–917.

Perry, R. J., Rosen, H. R., Kramer, J. H., Beer, J. S., Levenson, R. L., & Miller, B. L. (2001). Hemispheric dominance for emotions, empathy and social behaviour: Evidence from right and left handers with frontotemporal dementia. *Neurocase*, 7, 145–160.

Pick, A. (1892). Über die Beziehungen der senilen Hirnatrophie zur Aphasie. *Prager medicinische Wochenschrift*, 17, 165–167.

Pick, A., Girling, D. M., & Berrios, G. E. (1997). On the symptomatology of left-sided temporal lobe atrophy. Classic Text No. 29. (Translated and annotated by D. M. Girling and G. E. Berrios.). *History of Psychiatry*, 8, 149–159.

Piguet, O., Hornberger, M., Mioshi, E., & Hodges, J. R. (2011) Behavioural-variant frontotemporal dementia: Diagnosis, clinical staging, and management. *Lancet Neurology*, 10, 162–172.

Piguet, O., Petersen, A., Yin Ka Lam, B., Gabery, S., Murphy, K., Hodges, J. R., & Halliday, G. M. (2011) Eating and hypothalamus changes in behavioral-variant frontotemporal dementia. *Annals of Neurology* 69, 312–319.

Poorkaj, P., Bird, T. D., Wijsman, E., Nemens, E., Garruto, R. M., Anderson, L., ...Schellenberg, G. D. (1998). Tau is a candidate gene for chromosome 17 frontotemporal dementia. *Annals of Neurology*, 43, 815–825.

Quaid, K. A. (2011). Genetic counseling for frontotemporal dementias. *Journal of Molecular Neuroscience*, 45, 706–709.

Rabinovici, G. D., Jagust, W. J., Furst, A. J., Ogar, J. M., Racine, C. A., Mormino, E. C., ...Gorno-Tempini, M. L. (2008). Abeta amyloid and glucose metabolism in three variants of primary progressive aphasia. *Annals of Neurology*, 64, 388–401.

Rabinovici, G. D., Rosen, H. J., Alkalay, A., Kornak, J., Furst, A. J., Agarwal, N., ...Jagust, W. J. (2012). Amyloid vs FDG-PET in the differential diagnosis of AD and FTLD. *Neurology*, 77, 2034–2042.

Rademakers, R., Cruts, M., & van Broeckhoven, C. (2004). The role of tau (MAPT) in frontotemporal dementia and related tauopathies. *Human Mutation*, 24, 277–295.

Rankin, K. P., Kramer, J. H., & Miller, B. L. (2005). Patterns of cognitive and emotional empathy in frontotemporal lobar degeneration. *Cognitive and Behavioral Neurology*, 18, 28–36.

Rankin, K. P., Baldwin, E., Pace-Savitsky, C., Kramer, J. H., & Miller, B. L. (2005). Self awareness and personality change in dementia. *Journal of Neurology, Neurosurgery and Psychiatry*, 76, 632–639.

Rankin, K. P., Gorno-Tempini, M. L., Allison, S. C., Stanley, C. M., Glenn, S., Weiner, M. W., & Miller, B. L. (2006). Structural anatomy of empathy in neurodegenerative disease. *Brain*, 129, 2945–2956.

Rascovsky, K., Hodges, J. R., Kipps, C. M., Johnson, J. K., Seeley, W. W., Mendez, M. F., ...Miller, B. M. (2007). Diagnostic criteria for the behavioral variant of frontotemporal dementia (bvFTD): Current limitations and future directions. *Alzheimer Disease and Associated Disorders*, 21, S14–18.

Rascovsky, K., Hodges, J. R., Knopman, D., Mendez, M. F., Kramer, J. H., Neuhaus, J., ...Miller, B. L. (2011). Sensitivity of revised diagnostic criteria for the behavioural variant of frontotemporal dementia. *Brain*, 134, 2456–2477.

Ratnavalli, E., Brayne, C., Dawson, K., & Hodges, J. R. (2002). The prevalence of frontotemporal dementia. *Neurology*, 58, 1615–1621.

Renton, A. E., Majounie, E., Waite, A., Simón-Sánchez, J., Rollinson, S., Gibbs, J. R., ...Traynor, B. J. (2011). A hexanucleotide repeat expansion in C9ORF72 is the cause of chromosome 9p21-linked ALS-FTD. *Neuron*, 72, 257–268.

Rosen, H. J., Alcantar, O., Rothlind, J., Sturm, V., Kramer, J. H., Weiner, M., & Miller, B. L. (2010). Neuroanatomical correlates of cognitive self-appraisal in neurodegenerative disease. *Neuroimage*, 49, 3358–3364.

Rosen, H. J., Allison, S. C., Schauer, G. F., Gorno-Tempini, M. L., Weiner, M. W., & Miller, B. L. (2005). Neuroanatomical correlates of behavioural disorders in dementia. *Brain*, 128, 2612–2625.

Rosso, S. M., Roks, G., Stevens, M., de Koning, I., Tanghe, H. L. J., Kamphorst, W., ...van Swieten, J. C. (2001). Complex compulsive behaviour in the temporal variant of frontotemporal dementia. *Journal of Neurology*, 248, 965–970.

Rosso, S. M., Donker Kaat, L., Baks, T., Joosse, M., de Koning, I., Pijnenburg, Y., ...van Swieten, J. C. (2003). Frontotemporal dementia in The Netherlands: Patient characteristics and prevalence estimates from a population-based study. *Brain*, 126, 2016–2022.

Sapolsky, D., Bakkour, A., Negreira, A., Nalipinski, P., Weintraub, S., Mesulam,

M. M.,...Dickerson, B. C. (2010). Cortical neuroanatomic correlates of symptom severity in primary progressive aphasia. *Neurology, 75*, 358–366.

Schenk, V. W. (1959). Re-examination of a family with Pick's disease. *Annals of Human Genetics, 23*, 325–333.

Seeley, W. W., Bauer, A. M., Miller, B. L., Gorno-Tempini, M. L., Kramer, J. H., Weiner, M., & Rosen, H. J. (2005). The natural history of temporal variant frontotemporal dementia. *Neurology, 64*, 1384–1390.

Seeley, W. W., Carlin, D. A., Allman, J. M., Macedo, M. N., Bush, C., Miller, B. L., & Dearmond, S. J. (2006). Early frontotemporal dementia targets neurons unique to apes and humans. *Annals of Neurology, 60*, 660–667.

Shinagawa, S., Ikeda, M., Fukuhara, R., & Tanabe, H. (2006). Initial symptoms in frontotemporal dementia and semantic dementia compared with Alzheimer's disease. *Dementia and Geriatric Cognitive Disorders, 21*, 74–80.

Shnall, A., Agate, A., Grinberg, A., Huijbregts, M., Nguyen, M. Q., & Chow, T. W. (2013). Development of supportive services for frontotemporal dementias through community engagement. *International Review of Psychiatry, 25*, 246–252.

Skibinski, G., Parkinson, N. J., Brown, J. M., Chakrabarti, L., Lloyd, S. L., Hummerich, H.,...Collinge, J. (2005). Mutations in the endosomal ESCRTIII-complex subunit CHMP2B in frontotemporal dementia. *Nature Genetics, 37*, 806–808.

Small, G. W., Kepe, V., Ercoli, L. M., Siddarth, P., Bookheimer, S. Y., Miller, K. J.,...Barrio, J. R. (2006). PET of brain amyloid and tau in mild cognitive impairment. *New England Journal Medicine, 355*, 2652–2663.

Snowden, J. S., Neary, D., & Mann, D. M. (2004). Autopsy proven sporadic frontotemporal dementia due to microvacuolar-type histology, with onset at 21 years of age. *Journal of Neurology, Neurosurgery and Psychiatry 75*, 1337–1339.

Snowden, J. S., Bathgate, D., Varma, A., Blackshaw, A., Gibbons, Z. C., & Neary, D. (2001). Distinct behavioural profiles in frontotemporal dementia and semantic dementia. *Journal of Neurology, Neurosurgery and Psychiatry, 70*, 323–332.

Snowden, J. S., Pickering-Brown, S. M., Mackenzie, I. R., Richardson, A. M., Varma, A., Neary, D., & Mann, D. M. (2006). Progranulin gene mutations associated with frontotemporal dementia and progressive non-fluent aphasia. *Brain, 129*, 3091–3102.

Torralva, T., Roca, M., Gleichgerrcht, E., Bekinschtein, T., & Manes, F. (2009). A neuropsychological battery to detect specific executive and social cognitive impairments in early frontotemporal dementia. *Brain, 132*, 1299–1309.

Vance, C., Rogelj, B., Hortobágyi, T., De Vos, K. J., Nishimura, A. L., Sreedharan, J.,...Shaw, C. E. (2009). Mutations in FUS, an RNA processing protein, cause familial amyotrophic lateral sclerosis type 6. *Science, 323*, 1208–1211.

Whitwell, J. L., Sampson, E. L., Loy, C. T., Warren, J. E., Rossor, M. N., Fox, N. C., & Warren, J. D. (2007). VBM signatures of abnormal eating behaviours in frontotemporal lobar degeneration. *Neuroimage, 35*, 207–213.

Williamson, C., Alcantar, O., Rothlind, J., Cahn-Weiner, D., Miller, B. L., & Rosen, H. J. (2009). Standardised measurement of self-awareness deficits in FTD and AD. *Journal of Neurology, Neurosurgery and Psychiatry, 81*, 140–145.

Wood, E. M., Falcone, D., Suh, E., Irwin, D. J., Chen-Plotkin, A. S., Lee, E. B.,...Grossman, M. (2013). Development and validation of pedigree classification criteria for frontotemporal lobar degeneration. *Journal of the American Medical Association: Neurology, 70*(11), 1411–1417.

Woolley, J. D., Gorno-Tempini, M. L., Seeley, W. W., Rankin, K., Lee, S. S., Matthews, B. R., & Miller, B. L. (2007). Binge eating is associated with right orbitofrontal-insular-striatal atrophy in frontotemporal dementia. *Neurology, 69*, 1424–1433.

Wylie, M. A., Shnall, A., Onyike, C. U., & Huey, E. D. (2013). Management of frontotemporal dementia in mental health and multidisciplinary settings. *International Review of Psychiatry, 25*, 230–236.

Xie, S. X., Forman, M. S., Farmer, J., Moore, P., Wang, Y., Wang, X.,...Grossman, M. (2008). Factors associated with survival probability in autopsy-proven frontotemporal lobar degeneration. *Journal of Neurology, Neurosurgery and Psychiatry, 79*, 126–129.

Yoshimura, N. (1989). Topography of Pick body distribution in Pick's disease: A contribution to understanding the relationship between Pick's and Alzheimer's diseases. *Clinical Neuropathology, 8*, 1–6.

Zhukareva, V., Mann, D., Pickering-Brown, S., Uryu, K, Shuck, T., Shah, K.,...Lee, V. M. (2002). Sporadic Pick's disease: A tauopathy characterized by a spectrum of pathological tau isoforms in gray and white matter. *Annals of Neurology, 51*, 730–739.

9

Primary Progressive Aphasia
A Language-Based Dementia

Marsel Mesulam

Progressive aphasias have been recognized for more than 100 years through case reports by Pick, Sérieux, Dejerine, Franceschi, and Rosenfeld (Franceschi, 1908; Pick, 1892, 1904; Rosenfeld, 1909; Sérieux, 1893). The current interest in this condition can be traced to a 1982 report of six patients with a slowly progressive language disorder and to the subsequent delineation of the primary progressive aphasia (PPA) syndrome (Mesulam, 1982, 2007). Primary progressive aphasia is diagnosed when language is the only area of major dysfunction early in the disease; when other mental faculties such as memory for daily events, visuospatial skills, face and object knowledge, and basic comportment remain relatively intact; and when structural brain imaging does not reveal a specific lesion, other than atrophy, that can account for the language deficit (Mesulam, 2001, 2003; Mesulam & Weintraub, 1992). In some patients, the principal signs and symptoms are confined to the area of language for as many as 10–14 years. In others, impairments in other cognitive functions can emerge after the initial few years, but the language dysfunction tends to remain the most salient feature and to deteriorate the most rapidly throughout the course of disease (Weintraub et al., 1990). PPA is a form of dementia since it causes gradual cognitive decline to the point where daily living functions become compromised. It is also an unusual dementia since episodic memory functions remain largely preserved for many years. In contrast to patients with amnestic dementias of the Alzheimer-type (DAT), who tend to lose interest in recreational and social activities, some patients with PPA maintain and even intensify involvement in complex hobbies such as gardening, carpentry, sculpting, and painting.

Primary progressive aphasia should be differentiated from states of pure progressive dysarthria, speech apraxia, or phonological disintegration, where the formation, rather than usage, of words becomes disrupted (Broussolle et al., 1996). It should also be differentiated from DAT and behavioral variant frontotemporal dementia (bvFTD), where word-finding disturbances or a paucity of speech may arise, but on a background of more salient impairments of memory (in DAT) and behavior (in bvFTD).

Age of onset has ranged from the 40s to the 80s. However, the majority of patients have had onset before the age of 65 (Mesulam, Wieneke, Thompson, Rogalski, & Weintraub,

2012). Several ancillary features of secondary importance can arise in conjunction with the aphasia. *Dysarhria* is not uncommon and can contribute to loss of fluency. *Ideomotor apraxia*, sometimes in the form of "sympathetic dyspraxia" in the left hand, can be encountered. A more frequent occurrence is the presence of buccofacial apraxia so that the command to "cough" cannot be followed, even though the patient understands the instructions and can perform the action spontaneously when the need arises. *Dyscalculia* is common, reflecting the anatomical proximity of the brain areas necessary for language and calculations. Occasionally, all components of the Gerstmann syndrome can be present. A careful neurological examination can reveal subtle signs reflecting the dysfunction of motor pathways in the language-dominant (usually left) hemisphere. These signs include mild flattening of the nasolabial fold, widening of the palpebral fissure, asymmetrical posturing of the hand while walking on the heels or edge of the feet, and mild cogwheeling rigidity induced when the other hand is engaged in repetitive tapping movements.

An abrupt onset of the aphasia excludes the diagnosis of PPA. Additional exclusionary criteria include the *early salience* of motor deficits, amnesia, abnormal comportment, associative agnosia, or visuospatial disorientation. Patients with these features may have the phenotypes of motor neuron disease (MND), corticobasal degeneration (CBD), progressive supranuclear palsy (PSP), DAT, bvFTD, or the syndrome of posterior cortical atrophy (PCA), each of which can be accompanied by a nonprimary but progressive aphasia. The mere presence of an aphasia is thus not sufficient for the diagnosis of PPA. Brain imaging is part of the diagnostic workup since any finding other than atrophy that can account for the aphasia (such as neoplasm or ischemic lesions) rules out the diagnosis of PPA (Fig. 9.1).

Additional cognitive, behavioral, and motor deficits that independently influence daily living activities arise in the middle or late stages of the disease (Rogalski & Mesulam, 2009; Sapolsky et al., 2010). We have used the descriptive term "PPA-plus" (PPA+) to designate the fact that the patient had initially fulfilled the diagnostic criteria for PPA but that the aphasia is no longer the only major deficit (Mesulam & Weintraub, 2008). Personality changes (inappropriate familiarity, impaired problem solving, blunted judgment) or asymmetrical extrapyramidal deficits may emerge quite commonly as the disease progresses and reflect the close anatomical association of PPA-causing diseases with those causing bvFTD and CBD.

Diagnosing PPA is easiest when the patient is examined early so that core criteria can be fulfilled explicitly. Occasionally, the clinician will see a patient at a more advanced clinical stage, at a time when the selectivity of aphasia may no longer be ascertainable because of language comprehension deficits or because deficits in other domains have emerged. In such cases, a structured interview with informants can be used to establish whether the aphasia had in fact emerged in relative isolation. A retrospective diagnosis of "possible PPA" is made if such an interview suggests that the diagnostic criteria were likely to have been met during an earlier phases of the disease in a patient who has since acquired other major deficits as well.

Subtyping and Terminology in Primary Progressive Aphasia

The study of patients with cerebrovascular lesions has led to the delineation of several aphasia subtypes, each characterized by a distinctive cluster of signs and symptoms linked to the principal lesion site within the language network. The clustering of aphasic deficits and their clinicopathological correlates is slightly different in PPA, perhaps because the lesions are selective for specific neuronal types and also indolently progressive, leading to more complex dissociations of function and some reorganization of cortical circuitry. We are now subdividing our PPA cases into three variants: agrammatic, semantic, and logopenic (Gorno-Tempini et al., 2004, 2011; Leyton et al., 2011; Mesulam et al., 2009, 2012; Sapolsky et al., 2010). The agrammatic subtype (PPA-G) is characterized by impairments of grammar (syntax and morphology) but not of word comprehension; the semantic subtype (PPA-S), by impairment of word comprehension but not of grammar; and the logopenic subtype (PPA-L), by intermittent word-finding hesitations without impairments of comprehension or grammar. Fluency is consistently

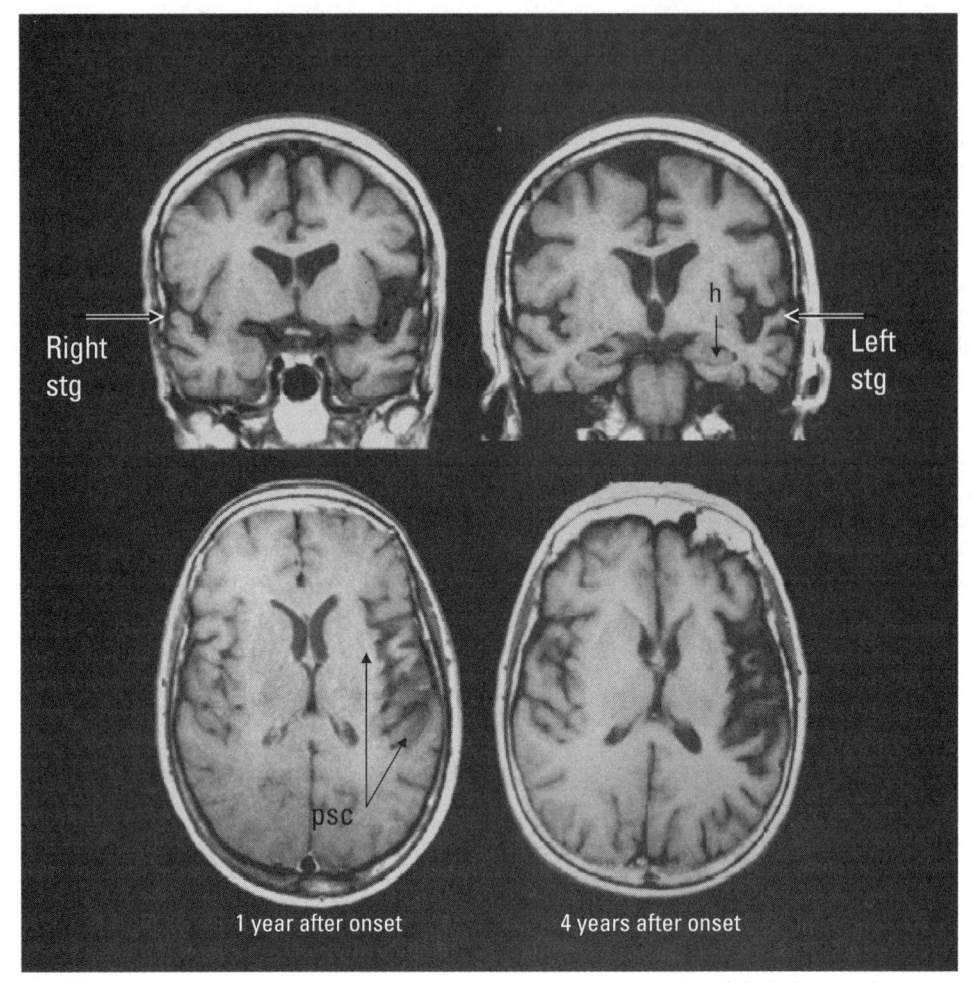

Figure 9.1 (Top) Two coronal sections, showing the asymmetric atrophy of the left perisylvian cortex in a patient with primary progressive aphasia. (Bottom) Two axial sections showing the progression of atrophy.

low in PPA-G, may be normal in PPA-S, and is highly variable in PPA-L. Repetition can be impaired in both PPA-G and PPA-L, but rarely in PPA-S. Some investigators consider repetition impairments as key components of PPA-L (Gorno-Tempini et al., 2008). In some patients grammar and comprehension are jointly impaired early in the disease. These patients can be said to have a mixed subtype of PPA, designated PPA-M. The PPA-G and PPA-L variants collectively account for what is also known as progressive nonfluent aphasia (PNFA), while the PPA-S variant designates the predominantly aphasic form of semantic dementia (SD).

Specific guidelines have been introduced by an international group of investigators for the classification of PPA into the PPA-G, PPA-L, and PPA-S subtypes (Gorno-Tempini et al., 2011). These guidelines have been implemented to select specific tests and quantitative parameters for the subtyping of patients at early and mild stages of disease (Mesulam et al., 2012). While the new system is rigorous, it is also burdensome. Table 9.1 offers a simpler descriptive set of guidelines that should be adequate for use in most clinical settings.

Neuropsychological Profiles

Standardized neuropsychological tests are helpful for reaching an early diagnosis

TABLE 9.1 Descriptive and Simplified Criteria for Classifying Primary Progressive Aphasia (PPA)

Diagnostic Criteria for PPA
The following three conditions must all be present:
1. A new and progressive language disorder (aphasia) as documented by neuropsychologically determined abnormalities in one or more of the following domains: grammaticality of sentence production, word retrieval in speech, object naming, word and sentence comprehension, spelling, reading, and repetition. Isolated impairments of articulation do not qualify
2. Relative preservation of episodic memory, executive functions, visuospatial skills, and comportment as documented by history, medical records, and/or neuropsychological testing
3. Imaging and other pertinent neurodiagnostic test results that rule out causes other than neurodegeneration

Agrammatic Subtype (PPA-G)
Impaired grammatical structure of spoken or written language in the absence of significant word comprehension impairments. Output is usually of low fluency but does not have to be dysarthric or apraxic.

Semantic Subtype (PPA-S)
Impaired word comprehension in the absence of significant impairment of grammar. Object naming is severely impaired. Output is motorically fluent but contains paraphasias, and circumlocutions.

Logopenic Subtype (PPA-L)
No significant grammar or word comprehension impairment. Fluency is variable with many word-finding hesitations and phonemic paraphasias. Object naming may be impaired and may constitute the only significant finding in the neuropsychological examination.

Mixed Subtype (PPA-M)
Impaired grammatical structure and word comprehension, even at the early stages of disease.

(Weintraub & Mesulam, 1993, 1996; Weintraub et al., 1990). However, a strict reliance on neuropsychological tests, most of which depend on verbal instructions, verbal responses, or covert verbal reasoning, may occasionally lead to the erroneous conclusion that areas other than language are also impaired. Scores on the Mini Mental State Examination (MMSE) (Folstein, Folstein, & McHugh, 1975), for example, can exaggerate the degree of disability (Osher, Wicklund, Rademaker, Johnson, & Weintraub, 2007). Although the language disorder in primary progressive aphasia may interfere with the ability to memorize word lists or solve reasoning tasks, the patient typically has no difficulty recalling daily events or behaving with sound judgment, indicating that explicit memory, reasoning, and social skills remain relatively intact.

The neuropsychological examination of the patient with suspected PPA should demonstrate the aphasia, characterize its subtype, and identify non-language cognitive domains that are relatively spared. Aphasia can be tested with one of the several clinical batteries designed for this purpose. The Western Aphasia Battery (WAB-R) includes subtests that measure spontaneous speech, word and sentence comprehension, naming, reading, and writing (Kertesz, 2006). An Aphasia Quotient, derived from the WAB-R, provides a measure of aphasia severity that can be tracked over time. Based on a subtyping algorithm previously described (Mesulam et al., 2009, 2012), grammatical production can be tested with the Northwestern Anagram Test (NAT), a measure of sentence construction that does not place demands on working memory or speech output (Weintraub et al., 2009). Single-word comprehension can be tested with items from the Peabody Picture Vocabulary Test (PPVT-IV), which provides a range of item difficulty (Dunn & Dunn, 2006). The Boston Naming Test (BNT) provides a standardized measure of object naming (Kaplan, Goodglass, & Weintraub, 1983).

Nonverbal functions should be tested with instruments that minimize interference from aphasia. Episodic memory can be tested with the Three Words Three Shapes (3W3S) test, a measure we previously designed to differentiate DAT from healthy cognitive aging (Weintraub & Mesulam, 1985; Weintraub et al., 2000). The 3W3S test showed that PPA patients have a selective retrieval impairment for words but not for shapes (Weintraub et al., 2012). PPA patients are therefore likely to forget words they hear or read but not events they experience. This pattern is different from the typical pattern of DAT where patients forget recent experiences. The relative preservation of reasoning skills in PPA can be documented with the Visual Verbal Test, a nonverbal test of cognitive flexibility (Wicklund, Johnson, & Weintraub, 2004). Visuoperceptual functions can be tested with Judgment of Line Orientation (Benton, Hamsher, Varney, & Speen, 1998). Behavioral changes, salient in early stages of bvFTD, but not typically apparent until later stages of illness in PPA, can be assessed with the Frontal Behavior Inventory (Kertesz, Nadkarni, Davidson, & Thomas, 2000).

Functional and Structural Neuroanatomy

Quantitative morphometry shows that the PPA-G subtype is most closely associated with atrophy in the posterior frontal lobe, including Broca's area; the PPA-S subtype with atrophy in the anterior temporal components of the language network, including the temporal pole; and the PPA-L subtype with atrophy in the temporo-parietal component of the language network (Gorno-Tempini et al., 2004; Mesulam et al., 2009, 2012; Sapolsky et al., 2010).

Abnormalities of blood flow and metabolism may emerge prior to the detectable atrophy. Single-photon emission tomography (SPECT) or positron emission tomography (PET) may therefore provide more sensitive diagnostic information than structural magnetic resonance imaging (MRI) or computed tomography (CT) scans. However, structural and metabolic imaging may be uninformative during the first several years of disease and the diagnosis may need to be based on the clinical examination alone (Mesulam et al., 2012). Functional imaging helps to explore the physiological bases of the language impairment. When asked to identify homonyms or synonyms in the course of functional MRI experiments, PPA patients and age-matched controls activate the same components of the language network, including Broca's and Wernicke's areas (Sonty et al., 2003). However, the functional connectivity between these two major nodes of the language network becomes disrupted (Sonty et al., 2007). It appears, therefore, that disrupted language processing in PPA may initially reflect an impairment of information transfer within the language network rather than a failure of activation at the network nodes. In comparison to neurologically intact subjects, the PPA patients also display additional aberrant activations within regions of the brain outside of the classic language network (Sonty et al., 2003). It is not yet clear whether these aberrant activations reflect compensatory processes or abnormal disinhibition. The latter possibility is supported by the fact that the intensity of the aberrant activations is inversely correlated with performance on a naming test (Sonty et al., 2003).

Neuropathology

Postmortem examinations show that the vast majority of PPA patients have the pathology of either frontotemporal lobar degeneration (FTLD) or of Alzheimer's disease (AD). Both major types of FTLD, FTLD-TAU and FTLD-TDP, have been reported (Mesulam et al., 2008). In the majority of PPA-G the neuropathology is of the FTLD type, mostly with tauopathy of the Pick or CBD/PSP types. In the majority of PPA-S, the neuropathology is also of the FTLD type but most frequently with TDP-43 inclusions of type C. Approximately 20%–30% of patients in these two variants show the neuropathology of AD (Knibb, Xuereb, Patterson, & Hodges, 2006; Mesulam et al., 2008). In PPA-L, more than half of the cases have AD pathology and the rest FTLD (Leyton et al., 2011; Mesulam et al., 2008). Quantitative analyses of postmortem cases showed that PPA patients with AD pathology had higher neocortical-to-entorhinal and left-to-right ratios of neurofibrillary tangles than patients who had the typical combination of AD pathology with an amnestic (rather than aphasic) dementia (Gefen et al., 2012). This atypical distribution of neurofibrillary degeneration is consistent with the anatomy of the clinical phenotype in PPA.

Determining whether an individual PPA patient has AD versus FTLD pathology is always challenging. *APOE* genotyping or F18-DG PET metabolic scans do not help in this differentiation. In fact, the ε4 allele of *APOE*, which is a major risk factor for the typical form of AD, is not a risk factor for the type of AD that causes PPA (Gefen et al., 2012; Rogalski et al., 2011). Amyloid imaging with PET and cerebrospinal fluid evaluations for phosphotau and beta amyloid may be helpful for the identification of patients with AD pathology, but this remains to be proven in neuropathologically verified cases (Rabinovici et al., 2008). A rapidly progressive language disorder with all the initial characteristics of PPA has been described in conjunction with Jacob-Creutzfeldt disease. However, the course is much more rapid than in the usual cases (Mandell, Alexander, & Carpenter, 1989).

Genetics and Risk Factors of Primary Progressive Aphasia

The vast majority of PPA is sporadic. However, PPA has also been reported in dominantly inherited forms of FTLD caused by mutations in *MAPT, GRN,* or *C9orf72* (Munoz, Ros, Fatas, Bermejo, & Yebenes, 2007; Rademakers et al., 2007; Simón-Sánchez et al., 2012). In the group of dominantly inherited FTLD kindreds, the PPA phenotype has been described most frequently in families with *GRN* mutations. In two families, *GRN* mutations consistently resulted in the PPA phenotype (Mesulam et al., 2007). In the PPA1 family, three of four siblings had PPA. The mutation consisted of a single nucleotide deletion in exon 9. In the PPA3 family, two of three siblings had PPA. The mutation was a C>T transition in exon 11. Both mutations resulted in a premature termination codon and a haploinsufficiency of progranulin. The neuropathological examination in affected members of both families showed FTLD pathology with inclusions containing TDP-43 of type A. In one member of the PPA3 family unbiased stereology showed that the number of TDP-43 inclusions was higher in neocortex than in memory-related mediotemporal limbic areas, and higher in language-related neocortices of the left hemisphere than in contralateral areas on the right (Gliebus et al., 2010). The distribution of inclusions was thus concordant with the PPA profile of impaired language with relatively spared memory function.

The fit between the clinical picture and the distribution of lesions may give the impression that progranulin deficiency and the resultant TDP-43 abnormalities selectively target components of the language network.

However, it is also well known that similar mutations can cause entirely different phenotypes in other families. Even within single families with *GRN* mutations, some members may have PPA and others, bvFTD. The fact that identical neuropathological entities can cause PPA in some patients while causing bvFTD or amnestic dementias in others justifies the search for patient-specific susceptibility factors that interact with the neurodegenerative disease by determining its primary anatomical location.

No such susceptibility factor has yet been identified in PPA or any of the other dementia syndromes. The strongest lead thus far is the high incidence of learning disabilities. We reported that learning disabilities, including dyslexia, were overrepresented in patients with PPA and their first-degree relatives when compared to controls and AD patients (Mesulam & Weintraub, 1992; Rogalski, Johnson, Weintraub, & Mesulam, 2008). In some of these families, the concentration of dyslexia was striking, affecting the majority of children or siblings. Furthermore, two patients with PPA onset in their 60s were found to have left hemi-craniosynostosis, a mild developmental abnormality that interferes with the normal growth of the underlying cortex. In these two patients, the left hemisphere hypoplasia was functionally compensated throughout most adulthood but appears to have provided the neural background for the emergence of PPA in the seventh decade of life (Alberca, Montes, Russell, & Mesulam, 2004). These observations have led us to wonder whether some cases of PPA could represent the tardive manifestation of genetic or acquired vulnerabilities of the language network that remain functionally compensated during most of adulthood but that become the locus of least resistance for the distribution of neurodegeneration. In other patients with a different set of prior vulnerabilities the same neurodegenerative process would be expected to have a different distribution and therefore different clinical manifestations.

Contributions of Primary Progressive Aphasia to Neurolinguistics and Cognitive Neuroscience

The contributions to classic aphasiology were based mostly on observations in patients with focal cerebrovascular lesions where the injury site, usually including cortical as well as subcortical areas, is abruptly and completely destroyed. In primary progressive aphasia, the gradual and selective loss of cortical neurons in the language network leads to more specific and subtle perturbations of language function. Research on PPA has already led to several new insights concerning language function. One of the most consequential new insights has been the realization that the classic neurological account of language is incomplete and that the anterior temporal lobe of the left hemisphere needs to be inserted into the language network as a third major hub with a critical role in language comprehension, especially of words denoting concrete entities (Gitelman, Nobre, Sonty, Parrish, & Mesulam, 2005; Hodges, Graham, & Patterson, 1995; Lambon Ralph, Cipolotti, Manes, & Patterson, 2010; Mesulam et al., 2009). In fact, some of these observations have cast serious doubts on existing characterizations of Wernicke's area and its role in language comprehension (Schwartz et al., 2009). Another equally important insight has been the realization that grammatical ability and fluency can be dissociated neuropsychologically as well as anatomically (Rogalski et al., 2011; Thompson et al., 2011). It is quite likely that future research in PPA will lead to additional insights into the functional organization of the language network.

Patient Care

The manifestations of PPA are distinctly different from those of typical Alzheimer's disease dementia. Different aspects of daily living activities are impaired and require different sorts of intervention. Some patients can learn sign language, others find it useful to carry laminated cards with specific messages, and still others benefit from voice synthesizers or laptops containing digitally stored words and phrases. An evaluation by a speech therapist is useful for exploring alternative communication strategies. In contrast to DAT, where new information cannot be retained in memory, the recall and evaluation of recent events remains intact, although the patient may not be able to express this knowledge verbally. Explaining this phenomenon to the family and offering an objective assessment of how the aphasia interferes with verbal expression and language comprehension tends to help caregivers cope with the patient's impairments. We find that psychosocial interventions, support groups, and targeted educational programs are necessary components of a comprehensive approach to patients and families (Weintraub & Morhardt, 2005).

In the absence of effective treatments that can prevent, reverse, or slow down the progression of AD or FTLD, there is currently no effective disease-modifying intervention for PPA. Controlled trials with bromocriptine and memantine have not yielded positive results (Johnson et al., 2010; Reed, Johnson, Thompson, Weintraub, & Mesulam, 2004). Although many patients with PPA may have atypical AD, cholinesterase inhibitors have not been particularly useful. However, a new trial of these agents, specifically in patients with the in vivo biomarkers of AD, would be useful to initiate. Anecdotal reports of success with omental transplants, intraspinal ethanercept, steroids, and transcranial magnetic stimulation have appeared but need to be confirmed. A very special feature of PPA is the relative sparing of the right hemisphere for many years during the course of the disease. Stimulating the plasticity of the right hemisphere so that it can take over some of the impaired language functions remains a major and futuristic goal for treatment.

Acknowledgments

This work was supported by grants DC008552 from the National Institute on Deafness and other Communication Disorders and AG13854 from the National Institute on Aging.

References

Alberca, R., Montes, E., Russell, E., & Mesulam, M-M. (2004). Left hemicranial hypoplasia in two patients with primary progressive aphasia. *Archives of Neurology, 61,* 265–268.

Benton, A., Hamsher, K., Varney, N., & Speen, O. (1998). *Contributions to neuropsychological assessment* (2nd ed.). New York, NY: Oxford University Press.

Broussolle, E., Bakchine, S., Tommasi, M., Laurent, B., Bazin, B., Cinotti, L.,...Chazot, G. (1996). Slowly progressive anarthria with late anterior opercular syndrome: A variant form of frontal cortical atrophy syndromes. *Journal of the Neurological Sciences, 144,* 44–58.

Dunn, L. A., & Dunn, L. M. (2006). *Peabody picture vocabulary test-4.* Pearson.

Folstein, M., Folstein, S., & McHugh, P. R. (1975). Mini-mental state: A practical method for grading the cognitive state of patients for the clinician. *Journal of Psychiatric Research, 12,* 189–198.

Franceschi, F. (1908). Gliosi perivasculare in un caso de demenza afasica. *Annali di Neurologia, 26,* 281–290.

Gefen, T., Gasho, K., Rademaker, A., Lalehzari, M., Weintraub, S., Rogalski, E.,…Mesulam, M-M. (2012). Clinically concordant variations of Alzheimer patology in aphasic versus amnestic dementia. *Brain, 135,* 1554–1565.

Gitelman, D. R., Nobre, A. C., Sonty, S., Parrish, T. B., & Mesulam, M-M. (2005). Language network specializations: An analysis with parallel task design and functional magnetic resonance imaging. *NeuroImage, 26,* 975–985.

Gliebus, G., Bigio, E., Gasho, K., Mishra, M., Caplan, D., Mesulam, M-M., & Geula, C. (2010). Asymmetric TDP-43 distribution in primary progressive aphasia with progranulin mutation. *Neurology, 74,* 1607–1610.

Gorno-Tempini, M. L., Brambati, S. M., Ginex, V., Ogar, J., Dronkers, N. F., Marcone, A.,…Miller, B. L. (2008). The logopenic/phonological variant of primary progressive aphasia. *Neurology, 71,* 1227–1234.

Gorno-Tempini, M. L., Dronkers, N. F., Rankin, K. P., Ogar, J. M., Phengrasamy, L., Rosen, H. J.,…Miller, B. L. (2004). Cognition and anatomy in three variants of primary progressive aphasia. *Annals of Neurology, 55,* 335–346.

Gorno-Tempini, M. L., Hillis, A., Weintraub, S., Kertesz, A., Mendez, M. F., Cappa, S. F.,…Grossman, M. (2011). Classification of primary progressive aphasia and its variants. *Neurology, 76,* 1006–1014.

Hodges, J., Graham, N., & Patterson, K. (1995). Charting the progression in semantic dementia: Implications for the organization of semantic memory. *Memory, 3,* 463–495.

Johnson, N. A., Rademaker, A., Weintraub, S., GItelman, D., Wieneke, C., & Mesulam, M-M. (2010). Pilot trial of memantine in primary progressive aphasia. *Alzheimer's Disease and Associated Disorders, 24,* 308.

Kaplan, E., Goodglass, H., & Weintraub, S. (1983). *The Boston naming test.* Philadelphia, PA: Lea & Febiger.

Kertesz, A. (2006). *Western Aphasia Battery-Revised (WAB-R).* Austin, TS: Pro-Ed.

Kertesz, A., Nadkarni, N., Davidson, W., & Thomas, A. W. (2000). The Frontal Behavioral Inventory in the differential diagnosis of frontotemporal dementia. *Journal of the International Neuropsychological Society, 6,* 460–468.

Knibb, J. A., Xuereb, J. H., Patterson, K., & Hodges, J. R. (2006). Clinical and pathological characterization of progressive aphasia. *Annals of Neurology, 59,* 156–165.

Lambon Ralph, M. A., Cipolotti, L., Manes, F., & Patterson, K. (2010). Taking both sides: Do unilateral anterior temporal lobe lesions disrupt semantic memory? *Brain, 133,* 3243–3255.

Leyton, C. E., Villemange, V. L., Savage, S., Pike, K. E., Ballard, K. J., Piguet, O.,…Hodges, J. (2011). Subtypes of progressive aphasia: Application of the international consensus criteria and validation using β-amyloid imaging. *Brain, 134,* 3030–3043.

Mandell, A. M., Alexander, M. P., & Carpenter, S. (1989). Creutzfeldt-Jacob disease presenting as isolated aphasia. *Neurology, 39,* 55–58.

Mesulam, M., Wieneke, C., Rogalski, E., Cobia, D., Thompson, C., & Weintraub, S. (2009). Quantitative template for subtyping primary progressive aphasia. *Archives of Neurology, 66,* 1545–1551.

Mesulam, M., Wicklund, A., Johnson, N., Rogalski, E., Leger, G. C., Rademaker, A.,…Bigio, E. H. (2008). Alzheimer and frontotemporal pathology in subsets of primary progressive aphasia. *Annals of Neurology, 63,* 709–719.

Mesulam, M., Johnson, N., Krefft, T. A., Gass, J. M., Cannon, A. D., Adamson, J. L.,…Graff-Radford, N. R. (2007). Progranulin mutations in primary progressive aphasia. *Archives of Neurology, 64,* 43–47.

Mesulam, M. M. (1982). Slowly progressive aphasia without generalized dementia. *Annals of Neurology, 11*(6), 592–598.

Mesulam, M-M. (2001). Primary progressive aphasia. *Annals of Neurology, 49,* 425–432.

Mesulam, M-M. (2003). Primary progressive aphasia: A language-based dementia. *New England Journal of Medicine, 348,* 1535–1542.

Mesulam, M-M. (2007). Primary progressive aphasia: A 25 year retrospective. *Alzheimer Disease and Associated Disorders, 21,* S8–S11.

Mesulam, M-M., & Weintraub, S. (1992). Spectrum of primary progressive aphasia. In M. N. Rossor (Ed.), *Unusual dementias* (pp. 583–609). London, UK: Baillière Tindall.

Mesulam, M-M., & Weintraub, S. (2008). Primary progressive aphasia and kindred disorders. In C. Duyckaerts & I. Litvan (Eds.), *Handbook of clinical neurology* (pp. 573–587). New York, NY: Elsevier.

Mesulam, M-M., Wieneke, C., Thompson, C., Rogalski, E., & Weintraub, S. (2012). Quantitative classification of primary progressive aphasia at early and mild impairment stages. *Brain, 135,* 1537–1553.

Mesulam, M-M., Rogalski, E., Wieneke, C., Cobia, D., Rademaker, A., Thompson, C., & Weintraub, S. (2009). Neurology of anomia in the semantic subtype of primary progressive aphasia. *Brain*, *132*, 2553–2565.

Munoz, D. G., Ros, R., Fatas, M., Bermejo, F., & Yebenes, J. G. (2007). Progressive nonfluent aphasia associated with a new mutation V363I in tau gene. *American Journal of Alzheimer's Disease and Other Dementias*, *22*, 294–299.

Osher, J., Wicklund, A., Rademaker, A., Johnson, N., & Weintraub, S. (2007). The Mini-Mental State Examination in behavioral variant frontotemporal dementia and primary progressive aphasia. *American Journal of Alzheimer's Disease and Other Dementias*, *22*, 468–473.

Pick, A. (1904). Zur Symptomatologie der linksseitigen Schlaffenlappenatrophie. *Monatsschrift für Psychiatrie und Neurologie*, *16*, 378–388.

Pick, A. (1982). Ueber die Beziehungen der senilen Hirnatrophie zur Aphasie. *Prager Medizinische Wochenschrift*, *17*, 165–167.

Rabinovici, G. D., Jagust, W. J., Furst, A. J., Ogar, J. M., Racine, C. A., Mormino, E. C.,...Gorno-Tempini, M. L. (2008). Aß amyloid and glucose metabolism in three variants of primary progressive aphasia. *Annals of Neurology*, *64*, 388–401.

Rademakers, R., Baker, M., Gass, J., Adamson, J., Huey, E. D., Momeni, P.,...Hutton, M. (2007). Phenotypic variability associated with progranulin haploinsufficiency in patients with the common 1477C-T (Arg493X) mutation: An international initiative. *Lancet Neurology*, *6*, 857–868.

Reed, D. A., Johnson, N. A., Thompson, C., Weintraub, S., & Mesulam, M-M. (2004). A clinical trial of bromocriptine for tretment of primary progressive aphasia. *Annals of Neurology*, *56*, 750.

Rogalski, E., Johnson, N., Weintraub, S., & Mesulam, M-M. (2008). Increased frequency of learning disability in patients with primary progressive aphasia and their first degree relatives. *Archives of Neurology*, *65*, 244–248.

Rogalski, E., Cobia, D., Harrison, T. M., Wieneke, C., Thompson, C., Weintraub, S., & Mesulam, M-M. (2011). Anatomy in language impairments in primary progressive aphasia. *Journal of Neuroscience*, *31*, 3344–3350.

Rogalski, E., Rademaker, A., Helenewski, I., Johnson, N., Bigio, E., Mishra, M.,...Mesulam, M. (2011). APOE e4 is a susceptibility factor in amnestic but not aphasic dementias. *American Journal of Alzheimer's Disease and Other Dementias*, *25*, 159–163.

Rogalski, E. J., & Mesulam, M-M. (2009). Clinical trajectories and biological features of primary progressive aphasia (PPA). *Current Alzheimer Research*, *6*, 331–336.

Rosenfeld, M. (1909). Die partielle Grosshirnatrophie. *Journal of Psychology and Neurology*, *14*, 115–130.

Sapolsky, D., Bakkour, A., Negreira, A., Nalipinski, P., Weintraub, S., Mesulam, M-M.,...Dickerson, B. C. (2010). Cortical neuroanatomic correlates of symptom severity in primary progressive aphasia. *Neurology*, *75*, 358–366.

Schwartz, M. F., Kimberg, D. Y., Walker, G. M., Faseyitan, O., Brecher, A., Dell, G. S., & Coslett, H. B. (2009). Anterior temporal involvement in semantic word retrieval: Voxel-based lesion-symptom mapping evidence from aphasia. *Brain*, *132*, 3411–327.

Sérieux, P. (1893). Sur un cas de surdité verbale pure. *Revue de Medecine*, *13*, 733–750.

Simón-Sánchez, J., Dopper, E. G. P., Cohn-Hokke, P. E., Hukema, R. K., Nicolau, N., Seelar, H.,...van Swieten, J. C. (2012). The clinical and pathological phenotype of C9ORF72 hexanucleotide repeat expansions. *Brain*, *135*, 723–735.

Sonty, S. P., Mesulam, M-M., Weintraub, S., Johnson, N. A., Parrish, T. P., & Gitelman, D. R. (2007). Altered effective connectivity within the language network in primary progressive aphasia. *Journal of Neuroscience*, *27*, 1334–1345.

Sonty, S. P., Mesulam, M-M., Thompson, C. K., Johnson, N. A., Weintraub, S., Parrish, T. B., & Gitelman, D. R. (2003). Primary progressive aphasia: PPA and the language network. *Annals of Neurology*, *53*, 35–49.

Thompson, C. K., Cho, S., Hsu, C-J., Wieneke, C., Rademaker, A., Weitner, B. B.,...Weintraub, S. (2011). Dissociations between fluency and agrammatism in primary progressive aphasia. *Aphasiology*, *26*, 20–43.

Weintraub, S., & Mesulam, M-M. (1985). Mental state assessment of young and elderly adults in behavioral neurology. In M-M. Mesulam (Ed.), *Principles of behavioral neurology* (pp. 71–123). Philadelphia, PA: FA Davis.

Weintraub, S., & Mesulam, M-M. (1993). Four neuropsychological profiles in dementia. In F. Boller & J. Grafman (Eds.), *Handbook of neuropsychology* (pp. 253–281). Amsterdam, The Netherlands: Elsevier.

Weintraub, S., & Mesulam, M-M. (1996). From neuronal networks to dementia: Four clinical profiles. In F. Fôret, Y. Christen, & F. Boller (Eds.), *La demence: Pourquoi?* (pp. 75–97).

Paris, France: Foundation Nationale de Gerontologie.

Weintraub, S., Mesulam, M-M., Wieneke, C., Rademaker, A., Rogalski, E. J., & Thompson, C. K. (2009). The Northwestern Anagram Test: Measuring sentence production in primary progressive aphasia. *American Journal of Alzheimer's Disease and Other Dementias, 24,* 408–416.

Weintraub, S., & Morhardt, D. J. (2005). Treatment, education and resources for non Alzheimer dementia: One size does not fit all. *Alzheimer Care Quarterly, 2005* (July/September), 201–214.

Weintraub, S., Peavy, G. M., O'Connor, M., Johnson, N. A., Acar, D., Sweeney, J., & Janssen, I. (2000). Three words—three shapes: A clinical test of memory. *Journal of Clinical and Experimental Neuropsychology, 22,* 267–278.

Weintraub, S., Rogalski, E., Shaw, E., Salwani, S., Rademaker, A., Wieneke, C., & Mesulam, M-M. (2012). Verbal and nonverbal memory in primary progressive aphasia: The Three Words-Three Shapes Test. *Behavioral Neurology, 26,* 67–76.

Weintraub, S., Rubin, N. P., & Mesulam, M. M. (1990). Primary progressive aphasia. Longitudinal course, neuropsychological profile, and language features. *Archives of Neurology, 47*(12), 1329–1335.

Wicklund, A., Johnson, N., & Weintraub, N. (2004). Preservation of reasoning in primary progressive aphasia: Further differentiation from Alzheimer's disease and the behavioral presentation of frontotemporal dementia. *Journal of Clinical and Experimental Neuropsychology, 26,* 347–355.

10

Posterior Cortical Atrophy

David F. Tang-Wai, Alison Lake, and Neill Graff-Radford

The first published reported case of posterior cortical atrophy (PCA) was by Arnold Pick in 1902 when he described a patient with a late-onset dementia that was characterized by a partial Balint's syndrome, alexia, aphasia, agraphia, and prosopagnosia. Over the subsequent 86 years, there have been few case reports that were described with autopsies demonstrating Alzheimer pathology (Table 10.1).

It was not until 1988 when Frank Benson et al. described five patients who developed a progressive dementia that presented with signs and symptoms of higher cortical visual dysfunction. All patients developed features of Balint's syndrome, Gertsmann's syndrome, visual agnosia, alexia, agraphia, and transcortical sensory aphasia (Benson, Davis, & Synder, 1988). Memory, insight, and judgment were relatively preserved until late in the course of the disorder. Both the observed cortical abnormalities and neuroimaging findings demonstrate dysfunction of the posterior association cortex (Benson et al., 1988; Giannakopoulos et al., 1999; Mendez, Mendez, Martin, Smyth, & Whitehouse, 1990; Rizzo et al., 2002). Benson suggested the descriptive term "posterior cortical atrophy (PCA)," to identify the disorder until a definitive cause could be identified.

Clinical Features

PCA is a rare, typically presenile (young-onset), dementia syndrome and can account for 5% of patients in a specialized dementia clinic (Snowden et al., 2007). However, the exact prevalence and incidence of PCA are unknown. The age of onset is usually in the mid-50s to 60s; however, patients in their 70s can also develop PCA. Both men and women can be affected; however, there appears to be an overrepresentation of affected women.

The presenting features of PCA are determined by the posterior cortical anatomical areas involved. Common presenting features include a partial Balint's syndrome (usually simultanagnosia), partial Gerstmann's syndrome, and visual field defects. Other less common features include a language disturbance and ideomotor apraxia.

Diagnosis may often be overlooked or delayed early in the course of the disorder because patients complain of visual difficulties (Table 10.2) (Tang-Wai et al., 2004) and usually have normal ophthalmological examinations. At times, patients are either given stronger lens prescriptions or even receive cataract extractions, but despite this, there is no improvement of visual symptoms. It is not until other symptoms and signs develop, such as a memory complaint, language

TABLE 10.1 Posterior Cortical Atrophy Review of the Literature From 1902 to 1988

Source	No. of Patients	Onset Before 65 years	Preserved Early Insight	Balint's Syndrome (all or partial)	Gerstmann's Syndrome (all or partial)	Other Cortical Dysfunctions	Longitudinal Follow-up	Pathology
Pick (1902)	1	N	?	Y (partial)	?	Alexia, aphasia, agraphia, prosopagnosia	?	N
Rosenfeld (1905)	1	N	?	N	?	Visual agnosia, topographagnosia,	?	Occipital atrophy
Grünthal (1926)	1	Y	?	N	?	Cortical blindness	?	AD
Pötzl (1928)	2	Y (1)	?	N	?	Visual agnosia, topographagnosia (1), agraphia (1), aphasia (1)	?	AD (1)
Grünthal (1928)	1	Y	?	Y (all)	Y	Topographagnosia, alexia, agraphia, aphasia	?	AD
Horn and Stengel (1930)	1	Y	?	Y (partial)	?	Alexia, agraphia, aphasia	?	AD
Von Hagen (1941)	1	Y	?	N	N	Visual agnosia, alexia, agraphia	?	N
Leuchtenberg (1942)	1	Y	?	Y (partial)	Y	Topographagnosia, alexia, aphasia, apraxia	?	N
Delay Nepveu, and Desclaux (1944)	1	Y	?	Y (all)	N	Alexia, agraphia, apraxia, aphasia, astereognosis	?	N
Morel (1945)	1	Y	?	Y (Sm, OcAp)	N	Alexia, aphasia, agraphia, color agnosia	N	AD
Ostenfeld (1963)	1	N	N	N	N	Visual agnosia, aphasia	?	Bioccipital atrophy
Taylor and Warrington (1971)	1	Y	?	N	N	Visual agnosia, aphasia, auditory agnosia, prosopagnosia	?	N
Bender and Feldmann (1972)	2	Y	?	N	N	Topographanosia (2), alexia (1), prosopagnosia, visual hallucinations	?	N
Flekkoy (1976)	1	N	?	Y (partial)	Y (acalculia)	Alexia, topographagnosia	?	N
Faden and Townsend (1976)	1	N	?	N	N	Cortical blindness, aphasia	?	AD
Cogan (1979)	2	Y	?	Y (partial in 1)	N	Visual agnosia, topographagnosia, alexia, apraxia, hemineglect (1), prosopagnosia (1)	?	AD (1)

(continued)

TABLE 10.1 Continued

Source	No. of Patients	Onset Before 65 years	Preserved Early Insight	Balint's Syndrome (all or partial)	Gerstmann's Syndrome (all or partial)	Other Cortical Dysfunctions	Longitudinal Follow-up	Pathology
Magnani et al. (1982)	1	Y	?	?		Visual agnosia, topographagnosia, alexia, agraphia, prosopagnosia	N	N
Cogan (1985)	3	Y	Y	N	Y (acalculia)	Dressing apraxia, alexia, topographic agnosia, visual agnosia, visual hallucination	Y	AD (1)
Nissen et al. (1985)	1	Y	?	N	Y (acalculia)	Visual agnosia, topographagnosia, alexia, agraphia, prosopagnosia	?	N
De Renzi (1986)	2	Y	?	N	Y (acalculia)	Visual agnosia, topographagnosia, alexia, apraxia, prosopagnosia		
Benson et al. (1988)	5	Y	Y	Y (all)	Y	Alexia, agraphia, visual agnosia, transcortical sensory aphasia	Y	N*

Y = yes or present; N = no or absent; ? = unknown or not clearly documented

TABLE 10.2 Samples of Complaints Expressed by Patients and/or Caregivers in Describing Their Visual Difficulty

Nonspecific complaints
- "I could see, but couldn't see"
- "…vision dimmed and blurred" and "…couldn't focus while reading"
- "[I] get dizzy when [I see] objects [are] moved in certain ways"
- "…when looking at letters, I can't see them together—better if larger print"

Complaints suggestive of simultanagnosia
- "…difficulty seeing things that are right in front of him"
- "I can see it, but I can't put it together"
- "…when she looks out at the panorama of view, she does not see items that she should see"
- "…having difficulty picking out one thing out of the many when she looked at a multitude of objects"
- "I get dizzy when I am in a store."
- "…can't tell where I sign on a cheque"

Complaints suggestive of optic ataxia
- ….with an upright vacuum…with a cord rolled around the handle…she would get confused and could not put the cord back [around the handle]

Complaints suggestive of visual tracking difficulties
- Difficulty tracking reading material horizontally; used a ruler under each line to help

Complaints suggestive of prosopagnosia
- Difficulty recognizing faces, geographical and landmark structures

disturbance, visual field cut, or symptoms suggestive of simultanagnosia, that patients are referred to a specialist. Even at this stage, diagnosis may still remain elusive because memory may be relatively preserved and simultanagnosia is difficult to demonstrate. Using a collage of items (e.g., animals) and asking patients to pick out the different items is helpful in detecting this problem. One set of diagnostic criteria has been established to help with identification and diagnosis (Table 10.3) (Tang-Wai et al., 2006).

Often patients present with anxiety in the absence of a prior psychiatric history (Crutch et al., 2012). This anxiety appears to be related to their preserved insight that there is

TABLE 10.3 Proposed Diagnostic Criteria of Posterior Cortical Atrophy

Core features
- Insidious onset and gradual progression
- Presentation with visual complaints, in the absence of significant primary ocular disease to explain the symptoms
- Absence of stroke or tumour
- Absence of early parkinsonism and hallucinations
- Relative preservation of anterograde memory and insight (early in the disorder)

Plus any of the following symptoms
- Simultanagnosia with or without optic ataxia or ocular apraxia
- Constructional dyspraxia
- Visual field defects
- Environmental disorientation
- Any of the elements of Gerstmann's syndrome

Supportive clinical features
- Alexia
- Presenile onset
- Ideomotor or dressing apraxia
- Prosopagnosia

Investigations
- Neuropsychological deficits relating to parietal and/or occipital regions
- Focal or asymmetric atrophy in parietal and/or occipital regions on structural imaging
- Focal or asymmetric hypoperfusion or hypometabolism in parietal and/or occipital regions on functional imaging

a cognitive dysfunction, which the patient is often unable to spontaneously describe. It is often not until the patient is questioned about which circumstances cause the anxiety that symptoms of higher order visual processing are described, such as being visually overwhelmed in grocery stores, which is suggestive of simultanagnosia.

Some specific symptoms related to higher order visual processing include the following:

- Reading difficulties are often reported, including letter-by-letter reading and using a ruler to help with tracking the line of print (without which the person may lose track of the sentence on the page)
- Inability to fill out forms because the individual elements on the form are difficult to process
- Ability to a see small portion of a picture but not the entire picture
- Inability to read the time on an analog watch but not a digital watch
- Inability to find static objects in front of the patient, such as a cluttered kitchen drawer, a refrigerator, or doorknobs or light switches
- Getting lost or disoriented in familiar areas
- Misjudging distances—especially while driving or parking a car (resulting in some cases in dents/scrapes or minor accidents)

Besides visual symptoms, early symptoms sometimes include difficulty performing calculations, writing, dressing, or using common objects or tools. Over time, patients with PCA progress into a generalized dementia as the other cognitive domains become affected.

The evolution of a patient's symptoms can help elucidate the underlying pathological process. The later development of REM sleep behavior disorder, parkinsonism, and visual hallucinations suggests concomitant dementia with Lewy bodies (Josephs et al., 2006; Tang-Wai et al., 2004). The development of asymmetric parkinsonism, dystonia, myoclonus, and apraxia suggests corticobasal degeneration (Tang-Wai et al., 2003).

Neuroimaging

Structural neuroimaging with either computed tomography (CT) or magnetic resonance imaging (MRI) of the brain often demonstrates parietal and occipital atrophy with some involvement of the temporal lobes when compared to persons with normal cognition (Fig. 10.1) (Tang-Wai et al., 2004). Findings are often similar to typical Alzheimer's disease (AD), with greater involvement of the parietal and occipital areas and relative preservation of the hippocampi among patients with PCA (Crutch et al., 2012). Diffusion tensor imaging (DTI) studies have demonstrated involvement in the white matter tracts in the posterior regions of the brain, including the bilateral inferior longitudinal fasciculus, inferior fronto-occipital fasciculus, and splenium of the corpus callosum (Migliaccio et al., 2012; Yoshida et al., 2004).

Functional neuroimaging with either single-photon emission computed tomography (SPECT) or positron emission tomography (PET) mirrors the structural imaging findings with either hypoperfusion or hypometabolism, respectively, of the parietal and occipital areas (Nestor, Caine, Fryer, Clarke, & Hodges, 2003) (Fig. 10.2). Bilateral hypometabolism of the frontal eye fields has also been found on PET studies and may

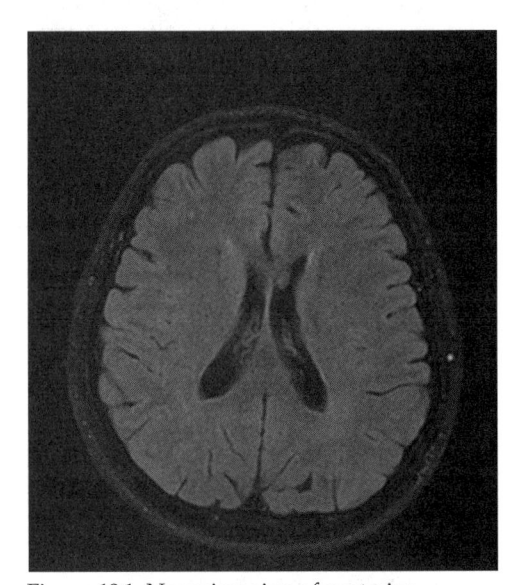

Figure 10.1 Neuroimaging of posterior cortical atrophy (PCA). Magnetic resonance imaging (MRI) axial FLAIR images of three patients: normal cognition (left panel), early stages of PCA (middle panel), and late stages of PCA (right panel) demonstrating parietal and occipital atrophy.

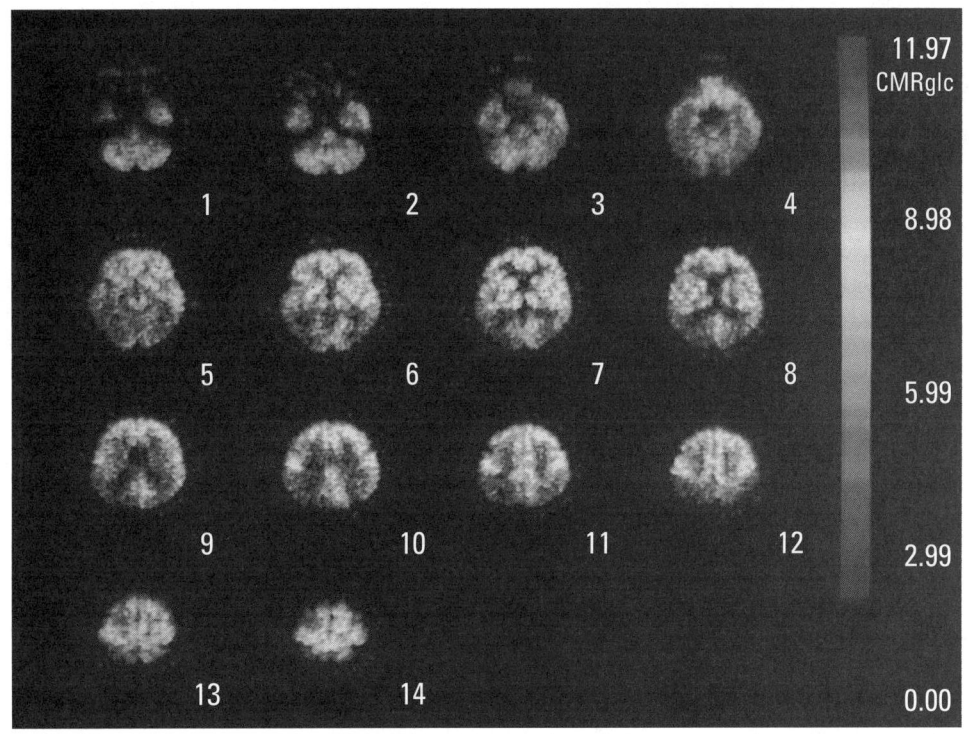

Figure 10.2 Positron emission tomography (PET) scan of a fourth patient with posterior cortical atrophy demonstrating parietal and occipital hypometabolism. (See color plate section)

represent the cause of ocular apraxia in PCA (Kas et al., 2011).

Individual case reports of patients with PCA undergoing amyloid-PET imaging with the Pittsburg B compound (PiB) have shown increased PiB binding in the occipital regions. However, when compared to typical AD, patients with PCA also showed similar diffuse PiB binding in the frontal, temporal, parietal, and occipital cortices despite the typical findings of additional hypometabolism posteriorly in the occipital regions on FDG-PET (Rosenbloom et al., 2011).

Genetics

There are two major findings thus far about the genetics of PCA. To date, there have not been any published cases of more than one person with PCA within a family with dementia (Crutch et al., 2012). There is no difference in the number of persons with a positive family history of dementia in PCA and persons with typical AD (Mendez, Ghajarania, & Perryman, 2002; Tang-Wai et al., 2004).

Examination of the frequency of apolipoprotein E (*APOE*) genotype between PCA and AD did not demonstrate any difference with typical AD or a significantly lower frequency than amnestic AD (Crutch et al., 2012). In our original series of the 40 patients where we had genetic samples, we did not identify a mutation in presenilin-1, presenilin-2, or amyloid precursor protein (unpublished data).

Biomarkers

Cerebrospinal fluid (CSF) biomarker analysis measuring Abeta-42, total tau, and phosphorylated tau among patients with PCA has shown that the profile is often consistent with typical AD with high total and phosphorylated-tau and low Abeta-42 levels (Baumann et al., 2010). In addition to functional neuroimaging, CSF biomarkers can help to discriminate AD from non-AD processes that cause PCA. In one study, three of twenty PCA patients were considered to have corticobasal degeneration, two of whom had normal CSF biomarkers while the rest had

CSF markers consistent with AD (Seguin et al., 2011).

Pathology

Although PCA is a reasonably clinically homogeneous syndrome, there is pathological heterogeneity. Corticobasal degeneration, dementia with Lewy bodies, subcortical gliosis, fatal familial insomnia, and Creutzfeld-Jacob disease have all been described as causing PCA (Renner et al., 2004). However, the most common reported pathological cause is AD with increased density of neurofibrillary tangles and in some studies amyloid plaques in the primary and association visual cortex compared to typical AD (Crutch et al., 2012). Hippocampal sparing is frequent pathological feature and accounts for the relatively preserved memory and insight of these patients at the start of the disease (Murray et al., 2011).

Management

Pharmacotherapy

As most of the cases of PCA are attributable to AD and some cases due to DLB, it is reasonable to prescribe cholinesterase inhibitors (donepezil, galantamine, or rivastigmine) and/or an NMDA-receptor antagonist (memantine). Although a few case studies have shown some benefit, however, the effectiveness of these medications for use in PCA remains largely unknown (Crutch et al., 2012).

For individuals who develop progressive and significant parkinsonism on examination, suggesting concomitant DLB or CBD, initiation of levodopa can be useful to manage the additional physical bradykinesia and rigidity.

Nonpharmacologic Therapy

One of the most valuable interventions that can be done for patients with PCA is to help them adapt their surroundings and activities to maintain their independence, which can result in clear improvement in quality of life, at least anecdotally. Since the visuospatial and visuoperceptual domains are predominantly affected in PCA, resources that benefit persons who have limited vision or who are blind would also benefit patients with PCA. General strategies include increasing the contrast of frequently used items from the background, such as light switches or doorknobs, increasing light levels within the home/environment, reducing clutter on floors and in drawers to allow easier identification of items, using a colored ruler's edge along a line of text to help with visual scanning when reading, and the use of talking books and watches. This is most beneficial in the earlier stages of the disorder while memory and insight are still relatively preserved. Ideally, referral to an occupational therapist aware of the issues regarding PCA who can perform a tailored home assessment can help the person and his or her family members. At the University of Toronto, our occupational therapist has performed several individualized home visits and has compiled a list of general recommendations (Box 10.1) for patients with PCA. Given the relative rarity of PCA, these recommendations have not been formally tested in studies but have appeared to help patients in our clinic.

BOX 10.1 Home Safety Recommendations for Patients With PCA

General Environment (Resource Center; CNIB; Chiu, Oliver, Marshall, & Letts, 2001)

- Simplify the environment
  - Remove clutter and objects no longer in use; keep pathways clear.
  - Remove unsafe furniture and accents (i.e., low-height stools, chairs, or tables).
  - Options to decrease the potential falls risk from scatter rugs and doormats:
    - Remove all unsafe scatter rugs/mats
    - Install nonslip underpadding

(continued)

- Replace with rugs/mats that have a rubber backing
    - Secure all edges with double sided carpet tape (not for outdoor use)
  - Relocate and secure trailing cords that are in high traffic areas.
  - Ensure there is adequate lighting: install extra lights fixtures, use night lights.
  - Leave lights on prior to nightfall.
  - Reduce glare in brightly lit areas by covering windows with sheer coverings.
  - Avoid using bare light bulbs; ensure light shades are in use.
  - Obtain a door alarm and/or safety lock.
  - Place stickers on large glass windows or large glass doors to prevent people from bumping or walking into them.
- Increase contrast
  - Label room doors; use yellow paper with black writing.
  - Paint doorframes and light switch plates in a contrasting color to the wall.
  - Use contrasting color dot (sticker, bumper dot, or tactile marker) to indicate the number/button to release an automatic door, on commonly used appliance settings, and for hot water taps.
  - Use contrasting color adhesive strips to mark pathways to important areas—bathroom, kitchen, living room, laundry.

Bathroom

- Reduce clutter on bathroom floor, countertop, in drawers and cabinets.
- Use high-contrast nonslip bath mat or strips.
- Safely install high-contrast grab bars in the shower or bathtub; use contrasting tactile strip on existing grab bars to differentiate from the tub or towel bar.
- Pick up bathmat when not in use and store appropriately to prevent falls.
- If there is noted difficulty accurately locating the toilet, consider obtaining a toilet seat in a contrasting bright color. Also consider obtaining a raised toilet seat with arms and taping the arms with a bright color in contrast against the toilet seat.
- Label important areas in the bathroom: toilet, sink, bathroom door (yellow paper with black writing).
- Tape handles (sink and toilet) with bright color contrasting tape to distinguish handles from the rest of the sink or the toilet.
- Use a contrasting colored tape or dot to indicate the hot water tap.
- Keep soap in a bright container (i.e., red) with contrasting color soap (i.e., white).
- Use signs as reminders to wash hands, flush toilet, brush teeth, etc.
- Keep frequently used items (toothbrush, paste) in small shallow basket or on a mat to contrast items against the counter.
- Use toothpaste that contrasts in color to the toothbrush and bristles (i.e., red toothpaste on white brush and bristles).
- Cover mirrors if necessary: often people with vision problems may not be able to recognize the item as a mirror.

Bedroom

- Use bright, contrasting color fitted sheet, top sheet, pillowcases. Each should be a different color to optimize identification and orientation to and within the bed.
- It may be easier for some to use a duvet rather then numerous sheets and blankets.
- Place a bright colored mat on nightstand to contrast against items placed on it.

Dressing

- Label drawers and shelves with high-contrast wording or pictures.
- Remove clothes that are no longer being used, including permanent removal of clothes no longer worn and temporary storage of out-of-season clothing.

(continued)

- Simplify and organize arrangement of clothing; for example, group similar items together, one drawer for shirts and another drawer for pants.
- Lay out clothing for the day.
- Minimize clothing requiring buttons and zippers and replace with elastic waists, pull-over/on, and loose clothing.
- Pin socks together when placing them in the laundry so they will stay matched.
- Ensure appropriate choice of footwear: flat, nonslip sole, enclosed toe and heel, Velcro fasteners.

Kitchen

- Indicate frequently used settings on appliances with a contrasting color bumper dot, tactile marker, bright tape, or nail polish (e.g., 350 degrees on the stove, normal cycle for the dishwasher, and the 1-minute button on the microwave).
- Dials at the front of the stove are more desirable than dials at the back of the stove in order to avoid reaching over the elements.
- Supervise the person while using the stove and, if necessary, disconnect the stove and other appliances when the person is at home alone.
- Consider using appliances with automatic shutoff (i.e., kettle).
- Place cleaning supplies away from food supplies.
- Dispose of hazardous substances that are no longer needed and store other potentially hazardous substances in a secure place (i.e., locked cupboard).
- Try to ensure that everything is put away in its routine place.
- Plan an appropriate organizational structure to the kitchen. Consider having one designated area of counter space for preferred and usual foods—an area that is both accessible and visible. Trial placing frequently used items on a contrasting mat or tray, located in the same place every day. This is in an attempt to increase independence in finding frequently used items and participating in meal preparation.
- Keep counters clear and minimize clutter.
- Other items to optimize safety, independence, and participation in the kitchen:
  - Elbow-length oven mitts to ensure maximum protection
  - Knife guard aid to enable safe use and pressure when cutting
  - Cutting board with a black side and a white side to enhance contrast while cutting
  - Gooseneck lamp above the cutting area may also assist with vision.
  - Large-print timer
  - Liquid measure tool to assist in pouring liquids and avoid spills
  - Relabel jars and canned goods using a thick black marker, white recipe card, single words, and elastic bands.

Eating

- Use brightly colored contrasting dishes and ensure they are all one solid color (no patterns and no ridged edges).
- Use a dark solid-colored placemat if using light-colored plates and use a light solid-colored placemat if using dark plates.
- Light-colored food will be easier to see on a solid dark-colored dish and dark food on a light dish.
- Avoid patterned table clothes.
- Maintain a strict pattern for mealtime setup. For example, always place the same utensils, drinking glass, and condiments in the same place for every meal.
- Avoid cluttering the eating area and only have necessary items within reach.
- Use verbal directions as reminders of where items are located (i.e., "Your glass is on your right," and "Salt and pepper is on your left.")
- Use plate guards if necessary during meal times.

(continued)

Stairs

- Ensure adequate lighting on the stairs; with switches at both the top and bottom.
- Install secure railings on at least one if not both sides.
- Install railing extensions that go further than the top and bottom of the stairs.
- Remove or replace unsafe flooring with a plain, nonslip surface.
- Contrasting color strips (paint or tape) on the edge of each individual step, as well as a tactile cue at the tope and the bottom of the stairs (both inside and outside).

Progression

- Install a lockable door or safety gate to prevent the use of stairs.
- Arrange living area that can be maintained on one level.

Medication Routine

- Supervision of medication routine is usually recommended.
- Store medications in a secure place.
- Remove and properly dispose of medications that are no longer needed or have expired.
- Inquire whether the medication routine can be simplified (i.e., to once a day instead of three times a day).
- Other ways to simplify a meds routine: prefilled blister packs; medication organizers and alarms; list of current medications; medication schedule.

Scheduling and Telephone Use

- Use a phone with large-print and high-contrast numbers, as well as one-touch programmable numbers.
- Program emergency and frequently used numbers into the phone and add tactile and/or high-contrast markers to increase ease of identification.
- Establish a dedicated communication area with needed items, including the phone, notepad, pen, whiteboard with large writing area, and a black marker.
- Place the telephone on a bright contrasting color mat.
- Use contrasting colored tape to outline phone cradle.
- If possible and necessary, utilize a voice activation service for phone dialing.
- Use talking watches or clocks to indicate the time and appointments.

Safety Issues

Driving is not recommended in persons with PCA. Management of finances will need supervision by family or trusted person. We often recommend, if not already done, that persons with PCA assign power of attorney for both health and financial decisions in the future event they become incapable of making decisions for themselves.

References

Baumann, T. P., Duyar, H., Sollberger, M., Kuhle, J., Regeniter, A., Gomez-Mancilla, B.,...Monsch, A. U. (2010). CSF-tau and CSF-Abeta (1-42) in posterior cortical atrophy. *Dementia and Geriatric Cognitive Disorders, 29*, 530–533.

Bender, M. B., & Feldmann, M. (1972). The so-called "visual agnosias." *Brain, 95*, 173–186.

Benson, F., Davis, J., & Synder, B. D. (1988). Posterior cortical atrophy. *Archives of Neurology, 45*, 789–793.

Canadian National Institute for the Blind. *Independent living*. Retrieved March 2014, from http://www.cnib.ca/en/living/independent-living/Pages/default.aspx

Chiu, T., Oliver, R., Marshall, L., & Letts, L. (2001). *Safety assessment of function and the environment for rehabilitation (SAFER) tool manual*. Toronto, ON: COTA Comprehensive Rehabilitation and Mental Health Services.

Cogan, D. G. (1985). Visual disturbances with focal progressive dementing disease. *American Journal of Opthalmology, 100*, 68–72.

Cogan, D. G. (1979). Visuospatial dysgnosia. *American Journal of Ophthalmology, 88,* 361–368.
Crutch, S. J., Lehmann, M., Schott, J. M., Rabinovici, G. D., Rossor, M. N., & Fox, M. C. (2012). Posterior cortical atrophy. *Lancet Neurology, 11,* 170–178.
De Renzi, E. (1986). Slowly progressive visual agnosia or apraxia without dementia. *Cortex, 22,* 171–180.
Delay, J., Nepveu, P., & Desclaux, P. (1944). La forme pariéto-occipitale de la maladie Pick. Etude de l'agnosie visuelle. *Revue Neurologique, 76,* 264–265.
Faden, A. I., & Townsend, J. J. (1976). Myoclonus in Alzheimer's disease. A confusing sign. *Archives of Neurology, 33,* 278–280.
Flekkoy, K. (1976). Visual agnosia and cognitive defects in a case of Alzheimer's disease. *Biological Pychiatry, 11,* 333–344.
Formaglio, M., Costes, N., Seguin, J., Tholance, Y., Le Bars, D., Roullet-Solignac, I., . . . Vighetto, A. (2011). In vivo demonstration of amyloid burden in posterior cortical atrophy: A case series with PET and CSF findings. *Journal of Neurology, 258,* 1841–1851.
Giannakopoulos, P., Gold, G., Duc, M., Michel, J. P., Hof, P. R., & Bouras, C. (1999). Neuroanatomic correlates of visual agnosia in Alzheimer's disease: A clinicopathologic study. *Neurology, 52,* 71–77.
Grünthal, E. (1926). Uber die Alzheimermersche Krankheit. Eine histopathologisch-klinische Studie. *Zeitschrift für die gesamte Neurologie und Psychiatrie, 101,* 128–157.
Grünthal, E. (1928). Zur hirnpathologischen Analyse der Alzheimerschen Krankheit. *Psychiatrisch-Neurologische Wochenschrift, 36,* 401–407.
Horn, L., & Stengel, E. (1930). Zur Klinik und Pathologie der Pickshen Atrophie. *Zeitschrift für die gesamte Neurologie und Psychiatrie, 128,* 265–273.
Josephs, K. A., Whitwell, J. L., Boeve, B. F., Knopman, D. S., Tang-Wai, D. F., Drubach, D. A., . . . Petersen, R. C. (2006). Visual hallucinations in posterior cortical atrophy. *Archives of Neurology, 63,* 1427–1432.
Kas, A., de Souza, L. C., Samri, D., Bartolomeo, P., Lacomblez, L., Kalafat, M., . . . Sarazin, M. (2011). Neural correlates of cognitive impairment in posterior cortical atrophy. *Brain, 134,* 1464–78.
Leuchtenberg, P. (1942). Ein klinischer Fall von Alzheimerscher Krankheit mit "akzentuierter" Atrophie der Parieto-Occipital-Region. *Allgemeine Zeitschrift für Psychiatrie, 121,* 97–123.
Mendez, M. F., Ghajarania, M., & Perryman, K. M. (2002). Posterior cortical atrophy: Clinical characteristics and differences compared to Alzheimer's disease. *Dement Geriatr Cogn Disord 2002*; 14: 33–40.
Mendez, M. F., Mendez, M. A., Martin, R., Smyth, K. A., & Whitehouse, P. J. (1990). Complex visual disturbances in Alzheimer's disease. *Neurology, 49,* 439–443.
Migliaccio, R., Agosta, F., Scola, E., Magnani, G., Cappa, S. F., Pagani, E., . . . Filippi, M. (2012). Ventral and dorsal streams in posterior cortical atrophy: A DT MRI study. *Neurobiology of Aging, 33,* 2572–2584.
Morel, F. (1945). Les aires striée, parastriée et peristriée dans les troubles de la fonction visuelle au cours de la maladie d'Alzheimer. *Confinia Neurologica, 6,* 238–242.
Murray, M. E., Graff-Radford, N. R., Ross, O. A., Petersen, R. C., Duara, R., & Dickson, D. (2011). W. Neuropathologically defined subtypes of Alzheimer's disease with distinct clinical characteristics: A retrospective study. *Lancet Neurology, 10,* 785–796.
Nestor, P. J., Caine, D., Fryer, T. D., Clarke, J., & Hodges, J. R. (2003). The topography of metabolic deficits in posterior cortical atrophy (the visual variant of Alzheimer's disease) with FDG-PET. *Journal of Neurology, Neurosurgery and Psychiatry, 74,* 1521–1529.
Nissen, M. J., Corkin, S., Buonanno, F. S., Growdon, J. H., Wray, S. H., & Bauer, J. (1985). Spatial vision in Alzheimer's disease. *Archives of Neurology, 42,* 667–671.
Ostenfeld, I. (1963). Et tilfaelde af visuel agnosi, forbundet med elektiv atrofi af okcipitallapperne. *Ugeskrift for Laeger, 125,* 954–957.
Pick, A. (1902). Über eine eigenthümliche Sehströng senile Dementer. *Jahrbucher für Psychiatrie und Neurologie, 22,* 35–44.
Pötzl, O. (1928). Die optisch-agnostischen Störungen. In O. Pötzl (Ed.), *Die Aphasielehre vom Standpunkte der klinischen Psychiatrie.* Leipzig, Germany: Wien.
Renner, J. A., Burns, J. M., Hou, C. E., McKeel, D. W. Jr., Storandt, M., & Morris, J. C. (2004). Progressive posterior cortical dysfunction: A clinicopathologic series. *Neurology, 63,* 1175–80.
Useful Home Adaptations for the Blind and Visually Impaired. (n.d.). *Your Low Vision Resource Center.* Retrieved October 20, 2009, http://www.lowvision.com/tips/useful-home-adaptations-for-the-blind-and-visually-impaired.
Rizzo, M., & Vecera, S. P. (2002). Psychoanatomical substrates of Bálint's syndrome. *Journal of Neurology, Neurosurgery and Psychiatry, 72,* 162–178.
Rosenbloom, M. H., Alkalay, A., Agarwal, N., Baker, S. L., O'Neil, J. P., Janabi, M., . . . Rabinovici, G. D. (2011). Distinct clinical and metabolic deficits in PCA and AD are

not related to amyloid distribution. *Neurology, 76*, 1789–1796.

Rosenfeld, M. (1905). Über Herdsymptome bei den zur Verblödung führenden Psychosen. *Zeitschrift für klinische Medicin, 56*, 59–68.

Seguin, J., Formaglio, M., Perret-Liaudet, A., Quadrio, I., Tholance, Y., Rouaud, O.,...Krolak-Salmon, P. (2011). CSF biomarkers in posterior cortical atrophy. *Neurology, 76*, 1782–1788.

Snowden, J. S., Stopford, C. L., Julien, C. L., Thompson, J. C., Gibbon, L., Pritchard, A.,...Mann, D. (2007). Cognitive phenotypes in Alzheimer's disease and genetic risk. *Cortex. 43*, 835–845.

Tang-Wai, D. F., Graff-Radford, N. R., Boeve, B. F., Dickson, D. W., Parisi, J. E., Crook, R.,...Petersen, R. C. (2004). Clinical, genetic, and neuropathologic characteristics of posterior cortical atrophy. *Neurology, 63*, 1168–1174.

Tang-Wai, D. F., Josephs, K. A., Boeve, B. F., Dickson, D. W., Parisi, J. E., & Petersen, R. C. (2003). Pathologically confirmed corticobasal degeneration presenting with visuospatial dysfunction. *Neurology, 61*, 1134–35.

Taylor, A., & Warrington, E. K. (1971). Visual agnosia: A single case report. *Cortex, 7*, 152–161.

von Hagen, K. O. (1941). Two clinical cases of mind blindness (visual agnosia) one due to carbon monoxide poisoning intoxication, one due to a diffuse degenerative process. *Bulletin of the Los Angeles Neurological Society, 6*, 191–195.

Yoshida, T., Shiga, K., Yoshikawa, K., Yamada, K., & Nakagawa, M. (2004). White matter loss in the splenium of the corpus callosum in a case of posterior cortical atrophy: A diffusion tensor imaging study. *European Neurology, 52*, 77–81.

11

Progressive Supranuclear Palsy and Corticobasal Degeneration

Stephanie Lessig and Irene Litvan

Parkinsonian disorders are defined by a clinical syndrome of akinesia associated with rigidity, tremor at rest, or gait difficulties. Patients with an "atypical" parkinsonism usually have rapid disease progression; no benefit from dopaminergic therapy; early gait, dysarthria, dysphagia, or autonomic symptomatology; and presence of oculomotor, cerebellar, or pyramidal signs. Among these disorders, progressive supranuclear palsy (PSP) and corticobasal degeneration (CBD) share similar pathology: abnormal deposition of the filamentous protein tau and association with the H1 tau genotype. In addition, they share clinical features of relatively rapid progression, poor response to levodopa, early dysarthria and dysphagia, and early frontal dementia. Moreover, PSP and CBD may have overlapping phenotypic clinical presentations. This chapter discusses the clinical features of these two tauopathies with a focus on the cognitive problems.

Progressive Supranuclear Palsy

PSP is one of the most common atypical parkinsonian disorders (Litvan et al., 1996). It was first described as a clinicopathological entity by Steele, Richardson, and Olszewski in the early 1960s (Steele, Richardson, & Olszewski 1964). Their description included patients with a gait disorder, supranuclear vertical gaze palsy, frontal cognitive dysfunction, and symmetric parkinsonism, though the definition of PSP has grown to include several other phenotypes (Imai, Nakamura, Kondo, & Narabavashi, 1993; Matsuo et al., 1991; Williams, Holton, Strand, Revesz, & Lees, 2007). Progress in the understanding of this disorder has been marked by identification of the key pathology, standardized diagnostic criteria, description of multiple phenotypes, study of genetic factors, neuroimaging, and recent development of biological therapies (Wenning, Litvan, & Tolosa, 2011).

Pathology

As there are no current diagnostic markers of PSP, pathology is the gold standard for its diagnosis. PSP is characterized by aggregates of tau protein in neurons forming neurofibrillary tangles and in glia as tufted astrocytes and oligodendroglial inclusions. These are particularly subcortical (including the basal ganglia and supranuclear oculomotor nuclei, with the most affected regions being the subthalamic nucleus and substantia nigra), though extension to the frontal cortex can occur (Barsottini, Felicio, DeAquino, & Pedoso, 2010; Dickson, Ahmed, Algom, Tsuboi, & Josephs, 2010). Pathological tau in PSP is composed of aggregates of 4 repeat (E10+) isoforms. Neurochemical studies show degeneration of the dopaminergic, cholinergic, and GABAergic systems in the striatum and other basal ganglionic and brainstem nuclei.

Clinical Features

The mean age of onset of PSP is between 55 and 75 years (Litvan et al., 1996; O'Sullivan et al., 2008). The most commonly recognized criteria for the diagnosis of "classical" PSP phenotype is the NINDS-SPSP criteria (Litvan et al., 1996, shown in Table 11.1). Using this set of criteria the estimated prevalence of PSP is 6.5 per 100,000 (Nath et al., 2001). The inclusion clinical criteria emphasize prominent postural instability with falls/tendency to falls within the first year of symptom onset and vertical supranuclear gaze palsy or slowing of vertical saccades (Litvan, 1998). These criteria were developed for high specificity, aimed at excluding features suggestive of other parkinsonian syndromes (Litvan, Agid, Calne, et al., 1996). The probable NINDS-SPSP criteria emphasizes accuracy of these criteria, when used by experienced clinicians, is about 75% (Osaki et al., 2004), with sensitivity of 75% and specficity of 98.5% (Lopez et al., 1999), as this set of criteria identifies the "classical," also called Richardson PSP phenotype.

The Neuroprotection and Natural History in Parkinson's Plus Syndromes (NNIPPS) Study Group adapted these criteria for use in large-scale clinical trials. Their criteria include an akinetic-rigid syndrome, present for 1–8 years, with an age of onset after age 30 years, although none of their patients were younger than 50. They required a supranuclear ophthalmoplegia and postural instability or falls within 3 years of disease onset in the absence of other conditions, including idiopathic Parkinson's disease, history of stroke or head trauma, or severe tremor at rest (Benismon et al., 2009).

TABLE 11.1 NINDS-SPSP Criteria for the Diagnosis of Progressive Supranuclear Palsy PSP (PSP-RS)

Possible PSP (Clinical Probable)
All three of these:
1. Gradually progressive disorder
2. Onset at age 40 or later
3. No evidence for competing diagnostic possibilities

Plus either of these:
4. Vertical gaze palsy

Or
5. Slowing of vertical saccades and prominent postural instability with falls or tendency to fall in the first year

Probable PSP (Clinical Definite)
All five of these:
1. Gradually progressive disorder
2. Onset at age 40 or later
3. No evidence for competing diagnostic possibilities
4. Vertical gaze palsy
5. Slowing of vertical saccades and prominent postural instability with falls or tendency to fall in the first year

Criteria That Exclude PSP-RS From Consideration
1. Recent encephalitis
2. Alien limb syndrome, cortical sensory deficits, or temporoparietal atrophy
3. Psychosis unrelated to dopaminergic treatment
4. Important cerebellar signs
5. Important unexplained dysautonomia
6. Severe, asymmetric parkinsonism
7. Relevant structural abnormality of basal ganglia on neuroimaging
8. Whipple's disease on CSF PCR, if indicated

PSP-RS (Richardson's Syndrome)

So-called Richardson's syndrome is the "classical" form of PSP. These patients present with early falls, axial rigidity, typically but rarely with retrocollis, and usually with the typical history of eye disturbances characterized by photophobia, blurred vision/diplopia, tearing, and on examination slowed and hypometric vertical saccades preceding the development of supranuclear vertical gaze palsy, as well as decreased convergence, square-wave jerks, and eyelid apraxia. Although vertical gaze palsy is the defining feature, it may occur several years after symptom onset. PSP-RS patients also have early slow and slurred speech, and dysphagia. Cognitive features, including intellectual slowing and early executive function impairment, are characteristic (see later discussion). Most patients become dependent within 3–4 years of diagnosis (Gerstenecker et al., 2013).

Motor Features

The first motor symptom of PSP is usually postural instability and tendency to fall, which is also a large source of morbidity and mortality. Other common early or presenting features include dysarthria, bradykinesia, and monotonous speech (Jankovic, Friedman, Pirozzolo, & McCrary, 1990; Litvan et al. 1996). Examination may show an akinetic-rigid syndrome, with prominent axial rigidity and symmetric bradykinesia. The neck may be held in abnormal position (most typical but infrequently retrocollis) (Litvan, Agid, et al., 1996). Gait may appear wide-based and unsteady. In addition to early falls, dysarthria and dysphagia may be prominent, which increases the risk of aspiration pneumonia, another source of morbidity and mortality in PSP. At times this phenotype is misdiagnosed initially as Parkinson's disease postural instability gait disorder (PIGD) variant.

Visual Symptoms

Symptoms of visual disturbance are an infrequent presenting symptom and can include diplopia, difficulties reading, and blurred vision (Pelak & Hall, 2004). Characteristc eye findings in PSP include supranuclear deficits in either downward or upward gaze preceded by slowness of vertical saccades and decreased or absence of vertical optokinetic nystagmus, later affecting horizontal gaze. Vertical supranuclear gaze palsy may be a presenting symptom in less than 10% of the cases; it often develops within 3–4 years of symptom onset but at times is never clinially manifested (Litvan et al., 1996). As upgaze abnormalities can occur in other neurodegenerative diseases as well as in the course of normal aging, limitations in downward gaze are considered more specific for PSP (Litvan, Campbell, et al., 1997); however, specificity increases when the upward gaze abnormalities are associated with absence of OKNs and slowing of saccades.

Cognitive Features

Up to 70% of patients with PSP have been reported as having a "frontal" or classically "subcortical" dementia (Kertesz & McMonagle, 2010). Initial descriptions of cognitive impairment in PSP were characterized as a "subcortical dementia" (Albert, Feldman, & Willis, 1974). This was defined by forgetfulness, slowness of mentation, personality or mood changes, and impaired ability to manipulate acquired knowledge, in the absence of "cortical" features of aphasia, agnosia, or apraxia. This was noted to be similar to patients with frontal lobe lesions, and frontal dysfunction does appear early in classical PSP (Ghosh et al., 2012; Grafman, Litvan, & Stark, 1995; Pillon, Dubois, Ploska, & Agid, 1991). Complex tasks, including planning, attention set shifting, abstraction, and reasononing, are significantly impaired in PSP (Grafman et al., 1995; Kertesz & Monagle, 2010). This includes decreased abilities on tests of verbal fluency (Maher, Smith, & Lees, 1985; Pillon, Dubois, Lhermitte, & Agid, 1986), attentional set shifting (Robbins et al., 1994), and initiation and perseveration (Brown et al., 2010).

In addition, other studies point to notable deficits in visual attention, slowed information processing, memory retrieval, parallel processing, and executive functions (Brown et al., 2010; Grafman et al., 1995; Kertesz & Monagle, 2010; Soliveri et al., 2000; Vanvoorst et al., 2008).

Visual attention difficulty has been idenfitied in several studies, when compared to controls or other parkinsonian disorders such a multiple systems atrophy (Esmonde, Giles, Gibson, & Jodges, 1996; Grafman et al., 1995; Soliveri et al., 2000). This includes tasks of visual search and line orientation (Soliveri et al., 2000). Recent studies suggest this deficit is a primary cognitive problem that correlates with the degree of disruption of eye movement abnormalities (DiFabio, Zampieri, Tuite, & Konczak, 2006).

Slowed information processing has been described as taking increased time to respond (up to several minutes to respond to a single question). This feature can be marked (Albert et al., 1974). This slowing also appears to be independent of motor slowing (Dubois, Pillon, Legault, & Lhermitte, 1988).

Memory is usually preserved, although retrieval is affected. Characteristically, in PSP-RS short-term storage seems preserved (Grafman et al., 1995), characterized by impaired free recall with preserved recognition memory (Kertesz & Monagle, 2010). Encoding is usually preserved in PSP-RS.

Behavioral changes are typically observed in patients with the PSP-RS phenotype. Usually, they present with significant apathy, frequently confused with depression (Litvan et al., 1996), impulsivity and less frequently disinhibition. There are cases reported of patients presenting with behavioral disturbance suggestive of frontotemporal dementia as well (Hassan, Parisi, & Josephs, 2011). In fact, frontotemporal dementia can also be a PSP phenotypic presentation.

PSP-P (Parkinsonism)

This phenotype occurs in about one third of patients and is more indolent, with initial PD-like features that include asymmetric bradykinesia and rigidity, rest tremor, and clear but eventually limited levodopa response. Falls and cognitive impairment occur at later stages than in PSP-RS. These patients have a slower progression, though may look similar to PSP-RS in about 6 years. Pathology is greater in the basal ganglia and brainstem, with less observed in the cortex than that seen with PSP-RS (Barsottini et al., 2010; Dickson et al., 2010).

PSP-PAGF (Pure Akinesia With Gait Freezing)

Pure akinesia with gait freezing is a rare phenotypic presentation of PSP initially described by Imai (Imai, 1996). It is characterized by a gradual onset of pure gait freezing, in the absence of limb rigidity or eye movement abnormalities for several years. Micrographia and hypophonia could also be present. The majority of the patients with this phenotype have postmortem PSP pathology. They also have a significantly slower progression than PSP-RS (Compta et al., 2007; Williams et al., 2007). Pathology is milder and similar to that seen in PSP-P (Barsottini et al., 2010; Dickson et al., 2010).

PSP-PNFA (Progressive Nonfluent Aphasia)

There are very few case reports of PSP patients presenting with progressive nonfluent aphasia (PSP-PNFA). However, most PSP patients have decreased spontaneous speech and verbal fluency, which as the retrieval deficits, are characteristic features of their significant executive dysfunction. PSP-PNFA patients eventually develop vertical supranuclear gaze palsy that allows the diagnosis of PSP later in the disease course. Patients with this phenotype have increased midbrain atrophy compared to those with pure PNFA (without a gaze palsy) (Rohrer et al., 2010).

PSP-CBS (Corticobasal Syndrome)

Recent studies have shown that patients with this phenotype may also have underlying PSP. They usually present with a unilateral ideomotor apraxia, alien limb phenomena, aphasia, and cortical sensory deficit in addition to unilateral parkinsonism, myoclonus, and dystonia. The disease spreads contralaterally. Some may develop eye movement abnormalities, usually increased latency of saccades affecting horizontal and vertical gaze (Zadikoff & Lang, 2005). Interestingly, review of the videos corresponding to the original cases described by Steele-Richardson-Olsewski show that one of their cases had a clearly asymmetric presentation. This phenotype is further discussed later in this chapter.

Genetics

PSP is typically a sporadic disorder (Jankovic et al., 1990), but familial aggregation has been recently reported by some investigators (Borroni, Agosti, Magnani, DiLuca, & Pakovani, 2011; Donker et al., 2009), although it remains controversial (Vidal, Vidailhet, Derkinderen, Tzourio, & Alpérovitch, 2010). There are patients with mutations in the gene responsible for tau protein production, microtubule associated protein tau (*MAPT*) that may present with the PSP phenotype. Approximately five mutations in *MAPT* are responsible for a few autosomal dominant familial cases (Borroni et al., 2011) with this phenotype. However, there has been a link in polymorphisms in the *MAPT* gene associated with PSP. In particular, eight polymorphisms have been identified, defining two haplotypes, H1 and H2. The H1 haplotype in particular has been linked to an increased risk of PSP in the Caucasian population (Baker et al., 1999). More recently, using GWAS (Genome Wide Association Study), in addition to the H1 *MAPT* haplotype, several genes (*STX6*, *EIF2AK3*, and *MOB*) have been identified that are more prevalent in PSP patients (Hoglinger et al., 2011).

Neuroimaging

Classic findings on conventional magnetic resonance imaging (MRI) scans for PSP include the "hummingbird sign" seen on sagittal images or "morning glory sign" seen on axial images, both due to midbrain atrophy (Fig. 11.1). However, these findings may occur in later stage disease or never appear. A recent study found the sensitivity of these findings to be 73%, though with specificity of 94% and accuracy of 86% (Massey et al., 2012).

^{123}I-Ioflupane/SPECT binding to striatal dopamine transporter (DAT) uptake has been used in PSP, and it has recently been approved for clinical use in Parkinson's disease in the United States. This form of imaging shows reduced DAT binding in the caudate and putamen in PSP (Antonini et al., 2003). However, this pattern is also observed in the other atypical parkinsonian disorders. Other investigations involving VBM (voxel-based morphology) and DTI (diffusion-tensor imaging) have variable results to date.

Therapeutics

There are no known therapies to stop or slow the progression of PSP. Current treatment options, therefore, remain symptomatic.

A few of the motor features, in particular rigidity and bradykinesia, can be treated to a degree by levodopa. The effects, however, are usually modest, and often, temporary. Retrospective studies report up to 30% of patients with PSP may have some benefit from high levodopa doses averaging 1000 mg (Constantinescu, Richard, & Kurlan, 2007). Unlike Parkinson's disease, however, PSP patients usually do not develop complications of levodopa, including dyskinesias, fluctuations, and hallucinations (Nieforth & Golbe, 1993).

Select eyelid abnormalities, including blepharospasm and eyelid apraxia, may be treated with local botulinum toxin injections.

Supportive care, including physical, speech, occupational, and swallow therapy, can also be of benefit in PSP. In particular, education about cognitive, behavioral, gait, and speech abnormalities can aid families to cope with these problems. Swallow evaluations can be useful in determining the appropriate food consistency as well as provide education to the patient in safe swallowing practices.

Recent therapeutic aims have focused on reduction of the accumulation of tau protein, aimed at altering disease progression. A double-blind placebo-controlled trial involving GSK β- inhibitors such as tideglusib (NP031112) has been completed, as well as a cytoskeleton stabilizer such as davunetide (AL 108), both being ineffective. A free-radical scavenger and enhancer of metabolism such as coenzyme Q-10 is being conducted. Unfortunately, to date the

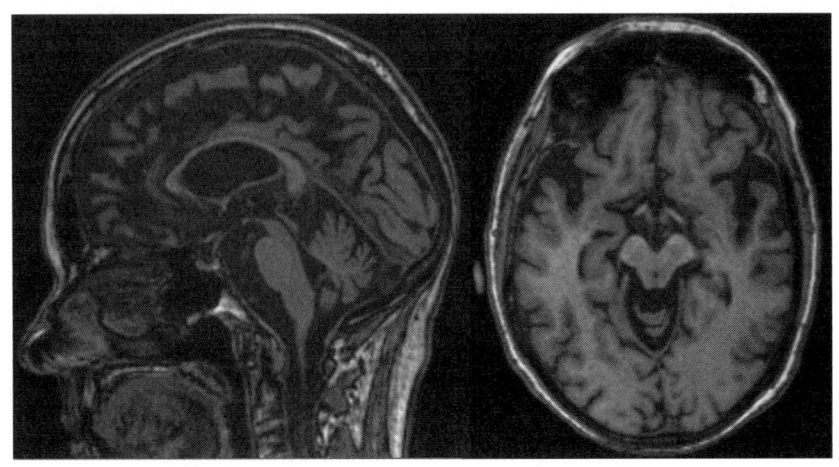

Figure 11.1 A 70-year-old woman with progressive supranuclear palsy, whose magnetic resonance imaging (MRI) scan illustrates mild brain atrophy as seen from sagittal (left) and axial (right) views.

completed trials have failed to meet primary outcome measures, but the infrastructure for conducting multicenter clinical trials continues to mature as a result of these initial attempts, facilitating next-generation trials.

Corticobasilar Degeneration

The least common atypical parkinsonian disorder, corticobasilar degeneration (CBD), was first described in 1968 (Rebeiz, Kolodny, & Richardson, 1968). This was initially described as asymmetric akinesia and rigidity, dystonia of the upper limb, apraxia, and myoclonus, now termed the corticobasal syndrome (CBS). Understanding of this complex disorder has included recognition of various clinical phenotypes and standardization of neuropathological criteria, and recently the standardization of clinical criteria (Armstrong et al., 2013). The various phenotypes include the corticobasal syndrome, primary progressive aphasia, and behavioral variant of frontotemporal dementia.

CBD typically occurs in the sixth and seventh decade, with a life expectancy of 7–9 years from symptom onset (Wenning, Litvan, & Tolosa, 2011).

Clinical Features

Corticobasal Syndrome

The classic features of CBS include asymmetric levodopa-nonresponsive parkinsonism (akinesia and rigidity) accompanied by cortical and basal ganglia dysfunction, including limb and oculomotor apraxia (loss of ability to perform these movements, despite lack of primary motor or sensory disturbances), cortical sensory deficits (extinction to double simultaneous stimulation, agraphesthesia, astereognosia), dystonic posturing of the limb, myoclonus (brief jerks), and alien limb phenomena (inability to recognize ownership of a limb) (Kouri et al., 2011). Of these symptoms, limb rigidity is observed most frequently (Armstrong et al., 2013). A large percentage of patients also develop cognitive dysfunction or frank dementia during the course of their illness.

Apraxia is a characteristic feature. Different types of apraxia are observed in CBS (Stover, Wainer, & Watts, 2004), including ideomotor, ideational, and limb-kinetic apraxia (see Chapter 5). Ideomotor apraxia is defined as impaired motor acts despite intact motor, sensory, and language function. Since patients with the CBS frequently show motor deficits, it is recommended to explore praxis in the most spared limb. Patients commit temporal and spatial errors, affecting timing, sequencing, amplitude, orientation, and limb position in space (Gross & Grossman, 2008). This is usually demonstrated by the inability to mimic activities such as brushing teeth or waving goodbye. Ideational apraxia is defined as the inability to carry out a complex, multistep task, such as making a cup of tea. Limb-kinetic apraxia causes gross difficulties with dexterity and fine motions of the affected limb, such as using scissors (Leiguarda et al., 2002).

Eye movement abnormalities can also be present, including increased latency of saccades and jerky smooth pursuit eye movements. Unlike PSP, however, range of movements is generally full. Blepharospasm and eyelid apraxia can also occur.

While CBS was traditionally thought to predict underlying CBD pathology, in recent years it has been increasingly recognized that CBD is just one of a broader set of underlying pathologies. In addition to PSP, posterior forms of Alzheimer's disease, Creutzfeld-Jakob disease, and frontotemporal lobar degeneration (usually tauopathy) can present with this phenotype.

In one series, over half of CBD cases had cognitive impairment and 70% during the disease course (Armstrong et al., 2013). This has included deficits in memory retrieval as well as other aspects of cognition. One study demonstrated patients with CBD had difficulties with word fluency, verbal comprehension, perceptual organization, and cognitive flexibility (Vanvoorst et al., 2008). Another study showed executive, language, and visuospatial deficits with relative preservation of episodic memory (Murray et al., 2007). Several series have also demonstrated prevalent memory loss, where patients with a clinical diagnosis of Alzheimer's disease proved to have CBD (Grimes, Lang, & Bergeron, 1999; Ling et al., 2010; Murray et al., 2007). See Table 11.2 for a list of clinical CBS phenotypes and Table 11.3 for current CBS diagnostic criteria.

TABLE 11.2 Proposed Clinical Phenotypes (Syndromes) Associated With the Pathology of Corticobasal Degeneration

Probable corticobasal syndrome
Asymmetric presentation of two of the following: (a) limb rigidity or akinesia, (b) limb dystonia, (c) limb myoclonus plus two of the following: (d) orobuccal or limb apraxia, (e) cortical sensory deficit, (f) alien limb phenomena (more than simple levitation)

Possible corticobasal syndrome
May be symmetric: one of the following: (a) limb rigidity or akinesia, (b) limb dystonia, (c) limb myoclonus plus one of (d) orobuccal or limb apraxia, (e) cortical sensory deficit, (f) alien limb phenomena (more than simple levitation)

Frontal behavioral-spatial syndrome
Two of the following: (a) executive dysfunction, (b) behavioral or personality changes, (c) visuospatial deficits

Nonfluent/agrammatic variant of primary progressive aphasia
Effortful, agrammatic speech plus at least one of (a) impaired grammar/sentence comprehension with relatively preserved single-word comprehension or (b) groping, distorted speech production (apraxia of speech)

Progressive supranuclear palsy syndrome
Three of the following: (a) axial or symmetric limb rigidity or akinesia, (b) postural instability or falls, (c) urinary incontinence, (d) behavioral changes, (e) supranuclear vertical gaze palsy or decreased velocity of vertical saccades

Progressive Nonfluent Aphasia

Patients with PNFA may initially present with anomia and eventually may develop a progressive loss of expressive language, including word processing, naming, and syntax. There is relative sparing of receptive and single-word comprehension. These patients may also exhibit progressive dysarthria and may eventually become mute.

Frontotemporal Dementia Phenotype Variant

Many patients with CBD present with behavioral disturbances. This can include apathy, disinhibition, irritability, personality changes, and anxiety (Grimes et al., 1999; Kertesz, Martinez-Lage, Davidson, & Munoz, 2000; Lee et al., 2011; Ling et al., 2010; Llado et al., 2008; McMonagle, Blair, & Kertesz, 2006; Murray et al., 2007). Agitation, aggressiveness, and emotional lability have also been reported (Murray et al., 2007). Social withdrawal can precede motor symptoms of CBD (described previously) by several years (Lee et al., 2011). These patients are thought to have a have a predominant frontal pathology at the outset (Lee et al., 2011). Formal assessment of these patients demonstrating apathy and disinhibition has been carried out using the Frontal Behavioral Inventory (Kertesz et al., 2000; McMonagle, Blair, & Kertesz, 2006).

PSP-RS

Patients with CBD can also present with the classical PSP phenotype described previously. Some of the series (Kouri et al., 2011) suggest that CBD patients may have more significant frontal disturbances than those observed in PSP, but future longitudinal studies are needed to identify features that could disentangle the underlying specific tauopathy.

Neuropathology

Gross findings in CBD patients with the CBS include asymmetric atrophy correlating with the onset of symptoms affecting the frontoparietal areas. Proposed criteria for pathological diagnosis (Dickson et al., 2002) emphasize tau-positive neuronal and glial lesions. Thread-like lesions in both gray and white matter, as well as astocytic plaques (as opposed to tufted astrocytes seen in PSP), are suggestive of CBD. These lesions seem to be more prominent in the primary motor and somatorsensory cortices and are at times accompanied by cortical atrophy, which may be asymmetric in the CBS (Kouri et al., 2011).

Therapeutics

There has been little advancement in therapeutics in CBD. This has been compounded

TABLE 11.3 Diagnostic Criteria for Corticobasal Degeneration (CBD)

	Clinical Research Criteria for Probable Sporadic CBD	Clinical Criteria for Possible CBD
Presentation	Insidious onset and gradual progression	Insidious onset and gradual progression
Minimum duration of symptoms, y	1	1
Age at onset, y	50	No minimum
Family history (two or more relatives)	Exclusion	Permitted
Permitted phenotypes	(1) Probable CBS or (2) FBS or NAV plus at least one CBS criteria	(1) Possible CBS or (2) FBS or NAV or (3) PSPS plus at least one CBS feature
Genetic mutation affecting tau (e.g., MAPT)	Exclusion	Permitted

CBS, corticobasal syndrome; FBS, frontal behavioral-spatial syndrome; NAV, nonfluent/agrammatic variant of primary progressive aphasia; PSPS, progressive supranuclear palsy syndrome.

by the heterogeneity of this disorder. As mentioned previously, motor symptoms respond little to parkinsonian medications such as levodopa, if at all. Clonazepam has been the most beneficial for action tremor and myoclonus, as well as for sleep in small doses.

Like PSP, supportive therapies such as swallow evaluations can determine the most appropriate food consistency. Physical therapy can help maintain mobility and prevent contractures. Occupational therapy can be helpful for daily activities such as use of utensils.

In summary: PSP and CBD present with multiple clinical phenotypes, some of which overlap such as the CBS, classical PSP, and frontotemporal behavioral variant dementia. The diagnosis of classical PSP is usually accurate, but the diagnosis of CBD is much more challenging. Biomarkers for the diagnosis are needed to diagnose these disorders early and more accurately now that biological therapies are being translated to the clinic.

References

Albert, M. L., Feldman, R. G., & Willis, A. L. (1974). The 'subcortical dementia' of progressive supranuclear palsy. *Journal of Neurology, Neurosurgery and Psychiatry, 37*, 121–130.

Antonini, A., Benti, R., & DeNotaris, R., Tesei, S., Zecchinelli, A., Sacilotto, G.,...Gerundini, P. (2003). I-Ioflupane/SPECT binding to striatal dopamine transporter (DAT) uptake in patients with Parkinson's disease, multiple system atrophy, and progressive supranuclear palsy. *Neurological Sciences, 24*, 1–2.

Armstrong, M., Litvan, I., Lang, A. E., Bak, T. H., Bhatia, K. P., Borroni, B.,...Weiner, W. J. (2013). Criteria for the diagnosis of corticobasal degeneration. *Neurology, 80*(5), 496–503.

Baker, M., Litvan, I., Houlden, H., Adamson, J., Dickson, D., Perez-Tur, J.,...Hutton, M. (1999). Association of an extended haplotype in the tau gene with progressive supranuclear palsy." *Human Molecular Genetics, 8*(4), 711–715.

Barsottini, O. G. P., Felicio, A. C., DeAquino, C. C. H., & Pedoso, J. L. (2010). Progressive supranuclear palsy: New concepts. *Arqivos de Neuropsiquiatria, 68*(6), 938–946.

Benismon, G., Ludolph, A., Agid, Y., Vidailhet, M., Payan, C., & Leigh, P. N. (2009). Riluzole treatment, survival, and diagnostic criteria in Parkinson plus disorders: The NNIPPS Study. *Brain, 132*, 156–171.

Borroni, B., Agosti, C., Magnani, E., DiLuca, M., & Pakovani, A. (2011). Genetic bases of progressive supranuclear palsy: The MAPT tau disease. *Current Medicinal Chemistry, 18*, 2655–2660.

Brown, R. C., Locomblez, L., Landwehrmeyer, B. G., Bak, T., Uttner, I., Dubois, B.,...Leigh, N. P. (2010). Cognitive impairment in patients with multiple system atrophy and progressive supranuclear palsy. *Brain, 133*(8), 2382–2393.

Compta, Y., Valldeioriola, F., Tolosa, E., Rey, M. J., Martí, M. J., & Valls-Solé, J. (2007). Long lasting pure freezing of gait preceding progressive supranuclear palsy: A clinicopathological study. *Movement Disorders, 22*(13), 1954–1958.

Constantinescu, R., Richard, I., & Kurlan, R. (2007). Levodopa responsiveness in disorders with Parkinsonism: A review of the literature. *Movement Disorders, 22*(15), 2141–2148.

Dickson, D. W., Bergeron, C., Chin, S. S., Duyckaerts, C., Horoupian, D., Ikeda, K., & Litvan, I. (2002). Office of rare diseases neuropathologic criteria for corticobasal degeneration. *Journal of Neuropathology and Experimental Neurology, 61*(11), 935–946.

Dickson, D. W., Ahmed, Z., Algom, A. A., Tsuboi, Y., & Josephs, K. A. (2010). Neuropathology of variants of progressive supranuclear palsy. *Current Opinion in Neurology, 23,* 394–400.

DiFabio, R. P., Zampieri, C., Tuite, P., & Konczak, J. (2006). Association between vestibuloocular reflex suppression during smooth pursuit movmeents of the head and attention deficit in progressive supranuclear palsy. *Movement Disorders, 21*(7), 910–915.

Donker, K. L., Boon, A. J., Azmani, A., Kamphorst, W., Breteler, M. M., Anar, B., . . . van Swieten, J. C. (2009). Familial aggregation of Parkinsonism in progressive supranuclear palsy. *Neurology, 73*(2), 98–105.

Dubois, B., Pillon, B., Legault, F., & Lhermitte, F. (1988). Slowing of cognitive processing in progressive supranuclear palsy. *Arch Neurol, 45,* 1194–1199.

Esmonde, T., Giles, E., Gibson, M., & Jodges, J. R. (1996). Neuropsychological performance, disease severity, and depression in progressive supranuclear palsy. *Journal of Neurology, 243,* 638–643.

Gerstenecker, A., Mast, B., Duff, K., Ferman, T. J., Litvan, I., & ENGENE-PSP study group. (2013). Executive dysfunction is the primary cognitive impairment in progressive supranuclear palsy. *Neurology, 28*(2), 104–113.

Ghosh, B. C. P., Calder, A. J., Peers, P. V., Lawrence, A. D., Acosta-Cabronero, J., Pereira, J. M., . . . Rowe, J. B. (2012). Social cognitive deficits and their neural correlates in progressive supranuclear palsy. *Brain, 135*(7), 2089–2102.

Grafman, J., Litvan, I., & Stark, M. (1995). Neuropsychological features of progressive supranuclear palsy. *Brain and Cognition, 28,* 311–320.

Grimes, D. A., Lang, A. E., & Bergeron, C. B. (1999). Dementia as the most common presentation of cortical-basal ganglionic degeneration. *Neurology, 53,* 1969–1974.

Gross, R. G., & Grossman, M. (2008). Update on apraxia. *Current Neurology and Neuroscience Reports, 8*(6), 490–496.

Hassan, A., Parisi, J. E., & Josephs, K. A. (2011). Autopsy-proven progressive supranuclear palsy presenting as behavioral variant frontotemporal dementia. *Neurocase, 18*(6), 478–488.

Hoglinger, G. U., Melhem, N. M., Dickson, D. W., Sleiman, P. M., Wang, L. S., Klei, L., . . . Schellenberg, G. D. (2011). Identification of common variants influencing risk of tauopathy progressive supranuclear palsy. *Nature Genetics, 43*(7), 699–705.

Imai, H. (1996). Clinicophysiological features of akinesia. *European Neurology, 36*(Suppl 1), 9–12.

Imai, H., Nakamura, T., Kondo, T., & Narabavashi, H. (1993). Dopa-unresponsive pure akinesia or freezing: A condition within a wide spectrum of PSP? *Advances in Neurology, 60,* 622–625.

Jankovic, J., Friedman, D. I., Pirozzolo, F. J., & McCrary, J. A. (1990). Progressive supranuclear palsy: Motor, neurobehavioral, and neuro-opththalmic findings. *Advances in Neurology, 53,* 293–304.

Kertesz, A., & Monagle, P. (2010). Behavior and cognition in corticobasilar degeneration and progressive supranuclear palsy. *Journal of Neurological Sciences, 289,* 138–143.

Kertesz, A., Martinez-Lage, P., Davidson, W., & Munoz, D. G. (2000). The corticobasal degeneration syndrome overlaps progressive aphasia and frontotemporal dementia. *Neurology, 55,* 1368–1375.

Kouri, N., Murray, M. E., Hassan, A., Rademakers, R., Uitti, R. J., Boeve, B. F., . . . Dickson, D. W. (2011). Neuropathologic features of corticobasal degeneration presenting as corticobalas syndrome or Richardson syndrome. *Brain, 134*(Pt 11), 3264–3275.

Lee, S. E., Rabinovici, G. D., Mayo, M. C., Wilson, S. M., Seeley, W. W., DeArmond, S. J., . . . Miller, B. L. (2011). Clinicopathological correlations in corticobasal degeneration. *Annals of Neurology, 70,* 327–240.

Leiguarda, R. C., Merello, M., Nouzeilles, M. I., Balej, J., Rivero, A., & Nogues, M. (2002). Limb-kinetic apraxia in corticobasal degeneration: Clinical and kinematic features. *Movement Disorders, 18*(1), 49–59.

Ling, H., O'Sullivan, S. S., Hoton, J. L., Revesz, T., Massey, L. A., Williams, D. R., . . . Lees, A. J. (2010). Does corticobasal degeneration exist? A clinicopathological re-evaluation. *Brain, 133,* 2045–2057.

Litvan, I. (1998). Progressive supranuclear palsy: Staring into the past, moving into the future. *Neurologist, 4,* 13–20.

Litvan, I., Campbell, G., Mangone, C. A., Verny, M., McKee, A., Chaudhuri, K. R., . . . D'Olhaberriague, L. (1997). Which clinical features differentiate progressive supranuclear palsy (Steele-Richardson-Olszewski syndrome) from related disorders? A clinipathological study. *Brain, 120,* 65–74.

Litvan, I., Agid, Y., Goetz, C. G., Jankovic, J., Wenning, G. K., Brandel, J. P., . . . Bartko, J. J. (1997). Accuracy of the clinical diagnosis of corticobasal degeneration: A clinicopathologic study. *Neurology, 48,* 119–125.

Litvan, I., Agid, Y., Calne, D., Campbell, G., Dubois, B., Duvoisin, R. C.,...Zee, D. S. (1996). Clinical research criteria for the diagnosis of progressive supranuclear palsy (Steele-Richardson-Olszewski syndrome): Report of the NINDS-SPSP international workshop. *Neurology*, 47, 1–9.

Llado, A., Sanchez-Valle, R., Rey, M. J., Ezquerra, M., Tolosa, E., Ferrer, I., & Molinuevo, J. L. (2008). Clinicopathological and genetic correlates of frontotemporal lobar degeneration and corticobasal degeneration. *Journal of Neurology*, 255, 488–494.

Lopez, O. L., Litvan, I., Catt, K. E., Stowe, R., Klunk, W., Kaufer, D. I.,...DeKosky, S. T. (1999). Accuracy of four clinical diagnostic criteria for the diagnosis of neurodegenerative dementias. *Neurology*, 53(6), 1292–1299.

Maher, E. R., Smith, E. M., & Lees, A. J. (1985). Cognitive deficits in the Steele-Richardson-Olszewski syndrome (progressive supranuclear palsy). *Journal of Neurology, Neurosurgery and Psychiatry*, 48, 1234–1239.

Massey, L. A., Micallef, C., Paviour, D. C., O'Sullivan, S. S., Ling, H., Williams, D. R.,...Jäger, H. R. (2012). Conventional magnetic resonance imaging in confirmed progressive supranuclear palsy and multiple systems atrophy. *Movement Disorders*, 27(14), 1754–1762.

Matsuo, H., Takashima, H., Kishikawa, M., Kinoshita, I., Mori, M., Tsujihata, M., & Nagataki, S. (1991). Pure akinesia: An atypical manifestation of progressive supranuclear palsy. *Journal of Neurology, Neurosurgery and Psych*, 54(5), 397–400.

McMonagle, P., Blair, M., & Kertesz, A. (2006). Corticobasal degeneration and progressive aphasia. *Neurology*, 67, 1444–1451.

Murray, R., Neumann, M., Forman, M. S., Farmer, J., Massimo, L., Rice, A.,...Grossman, M. (2007). Cognitive and motor assessment in autopsy-proven corticobasal degeneration. *Neurology*, 68, 1274–1283.

Nath, U., Ben-Shlomo, Y., Thomson, R. G., Morris, H. R., Wood, N. W., Lees, A. J., & Burn, D. J. (2001). The prevalence of progressive supranuclear palsy (Steele-Richardson-Olswekski syndrome) in the UK. *Brain*, 124(7), 1438–1449.

Nieforth, K. A., & Golbe, L. I. (1993). Retrospective study of drug response in 87 patients with progressive supranuclear palsy. *Clinical Neuropharmacology*, 16(4), 338–346.

Osaki, Y., Ben-Shlomo, Y., Lees, A. J., Daniel, S. E., Colosimo, C., Wenning, G., & Quinn, N. (2004). Accuracy of clinical diagnosis of progressive supranuclear palsy. *Movement Disorders*, 19(2), 181–189.

O'Sullivan, S. S., Massey, L. A., Williams, D. R., Silveira-Moriyama, L., Kempster, P. A., Holton, J. L.,...Lees, A. J. (2008). Clinical outcomes of progressive supranuclear palsy and multiple systems atrophy. *Brain*, 131(5), 1362–1372.

Pelak, V. S., & Hall, D. A. (2004). Neuro-ophthalmic manifestations of neurodegenerative disease. *Ophthalmology Clinics of North America*, 17(3), 311–320.

Pillon, B., Dubois, B., Ploska, A., & Agid, Y. (1991). Severity and specificity of cognitive impairment in Alzheimer's, Huntington's, Parkinson's diseases and progressive supranuclear palsy. *Neurology*, 41, 634–643.

Pillon, B., Dubois, B., Lhermitte, F., & Agid, Y. (1986). Heterogeneity of cognitive impairment in progressive supranuclear palsy, Parkinson's disease, and Alzheimer's disease. *Neurology*, 36, 1179–1185.

Rebeiz, J. J., Kolodny, E. H., & Richardson, E. P. (1968). Corticodentatonigral degeneration with neuronal achromasia. *Archives of Neurology*, 18, 20–33.

Robbins, T. W., James, M., Owen, A. M., Lange, K. W., Lees, A. J., Leigh, P. N.,...Summers B. A. (1994). Cognitive deficits in progressive supranuclear palsy, Parkinson's disease, and multiple system atrophy in tests sensitive to frontal lobe dysfunction. *Journal of Neurology, Neurosurgergy and Psychiatry*, 57, 79–88.

Rohrer, J. D., Paviour, D., Bronstein, A. M., O'Sullivan, S. S., Lees, A., & Warren, J. D. (2010). Progressive supranuclear palsy syndrome presenting as progressive nonfluent aphasia: A neuropsychological and neuroimaging analysis. *Movement Disorders*, 25(2), 179–188.

Soliveri, P., Monza, D., Paridi, D., Carella, F., Genitrini, S., Testa, D., & Girotti, F. (2000). Neuropsychological follow up in patients with Parkinson's disease, striatonigral degeneration-type multiple systems atrophy, and progressive supranuclear palsy. *Journal of Neurology, Neurosurgery and Psychiatry*, 69, 313–318.

Steele, J. C., Richardson, J. C., & Olszewski, J. (1964). Progressive supranuclear palsy. *Archives of Neurology*, 10, 333–359.

Stover, N. P., Wainer, B. H., & Watts, R. L. (2004). Corticobasal degeneration. In R. L. Watts & W. C. Koller (Eds.), *Movement disorders: Neurologic principles and practice* (2nd ed., pp. 763–778). San Francisco, CA: McGraw-Hill

Vanvoorst, W. A., Greenaway, M. C., Boeve, B. F., Ivnik, R. J., Parisi, J. E., Eric Ahlskog, J.,...Josephs, K. A. (2008). Neuropsychological findings in clinically atypical autopsy confirmed corticobasal degeneration and progressive supranuclear palsy. *Parkinsonism and Related Disorders, 14,* 376–378.

Vidal, J. S., Vidailhet, M., Derkinderen, P., Tzourio, C., & Alpérovitch, A. (2010). Familial aggregation in atypical Parkinson's disease: A case control study in multiple system atrophy and progressive supranuclear palsy. *Journal of Neurology, 257*(8), 1388–1393.

Wenning, G., Litvan, I., & Tolosa, E. (2011). Milestones in atypical and secondary Parkinsonisms. *Movement Disorders, 26,* 1083–1095.

Williams, D. R., Holton, J. L., Strand, K., Revesz, T., & Lees, A. J. (2007). Pure akinesia with gait freezing: A third clinical phenotype of progressive supranuclear palsy. *Movement Disorders,* 2007: 22(15), 2235–2241.

Zadikoff, C., & Lang, A. E. (2005). Apraxia in movement disorders. *Brain, 128*(7), 1480–1497.

12

Dementia With Lewy Bodies and Parkinson's Disease Dementia

Haşmet A. Hanağası, Başar Bilgiç, and Murat Emre

Dementia with Lewy bodies (DLB) and Parkinson's disease dementia (PD-D) are neurodegenerative disorders that affect cognition, behavior, movement, and autonomic function. Both DLB and PD-D are members of the class of neurodegenerative diseases collectively referred to as synucleinopathies; they are believed to represent two entities on the same disease spectrum with overlapping clinical, neurochemical, and pathological findings.

Dementia With Lewy Bodies

Several other terms have been used to describe DLB in the past, including diffuse Lewy body disease, Lewy body dementia, the Lewy-body variant of Alzheimer's disease, senile dementia of Lewy-body type, and dementia associated with cortical Lewy bodies. The term "DLB" was proposed at a consensus meeting (the First International Workshop of the Consortium on dementia with Lewy bodies) in 1996 (I. G. McKeith, 2006) and is now widely used.

Although the term itself presumes the presence of a particular pathology (i.e., Lewy bodies), clinical diagnostic criteria with reasonable predictive accuracy for the pathological entity have been developed by the Consortium on Dementia With Lewy Bodies (McKeith, Perry, & Perry, 1999; McKeith et al., 2005). Subsequently diagnostic criteria for PD-D were also published (Emre et al., 2007). DLB and PD-D have grossly overlapping clinical features except for the chronology and temporal course of symptoms. In the consensus guidelines, an arbitrary cut point was proposed with regard to chronology of symptoms to distinguish these two disorders. Thus, patients who develop dementia after 1 year following the onset of parkinsonian symptoms should be diagnosed as PD-D, whereas those who develop dementia and parkinsonism concomitantly or within 1 year of each other should be diagnosed as DLB. This so-called 1-year rule is largely meant for research purposes. In practice, patients who are diagnosed with Parkinson's disease (PD) first and subsequently develop dementia should be given the diagnosis of PD-D, whereas those who develop dementia first followed by parkinsonism should be designated as DLB.

Epidemiology of Dementia With Lewy Bodies

The first pathological description of the entity now known as DLB was made by Okazaki et al. in 1961. It is the second most common cause of neurodegenerative dementias after Alzheimer's disease (AD), accounting for 15% to 30% of all dementia cases at autopsy series (Barker et al., 2002; Hulette et al., 1995; Lim et al., 1999; Okazaki, Lipkin, & Aronson, 1961). Only a few studies have assessed the prevalence and incidence of DLB in patients with dementia or in the general population. Most of these studies have not applied the new clinical diagnostic criteria. In a systematic review of studies using the consensus diagnostic criteria, prevalence estimates were found to vary widely between <1% to 5% in the general population, and <1% to 30.5% in dementia patients (Zaccai, McCracken, & Brayne, 2005). The Cache County study revealed an incidence rate of 3.2% among all new dementia cases and 0.1% in the general population (Miech et al., 2002). In a large Finnish community study including 601 adults aged 75 years or older, the prevalence of DLB was reported to be 21.9% among all demented cases (Rahkonen et al., 2003). Lower prevalence rates were reported in Asian countries (Chan, Chiu, Lam, & Leung, 2002; Kobayashi et al., 2011; Yamada, Hattori, Miura, Tanabe, & Yamori, 2001).

DLB usually appears later in life, with a mean age of onset between 60 and 80 years (McKeith et al., 2005); onset before age 60 is rare. Mean survival time (8–10 years; range 2–20 years) and rate of cognitive decline are similar to that seen in AD. However, several case series have reported patients with a more rapid progression than that in AD (Olichney et al., 1998; Walker, Allen, Shergill, Mullan, & Katona, 2000; Williams, Xiong, Morris, & Galvin, 2006). Rarely, patients with DLB may show rapid progression to death within 1 to 2 years (Gaig et al., 2011). Relative risk factors for increased mortality in DLB include older age, neuroleptic sensitivity, the presence of parkinsonism, fluctuating cognition, and hallucinations. DLB patients with neuroleptic sensitivity show a two-fold to three-fold increase in mortality (McKeith, Fairbairn, Perry, Thompson, & Perry, 1992). Compared to AD, patients with DLB have been reported to have a greater risk of hospital admission (or death), often due to fall-related injuries and bronchopneumonia (Hanyu et al., 2009).

Genetics of Dementia With Lewy Bodies

Family studies have reported a higher frequency of DLB among persons having a positive family history of dementia compared to those who do not (Papapetropoulos et al., 2006; Woodruff et al., 2006). Nervi et al. reported that DLB and core features of DLB aggregate in families (Nervi et al., 2011). Compared with siblings of probands with clinically diagnosed AD, siblings of probands with clinically diagnosed DLB were at increased risks of DLB and visual hallucinations (Nervi et al., 2011).

The first chromosomal locus for DLB was mapped at 2q35-q36 in an autopsy-confirmed Belgian family across three generations with different phenotypes including dementia and/or parkinsonism (Bogaerts et al., 2007). Molecular genetic analysis, including comprehensive sequencing of all candidate genes and analyses of copy number variations, did not reveal a simple pathogenic or gene dosage mutation that cosegregated with DLB in this pedigree (Meeus et al., 2010).

The findings on APOE polymorphisms in DLB are inconclusive. In some studies an increased APOE4 allele frequency was reported, whereas others found no such difference (Borroni et al., 2006; Engelborghs et al., 2003; Singleton et al., 2002). No association between APOE4 allele and brain atrophy was found in DLB patients; however, APOE4 may be associated with a more accelerated progression of cognitive decline.

Duplications or triplications of the alpha-synuclein gene are known to cause familial forms of PD, PD-D, or DLB; mutations in the gene itself are very rare. It has been suggested that gene multiplications lead to a gene dose-dependent increase in the expression of alpha-synuclein with a concomitant increase in the severity of the disease and a decrease in the age of onset (Chartier-Harlin et al., 2004; Farrer et al., 2004). Glucoserebrosidase (GBA) mutations have also been associated with pathologically "pure" Lewy body disorders, characterized by more extensive, cortical Lewy body pathology (Clark et al., 2009). Nishioka et al. reported the presence of GBA mutations in 6.8% (4/59) of cases with a pathological diagnosis of diffuse Lewy body disease (Nishioka et al., 2011). Mutations or variants of autosomal dominant AD genes (PSEN1, PSEN 2), genes associated with frontotemporal dementia (MAPT, GRN), and autosomal recessive PD genes (Parkin and PINK1) may also have a role (Meeus et al., 2012).

Clinical Features of Dementia With Lewy Bodies

Clinical features of DLB include cognitive, psychiatric, neurological, sleep, and autonomic symptoms.

Cognitive Features

The central clinical feature required for the diagnosis of DLB is progressive cognitive decline that interferes with normal social and occupational function (McKeith et al., 2005). The cognitive profile of DLB is characterized by significant deficits in executive and visuospatial functions as well as attention (Calderon et al., 2001; Walker, Allen, Shergill, & Katona, 1997). Prominent memory impairments may be absent in the early stages of DLB, but they usually appear as the disease progresses. On the other hand, DLB patients with concurrent Alzheimer-type tau pathology may show prominent memory deficits, more characteristic of AD, even in the early stage.

A core feature of DLB is the fluctuation in cognitive function, which is an early and prominent symptom, occurring in 50% to 75% of patients during the course of the disease (McKeith et al., 2005). Fluctuation has been defined as pronounced variations in attention and alertness that may vary from hour to hour or day to day and has been found to occur regardless of the severity of cognitive disturbances (Ferman et al., 2004). There is no consistent fluctuation pattern for the same patient. Fluctuations in cognition and attention interfere with neuropsychological evaluation and lead to high variability of cognitive performance. Fluctuations in cognition are reported to be associated with cholinergic deficits (Ferman et al., 2004); they can be identified in the electroencephalogram and can be measured with neuropsychological evaluations using timed or paced computerized tests such as choice reaction time or digit vigilance, or using fluctuation rating scales (The Clinician Assessment of Fluctuation, The Mayo Fluctuations Composite Scale, and the One Day Fluctuation Assessment Scale) (Walker et al., 2000a, 2000b).

Behavioral Features

Persistent visual hallucinations are the most common psychiatric symptom and at least two thirds of patients report visual hallucinations (McKeith et al., 2005). Hallucinations are usually present early in the course of illness; they are often recurrent, well formed, detailed, and consist of mute images (Mosimann et al., 2006). They may be nondisturbing to patients, but they are usually stressful for the family and caregivers. Patients may have preserved insight into hallucinations. Loss of vision and a decreased level of consciousness can exacerbate visual hallucinations. Visual illusions are also common where patients perceive objects differently from their true identity. Auditory, olfactory, and tactile hallucinations appear less common, and they usually occur together with concomitant visual hallucinations. Delusions are less prevalent; they constitute a supportive feature for diagnosis of DLB (McKeith et al., 2004). They are commonly in the form of belief of strangers living in the home (phantom boarder) or delusions of persecution; delusions of theft and infidelity may also occur. Three classes of psychotic symptoms were found to be associated with dissociable perfusion abnormalities on single-photon emission computed tomography (SPECT) imaging: visual hallucinations with dysfunction of the parietal and ventral occipital cortices, misidentifications with dysfunction of the limbic-paralimbic structures, and delusions with dysfunction of the frontal cortices (Nagahama, Okina, Suzuki, & Matsuda, 2010). Depression and anxiety may appear years before the onset of dementia and up to 40% of DLB patients experience a major depressive episode in the course of their illness (Auning et al., 2011).

Motor, Autonomic, and Other Associated Features

Another core feature of DLB is the presence of spontaneous (i.e., non-drug-induced) parkinsonism and has a prevalence ranging from 70% to 100% (McKeith et al., 2005). Some pathological series indicate that 25% of DLB cases may have no parkinsonism. In a prospective clinicopathological study, the absence of parkinsonism was found to be the most common reason for misdiagnosis of DLB (McKeith et al., 2000). Parkinsonism varies in severity; patients usually have rigidity and bradykinesia, shuffling gait, stooped posture, and masked faces while resting tremor is infrequent. Postural instability can be profound early in the illness. McKeith et al. reported that more than 50% of DLB patients have severe sensitivity to neuroleptics (Keith et al., 1992). Neuroleptic sensitivity is not dose related; it may may appear as rapid and irreversible worsening of parkinsonism, cognitive decline, drowsiness, and occasionally with a neuroleptic malignant syndrome–like presentation with autonomic instability. Severe sensitivity to neuroleptics increases morbidity and mortality in DLB patients.

Other Clinical Features

Other features suggestive or supportive of diagnosis include sleep or sleep-wake cycle disturbances. REM sleep behavior disorder is a parasomnia characterized by loss of normal skeletal muscle atonia during REM sleep, with associated motor activity, resulting in vivid dreams with simple or complex motor behavior (Postuma, Gagnon, & Montplaisir, 2012). It predominately occurs in males and has an onset after the age of 50–60. It is present in nearly 70% of DLB patients and may occur many years before the onset of dementia or parkinsonism. It may be the first symptom of DLB or other synucleinopathies such as Parkinson's disease or multiple system atrophy (Postuma et al., 2012). As the disease progresses, it may become less frequent or less symptomatic (Postuma, Gagnon, Vendette, & Montplaisir, 2009). The inclusion of RBD as a core clinical feature improves the diagnostic accuracy of autopsy-confirmed DLB patients (Ferman et al., 2011). Excessive daytime somnolence, a disturbance of sleep-wake cycle, is also common.

Autonomic abnormalities are frequent in DLB patients (Horimoto et al., 2003). Autonomic dysfunction may include orthostatic hypotension, impotence, urinary incontinence, or constipation. Urinary incontinence is the most frequent autonomic symptom and constipation is the second (McKeith et al., 2005). These symptoms are thought to be due to the presence of Lewy body pathology and neuronal loss in the central and likely also peripheral autonomic nervous system (McKeith et al., 2005).

Other supporting features of DLB include repeated falls, syncope, and transient loss of consciousness. DLB patients often report frequent unexplained falls; these may be related to postural instability or autonomic dysfunction. Transient and otherwise unexplained lapses of consciousness, with or without falls, may represent orthostatic syncope.

Neuropathological and Biochemical Correlates of Dementia With Lewy Bodies

The pathologic diagnosis of DLB mandates the presence of Lewy bodies (LBs) in neuronal cytoplasma; Lewy neurites are also common. They can be seen in the brainstem nuclei, amygdala, limbic-paralimbic cortices, basal ganglia, and cerebral cortex (Hansen et al., 1990). Gliosis and neuronal loss are also present in these regions. LBs are usually found in the deeper layers of the neocortex and tend to be widespread; they also involve medulla and peripheral autonomic nervous system. Alpha-synuclein is the major protein component of LBs and Lewy neurites (Spillantini, Crowther, Jakes, Hasegawa, & Goedert, 1998); neurofilaments, ubiquitin, torsin A, and parkin appear to be minor structural components (Beyer, Domingo-Sàbat, & Ariza, 2009). Morphologically, LBs may be divided into brainstem and cortical types (Hansen et al., 1990). "Brainstem" type LBs are easily seen using standard histological methods: They are spherical intraneuronal cytoplasmic inclusions characterized by a hyaline eosinophilic core, concentric lamellar band, and a narrow pale halo. Hematoxylin and eosin staining is usually sufficient to detect brainstem-type LBs. Cortical LBs may occur in limbic and neocortical regions, mainly in the small neurons of the cortex. Due to their small size and lack of halo, they are not readily identifiable with classical histological stains; immunohistochemistry with anti-alpha-synuclein antibodies is required to detect them. The last revision of the DLB Consortium criteria proposed a revised pathologic classification using alpha-synuclein immunohistochemistry with semiquantitative grading of Lewy-related pathology (mild, moderate, severe, very severe) in brainstem, limbic, and diffuse neocortical areas rather than counting LBs in various brain regions (McKeith et al., 2005). However, the validation of this pathologic classification is as yet limited (Nelson et al., 2010).

In addition to Lewy body pathology, 75% to 90% of DLB patients have concomitant amyloid plaques and many patients meet the pathological criteria for Alzheimer's disease according to "Consortium to establish a registry for Alzheimer's disease (CERAD) criteria" ("Consensus recommendations for the postmortem diagnosis of Alzheimer's disease," 1997; Lopez et al., 2002; Mirra et al., 1991). Concomitant amyloid plaques are common, whereas neurofibrillary tangles are rare. In addition, vascular pathology can be found in up to 30% of DLB patients (Jellinger, 2003). Concomitant AD-type or vascular pathology may have an impact on the clinical presentation (Merdes et al., 2003). The presence of concomitant AD pathology may be associated with more severe memory impairment and atrophy in the medial temporal lobe compared to "pure" DLB patients, whereas LB pathology may be associated with more severe executive and visuospatial dysfunction. It was suggested that the presence or absence of AD pathology may determine the premortem DLB diagnosis, rather than the distribution of LBs (Nelson et al., 2009).

Biochemically DLB is associated with profound cholinergic and dopaminergic deficits (Perry, Irving, Blessed, Fairbairn, & Perry, 1990). A cholinergic deficit is more prominent in DLB than in AD and tends to occur early in the disease course (Samuel, Alford, Hofstetter, & Hansen, 1997). There is loss of cholinergic neurons in the nucleus basalis of Meynert (Perry et al., 1994), deficits in choline acetyltransferase levels are found in temporal and parietal cortex, and reduction of choline acetyltransferase activity in temporal lobe is correlated with the degree of the cognitive impairment (Lippa, Smith, & Perry, 1999). A higher LB density in the limbic system (amygdala) is associated with visual hallucinations (Harding, Broe, & Halliday, 2002). Cholinergic deficits are greater in temporal cortex of those with visual hallucinations as compared to those without (Gómez-Isla et al., 1999). Muscarinic M1 postsynaptic receptor binding in the temporal lobe may be increased in patients with delusional thinking (Ballard et al., 2000).

A dopaminergic deficit is the other important neurochemical feature of DLB. The reduction in postsynaptic D2 receptor density in the striatum is greater in DLB than in PD or healthy controls, which may contribute to the weak response to dopaminergic drugs or neuroleptic sensitivity seen in DLB patients (Piggott et al., 1999). Deficits in the serotoninergic and noradrenergic systems may also be related to cognitive-behavioral impairment. LBs occur in the dorsal raphe nucleus, and marked reduction of serotonin levels have been reported in the basal ganglia and cerebral cortices of patients with DLB (Perry et al., 1990).

Neuroimaging Features of Dementia With Lewy Bodies

Relative preservation of the hippocampus and medial temporal lobes compared with AD patients has been described in pathologically confirmed DLB patients (Burton et al., 2009). Sabattoli et al. found that there was mild hippocampal atrophy (10%–20%) in DLB patients compared to a control group, but it was less than that seen in AD (Sabattoli et al., 2008). There is, however, considerable overlap between AD and DLB, and the utility of magnetic resonance imaging (MRI) for differential diagnosis is limited. In pathologically verified DLB cases, LBs but not AD pathology was associated with reduced amygdala volume, while neither LB nor AD pathology was associated with volume loss in hippocampus or entorhinal cortex, suggesting that other neuropathological factors account for atrophy in these structures (Burton et al., 2012). Others have found that hippocampal atrophy on MRI may be associated with neurofibrillary tangle pathology in patients with LB pathology (Kantarci et al., 2012). Atrophy in other cortical and subcortical structures has also been reported in DLB, including the striatum, substantia innominata, hypothalamus, and dorsal midbrain

(Kantarci et al., 2012). The rate of overall cerebral atrophy in longitudinal MRI studies has been reported to be 1.4% per year, three times more than that seen in controls, but less than that seen in AD (2% per year) (O'Brien et al., 2001).

In an MR spectroscopy (MRS) study, Molina et al. found no changes in the gray matter N-asetyl aspartat/Creatinin (NAA/Cr) levels in DLB patients compared to healthy controls (Molina et al., 2002). In another MRS study using a single voxel spanning the right and left posterior cingulate gyri and inferior precunei, Kantarci et al. reported that NAA/Cr levels were reduced in subjects with AD, vascular dementia, and frontotemporal lobar degeneration compared with healthy controls but were not reduced in DLB (Kantarci et al., 2004). In a diffusion tensor imaging study, changes (increased diffusivity [D] and decreased fractional anisotropy [FA] values) in corpus callosum and pericallosal areas were found in DLB patients as compared to normal controls (Bozzali et al., 2005). White matter was also affected in the frontal, parietal, and occipital areas with less involvement of the temporal lobe. The authors suggested that these white matter changes may reflect the pathophysiological process that eventually affects neurons in the association cortices. In another DTI study, the DLB group had reduced FA in the precuneus area compared to controls and AD patients (Firbank, Colloby, Burn, McKeith, & O'Brien, 2003). Areas of reduced FA in DLB versus controls were also found primarily in parietooccipital white matter tracts where the changes were more diffuse in AD; compared to AD, DLB was also associated with reduced FA in pons and left thalamus (Watson et al., 2012). This study suggests that patterns of DTI changes in AD and DLB are significantly different and DTI may be a useful technique to investigate early changes in DLB. Finally, resting-state functional magnetic resonance imaging (fMRI) studies have reported increased functional connectivity between the right posterior cingulate and other brain areas (Galvin, Price, J. L., Yan, Morris, & Sheline, 2011; Kenny, Blamire, Firbank, & O'Brien, 2012).

SPECT and positron emission tomography (PET) studies have demonstrated decreased glucose metabolism and perfusion deficits in parietal and occipital areas in DLB (Albin et al., 1996; Lobotesis et al., 2001). However, occipital hypometabolism is not always present and FDG-PET changes may be similar to that seen in AD. Reduced uptake of 18 F-fluorodopa in the striatum may distinguish DLB from AD with high sensitivity and specificity (Hu et al., 2000). Several studies, using 123I-beta-CIT SPECT, demonstrated reduced dopamine transporter binding in the caudate and posterior putamen in DLB compared to AD patients (McKeith et al., 2007; O'Brien et al., 2009), but no difference between DLB and PD patients. Similarly, thoracic SPECT imaging using 123-I metaiodobenzylguanidine (MIBG), a marker of postganglionic cardiac sympathetic innervation, shows reduced cardiac MIBG uptake in DLB and PD patients as opposed to normal findings in AD (Yoshita et al., 2001). It was suggested that combining SPECT and MIBG scintigraphy could increase the diagnostic accuracy for DLB (Tateno et al., 2011). In studies using amyloid PET imaging, 80% of DLB cases were found to have increased amyloid load, whereas only 20% of patients with PD-D have this finding (Edison et al., 2008; Foster et al., 2010; Gomperts et al., 2008).

Standard electroencephalography (EEG) may show early slowing of background activity in DLB patients compared with AD as well as epoch-by-epoch fluctuations. Frontal intermittent delta activity and transient temporal slow waves are other changes that are more common in DLB than in AD (Bonanni et al., 2008; Roks, Korf, van der Flier, Scheltens, & Stam, 2008).

Cerebrospinal Fluid Biomarkers in Dementia With Lewy Bodies

Currently, there are no blood or cerebrospinal fluid (CSF) markers that can be used for diagnosis, to follow disease progression, or as an outcome parameter for therapeutic interventions in DLB. Alpha-synuclein has been studied as a potential biomarker for DLB, but results have been controversial (Mollenhauer et al., 2008; Ohrfelt et al., 2009). Amyloid beta 40-42 in CSF, a biomarker for AD, has been found to be lower in DLB compared to controls and PD-D cases (Bibl et al., 2006; Parnetti et al., 2008). In addition, Mulugeta et al. suggested CSF amyloid β38 as a diagnostic biomarker for DLB (Mulugeta et al., 2011); the Aβ42/Aβ38 ratio discriminated

AD from DLB with a sensitivity of 78% and a specificity of 67%.

Diagnosis of Dementia With Lewy Bodies

The revised consensus criteria for clinical diagnosis of DLB are shown in Table 12.1 (McKeith et al., 2005). The central feature required for the diagnosis of DLB is progressive cognitive decline that interferes with the social and occupational functioning of the patient (i.e., dementia). Core features include fluctuation in cognition with pronounced variation in attention and alertness, recurrent and persistent visual hallucinations, and spontaneous parkinsonism. Consensus guidelines recommend that two of the core clinical features have to be present for a diagnosis of probable and one for a diagnosis of possible DLB. Suggestive and supportive features may increase diagnostic accuracy.

TABLE 12.1 Revised Criteria for the Clinical Diagnosis of Dementia With Lewy Bodies (DLB)

1. **Central feature (essential for a diagnosis of possible or probable DLB)**
   - Dementia defined as progressive cognitive decline that interferes with social and occupational function
   - Prominent or persistent memory impairment may not necessarily occur in the early stages but is usually evident with progression.
   - Deficits on tests of attention, executive function, and visuospatial ability may be especially prominent.
2. **Core features (two core features are sufficient for a diagnosis of probable DLB, one for possible DLB)**
   - Fluctuating cognition with pronounced variation in attention and alertness
   - Recurrent visual hallucinations
   - Spontaneous features of parkinsonism
3. **Suggestive features (1 or more + a core feature = probable DLB; any 1 alone = possible DLB)**
   - REM sleep behavior disorder
   - Severe neuroleptic sensitivity
   - Low dopamine transporter uptake in basal ganglia demonstrated by SPECT or PET imaging
4. **Supportive features (commonly present but lacking diagnostic value)**
   - Repeated falls and syncope
   - Transient, unexplained loss of consciousness
   - Severe autonomic dysfunction, e.g., orthostatic hypotension, urinary incontinence
   - Hallucinations in other modalities
   - Systematized delusions
   - Depression
   - Relative preservation of medial temporal lobe on CT or MRI scan
   - Decreased tracer uptake on SPECT or PET imaging in occipital regions
   - Abnormal (low-uptake) MIBG myocardial scintigraphy
   - Prominent slow waves on EEG with temporal lobe transient sharp waves
5. **A diagnosis of DLB is less likely**
   - In the presence of cerebrovascular disease evident as focal neurologic signs or on brain imaging
   - In the presence of any other physical illness or brain disorder sufficient to account in part or in total for the clinical picture
   - If parkinsonism only appears for the first time at a stage of severe dementia
6. **Temporal sequence of symptoms**
   - DLB should be diagnosed when dementia occurs before or concurrently with parkinsonism (if it is present). The term "Parkinson disease dementia (PD-D)" should be used to describe dementia that occurs in the context of well-established Parkinson disease. In a practice setting the term that is most appropriate to the clinical situation should be used and generic terms such as LB disease are often helpful. In research studies in which distinction needs to be made between DLB and PD-D, the existing 1-year rule between the onset of dementia and parkinsonism DLB continues to be recommended. Adoption of other time periods will simply confound data pooling or comparison between studies. In other research settings that may include clinicopathologic studies and clinical trials, both clinical phenotypes may be considered collectively under categories such as LB disease or alpha-synucleinopathy.

CT, computerized tomography; EEG, electroencephalography; MIBG, metaiodobenzylguanidine; MRI, magnetic resonance imaging; PET, positron emission tomography; SPECT, single-photon emission computerized tomography.

Source: From McKeith et al. (2005).

Suggestive features are significantly more frequent than in other dementing diseases, but their specificity is low. These are REM sleep behavior disorder, severe neuroleptic sensitivity, and decreased dopamine transporter binding in striatum. In situations in which there is one or more suggestive feature plus a core feature, a diagnosis of probable DLB can be made. Possible DLB can be diagnosed if one or more suggestive features are present in a patient with dementia even in the absence of any core features. Supportive features include repeated falls and syncope, transient or unexplained loss of consciousness, severe autonomic dysfunction, systematized delusions, hallucinations in other modalities (i.e., auditory and tactile), depression, relative preservation of medial temporal lobe on computed tomography (CT) or MRI scan, decreased tracer uptake on SPECT or PET imaging in occipital regions, abnormal 123-I MIBG scintigraphy, and prominent slow waves on EEG with transient sharp waves in temporal lobe.

The sensitivity and specificity of the first and second consensus clinical criteria for DLB have been examined in several autopsy studies, and while the specificity was found to be high, sensitivity was low (Galasko et al., 1994; Gómez-Isla et al., 1999; McKeith et al., 2000; Schneider, Arvanitakis, Bang, & Bennett, 2007). Large autopsy series on sensitivity and specificity of new DLB criteria are not yet available.

The diagnosis of DLB is principally based on clinical features and exclusion of other diagnoses. Confidence in the diagnosis is reduced by a history of stroke, focal neurological signs, or the presence of significant comorbid physical illness or other brain disorders.

Management of Patients With Dementia With Lewy Bodies

Management of DLB includes both nonpharmacologic and pharmacologic approaches. Nonpharmacologic approaches have the potential to reduce clinical symptoms and functional impairment. Recognition of potentially treatable sensory impairments such as impaired vision and environmental changes such as improving lighting may reduce hallucinations and falls. Behavioral symptoms may be relieved or reduced if caregivers employ behavioral modification strategies. Education and family support are also important parts of the management and can reduce undue use of antipsychotics.

All drugs with anticholinergic effects (e.g., tricyclic antidepressants, anticholinergics, antispasmodics) should be discontinued because they have the potential to further impair cognition, exacerbate psychotic symptoms, and may be associated with orthostatic hypotension in patients with DLB (McKeith et al., 2004). L-dopa is preferred to treat the motor symptoms of DLB, but it should be started at low doses and increased slowly to the minimum required dose. Patients with DLB may be less responsive to levodopa therapy than those with Parkinson's disease. Only 30%–50% of patients improve significantly (Lucetti et al., 2010; Molloy, McKeith, O'Brien, & Burn, 2005). Potential side effects of levodopa include visual hallucinations, delusions, orthostatic hypotension, and nausea. Other antiparkinsonian agents, including monoamine oxidase B inhibitors, amantadine, and dopamine agonists, are usually less tolerable in DLB patients.

Orthostatic hypotension can be treated with hydration, increased dietary salt intake or with salt tablets, avoidance of prolonged bed rest, thigh-high compression stockings, efforts to stand up slowly, and avoidance of medications that contribute to orthostasis. If these measures are ineffective, fludrocortisone and midodrine can be considered. Constipation may benefit from exercise, increased dietary fiber, increased water intake, and laxative drugs. REM sleep behavior disorder can be treated with low-dose clonazepam (0.25–1.0 mg) at bedtime; however, clonazepam has the potential to worsen the symptoms of obstructive sleep apnea (Postuma et al., 2012). Melatonin may also be effective at a dose of 3 to 12 mg, either as monotherapy or in conjunction with clonazepam. Although the evidence base in DLB is weak, drugs such as modafinil and methylphenidate can be considered to treat excessive daytime sleepiness. Serotonin reuptake inhibitors (SSRIs) and serotonin-norepinephrine reuptake inhibitors (SNRIs) can be used for the treatment of depressive symptoms or anxiety.

Visual hallucinations are often the most troubling neuropsychiatric feature in DLB, particularly to family members. They do not require drug treatment, however, if they are not frightening or otherwise distressing to the patient. Antipsychotics are used to treat psychotic symptoms, but neuroleptics should be used with great caution in DLB, as some patients may show severe neuroleptic sensitivity, which is not predictable in an individual patient (McKeith et al., 1992). In addition, antipsychotics may increase the risk of cerebrovascular events and death in elderly patients with dementia (Raedler, 2010). As reductions in cholinergic activity correlate with hallucinations, cholinesterase inhibitors may be considered for management of hallucinations and delusions, if they are not severe, before using a neuroleptic (McKeith et al., 2000; Mori, Ikeda, & Kosaka, 2012). If the symptoms are refractory, cause significant impairment or severe burden for caregivers, quetiapine and clozapine can be considered. Initial doses should be low and the dose should be titrated slowly while monitoring for functional decline. Neuroleptics can cause orthostatic hypotension, and blood pressure monitoring may be necessary in some patients.

Since patients with DLB have severe cholinergic deficits, several studies have been performed with cholinesterase inhibitors. Results from randomized controlled trials with rivastigmine and donepezil indicated improvements in cognitive function and behavioral symptoms (McKeith et al., 2000; Mori et al., 2012). McKeith et al. reported a multicenter, randomized, controlled study of 120 patients with DLB using rivastigmine or placebo for 20 weeks (McKeith et al., 2000). Patients with a diagnosis of probable DLB and a Mini Mental State Examination (MMSE) score of greater than 10 were treated with 6–12 mg/day of rivastigmine or placebo. Although there was a slight improvement in mean MMSE score in the rivastigmine group at week 20, this was not statistically significant compared to placebo. Clinician-assessed global status was also not significantly different between the two treatment groups. Change from baseline in mean Neuropsychiatric Inventory (NPI, 10 items) score was also not significantly different between the two groups in the intention-to-treat (ITT, last observation carried forward) analysis at week 20; the difference was, however, statistically significant in favor of rivastigmine in the observed cases (OC) analysis. More than twice as many patients on rivastigmine (63.4%) than on placebo (30.0%) showed at least a 30% improvement from baseline in their NPI-4 scores ($p ≤ .001$), with psychotic features resolving almost completely in over half of the treated patients. Apathy, anxiety, delusions, and hallucinations were the symptoms to show the best response. There was also a significant improvement in a computerized test of attention, choice reaction time. During a 3-week washout period, improvements seen with rivastigmine returned to baseline. Nausea (37%), vomiting (25%), anorexia (19%), and somnolence (9%) were the most common side effects. Worsening of parkinsonism was not reported, although emergent tremor was noted in four rivastigmine-treated patients.

In another large randomized, placebo-controlled study, the effect of donepezil (3, 5, 10 mg/day) was assessed in 140 DLB patients for 12 weeks (Mori et al., 2012). Patients given 5 mg or 10 mg donepezil showed greater improvement in the majority of the cognitive and behavioral scales, including the MMSE and NPI. Donepezil treatment also led to improved global function, as measured by CIBIC-plus and reduced caregiver burden at the highest dose. Patients taking donepezil were less apathetic, less anxious, had less cognitive fluctuation, and had fewer delusions and hallucinations compared to placebo patients. Approximately 8% of the study population withdrew due to adverse events, and the prevalence of withdrawal or adverse events, including typical cholinergic side effects, did not differ among treatment groups.

Changes in glutamatergic activity have been reported in patients with DLB (Dalfó, Albasanz, Martin, & Ferrer, 2004). The N-methyl-D-aspartate antagonist memantine was tested in two randomized, placebo-controlled studies including DLB patients; however, the results were not consistent (Aarsland et al., 2009; Emre et al., 2010). The larger study in patients with Lewy-body-related dementias included 199 patients, of which 121 had PD-D and 78 had DLB (Emre et al., 2010). At week 24, patients treated with memantine had greater improvements in global status (as measured by the Alzheimer's Disease Cooperative Study [ADCS] clinical global impression of change [CGIC] score) than did patients who received placebo; improvements were predominantly in the DLB group.

Behavioral symptoms as assessed with NPI total score significantly improved in the DLB group only. Cognitive test scores, activities of daily living scores, motor symptoms, or caregiver burden scores did not show significant improvements in either patient group. Adverse events in the two treatment groups were similar, except for slightly more sedation in the memantine group. In another, smaller randomized trial of memantine in patients with Lewy-body-related dementias, including patients with DLB or PD-D, improved mean CGIC score was observed in the total population after 6 months of treatment; the difference was driven by a larger efficacy in the PD-D group (Aarsland et al., 2009). NPI scores showed a statistically significantly improvement in the memantine group as compared to placebo in the DLB group, but not in the PD-D sample. No statistically significant differences were observed for individual cognitive tests, ADCS-Activities of Daily Living or Zarit caregiver burden scores. The incidence of adverse events and number of discontinuations due to adverse events were similar in both groups.

In conclusion, cholinesterase inhibitors such as rivastigmine and donepezil should be considered in all patients with a diagnosis with DLB, taking into account potential benefits and risks. The data on benefits of memantine are less clear, although memantine may be considered in patients with prominent neuropsychiatric symptoms.

Parkinson's Disease Dementia

PD is one of the most common movement disorders, affecting 1% of people older than 60 years. Although considered primarily a motor disorder, nonmotor signs and symptoms may accompany PD from early stages onward and be present even before the manifestation of motor symptoms. Due in part to advances in the treatment and increased life expectancy, cognitive impairment in patients with PD has become increasingly well recognized and research in this field has tremendously accelerated.

Epidemiology of Parkinson's Disease Dementia

In the early stages of PD, when motor symptoms predominate, cognitive and behavioral symptoms may be overlooked. If appropriate neuropsychological tests are administered, subtle deficits can often be detected even in the early stages of PD. In the majority of patients, overt cognitive impairment tends to become manifest in the late stages of the disease. In a community-based study in the United Kingdom, 36% of newly diagnosed patients were found to have cognitive impairment at the time of diagnosis, while 57% of this cohort developed cognitive deficits within 3.5 (+/−0.7) years. In the same cohort, 21 incident dementia cases were identified over 5.2 years of follow-up, corresponding to a dementia incidence estimate of 38.7 per 1,000 person-years of observation (Williams-Gray et al., 2009). In another study, 24% of 115 newly diagnosed PD patients displayed impaired performance on at least three neuropsychological tests and were classified as cognitively impaired (Muslimovic, Post, Speelman, & Schmand, 2005). A pooled analysis comprising 1,346 nondemented PD patients from eight centers showed that 25.8% of patients had mild cognitive impairment (MCI) (Aarsland et al., 2010).

Both prevalence and incidence of dementia are increased in PD compared with age-matched controls. A systematic review of 12 selected studies found a point prevalence of 24%–31%. The prevalence of PD-D in the general population aged 65 years and over was calculated to be 0.3%–0.5% and 3%–4% of patients with dementia in the general population were estimated to be due to PD-D (Aarsland, Zaccai, & Brayne, 2005).

Incidence rates are more reliable than prevalence rates to estimate the true risk of dementia in PD, as demented patients are unlikely to survive as long as nondemented patients. The risk of dementia in PD has been reported to vary between 1.7 and 5.9 times that of controls (de Lau, Schipper, Hofman, Koudstaal, & Breteler, 2005; Marder, Tang, Cote, Stern, & Mayeux, 1995). In the Sydney cohort, 48% of surviving patients had developed dementia 15 years after the diagnosis (Hely, Morris, Reid, & Trafficante, 2005) and the cumulative incidence had risen to 83% 20 years after the diagnosis (Hely, Reid, Adena, Halliday, & Morris, 2008). In another study conducted in Norway, 8-year cumulative prevalence of dementia was 78.2%, with 26% of cases being demented already at baseline in this prevalence sample (Aarsland, Andersen, et al.,

2003). The 12-year frequency of dementia in this cohort was 60% at the end of the follow-up period (Buter et al., 2008). In the Rotterdam study, which employed a door-to-door survey, 15% of the PD patients developed dementia compared to the 4.9% of the control group, during a mean follow-up time of 4.3 years for the incident and 6.9 years for the prevalent PD group (de Lau et al., 2005).

A number of demographic and clinical features have been suggested to be associated with risk of dementia in PD patients (Table 12.2), but many have not been consistently replicated. The best established risk factors for dementia in PD include old age at disease onset or at the time of evaluation, severe motor disability, long disease duration, and atypical neurological features such as early autonomic failure, symmetrical disease presentation, and unsatisfactory response to dopaminergic treatment. Both cross-sectional and prospective studies have found advanced age as a prominent risk factor. The combination of more severe parkinsonian symptoms and old age conferred a 12-fold increased dementia risk compared to young patients with mild parkinsonism (Levy, Schupf, et al., 2002).

Low cognitive scores at baseline; early development of confusion, hallucinations, or psychosis on dopaminergic medication; axial involvement, including speech impairment and postural imbalance; presence of depression; smoking; and excessive daytime sleepiness may also be associated with increased risk of dementia in PD. Rapid eye movement (REM) sleep behavior disorder (RBD) is frequently seen in PD and may be more frequent in patients who eventually develop dementia. In one study, PD patients with RBD had a six-fold higher occurrence of dementia than those without (Marion, Qurashi, Marshall, & Foster, 2008). In a recent population-based cohort study, RBD was associated with a 2.2-fold increased risk of developing PD-MCI over 4 years (Boot et al., 2012). Dementia seems to be associated with the so-called postural instability and gait disorder phenotype of PD (PIGD type), while tremor predominant PD patients seem to have lower risk of developing dementia. Neuropsychological features such as poor verbal fluency as well as poor performance on verbal memory, and the presence of subtle impairment in executive functions at baseline were significantly associated with incident dementia (Woods & Tröster, 2003). It was suggested that not all patients with cognitive impairment would progress to dementia: Impairment in cognitive tests relying on frontal executive functions were associated with a lower risk of dementia, whereas impairment in those tests tapping more posterior cortical functions was associated with a higher risk (Williams-Gray et al., 2009). Reduced cerebrospinal fluid (CSF) β-amyloid levels, an established CSF biomarker in Alzheimer's disease (AD), was found to be related with cognitive decline in PD patients (Siderowf et al., 2010). In another study white matter hyperintensities were associated with cognitive decline in PD patients regardless of age, sex, education status, duration or severity of PD symptoms, and vascular risk factors (Lee et al., 2010).

In addition to constituting risk factors for dementia, the PIGD phenotype and longer disease duration were also found to be risk factors for mild cognitive impairment believed to be representing a predementia state in PD (Sollinger, Goldstein, Lah, Levey, & Factor, 2010).

Although several environmental risk factors have been associated with PD, less is known about their role in PD-D. Smoking was associated with a four-fold higher risk for dementia in PD (Ebmeier et al., 1990).

TABLE 12.2 Potential Risk Factors Reported to Be Associated With Cognitive Impairment and Dementia in Parkinson's Disease Dementia

- Age
- Duration of disease
- Severity of motor disability
- Autonomic dysfunction
- Symmetrical disease presentation
- Unsatisfactory response to dopaminergic treatment
- Postural instability and gait disorder (PIGD) phenotype
- Low cognitive scores at baseline
- Early development of confusion, hallucinations, or psychosis on dopaminergic medication
- Excessive daytime sleepiness
- Reduction in cerebrospinal fluid β-amyloid levels
- White matter hyperintensities in magnetic resonance imaging
- REM sleep behavior disorder

Another study with a mean follow-up of 3.6 ± 2.2 years found a two-fold increase in the risk of dementia in PD patients with a history of smoking. In the same study there was no significant association with head injury, diabetes mellitus, and incident dementia (Levy, Tang, et al., 2002). Estrogen replacement therapy was found to be protective in one study (Marder et al., 1998).

Genetics of Parkinson's Disease Dementia

In a community-based study, siblings of PD-D patients were found to have three-fold increased risk of history of AD (Marder et al., 1999). The data on the association of the apolipoprotein E ε4 (ApoE ε 4) allele with PD-D have been inconsistent (Huang, Chen, & Poole, 2004).

Variations in the tau (*MAPT*) gene seem to be a genetic risk factor: *MAPT* H1/H1 haplotype has been associated with a greater rate of cognitive decline and dementia in PD patients (Goris et al., 2007; Healy et al., 2004), being a strong predictor of dementia with an odd ratio of 12.1 in the CamPaIGN cohort. In a Spanish case-control study consisting of PD, PD-D, DLB, and AD patients and control subjects, the H1 haplotype was found to be strongly associated with PD and has a strong influence on the risk of dementia in PD patients but not in other neurodegenerative diseases such as DLB and AD (Setó-Salvia et al., 2011).

A significantly higher frequency of heterozygote mutations in the glucocerebrosidase gene (GBA) has been reported in PD and dementia with Lewy bodies (DLB) compared with control subjects. GBA mutations may exert a large effect on susceptibility for Lewy body disorders at the individual level, but they are associated with a modest (approximately 3%) population-attributable risk in individuals of European ancestry (Mata et al., 2008). Up to half of the PD patients heterozygous for GBA mutations developed cognitive impairment later in their disease in one series (Goker-Alpan et al., 2008). Recently PD patients with GBA mutations were found to be at higher risk of dementia with an odds ratio of 5.8 (Setó-Salvia et al., 2012).

Altered expression of or missense mutations in the alpha-synuclein gene have been linked to early-onset familial PD, sometimes associated with dementia. There is, however, a more robust relationship with cognitive decline and multiplication of alpha-synuclein gene such as its duplication, and more so with its triplication (Farrer et al., 2004; Sironi et al., 2010).

Mutations in parkin, PINK1, and DJ-1 genes cause autosomal recessive PD. Dementia rates seem to be lower in patients with PINK1 and DJ-1 mutations, whereas the rate in parkin mutations may be more similar to idiopathic PD patients. There are case reports of cognitive impairment associated with the G2019S LRRK2 mutations where the inheritance pattern is autosomal dominant (Wider, Dickson, & Wszolek, 2010). The frequency of dementia in monogenic forms of PD does not appear to be higher, and indeed it may be lower than in sporadic PD. Relatively younger age of patients, especially in recessive forms, may be one reason for this observation (Kasten et al., 2010).

Clinical Features of Parkinson's Disease Dementia

Clinical features of PD-D include cognitive, behavioral, or autonomic symptoms as well as disturbances of the sleep-wake cycle. In typical cases, the profile of dementia can be best described as a dysexecutive syndrome with prominent impairment of attention, executive and visuospatial functions, moderately impaired memory, and neuropsychiatric symptoms, including apathy and psychosis (Table 12.3).

Cognitive Features

Some degree of cognitive impairment is frequently seen already in nondemented PD patients, even at the onset of the disease. The most common deficits are in executive functions, visuospatial functions, memory, and attention (Table 12.4). Cognitive impairment without dementia can be designated as mild cognitive impairment of PD, or PD-MCI where the activities of daily living are largely preserved. Transition from MCI to dementia is gradual, both in terms of symptom severity as well as temporal course. The profile of cognitive deficits in PD-MCI is variable, but the most frequent subtype is single-domain

TABLE 12.3 Clinical Features of Dementia Associated With Parkinson's Disease

I. Core features
1. Diagnosis of Parkinson's disease according to Queen Square Brain Bank criteria
2. A dementia syndrome with insidious onset and slow progression, developing within the context of established Parkinson's disease and diagnosed by history, clinical, and mental examination, defined as follows:
   - Impairment in more than one cognitive domain
   - Representing a decline from premorbid level
   - Deficits severe enough to impair daily life (social, occupational, or personal care), independent of the impairment ascribable to motor or autonomic symptoms

II. Associated clinical features
1. Cognitive features:
   - Attention: Impaired. Impairment in spontaneous and focused attention, poor performance in attentional tasks; performance may fluctuate during the day and from day to day
   - Executive functions: Impaired. Impairment in tasks requiring initiation, planning, concept formation, rule finding, set shifting, or set maintenance; impaired mental speed (bradyphrenia)
   - Visuospatial functions: Impaired. Impairment in tasks requiring visuospatial orientation, perception, or construction
   - Memory: Impaired. Impairment in free recall of recent events or in tasks requiring learning new material, memory usually improves with cueing, recognition is usually better than free recall
   - Language: Core functions largely preserved. Word-finding difficulties and impaired comprehension of complex sentences may be present.
2. Behavioral features
   - Apathy: Decreased spontaneity; loss of motivation, interest, and effortful behavior
   - Changes in personality and mood, including depressive features and anxiety
   - Hallucinations: Mostly visual, usually complex, formed visions of people, animals, or objects
   - Delusions: Usually paranoid, such as infidelity or phantom boarder (unwelcome guests living in the home) delusions
   - Excessive daytime sleepiness

III. Features that do not exclude PD-D but make the diagnosis uncertain
- Coexistence of any other abnormality that may by itself cause cognitive impairment, but judged not to be the cause of dementia, e.g., presence of relevant vascular disease in imaging
- Time interval between the development of motor and cognitive symptoms not known

IV. Features suggesting other conditions or diseases as cause of mental impairment, which, when present, make it impossible to reliably diagnose PD-D
- Cognitive and behavioral symptoms appearing solely in the context of other conditions such as: Acute confusion due to
  a) Systemic diseases or abnormalities
  b) Drug intoxication
  Major depression according to *DSM-IV*
- Features compatible with "probable vascular dementia" criteria according to NINDS-AIREN (dementia in the context of cerebrovascular disease as indicated by focal signs in neurological exam such as hemiparesis, sensory deficits, and evidence of relevant cerebrovascular disease by brain imaging *and* a relationship between the two as indicated by the presence of one or more of the following: onset of dementia within 3 months after a recognized stroke, abrupt deterioration in cognitive functions, and fluctuating, stepwise progression of cognitive deficits)

Source: From Emre et al. (2007).

nonamnestic MCI with a slightly higher frequency than single-domain amnestic MCI, both of which are more common than multi-domain MCI (Aarsland et al., 2010).

Impairment of attentional functions and working memory is an early and prominent feature of patients with PD-D. Reaction time and vigilance are impaired; fluctuating attention is similar to those seen in patients with DLB. PD-D patients tend to be more apathetic compared to AD patients. Impaired attention is an important determinant of activities of daily living (ADLs) in PD-D; in one study a measure of vigilance and focused attention was the single strongest cognitive predictor of ADL status, matching the strength of the effect of motor function on ADLs (Bronnick et al., 2006).

TABLE 12.4 Cognitive Features in Parkinson's Disease Dementia (PD-D)

Deficits in executive functions
- Impairment in planning, set shifting, abstract reasoning, mental flexibility

Memory impairment
- Impairment in episodic memory
  - Free recall impaired, may improve with cueing, recognition usually better
- Impaired working memory

Visuospatial dysfunction
- Both perception and constructional deficits
- Usually early and disproportionate to the level of overall cognitive impairment

Attentional deficits
- Impairment in focused and complex attention (e.g., choice reaction time, internally cued behavior)
- Fluctuating attention

Language
- Usually preserved except for word finding difficulties and understanding complex sentences

Impairment in executive functions is one of the core features of PD-D. In the Mattis Dementia Rating Scale, PD-D patients were found to have lower initiation, perseverance, and construction, but higher memory subscores compared to patients with AD (Aarsland, Litvan, et al., 2003). A dysexecutive syndrome typically presents early in the course of PD-D and is prominent throughout the disease course. Insight is usually preserved in PD-D, in contrast to patients with AD, where deficits are often at least partially denied.

Visual and verbal working memory and implicit memory such as procedural learning can all be impaired in PD-D. The relative severity of memory impairment, as compared to general level of cognitive dysfunction, and the profile of impairment usually differ from that seen in AD. In typical cases the memory impairment is characterized by a deficit in free recall with relatively preserved recognition, indicating that information is stored, but not readily retrieved; when structured cues or multiple choices are provided, retrieval improves. Memory scores in patients with PD-D were found to correlate with performance on executive function tests. Based on this observation, it was suggested that impairment of memory in PD-D, at least to some extent, may be due to difficulties in developing internally cued search strategies, although this view has been recently challenged (Brønnick, Alves, Aarsland, Tysnes, & Larsen, 2011). Memory impairment of the "temporolimbic type," similar to that seen in AD, can also be seen in a subpopulation of PD-D patients (Weintraub, Moberg, Culbertson, Duda, & Stern, 2004).

Another early cognitive deficit in PD-D is impairment in visuospatial functions. Impairment, especially in visuoperceptual abilities, is more severe compared with AD patients with similar global dementia severity. Visuospatial abilities such as object assembly are more impaired in PD-D, whereas visuospatial memory tasks are worse in AD. Deficits in visuospatial functions become more evident in more complex tasks, which require planning and sequencing of response or self-generation of strategies. These deficits may thus be, at least partly, due to problems in sequential organization of behavior or in executive functions.

Primary language functions are largely preserved in PD-D as compared to AD, and deficits usually consist of word-finding difficulties, pauses in spontaneous speech, and difficulty understanding complex sentences. In nondemented PD patients, verb generation is more impaired than generation of nouns, suggesting that deficits may preferentially affect the representation of actions.

Several structured scales, some specifically developed for PD, can be used for screening for cognitive impairment. The Montreal Cognitive Assessment (MoCA) can be used as a screening instrument; in one study a cutoff score of 21/30 yielded a sensitivity of 90% in PD-D patients (Dalrymple-Alford et al., 2010). Both the MoCA and cognitive screening instruments specifically developed for PD, including Mini Mental Parkinson and the Parkinson Neuropsychometric Dementia Assessment (PANDA), have been shown to be more sensitive than the MMSE in detecting cognitive impairment in PD. More elaborate cognitive scales for in-depth assessment include the general cognitive scales such as Mattis Dementia Rating Scale and the CAMCOG-R, as well as PD-specific scales such as SCales for Outcomes of PArkinson's disease-cognition (SCOPA-Cog) and PD Cognitive Rating Scale (PD-CRS) (Kulisevsky & Pagonabarraga, 2009).

Behavioral Features

While a wide range of neuropsychiatric symptoms are seen in PD, they are more frequent and more prominent in PD-D. The most common symptoms in PD-D are depression, apathy, anxiety, hallucinations, and insomnia; at least one neuropsychiatric symptom is present in more than 90% of patients (Aarsland et al., 2007). Hallucinations and delusions may follow treatment with dopaminergic agents, but they occur more frequently in PD-D than in PD. When minor forms such as feeling of presence are included, hallucinations occur in 70% of patients with PD-D, as compared to 25% of those with AD (Fénelon, Mahieux, Huon, & Ziégler, 2000). Delusional misidentification syndromes are found in 17% of PD-D patients and are associated with hallucinations and more severe memory and language deficits (Pagonabarraga et al., 2008). In PD-D, apathy is common in the earlier stages, while delusions increase with more severe motor and cognitive dysfunction. In a longitudinal study, patients with PD-D were discriminated by the presence of cognitive fluctuations, visual and auditory hallucinations, depression, and sleep disturbance from patients with AD; these features were identical to those observed in DLB patients, supporting the concept that these clinical phenotypes are part of the same spectrum (Galvin, Pollack, & Morris, 2006). Depression is more common in PD-D than in AD.

Motor, Autonomic, and Other Associated Features

In PD-D patients, motor symptoms are frequently described as being more symmetrical with predominance of bradykinesia, rigidity, and postural instability. Such features are also correlated with more rapid cognitive decline, whereas tremor dominance has been associated with relative preservation of mental status. In a cross-sectional study, the PIGD subtype was overrepresented with 88% in patients with PD-D in contrast to 38% in nondemented patients (Burn et al., 2003). It was also found that in nearly all dementia cases, dementia was preceded by PIGD-dominant PD or by a transition from tremor dominant to PIGD-type PD (Alves, Larsen, Emre, Wentzel-Larsen, & Aarsland, 2006). In the CamPaign study, severity of akinetic-rigid type was associated with a higher risk for dementia independent of age (Williams-Gray, Foltynie, Brayne, Robbins, & Barker, 2007). PD patients with falls are more likely to have lower MMSE scores than those without falls and also more likely to have dementia. L-dopa-responsiveness may diminish as cognitive impairment emerges, although this assumption is largely based on retrospective clinical data. Mechanisms underlying relative loss of L-dopa response may include development of alpha-synuclein pathology in striatum and loss of striatal dopamine D2 and D3 receptors. On the other hand, this may simply reflect the development or predominance of nondopaminergic axial features, such as postural instability.

Autonomic disturbances in PD, including constipation, urinary incontinence, orthostatic and postprandial hypotension resulting in syncope and falls, excessive sweating, reduced heart rate variability predisposing to ventricular arrhythmias, and sexual dysfunction are frequent and may significantly contribute to disability in patients with PD-D. In a comparative study using a battery of autonomic function tests and power spectral analysis of heart rate variability, cardiovascular autonomic dysfunction was found to be more frequent in patients with PD-D as compared to those with DLB, vascular dementia and AD, with PD-D patients (Allan et al., 2007).

REM sleep behavior disorder (RBD) is common in PD-D. Conversely, half of patients with primary RBD develop a neurodegenerative disease (usually PD or DLB) over a 10-year follow-up period. The presence of RBD in patients with PD is also associated with cognitive deficits: In nondemented patients with PD, only those with concomitant RBD had impaired performance on neuropsychological tests, specifically on measures of episodic verbal memory, executive function, and visuospatial and visuoperceptual processing (Vendette et al., 2007). In some patients, RBD can be an early indicator of incipient dementia and may antedate the onset of dementia for many decades. Excessive daytime sleepiness and poor sleep quality are more common in patients with PD, PD-D, and DLB as compared to AD.

Neuropathological and Biochemical Correlates of Parkinson's Disease Dementia

PD-D is characterized by variable combination of three types of pathological changes: degeneration in subcortical nuclei, cortical AD-type pathology, and Lewy body (LB)–type degeneration (Emre, 2003). In a recent study, the combination of LB-type and AD-type pathology was found to be a better predictive of dementia than the severity of the single pathology (Compta et al., 2011). As is the case in other neurodegenerative diseases, the topographical and temporal sequence of neuronal loss rather than the type of protein aggregation ultimately determines the clinical phenotype. AD-type and LB-pathology do not need to be mutually exclusive as there are interactions between different protein aggregations (i.e., accumulation of alpha-synuclein, tau, and beta-amyloid). For example, alpha-synuclein can induce phosphorylation and fibrilliation of tau, while beta-amyloid can promote formation of alpha-synuclein oligomers and polymers. Beta-amyloid deposits in cerebral cortex were found to enhance alpha-synuclein-induced damage, and the presence of beta-amyloid may promote the aggregation of alpha-synuclein further exacerbating alpha-synuclein-induced neuronal dysfunction (Pletnikova et al., 2005). Hence, protein aggregation may be synergistic in PD-D, with one protein promoting the aggregation of the other, although the consequences of these protein aggregations in terms of cellular function are uncertain.

Difficulties in defining the underlying substrate of dementia in PD also relate to methodological differences. As opposed to earlier studies that utilized ubiquitin staining, more recent studies performed using alpha-synuclein immunohistochemistry revealed that dementia best correlates with LB pathology, although AD-type pathology of variable extent (more plaques than tangles) usually coexists. The fact that families with alpha-synuclein gene duplications and moreso those with triplications develop dementia more often also supports a primary and possibly a "dose-dependent" role for synuclein-based pathology in development of PD-D.

Cell loss in subcortical nuclei projecting to areas involved in cognition or degeneration in subcortical structures involved in neuronal loops connecting with cortical areas, such as thalamic components of the limbic loop, are also prominent. Dementia in PD usually develops later in the disease course and may be related to an ascending order of pathological changes, as suggested by Braak et al. (Braak et al., 2003; Halliday, Hely, Reid, & Morris, 2008). Some support for this "bottom-up" hypothesis is also provided by other studies (Ballard et al., 2006): PD patients with relatively long disease duration prior to dementia onset had lower levels of cortical choline acetyltransferase than those with a short disease duration before dementia onset, implying greater loss of ascending cholinergic projections. In contrast, a more "top-down" pathological process, with greater burden of cortical pathology in PD patients with a more malignant disease course and short time before dementia onset has also been described (Ballard et al., 2006; Halliday et al., 2008). A clinicopathological study arising from the Sydney cohort suggested that there may be three types of pathological constellations associated with three different clinical phenotypes, in particular with regard to the temporal course of dementia. Younger patients who developed dementia late in the disease process seem to have a predominance of alpha-synuclein pathology with little amyloid pathology, whereas those patients with a late age of onset and rapid progression to dementia seem to have mixed alpha-synuclein and amyloid pathology: Such patients, which constituted 25% of the sample with dementia, had severe neocortical Lewy body disease, more consistent with a "DLB-like" phenotype, but also with a high amyloid burden (Halliday et al., 2008). It is unknown which factors determine this clinical and pathological variability, although age of onset is probably one of them. Further complicating are findings from another clinico-pathological study: Approximately 55% of subjects with widespread alpha-synuclein pathology (Braak PD stages 5-6) lacked clinical signs of dementia or extrapyramidal signs antemortem (Parkkinen, Pirttilä, & Alafuzoff, 2008); it is unclear why these subjects could "tolerate" high levels of synuclein deposition without having symptoms.

Biochemically, degeneration of the subcortical nuclei results in various neurochemical deficits, including cholinergic, dopaminergic, serotoninergic, and noradrenergic. The most profound is the cholinergic deficit, although the others may contribute to some aspects of mental dysfunction. Loss of cholinergic cells in the nucleus basalis of Meynert (nbM) greater than that observed in AD occurs in patients with PD-D LBs are frequently found in nbM cells. PD patients without dementia may also exhibit cell loss and alpha-synuclein pathology in the nbM, suggesting the degeneration of the nbM may precede the clinical features. Cholinacetyltransfarase activity is markedly decreased in the frontal cortex of PD and DLB when compared to normal controls and AD. In contrast to AD, PD-D is also associated with neuronal loss in the pedunculopontine cholinergic nuclei, which project to structures such as thalamus. Using vesicular acetylcholine transporter ($[^{123}I]$ iodobenzovesamicol (IBVM)) as a marker of cholinergic integrity, SPECT demonstrated reduction in IBVM binding in parietal and occipital cortices in nondemented PD patients, while demented PD cases have a more extensive decrease in cortical binding, similar to patients with early-onset AD (Kuhl et al., 1996). Functional imaging studies with PET demonstrated that compared with controls mean cortical AChE activity was lowest in patients with PD-D, followed by patients with PD without dementia and AD patients with equal severity of dementia (Bohnen et al., 2003). A subsequent study revealed that the degree of cortical cholinergic deficits correlated particularly well with typical cognitive deficits found in PD-D, for example, impaired performance on tests of attention and executive functions (Bohnen et al., 2006).

The locus coeruleus, the main source of noradrenergic input to the forebrain and cortex, also shows neuronal loss especially in demented and depressed PD patients (Jellinger, 2000). Degeneration in the serotonergic dorsal raphe nucleus was also reported and suggested to be related with symptoms of dementia (Jellinger, 1991). Neuronal loss was observed in ventral tegmental area as well, which provides dopaminergic input to mesolimbic and prefrontal cortex and medial substantia nigra. In one study degree of dementia was found to be associated with the neuronal loss in medial substantia nigra (Rinne, Rummukainen, Paljärvi, & Rinne, 1989).

Neuroimaging Features

In structural imaging there is frontal, occipital, and parietal gray matter loss and an increased rate of whole-brain atrophy in PD-D patients compared with control subjects. Atrophy of gray and white matter in PD-D is less prominent compared to DLB patients. A recent volumetric study revealed a relationship between decrease in caudate volume (but not in hippocampus) and cognitive decline (Apostolova et al., 2010). However, there are also studies showing an atrophy of medial temporal lobe structures such as hippocampus, enthorhinal cortex, and amydala, but these are not as prominent as found in AD. Supratentorial white-matter hyperintensities were also found to be independently associated with cognitive decline in PD-D patients (Lee et al., 2010).

Reduced fractional anisotrophy (FA) was found in the substantia nigra of the nondemented PD patients with diffusion tensor imaging. PD-D patients showed significant FA reduction in the bilateral posterior cingulate bundles compared with nondemented PD patients (Matsui et al., 2007); both FA and mean diffusivity values in cingulate and corpus callosum showed significant correlations with cognitive parameters (Matsui et al., 2007; Wiltshire et al., 2010). In a recent resting-state functional MRI study, corticostriatal connectivity was found to be selectively disrupted in PD-D patients (Seibert, Murphy, Kaestner, & Brewer, 2012).

Positron emission tomography in PD-D may reveal hypometabolism in parietal and temporal cortex similar to pattern seen in AD, and hypometabolism in visual areas and frontal lobe are additionally described, similar to findings seen in DLB. PET with N-[11C]-methyl-4-piperidyl acetate (MP4A) can be used to assess cholinergic innervation of cortex. PD-D patients exhibited a severe cholinergic deficit in various cortical regions, including frontal and temporo-parietal cortices (Hilker et al., 2005). Amyloid PET studies have generally demonstrated relatively low binding in PD-D, in contrast to DLB, where it is often elevated. In PD-D, the mean cortical amyloid load was comparable to controls and nondemented PD patients (Maetzler et al., 2008). In another study 83% (10/12) of PD-D patients had "normal" PIB uptake, whereas 85% (11/13) of DLB patients had significantly increased amyloid load in one or more cortical regions (Edison et al., 2008). In yet another study, increased cortical amyloid burden was found in DLB similar to AD, not in PD-D; striatal PiB retention in the DLB and PD-D groups was associated with less impaired motor function (Gomperts et al., 2008). These findings suggest that global cortical amyloid burden is low and infrequent in PD-D compared to DLB and AD.

A review of rCBF SPECT studies in PD-D found frontal hypoperfusion or bilateral temporoparietal deficits (Bissessur, Tissingh, Wolters, & Scheltens, 1997). Perfusion deficits in precuneus and inferior lateral parietal regions have also been described in PD-D. SPECT studies with Iodine-123 meta-iodobenzylguanidine (^{123}I-MIBG), a marker of postganglionic sympathetic cardiac innervation, demonstrate innervation deficits both in PD-D and DLBs, but not in AD. Similarly to DLB, reductions were found in dopamine transporter markers ((123)I-FP-CIT binding) in the caudate, anterior, and posterior putamens in subjects with PD-D compared to those with AD and controls. Both ^{123}I-MIBG and (123) I-FP-CIT SPECT methods can be used to differentiate patients with DLB or PD-D from those with AD.

Cerebrospinal Fluid Biomarkers in Parkinson's Disease Dementia

Cerebrospinal fluid levels of α-synuclein have been found to be decreased in patients with PD, PD-D, DLB, but increased in patients with AD. When combined with established AD biomarkers such as CSF levels of β-amyloid 1-42, CSF α-synuclein levels may be helpful in the differential diagnosis of AD versus PD-D (Hall et al., 2012). Developing a panel of markers seems a more promising strategy than using a single biomarker for differential diagnosis of PD-D.

Diagnosis of Parkinson's Disease Dementia

The clinical diagnostic criteria for PD-D have been established by a Movement Disorder Society Task Force (Emre et al., 2007), along with practical recommendations for diagnostic procedures (Dubois, Burn, et al., 2007). Clinical features of PD-D are shown in Table 12.3 and diagnostic criteria for Probable and Possible PD-D, representing two levels of diagnostic certainty, are given in Table 12.5. Recently diagnostic criteria for

TABLE 12.5 Diagnostic Criteria for Parkinson's Disease Dementia (PD-D)

Probable PD-D
A. Core features: Both must be present
B. Associated clinical features:
- Typical profile of cognitive deficits including impairment in at least two of the four core cognitive domains (impaired attention which may fluctuate, impaired executive functions, impairment in visuospatial functions, and impaired free recall memory, which usually improves with cueing)
- The presence of at least one behavioral symptom (apathy, depressed or anxious mood, hallucinations, delusions, excessive daytime sleepiness) supports the diagnosis of Probable PD-D; lack of behavioral symptoms, however, does not exclude the diagnosis.

C. None of the group III features present
D. None of the group IV features present

Possible PD-D
A. Core features: Both must be present
B. Associated clinical features:
- Atypical profile of cognitive impairment in one or more domains, such as prominent or receptive-type (fluent) aphasia, or pure storage-failure type amnesia (memory does not improve with cueing or in recognition tasks) with preserved attention
- Behavioral symptoms may or may not be present

OR

C. One or more of the group III features present

Source: From Emre et al. (2007).

mild cognitive impairment in PD (PD-MCI) have also been published by a Task Force of Movement Disorder Society. (Litvan et al., 2012).

The diagnosis of PD-D can be complicated by various factors, such as motor and speech dysfunction. Severe motor impairment may render it difficult to assess whether cognitive deficits are present and to what extent they contribute to functional impairment. Comorbid conditions such as depression, systemic disorders, or adverse effects of drugs may also mimic symptoms of dementia. The onset, course, and pattern of behavioral symptoms and cognitive deficits as well as the clinical context within which these symptoms occur can be helpful in differential diagnosis. Conditions that can mimic PD-D include cerebrovascular disease with dementia and parkinsonism, DLB, AD with drug-induced parkinsonism, and PD patients who develop acute confusion or depression. A detailed history with emphasis on features known to be associated with PD-D, an adequate neuropsychological assessment, and a review of current medication are helpful in diagnosis.

Management of Patients With Parkinson's Disease Dementia

As is the case for DLB and other dementias, both pharmacologic and nonpharmacologic approaches are used in the management of PD-D. As with all of these forms of cognitive impairment, medical and iatrogenic contributors to relatively more prominent cognitive or behavioral symptoms need to be assessed. Pharmacologic treatment modalities include both "specific" approaches based on neurotransmitter deficits and nonspecific drugs to treat behavioral symptoms.

Based on the prominent cholinergic deficits associated with PD-D, ChE-Is have been investigated in PD-D patients. There have been two large randomized, placebo-controlled trials, one with rivastigmine and the other with donepezil.

The rivastigmine trial included 541 PD-D patients with mild to moderate-stage dementia (Emre et al., 2004). At 6 months, both primary endpoints (ADAS-cog, a composite cognitive scale and CGIC, a scale for the assessment of change in global status) as well as all secondary endpoints (including NPI to assess behavioral symptoms, tests of attention and executive functions) showed improvements in favor of rivastigmine; activities of daily living scores showed minimal worsening in patients on rivastigmine, those on placebo worsening significantly more. Except for more patients with worsening of tremor (10% under rivastigmine, 4% under placebo), there were no effects on motor symptoms as compared to placebo. The beneficial effects seen during the first 6 months were maintained in the 6-month extension period, although there was a slight decline in efficacy (Poewe et al., 2006). A subgroup analysis showed that patients with visual hallucinations at baseline derived greater benefits in cognitive outcomes; this was mainly driven by a more rapid decline in the hallucinating group (Burn et al., 2006). Another subgroup analysis focusing on attention as assessed by a computerized test battery demonstrated that all aspects of attention (including focused attention, sustained attention, consistence of responding, and central processing speed) improved under rivastigmine treatment (Wesnes, McKeith, Edgar, Emre, & Lane, 2005). On the basis of this study rivastigmine was approved for treatment of patients with mild to moderate PD-D, both in the European Union and the United States. A patch form of rivastigmine has also become available, and it is approved for treatment of PD-D in several countries.

Donepezil, suggested to be beneficial in an initial small placebo-controlled, cross-over study (Ravina et al., 2005), was also tested in a large, randomized, double-blind, placebo-controlled trial. In total, 550 patients were included, comparing two doses of donepezil (5 mg and 10 mg) with placebo over 6 moths, ADAS-cog and CIBIC-plus being co-primary endpoints (Dubois, Tolosa, et al., 2007). The difference between placebo and donepezil groups in ADAS-cog was not statistically significant in the predefined statistical model, when treatment-by-country interaction was removed from the model; however, there was a significant, dose-dependent benefit with donepezil. The 10 mg group but not the 5 mg group had significantly better CIBIC-plus scores compared to placebo. Significant differences in favor of both donepezil doses were found on several secondary endpoints, including the MMSE, Brief Test of Attention and Verbal Fluency

Test, whereas there were no significant differences on ADL and behavioral scales. There was no worsening of motor symptoms. In another open-label study, the effects of donepezil on central processing speed and other attentional measures were tested over 20 weeks. Power of attention, continuity of attention, and reaction time variability were found to be improved as compared to baseline (Rowan et al., 2007).

In a few open-label studies galantamine was suggested to have beneficial effects in patients with PD-D (Aarsland, Mosimann, & McKeith, 2004). In a placebo-controlled, randomized, double-blind 16-week trial of galantamine, 16–24 mg in 69 nondemented PD patients, there were no beneficial effects on any of the cognitive functions assessed; dropouts due to gastrointestinal side effects and self-reported worsening of PD symptoms were greater in the galantamine group (Grace, Amick, & Friedman, 2009).

In a Cochrane meta-analysis evaluating the efficacy of ChE-Is in PD-D, 5.3% of patients were concluded to have benefits on outcome scales, whereas 10.1% patients on placebo demonstrated worsening, suggesting that the effect size is close to 15% (Maidment, Fox, & Boustani, 2006). In another, more recent Cochrane meta-analysis the authors concluded that the use of cholinesterase inhibitors in PD-D is associated with a positive impact on global assessment, cognitive function, behavioral disturbance, and activities of daily living rating scales (Rolinski, Fox, Maidment, & McShane, 2012). Based on two large randomized controlled trials and the results of meta-analysis, treatment with a ChEI such as rivastigmine or donepezil should be considered in patients with PD-D, taking into account expected benefits and risks.

In a randomized, placebo-controlled trial including patients either with DLB or PD-D, summarized previously in detail, there was a significant difference in favor of memantine in the global outcome scale, whereas there were no significant differences on MMSE and NPI. Patients with PD-D had more benefits as compared to those with DLB (Aarsland et al., 2009). In the largest ever randomized, placebo-controlled trial, however, which included 199 patients either with DLB or PD-D, there were no significant differences between memantine and placebo in the PD-D population. The ADL scale, caregiver burden scale, and a number of cognitive tests did not show significant differences between active and placebo in either population (Emre et al., 2010). These results suggest that memantine may have mild beneficial effects in patients with DLB but not clearly in PD-D.

Another NMDA antagonist, amantadine, was reported to delay the onset of dementia in PD and to attenuate its severity in a retrospective analysis (Inzelberg et al., 2006). These results should be interpreted with caution, however, until they are replicated in prospective, randomized, controlled trials.

Behavioral symptoms may improve with ChE-Is; therefore, patients with behavioral symptoms such as hallucinations should be first treated with these agents before considering neuroleptics (Emre et al., 2004). Neuroleptic treatment, however, may become necessary, especially in patients with severe psychosis or agitation. Classical neuroleptics are contraindicated as they worsen motor function and may result in life-threatening neuroleptic hypersensitivity. Studies with new generation ("atypical") neuroleptics in PD-D patients are few; most studies were performed in PD patients with hallucinations or psychosis, without indicating the presence or absence of dementia. In a systematic review of atypical neuroleptics for the treatment of psychosis in PD, clozapine was concluded to be the only drug with proven efficacy and acceptable tolerability provided that appropriate safety monitoring is performed (Goetz, Koller, & Poewe, 2002). Other atypical neuroleptics such as olanzapine and risperidone can worsen motor function; the efficacy of quetiapine is not well demonstrated, although it may be considered under careful monitoring for side effects.

There are no randomized, controlled studies of antidepressants in patients with PD-D. Tricyclic antidepressants such as amitriptyline and nortriptiline may be effective in PD depression; they should, however, not be administered in patients with PD-D, as they may worsen cognition due to their anticholinergic effects. The dopamine agonist pramipexole was shown to be effective in PD depression (Barone et al., 2010), but it has the potential to worsen hallucinations and confusion in PD-D patients and should not be considered in this population. Selective serotonin reuptake inhibitors such as paroxetine, or mixed serotonin and noradrenalin reuptake inhibitors such as venlafaxine, have been shown to be effective in PD depression (Richard et al., 2012) and they are preferred in patients with PD-D, taking into account their adverse effects and potential interaction with other medication such as monamine oxidase B inhibitors. Antidepressants with sedating properties such as trazodone can be considered to treat sleep disturbances. If RBD causes significant distress and is thought to warrant treatment, melatonin or very low doses of clonazepam may be used; daytime somnolence and confusion, however, should be monitored. Excessive daytime sleepiness may occur in PD-D patients, more frequently than in nondemented PD patients. Modafinil, a well-tolerated agent that promotes wakefulness, was tested in nondemented PD patients (Adler, Caviness, Hentz, Lind, & Tiede, 2003) but not in PD-D; it may be considered empirically. Atomoxetine, a highly selective noradrenaline reuptake inhibitor, may also be effective in the treatment of excessive daytime somnolence (Weintraub et al., 2010).

References

Aarsland, D., Andersen, K., Larsen, J. P., Lolk, A., & Kragh-Sørensen, P. (2003). Prevalence and characteristics of dementia in Parkinson disease: an 8-year prospective study. *Archives of Neurology, 60,* 387–392.

Aarsland, D., Ballard, C., Walker, Z., Bostrom, F., Alves, G., Kossakowski, K.,...Londos, E. (2009). Memantine in patients with Parkinson's disease dementia or dementia with Lewy bodies: A double-blind, placebo-controlled, multicentre trial. *Lancet Neurology, 8,* 613–618.

Aarsland, D., Brønnick, K., Ehrt, U., De Deyn, P. P., Tekin, S., Emre, M., & Cummings, J. L. (2007). Neuropsychiatric symptoms in patients with Parkinson's disease and dementia: Frequency, profile and associated care giver stress. *Journal of Neurology, Neurosurgery and Psychiatry, 78,* 36–42.

Aarsland, D., Bronnick, K., Williams-Gray, C., Weintraub, D., Marder, K., Kulisevsky, J.,...Emre, M. (2010). Mild cognitive impairment in Parkinson disease: A multicenter pooled analysis. *Neurology, 75,* 1062–1069.

Aarsland, D., Litvan, I., Salmon, D., Galasko, D., Wentzel-Larsen, T., & Larsen, J. P. (2003). Performance on the dementia rating scale in Parkinson's disease with dementia and dementia with Lewy bodies: Comparison with progressive supranuclear palsy and Alzheimer's disease. *Journal of Neurology, Neurosurgery and Psychiatry, 74,* 1215–1220.

Aarsland, D., Mosimann, U. P., & McKeith, I. G. (2004). Role of cholinesterase inhibitors in Parkinson's disease and dementia with Lewy bodies. *Journal of Geriatric Psychiatry and Neurology, 17,* 164–171.

Aarsland, D., Zaccai, J., & Brayne, C. (2005). A systematic review of prevalence studies of dementia in Parkinson's disease. *Movement Disorders, 20,* 1255–1263.

Adler, C. H., Caviness, J. N., Hentz, J. G., Lind, M., & Tiede, J. (2003). Randomized trial of modafinil for treating subjective daytime sleepiness in patients with Parkinson's disease. *Movement Disorders, 18,* 287–293.

Albin, R. L., Minoshima, S., D'Amato, C. J., Frey, K. A., Kuhl, D. A., & Sima, A. A. (1996). Fluoro-deoxyglucose positron emission tomography in diffuse Lewy body disease. *Neurology, 47,* 462–466.

Allan, L. M., Ballard, C. G., Allen, J., Murray, A., Davidson, A. W., McKeith, I. G., & Kenny, R. A. (2007). Autonomic dysfunction in dementia. *Journal of Neurology, Neurosurgery and Psychiatry, 78,* 671–677.

Alves, G., Larsen, J. P., Emre, M., Wentzel-Larsen, T., & Aarsland, D. (2006). Changes in motor subtype and risk for incident dementia in Parkinson's disease. *Movement Disorders, 21,* 1123–1130.

Apostolova, L. G., Beyer, M., Green, A. E., Hwang, K. S., Morra, J. H., Chou, Y-Y.,...Thompson, P. M. (2010). Hippocampal, caudate, and ventricular changes in Parkinson's disease with and without dementia. *Movement Disorders, 25,* 687–688.

Auning, E., Rongve, A., Fladby, T., Booij, J., Hortobágyi, T., Siepel, F. J.,...Aarsland, D. (2011). Early and presenting symptoms of dementia with Lewy bodies. *Dementia and Geriatric Cognitive Disorders, 32,* 202–208.

Ballard, C., Piggott, M., Johnson, M., Cairns, N., Perry, R., McKeith, I.,...Perry, E. (2000). Delusions associated with elevated muscarinic binding in dementia with Lewy bodies. *Annals of Neurology, 48,* 868–876.

Ballard, C., Ziabreva, I., Perry, R., Larsen, J. P., O'Brien, J., McKeith, I.,... Aarsland, D. (2006). Differences in neuropathologic characteristics across the Lewy body dementia spectrum. *Neurology, 67,* 1931–1934.

Barker, W. W., Luis, C. A., Kashuba, A., Luis, M., Harwood, D. G., Loewenstein, D.,...Duara, R. (2002). Relative frequencies of Alzheimer disease, Lewy body, vascular and frontotemporal dementia, and hippocampal sclerosis in the State of Florida Brain Bank. *Alzheimer Disease and Associated Disorders, 16,* 203–212.

Barone, P., Poewe, W., Albrecht, S., Debieuvre, C., Massey, D., Rascol, O., ... Weintraub, D. (2010). Pramipexole for the treatment of depressive symptoms in patients with Parkinson's disease: A randomised, double-blind, placebo-controlled trial. *Lancet Neurology, 9*, 573–580.

Beyer, K., Domingo-Sàbat, M., & Ariza, A. (2009). Molecular pathology of Lewy body diseases. *International Journal of Molecular Science, 10*, 724–745.

Bibl, M., Mollenhauer, B., Esselmann, H., Lewczuk, P., Klafki, H-W., Sparbier, K., ... Wiffang, J. (2006). CSF amyloid-beta-peptides in Alzheimer's disease, dementia with Lewy bodies and Parkinson's disease dementia. *Brain, 129*, 1177–1187.

Bissessur, S., Tissingh, G., Wolters, E. C., & Scheltens, P. (1997). rCBF SPECT in Parkinson's disease patients with mental dysfunction. *Journal of Neural Transmission Supplemental, 50*, 25–30.

Bogaerts, V., Engelborghs, S., Kumar-Singh, S., Goossens, D., Pickut, B., van der Zee, J., ... Van Broeckhoven, C. (2007). A novel locus for dementia with Lewy bodies: A clinically and genetically heterogeneous disorder. *Brain, 130*, 2277–2291.

Bohnen, N. I., Kaufer, D. I., Hendrickson, R., Ivanco, L. S., Lopresti, B. J., Constantine, G. M., ... Dekosky, S. T. (2006). Cognitive correlates of cortical cholinergic denervation in Parkinson's disease and Parkinsonian dementia. *Journal of Neurology, 253*, 242–247.

Bohnen, N. I., Kaufer, D. I., Ivanco, L. S., Lopresti, B., Koeppe, R. A., Davis, J. G., ... Dekosky, S. T. (2003). Cortical cholinergic function is more severely affected in parkinsonian dementia than in Alzheimer disease: An in vivo positron emission tomographic study. *Archives of Neurology, 60*, 1745–1748.

Bonanni, L., Thomas, A., Tiraboschi, P., Perfetti, B., Varanese, S., & Onofrj, M. (2008). EEG comparisons in early Alzheimer's disease, dementia with Lewy bodies and Parkinson's disease with dementia patients with a 2-year follow-up. *Brain, 131*, 690–705.

Boot, B. P., Boeve, B. F., Roberts, R. O., Ferman, T. J., Geda, Y. E., Pankratz, V. S., ... Petersen, R. C. (2012). Probable rapid eye movement sleep behavior disorder increases risk for mild cognitive impairment and Parkinson disease: A population-based study. *Annals of Neurology, 71*, 49–56.

Borroni, B., Grassi, M., Costanzi, C., Archetti, S., Caimi, L., & Padovani, A. (2006). APOE genotype and cholesterol levels in Lewy body dementia and Alzheimer disease: Investigating genotype-phenotype effect on disease risk. *American Journal of Geriatric Psychiatry, 14*, 1022–1031.

Bozzali, M., Falini, A., Cercignani, M., Baglio, F., Farina, E., Alberoni, M., ... Nemni, R. (2005). Brain tissue damage in dementia with Lewy bodies: An in vivo diffusion tensor MRI study. *Brain, 128*, 1595–1604.

Braak, H., Del Tredici, K., Rüb, U., de Vos, R. A. I., Jansen Steur, E. N. H., & Braak, E. (2003). Staging of brain pathology related to sporadic Parkinson's disease. *Neurobiology of Aging, 24*, 197–211.

Bronnick, K., Ehrt, U., Emre, M., De Deyn, P. P., Wesnes, K., Tekin, S., & Aarsland, D. (2006). Attentional deficits affect activities of daily living in dementia-associated with Parkinson's disease. *Journal of Neurology, Neurosurgery and Psychiatry, 77*, 1136–1142.

Brønnick, K., Alves, G., Aarsland, D., Tysnes, O-B., & Larsen, J. P. (2011). Verbal memory in drug-naive, newly diagnosed Parkinson's disease. The retrieval deficit hypothesis revisited. *Neuropsychology, 25*, 114–124.

Burn, D., Emre, M., McKeith, I., De Deyn, P. P., Aarsland, D., Hsu, C., & Lane, R. (2006). Effects of rivastigmine in patients with and without visual hallucinations in dementia associated with Parkinson's disease. *Movement Disorders, 21*, 1899–1907.

Burn, D. J., Rowan, E. N., Minett, T., Sanders, J., Myint, P., Richardson, J., ... McKeith, I. G. (2003). Extrapyramidal features in Parkinson's disease with and without dementia and dementia with Lewy bodies: A cross-sectional comparative study. *Movement Disorders, 18*, 884–889.

Burton, E. J., Barber, R., Mukaetova-Ladinska, E. B., Robson, J., Perry, R. H., Jaros, E., ... O'Brien, J. T. (2009). Medial temporal lobe atrophy on MRI differentiates Alzheimer's disease from dementia with Lewy bodies and vascular cognitive impairment: A prospective study with pathological verification of diagnosis. *Brain, 132*, 195–203.

Burton, E. J., Mukaetova-Ladinska, E. B., Perry, R. H., Jaros, E., Barber, R., & O'Brien, J. T. (2012). Neuropathological correlates of volumetric MRI in autopsy-confirmed Lewy body dementia. *Neurobiology of Aging, 33*, 1228–1236.

Buter, T. C., van den Hout, A., Matthews, F. E., Larsen, J. P., Brayne, C., & Aarsland, D. (2008). Dementia and survival in Parkinson disease: A 12-year population study. *Neurology, 70*, 1017–1022.

Calderon, J., Perry, R. J., Erzincliglu, S. W., Berrios, G. E., Dening, T. R., & Hodges, J. R. (2001). Perception, attention, and working memory are disproportionately impaired in dementia with Lewy bodies compared with

Alzheimer's disease. *Journal of Neurology, Neurosurgery and Psychiatry, 70,* 157–164.

Chan, S. S. M., Chiu, H. F. K., Lam, L. C. W., & Leung, V. P. Y. (2002). Prevalence of dementia with Lewy bodies in an inpatient psychogeriatric population in Hong Kong Chinese. *International Journal of Geriatric Psychiatry, 17,* 847–850.

Chartier-Harlin, M-C., Kachergus, J., Roumier, C., Mouroux, V., Douay, X., Lincoln, S.,...Destée, A. (2004). Alpha-synuclein locus duplication as a cause of familial Parkinson's disease. *Lancet, 364,* 1167–1169.

Clark, L. N., Kartsaklis, L. A., Wolf, G. R., Dorado, B., Ross, B. M., Kisselev, S.,...Marder, K. (2009). Association of glucocerebrosidase mutations with dementia with Lewy bodies. *Archives of Neurology, 66,* 578–583.

Compta, Y., Parkkinen, L., O'Sullivan, S. S., Vandrovcova, J., Holton, J. L., Collins, C.,...Revesz, T. (2011). Lewy- and Alzheimer-type pathologies in Parkinson's disease dementia: Which is more important? *Brain, 134,* 1493–1505.

Consensus recommendations for the postmortem diagnosis of Alzheimer's disease. The National Institute on Aging, and Reagan Institute Working Group on Diagnostic Criteria for the Neuropathological Assessment of Alzheimer's Disease. (1997). *Neurobiology of Aging, 18,* S1–S2.

Dalfó, E., Albasanz, J. L., Martin, M., & Ferrer, I. (2004). Abnormal metabotropic glutamate receptor expression and signaling in the cerebral cortex in diffuse Lewy body disease is associated with irregular alpha-synuclein/phospholipase C (PLCbeta1) interactions. *Brain Pathology, 14,* 388–398.

Dalrymple-Alford, J. C., MacAskill, M. R., Nakas, C. T., Livingston, L., Graham, C., Crucian, G. P.,...Anderson, T. J. (2010). The MoCA: Well-suited screen for cognitive impairment in Parkinson disease. *Neurology, 75,* 1717–1725.

Dubois, B., Tolosa, E., & Kulisevsky, J. (2007). Efficacy and safety of donepezil in the treatment of Parkinson's disease patients with dementia.

Dubois, B., Burn, D., Goetz, C., Aarsland, D., Brown, R. G., Broe Gerald, A.,...Emre, M. (2007). Diagnostic procedures for Parkinson's disease dementia: Recommendations from the movement disorder society task force. *Movement Disorders, 22,* 2314–2324.

Ebmeier, K. P., Calder, S. A., Crawford, J. R., Stewart, L., Besson, J. A., Mutch, W. J. (1990). Mortality and causes of death in idiopathic Parkinson's disease: Results from the Aberdeen whole population study. *Scottish Medical Journal, 35,* 173–175.

Edison, P., Rowe, C. C., Rinne, J. O., Ng, S., Ahmed, I., Kemppainen, N.,...Brooks, D. J. (2008). Amyloid load in Parkinson's disease dementia and Lewy body dementia measured with [11C]PIB positron emission tomography. *Journal of Neurology, Neurosurgery and Psychiatry, 79,* 1331–1338.

Emre, M., Aarsland, D., Albanese, A., Byrne, E. J., Deuschl, G., De Deyn, P. P.,...Lane, R. (2004). Rivastigmine for dementia associated with Parkinson's disease. *New England Journal of Medicine, 351,* 2509–2518.

Emre, M., Aarsland, D., Brown, R., Burn, D. J., Duyckaerts, C., Mizuno, Y.,...Dubois, B. (2007). Clinical diagnostic criteria for dementia associated with Parkinson's disease. *Movement Disorders, 22,* 1689–1707; quiz 1837.

Emre, M., Tsolaki, M., Bonuccelli, U., Destée, A., Tolosa, E., Kutzelnigg, A.,...Jones, R. (2010). Memantine for patients with Parkinson's disease dementia or dementia with Lewy bodies: A randomised, double-blind, placebo-controlled trial. *Lancet Neurology, 9,* 969–977.

Emre M. (2003). What causes mental dysfunction in Parkinson's disease? *Movement Disorders, 18*(Suppl 6), S63–S71.

Engelborghs, S., Dermaut, B., Goeman, J., Saerens, J., Mariën, P., Pickut, B. A., (2003). Prospective Belgian study of neurodegenerative and vascular dementia: APOE genotype effects. *Journal of Neurology, Neurosurgery and Psychiatry, 74,* 1148–1151.

Farrer, M., Kachergus, J., Forno, L., Lincoln, S., Wang, D-S., Hulihan, M.,...De Deyn, P. P. (2004). Comparison of kindreds with Parkinsonism and alpha-synuclein genomic multiplications. *Annals of Neurology, 55,* 174–179.

Fénelon, G., Mahieux, F., Huon, R., & Ziégler, M. (2000). Hallucinations in Parkinson's disease: Prevalence, phenomenology and risk factors. *Brain, 123*(Pt 4), 733–745.

Ferman, T. J., Boeve, B. F., Smith, G. E., Lin, S-C., Silber, M. H., Pedraza, O.,...Dickson, D. W. (2011). Inclusion of RBD improves the diagnostic classification of dementia with Lewy bodies. *Neurology, 77,* 875–882.

Ferman, T. J., Smith, G. E., Boeve, B. F., Ivnik, R. J., Petersen, R. C., Knopman, D.,...Dickson, D. W. (2004). DLB fluctuations: Specific features that reliably differentiate DLB from AD and normal aging. *Neurology, 62,* 181–187.

Firbank, M. J., Colloby, S. J., Burn, D. J., McKeith, I. G., & O'Brien, J. T. (2003). Regional cerebral blood flow in Parkinson's disease with and without dementia. *Neuroimage, 20,* 1309–1319.

Foster, E. R., Campbell, M. C., Burack, M. A., Hartlein, J., Flores, H. P., Cairns, N. J.,...Perlmutter, J. S. (2010). Amyloid imaging of Lewy body-associated disorders. *Movement Disorders, 25*, 2516–2523.

Gaig, C., Valldeoriola, F., Gelpi, E., Ezquerra, M., Llufriu, S., Buongiorno, M.,...Tolosa, E. (2011). Rapidly progressive diffuse Lewy body disease. *Movement Disorders, 26*, 1316–1323.

Galasko, D., Hansen, L. A., Katzman, R., Wiederholt, W., Masliah, E., Terry, R.,...Thal, L. J. (1994). Clinical-neuropathological correlations in Alzheimer's disease and related dementias. *Archives of Neurology, 51*, 888–895.

Galvin, J. E., Price, J. L., Yan, Z., Morris, J. C., & Sheline, Y. I. (2011). Resting bold fMRI differentiates dementia with Lewy bodies vs Alzheimer disease. *Neurology, 76*, 1797–1803.

Galvin, J. E., Pollack, J., & Morris, J. C. (2006). Clinical phenotype of Parkinson disease dementia. *Neurology, 67*, 1605–1611.

Goetz, C. G., Koller, W. C., & Poewe, W. (2002). Drugs to treat dementia and psychosis: Management of Parkinson's disease. *Movement Disorders, 17*(Suppl 4), S120–S127.

Goker-Alpan, O., Lopez, G., Vithayathil, J., Davis, J., Hallett, M., & Sidransky, E. (2008). The spectrum of Parkinsonian manifestations associated with glucocerebrosidase mutations. *Archives of Neurology, 65*, 1353–1357.

Gómez-Isla, T., Growdon, W. B., McNamara, M., Newell, K., Gómez-Tortosa, E., Hedley-Whyte, E. T.,...Hyman, B. T. (1999). Clinicopathologic correlates in temporal cortex in dementia with Lewy bodies. *Neurology, 53*, 2003–2009.

Gomperts, S. N., Rentz, D. M., Moran, E., Becker, J. A., Locascio, J. J., Klunk, W. E.,...Johnson, K. A. (2008). Imaging amyloid deposition in Lewy body diseases. *Neurology, 71*, 903–910.

Goris, A., Williams-Gray, C. H., Clark, G. R., Foltynie, T., Lewis, S. J. G., Brown, J.,...Sawcer, S. J. (2007). Tau and alpha-synuclein in susceptibility to, and dementia in, Parkinson's disease. *Annals of Neurology, 62*, 145–153.

Grace, J., Amick, M. M., & Friedman, J. H. (2009). A double-blind comparison of galantamine hydrobromide ER and placebo in Parkinson disease. *Journal of Neurology, Neurosurgery and Psychiatry, 80*, 18–23.

Hall, S., Ohrfelt, A., Constantinescu, R., Andreasson, U., Surova, Y., Bostrom, F.,...Hansson, O. (2012). Accuracy of a panel of 5 cerebrospinal fluid biomarkers in the differential diagnosis of patients with dementia and/or Parkinsonian disorders. *Archives of Neurology, 69*(11), 1445–1452.

Halliday, G., Hely, M., Reid, W., & Morris, J. (2008). The progression of pathology in longitudinally followed patients with Parkinson's disease. *Acta Neuropathologica, 115*, 409–415.

Hansen, L., Salmon, D., Galasko, D., Masliah, E., Katzman, R., DeTeresa, R.,...Klauber, M. (1990). The Lewy body variant of Alzheimer's disease: A clinical and pathologic entity. *Neurology, 40*, 1–8.

Hanyu, H., Sato, T., Hirao, K., Kanetaka, H., Sakurai, H., & Iwamoto, T. (2009). Differences in clinical course between dementia with Lewy bodies and Alzheimer's disease. *European Journal of Neurology, 16*, 212–217.

Harding, A. J., Broe, G. A., & Halliday, G. M. (2002). Visual hallucinations in Lewy body disease relate to Lewy bodies in the temporal lobe. *Brain, 125*, 391–403.

Healy, D. G., Abou-Sleiman, P. M., Lees, A. J., Casas, J. P., Quinn, N., Bhatia, K.,...Wood, N. W. (2004). Tau gene and Parkinson's disease: A case-control study and meta-analysis. *Journal of Neurology, Neurosurgery and Psychiatry, 75*, 962–965.

Hely, M. A., Morris, J. G. L., Reid, W. G. J., & Trafficante, R. (2005). Sydney Multicenter Study of Parkinson's disease: Non-L-dopa-responsive problems dominate at 15 years. *Movement Disorders, 20*, 190–199.

Hely, M. A., Reid, W. G. J., Adena, M. A., Halliday, G. M., & Morris, J. G. L. (2008). The Sydney multicenter study of Parkinson's disease: The inevitability of dementia at 20 years. *Movement Disorders, 23*, 837–844.

Hilker, R., Thomas, A. V., Klein, J. C., Weisenbach, S., Kalbe, E., Burghaus, L.,...Heiss, W. D. (2005). Dementia in Parkinson disease: Functional imaging of cholinergic and dopaminergic pathways. *Neurology, 65*, 1716–1722.

Horimoto, Y., Matsumoto, M., Akatsu, H., Ikari, H., Kojima, K., Yamamoto, T.,...Kosaka, K. (2003). Autonomic dysfunctions in dementia with Lewy bodies. *Journal of Neurology, 250*, 530–533.

Hu, X. S., Okamura, N., Arai, H., Higuchi, M., Matsui, T., Tashiro, M.,...Sasaki, H. (2000). 18F-fluorodopa PET study of striatal dopamine uptake in the diagnosis of dementia with Lewy bodies. *Neurology, 55*, 1575–1577.

Huang, X., Chen, P. C., & Poole, C. (2004). APOE-[epsilon]2 allele associated with higher prevalence of sporadic Parkinson disease. *Neurology, 62*, 2198–2202.

Hulette, C., Mirra, S., Wilkinson, W., Heyman, A., Fillenbaum, G., & Clark, C. (1995). The Consortium to Establish a Registry for Alzheimer's Disease (CERAD). Part IX. A prospective cliniconeuropathologic study of Parkinson's features in Alzheimer's disease. *Neurology, 45*, 1991–1995.

Inzelberg, R., Bonuccelli, U., Schechtman, E., Miniowich, A., Strugatsky, R., Ceravolo, R.,...Rabey, J. M. (2006). Association between amantadine and the onset of dementia in Parkinson's disease. *Movement Disorders, 21,* 1375–1379.

Jellinger, K. A. (1991). Pathology of Parkinson's disease. Changes other than the nigrostriatal pathway. *Molecular Chemistry and Neuropathology, 14,* 153–197.

Jellinger, K. A. (2000). Morphological substrates of mental dysfunction in Lewy body disease: an update. *Journal of Neural Transmission Supplemental, 59,* 185–212.

Jellinger, K. A. (2003). Prevalence of vascular lesions in dementia with Lewy bodies. A postmortem study. *Journal of Neural Transmission, 110,* 771–778.

Kantarci, K., Petersen, R. C., Boeve, B. F., Knopman, D. S., Tang-Wai, D. F., O'Brien, P. C.,...Jack, C. R., Jr. (2004). 1H MR spectroscopy in common dementias. *Neurology, 63,* 1393–1398.

Kantarci, K., Ferman, T. J., Boeve, B. F., Weigand, S. D., Przybelski, S., Vemuri, P.,...Dickson, D. W. (2012). Focal atrophy on MRI and neuropathologic classification of dementia with Lewy bodies. *Neurology, 79,* 553–560.

Kasten, M., Kertelge, L., Brüggemann, N., van der Vegt, J., Schmidt, A., Tadic, V.,...Klein, C. (2010). Nonmotor symptoms in genetic Parkinson disease. *Archives of Neurology, 67,* 670–676.

Kenny, E. R., Blamire, A. M., Firbank, M. J., & O'Brien, J. T. (2012). Functional connectivity in cortical regions in dementia with Lewy bodies and Alzheimer's disease. *Brain, 135,* 569–581.

Kobayashi, S., Tateno, M., Park, T. W., Utsumi, K., Sohma, H., Ito, Y. M.,...Saito, T. (2011). Apolipoprotein E4 frequencies in a Japanese population with Alzheimer's disease and dementia with Lewy bodies. *PLoS One, 6,* e18569.

Kuhl, D. E., Minoshima, S., Fessler, J. A., Frey, K. A., Foster, N. L., Ficaro, E. P.,...Koeppe, R. A. (1996). In vivo mapping of cholinergic terminals in normal aging, Alzheimer's disease, and Parkinson's disease. *Annals of Neurology, 40,* 399–410.

Kulisevsky, J., & Pagonabarraga, J. (2009). Cognitive impairment in Parkinson's disease: Tools for diagnosis and assessment. *Movement Disorders, 24,* 1103–1110.

de Lau, L. M. L., Schipper, C. M. A., Hofman, A., Koudstaal, P. J., & Breteler, M. M. B. (2005). Prognosis of Parkinson disease: Risk of dementia and mortality: the Rotterdam Study. *Archives of Neurology, 62,* 1265–1269.

Lee, S-J., Kim, J-S., Yoo, J-Y., Song, I-U., Kim, B-S., Jung, S-L.,... Lee, K. S. (2010). Influence of white matter hyperintensities on the cognition of patients with Parkinson disease. *Alzheimer Disease and Associated Disorders, 24,* 227–233.

Levy, G., Schupf, N., Tang, M-X., Cote, L. J., Louis, E. D., Mejia, H.,...Marder, K. (2002). Combined effect of age and severity on the risk of dementia in Parkinson's disease. *Annals of Neurology, 51,* 722–729.

Levy, G., Tang, M-X., Cote, L. J., Louis, E. D., Alfaro, B., Mejia, H.,...Marder, K. (2002). Do risk factors for Alzheimer's disease predict dementia in Parkinson's disease? An exploratory study. *Movement Disorders, 17,* 250–257.

Lim, A., Tsuang, D., Kukull, W., Nochlin, D., Leverenz, J., McCormick, W.,...Larson, E. B. (1999). Clinico-neuropathological correlation of Alzheimer's disease in a community-based case series. *Journal of the American Geriatric Society, 47,* 564–569.

Lippa, C. F., Smith, T. W., & Perry, E. (1999). Dementia with Lewy bodies: Choline acetyltransferase parallels nucleus basalis pathology. *Journal of Neural Transmission, 106,* 525–535.

Litvan, I., Goldman, J. G., Tröster, A. I., Schmand, B. A., Weintraub, D., Petersen, R. C.,...Emre, M. (2012). Diagnostic criteria for mild cognitive impairment in Parkinson's disease: Movement Disorder Society Task Force guidelines. *Movement Disorders, 27,* 349–356.

Lobotesis, K., Fenwick, J. D., Phipps, A., Ryman, A., Swann, A., Ballard, C.,...O'Brien, J. T. (2001). Occipital hypoperfusion on SPECT in dementia with Lewy bodies but not AD. *Neurology, 56,* 643–649.

Lopez, O. L., Becker, J. T., Kaufer, D. I., Hamilton, R. L., Sweet, R. A., Klunk, W., & DeKosky, S. T. (2002). Research evaluation and prospective diagnosis of dementia with Lewy bodies. *Archives of Neurology, 59,* 43–46.

Lucetti, C., Logi, C., Del Dotto, P., Berti, C., Ceravolo, R., Baldacci, F.,...Bonuccelli, U. (2010). Levodopa response in dementia with Lewy bodies: A 1-year follow-up study. *Parkinsonism and Related Disorders, 16,* 522–526.

Maetzler, W., Reimold, M., Liepelt, I., Solbach, C., Leyhe, T., Schweitzer, K.,...Berg, D. (2008). [11C]PIB binding in Parkinson's disease dementia. *Neuroimage, 39,* 1027–1033.

Maidment, I., Fox, C., & Boustani, M. (2006). Cholinesterase inhibitors for Parkinson's disease dementia. *Cochrane Database of Systematic Reviews,* CD004747.

Marder, K., Tang, M. X., Alfaro, B., Mejia, H., Cote, L., Jacobs, D.,...Mayeux, R. (1998). Postmenopausal estrogen use and Parkinson's disease with and without dementia. *Neurology, 50,* 1141–1143.

Marder, K., Tang, M. X., Alfaro, B., Mejia, H., Cote, L., Louis, E.,...Mayeux, R. (1999). Risk of Alzheimer's disease in relatives of Parkinson's disease patients with and without dementia. *Neurology, 52,* 719–724.

Marder, K., Tang, M. X., Cote, L., Stern, Y., & Mayeux, R. (1995). The frequency and associated risk factors for dementia in patients with Parkinson's disease. *Archives of Neurology*, 52, 695–701.

Marion, M-H., Qurashi, M., Marshall, G., & Foster, O. (2008). Is REM sleep behaviour disorder (RBD) a risk factor of dementia in idiopathic Parkinson's disease? *Journal of Neurology*, 255, 192–196.

Mata, I. F., Samii, A., Schneer, S. H., Roberts, J. W., Griffith, A., Leis, B. C.,...Zabetian, C. P. (2008). Glucocerebrosidase gene mutations: A risk factor for Lewy body disorders. *Archives of Neurology*, 65, 379–382.

Matsui, H., Nishinaka, K., Oda, M., Niikawa, H., Kubori, T., & Udaka, F. (2007). Dementia in Parkinson's disease: Diffusion tensor imaging. *Acta Neurologica Scandinavica*, 116, 177–181.

McKeith, I., Fairbairn, A., Perry, R., Thompson, P., & Perry, E. (1992). Neuroleptic sensitivity in patients with senile dementia of Lewy body type. *British Medical Journal*, 305, 673–678.

McKeith, I., Del Ser, T., Spano, P., Emre, M., Wesnes, K., Anand, R.,...Spiegel, R. (2000). Efficacy of rivastigmine in dementia with Lewy bodies: A randomised, double-blind, placebo-controlled international study. *Lancet*, 356, 2031–2036.

McKeith, I., Mintzer, J., Aarsland, D., Burn, D., Chiu, H., Cohen-Mansfield, J.,...Reid, W. (2004). Dementia with Lewy bodies. *Lancet Neurology*, 3, 19–28.

McKeith I., O'Brien, J., Walker, Z., Tatsch, K., Booij, J., Darcourt, J.,...Meyer, I. (2007). Sensitivity and specificity of dopamine transporter imaging with 123I-FP-CIT SPECT in dementia with Lewy bodies: A phase III, multicentre study. *Lancet Neurology*, 6, 305–313.

McKeith, I. G. (2006). Consensus guidelines for the clinical and pathologic diagnosis of dementia with Lewy bodies (DLB): Report of the Consortium on DLB International Workshop. *Journal of Alzheimers Disease*, 9, 417–423.

McKeith, I. G., Ballard, C. G., Perry, R. H., Ince, P. G., O'Brien, J. T., Neill, D.,...Perry, E. K. (2000). Prospective validation of consensus criteria for the diagnosis of dementia with Lewy bodies. *Neurology*, 54, 1050–1058.

McKeith, I. G., Dickson, D. W., Lowe, J., Emre, M., O'Brien, J. T., Feldman, H.,...Yamada, M. (2005). Diagnosis and management of dementia with Lewy bodies: Third report of the DLB Consortium. *Neurology*, 65, 1863–1872.

McKeith, I. G., Perry, E. K., & Perry, R. H. (1999). Report of the second dementia with Lewy body international workshop: Diagnosis and treatment. Consortium on Dementia with Lewy Bodies. *Neurology*, 53, 902–905.

Meeus, B., Nuytemans, K., Crosiers, D., Engelborghs, S., Peeters, K., Mattheijssens, M.,...Theuns, J. (2010). Comprehensive genetic and mutation analysis of familial dementia with Lewy bodies linked to 2q35-q36. *Journal of Alzheimers Disease*, 20, 197–205.

Meeus, B., Verstraeten, A., Crosiers, D., Engelborghs, S., Van den Broeck, M., Mattheijssens, M.,...Theuns, J. (2012). DLB and PDD: A role for mutations in dementia and Parkinson disease genes? *Neurobiology of Aging*, 33, 629.e5–629.e18.

Merdes, A. R., Hansen, L. A., Jeste, D. V., Galasko, D., Hofstetter, C. R., Ho, G. J.,... Corey-Bloom, J. (2003). Influence of Alzheimer pathology on clinical diagnostic accuracy in dementia with Lewy bodies. *Neurology*, 60, 1586–1590.

Miech, R. A., Breitner, J. C. S., Zandi, P. P., Khachaturian, A. S., Anthony, J. C., & Mayer, L. (2002). Incidence of AD may decline in the early 90s for men, later for women: The Cache County study. *Neurology*, 58, 209–218.

Mirra, S. S., Heyman, A., McKeel, D., Sumi, S. M., Crain, B. J., Brownlee, L. M.,...Berg, L. (1991). The Consortium to Establish a Registry for Alzheimer's Disease (CERAD). Part II. Standardization of the neuropathologic assessment of Alzheimer's disease. *Neurology*, 41, 479–486.

Molina, J. A., García-Segura, J. M., Benito-León, J., Gómez-Escalonilla, C., del Ser, T., Martínez, V., & Viaño, J. (2002). Proton magnetic resonance spectroscopy in dementia with Lewy bodies. *European Neurology*, 48, 158–163.

Mollenhauer, B., Cullen, V., Kahn, I., Krastins, B., Outeiro, T. F., Pepivani, I.,...Schlossmacher, M. G. (2008). Direct quantification of CSF alpha-synuclein by ELISA and first cross-sectional study in patients with neurodegeneration. *Experimental Neurology*, 213, 315–325.

Molloy, S., McKeith, I. G., O'Brien, J. T., & Burn, D. J. (2005). The role of levodopa in the management of dementia with Lewy bodies. *Journal of Neurology, Neurosurgery and Psychiatry*, 76, 1200–1203.

Mori, E., Ikeda, M., & Kosaka, K. (2012). Donepezil for dementia with Lewy bodies: A randomized, placebo-controlled trial. *Annals of Neurology*, 72, 41–52.

Mosimann, U. P., Rowan, E. N., Partington, C. E., Collerton, D., Littlewood, E., O'Brien, J. T.,...McKeith, I. G. (2006). Characteristics of visual hallucinations in Parkinson disease dementia and dementia with Lewy bodies. *American Journal of Geriatric Psychiatry*, 14, 153–160.

Mulugeta, E., Londos, E., Ballard, C., Alves, G., Zetterberg, H., Blennow, K.,...Aarsland, D. (2011). CSF amyloid β38 as a novel diagnostic marker for dementia with Lewy bodies. *Journal of Neurology, Neurosurgery and Psychiatry, 82*, 160–164.

Muslimovic, D., Post, B., Speelman, J. D., & Schmand, B. (2005). Cognitive profile of patients with newly diagnosed Parkinson disease. *Neurology, 65*, 1239–1245.

Nagahama, Y., Okina, T., Suzuki, N., & Matsuda, M. (2010). Neural correlates of psychotic symptoms in dementia with Lewy bodies. *Brain, 133*, 557–567.

Nelson, P. T., Kryscio, R. J., Jicha, G. A., Abner, E. L., Schmitt, F. A., Xu, L. O.,...Markesbery, W. R. (2009). Relative preservation of MMSE scores in autopsy-proven dementia with Lewy bodies. *Neurology, 73*, 1127–1133.

Nelson, P. T., Jicha, G. A., Kryscio, R. J., Abner, E. L., Schmitt, F. A., Cooper, G.,...Markesbery, W. R. (2010). Low sensitivity in clinical diagnoses of dementia with Lewy bodies. *Journal of Neurology, 257*, 359–366.

Nervi, A., Reitz, C., Tang, M-X., Santana, V., Piriz, A., Reyes, D.,...Mayeux, R. (2011). Familial aggregation of dementia with Lewy bodies. *Archives of Neurology, 68*, 90–93.

Nishioka, K., Ross, O. A., Vilariño-Güell, C., Cobb, S. A., Kachergus, J. M., Mann, D. M. A.,...Farrer, M. J. (2011). Glucocerebrosidase mutations in diffuse Lewy body disease. *Parkinsonism and Related Disorders, 17*, 55–57.

O'Brien, J. T., Paling, S., Barber, R., Williams, E. D., Ballard, C., McKeith, I. G.,...Fox, N. C. (2001). Progressive brain atrophy on serial MRI in dementia with Lewy bodies, AD, and vascular dementia. *Neurology, 56*, 1386–1388.

O'Brien, J. T., McKeith I. G, Walker, Z., Tatsch, K., Booij, J., Darcourt, J.,...Reininger, C. (2009). Diagnostic accuracy of 123I-FP-CIT SPECT in possible dementia with Lewy bodies. *British Journal of Psychiatry, 194*, 34–39.

Ohrfelt, A., Grognet, P., Andreasen, N., Wallin, A., Vanmechelen, E., Blennow, K., & Zetterberg, H. (2009). Cerebrospinal fluid alpha-synuclein in neurodegenerative disorders-a marker of synapse loss? *Neuroscience Letters, 450*, 332–335.

Okazaki, H., Lipkin, L. E., & Aronson, S. M. (1961). Diffuse intracytoplasmic ganglionic inclusions (Lewy type) associated with progressive dementia and quadriparesis in flexion. *J. Neuropathol. Experimental Neurology 1961*; 20: 237–244.

Olichney, J. M., Galasko, D., Salmon, D. P., Hofstetter, C. R., Hansen, L. A., Katzman, R., & Thal, L. J. (1998). Cognitive decline is faster in Lewy body variant than in Alzheimer's disease. *Neurology, 51*, 351–357.

Pagonabarraga, J., Llebaria, G., García-Sánchez, C., Pascual-Sedano, B., Gironell, A., & Kulisevsky, J. (2008). A prospective study of delusional misidentification syndromes in Parkinson's disease with dementia. *Movement Disorders, 23*, 443–448.

Papapetropoulos, S., Lieberman, A., Gonzalez, J., Singer, C., Laufer, D. Z., & Mash, D. C. (2006). Family history of dementia: Dementia with Lewy bodies and dementia in Parkinson's disease. *Journal of Neuropsychiatry and Clinical Neuroscience, 18*, 113–116.

Parkkinen, L., Pirttilä, T., & Alafuzoff, I. (2008). Applicability of current staging/categorization of alpha-synuclein pathology and their clinical relevance. *Acta Neuropathologica, 115*, 399–407.

Parnetti, L., Tiraboschi, P., Lanari, A., Peducci, M., Padiglioni, C., D'Amore, C.,... Calabresi, P. (2008). Cerebrospinal fluid biomarkers in Parkinson's disease with dementia and dementia with Lewy bodies. *Biological Psychiatry, 64*, 850–855.

Perry, E. K., Haroutunian, V., Davis, K. L., Levy, R., Lantos, P., Eagger, S.,... McKeith, I. G. (1994). Neocortical cholinergic activities differentiate Lewy body dementia from classical Alzheimer's disease. *Neuroreport, 5*, 747–749.

Perry, E. K., Marshall, E., Kerwin, J., Smith, C. J., Jabeen, S., Cheng, A. V., & Perry, R. H. (1990). Evidence of a monoaminergic-cholinergic imbalance related to visual hallucinations in Lewy body dementia. *Journal of Neurochemistry, 55*, 1454–1456.

Perry, R. H., Irving, D., Blessed, G., Fairbairn, A., & Perry, E. K. (1990). Senile dementia of Lewy body type. A clinically and neuropathologically distinct form of Lewy body dementia in the elderly. *Journal of Neurological Sciences, 95*, 119–139.

Piggott, M. A., Marshall, E. F., Thomas, N., Lloyd, S., Court, J. A., Jaros, E., (1999). Striatal dopaminergic markers in dementia with Lewy bodies, Alzheimer's and Parkinson's diseases: Rostrocaudal distribution. *Brain, 122*(Pt 8), 1449–1468.

Pletnikova, O., West, N., Lee, M. K., Rudow, G. L., Skolasky, R. L., Dawson, T. M.,...Troncoso, J. C. (2005). Abeta deposition is associated with enhanced cortical alpha-synuclein lesions in Lewy body diseases. *Neurobiology of Aging, 26*, 1183–1192.

Poewe, W., Wolters, E., Emre, M., Onofrj, M., Hsu, C., Tekin, S., & Lane, R. (2006). Long-term benefits of rivastigmine in dementia associated with Parkinson's disease: An active treatment extension study. *Movement Disorders, 21*, 456–461.

Postuma, R. B., Gagnon, J-F., & Montplaisir, J. Y. (2012). REM sleep behavior disorder: From dreams to neurodegeneration. *Neurobiological Diseases*, 46, 553–558.

Postuma, R. B., Gagnon, J-F., Vendette, M., & Montplaisir, J. Y. (2009). Idiopathic REM sleep behavior disorder in the transition to degenerative disease. *Movement Disorders*, 24, 2225–2232.

Raedler, T. J. (2010). Cardiovascular aspects of antipsychotics. *Current Opinion in Psychiatry*, 23, 574–581.

Rahkonen, T., Eloniemi-Sulkava, U., Rissanen, S., Vatanen, A., Viramo, P., & Sulkava, R. (2003). Dementia with Lewy bodies according to the consensus criteria in a general population aged 75 years or older. *Journal of Neurology, Neurosurgery and Psychiatry*, 74, 720–724.

Ravina, B., Putt, M., Siderowf, A., Farrar, J. T., Gillespie, M., Crawley, A.,...Simuni, T. (2005). Donepezil for dementia in Parkinson's disease: A randomised, double blind, placebo controlled, crossover study. *Journal of Neurology, Neurosurgery and Psychiatry*, 76, 934–939.

Richard, I. H., McDermott, M. P., Kurlan, R., Lyness, J. M., Como, P. G., Pearson, N.,...McDonald, W. (2012). A randomized, double-blind, placebo-controlled trial of antidepressants in Parkinson disease. *Neurology*, 78, 1229–1236.

Rinne, J. O., Rummukainen, J., Paljärvi, L., & Rinne, U. K. (1989). Dementia in Parkinson's disease is related to neuronal loss in the medial substantia nigra. *Annals of Neurology*, 26, 47–50.

Roks, G., Korf, E. S. C., van der Flier, W. M., Scheltens, P., & Stam, C. J. (2008). The use of EEG in the diagnosis of dementia with Lewy bodies. *Journal of Neurology, Neurosurgery and Psychiatry*, 79, 377–380.

Rolinski, M., Fox, C., Maidment, I., & McShane, R. (2012). Cholinesterase inhibitors for dementia with Lewy bodies, Parkinson's disease dementia and cognitive impairment in Parkinson's disease. *Cochrane Database of Systematic Reviews*, 3, CD006504.

Rowan, E., McKeith, I. G., Saxby, B. K., O'Brien, J. T., Burn, D., Mosimann, U.,...Wesnes, K. (2007). Effects of donepezil on central processing speed and attentional measures in Parkinson's disease with dementia and dementia with Lewy bodies. *Dementia and Geriatric Cognitive Disorders*, 23, 161–167.

Sabattoli, F., Boccardi, M., Galluzzi, S., Treves, A., Thompson, P. M., & Frisoni, G. B. (2008). Hippocampal shape differences in dementia with Lewy bodies. *Neuroimage*, 41, 699–705.

Samuel, W., Alford, M., Hofstetter, C. R., & Hansen, L. (1997). Dementia with Lewy bodies versus pure Alzheimer disease: Differences in cognition, neuropathology, cholinergic dysfunction, and synapse density. *Journal of Neuropathology and Experimental Neurology*, 56, 499–508.

Schneider, J. A., Arvanitakis, Z., Bang, W., & Bennett, D. A. (2007). Mixed brain pathologies account for most dementia cases in community-dwelling older persons. *Neurology*, 69, 2197–2204.

Seibert, T. M., Murphy, E. A., Kaestner, E. J., & Brewer, J. B. (2012). Interregional correlations in Parkinson disease and Parkinson-related dementia with resting functional MR imaging. *Radiology*, 263, 226–234.

Setó-Salvia, N., Clarimón, J., Pagonabarraga, J., Pascual-Sedano, B., Campolongo, A., Combarros, O.,...Kulisevsky, J. (2011). Dementia risk in Parkinson disease: Disentangling the role of MAPT haplotypes. *Archives of Neurology*, 68, 359–364.

Setó-Salvia, N., Pagonabarraga, J., Houlden, H., Pascual-Sedano, B., Dols-Icardo, O., Tucci, A.,...Clarimón, J. (2012). Glucocerebrosidase mutations confer a greater risk of dementia during Parkinson's disease course. *Movement Disorders*, 27, 393–399.

Siderowf, A., Xie, S. X., Hurtig, H., Weintraub, D., Duda, J., Chen-Plotkin, A.,...Clark, C. (2010). CSF amyloid {beta} 1-42 predicts cognitive decline in Parkinson disease. *Neurology*, 75, 1055–1061.

Singleton, A. B., Wharton, A., O'Brien, K. K., Walker, M. P., McKeith, I. G., Ballard, C. G.,...Morris, C. M. (2002). Clinical and neuropathological correlates of apolipoprotein E genotype in dementia with Lewy bodies. *Dementia and Geriatric Cognitive Disorders*, 14, 167–175.

Sironi, F., Trotta, L., Antonini, A., Zini, M., Ciccone, R., Della Mina, E.,...Goldwurm, S. (2010). alpha-Synuclein multiplication analysis in Italian familial Parkinson disease. *Parkinsonism and Related Disorders*, 16, 228–231.

Sollinger, A. B., Goldstein, F. C., Lah, J. J., Levey, A. I., & Factor, S. A. (2010). Mild cognitive impairment in Parkinson's disease: Subtypes and motor characteristics. *Parkinsonism and Related Disorders*, 16, 177–180.

Spillantini, M. G., Crowther, R. A., Jakes, R., Hasegawa, M., & Goedert, M. (1998). alpha-Synuclein in filamentous inclusions of Lewy bodies from Parkinson's disease and dementia with Lewy bodies. *Proceedings of the National Academy of Science USA*, 95, 6469–6473.

Tateno, F., Sakakibara, R., Kishi, M., Ogawa, E., Terada, H., Ogata, T., & Haruta, H. (2011). Sensitivity and specificity of metaiodobenzylguanidine (MIBG) myocardial accumulation in the diagnosis of Lewy body diseases in a movement disorder clinic. *Parkinsonism and Related Disorders, 17,* 395–397.

Vendette, M., Gagnon, J-F., Décary, A., Massicotte-Marquez, J., Postuma, R. B., Doyon, J.,...Montplaisir, J. (2007). REM sleep behavior disorder predicts cognitive impairment in Parkinson disease without dementia. *Neurology, 69,* 1843–1849.

Walker, M. P., Ayre, G. A., Cummings, J. L., Wesnes, K., McKeith, I. G., O'Brien, J. T., & Ballard, C. G. (2000a). Quantifying fluctuation in dementia with Lewy bodies, Alzheimer's disease, and vascular dementia. *Neurology, 54,* 1616–1625.

Walker, M. P., Ayre, G. A., Cummings, J. L., Wesnes, K., McKeith, I. G., O'Brien, J. T.,...Ballard, C. G. (2000b). The Clinician Assessment of Fluctuation and the One Day Fluctuation Assessment Scale. Two methods to assess fluctuating confusion in dementia. *British Journal of Psychiatry, 177,* 252–256.

Walker, Z., Allen, R. L., Shergill, S., & Katona, C. L. (1997). Neuropsychological performance in Lewy body dementia and Alzheimer's disease. *British Journal of Psychiatry, 170,* 156–158.

Walker, Z., Allen, R. L., Shergill, S., Mullan, E., & Katona, C. L. (2000). Three years survival in patients with a clinical diagnosis of dementia with Lewy bodies. *International Journal of Geriatric Psychiatry, 15,* 267–273.

Watson, R., Blamire, A. M., Colloby, S. J, Wood, J. S., Barber, R., He, J., & O'Brien, J. T. (2012). Characterizing dementia with Lewy bodies by means of diffusion tensor imaging. *Neurology, 79,* 906–914.

Weintraub, D., Mavandadi, S., Mamikonyan, E., Siderowf, A. D., Duda, J. E., Hurtig, H. I.,...Stern, M. B. (2010). Atomoxetine for depression and other neuropsychiatric symptoms in Parkinson disease. *Neurology, 75,* 448–455.

Weintraub, D., Moberg, P. J., Culbertson, W. C., Duda, J. E., & Stern, M. B. (2004). Evidence for impaired encoding and retrieval memory profiles in Parkinson disease. *Cognitive and Behavioral Neurology, 17,* 195–200.

Wesnes, K. A., McKeith, I., Edgar, C., Emre, M., & Lane, R. (2005). Benefits of rivastigmine on attention in dementia associated with Parkinson disease. *Neurology, 65,* 1654–1656.

Wider, C., Dickson, D. W., & Wszolek, Z. K. (2010). Leucine-rich repeat kinase 2 gene-associated disease: Redefining genotype-phenotype correlation. *Neurodegenerative Diseases, 7,* 175–179.

Williams, M. M., Xiong, C., Morris, J. C., & Galvin, J. E. (2006). Survival and mortality differences between dementia with Lewy bodies vs Alzheimer disease. *Neurology, 67,* 1935–1941.

Williams-Gray, C. H., Foltynie, T., Brayne, C. E. G., Robbins, T. W., & Barker, R. A. (2007). Evolution of cognitive dysfunction in an incident Parkinson's disease cohort. *Brain, 130,* 1787–1798.

Williams-Gray, C. H., Evans, J. R., Goris, A., Foltynie, T., Ban, M., Robbins, T. W.,...Barker, R. A. (2009). The distinct cognitive syndromes of Parkinson's disease: 5 year follow-up of the CamPaIGN cohort. *Brain, 132,* 2958–2969.

Wiltshire, K., Concha, L., Gee, M., Bouchard, T., Beaulieu, C., & Camicioli, R. (2010). Corpus callosum and cingulum tractography in Parkinson's disease. *Canadian Journal Neurological Sciences, 37,* 595–600.

Woodruff, B. K., Graff-Radford, N. R., Ferman, T. J., Dickson, D. W., DeLucia, M. W., Crook, J. E.,...Duara, R. (2006). Family history of dementia is a risk factor for Lewy body disease. *Neurology, 66,* 1949–1950.

Woods, S. P., & Tröster, A. I. (2003). Prodromal frontal/executive dysfunction predicts incident dementia in Parkinson's disease. *Journal of the International Neuropsychology Society, 9,* 17–24.

Yamada, T., Hattori, H., Miura, A., Tanabe, M., & Yamori, Y. (2001). Prevalence of Alzheimer's disease, vascular dementia and dementia with Lewy bodies in a Japanese population. *Psychiatry and Clinical Neuroscience, 55,* 21–25.

Yoshita, M., Taki, J., & Yamada, M. (2001). A clinical role for [(123)I]MIBG myocardial scintigraphy in the distinction between dementia of the Alzheimer's-type and dementia with Lewy bodies. *Journal of Neurology, Neurosurgery and Psychiatry, 71,* 583–588.

Zaccai, J., McCracken, C., & Brayne, C. (2005). A systematic review of prevalence and incidence studies of dementia with Lewy bodies. *Age and Ageing, 34,* 561–566.

13

Vascular Cognitive Impairment

Charles DeCarli

While Alzheimer's disease (AD) is the most common cause of dementia among older individuals (Evans et al., 1989; Sayetta, 1986), the lifetime risk for stroke equals and may exceed the risk of AD in some circumstances (Seshadri et al., 2006). In addition, magnetic resonance imaging (MRI) evidence of asymptomatic cerebrovascular disease (CVD) occurs in one third of older individuals (Decarli et al., 2005). It is, therefore, not surprising that concurrent CVD is often seen in older dementia patients, even though they may have a slowly progressive dementing illness most consistent with AD (Mungas, Reed, Ellis, & Jagust, 2001). This chapter reviews the definition of vascular cognitive impairment as it relates to dementia after stroke, slowly progressive dementia, and the interaction of clinically silent CVD with AD.

Vascular Cognitive Impairment Defined

As our understanding of the relationship between vascular disease and cognition continues to evolve, so does our terminology. In fact, over the last 5 years, two separate consensus conference statements have been published (Hachinski et al., 2006; Gorelick et al., 2011), although the aim of the two statements differed slightly. The interested reader is encouraged to review both for further details. Evolving consensus, however, has moved toward defining vascular cognitive impairment (VCI) as encompassing all forms of cognitive impairment associated with CVD, ranging from subtle impairments in otherwise cognitively normal individuals through mild cognitive impairment to dementia (O'Brien et al., 2003). In fact, the most recent consensus specifically states that "the term *VCI* characterizes all forms of cognitive deficits from VaD to MCI of vascular origin" (Gorelick et al., 2011, p. 2673) and vascular dementia (VaD) is considered to be the extreme end of the spectrum of VCI (Gorelick et al., 2011; Hachinski et al., 2006), where vascular disease is felt to be the sole cause for the cognitive impairment (Fig. 13.1).

VCI also encompasses dementias where both CVD and AD processes are thought to co-occur (Gorelick et al., 2011; Hachinski et al., 2006). As noted by Gorelick et al.: "VCI encompasses all the cognitive disorders associated with cerebrovascular disease, from frank dementia to mild cognitive deficits. Simply put, VCI is a syndrome with evidence of clinical stroke or subclinical vascular brain injury and cognitive impairment affecting at least one cognitive domain. The most severe form of VCI is VaD" (Gorelick et al., 2011, p. 2673).

VaD   AD

Figure 13.1 Spectrum of vascular and Alzheimer's disease pathologies in dementia.

Definition of Vascular Dementia

The most current consensus statement defines VaD in a manner similar to current consensus diagnoses of AD (McKhann et al., 1984) using designations of clinically probable and clinically possible VaD as noted in Table 13.1 from Gorelick et al. (2011). Importantly, unlike previous diagnostic criteria (Roman et al., 1993), the definition of dementia is more inclusive and the methods to detect dementia are specified. Although VaD may result from many forms of CVD, VaD is most clearly delineated by the presence of symptomatic CVD, usually due to atherothrombotic stroke, in association with stepwise declines in cognition (Roman et al., 1993) or evidence of multiple, bilateral gray-matter infarcts (Knopman et al., 2003).

An accurate diagnosis for VaD is important to clinical practice. For example, stroke is associated with increased mortality (Sacco, Wolf, Kannel, & McNamara, 1982), and stroke patients with cognitive impairment have poorer ADL recovery (Wagle et al., 2011). Most important, the diagnosis of VaD

TABLE 13.1 Diagnostic Criteria for Vascular Dementia

Dementia
1. The diagnosis of dementia should be based on a decline in cognitive function from a prior baseline and a deficit in performance in cognitive domains that are of sufficient severity to affect the subject's activities of daily living.
2. The diagnosis of dementia must be based on cognitive testing, and a minimum of four cognitive domains should be assessed: executive/attention, memory, language, and visuospatial functions.
3. The deficits in activities of daily living are independent of the motor/sensory sequelae of the vascular event.

Probable vascular dementia
1. There is cognitive impairment and imaging evidence of cerebrovascular disease and
   a. There is a clear temporal relationship between a vascular event (e.g., clinical stroke) and onset of cognitive deficits, or
   b. There is a clear relationship in the severity and pattern of cognitive impairment and the presence of diffuse, subcortical cerebrovascular disease pathology (e.g., as in CADASIL).
2. There is no history of gradually progressive cognitive deficits before or after the stroke that suggests the presence of a nonvascular neurodegenerative disorder.

Possible vascular dementia
There is cognitive impairment and imaging evidence of cerebrovascular disease but:
1. There is no clear relationship (temporal, severity, or cognitive pattern) between the vascular disease (e.g., silent infarcts, subcortical small-vessel disease) and the cognitive impairment.
2. There is insufficient information for the diagnosis of vascular dementia (e.g., clinical symptoms suggest the presence of vascular disease, but no CT/MRI studies are available).
3. Severity of aphasia precludes proper cognitive assessment. However, patients with documented evidence of normal cognitive function (eft annual cognitive evaluations) before the clinical event that caused aphasia could be classified as having probable vascular dementia
4. There is evidence of other neurodegenerative diseases or conditions in addition to cerebrovascular disease that may affect cognition, such as:
   a. A history of other neurodegenerative disorders (e.g., Parkinson disease, progressive supranuclear palsy, dementia with Lewy bodies);
   b. The presence of Alzheimer disease biology is confirmed by biomarkers (e.g., positron emission tomography, cerebrospinal fluid, amyloid ligands) or genetic studies (e.g., 11,91 mutation); or
   c. A history of active cancer or psychiatric or metabolic disorders that may affect cognitive function.

suggests the presence of systemic vascular disease that may require medical treatment.

The diagnosis of VaD is based on two factors: demonstration of the presence of a cognitive disorder (dementia or MCI) by neuropsychological testing *and* presence of vascular disease by neuroimaging. The second critical clinical feature of VaD is determining the relationship of the CVD to the cognitive symptoms. To appropriately diagnose VaD, it is critical to identify the presence of cortical or subcortical infarcts or other stroke lesions, and these should be associated with clinical symptomatology. Although some authors propose that the symptoms should appear within 3 months after a stroke, this is an arbitrary time and symptoms may develop after this time frame. Studies of the sensitivity of this diagnostic approach note that it is quite specific (Gold et al., 2002), but not sensitive to the presence of CVD in combination with AD pathology, which will be discussed later.

Clinical Components of the Vascular Dementia Diagnosis

Probable Vascular Dementia Diagnosis in the Setting of Stroke

The diagnosis of VaD involves considering the clinical syndrome as well as the relationship between the clinical syndrome and cognitive impairment. The diagnosis of VaD is most certain in the setting of stroke. The stroke symptoms can comprise any of a host of common disabilities, including aphasia, agraphia, or agnosia, but *must* include impairment of cortical function beyond primary sensation and *must* include a decline in cognitive ability below that of a previously attained state in more than one area of cognitive ability. Therefore, primary aphasic disorders, for example, after stroke are generally not considered dementias even though the affected individual may have substantial functional impairment. The modified diagnosis of VaD, however, does allow for dementia diagnosis when the functional impairment exceeds that due to motor and sensory deficits due to the stroke (Gorelick et al., 2011). For example, an individual with a posterior aphasia without serious motor disabilities may be considered demented under the new criteria. In cases of cortical injury, the cognitive syndrome generally follows immediately from the stroke, thereby assuring a causal relationship. All symptoms months to years after a stroke should cause the clinician to suspect a secondary cause unless new, clinically silent brain infarction (e.g., frontal lobe infarct) involving cortex or subcortical white matter can be identified with imaging.

It is important that the clinician recognize that the occasional "strategic" infarct can cause an abrupt dementia syndrome (Roman, 2003). Examples include thalamic infarction, which can cause a dense amnesia and executive function impairments, or infarction of the angular gyrus, which can cause Gertsmann's syndrome (agraphia, acalculia, finger agnosia, and right-left confusion).

Probable Vascular Dementia With Extensive Subcortical Cerebrovascular Disease

While subcortical VaD is commonly suspected in clinical practice, it is often difficult to assess the extent of subcortical disease necessary to be the sole cause of a dementia syndrome. Cerebral autosomal dominant arteriopathy with subcortical infarcts and leukoencephalopathy (CADASIL), although rare, is one pathological entity in which subcortical disease is strictly sufficient for the dementia (Andre, 2010) and serves as an ideal example.

CADASIL is characterized by a history of migraine headaches, mid-adult onset of cerebrovascular disease progressing to dementia, and diffuse white matter lesions and subcortical infarcts as seen on neuroimaging. The pathologic hallmark of CADASIL is electron-dense granules in the media of arterioles that can often be identified by electron microscopic (EM) evaluation of skin biopsies. More than 90% of individuals have mutations in *NOTCH3*, the only gene known to be associated with CADASIL. Molecular genetic testing is available on a clinical basis. Supportive care and possibly platelet aggregation inhibitors are the only treatment beyond genetic counseling. Angiography and anticoagulants may provoke cerebrovascular accidents and smoking increases the risk of stroke in those affected by this disease. There are no formal diagnostic criteria, but typical signs and symptoms include the following: migraine with aura, stroke-like episodes before age 60,

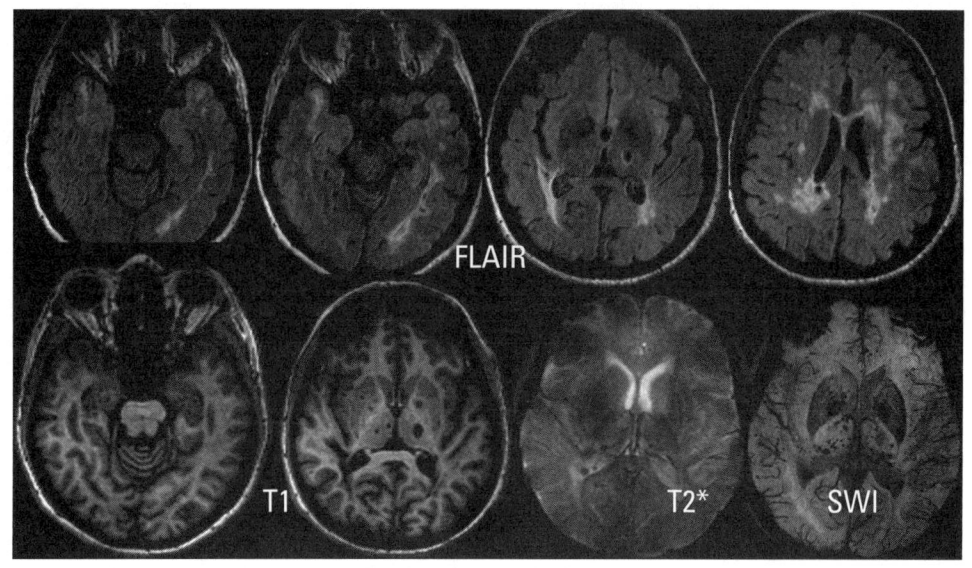

Figure 13.2 Magnetic resonance imaging (MRI) in cerebral autosomal dominant arteriopathy with subcortical infarcts and leukoencephalopathy (CADASIL).

cognitive decline, and behavioral changes. Clinical diagnostic studies that support the diagnosis of CADASIL include MRI white matter changes in the anterior aspect of the temporal poles bilaterally and white matter changes in the external capsule (Fig. 13.2). Additionally, subcortical lacunar infarcts and microhemorrhages are often common. Recent publications note that anterior temporal white matter changes may occur as early as age 20 years (Lesnik Oberstein et al., 2003; van den Boom et al., 2003). Cerebral microbleeds, located in the thalamus, can also occur (Lesnik Oberstein et al., 2003).

The pattern of cognitive dysfunction is characterized by deficits in executive function (timed measures and measures of error monitoring), verbal fluency, and memory with benefit from cues. In most cases, cognitive decline is slowly progressive with additional stepwise deterioration and is associated with repeated lacunar infarcts noted by MRI (Liem et al., 2007). Some have observed deterioration of working memory and executive function in individuals with *NOTCH3* mutations in the prestroke phase, and infer that cognitive decline may start insidiously before the onset of symptomatic ischemic episodes. Importantly, about thirty percent of individuals with CADASIL experience psychiatric disturbances, varying from personality changes to severe depression (Dichgans et al., 1998). Individuals with CADASIL presenting with psychiatric problems also have been described.

CADASIL, however, is a unique disease that often begins before 30 years of age with dementia onset by age 55, on average. As a consequence, "contamination" by AD is relatively rare. In the common clinical setting of dementia, individuals are often mistakenly diagnosed as "mixed dementia" or "subcortical ischemic vascular dementia" when findings of modest white matter disease in the absence of subcortical infarcts. In these settings, AD pathology is generally the leading cause of the dementia (Chui et al., 2006). It, therefore, is difficult to assess the extent of subcortical vascular injury necessary to be sufficient for dementia. Criteria have been developed that attempt to codify the extent of subcortical pathology necessary to cause dementia in SIVD (Roman et al., 1993) but have generally failed (van der Flier, van Straaten, Barkhof, & Scheltens, 2005). The strongest pathological evidence for subcortical vascular injury sufficient to contribute to dementia (Knopman et al., 2003) suggests that more than four lacunas are necessary with or without extensive white matter pathology, particularly if these lacunas occur in strategic areas such as the thalamus (Van der Werf et al., 2003). Neuroimaging, therefore, is an important tool in the assessment of VCI.

Imaging of Vascular Cognitive Impairment

Early attempts to compare MRI measures among clinically diagnosed AD and VaD subjects were relatively small and inconclusive. More recent reports of the qualitative assessment of MRI differences between AD and VaD patients with larger samples have suggested that medial-temporal atrophy (MTA), particularly hippocampal atrophy, is uniquely associated with clinical AD as opposed to VaD (Du et al., 2002). In fact, hippocampal atrophy is considered the imaging hallmark of clinical AD and is strongly associated with AD pathology (Jack et al., 1997, 1999, 2002). Bastos-Leite et al., however, reported a high rate of MTA in a well-characterized sample of VaD patients and an association of MTA with cognitive functioning in the same group (Bastos-Leite et al., 2007); similarly other MRI studies have found extensive hippocampal atrophy in patients with suspected VaD (Fein et al., 2000), and hippocampal sclerosis has been associated with severe hippocampal atrophy on MRI (Jagust et al., 2008). Global cerebral atrophy also has been associated with cognitive performance in both AD and VaD patients (Scheltens et al., 1992). While VaD characteristically has been associated with white matter hyperintensities (WMH) in addition to infarction, WMH have been negatively correlated with cognitive functioning in persons with normal cognition (Au et al., 2006), VaD (Gootjes et al., 2004), MCI (Nordahl et al., 2005), and AD (Yoshita et al., 2006), suggesting that the effect of this pathology transcends clinical diagnosis.

Recently, Logue et al. (2011) performed a semiquantitative assessment of MRI measures from a clinical trial of donepezil in VaD and a genetic study of AD. A total of 2,237 individual MRI datasets were assessed with nearly equal distribution between cognitively normal older individuals (CN), VaD, and AD. Measures of cerebral atrophy, medial temporal atrophy, extent of WMH and the presence, size, and location of cerebral infarcts were obtained for each individual scan.

For all MRI ratings, the CN group was lowest with the VaD group showing the highest scores on cerebral atrophy, white matter hyperintensities, and number of infarcts. The AD group showed the greatest MTA. Differences between the VaD and AD group were significant for CN, WMH, and MTA with CN and WMH being significantly worse in the VaD group, whereas MTA was significantly worse for the AD group. While AD subjects generally had worse MTA ratings and CN had low ratings, the VaD group showed a substantial proportion of subjects at each MTA rating level except 0.

As expected, VaD had a substantially higher prevalence of large infarcts (39%) compared to AD (5%) and CN (2%). Significant differences in the prevalence of both large and small infarcts between VaD and AD subjects were also noted.

Regression models comparing the pathological processes underlying these two samples found both similarities and differences. For example, among VaD patients, age, sex, infarcts, WMH, and MTA were significantly related to cerebral atrophy. Conversely, only age, WMH, and MTA were significantly associated with cerebral atrophy in the AD group. In addition, the regression model accounted for more variance of cerebral atrophy in VaD patients ($R^2 = 0.36$) than for AD patients ($R^2 = 0.27$).

The authors next explored the relationship between MTA and vascular markers (WMH and stroke [yes/no]). Among VaD patients, both presence of stroke and WMH contributed significantly to MTA, but in opposing directions with increasing WMH associated with worsening MTA scores, but the presence of stroke associated with improved MTA scores. Conversely, among AD patients, only age and WMH contributed significantly to the model predicting MTA.

Finally, the authors investigated the relationship between MRI measures and cognitive ability (MMSE) to test the hypothesis that various MRI measures would show different associations with cognition due to the different etiologies of dementia. Surprisingly, MMSE scores were related to MTA in both VaD ($R^2 = 0.131$) and AD ($R^2 = 0.123$) with a similar magnitude. Examining vascular factors in relation to MMSE scores, associations were found between MMSE and WMH in the VaD group, but this association explained only a limited amount of additional variance ($R^2 = 0.039$) in MMSE. There was no association between WMH and MMSE for the AD group.

In summary, this study finds that vascular injury is apparent in patients believed to have VaD with significantly greater WMH and multiple infarcts. In VaD the vascular injury also leads to both cerebral and hippocampal atrophy. However, the cognitive aspects of the dementia syndrome appear most strongly correlated with the atrophy measures. Because of this, the authors conclude that MRI data from two dementia cohorts with differing etiologies find that dementia symptoms are most strongly associated with cerebral atrophy suggesting that tissue loss is the major substrate of the dementia syndrome. Therefore, we are left to conclude that there is no specific MRI measure to date that reliably predicts VaD, and we can only conclude that MRI is sensitive to vascular brain injury, but it cannot predict the impact on cognition. Further studies on this topic are in progress, and recently published standards for these investigations should hopefully improve the harmonization of methods and reporting of results across laboratories.

Positron emission tomography (PET) will likely prove to be a valuable tool for generating new insights into the dissociable and synergistic aspects of CVD and AD. For example, a recent fluorodeoxyglucose PET investigation in individuals with mild cognitive impairment (MCI) who converted to dementia demonstrated that frontal hypometabolism was associated with WMH but temporoparietal hypometabolism was associated with cerebrospinal fluid amyloid levels. The advent of cerebral amyloid PET imaging, however, may prove helpful to more precisely understanding the role of cerebrovascular disease in VCI. Preliminary studies suggest that cerebral amyloid retention is associated with vascular risk factors (Reed et al., 2011), but not WMH or cognition among older individuals (Marchant et al., 2011). Although preliminary, the combined use of MRI measures of vascular brain injury and amyloid PET may offer new insights into the pathophysiology of VCI.

Vascular Mild Cognitive Impairment

Cerebrovascular disease can also cause mild cognitive deficits that can affect multiple cognitive functions, and some authors have proposed the term *vascular mild cognitive impairment* (*VaMCI*) (DeCarli et al., 2001; Gorelick et al., 2011; Lopez et al., 2003; Nordahl et al., 2005). This is the "vascular" equivalent of MCI commonly used to identify subjects in the transition from normalcy to AD (Winblad et al., 2004).

According to the recent consensus statement by Gorelick et al. (2011), the same diagnostic criteria applied to VaD should be applied for the diagnosis of VaMCI with the exception that instrumental activities of daily living should be unaffected or only mildly affected. Most authors interpret this to imply that the clinical dementia rating scale (CDR) (Morris, 1993) should be no greater than 0.5. This new diagnostic criteria also includes the condition of "unstable" VaMCI. This term is used to designate individuals initially diagnosed with VaMCI who subsequently improve to normal cognitive ability. Reversibility may result from multiple causes such as treatment of concurrent medical illnesses, treatment of depression, or "poststroke" recovery. Importantly, this diagnostic approach brings VCI into a taxonomy similar to the AD community, emphasizing only differences in disease etiology.

The prevalence of VaMCI is likely to be substantial. For example, multiple studies find an increased prevalence of men in MCI studies (Petersen et al., 2005). Older men have substantially greater brain vascular burden (Wolf et al., 1991) and are at a greater lifetime risk for stroke as compared to AD (Seshadri & Wolf, 2007). Finally, nearly 40% of all patients diagnosed with amnestic MCI fail to show evidence of amyloid retention when using amyloid imaging (Pike et al., 2007). While many other non-AD dementias have prodromal states, most are not memory specific with the exception of vascular disease, suggesting that this may be the second most common form of MCI, although this remains to be studied.

Given the high prevalence of CVD in the elderly and evidence suggesting that CVD may strongly contribute to prevalent dementia, a number of studies have begun to explore the possible impact of CVD on cognitive impairment among the elderly (DeCarli et al., 2001; Lopez et al., 2003; Luchsinger et al., 2009; Rockwood et al., 1999, 2000). In these studies, evidence of vascular brain injury, primarily identified by risk factors or the presence of WMH on MRI, is increased in prevalence among individuals with MCI, including amnestic MCI (aMCI). In fact, at least one study has suggested that aMCI may result strictly from vascular disease alone (Nordahl et al., 2005). In addition, a more recent study found evidence that both WMH and silent brain infarcts are associated with *incident* MCI (Debette et al., 2010). Another intriguing finding of this study was that these same vascular markers were associated with increased mortality. Competitive mortality, therefore, may explain why fewer individuals with severe CVD progress onto dementia.

Although episodic memory has historically been linked to the hippocampus and surrounding cortices, evidence from neuropsychological and neuroimaging studies suggests that the prefrontal cortex plays a critical role in implementing executive control processes that contribute to normal episodic memory functioning (Ranganath, Johnson, & D'Esposito, 2003). Episodic memory failure in VaMCI, therefore, may be secondary to a more general impairment in executive control processes.

Impact of Cerebrovascular Disease on Cognition in Normal Individuals

Finally, to understand the full spectrum of VCI, it is important to understand how vascular brain injury can affect individuals who appear cognitively normal.

A number of epidemiological studies show strong associations between elevations in middle life blood pressure and the prevalence of later life cognitive impairment and dementia (Elias, 1993; Elias, D'Agostino, Elias, & Wolf, 1995; Elias et al., 2004; Launer, 1995). While the exact mechanism by which CVD leads to cognitive impairment remains unclear, a number of cross-sectional as well as longitudinal prospective studies suggest that CVD-related brain changes are associated with these cognitive changes (Longstreth et al., 1996, 1998; Swan et al., 1998, 2000; Vermeer et al., 2003).

In older individuals (Decarli et al., 2005; Longstreth et al., 1998) who have normal cognition, evidence of cerebrovascular injury is common. Epidemiological studies of cognitively normal older individuals find significant increases in WMH burden and silent cerebral infarcts detected by MRI with increasing age (Decarli et al., 2005; Longstreth et al., 1998; van Dijk, Prins, Vermeer, Koudstaal, & Breteler, 2002; Vermeer, Koudstaal, Oudkerk, Hofman, & Breteler, 2002; Vermeer, Longstreth, & Koudstaal, 2007). Moreover, reports from the Framingham Heart Study support the notion that WMH, silent cerebral infarcts, and cerebral atrophy increase substantially in prevalence with increasing age and are all related to vascular risk factors within a community population (Decarli et al., 2005; Jeerakathil et al., 2004; Seshadri et al., 2004).

These studies have also explored the relationship between CVD and cognition. Much of the results from these studies can be summarized by noting that frontal lobe–mediated cognitive domains of attention, concentration, and psychomotor speed are most affected (Au et al., 2006; Elias et al., 2004; Seshadri et al., 2004; Swan et al., 1998, 2000). Evidence of frontal lobe dysfunction, particularly by WMH, is supported by PET imaging, which finds reduced frontal metabolism in association with vascular-related brain injury, particularly WMH (DeCarli et al., 1995; Tullberg et al., 2004) as well as significant associations between frontal lobe metabolism, memory impairment, and future cognitive decline in patients with dementia and WMH (Reed, Eberling, Mungas, Weiner, & Jagust, 2000, 2001).

In summary, community-based studies of predominately healthy individuals find a significant inverse relationship between vascular brain injury and cognitive performance. It is important to remember, however, that while these differences are significant at the population level, they are generally asymptomatic to the individual, although one study (de Groot et al., 2001) found that individuals with WMH complain more frequently of memory loss.

Interaction of Cerebrovascular and Alzheimer's Disease

The relative impact of CVD on dementia occurrence has a long and debatable history (Brust, 1988; O'Brien, 1988). While there is a well-developed literature with regard to dementia after stroke (Henon et al., 2001; Moroney et al., 1996, 1997a, 1997b; Tatemichi, 1990; Tatemichi et al., 1990, 1992; Tatemichi, Desmond, & Prohovnik,

1995; Tatemichi, Desmond, Prohovnik, & Eidelberg, 1995), it remains quite common to identify individuals who have a slowly progressive dementing illness, multiple vascular risk factors, and extensive WMH or lacunar infarction detected by brain imaging. The impact of this cerebrovascular brain injury in asymptomatic individuals on dementia incidence remains unclear, but accumulating evidence suggests that CVD-related brain injury may significantly increase the likelihood of developing dementia, possibly through an additive interaction with AD (Esiri, Nagy, Smith, Barnetson, & Smith, 1999; Jagust, 2001; Schneider et al., 2003, 2004; Snowdon et al., 1997), although individuals for whom their vascular disease is limited to WMH generally have substantial AD pathology at autopsy (Chui et al., 2006).

Vascular Risk Factors and Incident Dementia

In a seminal work, Launer and colleagues studied the relationship between middle-life blood pressure measures and late-life cognition in a group of Asian Americans living in Hawaii (Launer, 1995). This study found an inverse relationship between the pattern of middle-life systolic blood pressure and a measure of general cognition (CASI scores) at later life. Unfortunately, this study could not determine dementia incidence nor did it identify prevalent dementia types at follow-up examination. Since this initial observation, however, a number of studies have examined these relationships further. For example, Whitmer and colleagues (Whitmer, 2007 Whitmer, Gunderson, Barrett-Connor, Quesenberry, & Yaffe, 2005; Whitmer, Sidney, Selby, Johnston, & Yaffe, 2005; Whitmer et al., 2008) conducted a retrospective cohort study of 8,845 participants of a health maintenance organization who underwent health evaluations from 1964 to 1973 when they were between the ages of 40 and 44. Midlife cardiovascular risk factors included total cholesterol, diabetes, hypertension, and smoking. Diagnoses of dementia were then ascertained by medical records review between 1994 and 2003. The authors identified 721 participants (8.2%) with incident dementia. Smoking, hypertension, high cholesterol, and diabetes at midlife were each associated with a 20% to 40% increase in risk of dementia. A composite cardiovascular risk score was created using all four risk factors and was associated with dementia in a dose-dependent fashion. Compared with participants having no risk factors, the risk for dementia increased from 1.27 for having one risk factor to 2.37 for having all four risk factors. Not only did this study identify that the presence of multiple cardiovascular risk factors found at midlife substantially increases risk of late-life dementia but showed that this relationship occurred in a dose-dependent manner with increasing exposure.

Magnetic Resonance Imaging Measures of Cerebrovascular Disease and Incident Dementia

A number of studies have recently examined the role of vascular disease identified by MRI on progression to dementia. For example, Debette and colleagues (Debette et al., 2010), studied the relationship between WMH and SBI and risk of future stroke, dementia, and death. In their study, they noted that extensive WMH and SBI were significantly associated with future stroke, dementia, and death. A prior study by Vermeer colleagues (Vermeer et al., 2003) found that baseline thalamic infarcts were associated with memory deficits, whereas infarcts in other brain regions were most strongly associated with psychomotor speed. Importantly, in this nondemented group, future cognitive decline was only significantly associated with new infarction seen on repeat MRI, suggesting that repeated or multiple vascular events were necessary for cognitive decline. Our laboratory has also studied the impact of WMH and SBI on trajectories of cognitive decline. While we did not find a relationship between SBI and cognitive decline, we found that extensive WMH were associated with about a 4% drop in yearly cognitive ability (Carmichael et al., 2010). Moreover, similar measures in the Alzheimer's Disease Neuroimaging Initiative cohort (Carmichael et al., 2010) concluded that the presence of extensive WMH was associated with significant increases in MMSE and ADAS-Cog, measures commonly used to test medication effects on AD treatment.

In summary, these data suggest that both vascular risk factors and evidence of vascular brain injury are associated with both cognitive declines over 1–2 years and incident dementia over longer periods. Moreover, many of the individuals with incident dementia are diagnosed with AD. MRI measures, however, are not strictly tied to pathology. Fortunately, a number of pathological studies have been performed.

Interaction of Cerebrovascular Disease and Alzheimer's Disease Pathologies on Cognition

A particularly elegant series of pathological studies show evidence that postmortem infarction is associated with nearly twice the likelihood of incident dementia (Schneider et al., 2003). In addition, when adjusting for the extent of associated AD pathology, postmortem infarction significantly adds to the likelihood of dementia, particularly when AD pathology is relatively mild (Schneider et al., 2004). Interestingly, the presence of the apolipoprotein E ε4 (ApoE ε4) polymorphism increases the odds of postmortem infarction (Schneider et al., 2005) and mixed pathologies, primarily the combination of infarction and AD, are the strongest predictor of dementia within a community-based population (Schneider et al., 2007). Finally, diabetes, a very common vascular risk factor, is independently associated with postmortem evidence of vascular brain injury but not AD pathology (Arvanitakis et al., 2006). This series of studies emphasizes the additive role of CVD to AD in causing clinically expressed dementia. In addition, these data suggest that ApoE may function as a risk factor for both processes as previously hypothesized (Decarli, 2004), but that vascular risk factors may primarily contribute to dementia through vascular injury. Of course, not all published research supports this view. For example, a recent report that studied subjects recruited through memory disorders clinics failed to show a significant effect of CVD on dementia (Chui et al., 2006). Further work is clearly indicated in this area.

Future Diagnostic Methods

As noted in the previous section, WMH and MRI infarction appear to be reasonable in vivo markers of CVD. Amyloid imaging is an emerging technology that appears to be a reasonable measure of the AD process (Fagan et al., 2006; Ikonomovic et al., 2008). Amyloid imaging, therefore, may offer us the opportunity to better disentangle the independent and combined effects of AD and CVD pathologies. For example, amyloid imaging with Pittsburgh Compound B (PiB) finds that between 30% and 50% of individuals with MCI have normal PiB retention (Forsberg et al., 2007; Kemppainen et al., 2007; Lopresti et al., 2005; Rowe et al., 2007). Other studies find that PiB retention correlates with episodic memory impairment in MCI patients (Pike et al., 2007), that nonmemory MCI patients have normal PiB binding (Pike et al., 2007), and that PiB+ MCI patients convert to dementia at a significantly higher rate than nonmemory MCI (Forsberg et al., 2007; Kemppainen et al., 2007). These data, therefore, suggest that PiB imaging identifies individuals with differing etiologies for their MCI syndrome and that PiB- MCI subjects may include a subset of individuals with CVD as the predominant pathology. If correct, PiB imaging will provide a unique measure of AD pathology that can be applied to studies examining the relationship between cognition and the complex interaction of CVD and AD pathologies that commonly co-occur in older individuals. Early results support this assertion. Recent PiB studies find that amyloid retention is not associated with WMH and has little or no impact on cognition among cognitively normal individuals, whereas MRI measures of CVD have a negative impact on executive function in the same group of individuals (Marchant et al., 2011). Possibly even more interesting is the recent report that amyloid retention is related to the degree of vascular risk among cognitively normal individuals (Reed et al., 2011).

Conclusion

This review summarized a relatively large and growing literature that shows how CVD and AD processes combine to cause cognitive impairment ranging from subtle cognitive impairments in normal older individuals through MCI, and that CVD likely contributes additively to the cognitive effects of AD pathology. With the advent amyloid imaging it will be possible to assess the relative contributions of both pathologies to brain function, thereby further elucidating the combined effects of these two processes on cognitive aging and dementia risk.

In conclusion, vascular cognitive impairment can be thought of as the spectrum of cognitive disorders due to symptomatic or asymptomatic cerebrovascular injury. The influence of cerebrovascular disease on brain function appears to begin relatively early in life, possibly decades before AD pathology. CVD appears to affect normal cognitive aging, can be the sole cause of MCI, and likely contributes much to late-life dementia, even in the presence of AD. Given that the progression of CVD pathophysiology is modifiable through various interventions, the possible public health benefits of fully understanding and remedying the impact of CVD on cognitive health is likely to be substantial.

References

Andre, C. (2010). CADASIL: Pathogenesis, clinical and radiological findings and treatment. *Arqivos de Neuropsiquiatria*, 68(2), 287–299.

Arvanitakis, Z., Schneider, J. A., Wilson, R. S., Li, Y., Arnold, S. E., Wang, Z., & Bennett, D. A. (2006). Diabetes is related to cerebral infarction but not to AD pathology in older persons. *Neurology*, 67(11), 1960–1965.

Au, R., Massaro, J. M., Wolf, P. A., Young, M. E., Beiser, A., Seshadri, S.,...DeCarli, C. (2006). Association of white matter hyperintensity volume with decreased cognitive functioning: The Framingham Heart Study. *Archives of Neurology*, 63(2), 246–250.

Bastos-Leite, A. J., van der Flier, W. M., van Straaten, E. C., Staekenborg, S. S., Scheltens, P., & Barkhof, F. (2007). The contribution of medial temporal lobe atrophy and vascular pathology to cognitive impairment in vascular dementia. *Stroke*, 38(12), 3182–3185.

Brust, J. C. M. (1988).Vascular dementia is overdiagnosed. *Archives of Neurology*, 45, 799–801.

Carmichael, O., Mungas, D., Beckett, L., Harvey, D., Tomaszewski Farias, S., Reed, B.,...Decarli, C. (2012). MRI predictors of cognitive change in a diverse and carefully characterized elderly population. *Neurobiology of Aging*, 33(1), 83–95.

Carmichael, O., Schwarz, C., Drucker, D., Fletcher, E., Harvey, D., Beckett, L.,...DeCarli, C. (2010). Longitudinal changes in white matter disease and cognition in the first year of the Alzheimers Disease Neuroimaging Initiative. *Archives of Neurology*, 67(11), 1370–1378.

Chui, H. C., Zarow, C., Mack, W. J., Ellis, W. G., Zheng, L., Jagust, W. J.,...Vintners, H. V. (2006). Cognitive impact of subcortical vascular and Alzheimer's disease pathology. *Annals of Neurology*, 60(6), 677–87.

Debette, S., Beiser, A., Decarli, C., Au, R., Himali, J. J., Kelly-Hayes, M.,...Seshardi, S. (2010). Association of MRI markers of vascular brain injury with incident stroke, mild cognitive impairment, dementia, and mortality. The Framingham Offspring Study. *Stroke*, 41(4), 600–606.

Decarli, C. (2004). Vascular factors in dementia: An overview. *Journal of Neurological Sciences*, 226(1–2), 19–23.

Decarli, C., Massaro, J., Harvey, D., Hald, J., Tullberg, M., Au, R.,...Wolf, P. A. (2005). Measures of brain morphology and infarction in the framingham heart study: Establishing what is normal. *Neurobiology of Aging*, 26(4), 491–510.

DeCarli,C.,Miller,B. L.,Swan,G. E.,Reed,T.,Wolf, P. A., & Carmelli, D. (2001). Cerebrovascular and brain morphologic correlates of mild cognitive impairment in the National Heart, Lung, and Blood Institute Twin Study. *Archives of Neurology*, 58(4), 643–647.

DeCarli, C., Murphy, D. G., Tranh, M., Grady, C. L., Haxby, J. V., Gillette, J. A.,...Rappoport, S. I. (1995). The effect of white matter hyperintensity volume on brain structure, cognitive performance, and cerebral metabolism of glucose in 51 healthy adults. *Neurology*, 45(11), 2077–2084.

de Groot, J. C., de Leeuw, F. E., Oudkerk, M., Hofman, A., Jolles, J., & Breteler, M. M. (2001). Cerebral white matter lesions and subjective cognitive dysfunction: The Rotterdam Scan Study. *Neurology*, 56(11), 1539–1545.

Dichgans, M., Mayer, M., Uttner, I., Bruning, R., Muller-Hocker, J., Rungger, G.,...Gasser, T. (1998). The phenotypic spectrum of CADASIL: Clinical findings in 102 cases. *Annals of Neurology*, 44(5), 731–739.

Du, A. T., Schuff, N., Laakso, M. P., Zhu, X. P., Jagust, W. J., Yaffe, K.,...Weiner, M. W. (2002). Effects of subcortical ischemic vascular dementia and AD on entorhinal cortex and hippocampus. *Neurology*, 58(11), 1635–1641.

Elias, M. F., D'Agostino, R. B., Elias, P. K., & Wolf, P. A. (1995a). Neuropsychological test performance, cognitive functioning, blood pressure, and age: The Framingham Heart Study. *Experimental Aging Research*, 21(4), 369–391.

Elias, P. K., D'Agostino, R. B., Elias, M. F., & Wolf, P. A. (1995b). Blood pressure, hypertension, and age as risk factors for poor cognitive performance. *Experimental Aging Research,* 21(4), 393–417.

Elias, M. F., Sullivan, L. M., D'Agostino, R. B., Elias, P. K., Beiser, A., Au, R.,...Wolf, P. A. (2004). Framingham stroke risk profile and lowered cognitive performance. *Stroke,* 35(2), 404–409.

Elias, M. F., Wolf, P. A., D'Agostino, R. B., Cobb, J., & White, L. R. (1993). Untreated blood pressure level is inversely related to cognitive functioning: The Framingham Study. *American Journal of Epidemiology,* 138, 353–64.

Esiri, M. M., Nagy, Z., Smith, M. Z., Barnetson, L., & Smith, A. D. (1999). Cerebrovascular disease and threshold for dementia in the early stages of Alzheimer's disease. *Lancet,* 354(9182), 919–920.

Evans, D. A., Funkenstein, H. H., Albert, M. S., Scherr, P. A., Cook, N. R., Chown, M. J.,...Taylor, J. O. (1989). Prevalence of Alzheimer's disease in a community population of older persons. Higher than previously reported. *Journal of the American Medical Association,* 262(18), 2551–2556.

Fagan, A. M., Mintun, M. A., Mach, R. H., Lee, S. Y., Dence, C. S., Shah, A. R.,...Holtzman, D. M. (2006). Inverse relation between in vivo amyloid imaging load and cerebrospinal fluid Abeta42 in humans. *Annals of Neurology,* 59(3), 512–529.

Fein, G., Di Sclafani, V., Tanabe, J., Cardenas, V., Weiner, M. W., Jagust, W. J.,...Chui, H. (2000). Hippocampal and cortical atrophy predict dementia in subcortical ischemic vascular disease. *Neurology,* 55(11), 1626–1635.

Forsberg, A., Engler, H., Almkvist, O., Blomquist, G., Hagman, G., Wall, A.,...Nordberg, A. (2007). PET imaging of amyloid deposition in patients with mild cognitive impairment. *Neurobiology of Aging,* 29(10), 1456–1465.

Gold, G., Bouras, C., Canuto, A., Bergallo, M. F., Herrmann, F. R., Hof, P. R.,...Giannakopoulos, P. (2002). Clinicopathological validation study of four sets of clinical criteria for vascular dementia. *American Journal of Psychiatry,* 159(1), 82–7.

Gorelick, P. B., Scuteri, A., Black, S. E., Decarli, C., Greenberg, S. M., Iadecola, C.,...Seshadri, S. (2011). Vascular contributions to cognitive impairment and dementia: A statement for healthcare professionals from the American Heart Association/American Stroke Association. *Stroke,* 42(9), 2672–2713.

Gootjes, L., Teipel, S. J., Zebuhr, Y., Schwarz, R., Leinsinger, G., Scheltens, P.,...Hampel, H. (2004). Regional distribution of white matter hyperintensities in vascular dementia, Alzheimer's disease and healthy aging. *Dementia and Geriatric Cognitive Disorders,* 18(2), 180–188.

Hachinski, V., Iadecola, C., Petersen, R. C., Breteler, M. M., Nyenhuis, D. L., Black, S. E.,...Leblanc, G. G. (2006). National Institute of Neurological Disorders and Stroke-Canadian Stroke Network vascular cognitive impairment harmonization standards. *Stroke,* 37(9), 2220–22241.

Henon, H., Durieu, I., Guerouaou, D., Lebert, F., Pasquier, F., & Leys, D. (2001). Poststroke dementia: Incidence and relationship to prestroke cognitive decline. *Neurology,* 57(7), 1216–1222.

Ikonomovic, M. D., Klunk, W. E., Abrahamson, E. E., Mathis, C. A., Price, J. C., Tsopelas, N. D., (2008). Post-mortem correlates of in vivo PiB-PET amyloid imaging in a typical case of Alzheimer's disease. *Brain,* 131(Pt 6), 1630–1645.

Jack, C. R., Dickson, D. W., Parisi, J. E., Xu, Y. C., Cha, P. C., O'Brien, P. C.,...Petersen, R. C. (2002). Antemortem MRI findings correlate with hippocampal neuropathology in typical aging and dementia. *Neurology,* 58, 750–757.

Jack, C. R., Jr., Petersen, R. C., Xu, Y. C., O'Brien, P. C., Smith, G. E., Ivnik, R. J.,...Kokmen, E. (1999). Prediction of AD with MRI-based hippocampal volume in mild cognitive impairment. *Neurology,* 52(7), 1397–1403.

Jack, C. R., Jr., Petersen, R. C., Xu, Y. C., Waring, S. C., O'Brien, P. C., Tangalos, E. G.,...Kokmen, E. (1997). Medial temporal atrophy on MRI in normal aging and very mild Alzheimer's disease [see comments]. *Neurology,* 49(3), 786–794.

Jagust, W. (2001). Untangling vascular dementia. *Lancet,* 358(9299), 2097–2098.

Jagust, W. J., Zheng, L., Harvey, D. J., Mack, W. J., Vinters, H. V., Weiner, M. W.,...Chui, H. C. (2008). Neuropathological basis of magnetic resonance images in aging and dementia. *Annals of Neurology,* 63(1), 72–80.

Jeerakathil, T., Wolf, P. A., Beiser, A., Hald, J. K., Au, R., Kase, C. S.,...DeCarli, C. (2004). Cerebral microbleeds: Prevalence and associations with cardiovascular risk factors in the Framingham Study. *Stroke,* 35(8), 1831–1835.

Jeerakathil, T., Wolf, P. A., Beiser, A., Massaro, J., Seshadri, S., D'Agostino, R. B., & DeCarli, C. (2004). Stroke risk profile predicts white matter hyperintensity volume: The Framingham Study. *Stroke,* 35(8), 1857–1861.

Kemppainen, N. M., Aalto, S., Wilson, I. A., Nagren, K., Helin, S., Bruck, A.,...Rinne, J. O. (2007). PET amyloid ligand [11C]PIB uptake is increased in mild cognitive impairment. *Neurology,* 68(19), 1603–1606.

Knopman, D. S., Parisi, J. E., Boeve, B. F., Cha, R. H., Apaydin, H., Salviati, A.,...Rocca, W. A. (2003). Vascular dementia in a population-based autopsy study. *Archives of Neurology, 60*(4), 569–575.

Launer, L. J., Masaki, K., Petrovich, H., Foley, D., & Havlik, R. J. (1995). The association between mid-life blood pressure levels and late-life cognitive function. The Honolulu-Asia Aging Study. *Journal of the American Medical Association, 274,* 1846–1851.

Lesnik Oberstein, S. A., van den Boom, R., Middelkoop, H. A., Ferrari, M. D., Knaap, Y. M., van Houwelingen, H. C.,...Haan, J. (2003). Incipient CADASIL. *Archives of Neurology, 60*(5), 707–712.

Liem, M. K., van der Grond, J., Haan, J., van den Boom, R., Ferrari, M. D., Knaap, Y. M.,...Lesnik Oberstein, S. A. (2007). Lacunar infarcts are the main correlate with cognitive dysfunction in CADASIL. *Stroke, 38*(3), 923–928.

Logue, M. W., Posner, H., Green, R. C., Moline, M., Cupples, L. A., Lunetta, K. L.,...Decarli, C. (2011). Magnetic resonance imaging-measured atrophy and its relationship to cognitive functioning in vascular dementia and Alzheimer's disease patients. *Alzheimers Dementia, 7*(5), 493–500.

Longstreth, W. T., Jr., Bernick, C., Manolio, T. A., Bryan, N., Jungreis, C. A., & Price, T. R. (1998). Lacunar infarcts defined by magnetic resonance imaging of 3660 elderly people: The Cardiovascular Health Study. *Archives of Neurology, 55*(9), 1217–1225.

Longstreth, W. T., Jr., Manolio, T. A., Arnold, A., Burke, G. L., Bryan, N., Jungreis, C. A.,...Fried, L. (1996). Clinical correlates of white matter findings on cranial magnetic resonance imaging of 3301 elderly people. The Cardiovascular Health Study [see comments]. *Stroke, 27*(8), 1274–1282.

Lopez, O. L., Jagust, W. J., Dulberg, C., Becker, J. T., DeKosky, S. T., Fitzpatrick, A.,...Kuller, L. H. (2003). Risk factors for mild cognitive impairment in the cardiovascular health study cognition study: Part 2. *Archives of Neurology, 60*(10), 1394–1399.

Lopresti, B. J., Klunk, W. E., Mathis, C. A., Hoge, J. A., Ziolko, S. K., Lu, X., (2005). Simplified quantification of Pittsburgh Compound B amyloid imaging PET studies: A comparative analysis. *Journal of Nuclear Medicine, 46*(12), 1959–1972.

Luchsinger, J. A., Brickman, A. M., Reitz, C., Cho, S. J., Schupf, N., Manly, J. J.,...Brown, T. R. (2009). Subclinical cerebrovascular disease in mild cognitive impairment. *Neurology, 73*(6), 450–456.

Marchant, N. L., Reed, B. R., Decarli, C. S., Madison, C. M., Weiner, M. W., Chui, H. C., & Jagust, W. J. (2011). Cerebrovascular disease, beta-amyloid, and cognition in aging. *Neurobiology of Aging, 33*(5), 1006. e25-36.

McKhann, G., Drachman, D., Folstein, M., Katzman, R., Price, D., & Stadlan, E. M. (1984). Clinical diagnosis of Alzheimer's disease: Report of the NINCDS-ADRDA Work Group under the auspices of Department of Health and Human Services Task Force on Alzheimer's Disease. *Neurology, 34*(7), 939–944.

Moroney, J. T., Bagiella, E., Desmond, D. W., Paik, M. C., Stern, Y., & Tatemichi, T. K. (1996). Risk factors for incident dementia after stroke. Role of hypoxic and ischemic disorders. *Stroke, 27*(8), 1283–1289.

Moroney, J. T., Bagiella, E., Desmond, D. W., Paik, M. C., Stern, Y., & Tatemichi, T. K. (1997a). Cerebral hypoxia and ischemia in the pathogenesis of dementia after stroke. *Annals of the New York Academy of Sciences, 826*(3), 433–436.

Moroney, J. T., Bagiella, E., Tatemichi, T. K., Paik, M. C., Stern, Y., & Desmond, D. W. (1997b). Dementia after stroke increases the risk of long-term stroke recurrence. *Neurology, 48*(5), 1317–1325.

Morris, J. C. (1993). The Clinical Dementia Rating (CDR), current version and scoring rules. *Neurology, 43*(11), 2412–2414.

Mungas, D., Reed, B., Ellis, W. G., & Jagust, W. J. (2001). The effects of age on rate of progression of Alzheimer disease and dementia with associated cerebrovascular disease. *Archives of Neurology, 58,* 1243–1247.

Nordahl, C. W., Ranganath, C., Yonelinas, A. P., DeCarli, C., Reed, B. R., & Jagust, W. J. (2005). Different mechanisms of episodic memory failure in mild cognitive impairment. *Neuropsychologia, 43*(11), 1688–1697.

O'Brien, J. T., Erkinjuntti, T., Reisberg, B., Roman, G., Sawada, T., Pantoni, L.,...DeKosky, J. T. (2003). Vascular cognitive impairment. *Lancet Neurology, 2*(2), 89–98.

O'Brien, M. D. (1988). Vascular dementia is underdiagnosed. *Archives of Neurology, 45,* 797–798.

Reed, B. R., Eberling, J. L., Mungas, D., Weiner, M. W., & Jagust, W. J. (2000). Memory failure has different mechanisms in subcortical stroke and Alzheimer's disease. *Annals of Neurology, 48*(3), 275–284.

Reed, B. R., Eberling, J. L., Mungas, D., Weiner, M., & Jagust, W. J. (2001). Frontal lobe hypometabolism predicts cognitive decline in patients with lacunar infarcts. *Archives of Neurology, 58,* 493–7.

Petersen, R. C., Thomas, R. G., Grundman, M., Bennett, D., Doody, R., Ferris, S., (2005). Vitamin E and donepezil for the treatment of mild cognitive impairment. *New England Journal of Medicine, 352*(23), 2379–2388.

Pike, K. E., Savage, G., Villemagne, V. L., Ng, S., Moss, S. A., Maruff, P.,...Rowe, C. C. (2007). Beta-amyloid imaging and memory in non-demented individuals: Evidence for preclinical Alzheimer's disease. *Brain, 130*(Pt 11), 2837–2844.

Ranganath, C., Johnson, M. K., & D'Esposito, M. (2003). Prefrontal activity associated with working memory and episodic long-term memory. *Neuropsychologia, 41*(3), 378–389.

Reed, B. R., Marchant, N. L., Jagust, W. J., Decarli, C. C., Mack, W., & Chui, H. C. (2011). Coronary risk correlates with cerebral amyloid deposition. *Neurobiology of Aging, 33*(9), 1979–1987.

Rockwood, K., Howard, K., MacKnight, C., & Darvesh, S. (1999). Spectrum of disease in vascular cognitive impairment. *Neuroepidemiology, 18*(5), 248–254.

Rockwood, K., Wentzel, C., Hachinski, V., Hogan, D. B., MacKnight, C., & McDowell, I. (2000). Prevalence and outcomes of vascular cognitive impairment. Vascular Cognitive Impairment Investigators of the Canadian Study of Health and Aging. *Neurology, 54*(2), 447–451.

Roman, G. C. (2003). Vascular dementia: Distinguishing characteristics, treatment, and prevention. *Journal of the American Geriatric Society, 51*(5 Suppl Dementia), S296–S304.

Roman, G. C., Tatemichi, T. K., Erkinjuntti, T., Cummings, J. L., Masdeu, J. C., Garcia, J. H.,...Hofman, A. (1993). Vascular dementia: Diagnostic criteria for research studies. Report of the NINDS-AIREN International Workshop. *Neurology, 43*(2), 250–260.

Rowe, C. C., Ng, S., Ackermann, U., Gong, S. J., Pike, K., Savage, G.,...Villemagne, V. L. (2007). Imaging beta-amyloid burden in aging and dementia. *Neurology, 68*(20), 1718–1725.

Sacco, R. L., Wolf, P. A., Kannel, W. B., & McNamara, P. M. (1982). Survival and recurrence following stroke. The Framingham Study. *Stroke, 13*(3), 290–295.

Sayetta, R. B. (1986). Rates of senile dementia, Alzheimer's type, in the Baltimore Longitudinal Study. *Journal of Chronic Disease, 39*(4), 271–286.

Scheltens, P., Leys, D., Barkhof, F., Kuiper, M. A., Huglo, D., Weinstein, H. C.,...Valk, J. (1992). Atrophy of medial temporal lobes on MRI in 'probable' Alzheimer's disease and normal aging: Diagnostic value and neuropsychological correlates. *Journal of Neurology, Neurosurgery and Psychiatry, 55*, 967–972.

Schneider, J. A., Arvanitakis, Z., Bang, W., & Bennett, D. A. (2007). Mixed brain pathologies account for most dementia cases in community-dwelling older persons. *Neurology, 69*(24), 2197–2204.

Schneider, J. A., Bienias, J. L., Wilson, R. S., Berry-Kravis, E., Evans, D. A., & Bennett, D. A. (2005). The apolipoprotein E epsilon4 allele increases the odds of chronic cerebral infarction [corrected] detected at autopsy in older persons. *Stroke, 36*(5), 954–959.

Schneider, J. A., Wilson, R. S., Bienias, J. L., Evans, D. A., & Bennett, D. A. (2004). Cerebral infarctions and the likelihood of dementia from Alzheimer disease pathology. *Neurology, 62*(7), 1148–1155.

Schneider, J. A., Wilson, R. S., Cochran, E. J., Bienias, J. L., Arnold, S. E., Evans, D. A., (2003). Relation of cerebral infarctions to dementia and cognitive function in older persons. *Neurology, 60*(7), 1082–1088.

Seshadri, S., Beiser, A., Kelly-Hayes, M., Kase, C. S., Au, R., Kannel, W. B., & Wolf, P. A. (2006). The lifetime risk of stroke: Estimates from the Framingham Study. *Stroke, 37*(2), 345–350.

Seshadri, S., & Wolf, P. A. (2007). Lifetime risk of stroke and dementia: Current concepts, and estimates from the Framingham Study. *Lancet Neurology, 6*(12), 1106–1114.

Seshadri, S., Wolf, P. A., Beiser, A., Elias, M. F., Au, R., Kase, C. S., (2004). Stroke risk profile, brain volume, and cognitive function: The Framingham Offspring Study. *Neurology, 63*(9), 1591–1599.

Snowdon, D. A., Greiner, L. H., Mortimer, J. A., Riley, K. P., Greiner, P. A., & Markesbery, W. R. (1997). Brain infarction and the clinical expression of Alzheimer disease. The Nun Study. *Journal of the American Medical Association, 277*, 813–817.

Swan, G. E., DeCarli, C., Miller, B. L., Reed, T., Wolf, P. A., & Carmelli, D. (2000). Biobehavioral characteristics of nondemented older adults with subclinical brain atrophy. *Neurology, 54*(11), 2108–2114.

Swan, G. E., DeCarli, C., Miller, B. L., Reed, T., Wolf, P. A., Jack, L. M., & Carmelli, D. (1998). Association of midlife blood pressure to late-life cognitive decline and brain morphology. *Neurology, 51*(4), 986–993.

Tatemichi, T. K. (1990). How acute brain failure becomes chronic: A view of the mechanisms of dementia related to stroke. *Neurology, 40*, 1652–1659.

Tatemichi, T. K., Desmond, D. W., Mayeux, R., Paik, M., Stern, Y., Sano, M.,...Hauser, W. A. (1992). Dementia after stroke: Baseline frequency, risks, and clinical features in a hospitalized cohort. *Neurology, 42*, 1185–1193.

Tatemichi, T. K., Desmond, D. W., & Prohovnik, I. (1995). Strategic infarcts in vascular dementia. A clinical and brain imaging experience. *Arzneimittel-Forschung, 45*(3A), 371–385.

Tatemichi, T. K., Desmond, D. W., Prohovnik, I., & Eidelberg, D. (1995). Dementia associated with bilateral carotid occlusions: Neuropsychological and haemodynamic course after extracranial to intracranial bypass surgery. *Journal of Neurology, Neurosurgery and Psychiatry, 58*(5), 633–636.

Tatemichi, T. K., Foulkes, M. A., Mohr, J. P., Hewitt, J. R., Hier, D. B., Price, T. R., & Wolf, P. A. (1990). Dementia in stroke survivors in the stroke data bank cohort. Prevalence, incidence, risk factors, and computed tomographic findings. *Stroke, 21*, 858–866.

Tullberg, M., Fletcher, E., DeCarli, C., Mungas, D., Reed, B. R., Harvey, D. J.,...Jagust, W. J. (2004). White matter lesions impair frontal lobe function regardless of their location. *Neurology, 63*(2), 246–253.

van den Boom, R., Lesnik Oberstein, S. A., Spilt, A., Behloul, F., Ferrari, M. D., Haan, J.,...Buchen, M. A. (2003). Cerebral hemodynamics and white matter hyperintensities in CADASIL. *Journal of Cerebral Blood Flow and Metabolism, 23*(5), 599–604.

van der Flier, W. M., van Straaten, E. C., Barkhof, F., & Scheltens, P. (2005). NINDS AIREN neuroimaging criteria do not distinguish stroke patients with and without dementia. *Neurology, 65*(8), 1341.

Van der Werf, Y. D., Scheltens, P., Lindeboom, J., Witter, M. P., Uylings, H. B., & Jolles, J. (2003). Deficits of memory, executive functioning and attention following infarction in the thalamus: A study of 22 cases with localised lesions. *Neuropsychologia, 41*(10), 1330–1344.

van Dijk, E. J., Prins, N. D., Vermeer, S. E., Koudstaal, P. J., & Breteler, M. M. (2002). Frequency of white matter lesions and silent lacunar infarcts. *Journal of Neural Transmission Supplemental, 2002*(62), 25–39.

Vermeer, S. E., Longstreth, W. T., Jr., & Koudstaal, P. J. (2007). Silent brain infarcts: A systematic review. *Lancet Neurology, 6*(7), 611–619.

Vermeer, S. E., Koudstaal, P. J., Oudkerk, M., Hofman, A., & Breteler, M. M. (2002). Prevalence and risk factors of silent brain infarcts in the population-based Rotterdam Scan Study. *Stroke, 33*(1), 21–25.

Vermeer, S. E., Prins, N. D., den Heijer, T., Hofman, A., Koudstaal, P. J., & Breteler, M. M. (2003). Silent brain infarcts and the risk of dementia and cognitive decline. *New England Journal of Medicine, 348*(13), 1215–1222.

Wagle, J., Farner, L., Flekkoy, K., Bruun Wyller, T., Sandvik, L., Fure, B.,...Engedal, K. (2011). Early post-stroke cognition in stroke rehabilitation patients predicts functional outcome at 13 months. *Dementia and Geriatric Cognitive Disorders, 31*(5), 379–387.

Whitmer, R. A. (2007). Type 2 diabetes and risk of cognitive impairment and dementia. *Current Neurology and Neuroscience Reports, 7*(5), 373–380.

Whitmer, R. A., Gunderson, E. P., Barrett-Connor, E., Quesenberry, C. P., Jr., & Yaffe, K. (2005). Obesity in middle age and future risk of dementia: A 27 year longitudinal population based study. *British Medical Journal, 330*(7504), 1360.

Whitmer, R. A., Gustafson, D. R., Barrett-Connor, E., Haan, M. N., Gunderson, E. P., & Yaffe, K. (2008). Central obesity and increased risk of dementia more than three decades later. *Neurology, 71*(14), 1057–1064.

Whitmer, R. A., Sidney, S., Selby, J., Johnston, S. C., & Yaffe, K. (2005). Midlife cardiovascular risk factors and risk of dementia in late life. *Neurology, 64*(2), 277–281.

Winblad, B., Palmer, K., Kivipelto, M., Jelic, V., Fratiglioni, L., Wahlund, L. O.,...Petersen, R. C. (2004). Mild cognitive impairment—beyond controversies, towards a consensus: Report of the International Working Group on Mild Cognitive Impairment. *Journal of Internal Medicine, 256*(3), 240–246.

Wolf, P. A., D'Agostino, R. B., Belanger, A. J., & Kannel, W. B. (1991). Probability of stroke: A risk profile from the Framingham Study. *Stroke, 22*(3), 312–318.

Yoshita, M., Fletcher, E., Harvey, D., Ortega, M., Martinez, O., Mungas, D. M.,...DeCarli, C. S. (2006). Extent and distribution of white matter hyperintensities in normal aging, MCI, and AD. *Neurology, 67*(12), 2192–2198.

14

Cerebral Amyloid Angiopathy and Cognitive Impairment

Ellis S. van Etten, Steven M. Greenberg, and Anand Viswanathan

Cerebral amyloid angiopathy (CAA) is a cerebrovascular disorder that is commonly found in the brains of elderly people (Jellinger, 2002). CAA-related vascular dysfunction is caused by deposition of the amyloid-β (Aβ) peptide in small and medium-sized blood vessels (Vinters 1987; Vonsattel et al., 1991). CAA can lead to lesions typical of cerebral small-vessel disease (SVD). Indeed, all of the classic magnetic resonance imaging (MRI) markers of SVD can be seen in patients with CAA. These include small, punctate, microhemorrhages (or microbleeds) (Greenberg, Finklestein, & Schaefer, 1996; Greenberg et al., 2009), lacunar infarctions (Kimberly et al., 2009; Menon & Kidwell, 2009), and white matter hyperintensity (WMH) (Holland et al., 2008; Zhu et al., 2012). Although CAA classically presents with a lobar intracerebral hemorrhage (ICH), mounting evidence suggests that there are many patients with CAA without a major hemorrhage (Greenberg, Vonsattel, Stakes, Gruber, & Finklestein, 1993; Greenberg et al., 2009).

Epidemiology

CAA occurs in a highly prevalent sporadic form and a more rare hereditary form (Zhang-Nunes et al., 2006). Autopsy studies have suggested that the sporadic form is detectable in 10% to 40% of individuals above the age of 60 (Jellinger, 2002), and this figure increases to 50% in individuals above the age of 90 (McCarron & Nicoll, 2004). In patients with concomitant Alzheimer's disease (AD), CAA can be found in 80% or more of the affected brains (Ellis et al., 1996; Jellinger, 2002; Xu, Yang, & Wang, 2003). In patients with dementia, these two diseases often coexist and share the same neuropathologic finding of Aβ deposition (Selkoe, 2001; Smith & Greenberg, 2009). Cognitive impairment has, however, also been observed in CAA in the absence of extensive AD pathology (Grabowski, Cho, Vonsattel, Rebeck, & Greenberg, 2001; Natté et al., 2001), and CAA has been increasingly recognized as an independent cause of dementia (Arvanitakis et al., 2011; Greenberg, Gurol, Rosand, & Smith, 2004; Neuropathology Group, Medical Research Council Cognitive Function and Aging Study, 2001).

Pathophysiology

In its most common form, amyloid angiopathy results from Aβ deposition in the media and adventitia of cerebral small arteries and capillaries. After cleavage of the longer amyloid precursor protein (APP), Aβ species are formed consisting of 40 to 42 amino acids (Price, Tanzi, Borchelt, & Sisodia, 1998). Although the Aβ peptide is derived from APP in both sporadic CAA and in AD, certain hereditary forms of CAA are associated with accumulation of non-Aβ peptides (Zhang-Nunes et al., 2006).

It has been suggested that the Aβ peptide is primarily generated by neurons and is drained with interstitial fluid along perivascular spaces to cervical lymph nodes (Herzig, Van Nostrand, & Jucker, 2006; Roher et al., 2003; Weller et al., 1998). Aβ is likely actively cleared from the central nervous system across the blood–brain barrier through a variety of mechanisms (Bell et al., 2009; Deane et al., 2003, 2004). Impaired clearance may lead to amyloid deposits in the vessel wall (Fig. 14.1) and amyloid plaques in the brain parenchyma (Deane et al., 2003; Herzig et al., 2006). Overexpression of serum response factor (SRF) and myocardin in vascular smooth muscle cells can downregulate lipoprotein receptor-related protein (LRP-1) and initiate Aβ accumulation (Bell et al., 2009).

For reasons yet to be clarified, there is preferential Aβ deposition in the cerebral cortex, particularly the occipital lobe, with relative sparing of the deep hemispheric structures (e.g., thalamus and basal ganglia) and the brainstem (Herzig et al., 2004; Vinters, 1987).

The potential role of peripheral Aβ in the development of CAA has recently been highlighted in a transgenic mouse model, which showed acceleration of CAA and Aβ-related brain pathology after peripheral injection of Aβ-containing inoculates (Eisele et al., 2010). Peripheral Aβ may be an important precursor pool for brain Aβ, as several animal models have demonstrated that it can cross the blood–brain barrier (Ghilardi et al., 1996; Mackic et al., 1998, 2002; Martel, Mackic, McComb, Ghiso, & Zlokovic, 1996; Poduslo, Curran, Haggard, Biere, & Selkoe, 1997; Ujiie, Dickstein, Carlow, & Jefferies, 2003; Zlokovic et al., 1993).

Cerebrovascular deposition of Aβ in patients with sporadic and hereditary forms of CAA results in an array of vessel pathology. This includes loss of smooth muscle cells, thickening of the vessel wall with luminal narrowing, concentric splitting of the vessel wall ("vessel-in-vessel" appearance), microaneurysm formation, and perivascular microhemorrhage (Grabowski et al., 2001; Mandybur, 1986; Vinters, 1987; Vinters et al., 1994, 1998; Vonsattel et al., 1991; Zekry et al., 2003). These pathological findings can also be recapitulated in various animal models of CAA resulting from overexpression of the APP gene (Calhoun et al., 1999; Christie,

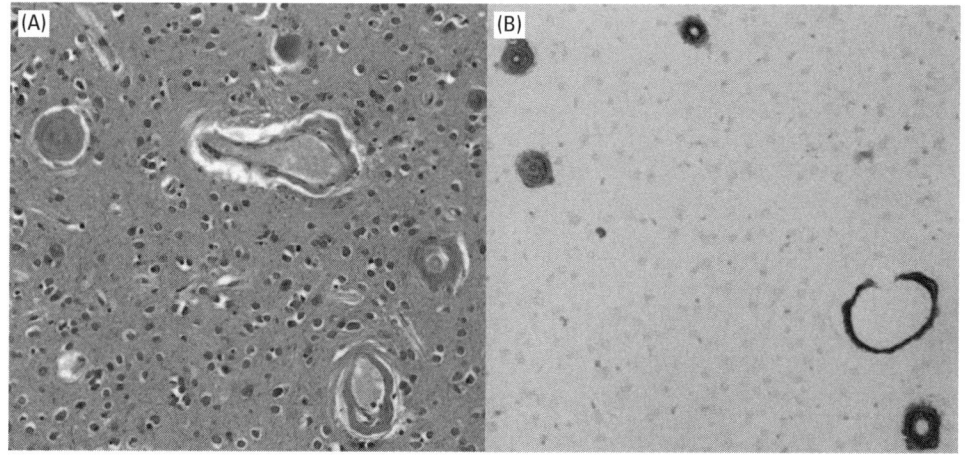

Figure 14.1 Pathologic appearance of cerebral amyloid angiopathy. (*A*) Amyloid deposits replace media and smooth muscle cells causing thickening of the vessel wall (hematoxylin & eosin; original magnification, 20×). (*B*) Immunoperoxidase staining for amyloid-β peptide showing circumferential staining of leptomeningeal blood vessels (original magnification, 20×). (Images courtesy of Dr. Matthew P. Frosch, MGH) (See color plate section)

Yamada, Moskowitz, & Hyman, 2001; Fryer et al., 2003; Van Dorpe et al., 2000; Winkler et al., 2001). Furthermore, deposition of Aβ has been shown to affect resting vessel diameter (Kimchi, Kajdasz, Bacskai, & Hyman, 2001; Mandybur, 1986) and modify cerebral vasoreactivity in animal models (Han et al., 2008; Niwa, Carlson, & Iadecola, 2000; Niwa, Younkin, et al., 2000; Shin et al., 2007) and in patients with CAA (Dumas et al., 2012; Smith et al., 2008). This vascular dysfunction may underlie the subcortical white matter damage seen in patients with advanced CAA (Gurol et al., 2006; Holland et al., 2008; Smith et al., 2004; Viswanathan et al., 2008). Although the distribution of white matter disease in CAA appears similar to patients with hypertensive vasculopathy (Smith et al., 2010), there is some suggestion that in at least a subgroup of CAA patients, the posterior white matter is predominantly affected (Zhu et al., 2012).

Genetics

In sporadic CAA, the only specific genetic risk factor consistently identified has been Apolipoprotein E (*APOE*) genotype. Possession of the *APOE* type ε2 and/or ε4 is associated with lobar hemorrhage (Biffi, Sonni, et al., 2010; Greenberg et al., 1998; Woo et al., 2002). The presence of either *APOE* ε2 or ε4 alleles possibly doubles the risk of a lobar ICH (odds ratio 2.3; 95% confidence interval 1.2–4.4) (Woo et al., 2002). Additionally, the *APOE* ε2 and ε4 alleles have been associated with an earlier age of onset of a lobar hemorrhage (Greenberg et al., 1998; Greenberg, Briggs, et al., 1996) and correlate with an increased risk of recurrent hemorrhages (O'Donnell et al., 2000).

The *APOE* ε2 allele alone predisposes patients with lobar ICH to hematoma expansion (Brouwers et al., 2012) and might have a role in the severity and clinical course of lobar ICH (Biffi et al., 2011). These studies are in line with the finding that *APOE* ε2 may promote splitting of the vessel wall, formation of microhemorrhages, and fibrinoid necrosis leading to vessel breakdown (Greenberg et al., 1998; McCarron et al., 1999). In contrast, the *APOE* ε4 allele is associated with an increase in the amount of vascular amyloid (Greenberg, Rebeck, Vonsattel, Gomez-Isla, & Hyman, 1995; Premkumar, Cohen, Hedera, Friedland, & Kalaria, 1996; Schmechel et al., 1993).

Interestingly, in AD the presence of the ε4 allele is associated with increased risk and a more rapid progression of the disease, whereas presence of the ε2 allele is associated with decreased risk (Corder et al., 1998). The effect of the different *APOE* genotypes in both diseases is likely to be mediated by the way amyloid accumulation is modulated (Olesen, Mikkelsen, Gerdes, & Jensen, 1997; Sanan et al., 1994; Verghese et al., 2011). For example, the ε4 allele is thought to increase Aβ aggregation and impair Aβ clearance (Verghese et al., 2011).

In addition to *APOE* as a risk factor for sporadic CAA, there are several genetic mutations that cause rare autosomal dominant familial forms of CAA. Patients with these hereditary forms of CAA usually have more severe clinical course and present at an earlier age (Bornebroek et al., 2003; De Jonghe et al., 1998; Palsdottir, Snorradottir, & Thorsteinsson, 2006; Van Nostrand, Melchor, Cho, Greenberg, & Rebeck, 2001). To date, several mutations have been described, most of which involve either missense mutations within the Aβ coding region or duplication of the *APP* gene. However, mutations in other genes unrelated to Aβ such as cystatin C and transthyretin have also been described (Ghiso, Pons-Estel, & Frangione, 1986; Jonsdottir & Palsdottir 1993; Palsdottir et al., 1988; Vidal et al., 1996).

The most common form of hereditary CAA is seen in families with autosomal dominant early-onset AD (ADEOAD). It has been suggested that in 2% to 18% of the individuals with ADEOAD, the disorder is caused by duplication of the *APP* locus, which often causes concomitant CAA (Cabrejo et al., 2006; Kasuga et al., 2009; Rovelet-Lecrux et al., 2006; Sleegers et al., 2006). A more rare form, hereditary cerebral hemorrhage with amyloidosis-Dutch type (HCHWA-D), the first hereditary CAA disorder to be discovered, is caused by a point mutation at codon 693 of *APP*, which results in modification of the Aβ peptide (Bakker et al., 1991; Levy et al., 1990; van Duinen et al., 1987; Wattendorff, Frangione, Luyendijk, & Bots, 1995). This is a dominantly inherited disorder where patients experience recurrent ICH, cognitive decline, and dementia. Although cognitive symptoms typically appear after initial stroke, they can manifest as the first symptom of the disease (Zhang-Nunes et al., 2006). Another hereditary CAA form, first discovered in an Iowa family, is caused by a point mutation in codon 694 of the *APP* gene (Grabowski et al., 2001; Van Nostrand et al., 2001). In this disorder, family members may have dramatically different clinical presentations, varying from recurrent ICH, to dementia and leukoaraiosis without ICH (Greenberg et al., 2003). Additionally, hereditary cerebral hemorrhage with amyloidosis-Icelandic type (HCHWA-I) is an autosomal dominant disorder seen in Icelandic families caused by a point mutation at codon 68 of the *cystatin C* gene. It causes cystatin C, a cysteine protein inhibitor, to form deposits in cerebral arteries leading to ICHs (Palsdottir et al., 2006).

Screening for hereditary CAA gene mutations among patient with sporadic CAA appears to have little clinical value because the familial and sporadic forms CAA are unlikely to share individual risk mutations. Therefore, systematic genetic screening in sporadic CAA patients lacking a strong family history of hemorrhage or dementia is not currently recommended (Biffi, Plourde, et al., 2010).

Diagnosis

Although a definitive diagnosis of sporadic CAA can only be made after histological investigation of affected brain tissue through biopsy or autopsy, clinical diagnostic criteria to identify patients with the disease, called the Boston Criteria, have been developed. Most reliably used in elderly patients presenting with lobar ICH, the Boston Criteria serve to identify those individuals likely to have pathologic evidence of advanced CAA (Table 14.1) (Greenberg, 1998; Knudsen, Rosand, Karluk, & Greenberg, 2001; van Rooden et al., 2009). *Probable* CAA is defined by the presence of multiple, strictly lobar hemorrhages (including microhemorrhages or microbleeds) detected by gradient-echo MRI with no other definite cause of ICH such as trauma, ischemic stroke, tumor, coagulopathy, or excessive anticoagulation (Fig. 14.2). Similarly, *possible* CAA is defined by the presence of a single lobar hemorrhage without other definite cause (Knudsen et al., 2001).

The Boston Criteria for diagnosis of CAA have been compared against the established

TABLE 14.1 Boston Criteria for Diagnosis of Cerebral Amyloid Angiopathy (CAA)–Related Hemorrhage

1. Definite CAA
Full postmortem examination demonstrating
 a. Lobar, cortical, or corticosubcortical hemorrhage
 b. Severe CAA with vasculopathy
 c. Absence of other diagnostic lesion
2. Probable CAA with Supporting Pathology
Clinical data and *pathologic tissue* (evacuated hematoma or cortical biopsy) demonstrating:
 a. Lobar, cortical, or corticosubcortical hemorrhage
 b. Some degree of CAA in specimen
 c. Absence of other diagnostic lesion
3. Probable CAA
Clinical data and *magnetic resonance imaging* or *computerized tomography* demonstrating:
 a. Multiple hemorrhages restricted to the lobar, cortical, corticosubcortical, or cerebellar region
 b. Age ≥55
 c. Absence of other cause of intracerebral hemorrhage*
4. Possible CAA
Clinical data and *magnetic resonance imaging* or *computerized tomography* demonstrating:
 a. Single lobar, cortical, or corticosubcortical hemorrhage
 b. Age ≥55
 c. Absence of other cause of intracerebral hemorrhage*

*Potential causes of intracerebral hemorrhage: excessive anticoagution (INR > 3.0); antecedent head trauma or ischemic stroke; central nervous system tumor, vascular malformation, or vasculitis; blood dyscrasia.

gold standard of pathologic diagnosis from specimens from autopsy, hematoma evacuation, or cortical biopsy (Knudsen et al., 2001). Of the 39 cases diagnosed with lobar ICH on clinical and radiologic grounds, all 13 cases with probable CAA also had a pathological diagnosis of CAA. Sixteen of the 26 cases with possible CAA had a pathological diagnosis of CAA. These data demonstrate the high specificity of the Boston Criteria to identify patients with lobar ICH and sporadic CAA (Table 14.2).

For further validation of the Boston Criteria and to refine their image components, they have recently been applied to patients who were diagnosed with hereditary CAA after genetic testing. In groups of symptomatic and asymptomatic patients with HCHWA-D, detection of lesions caused by CAA using the

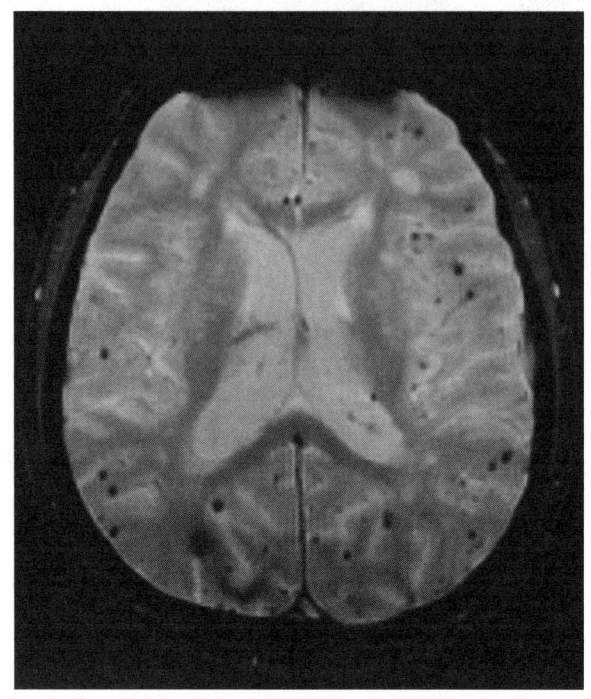

Figure 14.2 Axial slide of gradient recalled echo (GRE) magnetic resonance image (MRI) of patient with probable cerebral amyloid angiopathy demonstrating multiple punctate lobar areas of decreased intensity suggestive of cerebral microbleeds.

Boston Criteria was found to be highly sensitive, and including microbleeds in the assessment further increased the sensitivity (van Rooden et al., 2009).

Additionally, spontaneous subarachnoid hemorrhage localized to the convexity may be another radiographic manifestation of cerebral amyloid angiopathy. Also described as superficial siderosis, this finding was identified by one study in 60% (22 of 38) of pathologically verified cases of advanced CAA versus 0 of 22 ICHs due to other causes (Linn et al., 2010). Thus, superficial siderosis in elderly individuals with clinical and neuroimaging features consistent with CAA may be further suggestive of the diagnosis.

TABLE 14.2 Clinicopathologic Correlation in the Diagnosis of Cerebral Amyloid Angiopathy (CAA)

Clinical Diagnosis	Source of Pathologic Specimen	n	Pathologic Diagnosis + CAA	Pathologic Diagnosis − CAA
Probable CAA	All	13	13	0
	Postmortem brain	6	6	0
	Evacuated hematoma	5*	5	0
	Cortical biopsy	2	2	0
Possible CAA	All	26	16	10
	Postmortem brain	8	4	4
	Evacuated hematoma	16*	11	5
	Cortical biopsy	2	1	1
Total		39	29	10

*Three hematoma specimens (two probable CAA and one possible CAA) did not contain vessels and were not counted in these figures (Knudsen et al., 2001).

Whether sporadic CAA can reliably be recognized in patients without ICH and, if so, what degree of precision can be obtained remains uncertain and is an ongoing area of research. Establishing the predictive value of microbleeds detected in individuals without a major hemorrhage would be of considerable interest and could potentially identify patients with milder forms of the disease. Indirect evidence is suggestive that lobar microbleeds may be a reliable marker of cerebrobvascular amyloid deposition in subjects without ICH. Several population-based studies have found that cerebral microbleeds located in exclusively lobar regions are common in healthy elderly individuals (Mesker et al., 2011; Sveinbjornsdottir et al., 2008; Vernooij et al., 2008). Neuroimaging results from the Rotterdam study found that microbleeds were present in greater than 30% of healthy individuals over age 70 with the majority harboring microbleeds in a strictly lobar distribution (Mesker et al., 2011). Furthermore, in this study, individuals with the *APOE ε4* allele were more likely to have lobar microbleeds. Although further studies are needed, these data raise the possibility that there are a large number of asymptomatic elders in the general population with sporadic CAA. Criteria to reliably identify these individuals early in their clinical course, before they experience a devastating lobar ICH or cognitive impairment, need to be established.

Potential Emerging Techniques for Cerebral Amyloid Angiopathy Detection

Although the Boston criteria have been pathologically validated and have proven to strongly correlate with CAA-related pathology in patients with severe disease, the degree of reliability of these criteria in individuals with milder forms of the disease remains uncertain. Furthermore, these criteria still remain an indirect measure of the effects of Aβ-mediated pathology. This raises the question as to whether one can directly measure vascular Aβ burden during life, and if so, whether the methods involved reliably distinguish individuals with advanced CAA pathology from those with other Aβ pathologies such as AD. Several emerging techniques may serve as useful tools for more sensitive detection of CAA during life.

Positron emission tomography (PET)–based imaging using the amyloid binding ligand Pittsburgh Compound B has recently been developed (PiB-PET imaging). It is a noninvasive imaging technique to detect fibrillar Aβ deposits and has been used to quantify amyloid deposition in patients with Alzheimer's disease (Johnson et al., 2007; Klunk et al., 2004; Mathis et al., 2003). Several groups have applied this technique to study patients with probable/definite CAA or lobar ICH (Johnson et al., 2007; Ly et al., 2010). One study demonstrated that global PiB retention in nondemented CAA subjects was significantly increased in CAA relative to healthy control subjects, but lower in CAA than in AD. Importantly, there appears to be a greater proportion of PiB retention in the occipital cortex in patients with CAA compared to those with AD (Johnson et al., 2007; Ly et al., 2010). PiB appears to reliably detect vascular Aβ as has been shown in Iowa-type hereditary CAA (Greenberg et al., 2008). Further studies have suggested increased amyloid deposition occurs at sites of CAA-related microbleeds (Dierksen et al., 2010).

Other ligands for PET may include several ^{18}F-labeled tracers such as florbetapir, which was recently approved by the FDA (Anon, 2012). Although such ligands may potentially offer the advantage of more widespread use due to their longer half-lives (Herholz & Ebmeier, 2011), their utility in CAA diagnosis has not yet been reported.

Another approach to diagnose CAA may be to investigate the cerebrospinal fluid (CSF). It has been suggested that Aβ40 concentrations in CSF are decreased in CAA patients relative to controls and AD patients (Verbeek et al., 2009). Therefore, it is conceivable that the Aβ CSF profile could be used as another diagnostic tool in CAA detection. Finally, in vivo measures of abnormal vascular reactivity using transcranial Doppler ultrasound (TCD) (Smith et al., 2008) or functional MRI (Dumas et al., 2012) could function as another tool to help distinguish individuals with emerging CAA pathology.

Cerebral Amyloid Angiopathy–Related Cognitive Impairment

Cognitive dysfunction has been described in both sporadic (Greenberg et al., 1993; Silbert et al., 1995) and familial cases (Bornebroek, Haan, et al., 1996; Bornebroek, van Buchem, et al., 1996; Grabowski et al., 2001; Mead et al., 2000) of CAA, mostly in the absence of extensive Alzheimer pathology (Grabowski et al., 2001; Greenberg, Gurol, et al., 2004; Natté et al., 2001). Over 40% of patients with CAA-related ICH have some degree of cognitive decline during their life (Vinters, 1987). Interestingly, in very severe cases of CAA, cognitive impairment is a finding independent of a major hemorrhagic stroke (Grabowski et al., 2001; Greenberg, Gurol, et al., 2004; Natté et al., 2001). The MRC study demonstrated a significant association between severe CAA pathology and dementia independent for age, brain weight, neuritic and diffuse plaques, neocortical and hippocampal neurofibrillary tangles, Lewy bodies, and cerebrovascular disease (Neuropathology Group, Medical Research Council Cognitive Function and Aging Study, 2001). The Honolulu-Asia Aging Study (Pfeifer, White, Ross, Petrovitch, & Launer, 2002) found, after controlling for potential confounders, the accompanying presence of CAA in subjects with AD associated with significantly worse cognitive performance, although CAA was not significantly overrepresented in demented (55%) compared with nondemented (38%) brains. The recent Religious Orders cohort Study (Arvanitakis et al., 2011) showed that moderate to very severe CAA was associated with lower performance in specific cognitive domains, including lower perceptual speed and episodic memory. Whether cognition is affected in patients with less severe forms of CAA remains uncertain (Greenberg, Gurol, et al., 2004).

In a comprehensive review of the subject, Cordonnier and van der Flier (2011) concluded that while there is sufficient evidence to suggest that CMBs contribute to cognitive impairment in association with cerebrovascular disease, the evidence of an independent effect of CMBs on cognition among individuals with AD is less certain. One study suggested an independent effect (Goos et al., 2010), whereas another did not (Pettersen et al., 2008). The authors conclude that the evidence may be weak due to the low numbers of individuals in most studies (Cordonnier & van der Flier, 2011).

Although the exact mechanisms by which CAA may cause dementia are not fully elucidated, the brain parenchymal injuries resulting from the cerebrovascular pathology are likely to act as mediators of cognitive decline. Patients with a major hemorrhage can have abrupt cognitive decline accompanied with focal signs, but the cognitive function may recover over time (Korczyn, Vakhapova, & Grinberg, 2012). Interestingly, microbleeds have been shown to be associated independently with loss of cognitive functioning and functional dependence (van Es et al., 2011; Poels et al., 2012; Yakushiji et al., 2012), and more specifically with frontal executive dysfunction (Gregoire et al., 2012). Whether this is due to a direct contribution of CAA-related microbleeds to cognitive impairment as suggested in other pathologies (Viswanathan et al., 2010; Werring et al., 2004) or whether microbleeds are a marker of other CAA-related pathologies such as white matter hyperintensities (Gurol et al., 2006), changes in diffusion-tensor measurements (Salat et al., 2006; Viswanathan et al., 2008), small infarcts (Kimberly et al., 2009; Soontornniyomkij et al., 2010), or pathologies other than CAA like hypertension (Yakushiji et al., 2012) remains to be determined.

Small ischemic infarcts could also play an important role in developing cognitive impairment. Autopsy studies (Chui et al., 2006; Soontornniyomkij et al., 2010) and radiological studies (Gregoire et al., 2011; Kimberly et al., 2009) suggested that CAA-related dementia is associated with these small "silent" infarcts, in both gray and white matter areas, independent of AD pathology. These ischemic lesions are a frequent finding in sporadic CAA, ranging from 37% to nearly 100% of cases in autopsy studies (Haglund, Passant, Sjöbeck, Ghebremedhin, & Englund, 2006; Okamoto et al., 2009; Okazaki, Reagan, & Campbell, 1979; Olichney et al., 2000; Soontornniyomkij et al., 2010; Suter et al., 2002). Neuroimaging studies have demonstrated an occurrence of approximately 15% of hyperintense lesions on diffusion-weighted imaging (DWI) in ICH, suggestive of ischemic infarction (Garg et al., 2012; Gregoire et al., 2011; Kimberly et al., 2009; Lansberg et al., 2001; Menon et al., 2012; Prabhakaran et al., 2010). Their location, size, and radiological characteristics correspond to the ischemic lesions seen on pathologic examination in CAA patients (Haglund et al., 2006; Okamoto et al., 2009; Okazaki et al., 1979; Olichney et al., 2000; Suter et al., 2002).

Assuming these ischemic lesions are visually detectable on DWI 10 days after an ischemic stroke, the estimated prevalence would be 8 new infarctions per person-year (Kimberly et al., 2009). This estimate is strikingly high relative to the estimated incidence of new small hemorrhage (≈ 1.4 per year) or major, symptomatic ICH (≈ 0.14 per year) calculated from other cohorts with advanced CAA (Greenberg, Eng, Ning, Smith, & Rosand, 2004).

White matter damage is common in CAA (Gurol et al., 2006; Holland et al., 2008; Smith et al., 2004; Viswanathan et al., 2008) and has been associated with cognitive impairment in the disease prior to ICH (Smith, Rosand, Knudsen, Hylek, & Greenberg, 2002; Viswanathan et al., 2008). White matter damage is suggested to cause cognitive dysfunction by interrupting white matter fibers linking areas of association cortex, leading to difficulty with executive function and psychomotor speed (Au et al., 2006; Garde, Lykke Mortensen, Rostrup, & Paulson, 2005; Gupta et al., 1988; Schmidt, Petrovic, Ropele, Enzinger, & Fazekas, 2007; Smith et al., 2004). Patients with CAA have larger white matter hyperintensity burden on T2-weighted imaging compared to either healthy elderly subjects (Holland et al., 2008) or patients with AD (Gurol et al., 2006) and have evidence of tissue microstructural alterations on diffusion imaging (Salat et al., 2006; Viswanathan et al., 2008). These alterations in global diffusion tensor imaging measures using fractional anisotropy have been associated with cognitive impairment in CAA (Viswanathan et al., 2008).

Pathologic studies have suggested that CAA and AD often coexist. In AD patients CAA might have an additive effect by increasing dementia severity and, in patients with mild AD, it might aggravate cognitive impairment (Heyman et al., 1998; Petrovitch et al., 2005; Schneider, Arvanitakis, Bang, & Bennett, 2007; Snowdon et al., 1997). By contrast, CAA and AD can also present as distinct entities. Approximately 60%–80% of patients diagnosed with CAA-related lobar ICH did not show clinical symptoms of dementia before their initial ICH (Mandybur, 1986; Vinters, 1987). Similarly, only a minority of patients with AD demonstrates hemorrhages suggestive of advanced CAA (Atri et al., 2005; Cordonnier et al., 2006; Ellis et al., 1996; Hanyu, Tanaka, Shimizu, Takasaki, & Abe, 2003; Nakata et al., 2002; Pettersen et al., 2008).

Why certain patients develop CAA, while others develop AD or CAA and AD combined, is not fully understood, but it may in part be explained by differential accumulation of Aβ species. The cerebrovascular Aβ deposits in CAA mainly consist of the shorter, more soluble Aβ40 form (Herzig et al., 2004), whereas parenchymal plaques in AD show more Aβ42 species (Jankowsky et al., 2004; Johnson-Wood et al., 1997). Increase in the ratio between Aβ 40 and Aβ 42 may shift amyloid deposition from the parenchyma to the vessels (Herzig et al., 2006), and this balance between parenchymal and vascular amyloid deposits may be the key determinant in the pathogenesis of the two diseases (Fryer et al., 2005; Kumar-Singh, 2008; Love, Miners, Palmer, Chalmers, & Kehoe, 2009).

Interestingly, the presence of CAA may be a predisposing factor for inflammatory reaction against the active (Ferrer et al., 2004; Nicoll et al., 2003; Orgogozo et al., 2003) and passive (Black et al., 2010) Aβ vaccine studied in AD patients. The inflammation seen in some patients following Aβ42 immunization may resemble vasogenic edema seen in a subgroup of patients who develop inflammatory CAA (Salloway et al., 2009; Sperling et al., 2011, 2012). The inflammation is thought to be an immune response to the cerebrovascular amyloid deposits behaving as a foreign material (Greenberg & Frosch, 2011). This was hypothesized because of the location of the inflammatory reaction and the close relationship to inflammatory cells to cerebrovascular amyloid (Anders et al., 1997; Gray et al., 1990; Probst & Ulrich, 1985; Yamada et al., 1996). The finding of markers of CAA in AD patients may therefore have considerable implications for ongoing and future anti-amyloid trials.

Therapy Considerations and Future Directions

With no evidence-based treatment options available, optimal management of patients with CAA may be a challenge to many clinicians. Blood pressure control may serve as a strategy to reduce risk of CAA-related ICH recurrence (Arima et al., 2010). However, its impact on outcomes such as cognitive impairment or progression of small-vessel disease pathology remains to be determined. An important new therapeutic avenue to prevent major clinical consequences of CAA might be Aβ immunotherapy. As animal studies have shown, anti–Aβ therapy can reduce the Aβ burden in cerebral vessels (Prada et al., 2007; Schroeter et al., 2008; Thakker et al., 2009). Whether similar results could be obtained in patients with CAA and whether such therapy could modify clinical course in the disease remains to be investigated.

Summary

Over recent decades great progress has been made in determining the pathophysiology, genetics, and consequences of CAA. Mounting evidence is suggesting that CAA is an independent cause of cognitive impairment. Because this disease is highly prevalent in the elderly, its contribution to cognitive dysfunction could be substantial. Ongoing research aims to develop methods for early identification of patients with CAA and to reliably determine the burden of CAA in these individuals. Establishing criteria to reliably diagnose patients before they experience a lobar ICH or dementia will be a critical step in the development of new therapeutic strategies to prevent the major clinical consequences of this devastating disease.

References

Anders, K. H., Wang, Z. Z., Kornfeld, M., Gray, F., Soontornniyomkij, V., Reed, L. A.,...Vinters, H. V. (1997). Giant cell arteritis in association with cerebral amyloid angiopathy: Immunohistochemical and molecular studies. *Human Pathology*, 28(11), 1237–1246.

Anonymous. (2012). FDA approves 18F-florbetapir PET agent. *Journal of Nuclear Medicine*, 53(6), 15N.

Arima, H., Tzourio, C., Anderson, C., Woodward, M., Bousser, M. G., MacMahon, S.,...Chalmers, J. (2010). Effects of perindopril-based lowering of blood pressure on intracerebral hemorrhage related to amyloid angiopathy: The PROGRESS trial. *Stroke*, 41(2), 394–396.

Arvanitakis, Z., Leurgans, S. E., Wang, Z., Wilson, R. S., Bennett, D. A., & Schneider, J. A. (2011). Cerebral amyloid angiopathy pathology and cognitive domains in older persons. *Annals of Neurology*, 69(2), 320–327.

Atri, A., Locascio, J. J., Lin, J. M., Yap, L., Dickerson, B. C., Grodstein, F.,...Greenberg, S. M. (2005). Prevalence and effects of lobar microhemorrhages in early-stage dementia. *Neurodegenerative diseases*, 2(6), 305–312.

Au, R., Massaro, J. M., Wolf, P. A., Young, M. E., Beiser, A., Seshadri, S.,...DeCarli, C. (2006). Association of white matter hyperintensity volume with decreased cognitive functioning: The Framingham Heart Study. *Archives of Neurology*, 63(2), 246–250.

Bakker, E., van Broeckhoven, C., Haan, J., Voorhoeve, E., van Hul, W., Levy, E.,...Frangione, B, (1991). DNA diagnosis for hereditary cerebral hemorrhage with amyloidosis (Dutch type). *American Journal of Human Genetics*, 49(3), 518–521.

Bell, R. D., Deane, R., Chow, N., Long, X., Sagare, A., Singh, I.,...Zlokovic, B. V. (2009). SRF and myocardin regulate LRP-mediated amyloid-beta clearance in brain vascular cells. *Nature Cell Biology*, 11(2), 143–153.

Biffi, A., Anderson, C. D., Jagiella, J. M., Schmidt, H., Kissela, B., Hansen, B. M.,...Rosand, J. (2011). APOE genotype and extent of bleeding and outcome in lobar intracerebral haemorrhage: A genetic association study. *Lancet Neurology*, 10(8), 702–709.

Biffi, A., Plourde, A., Shen, Y., Onofrio, R., Smith, E. E., Frosch, M.,...Rosand, J. (2010). Screening for familial APP mutations in sporadic cerebral amyloid angiopathy. *PloS One*, 5(11), e13949.

Biffi, A., Sonni, A., Anderson, C. D., Kissela, B., Jagiella, J. M., Schmidt, H.,...Rosand, J. (2010). Variants at APOE influence risk of deep and lobar intracerebral hemorrhage. *Annals of Neurology*, 68(6), 934–943.

Black, R. S., Sperling, R. A., Safirstein, B., Motter, R. N., Pallay, A., Nichols, A., & Grundman, M. (2010). A single ascending dose study of bapineuzumab in patients with Alzheimer disease. *Alzheimer Disease and Associated Disorders*, 24(2), 198–203.

Bornebroek, M., De Jonghe, C., Haan, J., Kumar-Singh, S., Younkin, S., Roos, R., & Van Broeckhoven, C. (2003). Hereditary cerebral hemorrhage with amyloidosis Dutch type (AbetaPP 693): Decreased plasma amyloid-beta 42 concentration. *Neurobiology of Disease*, 14(3), 619–623.

Bornebroek, M., Haan, J., van Buchem, M. A., Lanser, J. B., de Vries-vd Weerd, M. A., Zoeteweij, M., & Roos, R. A. (1996). White matter lesions and cognitive deterioration in presymptomatic carriers of the amyloid precursor protein gene codon 693 mutation. *Archives of Neurology*, 53(1), 43–48.

Bornebroek, M., van Buchem, M. A., Haan, J., Brand, R., Lanser, J. B., de Bruïne, F. T., &

Roos, R. A. (1996). Hereditary cerebral hemorrhage with amyloidosis-Dutch type: Better correlation of cognitive deterioration with advancing age than with number of focal lesions or white matter hyperintensities. *Alzheimer Disease and Associated Disorders, 10*(4), 224–231.

Brouwers, H. B., Biffi, A., Ayres, A. M., Schwab, K., Cortellini, L., Romero, J. M.,...Goldstein, J. N. (2012). Apolipoprotein e genotype predicts hematoma expansion in lobar intracerebral hemorrhage. *Stroke, 43*(6), 1490–1495.

Cabrejo, L., Guyant-Maréchal, L., Laquerrière, A., Vercelletto, M., De la Fournière, F., Thomas-Antérion, C.,...Hannequin, D. (2006). Phenotype associated with APP duplication in five families. *Brain, 129*(Pt 11), 2966–2976.

Calhoun, M. E., Burgermeister, P., Phinney, A. L., Stalder, M., Tolnay, M., Wiederhold, K. H.,...Jucker, M. (1999). Neuronal overexpression of mutant amyloid precursor protein results in prominent deposition of cerebrovascular amyloid. *Proceedings of the National Academy of Sciences USA, 96*(24), 14088–14093.

Christie, R., Yamada, M., Moskowitz, M., & Hyman, B. (2001). Structural and functional disruption of vascular smooth muscle cells in a transgenic mouse model of amyloid angiopathy. *American Journal of Pathology, 158*(3), 1065–1071.

Chui, H. C., Zarow, C., Mack, W. J., Ellis, W. G., Zheng, L., Jagust, W. J.,...Vinters, H. V. (2006). Cognitive impact of subcortical vascular and Alzheimer's disease pathology. *Annals of Neurology, 60*(6), 677–687.

Corder, E. H., Lannfelt, L., Bogdanovic, N., Fratiglioni, L., & Mori, H. (1998). The role of APOE polymorphisms in late-onset dementias. *Cellular and Molecular Life Sciences, 54*(9), 928–934.

Cordonnier, C., van der Flier, W. M., Sluimer, J. D., Leys, D., Barkhof, F., & Scheltens. P. (2006). Prevalence and severity of microbleeds in a memory clinic setting. *Neurology, 66*(9), 1356–1360.

De Jonghe, C., Zehr, C., Yager, D., Prada, C. M., Younkin, S., Hendriks, L.,...Eckman, C. B. (1998). Flemish and Dutch mutations in amyloid beta precursor protein have different effects on amyloid beta secretion. *Neurobiology of Disease, 5*(4), 281–286.

Deane, R., Wu, Z., Sagare, A., Davis, J., Du Yan, S., Hamm, K.,...Zlokovic, B. V. (2004). LRP/amyloid beta-peptide interaction mediates differential brain efflux of Abeta isoforms. *Neuron, 43*(3), 333–344.

Deane, R., Du Yan, S., Submamaryan, R. K., LaRue, B., Jovanovic, S., Hogg, E.,...Zlokovic, B. (2003). RAGE mediates amyloid-beta peptide transport across the blood-brain barrier and accumulation in brain. *Nature Medicine, 9*(7), 907–913.

Dierksen, G. A., Skehan, M. E., Khan, M. A., Jeng, J., Nandigam, R. N., Becker, J. A.,...Greenberg, S. M. (2010). Spatial relation between microbleeds and amyloid deposits in amyloid angiopathy. *Annals of Neurology, 68*(4), 545–548.

Dumas, A., Dierksen, G. A., Gurol, M. E., Halpin, A., Martinez-Ramirez, S., Schwab, K.,...Greenberg, S. M. (2012). Functional MRI detection of vascular reactivity in cerebral amyloid angiopathy. *Annals of Neurology, 72*(1), 76–81.

Eisele, Y. S., Obermüller, U., Heilbronner, G., Baumann, F., Kaeser, S. A., Wolburg, H.,...Jucker, M. (2010). Peripherally applied Abeta-containing inoculates induce cerebral beta-amyloidosis. *Science, 330*(6006), 980–982.

Ellis, R. J., Olichney, J. M., Thal, L. J., Mirra, S. S., Morris, J. C., Beekly, D., & Heyman, A. (1996). Cerebral amyloid angiopathy in the brains of patients with Alzheimer's disease: The CERAD experience, Part XV. *Neurology, 46*(6), 1592–1596.

Ferrer, I., Boada Rovira, M., Sánchez Guerra, M. L., Rey, M. J., & Costa-Jussá, F. (2004). Neuropathology and pathogenesis of encephalitis following amyloid-beta immunization in Alzheimer's disease. *Brain Pathology (Zurich), 14*(1), 11–20.

Fryer, J. D., Taylor, J. W., DeMattos, R. B., Bales, K. R., Paul, S. M., Parsadanian, M., & Holtzman, D. M. (2003). Apolipoprotein E markedly facilitates age-dependent cerebral amyloid angiopathy and spontaneous hemorrhage in amyloid precursor protein transgenic mice. *Journal of Neuroscience, 23*(21), 7889–7896.

Fryer, J. D., Simmons, K., Parsadanian, M., Bales, K. R., Paul, S. M., Sullivan, P. M., & Holtzman, D. M. (2005). Human apolipoprotein E4 alters the amyloid-beta 40:42 ratio and promotes the formation of cerebral amyloid angiopathy in an amyloid precursor protein transgenic model. *Journal of Neuroscience, 25*(11), 2803–2810.

Garde, E., Lykke Mortensen, E., Rostrup, E., & Paulson, O. B. (2005). Decline in intelligence is associated with progression in white matter hyperintensity volume. *Journal of Neurology, Neurosurgery, and Psychiatry, 76*(9), 1289–1291.

Garg, R. K., Liebling, S. M., Maas, M. B., Nemeth, A. J., Russell, E. J., & Naidech, A. M. (2012). Blood pressure reduction, decreased diffusion on MRI, and outcomes after intracerebral hemorrhage. *Stroke, 43*(1), 67–71.

Ghilardi, J. R., Catton, M., Stimson, E. R., Rogers, S., Walker, L. C., Maggio, J. E., & Mantyh,

P. W. (1996). Intra-arterial infusion of [125I]A beta 1–40 labels amyloid deposits in the aged primate brain in vivo. *Neuroreport, 7*(15–17), 2607–2611.

Ghiso, J., Pons-Estel, B., & Frangione, B. (1986). Hereditary cerebral amyloid angiopathy: The amyloid fibrils contain a protein which is a variant of cystatin C, an inhibitor of lysosomal cysteine proteases. *Biochemical and Biophysical Research Communications, 136*(2), 548–554.

Grabowski, T. J., Cho, H. S., Vonsattel, J. P., Rebeck, G. W., & Greenberg, S. M. (2001). Novel amyloid precursor protein mutation in an Iowa family with dementia and severe cerebral amyloid angiopathy. *Annals of Neurology, 49*(6), 697–705.

Gray, F., Vinters, H. V., Le Noan, H., Salama, J., Delaporte, P., & Poirier, J. (1990). Cerebral amyloid angiopathy and granulomatous angiitis: Immunohistochemical study using antibodies to the Alzheimer A4 peptide. *Human Pathology, 21*(12), 1290–1293.

Greenberg, S. M. (1998). Cerebral amyloid angiopathy: Prospects for clinical diagnosis and treatment. *Neurology, 51*(3), 690–694.

Greenberg, S. M., Briggs, M. E., Hyman, B. T., Kokoris, G. J., Takis, C., Kanter, D. S., Kase, C. S., & Pessin, M. S. (1996). Apolipoprotein E epsilon 4 is associated with the presence and earlier onset of hemorrhage in cerebral amyloid angiopathy. *Stroke, 27*(8), 1333–1337.

Greenberg, S. M., Eng, J. A., Ning, M., Smith, E. E., & Rosand, J. (2004). Hemorrhage burden predicts recurrent intracerebral hemorrhage after lobar hemorrhage. *Stroke, 35*(6), 1415–1420.

Greenberg, S. M., Finklestein, S. P., & Schaefer, P. W. (1996). Petechial hemorrhages accompanying lobar hemorrhage: Detection by gradient-echo MRI. *Neurology, 46*(6), 1751–1754.

Greenberg, S. M., & Frosch, M. P. (2011). Life imitates art: Anti-amyloid antibodies and inflammatory cerebral amyloid angiopathy. *Neurology, 76*(9), 772–773.

Greenberg, S. M., Grabowski, T., Gurol, M. E., Skehan, M. E., Nandigam, R. N., Becker, J. A.,... Johnson, K. A. (2008). Detection of isolated cerebrovascular beta-amyloid with Pittsburgh compound B. *Annals of Neurology, 64*(5), 587–591.

Greenberg, S. M., Gurol, M. E., Rosand, J., & Smith, E. E. (2004). Amyloid angiopathy-related vascular cognitive impairment. *Stroke, 35*(11 Suppl 1), 2616–2619.

Greenberg, S. M., Rebeck, G. W., Vonsattel, J. P., Gomez-Isla, T., & Hyman, B. T. (1995). Apolipoprotein E epsilon 4 and cerebral hemorrhage associated with amyloid angiopathy. *Annals of Neurology, 38*(2), 254–259.

Greenberg, S. M., Shin, Y., Grabowski, T. J., Cooper, G. E., Rebeck, G. W., Iglesias, S.,... Baron, J. C. (2003). Hemorrhagic stroke associated with the Iowa amyloid precursor protein mutation. *Neurology, 60*(6), 1020–1022.

Greenberg, S. M., Vernooij, M. W., Cordonnier, C., Viswanathan, A., Al-Shahi Salman, R., Warach, S.,... Breteler, M. M. (2009). Cerebral microbleeds: A guide to detection and interpretation. *Lancet Neurology, 8*(2), 165–174.

Greenberg, S. M., Vonsattel, J. P., Segal, A. Z., Chiu, R. I., Clatworthy, A. E., Liao, A.,... Rebeck, G. W. (1998). Association of apolipoprotein E epsilon2 and vasculopathy in cerebral amyloid angiopathy. *Neurology, 50*(4), 961–965.

Greenberg, S. M., Vonsattel, J. P., Stakes, J. W., Gruber, M., & Finklestein, S. P. (1993). The clinical spectrum of cerebral amyloid angiopathy: Presentations without lobar hemorrhage. *Neurology, 43*(10), 2073–2079.

Gregoire, S. M., Charidimou, A., Gadapa, N., Dolan, E., Antoun, N., Peeters, A.,... Werring, D. J. (2011). Acute ischaemic brain lesions in intracerebral haemorrhage: Multicentre cross-sectional magnetic resonance imaging study. *Brain, 134*(Pt 8), 2376–2386.

Gregoire, S. M., Smith, K., Jäger, H. R., Benjamin, M., Kallis, C., Brown, M. M.,... Werring, D. J. (2012). Cerebral microbleeds and long-term cognitive outcome: Longitudinal cohort study of stroke clinic patients. *Cerebrovascular Diseases (Basel), 33*(5), 430–435.

Gupta, S. R., Naheedy, M. H., Young, J. C., Ghobrial, M., Rubino, F. A., & Hindo, W. (1988). Periventricular white matter changes and dementia. Clinical, neuropsychological, radiological, and pathological correlation. *Archives of Neurology, 45*(6), 637–641.

Gurol, M. E., Irizarry, M. C., Smith, E. E., Raju, S., Diaz-Arrastia, R., Bottiglieri, T.,... Greenberg, S. M. (2006). Plasma beta-amyloid and white matter lesions in AD, MCI, and cerebral amyloid angiopathy. *Neurology, 66*(1), 23–29.

Haglund, M., Passant, U., Sjöbeck, M., Ghebremedhin, E., & Englund, E. (2006). Cerebral amyloid angiopathy and cortical microinfarcts as putative substrates of vascular dementia. *International Journal of Geriatric Psychiatry, 21*(7), 681–687.

Han, B. H., Zhou, M. L., Abousaleh, F., Brendza, R. P., Dietrich, H. H., Koenigsknecht-Talboo, J.,... Zipfel, G. J. (2008). Cerebrovascular dysfunction in amyloid precursor protein transgenic mice: Contribution of soluble and insoluble amyloid-beta peptide, partial restoration via gamma-secretase inhibition. *Journal of Neuroscience, 28*(50), 13542–13550.

Hanyu, H., Tanaka, Y., Shimizu, S., Takasaki, M., & Abe, K. (2003). Cerebral microbleeds in Alzheimer's disease. *Journal of Neurology*, 250(12), 1496–1497.

Herholz, K., & Ebmeier, K. (2011). Clinical amyloid imaging in Alzheimer's disease. *Lancet Neurology*, 10(7), 667–670.

Herzig, M. C., Van Nostrand, W. E., & Jucker, M. (2006). Mechanism of cerebral beta-amyloid angiopathy: Murine and cellular models. *Brain Pathology (Zurich)*, 16(1), 40–54.

Herzig, M. C., Winkler, D. T., Burgermeister, P., Pfeifer, M., Kohler, E., Schmidt, S. D.,...Jucker, M. (2004). Abeta is targeted to the vasculature in a mouse model of hereditary cerebral hemorrhage with amyloidosis. *Nature Neuroscience*, 7(9), 954–960.

Heyman, A., Fillenbaum, G. G., Welsh-Bohmer, K. A., Gearing, M., Mirra, S. S., Mohs, R. C.,...Pieper, C. F. (1998). Cerebral infarcts in patients with autopsy-proven Alzheimer's disease: CERAD, part XVIII. Consortium to Establish a Registry for Alzheimer's Disease. *Neurology*, 51(1), 159–162.

Holland, C. M., Smith, E. E., Csapo, I., Gurol, M. E., Brylka, D. A., Killiany, R. J.,...Greenberg, S. M. (2008). Spatial distribution of white-matter hyperintensities in Alzheimer disease, cerebral amyloid angiopathy, and healthy aging. *Stroke*, 39(4), 1127–1133.

Jankowsky, J. L., Fadale, D. J., Anderson, J., Xu, G. M., Gonzales, V., Jenkins, N. A.,...Borchelt, D. R. (2004). Mutant presenilins specifically elevate the levels of the 42 residue beta-amyloid peptide in vivo: Evidence for augmentation of a 42-specific gamma secretase. *Human Molecular Genetics*, 13(2), 159–170.

Jellinger, K. A. (2002). Alzheimer disease and cerebrovascular pathology: An update. *Journal of Neural Transmission (Vienna)*, 109(5–6), 813–836.

Johnson, K. A., Gregas, M., Becker, J. A., Kinnecom, C., Salat, D. H., Moran, E. K.,...Greenberg, S. M. (2007). Imaging of amyloid burden and distribution in cerebral amyloid angiopathy. *Annals of Neurology*, 62(3), 229–234.

Johnson-Wood, K., Lee, M., Motter, R., Hu, K., Gordon, G., Barbour, R.,...McConlogue, L (1997). Amyloid precursor protein processing and A beta42 deposition in a transgenic mouse model of Alzheimer disease. *Proceedings of the National Academy of Sciences USA*, 94(4), 1550–1555.

Jonsdottir, S., & Palsdottir, A. (1993). Molecular diagnosis of hereditary cystatin C amyloid angiopathy. *Biochemical Medicine and Metabolic Biology*, 49(2), 117–123.

Kasuga, K., Shimohata, T., Nishimura, A., Shiga, A., Mizuguchi, T., Tokunaga, J.,...Ikeuchi, T. (2009). Identification of independent APP locus duplication in Japanese patients with early-onset Alzheimer disease. *Journal of Neurology, Neurosurgery, and Psychiatry*, 80(9), 1050–1052.

Kimberly, W. T., Gilson, A., Rost, N. S., Rosand, J., Viswanathan, A., Smith, E. E., & Greenberg, S. M. (2009). Silent ischemic infarcts are associated with hemorrhage burden in cerebral amyloid angiopathy. *Neurology*, 72(14), 1230–1235.

Kimchi, E. Y., Kajdasz, S., Bacskai, B. J., & Hyman, B. T. 2001. Analysis of cerebral amyloid angiopathy in a transgenic mouse model of Alzheimer disease using in vivo multiphoton microscopy. *Journal of Neuropathology and Experimental Neurology*, 60(3), 274–279.

Klunk, W. E., Engler, H., Nordberg, A., Wang, Y., Blomqvist, G., Holt, D. P.,...Långström, B. (2004). Imaging brain amyloid in Alzheimer's disease with Pittsburgh Compound-B. *Annals of Neurology*, 55(3), 306–319.

Knudsen, K. A., Rosand, J., Karluk, D., & Greenberg, S. M. (2001). Clinical diagnosis of cerebral amyloid angiopathy: Validation of the Boston criteria. *Neurology*, 56(4), 537–539.

Korczyn, A. D., Vakhapova, V., & Grinberg, L. T. (2012). Vascular dementia. *Journal of the Neurological Sciences*, 322(1–2), 2–10.

Kumar-Singh, S. (2008). Cerebral amyloid angiopathy: Pathogenetic mechanisms and link to dense amyloid plaques. *Genes, Brain, and Behavior*, 7(Suppl 1), 67–82.

Lansberg, M. G., Thijs, V. N., O'Brien, M. W., Ali, J. O., de Crespigny, A. J., Tong, D. C.,...Albers, G. W. (2001). Evolution of apparent diffusion coefficient, diffusion-weighted, and T2-weighted signal intensity of acute stroke. *American Journal of Neuroradiology*, 22(4), 637–644.

Levy, E., Carman, M. D., Fernandez-Madrid, I. J., Power, M. D., Lieberburg, I., van Duinen, S. G.,...Frangione, B. (1990). Mutation of the Alzheimer's disease amyloid gene in hereditary cerebral hemorrhage, Dutch type. *Science*, 248(4959), 1124–1126.

Linn, J., Halpin, A., Demaerel, P., Ruhland, J., Giese, A. D., Dichgans, M.,...Greenberg, S. M. (2010). Prevalence of superficial siderosis in patients with cerebral amyloid angiopathy. *Neurology*, 74(17), 1346–1350.

Love, S., Miners, S., Palmer, J., Chalmers, K., & Kehoe, P. (2009). Insights into the pathogenesis and pathogenicity of cerebral amyloid angiopathy. *Frontiers in Bioscience*, 14, 4778–4792.

Ly, J. V., Rowe, C. C., Villemagne, V. L., Zavala, J. A., Ma, H., O'Keefe, G.,...Donnan, G. A. (2010). Cerebral β-amyloid detected by Pittsburgh compound B positron emission topography predisposes to recombinant tissue plasminogen activator-related hemorrhage. *Annals of Neurology, 68*(6), 959–962.

Mackic, J. B., Weiss, M. H., Miao, W., Kirkman, E., Ghiso, J., Calero, M.,...Zlokovic, B. V (1998). Cerebrovascular accumulation and increased blood-brain barrier permeability to circulating Alzheimer's amyloid beta peptide in aged squirrel monkey with cerebral amyloid angiopathy. *Journal of Neurochemistry, 70*(1), 210–215.

Mackic, J. B., Bading, J., Ghiso, J., Walker, L., Wisniewski, T., Frangione, B., & Zlokovic, B. V. (2002). Circulating amyloid-beta peptide crosses the blood-brain barrier in aged monkeys and contributes to Alzheimer's disease lesions. *Vascular Pharmacology, 38*(6), 303–313.

Mandybur, T. I. (1986). Cerebral amyloid angiopathy: The vascular pathology and complications. *Journal of Neuropathology and Experimental Neurology, 45*(1), 79–90.

Martel, C. L., Mackic, J. B., McComb, J. G., Ghiso, J., & Zlokovic, B. V. (1996). Blood-brain barrier uptake of the 40 and 42 amino acid sequences of circulating Alzheimer's amyloid beta in guinea pigs. *Neuroscience Letters, 206*(2-3), 157–160.

Mathis, C. A., Wang, Y., Holt, D. P., Huang, G. F., Debnath, M. L., & Klunk, W. E. (2003). Synthesis and evaluation of 11C-labeled 6-substituted 2-arylbenzothiazoles as amyloid imaging agents. *Journal of Medicinal Chemistry, 46*(13), 2740–2754.

McCarron, M. O., & Nicoll, J. A. R. (2004). Cerebral amyloid angiopathy and thrombolysis-related intracerebral haemorrhage. *Lancet Neurology, 3*(8), 484–492.

McCarron, M. O., Nicoll, J. A., Stewart, J., Ironside, J. W., Mann, D. M., Love, S.,...Dewar, D. (1999). The apolipoprotein E epsilon2 allele and the pathological features in cerebral amyloid angiopathy-related hemorrhage. *Journal of Neuropathology and Experimental Neurology, 58*(7), 711–718.

Mead, S., James-Galton, M., Revesz, T., Doshi, R. B., Harwood, G., Pan, E. L.,...Plant, G. (2000). Familial British dementia with amyloid angiopathy: Early clinical, neuropsychological and imaging findings. *Brain, 123*(Pt 5), 975–991.

Menon, R. S., & Kidwell, C. S. (2009). Neuroimaging demonstration of evolving small vessel ischemic injury in cerebral amyloid angiopathy. *Stroke, 40*(12), e675–7.

Menon, R. S., Burgess, R. E., Wing, J. J., Gibbons, M. C., Shara, N. M., Fernandez, S.,...Kidwell, C. S. (2012). Predictors of highly prevalent brain ischemia in intracerebral hemorrhage. *Annals of Neurology, 71*(2), 199–205.

Mesker, D. J., Poels, M. M., Ikram, M. A., Vernooij, M. W., Hofman, A., Vrooman, H. A.,...Breteler, M. M. (2011). Lobar distribution of cerebral microbleeds: The Rotterdam Scan Study. *Archives of Neurology, 68*(5), 656–659.

Nakata, Y., Shiga, K., Yoshikawa, K., Mizuno, T., Mori, S., Yamada, K., & Nakajima, K. (2002). Subclinical brain hemorrhages in Alzheimer's disease: Evaluation by magnetic resonance T2*-weighted images. *Annals of the New York Academy of Sciences, 977*, 169–172.

Natté, R., Maat-Schieman, M. L., Haan, J., Bornebroek, M., Roos, R. A., & van Duinen, S. G. (2001). Dementia in hereditary cerebral hemorrhage with amyloidosis-Dutch type is associated with cerebral amyloid angiopathy but is independent of plaques and neurofibrillary tangles. *Annals of Neurology, 50*(6), 765–772.

Neuropathology Group, Medical Research Council Cognitive Function and Aging Study. (2001). Pathological correlates of late-onset dementia in a multicentre, community-based population in England and Wales. Neuropathology Group of the Medical Research Council Cognitive Function and Ageing Study (MRC CFAS). *Lancet, 357*(9251), 169–175.

Nicoll, J. A. R., Wilkinson, D., Holmes, C., Steart, P., Markham, H., & Weller, R. O. (2003). Neuropathology of human Alzheimer disease after immunization with amyloid-beta peptide: A case report. *Nature Medicine, 9*(4), 448–452.

Niwa, K., Carlson, G. A., & Iadecola, C. (2000). Exogenous A beta1-40 reproduces cerebrovascular alterations resulting from amyloid precursor protein overexpression in mice. *Journal of Cerebral Blood Flow and Metabolism, 20*(12), 1659–1668.

Niwa, K., Younkin, L., Ebeling, C., Turner, S. K., Westaway, D., Younkin, S.,...Iadecola, C. (2000). Abeta 1-40-related reduction in functional hyperemia in mouse neocortex during somatosensory activation. *Proceedings of the National Academy of Sciences USA, 97*(17), 9735–9740.

O'Donnell, H. C., Rosand, J., Knudsen, K. A., Furie, K. L., Segal, A. Z., Chiu, R. I.,...Greenberg, S. M. (2000). Apolipoprotein E genotype and the risk of recurrent lobar intracerebral hemorrhage. *New England Journal of Medicine, 342*(4), 240–245.

Okamoto, Y., Ihara, M., Fujita, Y., Ito, H., Takahashi, R., & Tomimoto, H. (2009). Cortical microinfarcts in Alzheimer's disease and subcortical vascular dementia. *Neuroreport, 20*(11), 990–996.

Okazaki, H., Reagan, T. J., & Campbell, R. J. (1979). Clinicopathologic studies of primary cerebral amyloid angiopathy. *Mayo Clinic Proceedings, 54*(1), 22–31.

Olesen, O. F., Mikkelsen, J. D., Gerdes, C., & Jensen, P. H. (1997). Isoform-specific binding of human apolipoprotein E to the non-amyloid beta component of Alzheimer's disease amyloid. *Brain Research Molecular Brain Research, 44*(1), 105–112.

Olichney, J. M., Hansen, L. A., Hofstetter, C. R., Lee, J. H., Katzman, R., & Thal, L. J. (2000). Association between severe cerebral amyloid angiopathy and cerebrovascular lesions in Alzheimer disease is not a spurious one attributable to apolipoprotein E4. *Archives of Neurology, 57*(6), 869–874.

Orgogozo, J-M., Gilman, S., Dartigues, J. F., Laurent, B., Puel, M., Kirby, L. C.,...Hock, C. (2003). Subacute meningoencephalitis in a subset of patients with AD after Abeta42 immunization. *Neurology, 61*(1), 46–54.

Palsdottir, A., Abrahamson, M., Thorsteinsson, L., Arnason, A., Olafsson, I., Grubb, A., & Jensson, O. (1988). Mutation in cystatin C gene causes hereditary brain haemorrhage. *Lancet, 2*(8611), 603–604.

Palsdottir, A., Snorradottir, A. O., & Thorsteinsson, L. (2006). Hereditary cystatin C amyloid angiopathy: Genetic, clinical, and pathological aspects. *Brain Pathology (Zurich), 16*(1), 55–59.

Petrovitch, H., Ross, G. W., Steinhorn, S. C., Abbott, R. D., Markesbery, W., Davis, D.,...White, L. R. (2005). AD lesions and infarcts in demented and non-demented Japanese-American men. *Annals of Neurology, 57*(1), 98–103.

Pettersen, J. A., Sathiyamoorthy, G., Gao, F. Q., Szilagyi, G., Nadkarni, N. K., St George-Hyslop, P.,...Black, S. E. (2008). Microbleed topography, leukoaraiosis, and cognition in probable Alzheimer disease from the Sunnybrook dementia study. *Archives of Neurology, 65*(6), 790–795.

Pfeifer, L. A., White, L. R., Ross, G. W., Petrovitch, H., & Launer, L. J. (2002). Cerebral amyloid angiopathy and cognitive function: The HAAS autopsy study. *Neurology, 58*(11), 1629–1634.

Poduslo, J. F., Curran, G. L., Haggard, J. J., Biere, A. L., & Selkoe, D. J. (1997). Permeability and residual plasma volume of human, Dutch variant, and rat amyloid beta-protein 1-40 at the blood-brain barrier. *Neurobiology of Disease, 4*(1), 27–34.

Poels, M. M. F., Ikram, M. A., van der Lugt, A., Hofman, A., Niessen, W. J., Krestin, G. P.,...Vernooij, M. W. (2012). Cerebral microbleeds are associated with worse cognitive function: The Rotterdam Scan Study. *Neurology, 78*(5), 326–333.

Prabhakaran, S., Gupta, R., Ouyang, B., John, S., Temes, R. E., Mohammad, Y.,...Bleck, T. P. 2010. Acute brain infarcts after spontaneous intracerebral hemorrhage: A diffusion-weighted imaging study. *Stroke, 41*(1), 89–94.

Prada, C. M., Garcia-Alloza, M., Betensky, R. A., Zhang-Nunes, S. X., Greenberg, S. M., Bacskai, B. J., & Frosch, M. P. (2007). Antibody-mediated clearance of amyloid-beta peptide from cerebral amyloid angiopathy revealed by quantitative in vivo imaging. *Journal of Neuroscience, 27*(8), 1973–1980.

Premkumar, D. R., Cohen, D. L., Hedera, P., Friedland, R. P., & Kalaria, R. N. (1996). Apolipoprotein E-epsilon4 alleles in cerebral amyloid angiopathy and cerebrovascular pathology associated with Alzheimer's disease. *American Journal of Pathology, 148*(6), 2083–2095.

Price, D. L., Tanzi, R. E., Borchelt, D. R., & Sisodia, S. S. (1998). Alzheimer's disease: Genetic studies and transgenic models. *Annual review of genetics, 32*, 461–493.

Probst, A., & Ulrich, J. (1985). Amyloid angiopathy combined with granulomatous angiitis of the central nervous system: Report on two patients. *Clinical Neuropathology, 4*(6), 250–259.

Roher, A. E., Kuo, Y. M., Esh, C., Knebel, C., Weiss, N., Kalback, W.,...Kokjohn, T. A. (2003). Cortical and leptomeningeal cerebrovascular amyloid and white matter pathology in Alzheimer's disease. *Molecular Medicine, 9*(3–4), 112–122.

Rovelet-Lecrux, A., Hannequin, D., Raux, G., Le Meur, N., Laquerrière, A., Vital, A.,...Campion, D. (2006). APP locus duplication causes autosomal dominant early-onset Alzheimer disease with cerebral amyloid angiopathy. *Nature Genetics, 38*(1), 24–26.

Salat, D. H., Smith, E. E., Tuch, D. S., Benner, T., Pappu, V., Schwab, K. M.,...Greenberg, S. M. (2006). White matter alterations in cerebral amyloid angiopathy measured by diffusion tensor imaging. *Stroke, 37*(7), 1759–1764.

Salloway, S., Sperling, R., Gilman, S., Fox, N. C., Blennow, K., Raskind, M.,...Grundman, M. (2009). A phase 2 multiple ascending dose trial of bapineuzumab in mild to moderate Alzheimer disease. *Neurology, 73*(24), 2061–2070.

Sanan, D. A., Weisgraber, K. H., Russell, S. J., Mahley, R. W., Huang, D., Saunders, A.,...Roses, A. D. (1994). Apolipoprotein E associates with beta amyloid peptide of Alzheimer's disease to form novel monofibrils. Isoform apoE4 associates more efficiently than apoE3. *Journal of Clinical Investigation, 94*(2), 860–869.

Schmechel, D. E., Saunders, A. M., Strittmatter, W. J., Crain, B. J., Hulette, C. M., Joo,

S. H., ... Roses, A. D. (1993). Increased amyloid beta-peptide deposition in cerebral cortex as a consequence of apolipoprotein E genotype in late-onset Alzheimer disease. *Proceedings of the National Academy of Sciences USA, 90*(20), 9649–9653.

Schmidt, R., Petrovic, K., Ropele, S., Enzinger, C., & Fazekas, F. (2007). Progression of leukoaraiosis and cognition. *Stroke, 38*(9), 2619–2625.

Schneider, J. A., Arvanitakis, Z., Bang, W., & Bennett, D. A. (2007). Mixed brain pathologies account for most dementia cases in community-dwelling older persons. *Neurology, 69*(24), 2197–2204.

Schroeter, S., Khan, K., Barbour, R., Doan, M., Chen, M., Guido, T., ... Games, D. (2008). Immunotherapy reduces vascular amyloid-beta in PDAPP mice. *Journal of Neuroscience, 28*(27), 6787–6793.

Selkoe, D. J. (2001). Alzheimer's disease: Genes, proteins, and therapy. *Physiological Reviews, 81*(2), 741–766.

Shin, H. K., Jones, P. B., Garcia-Alloza, M., Borrelli, L., Greenberg, S. M., Bacskai, B. J., ... Ayata, C. (2007). Age-dependent cerebrovascular dysfunction in a transgenic mouse model of cerebral amyloid angiopathy. *Brain, 130*(Pt 9), 2310–2319.

Silbert, P. L., Bartleson, J. D., Miller, G. M., Parisi, J. E., Goldman, M. S., & Meyer, F. B. (1995). Cortical petechial hemorrhage, leukoencephalopathy, and subacute dementia associated with seizures due to cerebral amyloid angiopathy. *Mayo Clinic Proceedings, 70*(5), 477–480.

Sleegers, K., Brouwers, N., Gijselinck, I., Theuns, J., Goossens, D., Wauters, J., ... Van Broeckhoven, C. (2006). APP duplication is sufficient to cause early onset Alzheimer's dementia with cerebral amyloid angiopathy. *Brain, 129*(Pt 11), 2977–2983.

Smith, E. E., & Greenberg, S. M. (2009). Beta-amyloid, blood vessels, and brain function. *Stroke, 40*(7), 2601–2606.

Smith, E. E., Gurol, M. E., Eng, J. A., Engel, C. R., Nguyen, T. N., Rosand, J., & Greenberg, S. M. (2004). White matter lesions, cognition, and recurrent hemorrhage in lobar intracerebral hemorrhage. *Neurology, 63*(9), 1606–1612.

Smith, E. E., Nandigam, K. R., Chen, Y. W., Jeng, J., Salat, D., Halpin, A., ... Greenberg, S. M. (2010). MRI markers of small vessel disease in lobar and deep hemispheric intracerebral hemorrhage. *Stroke, 41*(9), 1933–1938.

Smith, E. E., Rosand, J., Knudsen, K. A., Hylek, E. M., & Greenberg, S. M. (2002). Leukoaraiosis is associated with warfarin-related hemorrhage following ischemic stroke. *Neurology, 59*(2), 193–197.

Smith, E. E., Vijayappa, M., Lima, F., Delgado, P., Wendell, L., Rosand, J., & Greenberg, S. M. (2008). Impaired visual evoked flow velocity response in cerebral amyloid angiopathy. *Neurology, 71*(18), 1424–1430.

Snowdon, D. A., Greiner, L. H., Mortimer, J. A., Riley, K. P., Greiner, P. A., & Markesbery, W. R. (1997). Brain infarction and the clinical expression of Alzheimer disease. The Nun Study. *Journal of the American Medical Association, 277*(10), 813–817.

Soontornniyomkij, V., Lynch, M. D., Mermash, S., Pomakian, J., Badkoobehi, H., Clare, R., & Vinters, H. V. (2010). Cerebral microinfarcts associated with severe cerebral beta-amyloid angiopathy. *Brain Pathology, 20*(2), 459–467.

Sperling, R., Salloway, S., Brooks, D. J., Tampieri, D., Barakos, J., Fox, N. C., ... Grundman, M. (2012). Amyloid-related imaging abnormalities in patients with Alzheimer's disease treated with bapineuzumab: A retrospective analysis. *Lancet Neurology, 11*(3), 241–249.

Sperling, R. A., Jack, C. R., Jr., Black, S. E., Frosch, M. P., Greenberg, S. M., Hyman, B. T., ... Schindler, R. J. (2011). Amyloid-related imaging abnormalities in amyloid-modifying therapeutic trials: Recommendations from the Alzheimer's Association Research Roundtable Workgroup. *Alzheimer's and Dementia, 7*(4), 367–385.

Suter, O-C., Sunthorn, T., Kraftsik, R., Straubel, J., Darekar, P., Khalili, K., & Miklossy, J. (2002). Cerebral hypoperfusion generates cortical watershed microinfarcts in Alzheimer disease. *Stroke, 33*(8), 1986–1992.

Sveinbjornsdottir, S., Sigurdsson, S., Aspelund, T., Kjartansson, O., Eiriksdottir, G., Valtysdottir, B., ... Launer, L. J. (2008). Cerebral microbleeds in the population based AGES-Reykjavik study: Prevalence and location. *Journal of Neurology, Neurosurgery, and Psychiatry, 79*(9), 1002–1006.

Thakker, D. R., Weatherspoon, M. R., Harrison, J., Keene, T. E., Lane, D. S., Kaemmerer, W. F., ... Shafer, L. L. (2009). Intracerebroventricular amyloid-beta antibodies reduce cerebral amyloid angiopathy and associated micro-hemorrhages in aged Tg2576 mice. *Proceedings of the National Academy of Sciences USA, 106*(11), 4501–4506.

Ujiie, M., Dickstein, D. L., Carlow, D. A., & Jefferies, W. A. (2003). Blood-brain barrier permeability precedes senile plaque formation in an Alzheimer disease model. *Microcirculation, 10*(6), 463–470.

Van Dorpe, J., Smeijers, L., Dewachter, I., Nuyens, D., Spittaels, K., Van Den Haute, C., ... Van Leuven, F. (2000). Prominent cerebral amyloid angiopathy in transgenic mice overexpressing the London mutant of human

APP in neurons. *American Journal of Pathology*, 157(4), 1283–1298.

van Duinen, S. G., Castaño, E. M., Prelli, F., Bots, G. T., Luyendijk, W., & Frangione, B. (1987). Hereditary cerebral hemorrhage with amyloidosis in patients of Dutch origin is related to Alzheimer disease. *Proceedings of the National Academy of Sciences USA*, 84(16), 5991–5994.

van Es, A. C., van der Grond, J., de Craen, A. J., Westendorp, R. G., Bollen, E. L., Blauw, G. J.,...van Buchem, M. A. (2011). Cerebral microbleeds and cognitive functioning in the PROSPER study. *Neurology*, 77(15), 1446–1452.

Van Nostrand, W. E., Melchor, J. P., Cho, H. S., Greenberg, S. M., & Rebeck, G. W. (2001). Pathogenic effects of D23N Iowa mutant amyloid beta -protein. *Journal of Biological Chemistry*, 276(35), 32860–32866.

van Rooden, S., van der Grond, J., van den Boom, R., Haan, J., Linn, J., Greenberg, S. M., & van Buchem, M. A. (2009). Descriptive analysis of the Boston criteria applied to a Dutch-type cerebral amyloid angiopathy population. *Stroke*, 40(9), 3022–3027.

Verbeek, M. M., Kremer, B. P., Rikkert, M. O., Van Domburg, P. H., Skehan, M. E., & Greenberg, S. M. (2009). Cerebrospinal fluid amyloid beta(40) is decreased in cerebral amyloid angiopathy. *Annals of Neurology*, 66(2), 245–249.

Verghese, P.B., Castellano, J.M. & Holtzman, D.M., 2011. Apolipoprotein E in Alzheimer's disease and other neurological disorders. *Lancet Neurology*, 10(3), 241–252.

Vernooij, M. W., van der Lugt, A., Ikram, M. A., Wielopolski, P. A., Niessen, W. J., Hofman, A.,...Breteler, M. M. (2008). Prevalence and risk factors of cerebral microbleeds: The Rotterdam Scan Study. *Neurology*, 70(14), 1208–1214.

Vidal, R., Garzuly, F., Budka, H., Lalowski, M., Linke, R. P., Brittig, F.,...Wisniewski, T. (1996). Meningocerebrovascular amyloidosis associated with a novel transthyretin mis-sense mutation at codon 18 (TTRD 18G). *American Journal of Pathology*, 148(2), 361–366.

Vinters, H. V. (1987). Cerebral amyloid angiopathy. A critical review. *Stroke*, 18(2), 311–324.

Vinters, H. V., Natté, R., Maat-Schieman, M. L., van Duinen, S. G., Hegeman-Kleinn, I., Welling-Graafland, C.,...Roos, R. A. (1998). Secondary microvascular degeneration in amyloid angiopathy of patients with hereditary cerebral hemorrhage with amyloidosis, Dutch type (HCHWA-D). *Acta Neuropathologica*, 95(3), 235–244.

Vinters, H. V., Secor, D. L., Read, S. L., Frazee, J. G., Tomiyasu, U., Stanley, T. M.,...Akers, M. A. (1994). Microvasculature in brain biopsy specimens from patients with Alzheimer's disease: An immunohistochemical and ultrastructural study. *Ultrastructural Pathology*, 18(3), 333–348.

Viswanathan, A., Godin, O., Jouvent, E., O'Sullivan, M., Gschwendtner, A., Peters, N.,...Chabriat, H. (2010). Impact of MRI markers in subcortical vascular dementia: A multi-modal analysis in CADASIL. *Neurobiology of Aging*, 31(9), 1629–1636.

Viswanathan, A., Patel, P., Rahman, R., Nandigam, R. N., Kinnecom, C., Bracoud, L.,...Smith, E. E. (2008). Tissue microstructural changes are independently associated with cognitive impairment in cerebral amyloid angiopathy. *Stroke*, 39(7), 1988–1992.

Vonsattel, J. P., Myers, R. H., Hedley-Whyte, E. T., Ropper, A. H., Bird, E. D., & Richardson, E. P., Jr. (1991). Cerebral amyloid angiopathy without and with cerebral hemorrhages: A comparative histological study. *Annals of Neurology*, 30(5), 637–649.

Wattendorff, A. R., Frangione, B., Luyendijk, W., & Bots, G. T. (1995). Hereditary cerebral haemorrhage with amyloidosis, Dutch type (HCHWA-D): Clinicopathological studies. *Journal of Neurology, Neurosurgery, and Psychiatry*, 58(6), 699–705.

Weller, R. O., Massey, A., Newman, T. A., Hutchings, M., Kuo, Y. M., & Roher, A. E. (1998). Cerebral amyloid angiopathy: Amyloid beta accumulates in putative interstitial fluid drainage pathways in Alzheimer's disease. *American Journal of Pathology*, 153(3), 725–733.

Werring, D. J., Frazer, D. W., Coward, L. J., Losseff, N. A., Watt, H., Cipolotti, L.,...Jäger, H. R. (2004). Cognitive dysfunction in patients with cerebral microbleeds on T2*-weighted gradient-echo MRI. *Brain*, 127(Pt 10), 2265–2275.

Winkler, D. T., Bondolfi, L., Herzig, M. C., Jann, L., Calhoun, M. E., Wiederhold, K. H.,...Jucker, M. (2001). Spontaneous hemorrhagic stroke in a mouse model of cerebral amyloid angiopathy. *Journal of Neuroscience*, 21(5), 1619–1627.

Woo, D., Sauerbeck, L. R., Kissela, B. M., Khoury, J. C., Szaflarski, J. P., Gebel, J.,...Broderick, J. P. (2002). Genetic and environmental risk factors for intracerebral hemorrhage: Preliminary results of a population-based study. *Stroke*, 33(5), 1190–1195.

Xu, D., Yang, C., & Wang, L. (2003). Cerebral amyloid angiopathy in aged Chinese: A clinico-neuropathological study. *Acta Neuropathologica*, 106(1), 89–91.

Yakushiji, Y., Noguchi, T., Hara, M., Nishihara, M., Eriguchi, M., Nanri, Y.,...Hara, H. (2012). Distributional impact of brain microbleeds on global cognitive function in adults without neurological disorder. *Stroke*, *43*(7), 1800–1805.

Yamada, M., Itoh, Y., Shintaku, M., Kawamura, J., Jensson, O., Thorsteinsson, L., ... Otomo, E. 1996. Immune reactions associated with cerebral amyloid angiopathy. *Stroke*, *27*(7), 1155–1162.

Zekry, D., Duyckaerts, C., Belmin, J., Geoffre, C., Moulias, R., & Hauw, J. J. (2003). Cerebral amyloid angiopathy in the elderly: Vessel walls changes and relationship with dementia. *Acta Neuropathologica*, *106*(4), 367–373.

Zhang-Nunes, S. X., Maat-Schieman, M. L., van Duinen, S. G., Roos, R. A., Frosch, M. P., & Greenberg, S. M. (2006). The cerebral beta-amyloid angiopathies: hereditary and sporadic. *Brain Pathology (Zurich)*, *16*(1), 30–39.

Zhu, Y-C., Chabriat, H., Godin, O., Dufouil, C., Rosand, J., Greenberg, S. M., ... Viswanathan, A. (2012). Distribution of white matter hyperintensity in cerebral hemorrhage and healthy aging. *Journal of Neurology*, *259*(3), 530–536.

Zlokovic, B. V., Ghiso, J., Mackic, J. B., McComb, J. G., Weiss, M. H., & Frangione, B. (1993). Blood-brain barrier transport of circulating Alzheimer's amyloid beta. *Biochemical and Biophysical Research Communications*, *197*(3), 1034–1040.

15

The Differential Diagnosis of Rapidly Progressive and Rare Dementias
A Clinical Approach

Jeremy D. Schmahmann

This chapter presents a clinical perspective on the evaluation of a patient with impairment of cognitive function. The principal goal here is to establish a diagnosis. Determining what disease process is causing the dementia shapes the clinician's understanding of the pathophysiology of the process, provides insights into prognosis, and guides management.

It is useful to keep the profile of Alzheimer's disease in mind as one approaches the question of cognitive decline. Alzheimer's disease is characterized by the insidious development and progression of cognitive decline in a person usually in the seventh or eighth decades: initially, the signs are forgetfulness; then true memory loss for recently acquired information more than prior knowledge, and impaired new learning; followed by deficits in language, praxis, visual-spatial awareness, and loss of previously acquired skills required for functioning at home and at work. This occurs in the setting of generally preserved but vacuous social interactions and an essentially normal elementary neurological examination early in the course except for release phenomena. The presentation may be atypical, as occurs in primary progressive aphasia, or an apraxia-agnosia syndrome, but Alzheimer's disease has a profile sufficiently well defined that it can be strongly suspected on clinical grounds alone. When the clinical history and examination of a patient with cognitive decline do not conform to this rather stereotyped picture of Alzheimer's disease, the clinician's level of suspicion should be great that the diagnosis lies elsewhere.

Acute Confusion Versus Dementia

At the outset it is imperative to distinguish an acute or subacute (and often life-threatening) acute confusional state from dementia. Abrupt onset within hours to days of lethargy, confusion, and disorientation, or aphasia, memory loss, impaired concentration, and inability to perform complex functions such as driving, dressing, or taking care of personal hygiene need to be urgently assessed. The history of an acute or subacute onset may have a precipitant such as head trauma, or associated symptoms pointing to bacterial, fungal, or tuberculous meningitis; infectious endocarditis; Herpes simplex encephalitis; pneumonia; urinary tract infections; diabetic hyperglycemic nonketotic precoma; delirium tremens; the encephalopathy of acute intermittent porphyria; and others. The hallmark feature on examination is the presence of an impaired and fluctuating level of consciousness and inattention. This manifests as easy distractibility, wandering stream of conversation, inability to stick with the examiner's tasks, and illogical but not necessarily aphasic sentences. Agitation and restless fidgeting movements of the hands are common. Associated features on examination include fever, meningismus, autonomic instability (tachycardia and hypertension), the stigmata of chronic liver disease, or drug use. In this acute setting, one should not make a diagnosis of a neurodegenerative dementia as the cause of a patient's confusion unless there is a well-constructed history from reliable sources of a slow and insidious decline of cognitive function progressing over years that has been fully and appropriately evaluated on previous occasions. There are too many treatable causes of abrupt or subacute decline of cognition to accept a putative and possibly misleading diagnosis of "baseline dementia" as the working hypothesis for diagnosis and management in these cases.

Scope of the Problem

In a study of 178 cases referred to the University of California San Francisco with a working diagnosis of Creutzfeldt-Jakob disease (Geschwind, Shu, Haman, Sejvar, & Miller, 2008), 62% had prion disease, but 38% (67 patients) had nonprion causes, including autoimmune, infectious, psychiatric, malignant, toxic/metabolic, vascular, and neurodegenerative disorders generally considered insidious and slowly progressive but presenting in a fulminant form. Leukoencephalopathy and encephalopathy of unknown origin accounted for the 4.5% of patients who could not be definitively diagnosed. See Table 15.1

Stepwise Clinical Approach to the Diagnosis

The traditional approach to reaching a diagnosis rests upon the elicitation of a

TABLE 15.1 Nonprion Diagnoses of Patients in University of California, San Francisco, Cohort Initially Suspected of Having Creutzfeldt-Jakob disease

Condition	Cases (n)	Percentage of Nonprion RPDs
Neurodegenerative		
Corticobasal degeneration	8	
Frontotemporal dementia[a]	7	
Dementia with Lewy bodies	4	
Alzheimer's disease[b]	5	
Progressive supranuclear palsy	2	
Subtotal	26	39
Autoimmune		
Hashimoto's encephatopathy	4	
Multiple sclerosis	1	
Sarcoid	1	
Antibody mediated		
VGKC	2	
Yo and Hu	1	
Ma[c]	1	
CV2[c]	1	
GAD65	1	
Neuropil[c]	1	
Adenylate kinase 5	1	
Glial	1	
Subtotal	15	22
Unknown causative factor[d]	8	12
Infeetious[e]	4	6
Psychiatric	4	6
Malignancy[f]		
PCNSL	2	
Non-antibody-mediated paraneoplastic	2	
Subtotal	4	6
Toxic/metabolic		
Ethanol toxicity	1	
Methylmalonic academia	1	
Methotrexate toxicity	1	
Subtotal	3	4
Vascular	3	4
Total	67	100

[a] Includes two frontotemporal dementia/acute lateral sclerosis and one progressive subcortical gliosis PSG patient.
[b] Includes one familial subject.
[c] Includes one paraneoplastic patient.
[d] Includes one leukoencephalopathy, one pathology-proven astrogliosis, and one suspected cerebral anayloid angiopathy patient.
[e] Includes two pathology-proved meningoencephalitis and two viral encephalitis patients (unknown agent; patients recovered).
[f] Includes one thymoma and one systemic lymphoma with encephalopathy patient and two central nervous system lymphoma patients. RPD, rapidly progressive dementia; PCNSL, primary central nervous system lymphoma; VGKC, voltage-gated potassium channel antibody.
Source: From Geschwind, Shu, Haman, Sejvar, and Miller (2008); reproduced with permission.

comprehensive history, careful and directed examination, and consideration of appropriate special investigations. The general principles to be considered in the history are the background of the patient and family, who provides the history; the time course of the illness—its onset and duration; the principal defining features of the condition; its progression over time and the sequence of loss of function; and the associated neurological/medical/psychiatric issues. The examination includes a general medical examination, neurologic elementary examination, and mental status examination, including both neurologic and psychiatric aspects.

The first part of this chapter takes this clinical approach to the differential diagnosis of the many disorders under consideration (see Table 15.2). Accurate diagnosis is likely to be successful when the examiner adopts a systematic approach to each aspect of the exam, looking for clues to the core features of the case. These are elicited by methodical and hypothesis-driven exploration, allowing the examiner to select appropriate and targeted investigations. The importance of this diagnostic method cannot be overstated, particularly in the challenging scenario of the patient with cognitive decline, and even more so when the cognitive change is rapid.

The History

The ability of a patient to present a coherent, logical, and chronological account of himself or herself is an integral part of the mental state evaluation. Patients with acute confusion or dementia do not provide their own history. Major deficits or nonsequiturs in the history should be the tip-off that there is something amiss in the cognitive profile. Assuming that the history taker is compulsive, "poor histories" are given by poor historians, and usually for definable reasons.

What is the chief complaint? Is it memory loss and, if so, what is lost. Forgetfulness in later life is common and while interest in the earliest harbingers of Alzheimer's is growing, this complaint is not necessarily indicative of a major neurological disorder. "Forgetting what you went there for" and having trouble in dinner conversation coming up with names of people, but nevertheless remembering who they are, what they said, and to whom, may not be concerning, unless the patient is young (under 55 years) and there are other worrisome features such as a strong family history of dementia and changes in personality or lifestyle.

True loss of memory for important aspects of work, recent major events, and important family milestones, however, does raise concern. Are there associated features in the medical and neurological history that lead to suspicion of specific etiologic agents associated with memory loss such as new medications (beta blockers, sedatives, psychotropics), alcohol consumption, depression, metabolic disorders such as hypothyroidism, prior gastrectomy to suggest vitamin B12 or thiamine deficiency, or risk factors for human immunodeficiency virus (HIV) infection? Are there neighborhood symptoms and signs, such as early and prominent change in personality (frontotemporal dementia), focal weakness, paresthesia, or visual loss (focal brains lesions such as abscess or brain tumor), gait disturbance and incontinence (normal pressure hydrocephalus, Binswanger's disease), subacute onset of dementia with myoclonus and ataxia (Creutzfeldt-Jakob disease), or associated movement disturbances (Huntington's and Parkinson's diseases)?

Is the problem memory loss or a memory lapse? Is loss of memory transient, lasting seconds to minutes (as in seizures), or hours (as in partial complex status, or transient global amnesia)? Did headache occur around the time of the memory lapse (seen in complicated migraine)?

Does the family use the term "loss of memory" to mean aphasia or apraxia? Can the history differentiate between hemianopsia and a parietal neglect syndrome? Are there features suggestive of alien hand syndrome?

Are changes in personality the major or principal problems reported to the physician? Frontal lobe tumors such as meningiomas or gliomas, or frontotemporal dementia may present with changes in drive, ambition, judgment, and social and personal responsibility. These disorders may, for example, turn a pleasant, mild-mannered and hard-working individual into a stubborn, neglectful, apathetic, rigid, obsessional, and disinhibited person who engages in socially inappropriate and embarrassing behavior, but not associated with memory loss. The examiner needs to interpret changes in behavior in the

TABLE 15.2 Dementia: An Approach to Differential Diagnosis by Category and Disease

Trauma
    Diffuse axonal injury, hemorrhage
    Chronic subdural hematoma
    Postconcussion syndrome
    Chronic traumatic encephalopathy

Inflammation/Infection
    Herpes simplex encephalitis
    HIV and infectious complications
    Focal cerebritis/abscess
    Subacute bacterial endocarditis
    Prion disease—CJD, variant
    Progressive multifocal leukoencephalopathy
    Lyme encephalopathy (with or without meningitis)
    Subacute or chronic meningitis (tuberculosis, cryptococcus, cysticercosis, Listeria)
    Neurosyphilis (general paresis, gumma, meningovascular)
    Cerebral sarcoidosis
    Subacute sclerosing panencephalitis
    Whipple's disease of the brain

Neoplastic
    Tumor—benign (frontal meningioma, clivus chordoma invading medial temporal structures)
    Tumor—malignant, 1°/2°; presentation depends on location
    Intravascular lymphoma
    Paraneoplastic limbic encephalitis
    Radiation necrosis
    Postchemotherapy cognitive impairment (chemobrain)

Metabolic/Hormonal
    Renal—uremic encephalopathy (acute or chronic) and dialysis dementia
    Hepatic encephalopathy (acute or chronic)
    Hypercapnea/hyperviscosity/hypoxemia (acute or chronic)
    Vitamin B1 (thiamine) deficiency (Wernicke-Korsakoff)
    Vitamin B3 deficiency (nicotinic acid/niacin—Pellagra; dermatitis, diarrhea, dementia)
    Vitamin B12 deficiency (+/- pernicious anemia)
    Hypothroidism (myxedema madness)
    Vitamin E deficiency (neuropathy, ataxia, encephalopathy in Celiac disease)
    Acute intermittent porphyria

Vascular
    Focal vascular syndromes (thalamus, inferotemporal, anterior cingulate, bifrontal, triple border-zone watershed infarction, cerebellar posterior lobe)
    Multi-infarct dementia
    Binswanger progressive subcortical ischemic leukoencephalopathy
    Cerebral amyloid angiopathy +/− amyloid vasculitis
    Diffuse hypoxic/ischemic injury
    PRES (posterior reversible encephalopathy syndrome)
    Thrombotic thrombocytopenic purpura
    CADASIL (cerebral autosomal dominant arteriopathy with subcortical infarcts, leukoencephalopathy, migraine)
    MELAS (mitochondrial encephalopathy with lactic acidosis and stroke-like episodes)

Autoimmune
    Nonparaneoplastic limbic encephalitis
    Hashimoto encephalopathy (steroid-responsive encephalopathy syndrome [SREAT])
    Systemic lupus erythematosus
    Isolated angiitis of the nervous system
    Temporal arteritis
    Wegener's granulomatosis
    Polyarteritis nodosa
    Susac syndrome

(continued)

TABLE 15.2 Continued

Iatrogenic/Drugs/Toxins
    Medications: beta blockers, neuroleptics, antidepressants, anticonvulsants, histamine/dopamine blockade, methotrexate
    Alcohol (Wernicke-Korsakoff, Marchiafava-Bignami)
    Heroin: "chasing the dragon" leukoencephalopathy
    Mescaline, phencyclidine, cocaine
    Marijuana psychosis
    Toxic exposure: carbon monoxide, toluene, lead, mercury
    Poisoning: arsenic, cyanide

Demyelinating
    Acquired
        Multiple sclerosis, Schilder's, Balo's sclerosis
        ADEM (acute disseminated encephalomyelitis)
        Toxins
        Delayed posthypoxic leukoencephalopathy
        Electricity-induced demyelination
        Decompression sickness demyelination
    Genetic
        Adult-onset leukodystrophy with neuroaxonal spheroids
        X-linked adrenoleukodystrophy
        Metachromatic leukodystrophy
        Globoid cell leukodystrophy
        Vanishing white matter disease

Obstructive/Mechanical
    Obstructive hydrocephalus
    Normal pressure hydrocephalus
    Sagging brain syndrome—mimics frontotemporal dementia

Late-Life Degenerative Disorders
    Alzheimer's disease
    Frontotemporal dementia/Pick's disease
    Parkinson's disease
    Progressive supranuclear palsy
    Corticobasal degeneration
    Lewy body disease
    Huntington's disease
    ALS-dementia-Parkinson's complex
    Primary progressive aphasia as manifestation of diseases of progranulin, tau, TDP-43
    Posterior cortical atrophy as manifestation of Alzheimer's disease
    Wilson's disease
    Neurodegeneration with brain iron accumulation

Cerebellar Related
    Cerebellar cognitive affective syndrome in pure cerebellar disease—genetic or acquired
    Autosomal dominant spinocerebellar ataxias (SCAs)
    Recessively inherited ataxias and complex hereditary spastic paraplegias
    Fragile X tremor ataxia syndrome (FXTAS)
    Dentatorubropalidoluysian atrophy (DRPLA)
    Gordon Holmes syndrome
    Superficial siderosis
    Sagging brain syndrome
    Langerhans cell histiocytosis
    Cerebellar agenesis

Very Rare Pediatric Degenerative Disorders With Adult Presentations
    MERRF (mitochondrial encephalopathy with ragged red fibers)
    Niemann-Pick type C
    Gangliosidosis 2 (GM2/Adult Tay-Sachs)
    Alexander disease
    Lafora progressive myoclonus epilepsy
    Cerebrotendinous xanthomatosis
    PLO-SL (polycystic lipomembranous osteodysplasia with sclerosing leukoencephalopathy)
    Neuronal intranuclear inclusion disease

light of the patient's prior personality, lifestyle, and accomplishments, and then test cognitive functions in order to diagnose and treat the underlying disorder or behavioral abnormality.

Could there be depression of which both the family and the patient are unaware? What are the circumstances leading up to the evaluation? Is there a family history, or a past personal history, of depression? Is there evidence of the vegetative symptoms of depression—loss of weight, appetite, energy, interest, concentration? Is the sleep cycle reversed, or does the patient awake in the early hours of the morning for no apparent reason?

What is the time course of the illness? Is it an insidiously progressive constellation difficult to date precisely in its onset, lasting at least months, and probably years, as would be the case in most patients with degenerative dementias? Or is the course rapidly progressive and aggressively debilitating over weeks and months, as occurs in viral or prion diseases (progressive multifocal leukoencephalopathy, HIV, Creutzfeldt-Jakob [CJD]), subacute or chronic meningitides (tuberculosis, cryptococcus, neurocysticercosis, listeriosis), and limbic encephalitis (paraneoplastic, or non-tumor-related immune disorders including Hashimoto encephalopathy and voltage-gated potassium channel antibody [VGKC-Ab] syndrome)? Are there precise definable points of decompensation (stepwise progression) with perhaps some improvement but not a return to baseline, as occurs in patients with vascular dementias or multiple sclerosis? Is there a specific identifiable initiating event to the behavioral change, such as traumatic brain injury and repetitive closed head trauma, intracranial hemorrhage from arteriovenous malformation rupture, systemic illness, or cardiac bypass surgery?

Are there associated elementary neurological symptoms in the history, such as focal or transient deficits that accompany cerebrovascular disease, the dementia associated with multiple sclerosis, chronic hepatic encephalopathy, or alcohol-related dementia? Are there disturbances of gait and bladder function, suggesting normal pressure hydrocephalus, Binswanger's disease, or the cognitive changes seen in patients with inherited or acquired cerebellar ataxias? Is falling a prominent and early complaint, as may occur in progressive supranuclear palsy, or is there marked asymmetry to the motor presentation as occurs in corticobasal degeneration? Are there predominantly psychiatric symptoms such as auditory hallucinations, paranoia, delusional thinking, thought broadcasting, or anxiety and phobia that may be overwhelming and limiting the patient's activities, interests, and abilities? And are there circumstances in the history (injury at work, outstanding litigation) that would lead the examiner to suspect that secondary gain may play a role in the patient's complaints of disturbed memory, impaired concentration, and so on.

Is there a family history of dementia (Alzheimer's disease, Huntington's disease) or psychiatric illness (bipolar affective disorder, schizophrenia)? Is there a potentially relevant history of illness or risk factors such as HIV disease, systemic cancer (paraneoplastic limbic encephalitis), alcohol use, and previous surgery (thyroidectomy/ radiation, Bilroth II gastrectomy)?

What medications is the patient taking? Beta blockers, psychotropics, sedating antidepressants, anticonvulsants at high levels or in multiple combinations, H2-receptor blockers, dopamine blockers used for nonneurologic purposes such as metoclopramide, and many others agents can produce substantial cognitive impairment particularly in elderly patients, or in those whose coping mechanisms are already limited, as in those with borderline intellectual function at baseline.

The Examination

The examination may be diagnostic, or at least help limit the range of possible differential diagnoses. This includes a general medical examination, an elementary neurologic examination, and a detailed mental state evaluation.

General Medical Examination

A review of the list of diseases associated with changes in cognitive function underscores the need for a thorough general medical examination in order to detect the physical findings associated with these conditions. This includes the typical signs of an overactive or hypofunctioning thyroid gland; stigmata of chronic alcoholism, hepatic failure, or renal insufficiency; anemia and cachexia of acquired immunodeficiency syndrome (AIDS) or neoplasms; the cardiac and peripheral manifestations of endocarditis, atrial fibrillation, or congestive heart failure; and the hypertension, bruits, pulse asymmetries, and other peripheral evidence of risk factors for vascular dementia. The systemic illness suggested by these findings on the exam may be the cause of the cognitive impairment. If, however, there were an underlying dementing process, medical illnesses such as these or the fever of a urinary tract infection or pneumonia, or tender swollen calf of a deep vein thrombosis, could exacerbate the cognitive deficits.

Elementary Neurological Examination

There are a large number of neurologic diseases in which dementia is an integral part of the clinical scenario, and telltale features on a carefully performed neurologic examination will provide valuable pointers leading to the correct diagnosis.

Movement disorders are perhaps most readily discernible. Parkinson's disease is characterized by the triad of bradykinesia, rigidity, and tremor, but it does not always present classically, is often quite asymmetric, and is not infrequently heralded by depression. Cognitive decline generally occurs later in the course of the illness. Progressive supranuclear palsy (PSP) may present with falls and difficulty descending or ascending stairs. The examination shows supranuclear vertical gaze palsy (difficulty directing the eye downward on command), axial predominant rigidity, and intellectual decline. Corticobasal degeneration (CBD) usually includes asymmetric limb apraxia in the setting of an extrapyramidal bradykinesia. Lewy body disease should be in the differential diagnosis of dementia with early extrapyramidal features and visual hallucinations. The choreoathetoid movements of Huntington's disease may not present early, and instead one may only see minor movements that resemble simple tics. Psychiatric manifestations may herald the disease onset. Wilson's disease is said to present in adulthood, with dystonia, dysarthria, proximal wing-flapping tremor, and corneal Kayser-Fleischer rings best seen with the slit-lamp examination. Neurodegeneration with brain iron accumulation with dystonic and choreoathetoid features on examination may have an early adult presentation. All the inherited cerebellar ataxias (dominant and recessive) include a cognitive component; and multiple system atrophy, parkinsonian or cerebellar forms, may be associated with mental changes later in the course of the illness, as discussed further later in the chapter.

Retinal abnormalities in patients with dementia include optic atrophy in demyelinating disease; retinitis pigmentosa-like findings in mitochondrial diseases that cause dementia and loss of vision (e.g., mutation at position 8933); and focal pigmentary retinopathy with macular involvement in subacute sclerosing panencephalitis. Macular degeneration and cataracts that impair vision in a person with a clouded sensorium can lead to visual hallucinations (Charles Bonnet syndrome) and exaggeration of the clinical features of the dementia.

Visual field deficits are seen in focal brain lesions such as stroke, and in progressive multifocal leukoencephalopathy (PML) that has a predilection for the occipital lobes. Mass lesions in the pituitary gland or hypothalamus may cause visual field cuts (bitemporal hemianopsia), cognitive failure from hydrocephalus, and neuropsychiatric manifestations from damage to the hypothalamus and its limbic connections. Posterior cortical atrophy—a focal manifestation of Alzheimer's disease, can start with visual agnosia and progress to visual field cuts, and usually asymmetric quadrantanopsias.

Failure of vertical gaze is an early feature in PSP, along with gait instability and axial rigidity. Increased latency of saccadic eye movements (slowed initiation of saccades) or difficulty with volitionally directed gaze may be seen in CBD or frontotemporal dementia (FTD), whereas slowing of saccades and decreased saccade amplitude are seen in PSP. These tauopathies (PSP, FTD, and CBD) may manifest as the overlap disorder corticobasal syndrome (Armstrong et al., 2013) and thus are less distinguishable from each other on the basis of the oculomotor examination. Nystagmus indicates disease of the vestibulocerebellar system or possible drug effect, and similarly, failure of the vestibulo-ocular cancellation reflex indicates vestibulocerebellar impairment. An ocular stare occurs in Whipple's disease of the central nervous system caused by convergence failure and impoverishment of extraocular movements. This may be accompanied by the mouth and jaw movements of oculomasticatory myorhythmia, a striking constellation in this rare disorder.

Focal cranial mono- or polyneuropathies raise suspicion for life-threatening illnesses, including malignant meningeal infiltration, chronic basilar meningitides (e.g., cryptococcosis, tuberculosis), and infectious vasculopathies (e.g., syphilis) that may be associated with hydrocephalus, parenchymal brain involvement, or apparently silent subcortical strokes. Paget's disease of bone may cause compressive cranial neuropathies (mostly VIIIth nerve) and hydrocephalus. Superficial siderosis that produces progressive deafness and cerebellar dysfunction as a consequence of the insidious layering of blood products on the surface of the cerebellum and brainstem may also result in cognitive impairment. Susac syndrome is an inflammatory vasculopathy that produces multifocal brain demyelination, including the corpus callosum, along with hearing loss and visual loss from branch retinal artery occlusion. Hearing loss is also a relatively common occurrence in mitochondrial disorders such as mitochondrial encephalomyopathy, lactic acidosis, and stroke-like episodes (MELAS), which affects cognition and may lead to dementia.

The masked facies of parkinsonism, and rarely the trombone tremor of tertiary syphilis, may be evident. The nature of dysarthria is an important clue to the underlying diagnosis in dementia, as it can suggest extrapyramidal or cerebellar disease, or bulbar involvement as occurs in the ALS-dementia complex.

Peripheral neuropathy raises the possibility of vitamin B12 or multiple vitamin deficiency states, alcohol excess, hypothyroidism, neurosyphilis, HIV, and vasculitis (systemic lupus erythematosus, polyarterities nodosa), all of which can be associated with structural cerebral changes that cause dementia or altered behaviors. Neuropathy and dementia may also be seen as paraneoplastic effects of carcinoma, heavy metal intoxication (lead, mercury, arsenic), and adrenoleukodystrophy. Lyme disease may be associated with cognitive changes as well as peripheral neuropathy or polyradiculopathy. Lancinating radicular pains in the thoracic distribution occur in syphilis, diabetes, and Lyme disease.

Corticospinal tract signs occur late in primary degenerative dementias. If these features are evident early, they make diagnoses such as Alzheimer's, FTD, and Parkinson's disease less likely. Long tract signs are found in the amyotrophic lateral sclerosis–parkinsonism–dementia complex described initially in Guam, now recognized as part of a spectrum of the manifestations of the progranulin gene with brain deposits of the ubiquitinated TAR-DNA binding protein (TARDBP or TDP-43; Hasegawa et al., 2007; Yu et al., 2010). Corticospinal features raise the suspicion for focal structural disease such as occurs in vascular syndromes. Large arteriovenous malformations may produce a vascular steal phenomenon; intellectual decline becomes evident as the hemiparesis and hyperreflexia worsen over the years in the affected extremities. Multi-infarct dementia reflects the location, number, and size of strokes identified on the imaging studies. Multiple strokes on imaging studies are a prerequisite for this diagnosis. The dementia results from involvement of the multiple different cortical and subcortically based systems that subserve intellect, emotion, and memory. Binswanger's progressive subcortical leukoencephalopathy presents with cognitive decline and intellectual and emotional blunting, change in gait (slowing, falling), and often with incontinence, making it difficult to distinguish clinically from normal pressure hydrocephalus (NPH). The two are alike for good reason—the white matter adjacent to the ventricles is compromised in both, in Binswanger's by true ischemia, and in NPH presumably by compression of the descending corticospinal tracts and the intra- and interhemispheric association fibers by the slowly enlarging ventricles. The diagnosis is suggested by the clinical triad (ataxia, incontinence, and dementia). The radiographic studies, stroke risk (lipids, blood pressure, smoking, family history, coronary and/or peripheral vascular disease), and results of therapeutic spinal tap help determine which is the more likely diagnosis. Amyloid deposition in cerebral vessels is incriminated as a cause of massive lobar hemorrhage, but this entity also produces dementia in the absence of frank hemorrhage (Viswanathan & Greenberg, 2011), sometimes with superimposed episodes of transient unresponsiveness. Diagnosis in vivo is supported by susceptibility sequence magnetic resonance imaging (MRI) detection of multiple microhemorrhages at cortical–white matter boundaries. Autopsy findings show areas of microscopic and small macroscopic hemorrhage in the setting of amyloid-laden blood vessels throughout the brain.

Other entities associated with behavioral changes and long tract signs include diseases not generally considered high on the differential in elderly persons. Multiple sclerosis (MS) should be considered in a previously healthy young adult who presents with cognitive changes and long tract signs which may be related to concomitant myelopathy or involvement of the white matter in the cerebral hemispheres. Brainstem and optic nerve disease may be missing, and the telltale internuclear ophthalmoplegia and abnormal evoked responses may be absent. Cerebral predominant MS can present with depression, and the diagnosis can be missed until the course is advanced. The differential diagnosis of the leukoencephalopathies presenting with dementia includes degenerative diseases more usually seen in children. X-linked adrenoleukodystrophy manifests in adulthood in 3% of cases, with dementia accompanying long tract signs, hemianopsia, dysarthria, cortical blindness, and seizures. Autosomal recessive metachromatic leukodystrophy presents in adulthood as a white matter disorder with personality change and cognitive deficits. Krabbes's globoid cell leukodystrophy, also autosomal recessive, has rarely been described in adults, with hemiparesis and ataxia accompanying the demyelinating dementia. Subacute sclerosing panencephalitis (SSPE, a late complication of measles infection) also produces intense abnormalities in white matter as well as cortex, with long tract signs and cortical blindness accompanying the dementia. An elderly patient with episodic attacks of generalized weakness and fatigue associated with minor neurologic signs may suggest a pattern of ischemic disease such as Binswanger's. But if the stroke profile is unimpressive, and the episodes are too long to conform to transient ischemic attack, seizure, or migraine, then it is worthwhile considering late-life MS and its differential diagnosis, and investigating these entities with the appropriate studies (MRI, spinal fluid analysis, visual and somatosensory evoked potentials).

Extrapyramidal findings are expected in Parkinson's disease, neuroleptic-induced syndromes including confusion in the elderly, PSP, Lewy body disease, and the Parkinsonian variant of MSA. Patients with Alzheimer's disease have extrapyramidal features late in the course of the illness. In contrast, the young patient (30s) with early-onset autosomal dominant Alzheimer's disease from presenilin mutations can have marked extrapyramidal features of dystonia and bradykinesia, together with myoclonus that becomes marked as the illness rapidly evolves.

Patterns of sensory loss point to peripheral nerve disease, brainstem syndromes, or cerebral hemispheric lesions. Primary sensory loss (touch, pin, vibration, position) is unlikely to be present in degenerative dementias, but it may occur with lesions of the sensory thalamus and in diseases of white matter such as multi-infarct dementia and MS. Impaired graphesthesia and mislocalization of stimulus in the presence of intact primary sensation occur in degenerative dementias such as Alzheimer's disease, reflecting parietal lobe involvement.

Cerebellar features in a rapidly dementing illness, together with spontaneous myoclonus and/or stimulus-evoked startle myoclonus raise the possibility of Creutzfeldt-Jakob disease. The cerebellar features may be predominant, and the cerebellar variant of the illness has cerebellar features as the primary clinical manifestations until fairly late in the course (Brownell & Oppenheimer, 1965; Foley & Denny-Brown, 1955). Lesions of the cerebellum that affect the limbic and cognitive cerebellum in the vermis and posterior lobes, respectively, produce the cerebellar-cognitive affective syndrome (Schmahmann & Sherman, 1998). This includes deficits in executive function, visual-spatial disorganization, impaired verbal fluency, and blunted or inappropriate affect. If the lesion spares the sensorimotor cerebellum in the cerebellar anterior lobe, the patient will not be expected to have gait ataxia or extremity dysmetria.

Release phenomena are helpful in the examination. They are not specifically localizing unless asymmetric, but they usually implicate the prefrontal cortex and its connections. Palmar grasps and traction responses so strong as to allow the examiner to lift the patient off the examining table can be impressive, as are the root, snout, and suck reflexes and the palmar grasp. These can be the only hard neurologic findings in patients with Alzheimer's disease outside the mental state examination. The glabellar tap sign (failure to suppress the blink reflex with tapping the forehead) is not a "frontal-release" phenomenon but indicates extrapyramidal disturbance as occurs in Parkinson's disease. The palmomental reflex may be interesting to observe but also occurs in healthy individuals and is not particularly useful for diagnostic purposes.

Abulia is the neurologic equivalent of psychomotor retardation, with slowness, decreased responsiveness, and apathy (Fisher, 1983). The patient is slowed mentally and physically, may have paratonic rigidity (*geggenhalten*), does not generally initiate spontaneous conversation or action, and may produce accurate answers to mental state questions but usually after a disquietingly prolonged delay. This poverty of spontaneity is a hallmark of dorsolateral prefrontal pathology, the opposite of the gregarious and disinhibited, inappropriate jocularity that characterizes orbitofrontal cortex lesions. Apart from mass or other destructive lesions of the frontal lobes, many illnesses that result in widespread white matter damage produce a similar syndrome. This includes many of the white matter dementias that spare the cerebral cortex and the deep nuclei but devastate the long association fiber tracts that link cortical association areas. There are many causes of white matter dementia (see Table 15.3), but they often have a frontal lobe flavor that includes abulia as a hallmark of the presentation. Brain imaging is strikingly abnormal in these cases and helps direct the appropriate evaluation. Subcortical dementias, including Parkinson's disease, Huntington's disease, and PSP, among others, also produce slowness of response, but these entities are usually accompanied by overt movement disorders.

Brief lapses of consciousness may be discernible in the examination of a patient with frequent partial seizures. These can be so frequent as to interfere with the patient's ability to pay attention to his or her environment, learn new material, and keep track with ongoing activities. This could resemble a loss of memory, whereas in fact the patient is essentially "not there" when the memories are supposed to be laid down. Brief staring spells lasting moments, fluttering of the eyelids, smacking of the lips, an unexpected repetition of a movement or sentence, or apparent inattentiveness to the examiner's questions may be clues to the presence of an underlying complex partial seizure disorder. This needs to be differentiated from confused distractibility. The electroencephalogram is of particular benefit in this scenario.

We are reluctant as physicians to entertain the possibility of feigned physical signs, and sometimes the differentiation between neurologic disease, conversion disorder, and secondary gain can be difficult. A careful inquiry into the background circumstances and reliance upon the need for neurologic symptoms and signs to conform to known patterns of injury and deficit are helpful in sorting out the psychological/psychiatric/neurologic overlap.

Mental State Examination

The nature of the cognitive profile allows the examiner to draw upon structure-function correlations in the nervous system to localize the lesion in cortical and subcortical areas. The pattern of involvement of the affected regions generally reflects the underlying pathology, particularly in the neurodegenerative dementias such as Alzheimer's and FTD. Discussion of the mental state examination and of the neural substrates that subserve the different elements of cognition is found elsewhere in this volume.

Brain Imaging

Patterns of disease that cause dementia can be so distinctive on brain imaging that the radiographic findings help structure the diagnostic thoughts and the further approach to evaluation and management. MRI is the preferred and most sensitive method, but computerized tomography (CT) is an acceptable alternative when MRI is not available or contraindicated—as in the patient with a permanent cardiac pacemaker. Note that brain imaging is an extension of the clinical examination

TABLE 15.3 Cerebral White Matter Disorders

Genetic	Leukodystrophies (e.g., adrenoleukodystrophy, metachromatic leukodystrophy, globoid cell leukodystrophy)
	Vanishing white matter disease
	Alexander's disease
	Adult-onset leukodystrophy with neuroaxonal spheroids
	Mitochondrial encephalopathy with lactic acid and stroke (MELAS)
	Fragile X tremor-ataxia syndrome
	Polycystic lipomembranous osteodysplasia with sclerosing leukoencephalopathy
	Aminoacidurias (e.g., phenylketonuria)
	Phakomatoses (e.g., neurofibromatosis)
	Mucopolysaccharidoses
	Muscular dystrophy
	Callosal agenesis
Demyelinative	Multiple sclerosis
	Acute disseminated encephalomyelitis
	Acute hemorrhagic encephalomyelitis
	Schilder's disease
	Marburg's disease
	Balo's concentric sclerosis
Infectious	HIV and AIDS dementia complex
	Progressive multifocal leukoencephalopathy
	Subacute sclerosing panencephalitis
	Progressive rubella panencephalitis
	Varicella zoster encephalitis
	Cytomegalovirus encephalitis
	Lyme encephalopathy
Inflammatory	Systemic lupus erythematosus
	Behcet's disease
	Sjogren's syndrome
	Wegener's granulomatosis
	Temporal arteritis
	Ployarteritis nodosa
	Scleroderma
	Isolated angiitis of the central nervous system
	Sarcoidosis
Toxic	Cranial irradiation
	Therapeutic drugs (methotrexate, BCNU, cyclophosphamide)
	Drugs of abuse (e.g., toluene, heroin)
	Alcohol (Marchiafava Bignami disease)
	Environmental toxins (e.g., carbon monoxide)
Metabolic	Cobalamin deficiency
	Central pontine myelinolysis
	Hypoxic-ischemic injury
	Posterior reversible encephalopathy syndrome
	Hypertensive encephalopathy/eclampsia
	High-altitude cerebral edema
Vascular	Binswanger's disease
	CADASIL
	Leukoaraiosis
	Cerebral amyloid angiopathy
	Intravascular lymphoma
	White matter disease of prematurity
	Migraine
Traumatic	Traumatic brain injury (diffuse axonal injury)
	Shaken baby syndrome
	Corpus callosotomy
	Focal lesions of white matter tracts (e.g., fornix transection, splenium of CC tumor)

(*continued*)

TABLE 15.3 Continued

Neoplastic	Gliomatosis cerebri
	Diffusely infiltrative gliomas
	Lymphomatosis cerebri
	Langerhans cell histiocytosis
	Focal white matter tumors
Hydrocephalic	Early hydrocephalus
	Normal pressure hydrocephalus
Degenerative	White matter changes in Alzheimer's disease
	Effects of aging on myelin

Source: From Schmahmann, Smith, Eichler, and Filley, (2008).

and supplements, but does not replace the traditional clinical method. "MR-negative neurology" in the absence of a clearly formulated hypothesis derived from the history and examination (as in early Alzheimer's' disease prior to hippocampal atrophy) is both frustrating and misleading. On the other hand, obvious findings on MRI, ranging from butterfly glioma spreading across the corpus callosum, to multifocal lesions as in cerebral amyloid angiopathy and progressive multifocal leukoencephalopathy, or normal pressure hydrocephalus, help set the stage for the further workup and treatment.

Diseases That Cause Dementia, Developing Over Days to Weeks

The timing of disease onset and progression provides clues to the diagnosis. Acute life-threatening encephalopathies that develop into fulminant form in a matter of hours are not considered here, as these hyperacute diseases do not enter the differential diagnosis of dementia (e.g., bacterial meningitis, and encephalitides such as eastern equine, western equine, and West Nile virus). A number of illnesses with subacute progression over weeks to months may have an abrupt onset, and these are considered first before a discussion of more unusual forms of dementing disorders with a chronic course over years.

Differentiate Structural Disease From Nonfocal or Multifocal Brain Disease

The clinical approach generally allows the examiner to distinguish focal structural disorders from diffuse conditions such as toxic, metabolic, and infectious etiologies. Together with brain imaging and first-line laboratory tests, it should not be difficult to diagnose mental state changes from brain tumor, abscess, cerebritis, or hemorrhage, and a wide array of metabolic insults that can cause cognitive decline, or precipitate or worsen incipient or previously unrecognized cognitive impairment. Common metabolic abnormalities include those accompanying renal, hepatic, cardiac, and pulmonary failure; severe anemia; and dehydration (Table 15.2). Three particularly useful clinical signs pointing to a metabolic encephalopathy are fluctuating level of arousal, wandering of attention or easy distractibility with or without agitation, and asterixis—the sudden, brief, and repeated loss of power in antigravity muscles such as when the wrists are held in extension with the arms outstretched. Myoclonus, the brief, intermittent, positive contraction of groups of muscles in the limbs individually or together, occurs in a range of metabolic derangements such as magnesium deficiency and drug overdose with lithium, in hypoxemic ischemic encephalopathy, Hashimoto's encephalopathy, and in neurodegenerative disorders, including presenilin early-onset Alzheimer's and corticobasal degeneration, in addition to CJD.

Metabolic Disorders

Metabolic disorders not routinely evaluated will be missed unless the clinician develops the hypothesis and orders the appropriate confirmatory laboratory studies. The most common and important of these include the effects of alcohol, medications, drugs and toxins, vitamin deficiency states (B1, B3, B12, and E), and altered thyroid metabolism.

Alcohol

The older individual who may be alone, depressed, or forgetful can indulge in alcohol use which will cause confusion when taken in larger amounts, or exacerbate any underlying cognitive impairment even at levels that were previously tolerated. A history of alcoholism is not necessarily present. Apart from inebriation, neuropsychiatric complications of alcohol use are the alcohol withdrawal syndrome, which comes on usually within 1 to 3 days of cessation of alcohol and includes confusion, agitation, and autonomic features (McKeon, Frye, & Delanty, 2008). When left untreated (by benzodiazepines), the severe and persistent alcohol withdrawal syndrome progresses to full-blown delirium tremens, a potentially fatal disorder largely because of the cardiac manifestations of the autonomic storm (Kelly & Renner, 2008). Excessive alcohol use is also associated with thiamine deficiency, which causes Wernicke's encephalopathy, Korsakoff amnestic syndrome, and possibly Marchiafava-Bignami disease, discussed later.

Medications

The use of prescription medications for neuropsychiatric indications (psychotropics, tricyclic antidepressants, benzodiazepines), as well as a large number of medically indicated agents from beta blockers to histamine antagonists, can cause confusion in the elderly person, particularly if taken in higher doses or more frequently than prescribed. Inappropriate or incorrect use of hypoglycemic agents, for example, can produce episodes of confusion that are otherwise unexplained unless the history is carefully elicited. Polypharmacy in the older patient is an established reality because so many ailments in later years respond well to the judicious use of carefully selected therapeutic agents. The use of prescription medications targeted to each of these disorders sets up the higher likelihood of drug interactions and additive neuropsychiatric effects. Some of the common offending agents are those used for pain management, such as gabapentin and related compounds, anticonvulsant medications used for their analgesic properties, and narcotics that are considered mild in the younger individual but have disproportionate effects in the elderly. The key to prevention of confusion with these agents in the geriatric population is to use the smallest dose of medication possible, raising the dose in small increments over time depending on clinical response.

Thiamine Deficiency: Wernicke Korsakoff Syndrome and Marchiafava Bignami Disease

Most commonly occurring in the setting of prolonged alcohol use, thiamine (vitamin B1) deficiency is a treatable cause of confusion and a preventable form of dementia. Other clinical scenarios that place the patient at risk for thiamine deficiency are hyperemesis gravidarum because of the intractable vomiting that leads to decreased oral intake, and previous gastrectomy or gastric surgery for weight loss that can lead to impaired absorption of this essential vitamin in the small intestine. Wernicke syndrome is recognized by the tetrad of confusion, ataxia, nystagmus, and oculomotor impairments such as sixth nerve palsy (impaired lateral rectus movement). The percentage of patients who experience all these findings in the early stage of the syndrome is small. The recent onset of confusion is the most consistent feature, and it is the reason for the use of thiamine so liberally in confused patients in the emergency room. The metabolically active form of thiamine (thiamine pyrophosphate) is necessary for glucose metabolism, and therefore administering glucose to a patient with a clinical or subclinical thiamine deficiency exacerbates the thiamine deficiency and can either precipitate or worsen the clinical syndrome. This explains why thiamine is administered before dextrose is given intravenously to the acutely confused patient in the emergency room. The common practice of administering the thiamine-narcan-D50 "cocktail" to these patients also addresses the possibility of confusion and encephalopathy resulting from sedating narcotic drugs. Korsakoff syndrome is the long-term sequel of untreated thiamine deficiency, the clinical manifestation of hemorrhagic necrosis of the mammillary bodies, dorsomedial nucleus of thalamus, and periqueductal grey in the brainstem (Victor, Adams, & Collins, 1971). There is also involvement of the cerebellar dentate nuclei in the acute stage of Wernicke's (Bae, Lee, Lee, Choi, & Suh, 2001). The amnestic syndrome of Korsakoff syndrome is characterized by profound loss of the ability to lay down new memories, with preservation of prior knowledge and recall of events prior to the initiating illness. The anterograde amnesia occurs in isolation and is not associated with the penumbra of other cognitive domains as in Alzheimer's disease. Treatment of the syndrome is by prevention of the thiamine deficiency and early recognition of its appearance in the appropriate clinical context.

Marchiafava Bignami disease refers to the necrosis of the corpus callosum seen in the setting of excessive alcohol use, as well as in cases of malnutrition. It was originally described as a fatal disease affecting heavy consumers of red wine, but brain imaging has allowed premortem diagnosis, and not all patients succumb. The relationship to thiamine deficiency has been suggested, not least by improvement in the condition in patients treated promptly with vitamin B1, but this is not yet definitive. MRI shows acute demyelination in the splenium or the genu of the corpus callosum or the entire callosum, best seen on diffusion-weighted imaging but also on fluid attenuated inversion recovery sequence (FLAIR) and T2, or as a hypodensity on CT. Based on imaging features, type A is characterized by acute to subacute onset of impairment of consciousness and pyramidal tract syndromes, with imaging showing callosal edema, and a less favorable prognosis with considerable disability and fatality. Type B lacks major impairment of level of consciousness, is characterized by acute to subacute onset of cognitive impairment, dysarthria, gait disturbance and signs of interhemispheric disconnection, partial T2-hyperintense lesions on early MRI, and a generally favorable prognosis with treatment (Heinrich, Runge, & Khaw, 2004). The range of clinical manifestations includes confusion, delirium, unconsciousness, impaired memory and/or disorientation, with impaired gait, dysarthria, nystagmus, mutism, signs of disconnection or split brain syndrome, pyramidal sign with true weakness, primitive reflexes, rigidity, incontinence, sensory symptoms, and gaze palsy or diplopia. Seizures may occur. Cerebrospinal fluid (CSF) may show elevated protein, but leukocytosis in this setting generally reflects central nervous system (CNS) infection (Hillbom et al., 2013). Chronic cases have thinning of the corpus callosum and a cognitive profile that conforms to a frontal lobe syndrome, together with signs of interhemispheric disconnection.

Pellagra

Malnutrition and undernutrition occur worldwide, and developed nations are not immune to the neurological manifestations of a poor diet. Pellagra results from deficiency of nicotinic acid (niacin, vitamin B3) or tryptophan, which is converted to niacin. Poor diet, alcoholism, and gastrointestinal disorders with malabsorption are common precipitants. Hartnup disease, an autosomal recessive condition, prevents absorption of tryptophan and produces a pellagra-like disorder. Pellagra is known as the "three D's"—dermatitis, diarrhea, and dementia, with a fourth "D" (death) reflecting the unfortunate course if unrecognized. It is a particularly challenging diagnosis to make in cases in which the expected skin manifestations are absent, depriving the clinician of one of the didactic hallmarks of the illness. The dermatitis develops on exposed skin surfaces, but if the patient is not exposed to ultraviolet rays by virtue of habit and clothing, these features may be missing. In this circumstance, knowledge of the clinical background of the patient is paramount. In a Hungarian neuropathology surveillance program for CJD, 5 of 59 patients who came to autopsy showed neuropathological features of pellagra encephalopathy with widespread chromatolytic neurons. The course was between 2 and 24 months, with clinical signs manifesting as rapid-onset dementia, cerebellar ataxia, and corticospinal signs (Kapas et al., 2012). Pellagra encephalopathy is characterized clinically by rapidly progressive dementia, fluctuating cognition and frontal disinhibition, release phenomena, startle myoclonus, decreased arousal, a cerebellar motor syndrome, hyperreflexia, peripheral neuropathy, autonomic dysfunction, and cranial neuropathies (Ishii & Nishihara, 1981). In the alcoholic patient, it can be a challenge to distinguish the acute and persistent confusional state, disorientation, agitation, irritability, paranoia, and hallucinations of pellagra from alcohol withdrawal. Knowing of, and suspecting the disease, is the key to providing the appropriate therapy.

Vitamin B12 Deficiency

The myelopathy of pernicious anemia characteristically includes upper motor neuron findings from involvement of the lateral corticospinal tracts, and impaired position and vibration sense from damage to the posterior columns—subacute combined degeneration of the spinal cord (the differential diagnosis of which is HIV, neurosyphilis, and copper deficiency). Both the myelopathy and the dementia of vitamin B12 deficiency can occur in the absence of the hematological parameters of macrocytic megaloblastic anemia, which require associated folic acid deficiency. Reliance on the hematologic parameters for the suspicion of B12-deficient cognitive decline is a recipe for diagnostic failure. Cognitive impairment in B12 deficiency includes mania, depression, and psychosis, with deficits in memory, concentration, visuospatial performance, and executive functions (Osimani, Berger, Friedman, Porat-Katz, & Abarbanel, 2005). Relative or absolute B12 deficiency is implicated in exacerbation of cognitive failure in patients with other disorders, including Alzheimer's disease (Meins, Muller-Thomsen, & Meier-Baumgartner, 2000; Werder, 2010). Low normal levels of vitamin B12 appear to be prevalent in the population, and this is therefore an important entity to consider and test for in the appropriate clinical context. Elevated levels of methylmalonic acid and homocysteine will provide laboratory support for the suspicion of B12 deficiency when the B12 level itself is borderline. More specific tests for pernicious anemia causing B12 deficiency include antibodies to gastric parietal cells and intrinsic factor. These are indicated when there is no clear dietary basis of the disorder or a history of prior gastric or duodenal resection.

Vitamin E

The most common findings in vitamin E deficiency, seen in malabsorption syndromes such as celiac disease, poor diet, and some inherited disorders (ataxia with vitamin E deficiency; Schuelke, 2013) include the cerebellar motor syndrome of truncal and limb ataxia with dysarthria, loss of deep tendon reflexes, markedly diminished perception of vibration and position, ophthalmoplegia, ptosis, and muscle weakness (Schuelke, 2013; Sokol, 1988). Behavioral and personality disorders have been noted in the setting of vitamin E deficiency in patients with chronic liver disease, which of course is a confound in the evaluation of cognition. Burns and Holland (1986) reported that in their study of an elderly psychiatric population, nearly 60% of the patients with dementia had serum vitamin E levels below the accepted normal range, and they postulated that an absolute or relative deficiency of vitamin E could lower the age of onset or increase the rate of progression of dementia in Alzheimer's disease. A quarter century later, it appears that higher vitamin E levels are associated with reduced risk of cognitive impairment in non–cognitively impaired elderly adults (Mangialasche et al., 2013).

Thyroid Disorders

Myxedema madness is an old term referring to the cognitive deficits of apathy, inattention, and forgetfulness, and psychiatric symptoms of depression, mania, and psychosis with delusions and hallucinations that occur in the setting of frank hypothyroidism (Heinrich & Grahm, 2003). The presence of cognitive and affective impairments in patients with subclinical hypothyroidism as measured by elevated thyroid-stimulating hormone (Davis, Stern, & Flashman, 2003) is sufficient indication to ensure that thyroid levels are checked in patients with cognitive decline, be it acute or chronic. Patients with the hyperthyroidism of Grave's disease report emotional lability, irritability, insomnia, restlessness, agitation, depression, and anxiety as well as deficits in memory and concentration (Trzepacz, McCue, Klein, Levey, & Greenhouse, 1988; Vogel et al., 2007), and these improve markedly following treatment. When the associated medical features of thyroid dysfunction are evident, the diagnosis is readily suspected, but this is not always the case. Clinical suspicion and

Acute Intermittent Porphyria

This autosomal dominant disorder of enzymes in the haem biosynthetic pathway presents in acute crisis with gastrointestinal (abdominal pain, nausea, and vomiting), cardiac (hypertension and tachycardia), and neurological symptoms and signs. Neuropsychiatric manifestations range from anxiety and emotional lability to confusion and frank psychosis, while more widespread neurological involvement includes generalized seizures, painful motor neuropathy leading to flaccid quadriparesis, and bulbar involvement with aphonia, dysphagia, and respiratory paralysis. The diagnosis, once suspected, is made by detecting increased serum levels of delta aminolaevulinic acid and porphobilinogen (PBG), as well as elevated PBG in the urine (Disler & Eales, 1982; Whatley & Badminton, 2013). Acute intermittent porphyria has a high prevalence in individuals of Scandinavian descent. Variegate porphyria, which can also present with an acute neurological crisis, is common in southern Africa.

Rapidly Progressive Dementia (Other Than Metabolic Disorders)

Other than the metabolic disorders discussed previously, the following conditions should be at the top of the list of diseases to consider in a patient with a rapidly progressive dementing disorder, both because some are readily treatable, and because of the importance of the diagnosis for the patient and family. These are infections, limbic and other immune mediated encephalitides the prion diseases, stroke syndromes and vasculitides, focal lesions that produce new onset dementia, and cancers presenting in atypical ways such as stroke and meningeal infiltration.

Herpes Simplex Encephalitis

Viral encephalitides are not usually considered in the differential diagnosis of a subacute encephalopathy because these are catastrophic illnesses that develop over hours or days. The neurotropic double-stranded DNA Herpes simplex virus is a little different in that its course can be more indolent, coming on over days or weeks or more. Most cases are caused by HSV-1 (which cause cold sores) and are likely the result of retrograde transmission from the trigeminal ganglion, or from the olfactory nerve (Dinn, 1980). Early symptoms that include change in taste or smell may be dismissed; the apathy, irritability, and memory loss or confusion from involvement of the medial temporal and orbitofrontal cortices (Fig. 15.1) may not be striking at the outset; and the low-grade fever is nonspecific. Neurological deficits soon set in, however, with a range of language impairments reflecting the evolving aphasia from spread to the ventral prefrontal and temporal cortices and the language pathways that connect them. Confusion mounts, and the patient develops focal or generalized seizures or lapses directly into status epilepticus or coma. A high level of suspicion is needed to make the diagnosis urgently and initiate treatment with acyclovir as the agent of choice, as early treatment can stop the illness, limit further neuronal destruction, and improve prognosis for survival and recovery of neuropsychiatric function. Seizures are a major long-term complication, particularly when seizures are evident at the time of the acute illness (Sellner & Trinka, 2012). Persistent amnesia is a complication of damage to bilateral medial temporal structures critical to memory formation and consolidation. The triad of fever, confusion, and aphasia should be an instant tip-off to Herpes simplex encephalitis, but the differential diagnosis of this presentation includes diseases with very different etiologies and treatments—subacute infectious endocarditis, temporal arteritis, and thrombotic thrombocytopenic purpura.

In subacute infectious endocarditis (SBE) fever results from the systemic low-grade bacterial infection. Almost 30% of SBE patients experience neurological manifestations, the commonest of which is confusion (Jones & Siekert, 1989). Aphasia results from focal infarction in language cortex produced by the infectious vasculitis in the salient arterial supply—for example, inferior division of the middle cerebral artery or its posterior temporal branch.

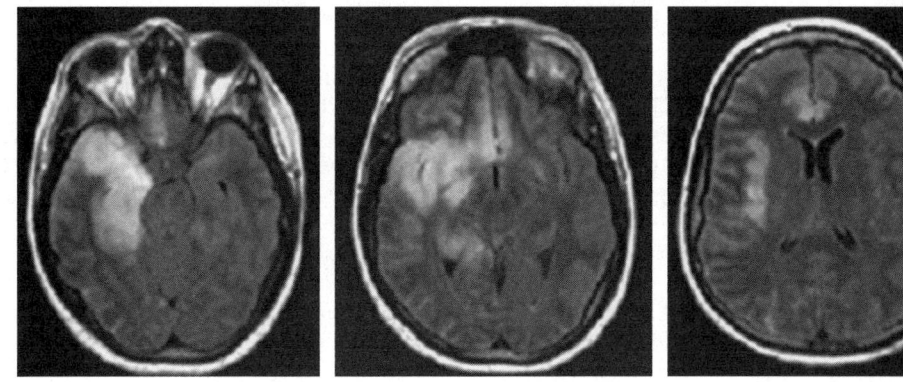

Figure 15.1 Axial fluid attenuated inversion recovery sequence (FLAIR)-weighted magnetic resonance imaging (MRI) scans (from ventral to dorsal, right to left) in a 36-year-old woman with Herpes simplex encephalitis involving the right anterior and medial temporal lobe, right insular cortex, and the orbital and medial prefrontal cortices bilaterally, R>L.

Temporal arteritis occurs in older individuals and may simulate an underlying neoplasm. Loss of appetite to the point of cachexia may occur, and intermittent fevers commonly accompany the illness together with a sense of overall systemic ill health and the laboratory finding of elevated erythrocyte sedimentation rate and C-reactive protein. The confusion and aphasia, like in the case of SBE, result from focal or multifocal cerebral infarction. Visual loss is a major risk in temporal arteritis from central retinal artery occlusion, and when suspected, should be treated urgently with corticosteroids even before the diagnosis has been established with certainty by temporal artery biopsy.

Thrombotic thrombocytopenic purpura is a thrombotic microangiopathy caused by inhibition of a metalloprotease that cleaves large multimers of von Willebrand factor into smaller units (George, 2006). Increased platelet adhesion leads to intravascular thrombosis. The illness can evolve over weeks, fever may be present, and accompanied by malaise. Neurological symptoms occur in approximately 65% of patients with TTP, with confusion, neuropsychiatric features such as hallucinations, focal neurologic deficits including aphasia, and seizures. Recognition (thrombocytopenia with microangiopathic hemolytic anemia) and urgent treatment with plasmapheresis prevents the life-threatening complications of stroke, myocardial infarction, and renal failure (Vesely et al., 2003).

Limbic Encephalitis

It was recognized in the 1960s that systemic cancer can present with neurobehavioral symptoms, with the focus of the degenerative and inflammatory pathology (neuronal loss, astrocytic proliferation with gliosis and perivascular infiltration) located in limbic structures particularly in the medial temporal regions—amygdala, hippocampus, and parahippocampal gyrus—but also in the cingulate gyrus and hypothalamus, hence limbic encephalitis (Corsellis, Goldberg, & Norton, 1968). Early reports established the principal clinical features of limbic encephalitis (LE) as the sudden or subacute onset over days and weeks of seizures, disorientation, confusion, anterograde and retrograde memory impairment, psychosis, hallucinations, and marked disturbance of affect such as anxiety or depression. Extralimbic involvement occurs in approximately half the cases, including brainstem findings and autonomic instability. It is imperative that the evaluation of a patient with subacute cognitive decline include the search for these underlying, often treatable, immune disorders.

New developments in immunology provide deeper understanding of the pathophysiology and treatment of these disorders (Asztely & Kumlien, 2012; Darnell & Posner, 2011; Graus & Dalmau, 2012; Lancaster & Dalmau, 2012). Antibodies directed against tumor antigens attack neural tissue, resulting in the clinical constellation. Limbic encephalitis may predate the symptoms of cancer by as much as 4 years. Many of the antibodies identified to date are linked with specific types and locations of tumors. There are instances of tumor-associated LE in which no antibodies have yet been identified; cases of LE with identified antibodies that may not be associated with underlying tumor; and cases of LE that respond to immunotherapy in which there is neither identified tumor nor an identified antibody.

Thus, LE may be categorized as follows:

- LE associated with antibodies from an identified tumor
- LE in which tumor is found but no antibodies are detected
- LE in which there are antibodies but no tumor (i.e., not a paraneoplastic phenomenon)
- LE (after a full diagnostic evaluation is otherwise negative) in which there is neither antibody identified nor a tumor detected, but the patient responds well to immunotherapy

Three different antigen-antibody scenarios have clinical relevance for the diagnosis and management of LE. The first is when antibodies produced in response to the tumor that target neuronal epitopes (the part of the antigen that is recognized by the immune system) are directed against nuclear or cytoplasmic proteins such as Hu, Yo, and Ma2. But antibodies have limited access to these neuronal antigens, and therefore the principal pathology is caused not by the antibody itself, but by the T-cell-mediated immune response against the neuronal antigen, leading to the inflammation and neurodegeneration that characterizes the disorder. These antibody-mediated disorders are associated principally with tumors of the lung, breast, ovaries, and testicles (see Table 15.4). Because of the neurodegeneration produced by the cell-mediated immune response, recovery of neurological function after treatment is only occasionally successful. The second is when antibodies target intracellular synaptic proteins (such as glutamic acid decarboxylase and amphiphysin) during synaptic vesicle fusion and reuptake, but T-cell mediated pathogenetic mechanisms may also be important. A third category of more recently described LE cases are defined by antibody attack against cell surface or synaptic proteins, including the N-methyl-D-aspartate (NMDA), α-amino-3-hydroxy-5-methyl-4-isoxazolepropionic acid (AMPA), gamma-aminobutyric acid-B (GABA-B), glycine, and the metabotropic glutmate receptor mGluR5, as well as two proteins previously thought to be VGKCs but are now known as leucine-rich glioma-inactivated protein 1 (LGI1) and contactin-associated protein-like 2 (Caspr2; see Table 15.5). In these disorders, the antibody directly attacks the cell-surface target producing the symptoms, and importantly, these disorders are usually not associated with an underlying malignancy (Irani et al., 2010). Seizures, psychosis, and confusion with memory loss are the hallmark of these disorders, which have a time course of onset over

TABLE 15.4 Well-Characterized Onconeuronal Antibodies and Paraneoplastic Neurological Syndromes

Antibody	Predominant Tumors	Most Common PNS
Hu (ANNAI)	SCLC	Encephalomyelitis, limbic encephalitis, brainstem encephalitis, PCD; sensory neuronopathy, gastrointestinal pseudoobstruction
CV2 (CRMP5)	SCLC, thymoma	Same as Hu, and chorea, optic neuropathy, isolated myelopathy, and mixed neuropathies
Amphiphysin	Breast SCLC	Stiff-person syndrome, myelopathy and myoclonus, encephalomyelitis, sensory neuronopathy
Ri (ANNA2)	Breast, SCLC	Brainstem encephalitis, opsoclonus myoclonus
Yo (PCA I)	Ovary, breast	PCD
Ma2	Testicular	Limbic and brainstem encephalitis
Tr	Hodgkin's	PCD

PCD, paraneoplastic cerebellar degeneration; PNS, paraneoplastic neurological syndromes; SCLC, small-cell lung cancer.
Source: From Graus and Dalmau (2012); reproduced with permission.

TABLE 15.5 Antibodies Against Cell Surface or Synaptic Antigens Associated With Paraneoplastic Neurological Syndromes

	Syndrome	Cancer
NMDAR	Encephalitis	Ovarian teratoma (rare in children, present in 58% older than 18 years)
GABA$_B$R	Limbic encephalitis	SCLC (70%)
CASPR2	Morvan's syndrome	Thymoma (38%)
AMPAR	Limbic encephalitis	SCLC, breast, thymus (60%)
VGCC	PCD	SCLC (>95%)
mGluR5	Limbic encephalitis	Hodgkin's disease (two cases reported only)

AMPAR, amino-3-hydroxy-5-methyl-4-isoxazolepropionic acid receptor; CASPR2, contactin-associated protein 2; GABA$_B$R, γ-aminobutyric acid-B receptor; mGluR5, metabotropic glutamate receptor type 5; NMDAR, N-methyl-D-aspartate receptor; PCD, paraneoplastic cerebellar degeneration; SCLC, small-cell lung cancer; VGCC, voltage-gated calcium channel.

Source: From Graus and Dalmau (2012); reproduced with permission.

days to weeks. Further, they often respond dramatically and completely to appropriate immune-based therapies. Morvan syndrome, associated with Caspr2 and with thymoma in about 50% of cases, is characterized by neuromyotonia with myokymia on electromyography (100%), neuropsychiatric features (insomnia, 89.7%; confusion, 65.5%; amnesia, 55.6%; hallucinations, 51.9%), dysautonomia (hyperhidrosis, 86.2%; cardiovascular, 48.3%), and neuropathic pain including painful muscle cramps (62.1%; Irani et al., 2012). This condition responds to thymectomy either alone or in combination with immune modulation (Abou-Zeid, Boursoulian, Metzer, & Gundogdu, 2012; Lancaster & Dalmau, 2012). The NMDA receptor antibody syndrome associated with ovarian teratomas includes psychiatric symptoms, catatonia, agitation, seizures, decreased level of consciousness, autonomic instability, and abnormal movements. Executive dysfunction and psychiatric symptoms endure after the acute phase has subsided. The glycine receptor antibody syndrome is a progressive encephalomyelitis with rigidity and myoclonus. And the mGluR5 antibody syndrome that occurs in the setting of Hodgkin's lymphoma produces a constellation of psychiatric symptoms, cognitive impairment, and memory loss termed the Ophelia syndrome (Lancaster et al., 2011).

The approach to the diagnosis involves a full clinical evaluation because the features that characterize limbic encephalitis are shared by other disorders as well. Investigations include brain MRI for the telltale FLAIR and T2 hyperintensities in limbic cortices; spinal tap for stigmata of inflammation; serum and CSF markers for the antibodies that have been indentified in these disorders; CT of neck, chest, abdomen, and pelvis; and ultrasound, if necessary, of the testicles. Whole-body positron emission tomography (PET) scan is necessary if the level of suspicion remains high but the first-line modalities do not identify tumor. Management includes definitive treatment of the underlying tumor when present, and immunotherapy with a combination, often in successive order, of corticosteroids, intravenous immunoglobulin, plasmapheresis, and more recently, cyclophosphamide and rituximab, managed by a team of physicians with the appropriate and necessary skill set to handle these complex cases. Psychiatric symptoms and seizures are all managed as indicated.

Hashimoto Encephalopathy

An acute or subacute cognitive and psychiatric syndrome occurs in the setting of antibodies directed against the thyroid gland (thyroglobulin, thyroid peroxidase) not necessarily associated at the same time with the symptoms or metabolic markers of thryotoxicosis or hypothyroidism (Brain, Jellinek, & Ball, 1966). The disorder disproportionately affects women (F:M, 4:1), and the constellation includes personality change, dementia, seizures, psychosis, myoclonus, altered consciousness, and sometimes gait impairment. The course may be relapsing and remitting. The manifestations can be varied, however, and a high level of suspicion is warranted to make the diagnosis of this treatable cause of a subacute and sometimes rapidly progressive dementia. A vasculitic form with stroke-like episodes has also been described (Kothbauer-Margreiter, Sturzenegger, Komor, Baumgartner, & Hess, 1996). Chong, Rowland, and Utiger (2003) reviewed the literature and identified 85 patients (69 women; mean age, 44 years) with encephalopathy and high serum antithyroid antibody concentrations. Findings included seizures in 66%, psychosis in 38%, and stroke-like signs in 27%. Subclinical hypothyroidism was noted in 35%, although some patients were overtly hypo- or hyperthyroid. Glucocorticoids produced improvement in 96% of the patients. In a retrospective review (Castillo et al., 2006) of 20 cases (14 females), median age at disease onset was 56 years and the most frequent clinical features were tremor (80%), transient aphasia (80%), myoclonus (65%), gait ataxia (65%), seizures (60%), and sleep abnormalities (55%). The electroencephalogram (EEG) is abnormal in >90% of cases, and there is elevated CSF protein in 80% of cases with inflammatory cells in approximately 25%. MRI abnormalities are noted in 25% of cases. The condition has prompted controversy as thyroid antibodies are found in the healthy population, and in patients with Hashimoto thyroiditis who do not have the neuropsychiatric constellation. The levels of antithyroid autoantibody titers also do not correlate with the severity or type of clinical presentation, and the pathogenetic role of antithyroid autoantibodies in this disorder is unknown. Some have preferred the term "steroid response encephalopathy associated with autoimmune thyroiditis" (Castillo et al., 2006), but the disease does not always melt away with steroids and may respond quite dramatically instead to intravenous immunoglobulin (Cornejo, Venegas, Goni, Salas, & Romero, 2010; Drulovic, Andrejevic, Bonaci-Nikolic, & Mijailovic, 2011) or other immune modulating agents (Marshall & Doyle, 2006).

The dementia, myoclonus, tremor, and ataxia of Hashimoto encephalopathy accompanied by an abnormal EEG and nonspecific abnormalities on the MRI thus mimic CJD in its earlier stages, and the evaluation of subacute dementia should include the appropriate tests in search of this entity: thyroid peroxidase and thyroglobulin antibodies. Similarly, the stroke-like episodes and MRI findings place it squarely in the differential of MELAS, discussed below, the acute stroke-like episodes of which can also respond to treatment with steroids (Walcott et al., 2012).

Vascular Diseases

Dementia occurs in the setting of cerebral autosomal dominant arteriopathy with strokes and ischemic leukoencephalopathy (CADASIL; Fig. 15.2), cerebral amyloid angiopathy, and Binswanger's progressive subcortical ischemic leukoencephalopathy (Fig. 15.3). Instant dementia follows stroke in cognitively relevant areas such as the anterior thalamus and the medial dorsal thalamus (Schmahmann, 2003); the hippocampal formation and entorhinal cortex in the setting of posterior cerebral artery strokes; the

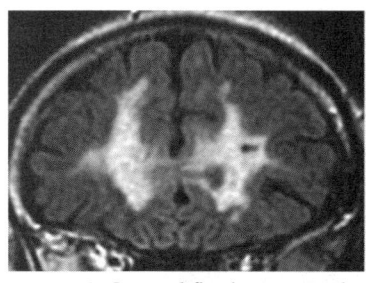

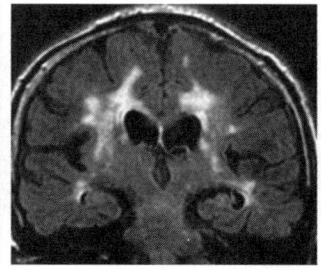

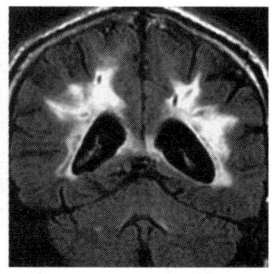

Figure 15.2 Coronal fluid attenuated inversion recovery sequence (FLAIR)-weighted magnetic resonance imaging (MRI) scans (from rostral to caudal, right to left) in a middle-aged man with cerebral autosomal dominant arteriopathy with strokes and ischemic leukoencephalopathy (CADASIL), showing diffuse subcortical ischemic leukoencephalopathy also characteristically involving the temporal stem.

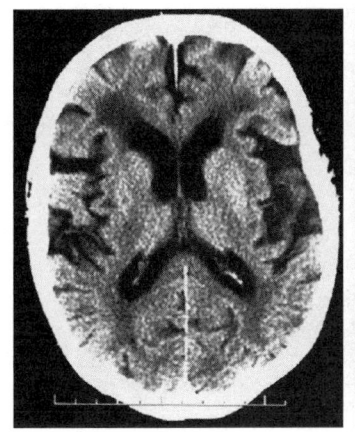

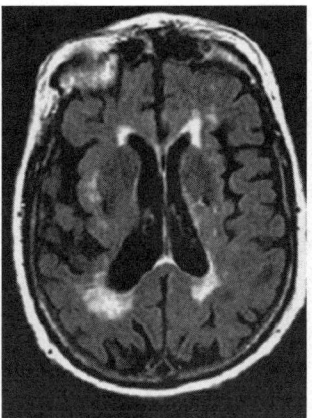

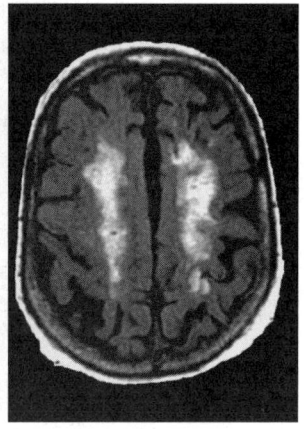

Figure 15.3 T1-weighted axial magnetic resonance imaging (MRI) (left) and fluid attenuated inversion recovery sequence (FLAIR)-weighted MRI images (middle and right) show white matter attenuation in an elderly man with Binswanger's progressive ischemic subcortical leukoencephalopathy.

anterior cingulate gyrus and cingulum bundle from infarctions in the territory of the anterior cerebral artery; and the multitude of behavioral syndromes following infarction in cortical and deep branches of the middle cerebral artery that damage cerebral association areas and their interconnected subcortical regions. These disorders and posterior reversible encephalopathy syndrome (PRES; Fig. 15.4) that can cause confusion, amnesia, and visual deficits are discussed elsewhere in this volume. In addition, rare inherited disorders that affect blood vessels such as Fabry's disease and Moya-Moya syndrome also produce cerebral infarction with consequences for cognition, and they are worth considering in the appropriate clinical and imaging contexts. Susac syndrome is a vasculopathy that mimics multiple sclerosis and is discussed below.

Trauma

Closed head trauma produces neurobehavioral and neuropsychiatric symptoms, either as a result of a single injury or as a consequence of multiple repeated insults over time. The symptoms of concussion, postconcussion syndrome, subacute and chronic subdural hematoma, chronic traumatic encephalopathy (previously known as dementia pugilistica), and direct effects of intraparenchymal hemorrhage on higher function are discussed elsewhere in this volume.

Focal Lesions

The location and extent of space-occupying lesions determine the nature of the clinical presentation. This is exemplified by butterfly gliomas that spread across the corpus callosum between the two frontal lobes (Fig. 15.5) and which present with a subacute neurobehavioral syndrome reflecting disintegration of frontal executive systems. Strokes in the tuberothalamic artery of thalamus infarct the anterior thalamic nuclei linked with limbic structures, producing anterograde amnesia, autobiographical memory impairment, and behavioral changes such as apathy; and infarction in the territory of the paramedian thalamic arteries produces amnestic and language deficits from damage to the medial dorsal thalamic nuclei that are tightly interconnected with the prefrontal cortex (Schmahmann, 2003). A less appreciated focal behavioral syndrome directly relevant to the determination of the subacute dementia results from mass lesions in the splenium of the corpus callosum also invading the adjacent retrosplenial cortex (Fig. 15.6) and likely involving the fornix and the hippocampal commissures that course immediately beneath the callosum. These lesions produce a profound amnestic syndrome (splenial amnesia; Osawa, Maeshima, Kubo, & Itakura, 2006; Rudge & Warrington, 1991; Schmahmann, unpublished observations in two cases) that are similar to those of lesions of the fornix

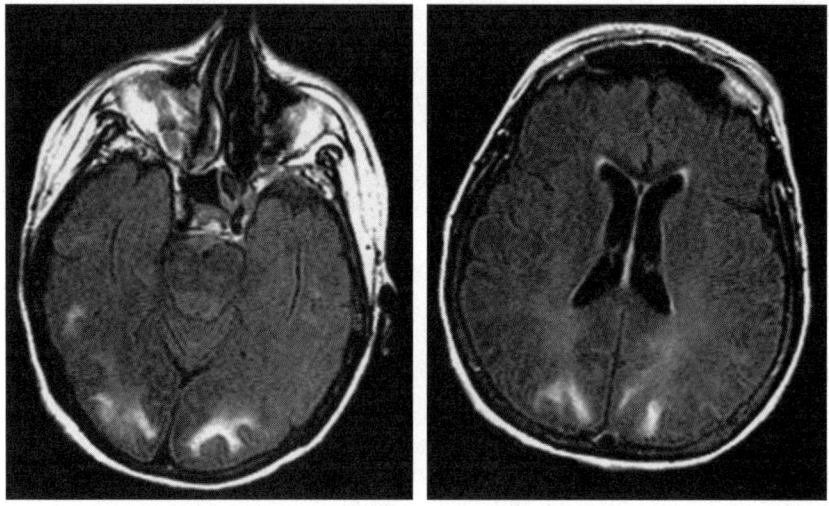

Figure 15.4 Axial fluid attenuated inversion recovery sequence (FLAIR)-weighted magnetic resonance imaging (MRI) (from ventral to dorsal, right to left) in a woman with posterior reversible encephalopathy syndrome (PRES) in the setting of severe hypertension, demonstrating the occipito-parietal location of the signal abnormality.

(D'Esposito, Verfaellie, Alexander, & Katz, 1995; Heilman & Sypert, 1977) and the anterior thalamus (Schmahmann, 2003)—subcortical nodes and pathways critical for declarative memory. The precise nature of a focal space-occupying lesion (tumor, sarcoidosis, tuberculoma, syphilitic gumma, and toxoplasmosis; Fig. 15.7) may be suggested by the clinical background and the imaging characteristics, but the diagnosis is not always evident from brain imaging, and biopsy may be indicated to determine optimal management. This approach is further necessitated in the case of brain tumors (primary or secondary) by the evolving sophistication of pharmocogenomics in targeting chemotherapeutic agents to different tumor types.

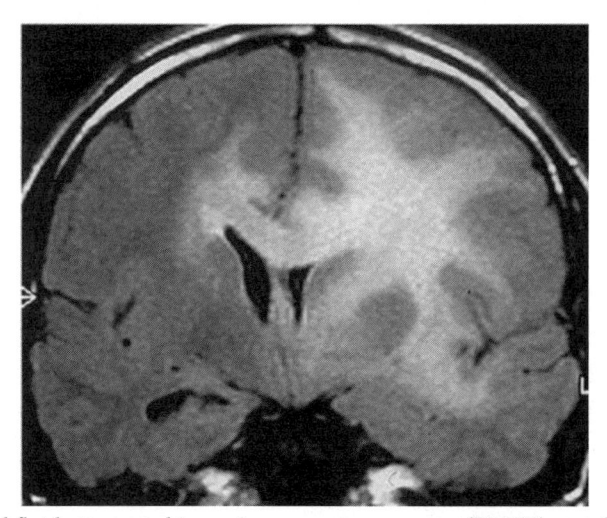

Figure 15.5 Coronal fluid attenuated inversion recovery sequence (FLAIR)-weighted magnetic resonance imaging (MRI) identifies an infiltrating high-grade astrocytoma distorting the left anterior hemisphere and spreading across the corpus callosum to the right side (butterfly glioma, gliomatosis cerebri).

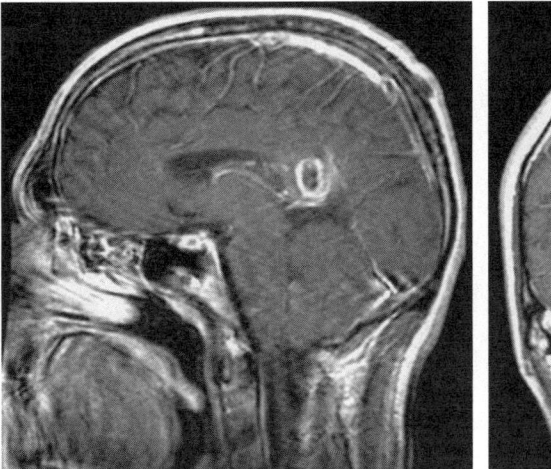

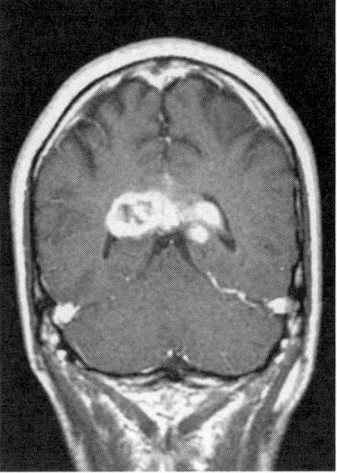

Figure 15.6 Postgadolinium sagittal T1-weighted magnetic resonance image (MRI) (left) and coronal image (right) identifying a contrast-enhancing mass (glioblastoma multiforme) centered in the splenium of the corpus callosum.

AIDS and HIV

The epidemic of dementia seen in the 1980s and early 1990s as part of the acquired immunodeficiency syndrome (AIDS) dementia complex (ADC) has largely abated in the developed work that has ready access to combination antiretroviral therapy (CART). It is still rampant, however, in large swaths of the developing world in which there is suboptimal acknowledgment and recognition of the disease, and a combination of inadequate neuroimaging, laboratory facilities, and limited access to drugs (Alkali, Bwala, Nyandaiti, & Danesi, 2013). NeuroAIDS affects half of the 22 million people currently living with the disease in sub-Saharan Africa. The commonest neuroAIDS syndrome is HIV-associated neurocognitive disorders (HAND), which affects over 1.5 million Africans yearly. Patients suffer progressive dementia accompanied by motor and behavioral dysfunction. Impaired memory and concentration with psychomotor slowing are the most common early presentation. Motor disturbances include ataxia, leg weakness, tremor, and loss of fine-motor coordination. Behavioral features commence

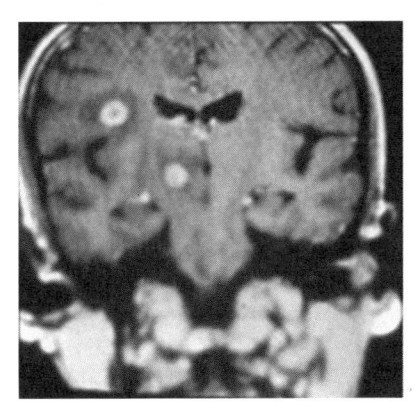

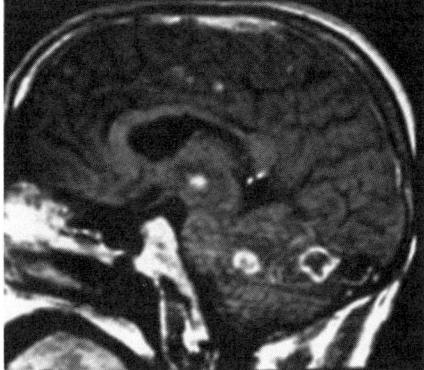

Figure 15.7 Coronal T1-weighted magnetic resonance imaging (MRI) scans in the coronal plane (left) and sagittal plane (right) following administration of gadolinium in a patient with HIV and cerebral toxoplasmosis. Multiple contrast enhancing lesions are identified, some of which are ring enhancing.

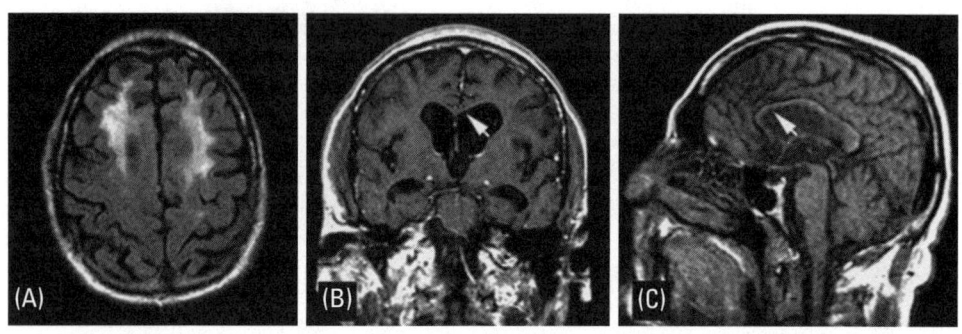

Figure 15.8 Axial fluid attenuated inversion recovery sequence (FLAIR)-weighted magnetic resonance imaging (MRI) (A), coronal T1-weighted MRI (B), and midsagittal T1-weighted MRI (C) in a young man with HIV showing frontal predominant leukoencephalopathy. Thinning of the corpus callosum (arrows) is identified in the coronal and midsagittal views.

with apathy, withdrawal, and then psychosis. The advanced disease is characterized by a stereotyped picture of severe multidomain dementia, mutism, incontinence, paraplegia, and myoclonus (Harris, Jeste, Gleghorn, & Sewell, 1991; Navia, Jordan, & Price, 1986; Schmahmann, 1997; 1998). Note that the paraplegia may arise either from severe bilateral cerebral disease or from the associated finding of vacuolar myelopathy (Gabuzda & Hirsch, 1987). White matter pathology in patients with HIV raises the specter of PML (Schutte, Ranchhod, Kakaza, & Pillay, 2013), but HIV encephalopathy in the absence of the full AIDS spectrum includes a clinically relevant leukoencephalopathy (Fig. 15.8), as well as axonal damage and neuronal loss induced directly by the human immunodeficiency virus (Gray et al., 2001), the neurobehavioral manifestations of which include slowing of information processing, forgetfulness, executive dysfunction, and affective changes, including notably, depression. It now also appears that even in the setting of chronic HIV infection managed successfully with CART, progressive changes in the brain, including white matter changes in the frontal lobes and neuronal damage to the basal ganglia, can lead to progressive neurocognitive decline (Gongvatana et al., 2013).

Neurosyphilis

This sexually transmitted disease is caused by the spirochete *Treponema pallidum*. Tertiary syphilis patients suffering from general paresis of the insane (GPI) hold a pivotal niche in the history of cognitive and behavioral neuroscience. According to Pearce (2012), GPI was a crucial starting point in which the causes of mental illness were slowly transformed from psychogenic disturbances of mind and spirits to organically determined diseases. Once a major cause of long-term neurological disability, including dementia, GPI remains an important consideration in the patient with atypical and rapidly progressive dementia, both in the era of global health and easy access to international travel from countries where the disease incidence is high, and in developed countries in the setting of the immunocompromised host with HIV (Knudsen, 2013). Tertiary syphilis is characterized by a subacute onset of disorientation, forgetfulness, and impaired judgment, together with psychiatric symptoms, including depression, mania, and psychosis (Stefani et al., 2013). In addition to the dementia, behavioral abnormalities, and chronic psychosis, tertiary syphilis patients may also experience acute transverse myelitis, chronic myelopathy, and syphilitic amyotrophy (Kayal, Goswami, Das, & Paul, 2011). In a recent study of 116 patients in China (Zheng et al., 2011), manifestations included progressive cognitive and behavioral deterioration, accompanied by psychotic and/or affective behavioral disorders, hyper-reflexia, frontal release signs (suck reflex), the Argyll-Robertson pupil, and focal or multifocal brain atrophy on imaging. This description is consistent with classical accounts (see Pearce, 2012) of disease onset 12 to 20 years after primary infection of a progressive mainly frontotemporal meningoencephalitis characterized by pyramidal weakness, impaired personality and memory, mania, erratic judgment, apathy, violence, "congestive attacks," and epilepsy, together with Argyll-Robertson pupils and concurrent tabes dorsalis. The pattern of presentation of GPI may not always be discretely different from the pattern of cognitive decline in Alzheimer's disease. Wang et al. (2011) found that patients with mild GPI had a pattern of cognitive impairment that resembled the memory, language, and executive deficits in mild Alzheimer's disease together with atrophy of the medial temporal lobes. The GPI patients had more abnormal signs on neurological examination, however. Diagnosis is established only if there is clinical suspicion that motivates the further investigation, or a standard approach to testing that is designed to detect and not miss the disease. Meningovascular syphilis can cause stroke at cerebral and spinal levels, and falls within the differential diagnosis of ischemic disorders with or without cognitive manifestations. Diagnosis of syphilis is supported by CSF lymphocytic pleocytosis and high protein levels, and serological tests, including the CSF nontreponemal Venereal Disease Reference Laboratory (VDRL) test and the serum treponemal *T. pallidum* particle agglutination assay (TPPA), *T. pallidum* haemagglutination assay (TPHA), and enzyme immunosorbent assay (EIA) IgG/IgM. Treatment with appropriate doses and durations of antibiotics (penicillin remains the drug of choice for all stages) cures the illness. The diagnosis should be suspected and tested for in any patient whose course is remotely atypical for Alzheimer's disease, particularly if there are both cognitive and psychiatric features.

Other Subacute and Chronic Meningitides

Neurocysticercosis is endemic in parts of the developing world and is one of the commonest causes of epilepsy worldwide. It is a chronic parasitic disease caused by invasion of the CNS by the larvae of the *Taenia solium* worm. It can also result in a spectrum of cognitive abnormalities, ranging from impairment in a single domain, to mild cognitive impairment, and dementia. The neurocognitive manifestations (Rodrigues et al., 2012) are evident mostly during the phase of active infection, during which 12.5% of the 40 patients studied met criteria for dementia. Cognitive decline was less prominent in patients in whom the cysts had calcified, and whereas these patients did not meet criteria for dementia, more than 50% of this group of 40 patients evaluated was impaired on tests of memory, attention, executive functions, language, and visuospatial skills.

Listeria monocytogenes, a gram-positive bacterium that is spread by contaminated food, is a concern in patients chronically immunosuppressed on steroids. The meningoencephalitis produces focal neurological deficits (Pollock, Pollock, & Harrison, 1984), and it has been associated with persistent cognitive decline, with impaired short-term memory, concentration, and apathy, as well as catatonia (Kellner, Sonntag, & Strian, 1990), mania, depression, and psychosis (Duncan, 1989).

Cryptococcal meningitis may affect immunocompetent hosts but is more prevalent in immune-compromised individuals, notably those with long-term corticosteroid use, but most dramatically in individuals infected with HIV (Pyrgos, Seitz, Steiner, Prevots, & Williamson, 2013). After the acute illness has been treated, its principal mechanism for causing long-term cognitive change is through noncommunicating hydrocephalus from obstruction of CSF flow at the foramina of Luschka and Magendie, or communicating hydrocephalus by prevention of CSF resorption through the Pacchionian granulations at the vertex. During the active infection, the problem of elevated ICP without hydrocephalus produces a combination of headache as well as confusion and obtundation that can be life-threatening and which requires ventriculoperitoneal shunting (Petrou et al., 2012).

Lyme Encephalopathy

Lyme disease is the most common tick-borne disease in the United States (highest prevalence in the coastal Northeast, northwest California, and the Great Lakes region) and Europe. It is caused by the spirochaete *Borrelia burgdorferi* and transmitted to humans through the bite of the deer tick, *Ixodes scapularis*, and the Western black-legged tick, *Ixodes pacificus*. There are three stage of the illness. Early localized infection causes erythema migrans, fever, malaise, fatigue, headache, myalgias, and arthralgias. Early disseminated infection occurring days to weeks later causes neurologic, musculoskeletal, or cardiovascular symptoms and multiple erythema migrans lesions. Late disseminated infection produces migratory polyarthritis with intermittent swelling and pain of one or more joints, particularly the knees, along with neurologic manifestations (Bratton, Whiteside, Hovan, Engle, & Edwards, 2008). The neurology of Lyme (neuroborreliosis) includes lymphocytic meningitis, cranial mononeuropathies such as facial paralysis, hearing loss, and occasionally oculomotor palsies, and lumbosacral polyradiculoneuropathy, which can be painful. A range of encephalitic presentations from confusion and fatigue to cognitive decline and neuropsychiatric symptoms have been reported, but in the chronic posttreatment stage of the illness these are often not associated with laboratory evidence of active CNS borreliosis (Halperin, 2010). Laboratory diagnosis is made by antibody testing and confirmed with Western blot analysis. In active neurological manifesting Lyme disease the CSF shows lymphocytic pleocytosis (<100–200 cells/mm^3) with B cell predominance, elevated protein, and normal to minimally decreased glucose.

First-line antibiotics used to treat Lyme include doxycycline and amoxicillin; cefuroxime and erythromycin are also used. Late or severe disease requires intravenous ceftriaxone or penicillin G. Lyme-associated vasculitis may rarely cause focal cerebral ischemic insults and a marked encephalopathy (Back et al., 2013), and treatment regimens include both the appropriate antibiotic regimen as well as immunosuppressant therapy with mineralocorticoids. This can be lifesaving (author's personal experience of one case).

Controversy has arisen about the length of treatment of the late-stage neurologic manifestations of Lyme and about the entity of post-Lyme encephalopathy. Patients may report persistent symptoms after the standard 3 weeks of IV antibiotic therapy for Lyme disease, including fatigue, myalgia, arthralgia, sensory disturbances, and neurocognitive dysfunction. In a study of IV antibiotics for 10 weeks to treat post-Lyme "mild to moderate cognitive impairment and marked levels of fatigue, pain, and impaired physical functioning," improvement was reported 2 weeks after course completion but was not sustained 3 months later (Fallon et al., 2008). The results of this study, like others that took a similar approach, were regarded as negative, demonstrating "the absence of any lasting improvement in cognitive function" by the prolonged use of antibiotics for this entity (Halperin, 2008). Sjowall, Ledel, Ernerudh, Ekerfelt, and Forsberg (2012) found that 3 weeks of oral doxycycline treatment did not lead to any improvement of either the persistent symptoms or quality of life in postneuroborreliosis patients. Given the vested interests, financial and others, in the Lyme testing industry, and patients with ill-defined neurocognitive and systemic symptoms thought to be "persistent Lyme encephalopathy" (Fallon, Petkova, Keilp, & Slavov, 2009) desperate for answers and intervention, it is unlikely that this controversy will resolve any time soon. On a cautionary note, about 25% of patients with long-term IV access develop complications (Fallon et al., 2008). Personal experience of a patient with a remote history of Lyme disease and the cerebellar form of multiple system atrophy being treated elsewhere with intravenous and intrathecal ceftriaxone for over 2 years in the hope of clinical improvement is both sobering and disturbing.

Central Nervous System Vasculitis

Multifocal cerebral cortical and subcortical infarcts in the absence of major risk factors or laboratory evidence for extracranial or intracranial cerebrovascular disease can present with subacute confusion and raise the differential diagnosis of the inflammatory vasculopathies of the central nervous system. These disorders include primary angiitis of the central nervous system (PANCS) that produces inflammation and destruction of CNS vessels without evidence of vasculitis outside the CNS, and cerebral involvement by systemic lupus erythematosus that is usually accompanied by systemic markers of disease.

PACNS is more common in men, with a peak at age 50. The course is variable, ranging from acutely presenting to chronic and insidious. The diagnostic requirements for PANCS are the presence of an acquired otherwise unexplained neurological or psychiatric deficit, with either classic angiographic appearance (beading of blood vessels from alternating vasoconstriction and focal dilation) or histopathological features of angiitis within the CNS, and no evidence of systemic vasculitis or any disorder that could cause or mimic the angiographic or pathological features of the disease (see Hajj-Ali, Singhal, Benseler, Molloy, & Calabrese, 2011 for further review and discussion). There are no associated constitutional symptoms, weight loss, or non-CNS disease. Headache occurs in the granulomatous form of the illness, together with diffuse and focal neurological deficits, multiple bilateral ischemic foci on brain MRI, and aseptic meningitis documented by chronic meningeal inflammation in the CSF. One can be alerted to the possibility of CNS vasculitis when the patient has at least three features of a clinical tetrad of headache, seizures, psychosis, and stroke. The headache may be nonspecific or have a vascular flavor (throbbing, light and noise sensitivity). Seizures may be focal, partial, or manifest only with irritable eletroencephalograhy in the absence of overt clinical seizures. Psychosis can manifest with a myriad of cognitive and emotional symptoms. The stroke syndromes may be transient ischemic events or fixed small vessel ischemia or large vessel infarction that is the proximate cause of the neurological presentation. Diagnosis is made on the grounds of clinical suspicion and angiographic evidence of beading of small- and medium-sized vessels. Diagnostic uncertainty arises commonly, however, particularly in those instances in which the vasculitis manifests as a focal brain mass, a condition encountered more commonly when the inflammation occurs in the setting of an underlying cerebral amyloid angiopathy (Hajj-Ali, Singhal, Benseler, Molloy, & Calabrese, 2011; Molloy, Singhal, & Calabrese, 2008). When brain biopsy is required, the diagnosis is established with the combination of normal brain parenchyma (apart from areas that have sustained ischemic infarction), together with an inflammatory vasculopathy. Biopsy also differentiates this condition from mimics such as Wegener's granulomatosis and sarcoidosis.

Wegener's granulomatosis is an autoimmune granulomatous inflammatory disorder with vasculitis associated with an antineutrophil cytoplasmic antibody (Holle & Gross, 2011). It affects the lung with alveolar hemorrhage and the kidneys with necrotizing glomerulonephritis. In addition to peripheral neuropathy, Wegener's causes CNS infiltrating granulomas of the meninges and within CNS, with symptoms that resemble those seen in other vasculitides.

Sarcoidosis is a multisystem granulomatous disease of unknown etiology with wide-ranging effects on the nervous system. It produces cranial mono or polyneuropathies, peripheral neuropathy, myopathy, and meningeal infiltration, and occasionally causes cerebral granulomas with confusion, psychosis, memory loss, and seizures (Sharma, 1997; Terushkin et al., 2010). The diagnosis is made by finding lymphadenopathy on chest X-ray or CT, elevated serum angiotensin-converting enzyme, gallium uptake in lymph nodes, and enhancing lesions in meninges and brain, and treatment is with corticosteroids and steroid-sparing immune modulating agents.

Systemic lupus erythematosus (SLE) has protean manifestations in the central nervous system, including focal neurologic and debilitating neuropsychiatric features (see Joseph, Lammie, & Scolding, 2007; ACR Ad Hoc Committee, 1999; Sciascia et al., 2013). As stated above, the tetrad of headache, seizure, psychosis, and stroke is helpful in determining whether CNS lupus could be the basis of a patient's subacute cognitive and/or neuropsychiatric decline. Strokes may be small or large vessel, and cortical or subcortical. The term *psychosis* here is used loosely to include a range of manifestations such as confusion, anxiety, depression, mania, and mild cognitive impairment. Cognitive defects may have some relation to the presence of antiphospholipid antibodies, disease activity, and chronic damage (Sciascia et al., 2013). Seizures may be focal or generalized, and headache can be a minor or predominant aspect of the constellation. The diagnosis poses a challenge, and clinical suspicion leads the practitioner to obtain the appropriate laboratory tests to establish the diagnosis with sufficient certainty to warrant targeted therapy. Management is optimally undertaken together with colleagues in rheumatology and allied fields, such as in the setting of stroke in lupus, with antiphospholipid antibodies (Kitagawa, Gotoh, Koto, & Okayasu, 1990) and noninfectious endocarditis (Libman-Sacks).

Acute Disseminated Encephalomyelopathy

This postinfectious immune-based disorder occurs as a monophasic illness, is less common in adults than in children, and can be devastating and life-threatening unless recognized and promptly treated. The disease is located in the cerebral white matter, causes marked edema in the area of demyelination and necrosis, is multifocal and asymmetric (Fig. 15.9), and can spread to contiguous or unconnected brain regions within a matter of days. The early manifestations depend on the location of the initial insult and can include cortical sensory syndromes of the parietal lobe (neglect, alien limb) among its early features. Headache may be part of the early clinical syndrome, but this is not invariable. As the illness progresses, cognitive and sensorimotor deficits mount to the point of decreased arousal, leading to coma from brain edema and herniation. MRI shows the dramatic and progressive multifocal demyelination with necrosis, sometimes with hemorrhagic transformation. CSF (obtained prior to the brain swelling that would be a contraindication to lumbar puncture) shows lymphocytic pleocytosis. These cases can resolve dramatically within days when treated with intravenous immunoglobulin (IVIG). Corticosteroids are reported to be first-line treatment (e.g., Sonneville, Klein, de Broucker, & Wolff, 2009) but in our experience in two dramatic adult cases were ineffective and delayed time to initiation of the effective IVIG therapy. Recognition of the early features of the clinical scenario, including recent viral infection within the preceding 2 to 30 days, cognitive and or neuropsychiatric manifestations with multifocal demyelination associated with edema and prominent gadolinium enhancement on brain image, can lead to a gratifying outcome.

Mitochondrial Encephalopathy With Lactic Acidosis and Stroke-Like Episodes

Mitochondrial encephalopathy with lactic acidosis and stroke-like episodes (MELAS) is a multisystem progressive neurodegenerative disorder associated with polygenetic, maternally inherited, mitochondrial

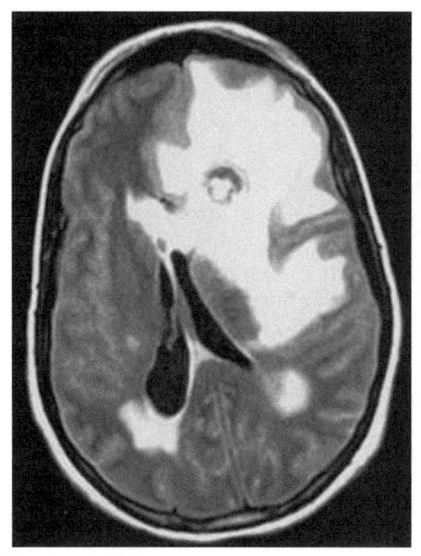

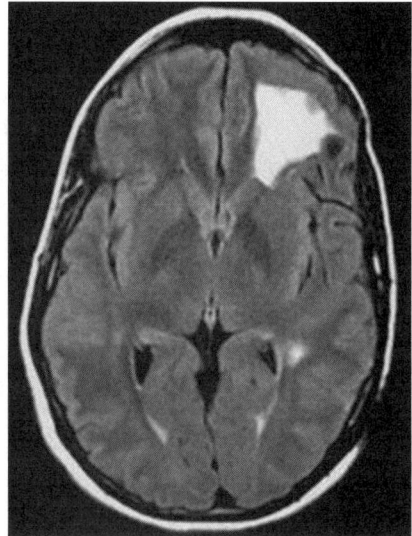

Figure 15.9 Axial fluid attenuated inversion recovery sequence (FLAIR)-weighted magnetic resonance imaging (MRI) scans in a 23-year-old woman with acute disseminated encephalomyelitis, during the acute life-threatening stage (left) and after recovery following treatment with intravenous immunoglobulin (right).

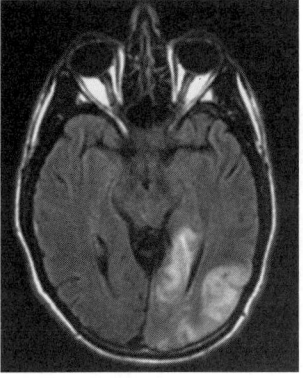

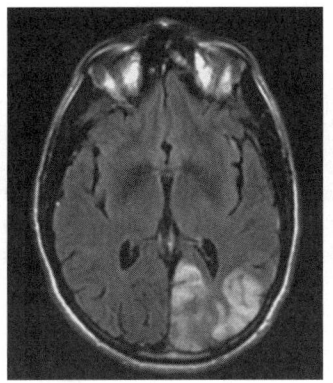

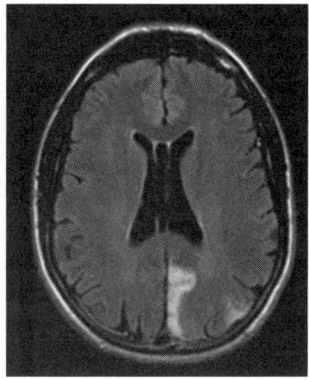

Figure 15.10 Axial fluid attenuated inversion recovery sequence (FLAIR)-weighted magnetic resonance imaging (MRI) scans (from ventral to dorsal, right to left) in a middle-aged man with mitochondrial encephalomyopathy, lactic acidosis, and stroke-like episodes (MELAS) showing signal abnormality and mild vasogenic edema in the left cerebral cortex and subjacent white matter of the posteromedial temporal lobe, occipital lobe, and medial and lateral parietal convexities. These findings resolved radiographically and clinically following treatment with intravenous high-dose methylprednisolone. (From Walcott et al., 2012)

DNA mutations (DiMauro & Hirano, 2001; Sproule & Kaufmann, 2008). It is characterized by headache, depression, seizure, encephalopathy, and recurrent neurological deficits labeled stroke-like because of their abrupt onset and focal manifestation. Other systemic manifestations include cardiomyopathy, diabetes mellitus, and sensorineural hearing loss. The diagnosis is suggested by the combination of stroke-like episodes, progressive encephalopathy leading to dementia, and convulsive or noconvulsive seizures. The range of clinical manifestations reflects the phenomenon of heteroplasmy, with variable penetrance occurring in different cells. The most frequent causative genetic mutation is the A-to-G transition at position 3243 of the mitochondrial genome, which can be tested in commercial laboratories. Psychiatric presentations are described, including confusion, aggression, hallucinations, and paranoia (Kaufman, Zuber, Rueda-Lara, & Tobia, 2010; Kim, Schmahmann, Falk, Stern, & Norris, 1999). The progressive elaboration of structural deficits over time leads to a multi-domain dementia. The location of the lesions in the acute episodes determines the nature of the clinical presentation, and the key feature on brain imaging is that the lesion is not confined to vascular territories (Fig. 15.10). The stroke-like episodes may be principally located in the cerebral cortex, but they can also involve white matter, independently or together with the cortical injury. The precise cause of the acute event and its pathophysiology is not fully established, although hypotheses have been offered together with evidence that the acute episodes can resolve with the use of corticosteroids (Walcott et al., 2012). Other therapeutic approaches have met with variable success, including the use of coenzyme Q-10, arginine, and succinate. One may be alerted to test for this unusual disorder when a relatively young person presents with recurrent episodes of confusion and focal neurological deficits, and brain imaging shows acute ischemic injury in the atypical pattern of being confined to the cortex but in a distribution that does not match a known vascular territory. The serum lactic acid is elevated, muscle biopsy shows the expected ragged red fibers (subsarcolemmal aggregates of enlarged and abnormal mitochondria on the Gomori trichome stain), and gene testing identifies the mitochondria mutation. When the case is rapidly evolving, one does not have the luxury of time to wait for the genetic diagnosis to be established; in these cases, muscle biopsy to confirm the clinical suspicion is a defensible approach.

Prion Disease

This group of disorders is presented last in this category only because it is presently incurable, but it is of great clinical and neurobiological importance and is always to be considered in the differential diagnosis of rapidly progressive dementia. Prion protein C is a normal alpha helical, transmembrane protein encoded by PRNP gene on chromosome 20. Diseases of human prions include Creutzfeldt-Jakob disease (CJD), fatal familial insomnia, Gerstmann-Straussler-Scheinker syndrome (GSS), and kuru. A brain disease in sheep, scrapie, was described in 1732 and was subsequently recognized as a transmissible spongiform encephalopathy (Alper, Cramp, Haig, & Clarke, 1967; Prusiner, 1982). Kuru was the first transmissible spongiform encephalopathy (TSE) recognized in humans, described in the Fore tribes of Papau, New Guinea who engaged in ritual endocannibalism (Brown, 1954; Gajdusek, Gibbs, & Alpers, 1966; Zigas & Gajdusek, 1957). Kuru affected the women and children of the tribe who ingested brain tissue. Tremor (shivering = kuru) and cerebellar ataxia, with dementia and myoclonus commenced within 9–24 months (Collinge et al., 2008). The hypothesis that TSE was caused by an infectious agent consisting solely of proteins without nucleic acid was developed when Alper, Cramp, Haig, and Clarke (1967) showed that scrapie was very resistant to radiation, and Griffith (1967) proposed mechanisms whereby this may happen. The emerging biology of these noninfectious particles later named prions (Prusiner, 1982) initiated the study of protein misfolding or conformational change as the cause of the spongiform encephalopathy characteristic of CJD, and which has become recognized as the basis for a wide range of neurodegenerative diseases (e.g., Takalo, Salminen, Soininen, Hiltunen, & Haapasalo, 2013). The brain pathology of kuru was subsequently shown to include plaques reactive to the prion protein in sheep with scrapie (PrPSc). The PrPSc is a beta-helical, intracellular protein that is protease resistant and polymerizes into fibrils or rods. In humans, mutations in different regions of the prion protein are associated with infectious neurodegenerative diseases that have very different clinical manifestations and neuropathological lesions, a phenomenon that is now being explored in the knock-in mouse model, which shows that single codon differences in a single gene in an otherwise normal genome can cause remarkably different neurodegenerative diseases and are sufficient to create distinct protein-based infectious elements (Jackson et al., 2013). It is therefore important for the clinician to consider prion diseases as more than just an academic exercise about rare conditions, because the biological principles governing prions may have direct relevance for some of the most pervasive and presently intractable neurodegenerative disorders in clinical practice.

Creutzfeldt-Jakob Disease

A common polymorphism at codon 129 of the prion protein (PrP) gene encodes methionine (Met) or valine (Val) and influences susceptibility in familial cases of Creutzfeldt-Jakob disease (CJD), and the specific genotype at codon 129 influences the phenotype of sporadic CJD (Palmer, Dryden, Hughes, & Collinge, 1991). Five phenotypically distinct subtypes of the PrP have been identified in the more common sporadically presenting cases of CJD, based on the Met/Val polymorphic genotype of codon 129 of the PrP gene (the great majority of which are homozygous for either Met or Val) and the presence of either one of the two protease K-resistant PrPSc types identified as 1 and 2 (Cali et al., 2009).

Creutzfeldt-Jakob disease has an incidence of about 1 case per million. In medical centers that serve large populations, it is not unreasonable to expect to see a patient with this disorder a few times annually. Sporadic CJD accounts for 85%–95% of cases, familial transmission occurs in 5%–15%, and iatrogenic transmission in <5% of cases (from human-derived pituitary hormone therapy, dural grafts and dural material for embolization, cornea and liver transplants, neurosurgical instruments, and depth electrodes). The mean age of onset is in the early 60s. The mean duration of the illness is 4–5 months and rarely more than 2 years. The disease presents with the triad of ataxia, dementia, and myoclonus, in varying combinations and in varying degrees. The dementia may include problems with concentration, memory, judgment, personality, and depression or disinhibition. The ataxia is not necessarily typical of cerebellar gait impairment, as the gait may fail for reasons related to noncerebellar systems engaged in the complex act of walking. Myoclonus occurs commonly,

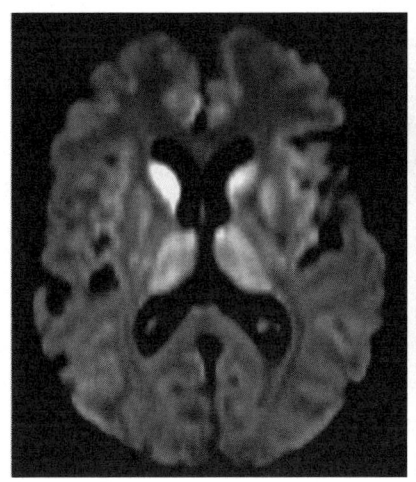

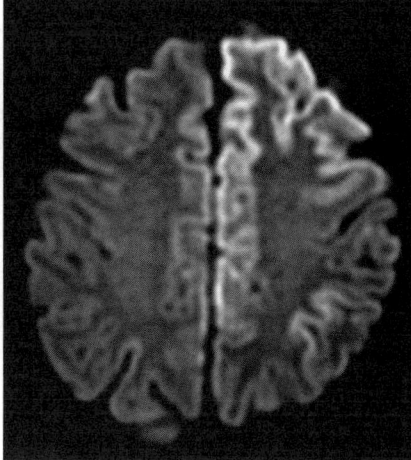

Figure 15.11 Axial diffusion-weighted magnetic resonance imaging (MRI) scans in two patients with Creutzfeldt-Jakob disease. Signal abnormality is seen maximally in the thalamus and caudate nucleus with mild involvement of the putamen and insular cortices in one case (left). Asymmetric L>R cortical ribbon signal hyperintensity is evident in the second case (right).

provoked by acoustic, tactile, or visual startle in 90% of cases. Approaching the patient with an ophthalmoscope may be sufficient to provoke a truncal myoclonic jerk. Early visual loss reflects occipital location of the pathology in the Heidenhain variety (Cooper, Murray, Heath, Will, & Knight, 2005), and cerebellar ataxia and oculomotor abnormalities in the Brownwell-Oppenheimer variant (1965) reflecting the cerebellar predominant location of the disease. Extrapyramidal (bradykinesia, rigidity) and corticospinal findings such as spasticity and hyperreflexia (40%–80%) reflect the basal ganglia and motor cortical involvement, and thalamic pathology adds to the complexity of the cognitive, affective, and sensorimotor phenomena. The diagnosis is supported by finding periodic triphasic waves on EEG in 67%–95% of cases, with a sensitivity of 67% and specificity of 86%. CSF analysis includes elevated protein and a modest leukocytosis with the presence of 14-3-3 protein, which has a sensitivity of 53% to 85% and specificity of 95%. The pathology is spongiform degeneration and astrogliosis diffusely distributed throughout the cortex, basal ganglia, thalamus, and cerebellum. The diagnostic procedure of choice is MRI that shows hyperintense signal on diffusion-weighted imaging (DWI) and FLAIR imaging in the locations most affected, including the cerebral cortical ribbon, thalamus, and basal ganglia (Fig. 15.11). Treatment trials have been disappointing, and successful therapies are yet to be developed. Management of seizures with antiepileptic agents and of myoclonus with benzodiazepines and levetiracetam can be effective as symptom-based interventions.

Variant CJD is the human counterpart to bovine spongiform encephalopathy (BSE) acquired by ingesting contaminated beef or beef products with BSE. It is exceedingly rare. Described in 1996 (World Health Organization, 1996), it affects younger individuals (mean age 29), has a relatively slower progression (mean 14 months), and is marked by the psychiatric presentation with depression, anxiety, and psychosis, followed 4–6 months later by ataxia, dysarthria, and dementia. Sensory abnormalities are notable, myoclonus is occasionally observed, diffuse slowing is detected on EEG (not triphasic waves), and unlike CJD, the MRI is not definitive. The PrPSc subtype 4 may be identified on biopsy of lymph tissue such as the tonsil, but this raises considerable issues of sterility and transmissibility for personnel and equipment. The brain pathology includes diffuse spongiform changes and kuru-like plaques—dense amyloid deposition surrounded by a halo of vacuolation (Ironside, 1998; Mastrianni, 2003).

Fatal familial insomnia is an autosomal dominant disorder caused by a D178N mutation of the prion protein gene on chromosome

20 in conjunction with methionine at codon 129 mutation of the prion protein gene (Tian et al., 2013). The disease rarely presents as a nonfamilial case. It has a mean age of onset of 35 to 61 years and a mean duration of 13 months. Pathological findings include neuronal dropout and gliosis primarily within the thalamus and inferior olivary nucleus, with relative lack of spongiform degeneration in the cerebral cortex (DeArmond & Prusiner, 1997). The illness is characterized by rapidly progressive insomnia, abnormal sleep architecture on EEG, prominent autonomic alterations (hypertension, episodic hyperventilation, excessive lacrimation, sexual and urinary tract dysfunction, change in basal body temperature), and dementia with confusion, impaired concentration, poor memory, and hallucinations. Brainstem and cerebellar involvement manifest as vertical gaze palsy, nystagmus, dysarthria, and ataxia. Myoclonus, spasticity, and extrapyramidal features are also described (Brown & Mastrianni, 2010; Lugaresi et al., 1986; Xie et al., 2013).

Gerstmann-Straussler-Scheinker is an extremely rare, autosomal dominant disorder caused by mutations in the prion protein gene. Insidious onset commences around age 30 to 50, and the course averages about 3 to 7 years. Some patients have a predominantly cerebellar motor presentation; others have a cognitive decline with features suggestive of a frontotemporal dementia. Pyramidal involvement is heralded by spasticity; extrapyramidal involvement manifests with bradykinesia, increased muscle tone with or without cogwheeling, and masked facies. The pathology includes kuru-like amyloid plaques, which bind to PrP, and AD-like tangles (Brown & Mastrianni, 2010; DeArmond & Prusiner, 1997).

Uncommon Disorders With Multidomain Subacute Cognitive Decline

Progressive Multifocal Leukoencephalopathy

Depending on the location of the pathology in progressive multifocal leukoencephalopathy (PML), this disorder may present with subacute cognitive decline in up to one half of affected patients rather than sensorimotor impairment, or visual loss that occurs with posterior brain lesions. PML is the result of infection of CNS myelin-producing oligodendroglia by the JC polyomavirus. It occurs in the immunocompromised host, most commonly in the setting of HIV disease with CD4 lymphocyte count <200 cells/mm^3, nonsolid malignancies such as Hodgkin's disease and other lymphomas, chronic corticosteroid or immunosuppressive therapy following organ transplantation, and more recently, in the setting of treatment with natalizumab for autoimmune disorders such as multiple sclerosis, rheumatoid arthritis, and systemic lupus erythematosis. Brain MRI is strongly suggestive, revealing multifocal, nonconfluent, bilateral, asymmetric white matter hyperintensities in juxta-cortical white matter on FLAIR and T2-weighted imaging (Fig. 15.12). These only occasionally enhance with gadolinium; about 15% in HIV-associated PML, up to 40% in natalizumab-associated disease (Berger et al., 2013). Confluent areas of white matter abnormality may extend across the corpus callosum and down into deep regions as well, including the white matter tracts that traverse subcortical nuclei such as thalamus. It can extend into the cerebral peduncle, and when PML involves cerebellum it can envelope the deep nuclei with a curved appearance (shrimp sign, N. Venna, personal communication; Sahraian, Radue, Eshaghi, Besliu, & Minagar, 2012; Schmahmann, 1998; Schutte, Ranchhod, Kakaza, & Pillay, 2013). The leukoencephalopathy of PML differs from that of HIV leukoencephalopathy, which tends to be diffuse, bilateral, symmetric, and predominantly in the periventricular white matter. Diagnosis of PML can be established from the clinical setting, the brain imaging findings, and the presence of JC virus in the CSF detected by polymerase chain reaction. Brain biopsy is seldom required, and when performed, it shows the characteristic triad of multifocal demyelination, hyperchromatic, enlarged oligodendroglial nuclei with nuclear inclusions (JC virus), and enlarged bizarre astrocytes with lobulated hyperchromatic nuclei (Berger et al., 2013). The illness has a mortality rate of 30% to 50% in the first few months without treatment, but this has improved in patients with HIV since the introduction of combination antiretroviral therapy (CART), and in the case of natalizumab, removal of the inciting agent hastened by the use of plasmapheresis and corticosteroids to manage the immune

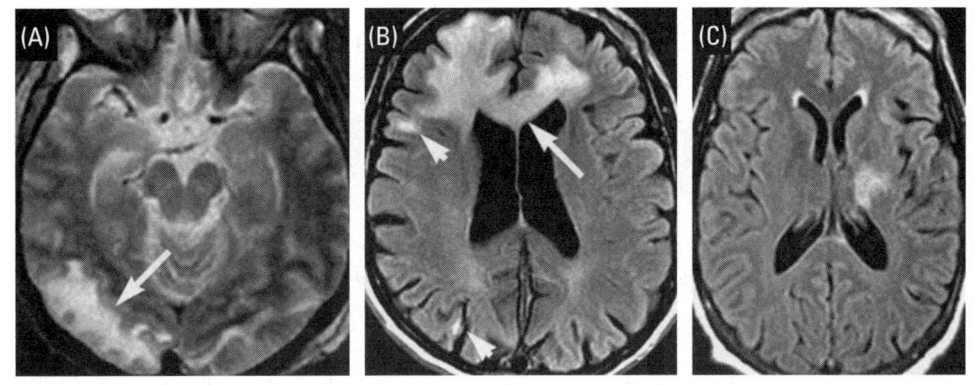

Figure 15.12 Brain magnetic resonance imaging (MRI) scans in two young men with progressive multifocal leukoencephalopathy in the setting of HIV. Hyperintense signal is seen in the right occipital cortex and white matter in the axial T2-weighted image in one case who presented with a left homonymous hemianopsia (*A*). The other patient with prominent abulia has multiple areas of signal hyperintensity on fluid attenuated inversion recovery sequence (FLAIR)-weighted axial images; bilaterally in the frontal lobes straddling the corpus callosum, in the right posterior parietal cortex (*B*), and in the deep white matter of the left hemisphere including the thalamus (*C*).

reconstitution inflammatory syndrome (Berger, 2011; Tan, McArthur, Clifford, Major, & Nath, 2011).

Intravascular Lymphoma

This rare (1 per million) subtype of extranodal diffuse large B-cell lymphoma affects elderly patients (median age 70) and is characterized by proliferation of clonal lymphocytes within small vessels with relative sparing of the surrounding tissue. It has a predilection for the central nervous system (see Ferreri et al., 2004; Zuckerman, Seliem, & Hochberg, 2006). It causes progressive cognitive and motor decline associated with focal areas of ischemia in cortical and subcortical regions on brain imaging, but without overt imaging evidence of vascular abnormality. Systemic manifestations include B symptoms (fever, night sweats, and weight loss) and anemia, with focal sensory or motor deficits, generalized weakness, confusion, rapidly progressive dementia, seizures, hemiparesis, dysarthria, ataxia, vertigo, and transient visual loss. It mimics other central nervous system diseases, the prominent subcortical white matter lesions (Fig. 15.13) reminiscent of cerebral vasculitis and the demyelination of multiple sclerosis. Patients may have high serum lactate dehydrogenase levels and lymphocytosis in the CSF, although cytopathology is rarely positive for malignant cells (Baehring, Longtine, & Hochberg, 2003). The diagnosis can only be made with certainty on brain biopsy, showing large malignant lymphocytes filling the lumina of small vessels. If diagnosed premortem, the disease may be cured by aggressive chemotherapy.

Subacute Sclerosing Panencephalitis

Subacute sclerosing panencephalitis (SSPE), a late complication of the measles virus, is rarely encountered in the United States, but it is not uncommon in developing countries like India (e.g., Chakor & Santosh, 2013). The ease of international travel, and international adoption, make it imperative to have a passing knowledge of this condition. SSPE has a latency after active measles infection of approximately 6 to 15 years. Its manifestations include personality change with confusion, agitation, and memory loss. Cortical blindness from the posterior location of the lesions may be a heralding sign. Myoclonus is common and can be incapacitating when generalized. Convulsive or noconvulsive status epilepticus occur. Ataxia and spasticity result from damage to motor pathways. The EEG shows generalized slowing with periodic complexes; serum and CSF analysis reveals the presence of IgG measles antibodies. The course is relentlessly progressive and rapid (18 months), leading to severe dementia 1 to 2 years after clinical onset. Involvement

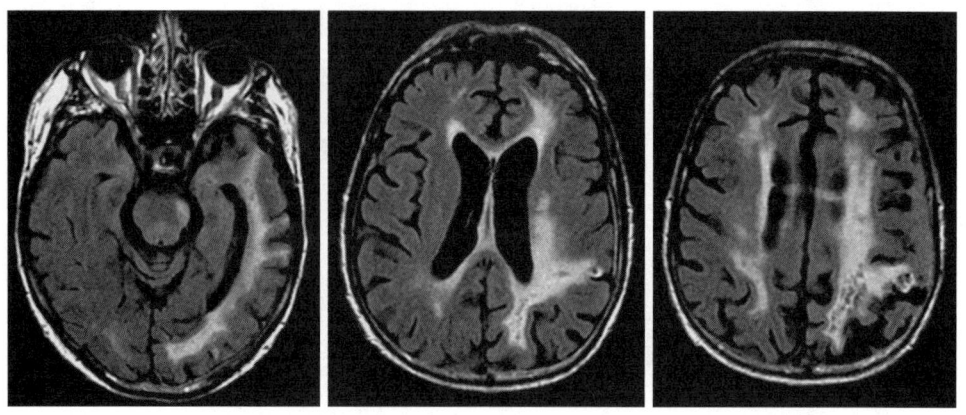

Figure 15.13 Axial fluid attenuated inversion recovery sequence (FLAIR)-weighted magnetic resonance imaging (MRI) scans (from ventral to dorsal, right to left) in an elderly man with subacute progression over weeks of cognitive change and right hemiparesis. Brain biopsy confirmed intravascular lymphoma.

of the brainstem results in dysautonomia, coma, and a vegetative stage. There is no effective cure at this time. Brain MRI findings range from normal initially, to hyperintensities on FLAIR and T2 images asymmetrically in parieto-occipital cortical-subcortical regions, symmetrically in the periventricular white matter (Ozturk, Gurses, Baykan, Gokyigit, & Eraksoy, 2002), and in the basal ganglia (Turaga, Kaul, Haritha Chowdary, & Praveen, 2012) and cerebellum (Fig. 15.14). As the disease progresses, there is increasing loss of white matter with cortical atrophy, and in the final stage most of the white matter is lost, the ventricles and extracerebral CSF spaces are severely widened, and posterior fossa structures show marked atrophy (Brismar, Gascon, von Steyern, & Bohlega, 1996; Turaga, Kaul, Haritha Chowdary, & Praveen, 2012).

Whipple's Disease of the Nervous System

Whipple disease (WD) is a chronic, relapsing, multisystem infection caused by the gram-positive bacillus *Tropheryma whippelii*. Systemic symptoms include fever and weight loss with gastrointestinal, arthritic, cardiac, ocular, and cutaneous manifestations (Schmahmann, 2006). Isolated CNS involvement occurs in about 5% of cases, has

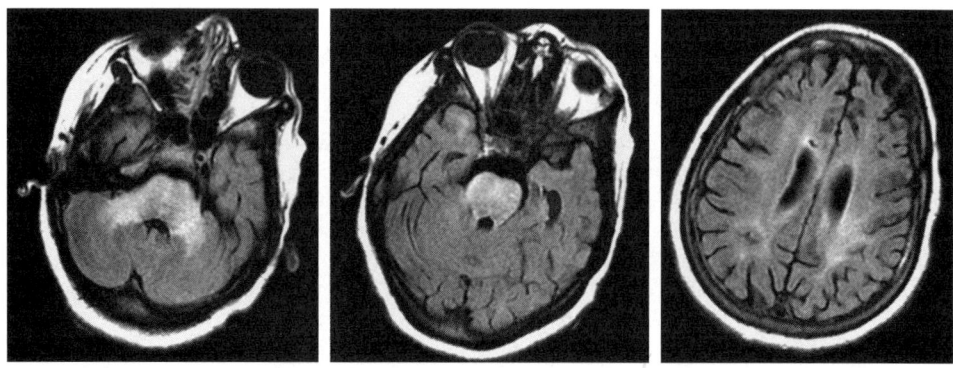

Figure 15.14 Axial fluid attenuated inversion recovery sequence (FLAIR)-weighted magnetic resonance imaging (MRI) scans (from ventral to dorsal, right to left) of a young woman with confusion, lethargy, and gait impairment, showing signal abnormality in the pons, middle cerebellar peduncles, and to a lesser extent in the cerebral white matter. A clinical diagnosis of subacute sclerosing panencephalitis was confirmed at autopsy.

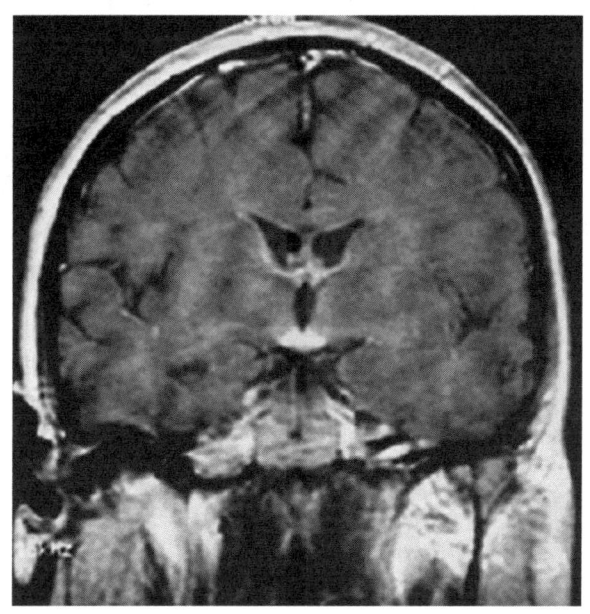

Figure 15.15 Coronal contrast enhanced T1-weighted magnetic resonance imaging (MRI) in a middle-aged woman with subacute confusion, memory loss, vertical gaze palsy, syndrome of inappropriate antidiuretic hormone secretion, and amenorrhea. Biopsy of the enhancing hypothalamic lesion confirmed central nervous system Whipple's disease.

a predilection for the midbrain and hypothalamus (Fig. 15.15), and has four main clinical presentations (Gerard et al., 2002; Smith, French, Gottsman, Smith, & Wakes-Miller, 1965). (1) Oculomasticatory myorhythmia consists of pendular convergent oscillations of both eyes with concurrent contractions of the jaw and tongue, occurring at a rate of 1 to 2 Hz, associated also with semirhythmic blinking, and movements of the proximal upper and lower extremities (oculo-facial-skeletal-myorhythmia). (2) Supranuclear vertical ophthalmoplegia may be accompanied by horizontal gaze palsy, with absent pupil response with attempted convergence but preserved with light (the opposite of the Parinaud syndrome). (3) Cognitive changes evolving over weeks or months include an amnestic syndrome with confabulation, delusional thinking, confusion, apathy, and disorientation, and personality changes include irritability, depression, paranoia, and hallucinations. (4) Hypothalamic involvement produces sleep disruption, polydipsia, hyperphagia, hypothermia, syndrome of inappropriate antidiuretic hormone secretion, and amenorrhea. MRI reveals T-2 and FLAIR hyperintense lesions in hypothalamus, rostral brainstem, medial temporal regions, and the basal ganglia. The diagnosis is confirmed by polymerase chain reaction on blood and CSF, which may also reveal foamy PAS-positive mononuclear cells. Diagnosis may require duodenal biopsy, and in extraordinary cases when clinical suspicion is high, brain biopsy may be necessary looking for granulomatous inflammation with granular ependymitis, microglial nodules, neuronal loss, and rod-shaped bacilli within macrophages and glia demonstrable with silver stains. Cephalosporins are the treatment of choice.

Dementia From Diseases Predominantly Affecting Cerebral White Matter

The concept of white mater dementia introduced in 1998 (Filley, 1998, 2012; Filley, Franklin, Heaton, & Rosenberg, 1988) rests on the fact that the cerebral white matter conveys the association fiber tracts linking cerebral cortical association areas with each other, as well as the striatal and projection fibers that link the association cortices with their interconnected subcortical nodes in the basal ganglia, thalamus, and cerebrocerebellar circuits (Schmahmann & Pandya, 2006,

2007, 2008). These fiber pathways are critical anatomical substrates of the distributed neural circuits (Goldman-Rakic, 1988; Jones & Powell, 1970; Mesulam, 1981; Nauta, 1964; Pandya & Kuypers, 1969; Schmahmann & Pandya, 2006) that provide the anatomical underpinning of cognition along with all neurological function. The notion that hemiparesis or visual loss arises from interruption of the corticospinal tracts or the optic radiation, respectively, provides historical empiric support for the importance of the white matter for neurological function. The description of disconnection syndromes resulting from disruption of these white matter pathways (Geschwind, 1965a, b) introduced behavioral neurology and neuropsychiatry as a rigorous intellectual discipline. It is now clear that whereas focal white matter lesions can lead to focal neurobehavioral syndromes, large-scale devastation of cerebral white matter leads to large scale devastation of cognitive function—hence, white matter dementia (WMD).

The clinical pattern seen in WMD includes disorders of executive function, together with deficits in memory, visuospatial impairment, and psychiatric presentations, ranging from disinhibition to paranoia, obsessive-compulsive behaviors, delusions, and hallucinations (Filley, 2001; Schmahmann, Smith, Eichler, & Filley, 2008). Depending on the exact nature and extent of the pathology, there may be preserved language, procedural memory, and extrapyramidal function (Filley, Heaton, Nelson, Burks, & Franklin, 1989). WMD is thus distinct from the cortical dementias in which memory encoding and language are usually impaired, and from the cognitive decline arising from lesions of the deep nuclei (basal ganglia and thalamus) in which extrapyramidal function and/or procedural memory are typically affected (Lafosse, Corboy, Leehey, Seeberger, & Filley, 2007; Schmahmann, 2003). For a list of diseases that affect the cerebral white mater disproportionately or primarily, see Table 15.3, Schmahmann, Smith, Eichler, and Filley (2008), and Filley (2012). Selected examples are highlighted later in the chapter, and others that may rightly be considered together with the WMDs (such as SSPE, PML, ADEM, SLE, MELAS, and HIV) are described elsewhere in this chapter.

Demyelinating Diseases

Multiple Sclerosis

Perhaps the paradigmatic white matter disease, MS is now known to cause destruction not only of myelin, but it also affects axons (Medana & Esiri, 2003), the gray matter of cerebral cortex (Stadelmann, Albert, Wegner, & Bruck, 2008), and subcortical areas, including thalamus (Minagar et al., 2013). Much is written about this frequently occurring nervous system illness, but less attention has been paid to the fact that cognitive impairment occurs in 40%–65% of affected individuals (Jongen, Ter Horst, & Brands, 2012; Rao, Leo, Bernardin, & Unverzagt, 1991), and dementia has an estimated prevalence as high as 23% (Boerner & Kapfhammer, 1999). Cognitive problems are seen in the subclinical radiologically isolated syndrome, clinically isolated syndrome (Fig. 15.16), and all phases of clinical MS, and can be prominent in pediatric-onset MS (Jongen, Ter Horst, & Brands, 2012). A wide range of focal neurobehavioral syndromes and neuropsychiatric disturbances are reported, including disorders of complex attention, information processing speed, episodic memory, and executive functions (Filley, 2001). Recognition of these nonmotor manifestations is important because disease-modifying agents may halt the clinical progression or lead to clinical improvement.

Susac Syndrome

Susac syndrome is an autoimmune endotheliopathy affecting the precapillary arterioles of the brain, retina, and inner ear (Rennebohm, Susac, Egan, & Daroff, 2010; Susac, 1994). It occurs across the age spectrum, with women (20–40 years) most vulnerable. The inflammatory vasculopathy produces multifocal brain demyelination, including the corpus callosum, and a clinical triad of sensorineural hearing loss, visual loss from branch retinal artery occlusion, and encephalopathy. Headache is a constant feature of the presentation and occurs particularly along with the encephalopathy. This rare disorder (304 cases in the published literature; Dorr et al., 2013) has a wide differential, including MS and other vasculitides, given that it can manifest with

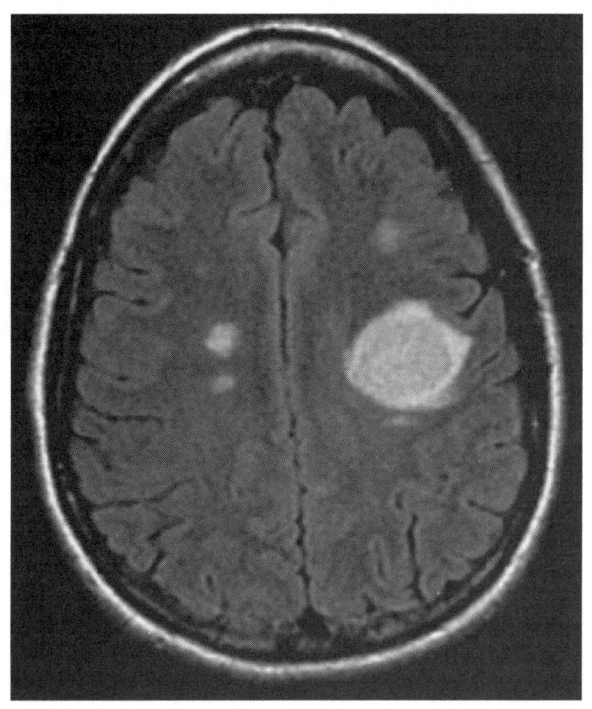

Figure 15.16 Axial T1-weighted magnetic resonance imaging (MRI) following gadolinium administration in a young woman with impaired speech shows enhancing cerebral white matter lesions L>R. The pattern of the demyelinating injury is consistent with Balos's concentric sclerosis.

cognitive and psychiatric features. Hearing loss is reported in 86% of cases, but at disease onset the expected triad of impaired vision, hearing, and mentation occurs in only 13% of cases. The encephalopathy occurs in 76% of cases over the course of the illness and is characterized by cognitive impairment, mainly deficits in memory, concentration, and executive functions; confusion with disorientation; and changes in behavior and personality with apathy, psychosis, and decreased arousal. Personal experience of one case was a severe amnestic dementia in a man in his 30s, associated with hearing loss, cerebellar motor findings, and branch retinal artery occlusions on the diagnostic test of fluorescein angiography. The brain MRI is very suggestive, if not pathognomonic, showing what have been called snowball lesions in the corpus callosum (Fig. 15.17), with multiple lesions—string of pearls—in the internal capsule (bright on diffusion-weighted imaging). The diagnosis can be established by a combination of clinical features, MRI findings, and fluorescein angiography and audiology testing. Treatment is with aggressive and prolonged immunosuppressants to prevent the multiphasic form of the illness.

Acquired Leukodystrophies

In delayed posthypoxic leukoencephalopathy, massive cerebral demyelination with delayed onset occurs in the setting of a unique combination of factors precipitating a hypoxemic ischemic event. The sequence of events most commonly described is an onset over hours of a sublethal dose of the three main forms of cerebral hypoxemia described by Plum and Posner (1966). Namely, anoxic anoxia (low environmental tension, depressed respirations, impaired pulmonary function), anemic anoxia (the oxygen-carrying capacity of blood is depleted as occurs with carbon monoxide), and ischemic anoxia (poor cerebral blood flow as in cardiac failure). Common scenarios include overdose of medication that both depress respiration and blood pressure such as hydrocodone, exposure to carbon monoxide (Lee & Marsden,

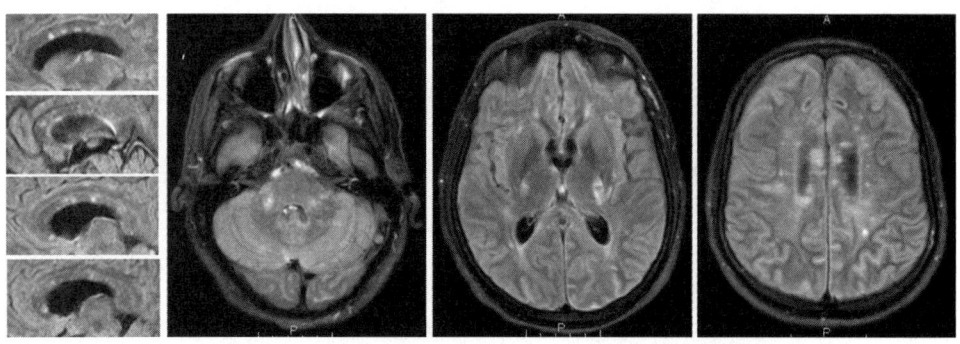

Figure 15.17 Fluid attenuated inversion recovery sequence (FLAIR)-weighted magnetic resonance imaging (MRI) in a young man with impaired gait, profound anterograde memory loss, and confusion in the setting of Susac syndrome. Sagittal images at left show the snowball appearance of lesions of the corpus callosum. The axial images (from ventral to dorsal, right to left) show signal hyperintensities in the middle cerebellar peduncles, posterior limb of the internal capsule L>R, and coronal radiata.

1994), slow and prolonged hypoxemia with hypotension as occurs in strangulation with attempted suicide, partial airway obstruction or prolonged respiratory arrest, and hemorrhagic shock. The characteristic feature is the near-death experience of the patient (Chen-Plotkin, Pau, & Schmahmann, 2008) with unresponsiveness or coma for a period of minutes to hours, followed by complete or near-complete recovery to full motor and cognitive health for a period of 2–3 weeks. The patient then slides into a neuropsychiatric decline of altered behavior, forgetfulness, inattention, confusion, gait impairment, bradykinesia, and incontinence, progressing to hypokinesia and immobility to the point of akinetic mutism with striking generalized rigidity and cortical blindness (Chen-Plotkin, Pau, & Schmahmann, 2008; Shprecher & Mehta, 2010; Schmahmann, other unpublished cases). The brain MRI typically shows symmetric white matter T2 and FLAIR hyperintensities, with diffusion-weighted imaging showing restricted diffusion of the white matter confirmed on apparent diffusion coefficient mapping. Over a matter of weeks, and more notable some months later, is a dramatic loss of volume of cerebral white matter with ex vacuo hydrocephalus (Fig. 15.18). Recovery is variable. Some patients may return to a more functional baseline, although psychiatric features and executive failure persist (Shprecher & Mehta, 2010; Schmahmann, unpublished data), while in other cases the rigid akinetic state persists with only minimal improvement over time. It is important to recognize this rare but essentially pathognomonic narrative of the acute initiating event followed by a period of near normalcy and then the subacute slide (days to a week or two) into the rigid akinetic mute state accompanied by new, diffuse leukoencephalopathy. This entity needs to be differentiated from acute disseminated encephalomyelitis (ADEM) and other toxic leukoencephalopathies that have a different history and imaging pattern, so as to avoid invasive diagnostic procedures such as brain biopsy. Hyperbaric oxygen treatment for acute carbon monoxide poisoning appears warranted (Weaver, Valentine, & Hopkins, 2007), but there are no studies of this approach in the patient with hypoxic ischemic injury entering phase 2 of the illness (the decline after recovery). The predilection for this complication of hypoxia is not known, and the suggestion that partial arylsulfatase deficiency is responsible in susceptible individuals (Weinberger, Schmidley, Schafer, & Raghavan, 1994) has not been borne out by subsequent studies.

Professional underwater divers report problems with long- and short-term memory and impaired concentration (Todnem, Nyland, Kambestad, & Aarli, 1990). Divers who have experienced decompression sickness (Caisson disease, nitrogen gas embolism after surfacing too rapidly from depths greater than 10 meters) have impairments in thinking, visualspatial function, and memory, along with subcortical white matter abnormalities on brain MRI (Levin et al., 1989). Seven of 19 divers studied with a battery of neuropsychological

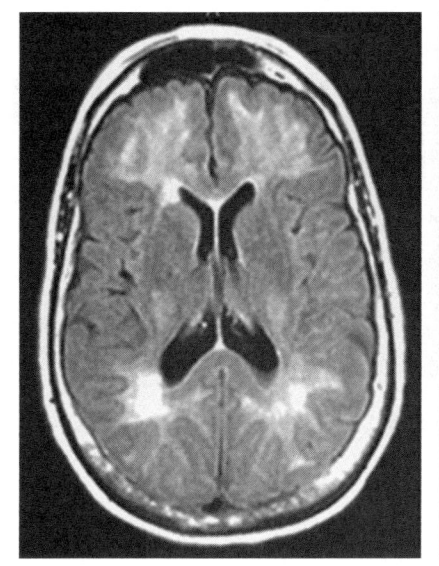

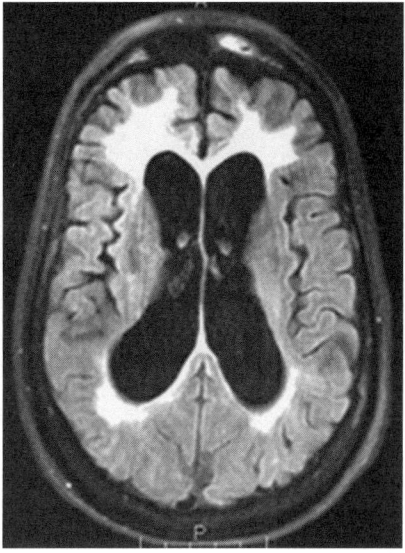

Figure 15.18 Axial fluid attenuated inversion recovery sequence (FLAIR)-weighted magnetic resonance imaging (MRI) in an elderly woman with delayed posthypoxic leukoencephalopathy. The left image was taken at the time she presented 2 weeks after recovery from the acute hypoxic event, with increasing confusion, amnesia, and bradykinesia. The right image was taken 2 years later and shows the loss of cerebral white matter with signal hyperintensity and ex vacuo ventriculomegaly.

tests (Peters, Levin, & Kelly, 1977) performed significantly below a control group on verbal and nonverbal tests, and they had impaired memory with marked disruption of storage of new information, reduced attention span (tested with forward digit span), slowed processing speed (Trails A test), and deficient mental flexibility (Trails B test; Peters, Levin, & Kelly, 1977). These cognitive features may occur together with or independent of the acute sequelae of decompression sickness, ranging from spinal cord lesions with paralysis, to hemianopsia, confusion, and coma, and more chronic neurological findings such as cerebellar ataxia and facial paralysis (Peters, Levin, & Kelly, 1977). Further, elderly recreational compressed-air divers who have not experienced decompression sickness ("the bends") have white matter hyperintensities on brain MRI greater in number and size than controls, which correlate with the number of hours of diving and are associated with decreased mental flexibility and poorer performance on tasks of visual tracking (Tetzlaff et al., 1999).

Electrical injury produces long-term cognitive and neuropsychiatric sequelae following lightning strikes, and industrial or residential accidents. These include deficits in attention, concentration, and verbal learning and recall as well as anxiety and somatic preoccupations (Duff & McCaffrey, 2001). Psychiatric diagnoses including depression with or without posttraumatic stress disorder were reported in 78% of a sample of 86 patients who suffered electrical injury, and these patients also showed impairments on tests of attention, verbal memory, and executive function (Ramati et al., 2009).

Toxic leukoencephalopathies result from exposure to agents that have a predilection for the cerebral white matter. Toluene (methylbenzene) is a household and industrial organic solvent used in glue and spray paint. It produces euphoria when inhaled and is a major drug of abuse. It produces an essentially pure leukoencephalopathy with selective myelin loss that spares the cerebral cortex, neurons, and axons in all but the most severe cases (Filley, Heaton, & Rosenberg, 1990; Rosenberg et al., 1988). The clinical manifestation is a syndrome of dementia, ataxia, dysarthria, and spasticity. Brain MRI reveals diffuse cerebral and cerebellar white matter hyperintensity. The degree of cerebral involvement strongly correlates with the severity of dementia. Autopsy reveals selective myelin loss that spares the cerebral cortex.

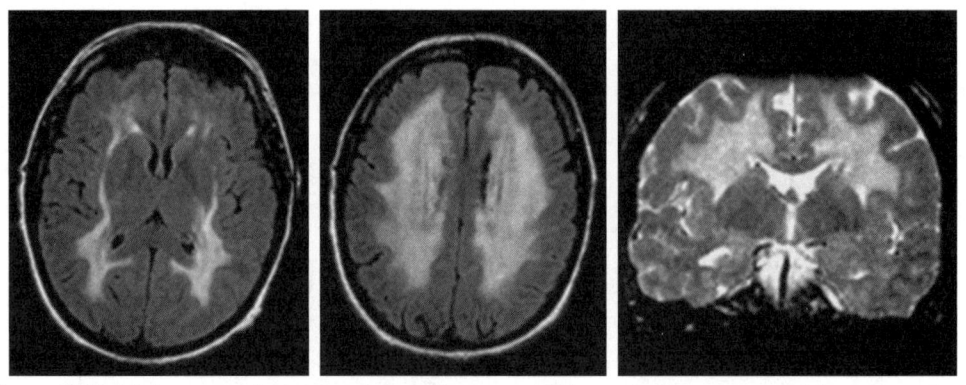

Figure 15.19 Methotrexate leukoencephalopathy in a middle-aged man seen on fluid attenuated inversion recovery sequence (FLAIR)-weighted magnetic resonance imaging (MRI). Left and middle: axial plane; right: coronal plane.

Methotrexate (MTX) chemotherapy may produce diffuse hemispheric demyelination (Fig. 15.19) and a clinical syndrome of cognitive slowing, executive dysfunction, and forgetfulness, although this adverse consequence is not universal and patients may experience only mild cognitive slowing (Fliessbach et al., 2005). Focal and sometimes reversible neurological syndromes caused by MTX are associated with discrete white matter lesions (Salkade & Lim, 2012), in addition to its recognized causative link to the posterior reversible encephalopathy syndrome (Henderson, Rajah, Nicol, & Read, 2003; Matsuda et al., 2011). The pathology of MTX toxicity includes a disseminated necrotizing leukoencephalopathy with prominent spheroids involving frontal and temporal lobes disproportionately, a disseminated demyelinating leukoencephalopathy with widespread demyelinated foci without significant axonal changes localized mainly in the occipital lobe (Matsubayashi, Tsuchiya, Matsunaga, & Mukai, 2009), and a severe demyelinating, partially liquefactive necrosis-like lesion symmetrically in the cerebral hemispheres, internal capsule, cerebral peduncle, pons, and pontocerebellar fibers but sparing the temporal lobes and the rostral parts of the frontal lobes (Yokoo et al., 2007).

Cranial irradiation has direct effect on cerebral white matter, producing a leukoencephalopathy in about one third of patients followed for more than 6 months. The clinical disorder is more severe in patients greater than 65 years of age (Ebi, Sato, Nakajima, & Shishido, 2013). The likely basis is radiation-induced vasculopathy leading to slowly evolving ischemic damage to the white matter.

Postchemotherapy cognitive impairment, referred to as chemo-brain or chemo-fog by patient support groups, occurs after systemic chemotherapy, particularly for breast cancer. Deficits are reported in verbal and visual spatial abilities, executive function, and mood (Ganz et al., 2013; Jim et al., 2012). The risk of this disorder is greater in patients who are older and have less cognitive reserve, and genetic factors appear to play a role (Rodin & Ahles, 2012). The underlying mechanism is not established, although preliminary data correlate changes in attention and executive function with decreased connectivity in dorsal attention and default mode networks on resting-state functional connectivity MRI (Dumas et al., 2013).

Inhalation of heated heroin vapor ("chasing the dragon") produces a progressive spongiform leukoencephalopathy with a cerebellar motor syndrome (ataxia, dysmetria, and dysarthria), bradykinesia, rigidity, and hypophonia, progressing over weeks to pseudobulbar palsy, akinetic mutism, decorticate posturing, and spastic quadriparesis. Death occurs in approximately 20% of cases. MRI reveals symmetric and widespread involvement of the white matter of the posterior cerebral hemispheres, corpus callosum, cerebellum, and brainstem. MR spectroscopy demonstrates depressed N-acetyl aspartic acid (NAA) indicating neuronal loss as well as a lactate peak (Fig. 15.20; Bartlett & Mikulis, 2005; Kriegstein et al., 1999; Offiah &

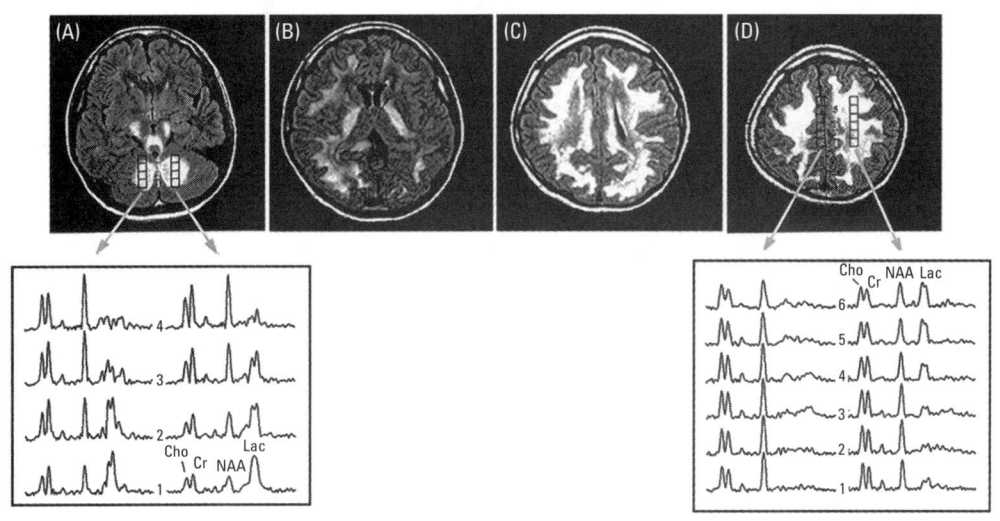

Figure 15.20 Axial fluid attenuated inversion recovery sequence (FLAIR)-weighted magnetic resonance imaging (MRI) in the axial plane (*A* through *D*, ventral to dorsal) in a young man following heroin inhalation, or chasing the dragon. Corresponding 1H magnetic resonance spectrography imaging in two of the images shows characteristic lactate peak and decreased N-acetyl aspartic acid (NAA). (From Kriegstein et al. 1999 reproduced with permission)

Hall, 2008). Clinical and MRI findings can progress after cessation of drug use. The brain shows spongiform degeneration of white matter with relative sparing of U-fibers (Kriegstein et al., 1999). The MRS evidence of lactate peak, mitochondrial swelling and distended endoplasmic reticulum in oligodendrocytes, and apparent benefit of antioxidants and mitochondrial cofactors suggest mitochondrial dysfunction (impaired energy metabolism at the cellular level) as a basis for this disorder (Bartlett & Mikulis, 2005; Kriegstein et al., 1999; Wolters et al., 1982). Notably, cocaine use can produce a similar syndrome, sometimes with good recovery. The precise pathophysiology is unknown (Bartlett & Mikulis, 2005; Bianco, Iacovelli, Tinelli, Lepre, & Pauri, 2011).

Genetic Diseases

The leukodystrophies are a heterogeneous group of genetic diseases involving dysmyelination, and some are a result of substrate accumulation due to enzymatic defects. This group includes adult-onset leukodystrophy with neuroaxonal spheroids, metachromatic leukodystrophy, globoid cell leukodystrophy, and vanishing white matter disease that are autosomal recessive, and X-linked adrenoleukodystrophy. Collectively, the incidence of these conditions rivals that of MS. The incidence of adrenoleukodystrophy alone is 1 in 17,000, or 20,000 patients annually in the United States (Bezman et al., 2001). (For further discussion of these disorders, see Costello, Eichler, & Eichler, 2009; Kohlschutter & Eichler, 2011; Schmahmann, Smith, Eichler, & Filley, 2008.) Related genetic white matter predominant disorders include MELAS and FXTAS, and they are described elsewhere in this chapter.

Adult-onset leukodystrophy with neuroaxonal spheroids (AOLNAS) is a familial or sporadic disorder characterized radiographically by symmetric, bilateral, T2 hyperintense and T1 hypointense MRI signal involving frontal lobe white matter. Neuropathological examination demonstrates a severe leukodystrophy with myelin and axonal loss, gliosis, macrophages, and axonal spheroids, with early and severe frontal white matter involvement, and complete sparing of cerebral cortical neurons (Freeman et al., 2009; Marotti, Tobias, Fratkin, Powers, & Rhodes, 2004). Freeman et al. (2009) detected abnormalities in mitochondrial enzymes and complex 1 deficiency in one case suggesting mitochondrial dysfunction. The genetic basis at least in a subset of cases has been defined in a recent report (Kleinfeld et al., 2013) showing a disease-causing mutation in the colony-stimulating factor 1 receptor (CSF1R) gene. The disorder presents with executive system dysfunction and other neurobehavioral deficits, progressing to dementia. The extent and degree of change outside the frontal lobe correlates with disease duration. The white matter containing long association tracts interconnecting parietal, temporal, and occipital lobes with the frontal lobe are affected early and most severely. The rostral and caudal parts of the corpus callosum are also involved early in the course, reflecting loss of white matter, particularly in the prefrontal and posterior parietal association areas. In contrast, projection pathways are spared until late in the illness, as exemplified in a patient whose cortical blindness corresponded to the late pathological changes in the sagittal stratum that contains the optic radiations (Freeman et al., 2009). This dichotomy of early dementia, but late failure of gait, strength, dexterity, and sensation, provides an interesting glimpse into the clinicopathological distinction between association and projection fiber tract involvement in AOLNAS, and the functional contributions of these different white matter tracts (Schmahmann, Smith, Eichler, & Filley, 2008).

X-linked adrenoleukodystrophy (X-ALD) is characterized by impaired ability to degrade very long chain fatty acids (VLCFA) that causes malfunction of the adrenal cortex and nervous system myelin (Moser, Smith, Watkins, Powers, & Moser, 2000). It presents in childhood in approximately 35% of patients. Affected boys develop normally until 4 to 8 years of age, then suffer dementia and progressive neurologic decline that leads to a vegetative state and death. More than 90% have adrenal insufficiency. It presents as adrenomyeloneuropathy in young adulthood in 35% to 40% of patients, with progressive paraparesis and sphincter disturbances leading to death in 20% of these patients in <2 years from rapidly progressive inflammatory demyelination (Eichler et al., 2007; van Geel, Bezman, Loes, Moser, & Raymond, 2001). Cerebral X-ALD in adulthood manifests with impaired psychomotor speed, spatial cognition, memory, and executive functions. This can lead to a presentation characterized in one man in his sixth decade by relentlessly progressive dementia with inattention, amnesia, impaired cognitive flexibility, problem-solving skills, and visual spatial disorganization. This progressed to stereotyped nonmeaningful but complex behaviors, relentless wandering, perseveration, apraxia, and posterior aphasia with fluent jargon, impaired comprehension, and poor repetition. In this case there was relative sparing of elementary motor features, normal reflexes, and plantar responses, but striking release phenomena were present, including palmar grasp, snout, root, and suck reflexes (Schmahmann & Eichler in Schmahmann, Smith, Eichler, & Filley, 2008). These very severe cases of global impairment including aphasias (Edwin et al., 1996) have marked brain atrophy on MRI along with the white matter damage. The characteristic finding is symmetric, posterior parietal and occipital periventricular white matter lesions, with a garland of gadolinium contrast enhancement (Melhem, Barker, Raymond, & Moser, 1999; Melhem, Loes, Georgiades, Raymond, & Moser, 2000) reflecting inflammatory demyelination (Fig. 15.21A). MRI spectroscopy in normal-appearing white matter on conventional MRI (Eichler, Barker, et al., 2002; Eichler, Itoh, et al., 2002) shows increased choline and decreased N-acetylaspartate.

Metachromatic leukodystrophy (MLD) is a lysosomal storage disorder resulting from a deficiency of aryl sulfatase A leading to intracellular accumulation of sulfatides. Adult onset is rare and includes psychosis, behavioral disturbances, and dementia (Austin et al., 1968; Hyde, Ziegler, & Weinberger, 1992). MRI reveals diffuse white matter lesions (periventricular, centrum semiovale, corpus callosum, internal capsule, cerebellum; Fig. 15.21B). Punctuate striated (tigroid) enhancement corresponds to patchy areas of preserved myelin (Faerber, Melvin, & Smergel, 1999).

Globoid cell leukodystrophy (GLD), or Krabbe's disease, is caused by deficiency of the enzyme galactosyl ceramidase (GALC) that is responsible for converting galactosylceramide into galactose and ceramide, leading to accumulation of galactosylceramide that prompts a macrophagocytic response, and psychosine that leads to death of myelin-producing oligodendrocytes (see Kohlschutter & Eichler, 2011). Rare adult-onset cases manifest slowly evolving hemiparesis, intellectual

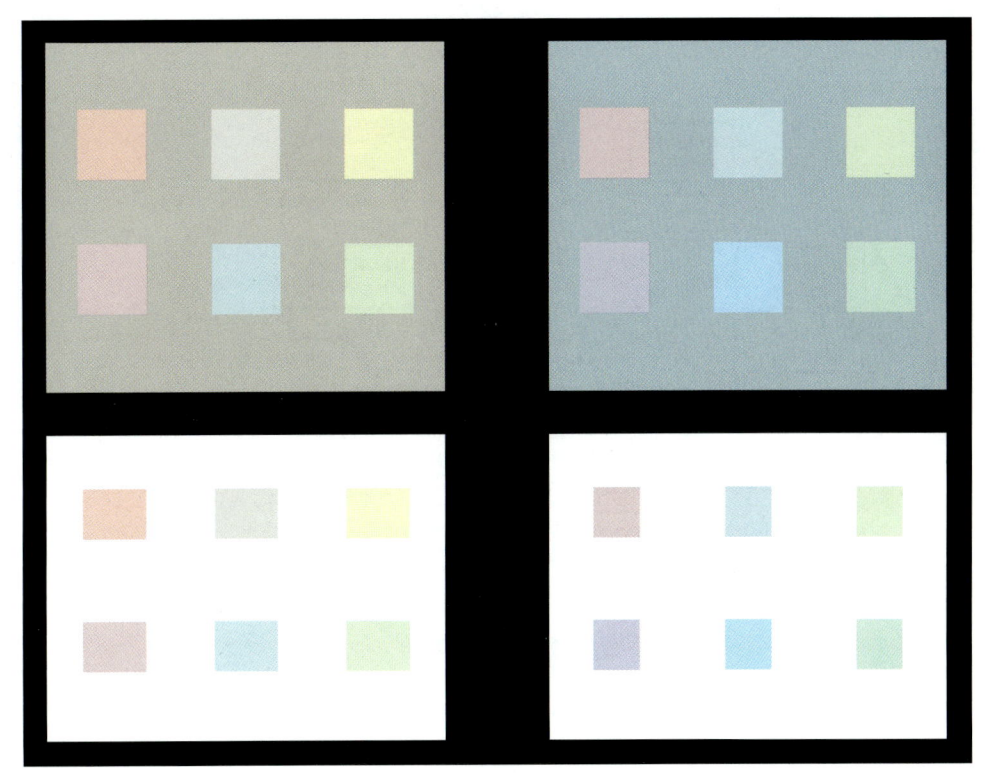

Figure 1.1 Color constancy. The color patches in the top and bottom figures are the same but are matched differently across the left and right rectangles as a function of the color of the background.

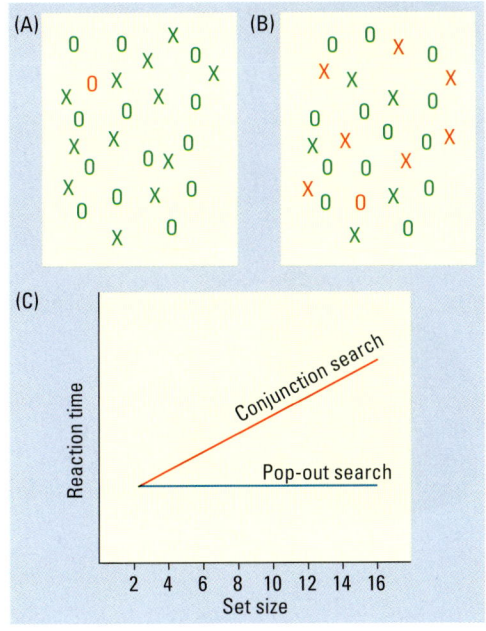

Figure 1.18 Conjunction and pop-out search. In both *A* and *B*, the task is to determine whether a red circle is present. In *A*, the target is defined as the feature in red; in *B*, the target is defined by the conjunction of red and circle. In *C* reaction time is shown for correct detections of present stimuli as a function of set size, consistent with parallel search not requiring serial deployment of attention in *A* and requiring serial deployment of attention in *B*.

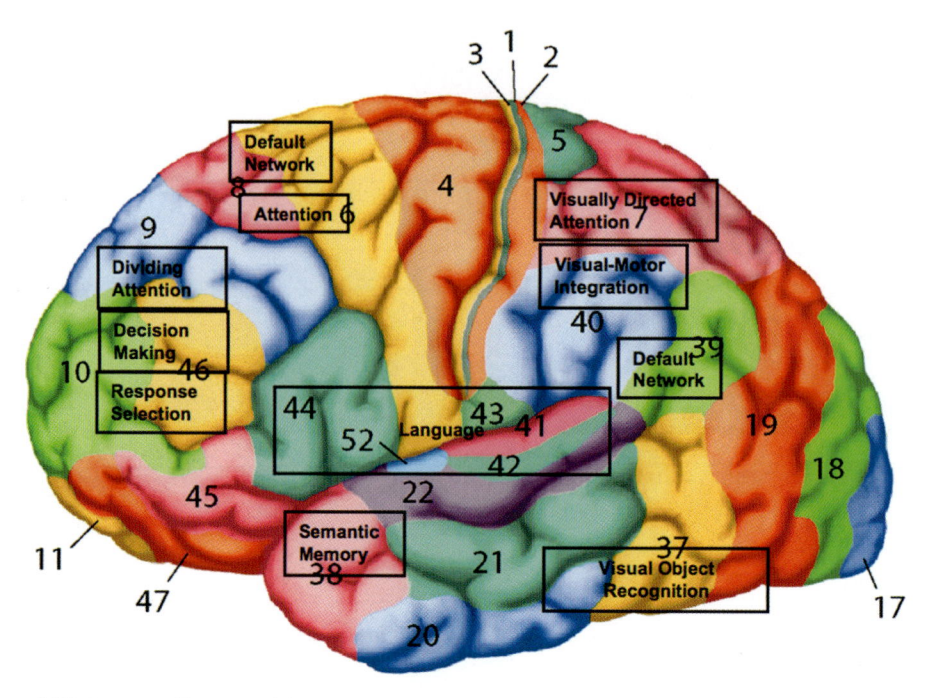

Figure 1.19 Cartoon of location of the major cognitive systems in the lateral human cortex.

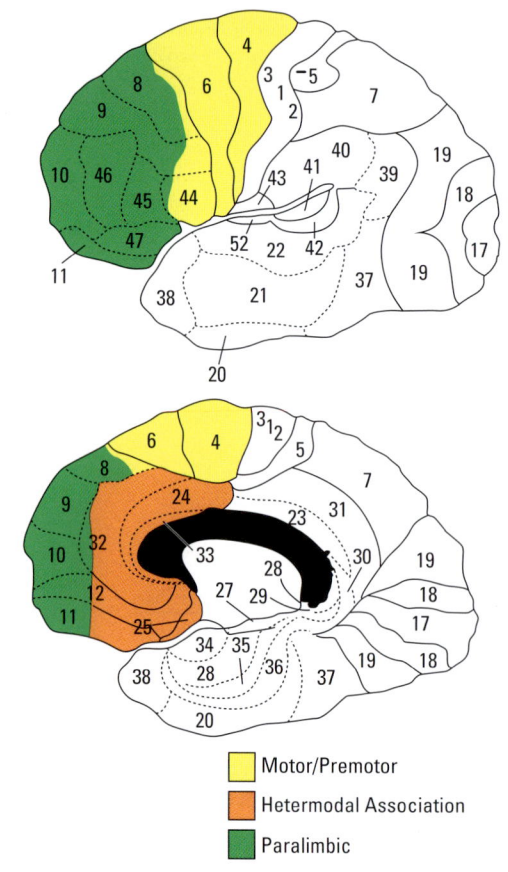

Figure 3.1 Divisions of the frontal lobe. Figure adapted from Mesulam (1986).

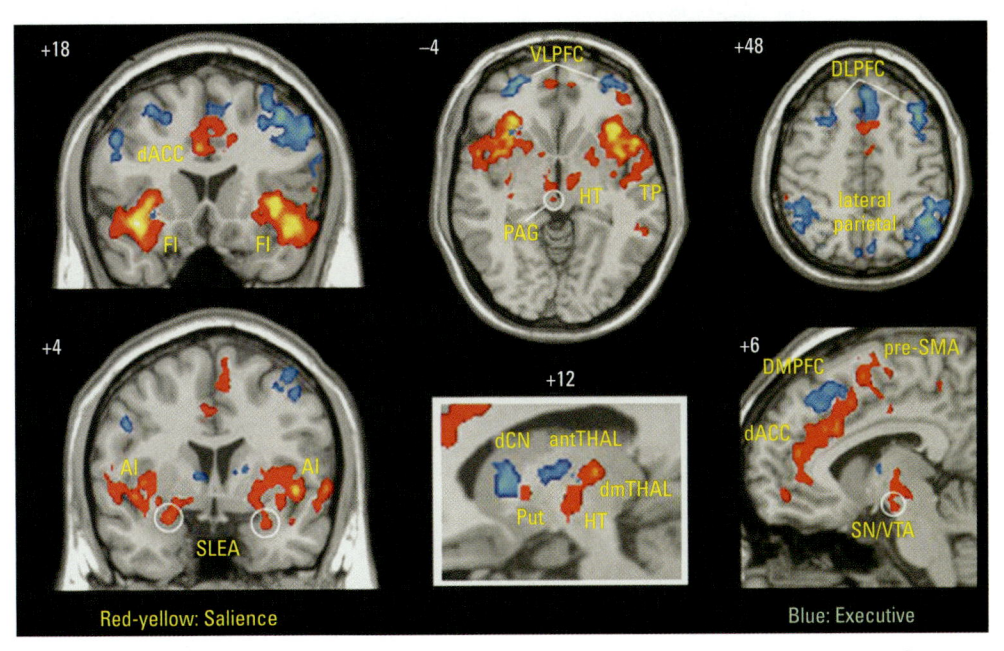

Figure 3.3 Salience and executive control networks revealed through intrinsic connectivity mapping. Image adapted from Seeley et al., 2007.

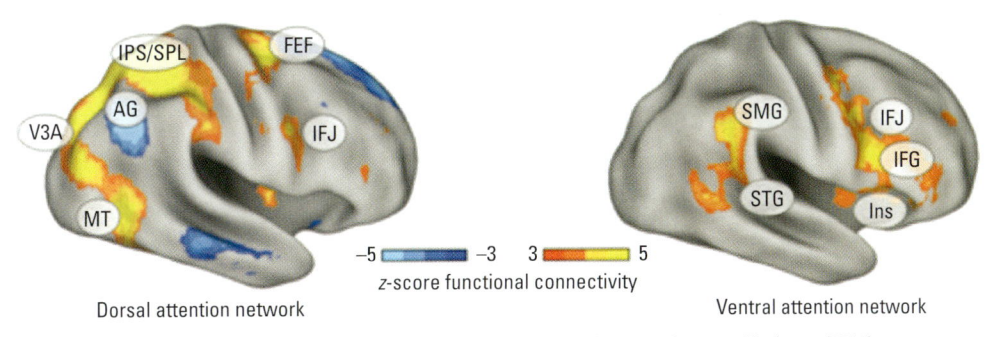

Figure 3.4 Dorsal and ventral attention networks. Image adapted from Corbetta & Shulman (2011).

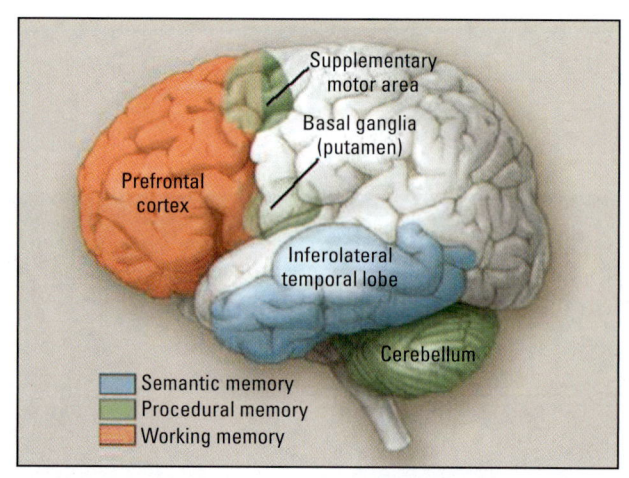

Figure 4.9 Semantic, Procedural, and Working Memory. The inferolateral temporal lobes are important in the naming and categorization tasks by which semantic memory is typically assessed. However, in the broadest sense, semantic memory may reside in multiple and diverse cortical areas that are related to various types of knowledge. The basal ganglia, cerebellum, and supplementary motor area are critical for procedural memory. The prefrontal cortex is active in virtually all working memory tasks; other cortical and subcortical brain regions will also be active, depending on the type and complexity of the working memory task. In addition to being involved in procedural memory, the cerebellum is also important for the motoric conditioning. (From Budson and Price, 2005; permission granted by the *New England Journal of Medicine*.) (See color plate section)

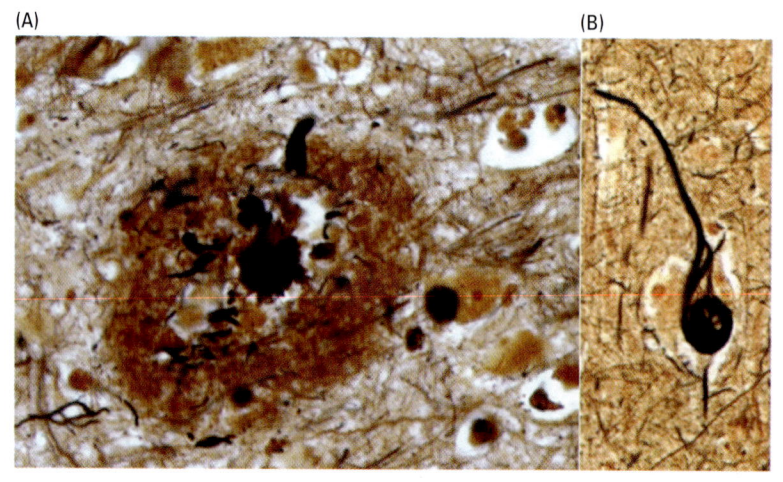

Figure 6.4 Hallmarks of Alzheimer's disease neuropathology: (*A*) neuritic plaques (about 180 μm in diameter; each one replaces an estimated 10^6 synapses and about 100 neurons). The centrally located core is made up of aggregates of amyloid-β, which results from incomplete degradation of a trans-membrane protein present in nerve terminals called amyloid-β precursor protein (APP). The gene for APP is located on chromosome 21. (*B*) Neurofibrillary tangles of Alzheimer and neuropil threads (argyrophilic neurons and threads) consist of intracellular accumulation of paired helical filaments caused by the hyperphosphorylation of tau. Tau protein is a phosphoprotein that binds to and promotes polymerization and stability of microtubules. The tau gene is located on chromosome 17. (Bielschowsky silver stain; original magnification, 630×)

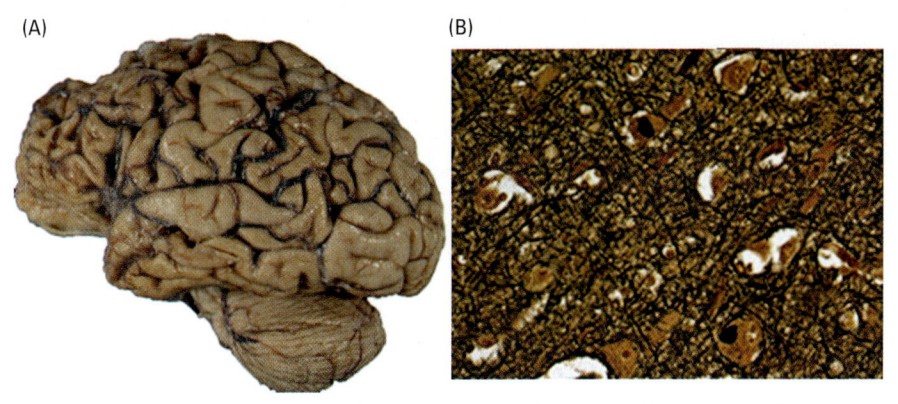

Figure 6.5 (*A*) Formalin fixed, lateral aspect of the left half brain of a 53-year-old patient with frontotemporal lobar degeneration (classical Pick's disease). Note the prominent circumscribed atrophy involving the frontal lobe, rostral temporal lobe, and the inferior parietal lobule. Although atrophic, the pre- and postcentral gyri, the caudal two thirds of the superior temporal gyrus, and occipital lobe are relatively preserved. (*B*) Microphotograph of Pick body containing pyramidal neurons of the third layer of the motor cortex. Pick bodies are argyrophilic, are labeled with AT8 antibodies directed against phosphorylated tau, or with antibodies directed against ubiquitinated proteins. They are not labeled with antibodies directed against α-synuclein aggregates, which is in contrast to Lewy bodies. (Bielschowsky silver stain; original magnification, 400×)

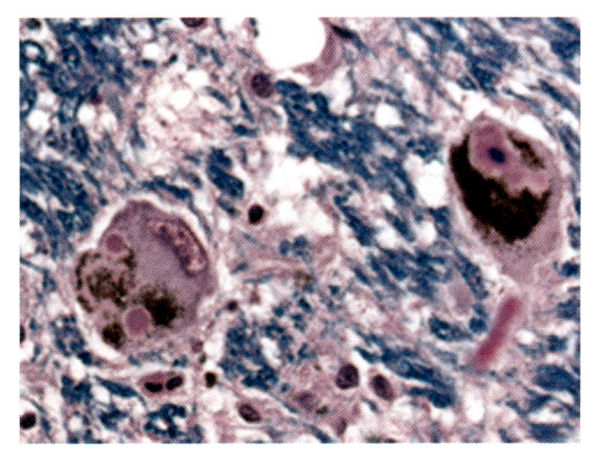

Figure 6.8 Lewy body (brainstem type) is usually round, 8–30 μm in diameter, and consists of a cytoplasmic, hyaline core with or without concentric lamellar bands, and with a peripheral, pale halo. These two Lewy body–containing neurons are from the nucleus coeruleus. One of them has two round Lewy bodies (lower left). The other has a somewhat bilobulated Lewy body with a visible, basophilic, and dark core (upper right). (LHE stain; original magnification, 630×)

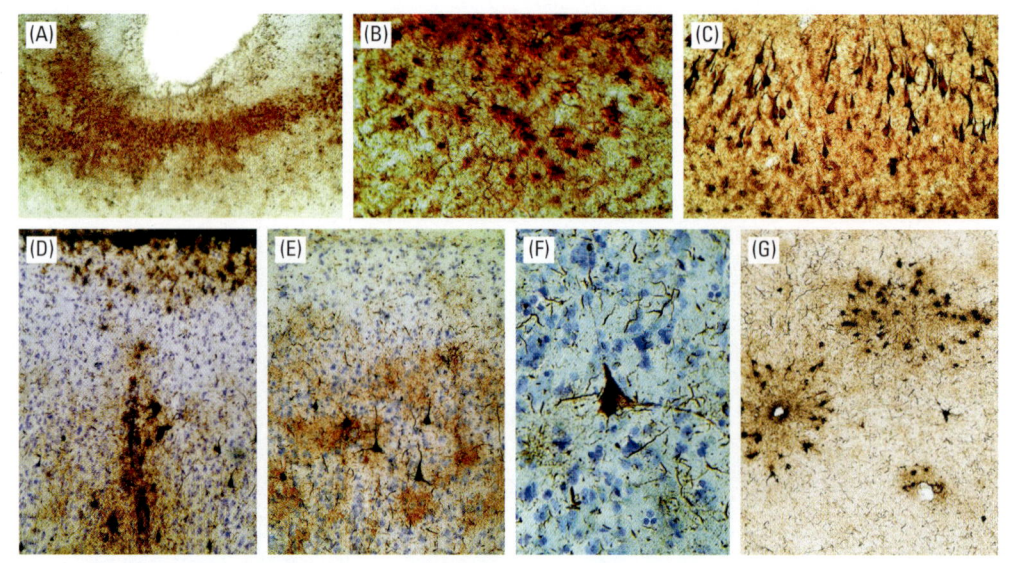

Figure 7.2 Distinctive pattern and morphology of tau immunoreactive neurofibrillary pathology in chronic traumatic encephalopathy. (*A*) Tau immunoreactive neurofibrillary degeneration is often most striking at depths of the sulci accompanied by focal thinning of the cortical ribbon (AT8 immunostain, original magnification, 60×). (*B*) Subpial tau immunoreactive tangles are found in both neurons and astrocytes (double immunostained section for GFAP [red] and AT8 [brown] showing colocalization of tau and GFAP [arrow]; original magnification, 350×). (*C*) Extremely dense NFTs and neuropil neurites are found in the medial temporal lobe structures, including CA1 of the hippocampus, shown here. Senile plaques are absent (AT8 immunostain, original magnification, 150×). (*D*) NFTs and astrocytic tangles tend to be centered around small blood vessels and in subpial patches (AT8 immunostain, original magnification, 150×). (*E*) NFTs characteristically involve cortical layers II and III in association with clusters of tau-positive astrocytic processes (AT8 immunostain, original magnification, 150×). (*F*) NFT in a Betz cell of primary motor cortex (AT8 immunostain, original magnification, 350×). (*G*) There is often a striking perivascular clustering of NFTs around small blood vessels (AT8, original magnification, 150×).

ALZHEIMER'S DISEASE

CHRONIC TRAUMATIC ENCEPHALOPATHY

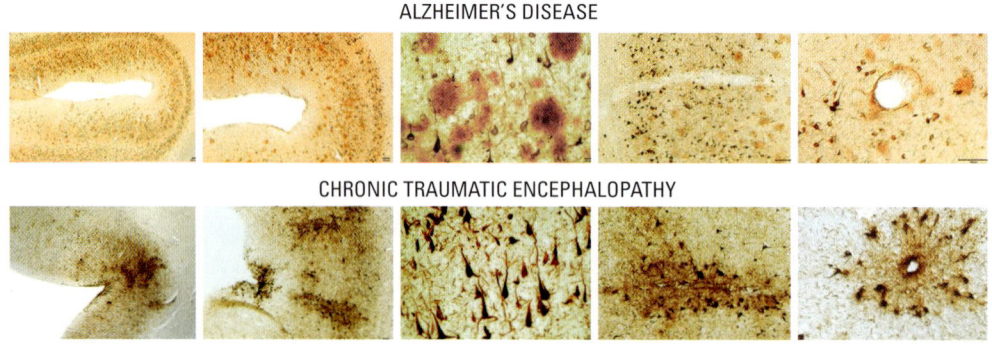

Figure 7.3 How the p-tau pathology of chronic traumatic encephalopathy is distinctive from Alzheimer's disease. (Top row) Alzheimer's disease: Double immunostained sections for Aß (red) and PHF-1 (brown) show diffuse, relatively uniform cortical distribution of NFTs preferentially involving laminae III and V, without accentuation at depths of sulci. Small blood vessels at sulcal depths show no clustering of neurofibrillary pathology perivascularly. There is also no clustering of neurofibrillary pathology in subpial or periventricular regions. (Bottom row) Chronic traumatic encephalopathy: Sections immunostained for AT8 showing irregular cortical distribution of p-tau pathology with prominent subpial clusters of p-tau astrocytic tangles, focal accentuation at depths of sulci, and distribution of NFTs in superficial cortical laminae I–III. Small blood vessels at bottom of cortical sulcus show prominent perivascular distribution of astrocytic tangles and NFTs (AT8). Double immunostained section for Aß (red) and PHF-1 (brown) (center panel) shows dense NFTs without Aß deposition.

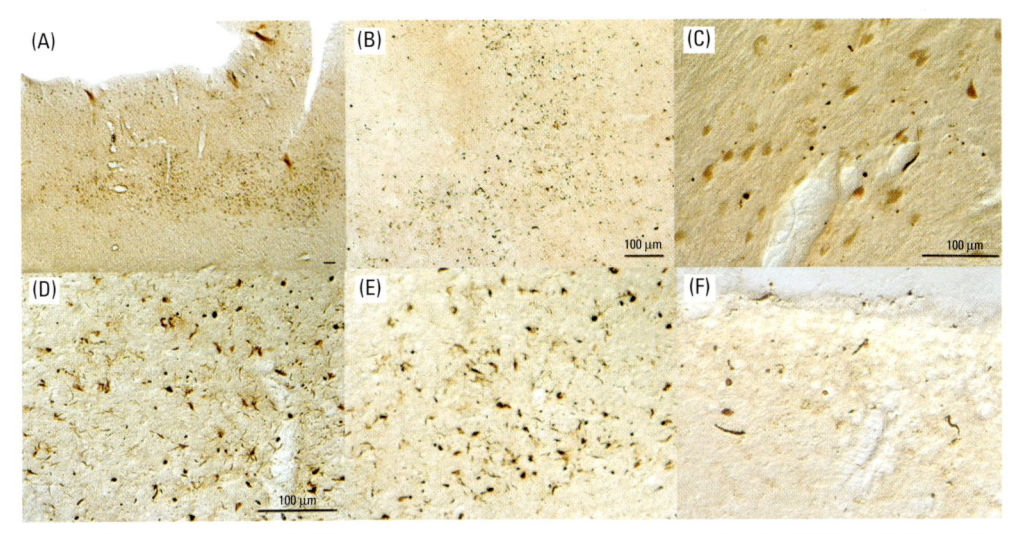

Figure 7.4 The phosphorylated TDP43 pathology of chronic traumatic encephalopathy (CTE). (*A, B, D,* and *E*) Dense pTDP-43 abnormalities are found in the cerebral cortex of stage IV CTE. (*C*) Dense pTDP-43 pathology in substantia nigra pars compacta. (*F*) Pronounced pTDP-43 immunopositive pathology in the periventricular region of the third ventricle. (All images: 50 µm tissue sections; all scale bars, 100 µm)

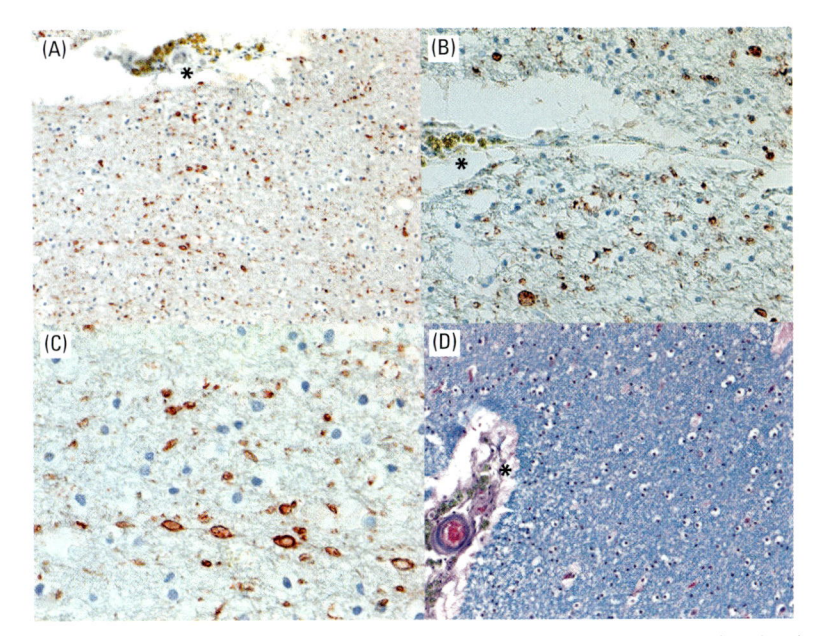

Figure 7.5 The axonal pathology of chronic traumatic encephalopathy (CTE). (*A–C*) Phosphorylated neurofilament staining (SMI-34) in cerebral white matter of stage III CTE shows marked reduction in axonal staining and numerous large, irregular axonal varicosities. A small arteriole shows marked infiltration with hemosiderin-laden macrophages (asterisks). (*D*) Luxol fast hematoxylin blue-stained section of white matter shows brisk astrocytosis, loss of myelinated fibers, and macrophages around vessel (asterisk). (10 µm tissue sections; scale bars: 100 µm)

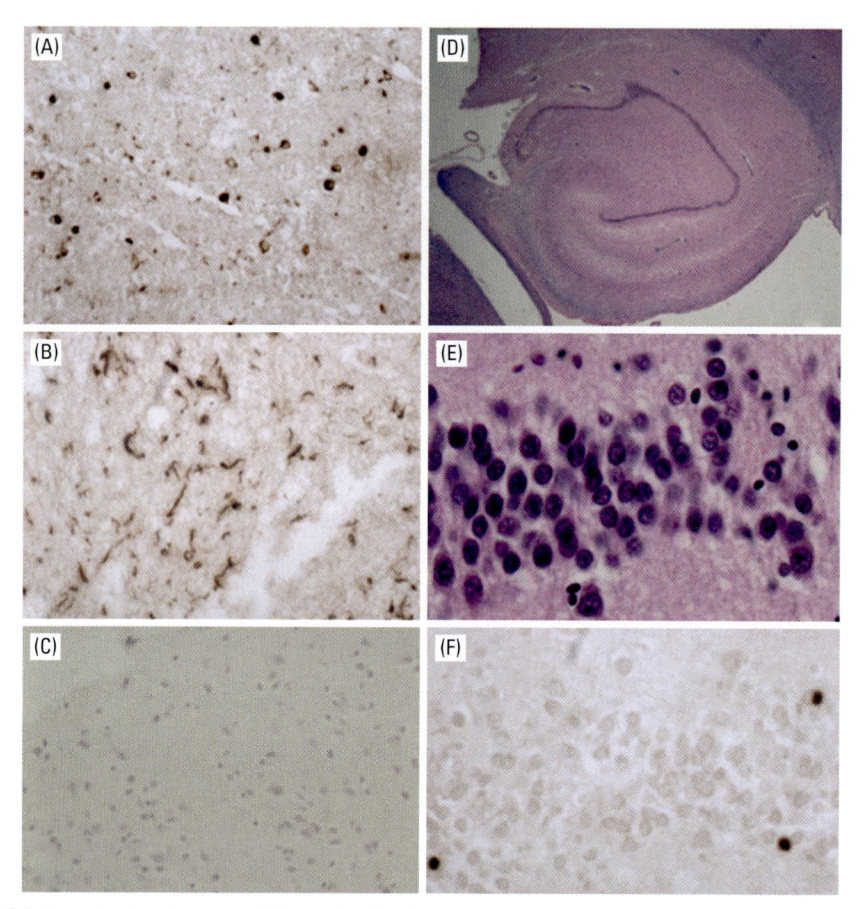

Figure 8.1 Tau pathology in a case of classical Pick's disease prominently affects neuronal and glial cells in gray matter (*A*, labeling with AT8 [phosphorylated tau] immunohistochemistry) and also usually demonstrates prominent abnormalities in white matter (*B*, labeling with AT8 immunohistochemistry) of frontal and temporal cortices, including the dentate gyrus of the hippocampus, with sparing of primary cortices particularly Heschl's and calcarine cortex (*C*, absent labeling with AT8 immunohistochemistry). The hippocampus (*D*, low-power hematoxylin and eosin stain) also classically shows dense, smooth-contoured rounded cytoplasmic inclusions in granule cells of the dentate gyrus (*E*, high-power hematoxylin and eosin stain), which are labeled with AT8 immunohistochemistry (*F*).

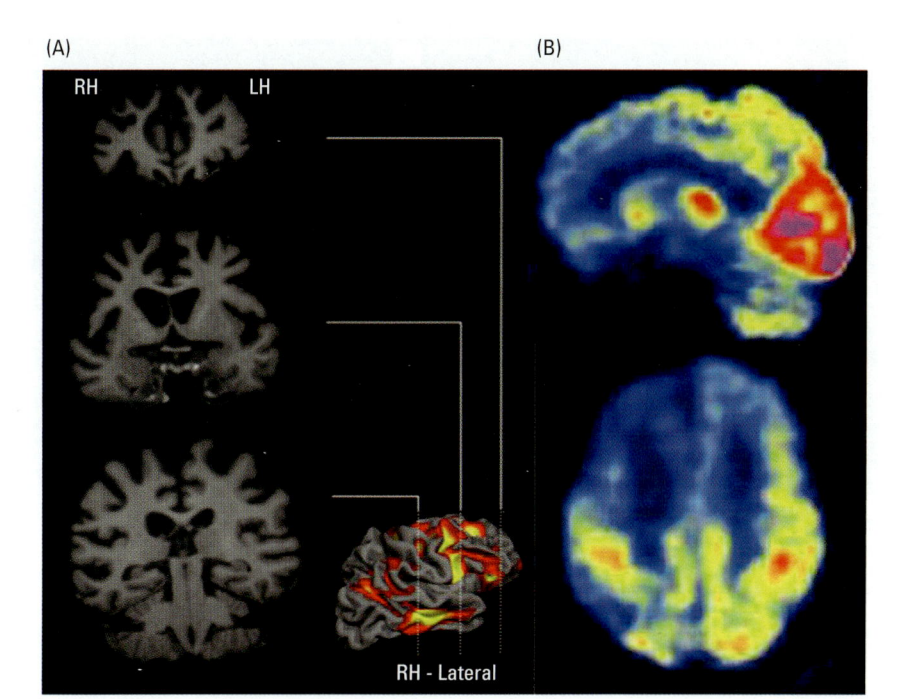

Figure 8.3 A 58-year-old man presented with behavioral symptoms (including apathy, impulsive eating) and executive dysfunction. (A) Magnetic resonance imaging (MRI) demonstrated bilateral (right greater than left) frontal, temporal, and parietal atrophy, quantified with a map of cortical thickness compared to controls. (B) Fludeoxyglucose positron emission tomography (FDG-PET) showed prominent bilateral (right greater than left) frontal and temporal hypometabolism. This man was found to have a Q300X (premature termination) mutation in *GRN*. He exhibited a 5-year clinical course from first symptoms to death. Postmortem examination revealed the expected TDP-43 pathology.

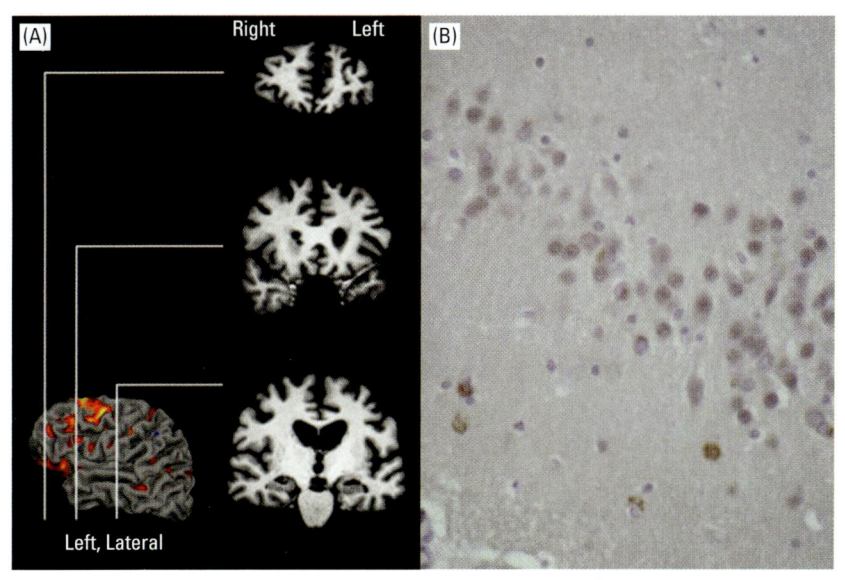

Figure 8.4 A 59-year-old man presented with behavioral symptoms (including loss of empathy, aggression, lack of insight), executive dysfunction, and word-finding difficulties. Shortly thereafter he developed dysarthria and dysphagia and was found to have clinical evidence of motor neuron disease with bulbar predominance (tongue weakness, fasciculations, lip weakness, as well as mild shoulder weakness and fasciculations with lower extremity hyperreflexia and extensor plantar responses). Electromyography showed sharp waves, fibrillation potentials, and fasciculation potentials in cervical, thoracic, and lumbar myotomes with long-duration, high-amplitude polyphasic potentials with reduced recruitment and rapid firing. (A) Magnetic resonance imaging (MRI) demonstrated bilateral (left greater than right) frontal atrophy, quantified with a map of cortical thickness compared to controls. He exhibited a 3.5-year clinical course from first symptoms to death. (B) Postmortem examination revealed the expected TDP-43 pathology (TDP-43 immunohistochemistry of dentate gyrus of hippocampus).

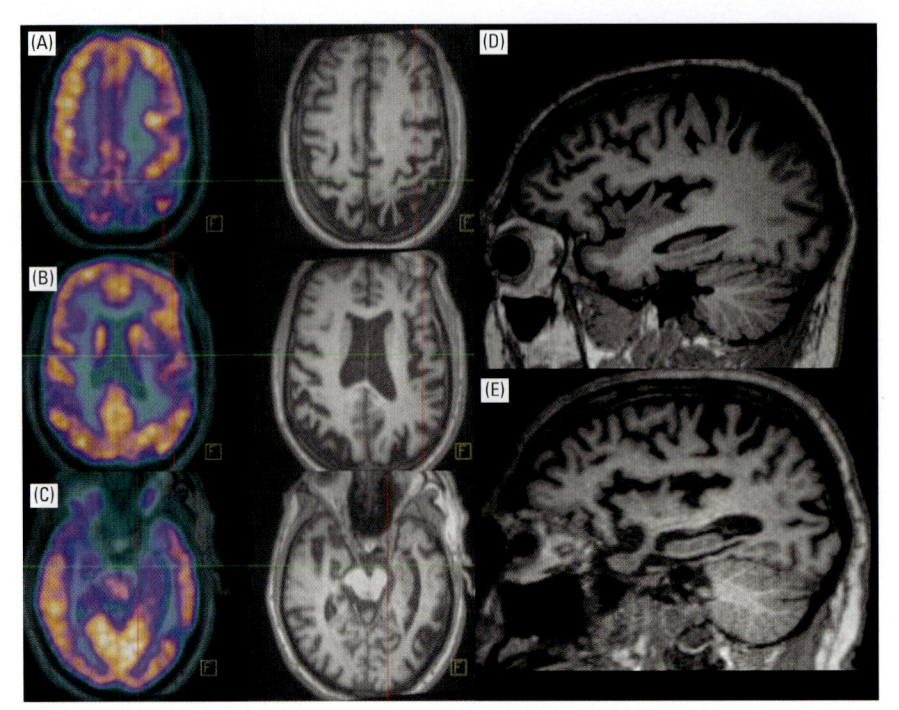

Figure 8.5 A 50-year-old man presented with unilateral dominant hand apraxia and depression without rigidity, alien hand syndrome, or eye movement abnormalities, followed shortly by executive dysfunction, word-finding difficulty, and memory loss. The initial neuroimaging examination revealed markedly asymmetric dominant hemisphere fludeoxyglucose positron emission tomography (FDG-PET) hypometabolism (*A, B, C,* left column) and atrophy (*A, B, C,* right column) extending from perirolandic and dorsal parietal cortex (*A*) into perisylvian cortex (*B*) and ventral temporal cortex (*C*) with relative preservation of frontal cortex and striatum. His symptoms progressed to include marked upper extremity apraxia with the eventual development of rigidity, aphasia, dysarthria, episodic and semantic memory impairment, compulsive behavior, impulsive eating, and agitation. Along with the progression of symptoms, atrophy progressed from (*D*) parietal and posterolateral temporal over a 4-year interval to include (*E*) ventral and anterior temporal, insular, and posterior frontal cortex.

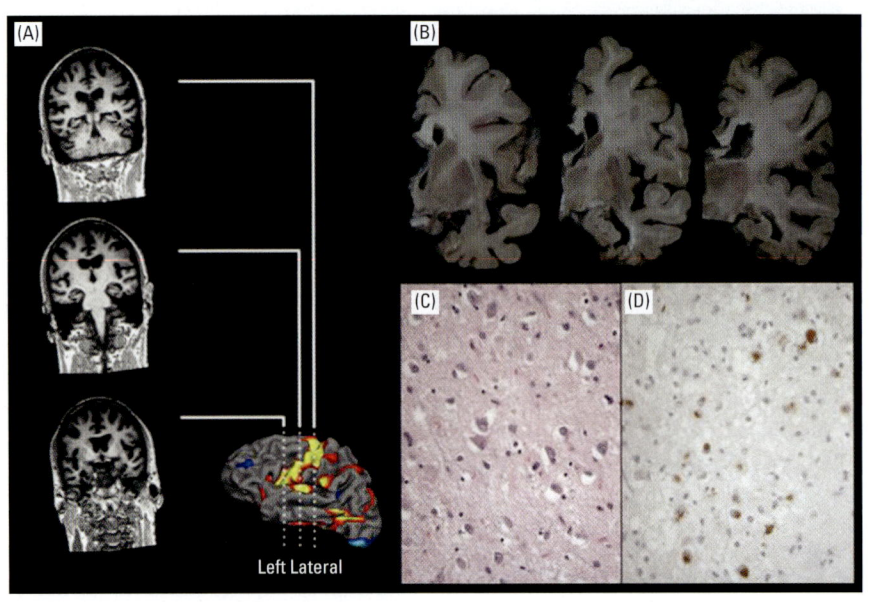

Figure 8.6 The 50-year-old man described in Figure 8.5 exhibited an 8-year clinical course from first symptoms to death. Despite (*A*) the clear magnetic resonance imaging (MRI) evidence of initial perirolandic and parietotemporal atrophy (left greater than right), quantified with a map of cortical thickness compared to controls with (*B*) postmortem support for these gross findings, histological examination revealed (*C*) Pick bodies and (*D*) tau immunoreactive pathology consistent with pathological Pick's disease.

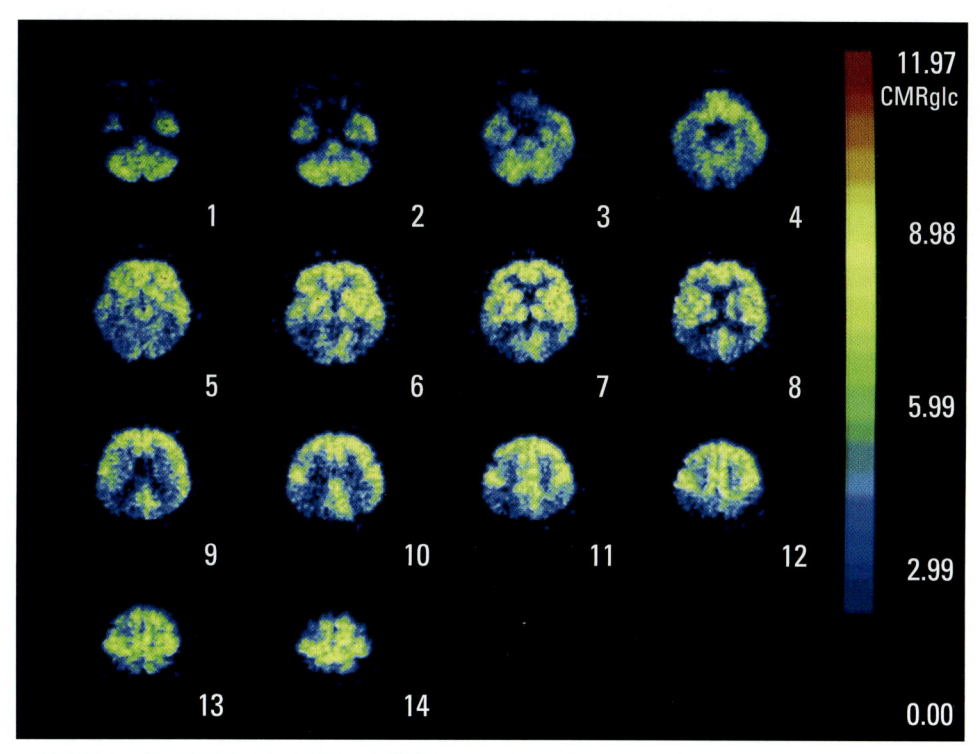

Figure 10.2 Positron emission tomography (PET) scan of a fourth patient with posterior cortical atrophy demonstrating parietal and occipital hypometabolism.

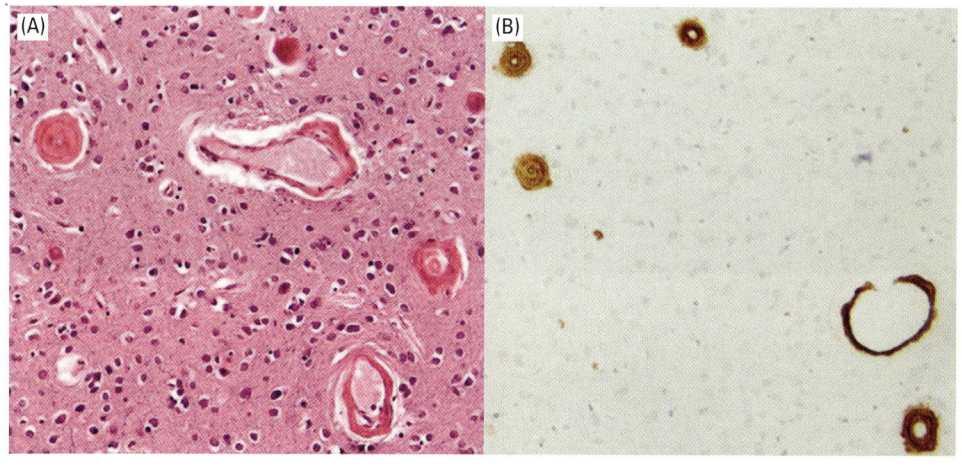

Figure 14.1 Pathologic appearance of cerebral amyloid angiopathy. (A) Amyloid deposits replace media and smooth muscle cells causing thickening of the vessel wall (hematoxylin & eosin; original magnification, 20×). (B) Immunoperoxidase staining for amyloid-β peptide showing circumferential staining of leptomeningeal blood vessels (original magnification, 20×). (Images courtesy of Dr. Matthew P. Frosch, MGH)

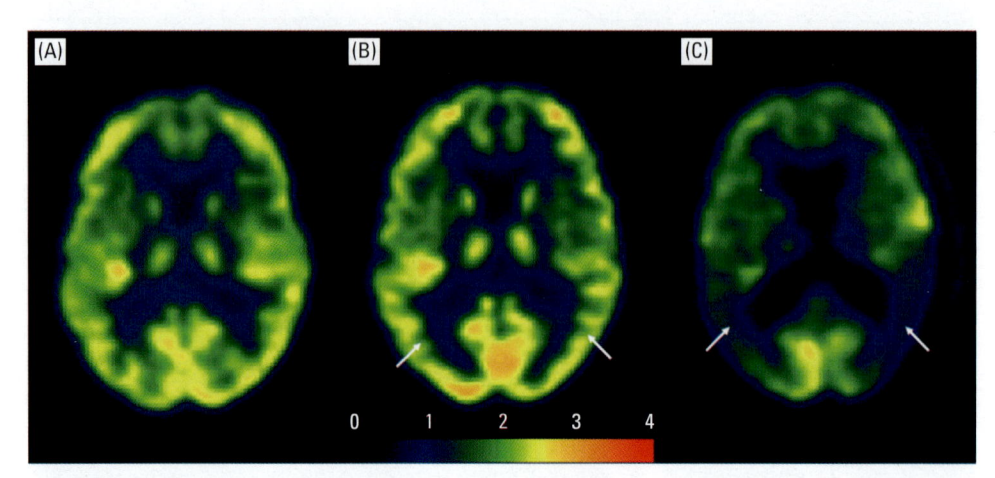

Figure 17.4 Fludeoxyglucose positron emission tomography (FDG-PET) in mild cognitive impairment (MCI). Axial section of FDG-PET scans in a cognitively normal individual (A) and individuals with MCI (B) and dementia (C). Red indicates the greatest areas of metabolism, while blue and black are the least. FDG-PET hypometabolism is a marker of neuronal injury and dysfunction. Bilateral temporoparietal hypometabolism is noted in MCI (B, white arrows) and even more so in dementia (C, white arrows) due to Alzheimer's disease and is indicative of an increased rate of progression from MCI to dementia.

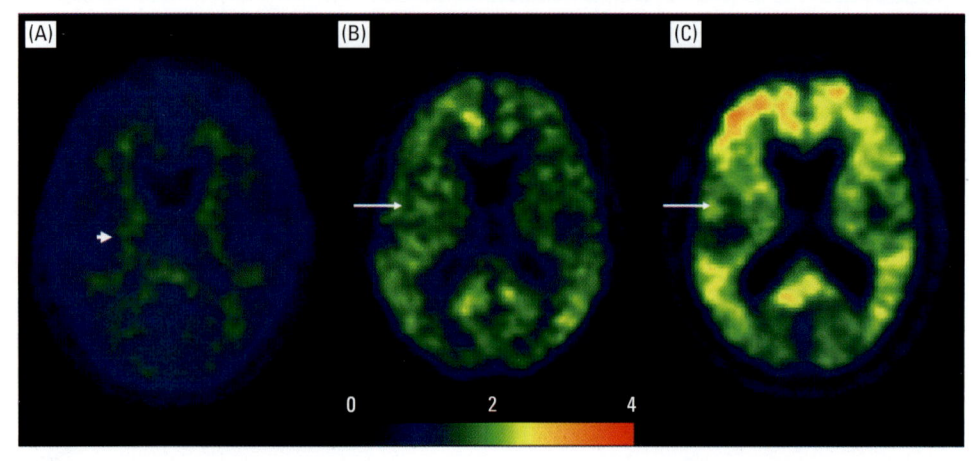

Figure 17.5 Amyloid imaging in mild cognitive impairment (MCI). Axial section of PiB-PET scans in a cognitively normal individual (A) and individuals with MCI (B) and dementia (C). PiB is a positron emission tomography (PET) tracer useful for detecting amyloid deposition in the brain. Brain areas where amyloid is absent appear blue; brain areas with the greatest tracer uptake appear red, while areas with less tracer uptake appear green or yellow. Amyloid deposition of the white matter, but not gray matter, is seen in cognitively normal individuals, creating a clear contrast in radioactivity between gray and white matter (A, short arrow). When amyloid is deposited in the cortices, as occurs in MCI (B, long arrow) and dementia (C, long arrow) due to Alzheimer's disease, diffuse reduction or loss of the normal gray-white contrast is noted. Amyloid deposition occurs early in the pathological cascade and before development of symptoms, creating relatively similar distribution and concentration of deposition between the MCI and dementia subjects.

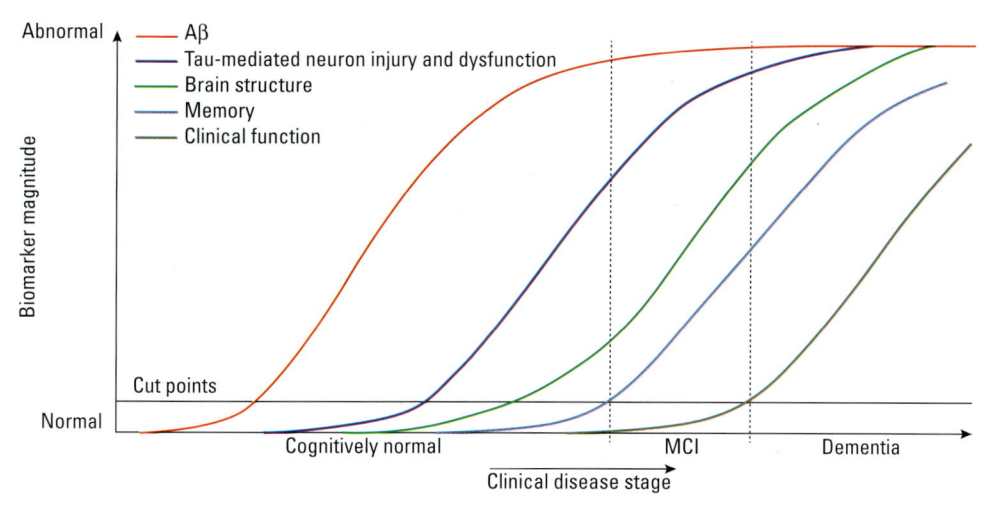

Figure 17.6 The evolution of biomarkers in the Alzheimer's pathological cascade. With the early deposition of amyloid in the pathological cascade, corresponding biomarkers (low cerebrospinal fluid [CSF], Aβ declines, and positive amyloid imaging) are detected before the development of clinical symptoms. Following this, there is a sequence of events characterizing neurodegeneration where evidence of brain dysfunction can be measured through CSF tau levels or fludeoxyglucose positron emission tomography (FDG-PET). As memory and clinical function decline, structural changes of the brain are noted on magnetic resonance imaging (MRI). MCI, mild cognitive impairment. (Reprinted from *The Lancet Neurology*, Vol. number 9, Clifford R Jack, David S Knopman, William J Jagust, Leslie M Shaw, Paul S Aisen, Michael W Weiner, Ronald C Petersen, John Q Trojanowski. Hypothetical model of dynamic biomarkers of the Alzheimer's pathological cascade, pages 119–128. Copyright (2010), with permission from Elsevier)

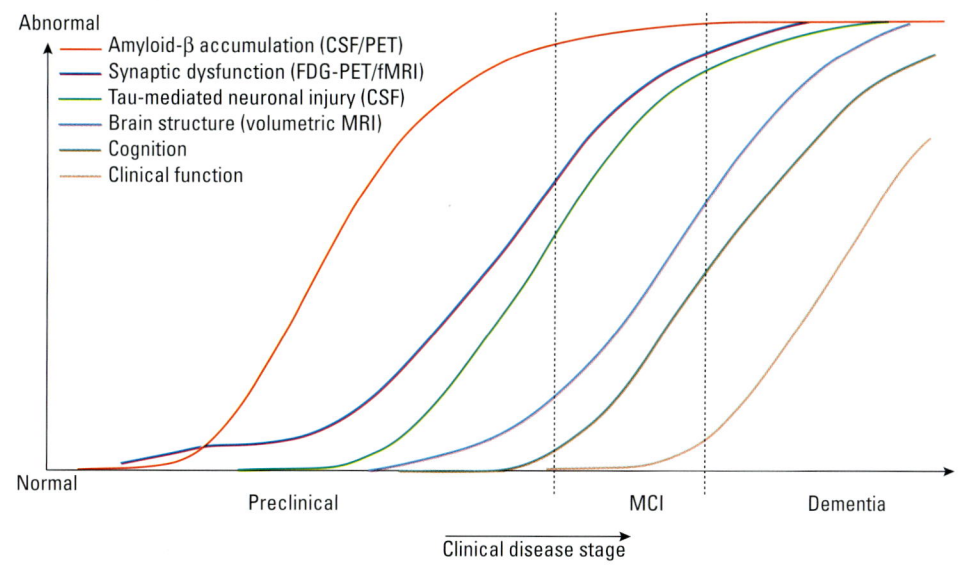

Figure 18.2 Hypothetical model of dynamic biomarkers of Alzheimer's disease (AD) expanded to explicate the preclinical phase: Aβ accumulation detected by cerebrospinal fluid (CSF) Aβ$_{42}$ assays or positron emission tomography (PET) amyloid imaging. Synaptic dysfunction evidenced by fludeoxyglucose (FDG)-PET or functional magnetic resonance imaging (MRI), with a dashed line to indicate that synaptic dysfunction may be detectable in carriers of the ε4 allele of the apolipoprotein E gene (*APOE*) prior to detectable Aβ deposition. Neuronal injury evidenced by CSF tau or phospho-tau. Brain structure by structural MRI. Biomarkers change from maximally normal to maximally abnormal (y axis) as a function of disease stage (x axis). The temporal trajectory of two key indicators used to stage the disease clinically, cognition and clinical function, are also illustrated. MCI, mild cognitive impairment. (Figure adapted with permission from Cliff Jack [Jack et al., 2010])

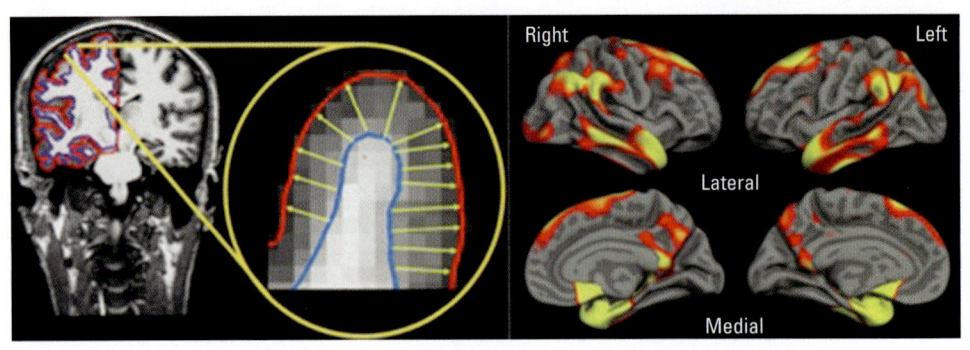

Figure 22.3 Computational neuroscience now offers methods to quantify aspects of brain structure from magnetic resonance imaging (MRI) scans. The left image depicts cortical thickness measurement from a T1-weighted MRI scan. The right image shows a map of the areas in yellow and red where the cerebral cortex is thinner in a group of mild Alzheimer's disease dementia patients compared to controls.

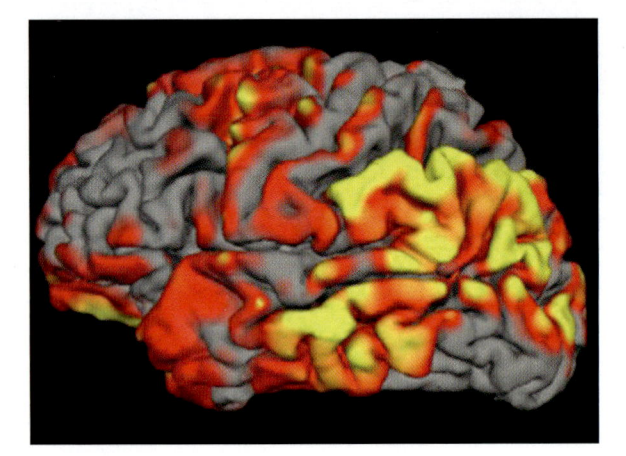

Figure 22.6 In mild Alzheimer's disease, cortical glucose metabolism is typically reduced in the temporoparietal region, as well as posterior midline and orbitofrontal regions. This now classic finding is useful clinically in differential diagnosis and may be valuable as an imaging biomarker for early detection of the metabolic signature of the disease in patients with minimal or no symptoms. This figure shows the largest reduction in metabolism in yellow, with lesser reductions in red hues from a single patient with mild AD, displayed on that patient's cortical surface as reconstructed from the anatomic magnetic resonance image. Areas without color exhibited normal metabolism compared to age-matched cognitively intact individuals.

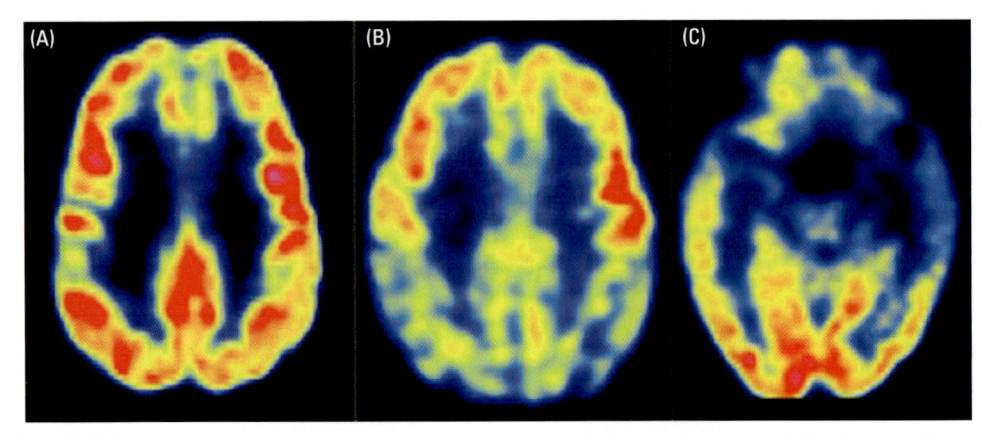

Figure 22.7 Fludeoxyglucose positron emission tomography (FDG-PET) can be very useful in the clinical evaluation of patients with dementia, particularly for the differentiation of Alzheimer's disease (AD) versus frontotemporal dementia (FTD). (A) Cognitively normal older adult; (B) mild AD dementia patient; (C) mild FTD dementia patient. (Images courtesy of Dr. Keith Johnson, Massachusetts General Hospital)

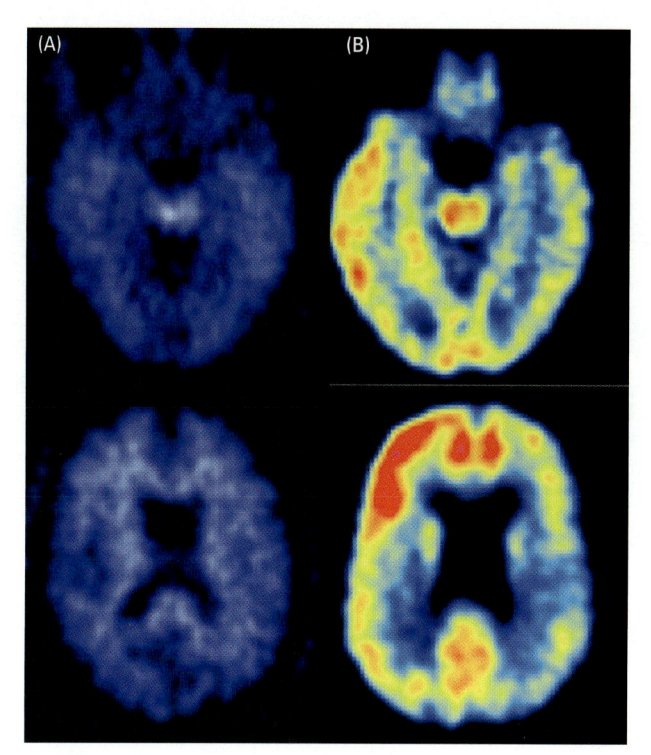

Figure 22.8 Amyloid positron emission tomography (PET) imaging is revolutionizing dementia research. Pittsburgh compound B (PiB) scan of (A) a cognitively intact 74-year-old adult demonstrates nonspecific binding ("negative"), while a scan of (B) a 73-year-old patient with mild Alzheimer's dementia shows robust signal throughout multiple cortical areas ("positive"). (Images courtesy of Dr. Keith Johnson, Massachusetts General Hospital)

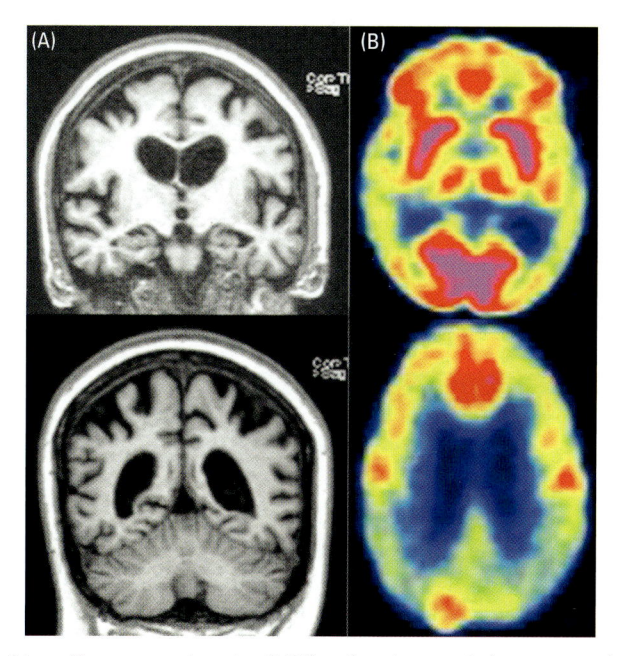

Figure 22.10 Case 1. Magnetic resonance imaging (MRI) and positron emission tomography (PET) often provide a reasonably convincing set of biomarkers in early-onset or atypical dementia patient evaluations. In this 39-year-old woman with familial dementia initially thought to be frontotemporal dementia, (A) an MRI scan showed relatively mild medial temporal lobe atrophy but prominent bilateral parietal atrophy, and (B) a fludeoxyglucose positron emission tomography (FDG-PET) scan showed prominent bilateral temporoparietal hypometabolism, supporting the diagnosis of Alzheimer's disease (AD). She was later found to carry a *PSEN1* mutation and ultimately was determined to have AD pathology at autopsy.

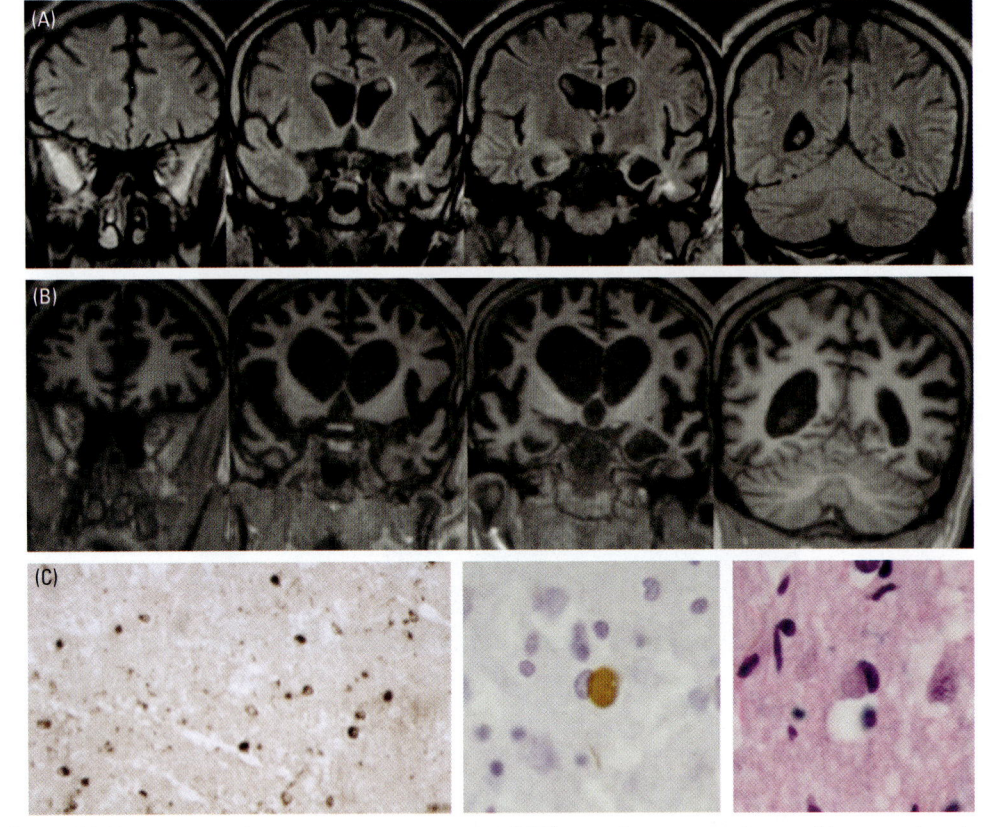

Figure 22.11 Case 2. Serial magnetic resonance imaging (MRI) scans 3 years apart show rapid progression of frontotemporal atrophy in this 31-year-old man who died of frontotemporal dementia at age 33. (*A*) A series of coronal FLAIR MRI images demonstrates left greater than right temporal lobe atrophy at a time when symptoms were clearly present but overall function was mildly impaired. (*B*) A similar series of coronal T1-weighted MRI images demonstrates marked progression of frontal, insular, and temporal atrophy with parietal involvement at a time when the patient was minimally communicative and dependent for most activities of daily living. (*C*) Postmortem histology demonstrated neuronal and glial cell loss with prominent tau immunohistochemical abnormalities (left), including Pick bodies (middle). The hematoxylin and eosin stained sections (right) also clearly demonstrated cellular inclusions typical of Pick-type tauopathy.

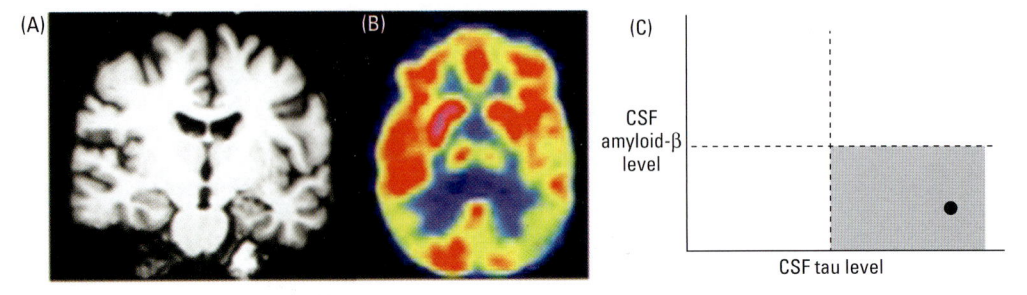

Figure 22.12 Case 3. Biomarkers in a 54-year-old woman with mild cognitive impairment with a clinical presentation suggestive of frontotemporal dementia. (*A*) Magnetic resonance imaging (MRI) showed a hint of hippocampal atrophy unilaterally but was otherwise normal. (*B*) Fludeoxyglucose positron emission tomography (FDG-PET) demonstrated bilateral (left greater than right) temporoparietal hypometabolism suggestive of Alzheimer's disease (AD) pathobiology. (*C*) Cerebrospinal fluid biomarkers were strongly consistent with AD pathobiology.

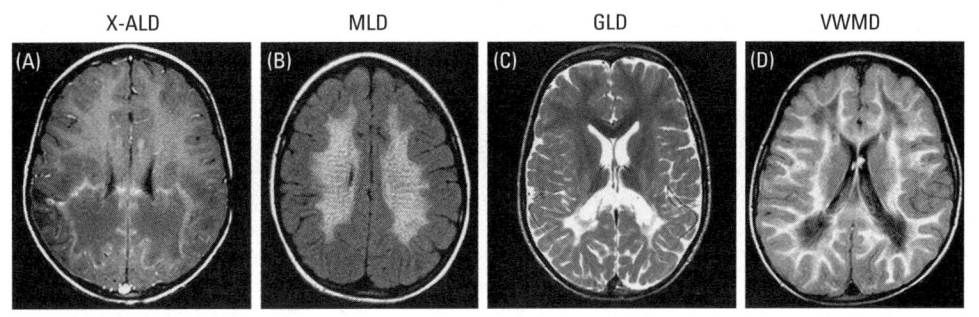

Figure 15.21 Magnetic resonance imaging (MRI) appearance of (A) X-linked adrenoleukodystrophy (X-ALD), T1-weighted image postgadolinium; (B) metachromatic leukodystrophy (MLD), fluid attenuated inversion recovery sequence (FLAIR)-weighted image; (C) globoid cell leukodystrophy (GLD), T2-weighted image; and (D) vanishing white matter disease (VWMD), T1-weighted image. (From Schmahmann, Smith, Eichler, & Filley, 2008, reproduced with permission)

impairment, cerebellar ataxia, visual failure, and spastic paraplegia. Brain imaging reveals symmetrical involvement of the basal ganglia, thalami, and posterior aspect of the centrum semiovale (Fig. 15.21C; Baram, Goldman, & Percy, 1986) leading to marked cerebral and cerebellar atrophy.

Vanishing white matter disease, also known as CNS hypomyelination, is caused by a defect in any one of the five subunits of eukaryotic initiation factor 2B (eIF2B) (van der Knaap, Pronk, & Scheper, 2006), a highly conserved, ubiquitously expressed protein that plays an essential role in the initiation of protein synthesis. Manifestations range from prenatal-onset white matter disease to juvenile or rarely, adult-onset ataxia, dementia, seizures, and ovarian insufficiency (Schiffmann & Elroy-Stein, 2006; Schiffmann et al., 1994). The course is chronic and progressive, with episodic declines following stressors such as fever, head trauma, or periods of fright. MRI is striking and shows vanishing white matter over time (Fig. 15.21D), with variable involvement of cerebellum and brainstem. Neuropathological abnormalities indicate a unique and selective disruption of oligodendrocytes and astrocytes with sparing of neurons. Autopsy confirms white matter rarefaction and cystic degeneration. There is no inflammatory response.

Cerebellar Related Disorders With Cognitive Change and Dementia

The fact that the cerebellum used to be regarded as purely a motor control device is, at this point in our understanding, an interesting quirk of medical history. The abundance of evidence from neuroanatomical studies, behavioral investigation in animals, clinical reports of patients suffering from a wide variety of disorders, task-based functional neuroimaging experiments, resting-state functional connectivity mapping, and most recently neuromodulation of cerebellum producing improvements in neuropsychiatric disorders makes it clear that the cerebellum, like basal ganglia and thalamus, is a noncerebral structure with a wide range of engagement in the neural control of sensorimotor function, intellect, and emotion (for review see Koziol et al., 2013; Schmahmann, 2004, 2010). In considering the dementias, there are two avenues of approach with respect to the cerebellum. The first is the nature of the cognitive and affective profile in patients with injuries confined to the cerebellum. The second is the range of cognitive and neuropsychiatric phenomena that occur either as a result of cerebellar injury or as a consequence of damage to noncerebellar structure in disorders that have a major cerebellar signature motorically and/or anatomico-pathologically (i.e., on brain imaging or at autopsy).

The Cerebellar Cognitive Affective Syndrome

This syndrome occurs following damage to the cerebellar posterior lobe and the vermis, and it comprises impairments of executive functions such as planning, set shifting, verbal fluency, abstract reasoning, and working memory; difficulties with spatial cognition, including visual-spatial organization and memory; personality change with blunting of affect or disinhibited and inappropriate behavior; and language deficits, including agrammatism and dysprosodia (Fig. 15.22; Levisohn, Cronin-Golomb, & Schmahmann, 2000; Schmahmann & Sherman, 1997, 1998). The cerebellar cognitive affective syndrome (CCAS) likely reflects disruption of the cerebellar modulation of neural circuits that link cerebellum in a bidirectional manner with the cerebral association and limbic/paralimbic areas that govern cognition and emotion (Schmahmann, 1991, 2010; Schmahmann & Sherman, 1998). Subsequent studies have provided confirmatory evidence for the existence of this syndrome and its anatomical basis (e.g., Baillieux et al., 2010; Tavano et al., 2007; Tedesco et al., 2011), and patients with cerebellar disorders ranging from near-total cerebellar agenesis (Fig. 15.23) to cerebellar hemorrhage (Fig. 15.24) continue to exemplify this constellation. The neuropsychiatric presentations of the CCAS reflect dysregulation of affect that occurs when lesions involve the "limbic cerebellum" (vermis and fastigial nucleus). In adults and children with congenital and acquired cerebellar lesions, observed behaviors include distractibility and hyperactivity, impulsiveness, disinhibition, anxiety, ritualistic and stereotypical behaviors, illogical thought and lack of empathy, and aggression and irritability (Schmahmann, Weilburg, & Sherman, 2007). Ruminative and obsessive behaviors, dysphoria and

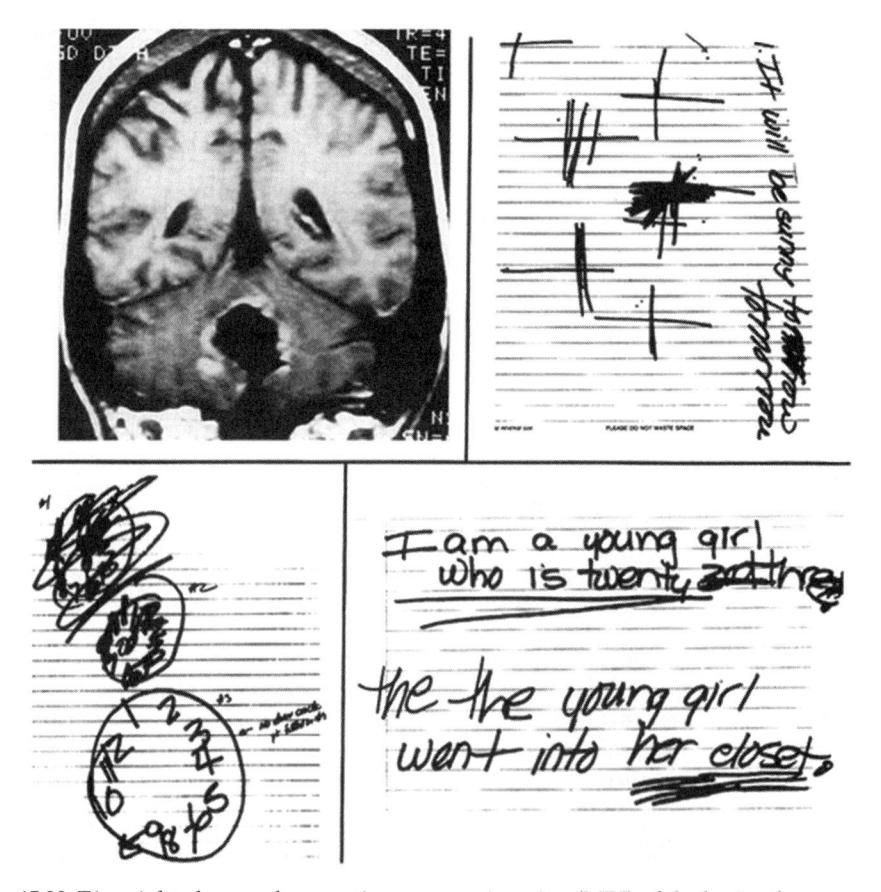

Figure 15.22 T1-weighted coronal magnetic resonance imaging (MRI) of the brain of a young woman performed following resection of a midline cerebellar ganglioglioma. Her responses when asked to draw a clock, bisect a line, and write a sentence reflect the executive dysfunction, visual spatial disorganization, and linguistic deficit (agrammatism) that characterize the cerebellar cognitive affective syndrome. (From Schmahmann and Sherman, 1998, reproduced with permission)

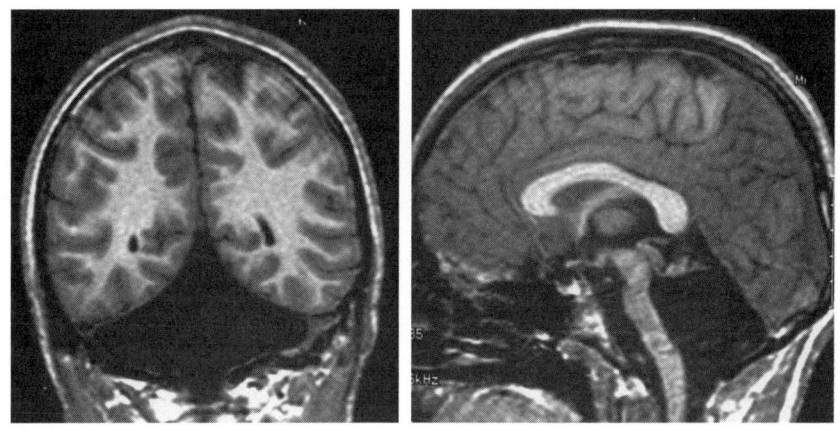

Figure 15.23 T1-weighted magnetic resonance imaging (MRI) showing near-total cerebellar agenesis with marked pontine base hypoplasia in a man now in his fourth decade (coronal image at left, midsagittal image on the right).

depression, tactile defensiveness and sensory overload, apathy, childlike behavior, and inability to appreciate social boundaries and assign ulterior motives can also be evident. These disparate neurobehavioral profiles cluster in five major domains, characterized broadly as disorders of attentional control, emotional control, and social skill set as well as autism spectrum disorders and psychosis spectrum disorders. Within the context of the dysmetria of thought theory (Schmahmann, 1991, 1996), the symptom complexes in each putative domain reflect either exaggeration (overshoot or hypermetria) or diminution (undershoot or hypometria) of responses to the internal or external environment, with some patients fluctuating between these two states. These observations and notions have implications for understanding and managing the patient with disorders of cognition and emotional modulation in the setting of cerebellar injury.

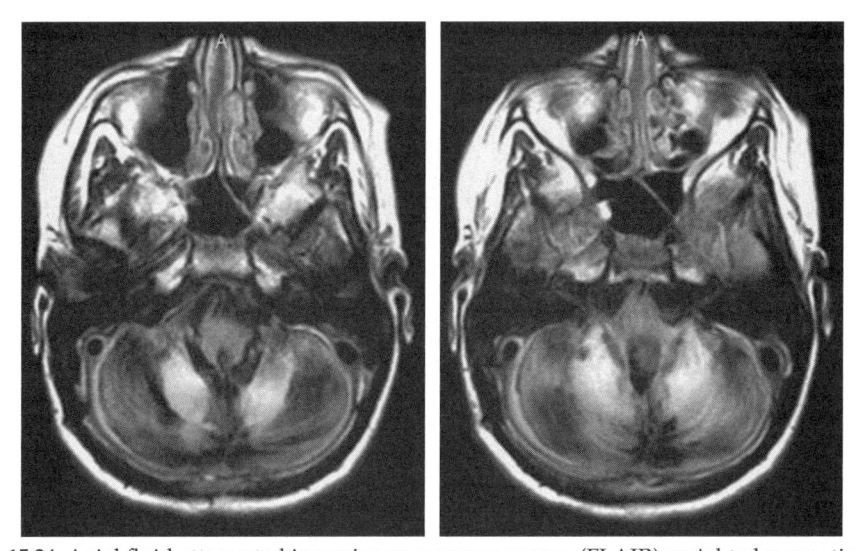

Figure 15.24 Axial fluid attenuated inversion recovery sequence (FLAIR)-weighted magnetic resonance imaging (MRI) scans through the cerebellum and brainstem (from ventral to dorsal, right to left) show signal hyperintensity and distortion of the cerebellum in a teenager 3 years following rupture of a cerebellar arteriovenous malformation. The clinical picture was overwhelmed by prolonged mutism, agitation, and aggression.

Cognition in the Ataxias

The occurrence of the CCAS in patients with the inherited spinocerebellar and other ataxias has also increasingly been recognized (Geschwind, 1999; Schmahmann, 1991). The ataxias in which pathology appears confined to cerebellum include SCA 5, SCA 6, and SCA 8. Studies in patients with SCA 6, for example, demonstrate impairments on tests of executive function involving skills of cognitive flexibility, inhibition of response, verbal reasoning, and abstraction (Cooper et al., 2010). Pathology is also confined to cerebellum in autosomal recessive cerebellar ataxia type 1 (ARCA 1) seen with greatest frequency in the French Canadian kindred. Cognition in these patients is characterized by deficits in attention, verbal working memory, and visuospatial/visuoconstructional skills (Laforce et al., 2010). Unlike the dementias that devastate memory storage, lesions confined to cerebellum often affect working memory to a substantially greater degree than declarative or episodic memory. Further, the visual and verbal memory impairment in patients with damage confined to cerebellum is characterized by difficulty with free or unstructured recall of previously embedded memories, rather than loss of the previously stored information as occurs in Alzheimer's disease. These deficits are aided by cognitive strategies that provide an external frame of reference to help organize access to long-term memory stores. Most of the spinocerebellar ataxias, including those with the highest prevalence such as SCA 1, 2, 3, and 7, as well as other neurological disorders that progressively debilitate cerebellum such as DRPLA (Tsuji, 2010) and Gordon Holmes syndrome (Margolin et al., 2013), are not confined to cerebellum, but often also involve the brainstem, basal ganglia, thalamus and cerebral cortex, and white matter. These ataxias with additional foci of neuropathology have cognitive deficits characteristic of CCAS, such as executive and visual spatial dysfunction (e.g. Braga-Neto et al., 2012), but their deficits also include impaired short- and long-term memory (Garrard, Martin, Giunti, & Cipolotti, 2008; Orsi et al., 2011), and some of the ataxias, such as SCA 2 (Fig. 15.25; Burk, 2007; Valis et al., 2011) and SCA 17 (De Michele et al., 2003; Toyoshima et al., 2012) manifest with multidomain dementia. Thus, when cerebellar injury and CCAS are accompanied by true amnestic dementia, suspicion should be high that the pathology includes noncerebellar structures.

Spinocerebellar ataxia type 17 (SCA 17), rare as it is having been reported in <100 families, is an important case in point. This autosomal dominant disorder, caused by an abnormal trinucleotide repeat expansion in *TBP* that encodes the TATA-box-binding protein (Toyoshima et al., 2012), can occur as a spontaneous mutation in up to 50%

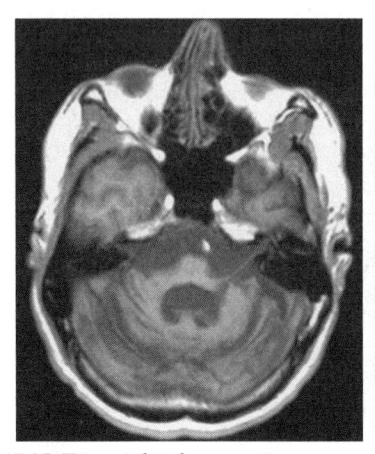

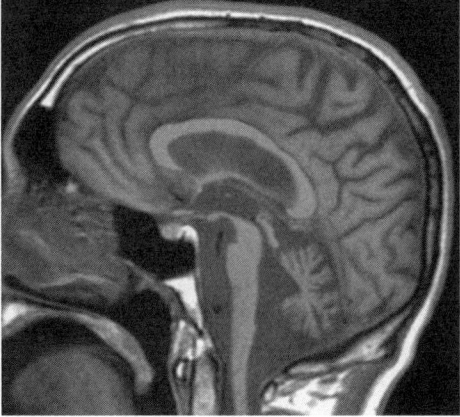

Figure 15.25 T1-weighted magnetic resonance imaging (MRI) scans (left axial, right midsagittal) in a teenager with spinocerebellar ataxia type 2. Clinical features were notable for cognitive failure as the earliest manifestation, followed by progressive dysarthria, ataxia, and extremity dysmetria as well as oculomotor paresis.

of cases. It may mimic Huntington's disease because in addition to the cerebellar motor syndrome of ataxia, dysarthria, and extremity dysmetria, patients experience choreiform or dystonic movements as well. The disorder often starts with cognitive or psychiatric impairment, however, sometimes in the teens with declining cognitive abilities or in later life (range 3 to 75 years, mean age of onset about 35 years) with disintegration of comportment, judgment, and social skills in a manner resembling frontotemporal dementia. The disease leads to a multidomain dementia with impairment of memory and language as well. Brain imaging shows atrophy of the cerebellum, striatum (putamen, caudate nucleus, and nucleus accumbens), frontal and temporal lobes, and the cuneus and cingulate gyrus (Lasek et al., 2006). Personal experience of this disease includes two intellectually gifted individuals, one whose illness commenced in adolescence with school failure, the other, a man in his mid-30s, with dissolution of family and personal life because of change in personality. Both progressed over one to two decades to severe multidomain dementia with complex motor impairments. For the clinician facing a patient with slowly evolving cognitive decline or psychiatric illness with concomitant motor features, knowing that such conditions exist is the first step to recognition, referral to specialty centers, and diagnosis—a critical step in management, counseling, and research.

Fragile X–Associated Tremor Ataxia Syndrome

Fragile X–associated tremor ataxia syndrome (FXTAS) is an adult-onset neurodegenerative disorder that affects men (rarely women) with the premutation expansion of 55–200 CGG repeats of the fragile X mental retardation 1 gene (FMR1). The length of the CGG repeat is proportional to the degree of neurological and neuropathological involvement (Greco et al., 2006; Jacquemont et al., 2003; Leehey et al., 2003). Patients present in older adulthood primarily with gait ataxia and intention tremor. Progressive cognitive decline is characterized by impaired executive function, working memory, intelligence, declarative learning and memory, speed of information processing, temporal sequencing, and visuospatial functioning. Language is generally spared (Grigsby et al., 2008). Erectile dysfunction and urinary urgency are common, and peripheral neuropathy may develop (Hagerman & Hagerman, 2013). The diagnosis can be further suspected if there is a family history of developmental delay or autism (FMR1 mental retardation presentation) in male children of an FXTAS patient's sisters. The MRI pattern of white matter pathology in FXTAS is distinctive: increased T2 and FLAIR signal in the middle cerebellar peduncle (MCP), which is confluent with white matter change within the cerebellum (Fig. 15.26). There are also scattered and/or confluent T2 and FLAIR hyperintensities

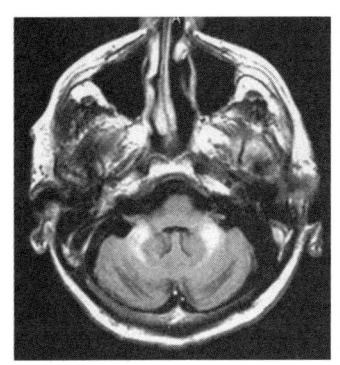

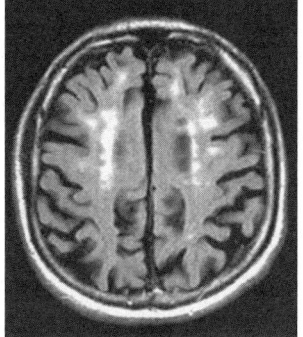

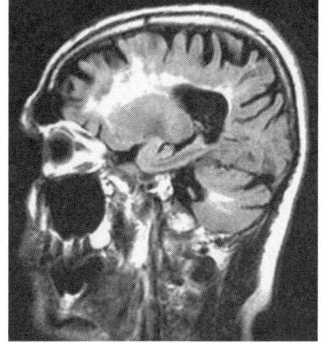

Figure 15.26 Axial fluid attenuated inversion recovery sequence (FLAIR)-weighted magnetic resonance imaging (MRI) scans in a middle-aged man with fragile X associated tremor ataxia syndrome (FXTAS). The characteristic imaging findings of signal hyperintensity in the middle cerebellar peduncles is seen in the axial image (left), with prominent cerebral and cerebellar atrophy and frontal predominant white matter signal hyperintensity on the axial (middle) and sagittal views (right).

predominantly within the frontal lobe along with generalized but frontal predominant cerebral atrophy (Jacquemont et al., 2003). Neuropathology reveals parenchymal pallor, spongiosis, and enlarged inclusion-bearing astrocytes in cerebral white matter, and widespread intranuclear and astroglial inclusions in brain, cranial nerve nuclei, and autonomic neurons of the spinal cord, with spongiosis in the MCPs (Greco et al., 2006). Cognitive decline likely reflects both the deafferentation of associative and paralimbic input to the cerebellum by the MCP lesions (Schmahmann, 1991, 2004; Schmahmann & Pandya, 1997) as well as the disruption of cerebral long association fiber tracts from the lesions of the cerebral white matter, particularly those within the prefrontal cortex.

Gordon Holmes Syndrome

This recessively inherited disorder is characterized by cerebellar ataxia, hypogonadotropic hypogonadism, and dementia (Holmes, 1908; Seminara, Acierno, Abdulwahid, Crowley, & Margolin, 2002). It was recently shown to be caused by mutations in genes engaged in ubiquitination (*RNF216* and *OTUD4*; Margolin et al., 2013) and in protein misfolding (*STUB* that encodes the protein *CHIP*; Shi et al., 2014). The hypogonadotropic hypogonadism presents in early adulthood, leading to progressive dysarthria and ataxia, with personality change, memory loss, and eventually mutism at end stage. Cerebellar and cortical atrophy are seen on brain imaging, with patchy areas of hyperintensity in cerebral white matter that may predate the ataxia and that evolve over time, together with T2 bright and T1 dark lesions of thalamus in the three cases personally followed by the author (Fig. 15.27). Neuropathological studies available to date show atrophy and severe neuronal loss and gliosis in the inferior olives, cerebellum, and areas CA3 and CA4 of the hippocampus (Holmes, 1908; Margolin et al., 2013).

Langerhans Cell Histiocytosis

Clonal proliferation of bone marrow–derived Langerhans cells or circulating plasmacytoid monocytes causes a granulomatous disorder, Langerhans cell histiocytosis (LCH). It occurs mostly in children but also in adulthood. CNS involvement may be a primary or a secondary phenomenon resembling paraneoplastic or immune-mediated processes. Primary brain involvement manifests as granulomas of the meninges, hypothalamic pituitary region with diabetes insipidus and anterior pituitary hormone deficiency, and multifocal intracerebral histiocytic granulomas with symptoms dependent on location (Prayer, Grois, Prosch, Gadner, & Barkovich, 2004). Secondary LCH is a neurodegenerative disorder (ND-LCH) with bilateral symmetric lesions in the cerebellum and basal ganglia, characterized by T-cell-dominated inflammation leading to neuronal and axonal destruction with secondary demyelination (Grois, Prayer, Prosch, &

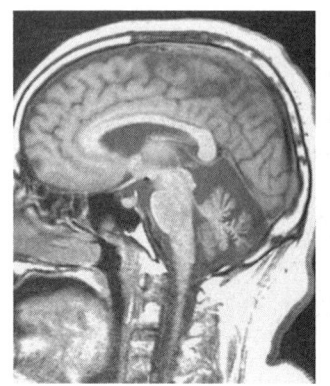

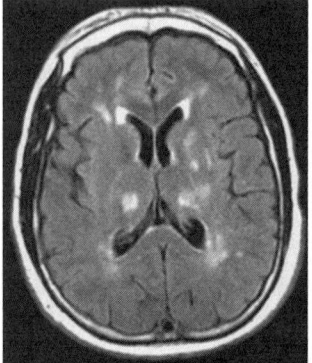

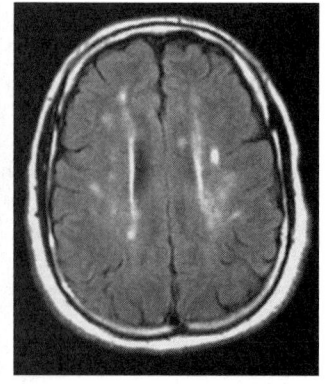

Figure 15.27 Midsagittal T1-weighted magnetic resonance imaging (MRI) scan (left) showing cerebellar volume loss in a young woman with Gordon Holmes syndrome as defined genetically in Margolin et al. (2013). The axial fluid attenuated inversion recovery sequence (FLAIR)-weighted MRI scans show white matter hyperintensities scattered bilaterally throughout the forceps minor and major, the corona radiata, and notably in the thalamus as well.

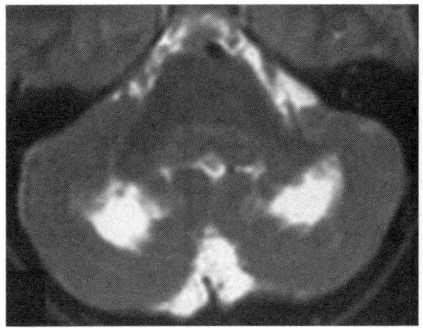

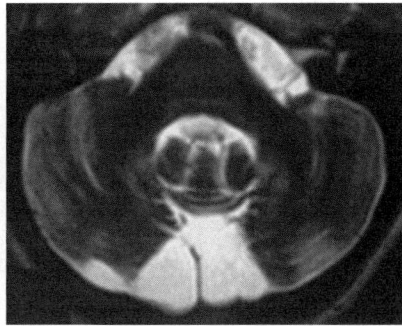

Figure 15.28 Axial T2-weighted magnetic resonance imaging (MRI) scans through the cerebellum in a young man with the neurodegenerative form of Langerhans cell histiocytosis. Hyperintense signal abnormality in the cerebellar white matter (left) on the MRI performed at age 8 years gives way to cerebellar atrophy when scanned at age 17 years (right). (From Schmahmann, Weilburg, & Sherman, 2007, reproduced with permission)

Lassmann, 2005; Prosch, Grois, Wnorowski, Steiner, & Prayer, 2007; van der Knaap, Pronk, & Scheper, 2008; Wnorowski et al., 2008). Brain MRI shows symmetrical, nonenhancing, T2-bright signal in the cerebellum. Similar abnormality can be seen in posterior periventricular cerebral white matter. Over time the imaging findings evolve to marked cerebellar and/or cerebral atrophy (Fig. 15.28; Prosch, Grois, Wnorowski, Steiner, & Prayer, 2007; van der Knaap, Pronk, & Scheper, 2008; Wnorowski et al., 2008). Cerebellar motor signs may be accompanied by cognitive impairment and neuropsychiatric features such as obsessive-compulsive disorder (Grois et al., 2010; Shuper et al., 2000). Children with ND-LCH have impaired attention, intellectual function, verbal and visual memory, linguistic skills, and mathematical skills, and those with hypothalamic damage may have abnormal eating patterns—binge eating, anorexia, or bulimia, with rage attacks, claustrophobia, agoraphobia, depression, and aggression (Nanduri et al., 2003). These cognitive and neuropsychiatric features are also described in adults in whom the cerebellar motor findings may be relatively modest but the brain imaging findings of cerebellar involvement are marked (Poretti, Boltshauser, & Schmahmann, 2012; Schmahmann, Weilburg, & Sherman, 2007).

Superficial Siderosis

This unusual condition results from repeated subarachnoid hemorrhage from such entities as dural arteriovenous fistulae, other vascular malformations, or prior trauma that cause deposition of hemosiderin over the superficial layers of the CNS (Fig. 15.29; Kumar et al., 2006). The cerebellum and eighth cranial nerves are the most severely affected, with involvement to a lesser extent of the orbital and medial prefrontal cortices, sometimes with layering of hemorrhage also over the cerebral convexities. The typical presentation is with cerebellar ataxia, hearing loss, and anosmia, although chronic recurrent spinal location of the hemorrhage can have clinical features in common with amyotrophic lateral sclerosis (Payer, Sottas, & Bonvin, 2010). Cognitive and affective changes are routinely reported. These generally conform to the CCAS and include impairments of visual recall and executive functions, together with deficits in theory of mind—the ability to represent other people's mental states (van Harskamp, Rudge, & Cipolotti, 2005).

Niemann-Pick Disease Type C

This rare autosomal recessive neurovisceral lipid storage disease resulting from mutations in NPC1 (95% of cases) or NPC2 presents in adulthood in about 5% of cases, at a mean age of 25 +/− 9.7 years (see Maubert, Hanon, & Metton, 2013; Mengel et al., 2013; Sevin et al., 2007). Neurological manifestations in adults are cerebellar ataxia (76%), vertical supranuclear ophthalmoplegia (75%), dysarthria, (63%), cognitive impairment with deficits in memory and executive

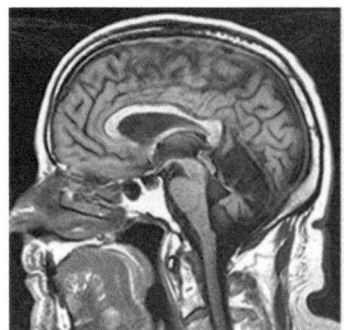

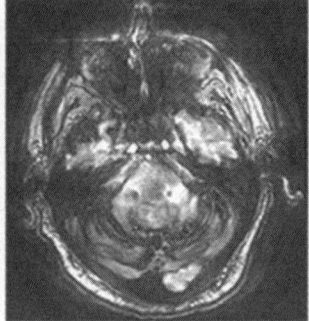

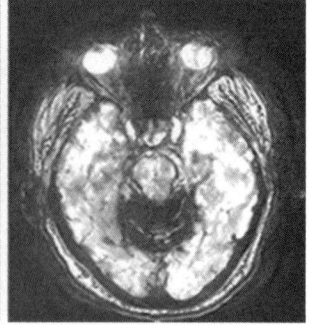

Figure 15.29 Magnetic resonance imaging (MRI) in a middle-aged man with superficial siderosis. Left, midsagittal T1-weighted MRI shows cerebellar volume loss and hypointense signal notably at the superior vermis. Middle and right images, axial gradient echo (susceptibility-weighted scans) show marked hypointense signal reflecting hemosiderin overlying the cerebellum at both the superior and inferior aspects.

function (61%), movement disorders (58%), splenomegaly (54%), psychiatric disorders (45%), and dysphagia (37%). Seizures and cataplexy are occasionally observed. The neuropsychiatric manifestations include schizophrenia-like psychosis with paranoia, auditory and visual hallucinations and disorganization, depression, bipolar disorder, obsessive-compulsive behaviors, confusion, sleep disorders, hyperactivity, agitation, aggression, and self-mutilation. The severity and nature of the symptoms may fluctuate and response to psychotropic agents may be poor. Whereas visceral manifestations with splenomegaly predominate in the perinatal through infantile ages of onset, neurological and psychiatric involvement is more prominent in the juvenile and adult-onset cases. The neurological findings of ataxia, dysarthria, dysphagia, and dystonia may develop after the cognitive and neuropsychiatric features have become established. The clinical tip-off is the presence of supranuclear vertical gaze palsy (note that this very helpful clinical sign is also seen in the tauopathy progressive supranuclear palsy, in CNS Whipple's disease, and in fatal familial insomnia). Routine laboratory tests in NP-C are normal, and therefore clinical suspicion is needed to make the diagnosis, which requires a skin biopsy for fibroblast culture to perform filipin staining, and then genetic confirmation by sequencing the NPC1 and NPC2 genes. The disease may respond to miglustat.

Epilepsy and Dementia

The vast topic of the many neurological disorders associated with both seizures and cognitive impairment is beyond the scope of this discussion. It is worth remembering, however, that long-term neurological diseases may be associated with impaired cognition for at least two separate, but related reasons. First, the cerebral cortical dysfunction leading to the epileptiform disorder is also the anatomical underpinning of the impaired cognition, as exemplified by the tuberous sclerosis complex (Chu-Shore, Major, Camposano, Muzykewicz, & Thiele, 2010), and other major disorders such as temporal lobe trauma, and the residual effects of Herpes simplex encephalitis that is highly epileptogenic and also affects structures in the medial temporal lobe critical for memory. Second, frequent or uncontrolled seizures may affect cognition directly. There are consequences of the epilepsy on the development of normal cognitive and social skills, particularly when the disease onset is early in life. Helmstaedter and Elger (2009) examined verbal learning and memory in 1,156 patients with chronic temporal lobe epilepsy (ages 6–68 years, mean epilepsy onset 14 +/- 11 years) and found that patients failed to build up adequate learning and memory performance during childhood and particularly during adolescence. Decline in performance over time ran in parallel in patients and controls, but because of the initial distance between the two groups, patients reached very poor performance levels much earlier. This increased the risk of premature "dementia" later on, even in the absence of an accelerated decline. These are relevant factors in assessing the cognitive state of a person with epilepsy who is thought to be undergoing cognitive decline. Knowledge of the patient's premorbid baseline is particularly relevant in this circumstance.

Sleep Deprivation and Cognition

Chronic sleep deprivation contributes to cognitive impairment. Primary snoring increases risk of neurocognitive impairment and lower intelligence in children; cognition in the setting of obstructive sleep apnea is more impaired in older than younger adults; and older adults, particularly women, with obstructive sleep apnea have an increased risk of minimal cognitive impairment or dementia when evaluated 5 years later (Grigg-Damberger & Ralls, 2012). These findings reflect the observation that sleep has measurable consequences on cognitive performance, and that sleep problems are intrinsically tied to common neuropsychological conditions. In their review of the topic, Waters and Bucks (2011) found that sleep loss decreases speed of information processing and attention/vigilance, and negatively impacts multiple aspects of cognition, including short-term memory, mental arithmetic, executive functions, memory, and language. Intraindividual variability is notable, both within a task and within a testing session, reflecting fluctuating vigilance and difficulty maintaining task instructions. Performance worsens as sleep debt accumulates in a dose-dependent manner. While moderate sleep reduction can have serious consequences for cognitive function, chronic sleep restriction of 6 hours or less per night produces cognitive impairments equivalent to that seen after two nights without sleep. Cognitive deficits may be reversed with return to normal sleep, highlighting the remediable nature of sleep-dependent cognitive dysfunction, and emphasizing the potential for positive effects of sleep intervention. This realization provides the clinician with a potentially powerful tool, both for diagnosing cognitive impairment in the setting of sleep deprivation and for the therapeutic opportunity to improve cognition in elderly patients by ensuring a good night's sleep. Note also that one needs to enquire specifically about the features of rapid eye movement (REM) sleep behavior disorder with thrashing movements of the arms and legs, and loud vocalization sometimes with terror, as this is a useful pointer to the early stages of neurodegenerative synucleinopathies manifesting as the extrapyramidal disorders Lewy body disease, Parkinson's disease, and multiple system atrophy (Ferini-Strambi, 2011).

Obstruction to Cerebrospinal Fluid Flow/Cerebrospinal Leak

Normal Pressure Hydrocephalus

Described by some of the preeminent neurologists and neurosurgeons of the late 20th century (Adams, 1966; Adams, Fisher, Hakim, Ojemann, & Sweet, 1965; Hakim & Adams, 1965), normal pressure hydrocephalus (NPH) has proven to be controversial (e.g., McGirr, Mohammed, Kurlan, & Cusimano, 2013). This is likely related to uncertainty about how to make the diagnosis, including the findings on brain imaging, the need for a single large volume spinal fluid drainage versus a lumbar drain over a few days, the time course of the onset of the expected immediate recovery and the duration of such improvement, and the presence of confounding features that either raise questions about the diagnosis or contribute to a complex clinical scenario in which NPH may be one contributing feature of the case, albeit a clinically significant one that may be amenable to treatment. This is not a dementing disease that should be missed. Erring on the side of caution in this treatable condition is reasonable. The diagnostic test of the cerebrospinal fluid tap, when successful, may provide the patient with an alternative to a progressive debilitating cognitive and motor decline.

There are ongoing attempts to better understand this condition. Prognostic factors for response to shunting now include the callosal angle, measured as the angle between the lateral ventricles on the coronal image through the posterior commissure, perpendicular to the anterior-posterior commissure plane (Ishii et al., 2008; Sjaastad & Nordvik, 1973). A significantly smaller callosal angle predicts response: 59° in responders versus 68° in nonresponders, and an angle below 63° is optimal for prognostic accuracy (Virhammar, Laurell, Cesarini, & Larsson, 2014). Additionally, the relative degree of CSF in the Sylvian fissures versus the high convexity fissures as measured by voxel-based morphometry distinguishes NPH from Alzheimer's disease with a high degree of specificity and sensitivity (Yamashita et al., 2013). In a study of 214 patients with NPH evaluated with diagnostic intracranial pressure (ICP) monitoring, those with increased ICP pulsatility had a response rate of 93% following VP shunt (Eide & Sorteberg, 2010). Three days of an external lumbar drain may supplement the single large volume spinal tap as a diagnostic test, and the use of lumboperitoneal (LP) shunts rather than ventriculoperitoneal (VP) shunts are being evaluated, with good success reported. In a study of 33 patients (Bloch & McDermott, 2012), all 33 (100%) NPH patients had preoperative gait dysfunction, 28 (85%) had incontinence, and 20 (61%) had memory deficits. At mean follow-up of 19 months after LP shunt, 100% of the patients demonstrated improved gait, 46% improved continence, and 55% improvement in memory. Shunt failure requiring revision occurred in 27% after an average of 11 months, but without neurologic complications.

For the clinician, it is imperative to recognize that the constellation of a change in cognition (with a wide range of manifestations), together with a change in gait (with many different possible presentations, and not just the classical magnetic or slipping clutch gait), and a change in sphincter control, mostly the bladder, is sufficient to warrant concern for this diagnosis. The suspicion is heightened if there is a history of prior head trauma, subarachnoid hemorrhage, or meningeal inflammation, infection, or tumor. The response to treatment with ventriculoperitoneal or lumboperitoneal shunt can be so dramatic even in relatively rapid onset cases that look like other disorders (e.g., Schwarzschild, Rordorf, Bekken, Buonanno, & Schmahmann, 1997) that it is incumbent upon the clinician to think of this diagnosis and, when the data point to its presence, treat it definitively and early. Personal experience, supported by the literature, indicates that even in the presence of other diseases, including Alzheimer's disease, the decline in function that accompanies the ventricular enlargement that is not ex vacuo but is a response to the primary issue of enlarged ventricles degrades quality of life. Further, VP shunt (and possibly LP shunt) in these cases can provide meaningful clinical improvement in a patient's overall quality of life.

The description by Raymond D. Adams (1966) of the phenotypic range of the behavioral, gait, and sphincter disturbances in his nine patients with NPH is extremely important. It is reproduced here verbatim with minor changes, as follows:

Disturbance in thinking and behaviour: Derangements in this sphere were the most common effect of mild hydrocephalus. Developing gradually or being left, as a syndrome of more severe proportions subsided (as in the cases of aneurysmal subarachnoid hemorrhage and trauma), a change in mental function was the complaint most frequently registered by the patient's family (all 9 cases) and was occasionally noted by the patient himself. Being forgetful (i.e. mild to severe impairment of retentive memory) was one feature, but observation also disclosed a paucity of thought and action. Less speech was initiated; the patient was less lively and spontaneous; the range and variety of activities was reduced. A decrease in quality of thinking was observed as well as a quantitative reduction and often it had resulted in unintelligent action. Emotional reactions likewise seemed less vivid; there was an indifference, an apathy, a lack of enduring affect. In only one case, an alcoholic woman, was excessive irritability noted, and this was principally in the nature of a lack of inhibition of impulse, with the immediate reaction conforming to her prevailing mood of depression and anxiety. Inner psychic life seemed impoverished; the patients were bereft of thought. When vaguely aware of their difficulty, reference was sometimes made to it as a trouble in thinking. One woman remarked upon being forgetful but seemed to overlook the fact that she had become completely incompetent to take care of her own affairs. Another spoke of herself as being 'scatty', meaning absentminded and easily distractable. At the earliest or mildest stages of illness examination revealed no aphasic disorder; calculation of varying degrees of complexity was possible though slow with the commission of many errors; no apraxic or agnosic abnormalities were noted; spatial orientation was intact though temporal orientation tended to be inexact. Other items of behaviour change consisted of inattentiveness and sporadic incontinence of sphincters, especially urinary, which appeared to embarrass others more than the patient. As the hydrocephalic symptomatology became more severe the patient would for long periods remain mute and relatively motionless, episodes that resembled catatonia or early parkinsonism. Questions tended to evoke action rather than reply, and verbal responses if made at all were usually monosyllabic. One patient sat for hours with a newspaper in hand or idly staring at a television set, rarely looking understandingly at either. Visual fixation and following movements of eyes would occur and at times all types of visual stimuli would seem to be equally attractive, thus revealing what might be termed a distractability of attention. Sphincteric incontinence was more frequent at this stage. The most advanced stages of the condition were attended by stupor with grasp and sucking reflexes and Babinski signs, but no paralysis of limbs. This could progress to coma.

Disturbance of gait and other neurological abnormalities: Difficulty in walking was noted in each of our cases but it was difficult to characterize. The mildest degree consisted of a slight uncertainty, a tendency to make a misstep in one or other direction which could lead to a fall. Tandem walking was difficult. Patients preferred to steady themselves and gain security by taking the arm of a companion or touching an article of furniture. More severe degrees of gait disturbance amounted to an unsteadiness reminiscent of what has been termed an 'apraxia of gait' or Brun's 'frontal lobe ataxia'. As the hydrocephalus worsened standing and walking became impossible. In contrast, limb movements were quite facile showing only slight hesitancy or slowness.

A tendency to suck and grasp was variably present in the more advanced stages of disease; the latter took more the form of an instinctual grasping than true grasp reflex, being bilateral and more easily evinced by attracting attention to something other than the hand. The tendon reflexes tended to be lively, especially in the legs, and were sometimes accompanied by extensor plantar reflexes on one or both sides, which were more frequent in states of mutism or stupor.

We came to recognize the clinical state as being different from that of other diseases which impair intellectual function in late life. We watched for it particularly amongst the patients suspected of having a dementing degenerative disease and found that those in whom poor memory, psychomotor impairment, uncertainty of gait and sphincteric incontinence were early symptoms, and where the evolution of the illness occurred over a few weeks to months and fluctuated, should be suspected as having hydrocephalus rather than presenile or senile brain atrophy.

Reversibility of the disorder of attention, memory, thinking and activity was more rapid than correction of the gait abnormality. In several instances a few weeks elapsed before locomotion became dependable, long after intellect had either been restored to normal or had reached a level of improvement from which it deviated little (page 1137).

Adams noted that the EEG was abnormal in all cases (generalized slowing is common; frontal intermittent rhythmic delta may occur late). As pointed out by the originators of the concept in 1965, the cognitive, gait, and bladder manifestations are likely the result of compression and stretching of brain tissue in frontocentral regions with involvement of the long association fiber tracts and the corpus callosum, explaining why NPH presents early on with a frontal lobe neurobehavioral syndrome. As the projection fibers and thalamocortical fibers become progressively involved, the pyramidal findings and alterations in level of arousal are affected.

Sagging Brain Syndrome

Intracranial hypotension results from occult or known sources of leakage of CSF from the subarachnoid space. Spontaneous intracranial hypotension has long been recognized as a cause of orthostatic headache (present in the erect position, abating with recumbency). Other symptoms include neck pain, nausea, vomiting, dizziness, hearing loss, diplopia, visual blurring, interscapular pain, and radicular upper extremity symptoms. Characteristic imaging features include diffuse pachymeningeal gadolinium enhancement, sinking of the brain, subdural fluid collections, enlargement of the pituitary, and engorgement of venous sinuses and the epidural venous plexus (Mokri, 2004). These findings together with CSF lymphocytic pleocytosis, elevated protein, normal glucose, and negative culture can lead to the mistaken diagnosis of aseptic meningitis (Balkan et al., 2012). Chronic CSF leak with downward displacement of the intracranial contents can mimic Chiari 1 malformation (Atkinson, Weinshenker, Miller, Piepgras, & Mokri, 1998) and produce distortion and expansion of the midbrain (Fig. 15.30) with few neurological signs, or patients may become drowsy and even lapse into coma due to central herniation (Savoiardo et al., 2007). It has recently been recognized that this constellation has a major impact on cognition with behavioral and cognitive dysfunction accompanied by daytime somnolence and headache, and all eight patients in the original report showed evidence on brain PET scan of hypometabolism of the frontotemporal regions—hence, the frontotemporal brain sagging syndrome (Wicklund et al., 2011). In the three cases followed by the author (Schmahmann, as yet unpublished), the sagging brain syndrome (SBS) produces motor slowing with cautious and unsteady gait, urinary incontinence, dysarthria, and dysphagia. There is change in personality characterized predominantly by disinhibited and (sexually) inappropriate behaviors coupled with apathy, lack of concern and empathy, and/or affective changes with depression and anxiety. Confusion, forgetfulness, executive dysfunction including impaired working memory, and obsessive-compulsive stereotypies are common features. Aphasias are notably absent. Identifying the CSF leak is the key to targeted intervention. Some patients improve with prolonged recumbency and autologous epidural blood patch. The acquired dementia of the SBS with its characteristic clinical and imaging features may be rare, but it is important to recognize because of the potential for improvement with treatment, and to avoid unnecessary investigations and misdiagnosis.

Other Rare Neurodegenerative Disorders With Cognitive Change

There are a number of rare neurodegenerative disorders that usually present in childhood but that can also manifest in adults and sometime with a subacute presentation (see Coker, 1991). These are exemplified by the following.

Wilson's disease (hepatolenticular degeneration; Wilson, 1912) is an autosomal recessive

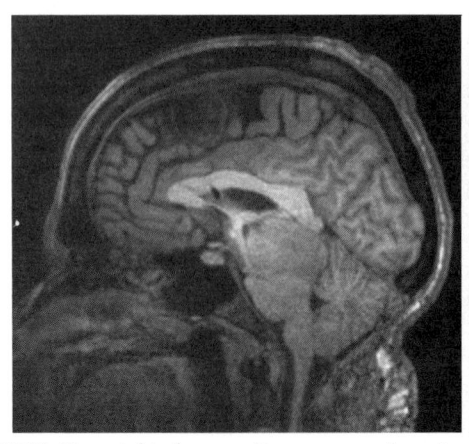

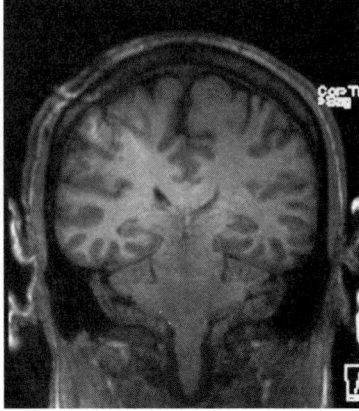

Figure 15.30 T1-weighted magnetic resonance imaging (MRI) scans in the midsagittal plane (left) and coronal plane (right) show the essential features of the sagging brain syndrome. There is sinking and distortion of the midbrain, diencephalon, and corpus callosum, and crowding of the posterior fossa. This middle-aged man presented as a case of frontotemporal dementia.

disorder of copper metabolism caused by mutations in the ATP7B gene. It manifests with prominent extrapyramidal signs, notably dysarthria, dystonia, tremor, and choreoathetosis. Cognitive and neuropsychiatric changes may be mild and include a frontal lobe syndrome with impulsivity, promiscuity, impaired social judgment, apathy, decreased attention, executive dysfunction with poor planning and decision making, and emotional lability, sometimes with pseudobulbar features; or a subcortical dementia with slowness of thinking, memory loss, and executive dysfunction, as well as depression (Lorincz, 2010 for review). It is important to make the diagnosis, looking for telltale signs on brain imaging, Kayser-Fleischer rings at the superior and inferior regions of the cornea, low serum ceruloplasmin, elevated 24-hour urine copper, and elevation of hepatic copper on liver biopsy, as the disease is treatable with copper chelating agents.

Neurodegeneration with brain iron accumulation (NBIA) refers to a group of inherited neurologic disorders characterized by abnormal accumulation of iron in the basal ganglia, most often in the globus pallidus and/or substantia nigra (for review, see Gregory & Hayflick, 2013). Nine genetic types are presently recognized. The hallmark clinical manifestations of NBIA are progressive dystonia and dysarthria, spasticity, and parkinsonism. Retinal degeneration and optic atrophy are common. Onset ranges from infancy to adulthood. Progression can be rapid or slow with long periods of stability. Brain imaging shows generalized cerebral and cerebellar atrophy. The neuropathological hallmark is axonal spheroids in the CNS and, in some types, in peripheral nerves. Neuropsychiatric features are more frequently seen in the adult-onset disease, as in pantothenate kinase associated neurodegeneration (PKAN), which also has the characteristic, if not pathognomonic, MRI finding of eye-of-the-tiger sign, T_2-weighted hypointense signal in the globus pallidus with a central region of hyperintensity.

Polycystic lipomembranous osteodysplasia with sclerosing leukoencephalopathy (PLO-SL) is an autosomal recessive disorder caused by mutations in *TYROBP (DAP12)* and *TREM*. It is characterized by fractures from radiologically demonstrable polycystic osseous lesions starting in the third decade, frontal lobe syndrome, and progressive dementia beginning in the fourth decade. Change of personality develops insidiously, with a frontal lobe syndrome, including impaired judgment, euphoria, loss of social inhibition, poor concentration, and lack of insight. Memory loss accompanies the personality changes, and seizures are common. Progressive pyramidal signs develop, leading to loss of mobility. Dementia eventually includes aphasia, agraphia, acalculia, and apraxia, and patients succumb before age 50. Generalized cerebral atrophy is present with frontal predominance, thin corpus callosum, severe reduction in cerebral white matter, and atrophy of the basal ganglia. Cortical neurons show chromatolysis, with neuronal loss in the caudate nuclei and thalamus, and cerebral white matter shows loss of axons and myelin with astrocytic proliferation and hypertrophy (see Paloneva, Autti, & Hakola, 2010 for review and references).

Rapid Onset of Late-Life Neurodegenerative Disorders

The genetic forms of Alzheimer's disease caused by the presenilin 1(PS1), presenilin 2, and amyloid precursor protein mutations have a clinical presentation quite different than the older onset AD, whether sporadic or familial. PS1-AD may include rapid onset dementia over months to a year or two, manifests as early as the third or early fourth decade, and often includes early psychiatric changes accompanying profound amnesia, myoclonus, dystonia, chorea, and cerebellar ataxia. The largest population of PS1-AD patients, about 5,000 individuals in Antioquia, Colombia, show memory impairments in the third decade of life, followed by progressive impairment of language and other cognitive processes, mild cognitive impairment at age 45, and dementia at age 50 (Sepulveda-Falla, Glatzel, & Lopera, 2012). The wide phenotypic heterogeneity in this PS1-AD cohort has not yet yielded any clear patterns of genotype-phenotype correlation (Larner, 2013). A young man with sporadically presenting PS1-AD personally examined (Kishore, Kimchi, Cunningham, Frosch, & Schmahmann, 2013) began having difficulties around age 32 with behavioral changes, paranoia, and irritability, followed by profound anterograde amnesia, lack of insight, and impaired gait, with ataxia, chorea, and progressively severe myoclonus leading to mutism and demise within 6 years. The combination of brain MRI and PET scan, CSF markers for Alzheimer's disease, and the PS1 gene testing permitted a diagnosis during life that was helpful in planning management and counseling.

This chapter concludes where it started, with the observations of the UCSF survey of patients referred for possible CJD. Fully 39% (26 patients out of 67) of these rapidly deteriorating cases were found at autopsy to be neurodegenerative (CBD, FTD, LBD, AD, and PSP; see Table 15.1). Personal experience provides anecdotal support for these empiric observations and makes the point that there are patients in whom these usually slowly evolving disorders have a more rapid, subacute onset. Two patients personally examined and followed to autopsy had Lewy body disease present in a precipitous manner, apparently fine one day, and confused and disoriented the next. The reason for these rapid declines has not been defined. Clues to the diagnosis are found in the motor and cognitive features on examination. That is, the case can be typical of the usual presentation in all respects but for the timing of the onset. Caution is warranted in reaching a diagnosis of these as-yet-untreatable disorders, given the multitude of potentially treatable conditions outlined before, and the possibility of intercurrent treatable illness such as a urinary tract infection exacerbating or precipitating the apparently sudden cognitive decline.

A practical list of disorders that should be foremost in the consideration of subacute and rapidly progressive dementias is in Table 15.6

TABLE 15.6 Subacute Dementia: A Working Approach to Differential Diagnosis (STOPIM)

Structural, **T**rauma, **O**bstructive, **P**araneoplastic, **I**nfectious, **M**etabolic—Toxic
Structural
    Strategic stroke (cortical and/or subcortical; location is critical)
    Multiple small strokes—subacute bacterial endocarditis, vasculitis, TTP
    Abscess or cerebritis (e.g., toxoplasma, seeded from lung, blood)
    Tumor—primary (focal, multicentric glioma, lymphoma), metastatic
    ADEM (acute demyelinating encephalomyelopathy)
    Multiple sclerosis and mimics, including sarcoidosis
    MELAS (mitochondrial encephalopathy, lactic acidosis, stroke-like episodes)
Trauma
    Subacute or chronic subdural hematoma (weeks to months)
    The concussion that does not resolve—intraparenchymal contusions
Obstructive
    Normal pressure hydrocephalus
    Obstructive hydrocephalus
    Sagging brain syndrome
Paraneoplastic
    Paraneoplastic limbic encephalitis
    Autoimmune (non-cancer-related) limbic encephalitis
Infectious
    Herpes simplex encephalitis
    Prion diseases—CJD, variant
    HIV and complications
    Progressive multifocal leukoencephalopathy (PML)
    Meningoencephalitis (Lyme, syphilis, TB, fungus, cryptococcus, cysticercosis, Whipple, SSPE)
Metabolic
    Encephalopathy with asterixis
        Hepatic, renal, hypoxemic encephalopathy
        Magnesium deficiency
        Lithium excess
    Vitamin deficiency—B1 (Wernicke), B3 (pellagra), B12, and E
    Thyroid—deficiency, excess, Hashimoto encephalopathy
    Toxins and poisons
Degenerative diseases with rapid onset—cannot stop them...yet

The acronym STOPIM is intended to convey the notion that many of these diseases and conditions, although not all, will respond to appropriate urgent intervention. A practical approach to the diagnostic laboratory workup of the causes of dementia is offered in Table 15.7

Acknowledgments

The valuable assistance of Jason MacMore, BA, is gratefully acknowledged. This work was supported in part by the Birmingham, MINDlink, Sidney R. Baer Jr. and National Ataxia Foundations, the National

TABLE 15.7 Laboratory Evaluations for the Cause of Dementia

Investigations are performed in a stepwise and logical sequence, determined by the degree of clinical suspicion.

First Level—For All Patients
A. CBC, ESR, BUN, creatinine, electrolytes, glucose, calcium, magnesium, LFTs, TSH, B12, RPR, chest X-ray, EKG, urinalysis and culture, MRI with gadolinium if suspect enhancing lesions; magnetic susceptibility study for microhemorrhages for amyloid (CT head +/- contrast, if MRI not available), neuropsychological testing
B. First level of evaluation if indicated based on the initial history and exam:
HIV, ANA, HbA1c, blood gas, blood culture, thiamine and red cell transketolase, Lyme titer and Western blot, vitamin E, FTA, PPD, lactate, pyruvate, ACE, porphyrins, methylmalonic acid, homocysteine, toxic screen (drugs, poisons, metals)
EEG

Second Level
Spinal tap—cells, protein, glucose, fungus, TB, virus, cytology, HSV-PCR, CSF aβ, tau, Lyme titer and Western blot, VDRL, oligoclonal banding, IgG, 14-3-3, glutamine, lactate, measles antibody
Vascular workup: lipid profile/anticardiolipin antibodies/carotid noninvasives/Holter monitor/echocardiogram
Quantitative plasma amino acids, quantitative urine organic acids
Vasculitis workup if ANA+ (anti-dsDNA, Ro, La, Sm, RNP, ANCA, C3, C4, CH50)
Limbic encephalitis paraneoplastic and autoimmune antibodies, CT chest, abdomen and pelvis, mammogram, testicular ultrasound
All-night sleep study, pO2

Third Level
PET/SPECT
Cerebral angiography for vasculitis, intravascular lymphoma
Fluorescein angiography
Gene testing—e.g., PS1, PS2, MAPT, TDP-43, CADASIL, MELAS, SCAs, FXTAS
Biopsy: brain/meninges, nerve/muscle, skin, liver, kidney

Diagnostic Evaluations in Extremely Rare Disorders
Low serum ceruloplasmin, high urine and liver copper levels in Wilson's disease
Very long chain fatty acids—ALD
WBC arylsulfatase A—MLD
Serum hexosaminidase A and B—Tay Sachs/Sandhoff
WBC for galactocerebroside beta-galactosidase—Krabbe's leukodystrophy
Serum cholestanol or urine bile acids—cerebrotendinous xanthomatosis
WBC beta-galactosidase—GM$_1$ gangliosidosis
Skin biopsy for biochemical testing of fibroblasts—Niemann-Pick type C
X-rays of hands for bone cysts, bone or skin biopsy for abnormal fat cells—polycystic lipomembranous osteodysplasia with sclerosing leukoencephalopathy
Urine mucopolysaccharides elevated, serum alpha-N-acetyl glucosaminidase-deficient, mucopolysaccharidoses

Indications for Brain Biopsy
Focal, relevant lesion(s) of undetermined cause, after extensive evaluation
Distinguish primary CNS lymphoma from PML and other entities if necessary
Central nervous system vasculitis
Rare pediatric neurodegenerative diseases presenting in adulthood: Krabbe's disease (PAS + histiocytes); Kuf's disease, intranuclear fingerprint pattern, and osmophilic granules on electron microscopy; Alexander's disease, Rosenthal fibers; neuronal intranuclear (eosinophilic) inclusion disease

Organization for Rare Disorders, and RO1 MH 64044 and MH 67980.

References

Abou-Zeid, E., Boursoulian, L. J., Metzer, W. S., & Gundogdu, B. (2012). Morvan syndrome: A case report and review of the literature. *Journal of Clinical Neuromuscular Disease, 13,* 214–227.

Adams, R. D. (1966). Further observations on normal pressure hydrocephalus. *Proceedings of the Royal Society of Medicine, 59,* 1135–1140.

Adams, R. D., Fisher, C. M., Hakim, S., Ojemann, R. G., & Sweet, W. H. (1965). Symptomatic occult hydrocephalus with "normal" cerebrospinal-fluid pressure. A treatable syndrome. *New England Journal of Medicine, 273,* 117–126.

ACR Ad Hoc Committee. (1999). The American College of Rheumatology nomenclature and case definitions for neuropsychiatric lupus syndromes. *Arthritis and Rheumatism, 42,* 599–608.

Alkali, N. H., Bwala, S. A., Nyandaiti, Y. W., & Danesi, M. A. (2013). NeuroAIDS in sub-Saharan Africa: A clinical review. *Annals of African Medicine, 12,* 1–10.

Alper, T., Cramp, W. A., Haig, D. A., & Clarke, M. C. (1967). Does the agent of scrapie replicate without nucleic acid? *Nature, 214,* 764–766.

Armstrong, M. J., Litvan, I., Lang, A. E., Bak, T. H., Bhatia, K. P., Borroni, B.,...Weiner, W. J. (2013). Criteria for the diagnosis of corticobasal degeneration. *Neurology, 80,* 496–503.

Asztely, F., & Kumlien, E. (2012). The diagnosis and treatment of limbic encephalitis. *Acta Neurological Scandinavica, 126,* 365–375.

Atkinson, J. L., Weinshenker, B. G., Miller, G. M., Piepgras, D. G., & Mokri, B. (1998). Acquired Chiari I malformation secondary to spontaneous spinal cerebrospinal fluid leakage and chronic intracranial hypotension syndrome in seven cases. *Journal of Neurosurgery, 88,* 237–242.

Austin, J., Armstrong, D., Fouch, S., Mitchell, C., Stumpf, D., Shearer, L., & Briner, O. (1968). Metachromatic leukodystrophy (MLD). 8. MLD in adults; diagnosis and pathogenesis. *Archives of Neurology, 18,* 225–240.

Back, T., Grunig, S., Winter, Y., Bodechtel, U., Guthke, K., Khati, D., & von Kummer, R. (2013). Neuroborreliosis-associated cerebral vasculitis: Long-term outcome and health-related quality of life. *Journal of Neurology, 260,* 1569–1575.

Bae, S. J., Lee, H. K., Lee, J. H., Choi, C. G., & Suh, D. C. (2001). Wernicke's encephalopathy: Atypical manifestation at MR imaging. *AJNR American Journal of Neuroradiology, 22,* 1480–1482.

Baehring, J. M., Longtine, J., & Hochberg, F. H. (2003). A new approach to the diagnosis and treatment of intravascular lymphoma. *Journal of Neurooncology, 61,* 237–248.

Baillieux, H., De Smet, H. J., Dobbeleir, A., Paquier, P. F., De Deyn, P. P., & Marien, P. (2010). Cognitive and affective disturbances following focal cerebellar damage in adults: A neuropsychological and SPECT study. *Cortex, 46,* 869–879.

Balkan, I. I., Albayram, S., Ozaras, R., Yilmaz, M. H., Ozbayrak, M., Mete, B.,...Tabak, F. (2012). Spontaneous intracranial hypotension syndrome may mimic aseptic meningitis. *Scandinavian Journal of Infectious Diseases, 44,* 481–488.

Baram, T. Z., Goldman, A. M., & Percy, A. K. (1986). Krabbe disease: Specific MRI and CT findings. *Neurology, 36,* 111–115.

Bartlett, E., & Mikulis, D. J. (2005). Chasing "chasing the dragon" with MRI: Leukoencephalopathy in drug abuse. *British Journal of Radiology, 78,* 997–1004.

Berger, J. R. (2011). The clinical features of PML. *Cleveland Clinic Journal of Medicine, 78*(Suppl 2), S8–12.

Berger, J. R., Aksamit, A. J., Clifford, D. B., Davis, L., Koralnik, I. J., Sejvar, J. J.,...Nath, A. (2013). PML diagnostic criteria: Consensus statement from the AAN Neuroinfectious Disease Section. *Neurology, 80,* 1430–1438.

Bezman, L., Moser, A. B., Raymond, G. V., Rinaldo, P., Watkins, P. A., Smith, K. D.,...Moser, H. W. (2001). Adrenoleukodystrophy: Incidence, new mutation rate, and results of extended family screening. *Annals of Neurology, 49,* 512–517.

Bianco, F., Iacovelli, E., Tinelli, E., Lepre, C., & Pauri, F. (2011). Recurrent leukoencephalopathy in a cocaine abuser. *Neurotoxicology, 32,* 410–412.

Bloch, O., & McDermott, M. W. (2012). Lumboperitoneal shunts for the treatment of normal pressure hydrocephalus. *Journal of Clinical Neuroscience, 19,* 1107–1111.

Boerner, R. J., & Kapfhammer, H. P. (1999). Psychopathological changes and cognitive impairment in encephalomyelitis disseminata. *European Archives of Psychiatry and Clinical Neuroscience, 249,* 96–102.

Braga-Neto, P., Pedroso, J. L., Alessi, H., Dutra, L. A., Felicio, A. C., Minett, T.,...Barsottini, O. G. (2012). Cerebellar cognitive affective syndrome in Machado Joseph disease: Core clinical features. *Cerebellum, 11,* 549–56.

Brain, L., Jellinek, E. H., & Ball, K. (1966). Hashimoto's disease and encephalopathy. *Lancet, 2,* 512–514.

Bratton, R. L., Whiteside, J. W., Hovan, M. J., Engle, R. L., & Edwards, F. D. (2008). Diagnosis and treatment of Lyme disease. *Mayo Clinic Proceedings, 83*, 566–571.

Brismar, J., Gascon, G. G., von Steyern, K. V., & Bohlega, S. (1996). Subacute sclerosing panencephalitis: Evaluation with CT and MR. *AJNR American Journal of Neuroradiology, 17*, 761–772.

Brown, K., Mastrianni, J. A. (2010). The prion diseases. *Journal of Geriatric Psychiatry and Neurology, 23*, 277–298.

Brown, W. T. (1954). *Papua New Guinea control reports.* [Kainantu Patrol Report No 8 of 1953/54], Department of District Services and Native Affairs, Australia New Guinea Administrative Unit.

Brownell, B., & Oppenheimer, D. R. (1965). An ataxic form of subacute presenile polioencephalopathy (Creutzfeldt-Jakob Disease). *Journal of Neurology, Neurosurgery and Psychiatry, 28*, 350–361.

Burk, K. (2007). Cognition in hereditary ataxia. *Cerebellum, 6*, 280–286.

Burns, A., & Holland, T. (1986). Vitamin E deficiency. *Lancet, 1*, 805–806.

Cali, I., Castellani, R., Alshekhlee, A., Cohen, Y., Blevins, J., Yuan, J.,...Gambetti, P. (2009). Co-existence of scrapie prion protein types 1 and 2 in sporadic Creutzfeldt-Jakob disease: Its effect on the phenotype and prion-type characteristics. *Brain, 132*, 2643–2658.

Castillo, P., Woodruff, B., Caselli, R., Vernino, S., Lucchinetti, C., Swanson, J.,...Boeve, B. (2006). Steroid-responsive encephalopathy associated with autoimmune thyroiditis. *Archives of Neurology, 63*, 197–202.

Chakor, R. T., & Santosh, N. S. (2013). Subacute sclerosing panencephalitis presenting as rapidly progressive young-onset dementia. *Journal of the Pakistan Medical Association, 63*, 921–924.

Chen-Plotkin, A. S., Pau, K. T., & Schmahmann, J. D. (2008). Delayed leukoencephalopathy after hypoxic-ischemic injury. *Archives of Neurology, 65*, 144–145.

Chong, J. Y., Rowland, L. P., & Utiger, R. D. (2003). Hashimoto encephalopathy: Syndrome or myth? *Archives of Neurology, 60*, 164–171.

Chu-Shore, C. J., Major, P., Camposano, S., Muzykewicz, D., & Thiele, E. A. (2010). The natural history of epilepsy in tuberous sclerosis complex. *Epilepsia, 51*, 1236–1241.

Coker, S. B. (1991). The diagnosis of childhood neurodegenerative disorders presenting as dementia in adults. *Neurology, 41*, 794–798.

Collinge, J., Whitfield, J., McKintosh, E., Frosh, A., Mead, S., Hill, A. F.,...Alpers, M. P. (2008). A clinical study of kuru patients with long incubation periods at the end of the epidemic in Papua New Guinea. *Philosophical Transactions of the Royal Society of London B: Biological Sciences, 363*, 3725–3739.

Cooper, F. E., Grube, M., Elsegood, K. J., Welch, J. L., Kelly, T. P., Chinnery, P. F., & Griffiths, T. D. (2010). The contribution of the cerebellum to cognition in Spinocerebellar Ataxia Type 6. *Behavioral Neurology, 23*, 3–15.

Cooper, S. A., Murray, K. L., Heath, C. A., Will, R. G., & Knight, R. S. (2005). Isolated visual symptoms at onset in sporadic Creutzfeldt-Jakob disease: The clinical phenotype of the "Heidenhain variant". *British Journal of Ophthalmology, 89*, 1341–1342.

Cornejo, R., Venegas, P., Goni, D., Salas, A., & Romero, C. (2010). Successful response to intravenous immunoglobulin as rescue therapy in a patient with Hashimoto's encephalopathy. *British Medical Journal Case Reports, 2010*. pii: bcr0920103332.

Corsellis, J. A., Goldberg, G. J., & Norton, A. R. (1968). "Limbic encephalitis" and its association with carcinoma. *Brain, 91*, 481–496.

Costello, D. J., Eichler, A. F., & Eichler, F. S. (2009). Leukodystrophies: Classification, diagnosis, and treatment. *Neurologist, 15*, 319–328.

D'Esposito, M., Verfaellie, M., Alexander, M. P., & Katz, D. I. (1995). Amnesia following traumatic bilateral fornix transection. *Neurology, 45*, 1546–1550.

Darnell, R., & Posner, J. (2011). *Paraneoplastic syndromes. Contemporary neurology series, Vol 79.* New York, NY: Oxford University Press.

Davis, J. D., Stern, R. A., & Flashman, L. A. (2003). Cognitive and neuropsychiatric aspects of subclinical hypothyroidism: Significance in the elderly. *Current Psychiatry Reports, 5*, 384–390.

De Michele, G., Maltecca, F., Carella, M., Volpe, G., Orio, M., De Falco, A.,...Bruni, A. (2003). Dementia, ataxia, extrapyramidal features, and epilepsy: Phenotype spectrum in two Italian families with spinocerebellar ataxia type 17. *Neurological Sciences, 24*, 166–167.

DeArmond, S., & Prusiner, S. (1997). Prion diseases. In P. Lantos & D. Graham (Eds.), *Greenfield's neuropathology* (6th ed., pp. 235–280). London, UK: Edward Arnold.

DiMauro, S., & Hirano, M. (2001). MELAS. In: Pagon RA, Adam MP, Bird TD, Dolan CR, Fong CT, Smith RJH, Stephens K, editors. GeneReviews® [Internet]. Seattle (WA): University of Washington, Seattle; 1993–2014.

Dinn, J. J. (1980). Transolfactory spread of virus in herpes simplex encephalitis. *British Medical Journal, 281*, 1392.

Disler, P. B., & Eales, L. (1982). The acute attack of porphyria. *South African Medical Journal, 61*, 82–84.

Dorr, J., Krautwald, S., Wildemann, B., Jarius, S., Ringelstein, M., Duning, T.,...Kleffner, I. (2013). Characteristics of Susac syndrome: A review of all reported cases. *Nature Reviews Neurology, 9*, 307–316.

Drulovic, J., Andrejevic, S., Bonaci-Nikolic, B., & Mijailovic, V. (2011). Hashimoto's encephalopathy: A long-lasting remission induced by intravenous immunoglobulins. *Vojnosanit Pregl, 68*, 452–454.

Duff, K., & McCaffrey, R. J. (2001). Electrical injury and lightning injury: A review of their mechanisms and neuropsychological, psychiatric, and neurological sequelae. *Neuropsychology Reviews, 11*, 101–116.

Dumas, J. A., Makarewicz, J., Schaubhut, G. J., Devins, R., Albert, K., Dittus, K., & Newhouse, P. A. (2013). Chemotherapy altered brain functional connectivity in women with breast cancer: A pilot study. *Brain Imaging and Behavior, 7*(4), 524–532.

Duncan, J. M. (1989). Listeria and psychiatric syndromes. *British Journal of Psychiatry, 154*, 887.

Ebi, J., Sato, H., Nakajima, M., & Shishido, F. (2013). Incidence of leukoencephalopathy after whole-brain radiation therapy for brain metastases. *International Journal of Radiation Oncology and Biological Physics, 85*, 1212–1217.

Edwin, D., Speedie, L. J., Kohler, W., Naidu, S., Kruse, B., & Moser, H. W. (1996). Cognitive and brain magnetic resonance imaging findings in adrenomyeloneuropathy. *Annals of Neurology, 40*, 675–678.

Eichler, F., Mahmood, A., Loes, D., Bezman, L., Lin, D., Moser, H. W., & Raymond, G. V. (2007). Magnetic resonance imaging detection of lesion progression in adult patients with X-linked adrenoleukodystrophy. *Archives of Neurology, 64*, 659–664.

Eichler, F. S., Barker, P. B., Cox, C., Edwin, D., Ulug, A. M., Moser, H. W., & Raymond, G. V. (2002). Proton MR spectroscopic imaging predicts lesion progression on MRI in X-linked adrenoleukodystrophy. *Neurology, 58*, 901–907.

Eichler, F. S., Itoh, R., Barker, P. B., Mori, S., Garrett, E. S., van Zijl, P. C.,...Melhem, E. R. (2002). Proton MR spectroscopic and diffusion tensor brain MR imaging in X-linked adrenoleukodystrophy: Initial experience. *Radiology, 225*, 245–252.

Eide, P. K., & Sorteberg, W. (2010). Diagnostic intracranial pressure monitoring and surgical management in idiopathic normal pressure hydrocephalus: A 6-year review of 214 patients. *Neurosurgery, 66*, 80–91.

Faerber, E. N., Melvin, J., & Smergel, E. M. (1999). MRI appearances of metachromatic leukodystrophy. *Pediatric Radiology, 29*, 669–672.

Fallon, B. A., Keilp, J. G., Corbera, K. M., Petkova, E., Britton, C. B., Dwyer, E.,...Sackeim, H. A. (2008). A randomized, placebo-controlled trial of repeated IV antibiotic therapy for Lyme encephalopathy. *Neurology, 70*, 992–1003.

Fallon, B. A., Petkova, E., Keilp, J. G., & Slavov, I. (2009). A randomized, placebo-controlled trial of repeated IV antibiotic therapy for Lyme encephalopathy prolonged lyme disease treatment: Enough is enough. Author Reply. *Neurology, 72*, 383–384.

Ferini-Strambi, L. (2011). Does idiopathic REM sleep behavior disorder (iRBD) really exist? What are the potential markers of neurodegeneration in iRBD? *Sleep Medicine, 12*(Suppl 2), S43–S49.

Ferreri, A. J., Campo, E., Seymour, J. F., Willemze, R., Ilariucci, F., Ambrosetti, A.,...Ponzoni, M. (2004). Intravascular lymphoma: Clinical presentation, natural history, management and prognostic factors in a series of 38 cases, with special emphasis on the 'cutaneous variant'. *British Journal of Haematology, 127*, 173–183.

Filley, C. M. (1998). The behavioral neurology of cerebral white matter. *Neurology, 50*, 1535–1540.

Filley, C. M. (2001). *The behavioral neurology of white matter*. New York, NY: Oxford University Press.

Filley, C. M. (2012). *Behavioral neurology of white matter*. New York, NY: Oxford University Press.

Filley, C. M., Franklin, G. M., Heaton, R. K., & Rosenberg, N. L. (1988). White matter dementia: Clinical disorders and implications. *Neuropsychiatry Neuropsychology and Behavioral Neurology, 1*, 239–254.

Filley, C. M., Heaton, R. K., Nelson, L. M., Burks, J. S., & Franklin, G. M. (1989). A comparison of dementia in Alzheimer's disease and multiple sclerosis. *Archives of Neurology* 1989; *46*, 157–161.

Filley, C. M., Heaton, R. K., & Rosenberg, N. L. (1990). White matter dementia in chronic toluene abuse. *Neurology, 40*, 532–534.

Fisher, C. M. (1983). Honored guest presentation: Abulia minor vs. agitated behavior. *Clinical Neurosurgery, 31*, 9–31.

Fliessbach, K., Helmstaedter, C., Urbach, H., Althaus, A., Pels, H., Linnebank, M.,...Schlegel, U. (2005). Neuropsychological outcome after chemotherapy for primary CNS lymphoma: a prospective study. *Neurology, 64*, 1184–1188.

Foley, J., & Denny-Brown, D. (1955). Subacute progressive encephalopathy with bulbar myoclonus. *Excerpta Medica (Amsterdam), Sect. VIII*, 782–784.

Freeman, S. H., Hyman, B. T., Sims, K. B., Hedley-Whyte, E. T., Vossough, A., Frosch,

M. P., & Schmahmann, J. D. (2009). Adult onset leukodystrophy with neuroaxonal spheroids: clinical, neuroimaging and neuropathologic observations. *Brain Pathology, 19*, 39–47.

Gabuzda, D. H., & Hirsch, M. S. (1987). Neurologic manifestations of infection with human immunodeficiency virus. Clinical features and pathogenesis. *Annals of Internal Medicine, 107*, 383–391.

Gajdusek, D. C., Gibbs, C. J., & Alpers, M. (1966). Experimental transmission of a Kuru-like syndrome to chimpanzees. *Nature, 209*, 794–796.

Ganz, P. A., Kwan, L., Castellon, S. A., Oppenheim, A., Bower, J. E., Silverman, D. H.,…Belin, T. R. (2013). Cognitive complaints after breast cancer treatments: Examining the relationship with neuropsychological test performance. *Journal of the National Cancer Institute, 105*, 791–801.

Garrard, P., Martin, N. H., Giunti, P., & Cipolotti, L. (2008). Cognitive and social cognitive functioning in spinocerebellar ataxia: A preliminary characterization. *Journal of Neurology, 255*, 398–405.

George, J. N. (2006). Clinical practice. Thrombotic thrombocytopenic purpura. *New England Journal of Medicine, 354*, 1927–1935.

Gerard, A., Sarrot-Reynauld, F., Liozon, E., Cathebras, P., Besson, G., Robin, C.,…Rousset, H. (2002). Neurologic presentation of Whipple disease: Report of 12 cases and review of the literature. *Medicine (Baltimore), 81*, 443–457.

Geschwind, D. H. (1999). Focusing attention on cognitive impairment in spinocerebellar ataxia. *Archives of Neurology, 56*, 20–22.

Geschwind, M. D., Shu, H., Haman, A., Sejvar, J. J., & Miller, B. L. (2008). Rapidly progressive dementia. *Annals of Neurology, 64*, 97–108.

Geschwind, N. (1965a). Disconnexion syndromes in animals and man. I. *Brain, 88*, 237–294.

Geschwind, N. (1965b). Disconnexion syndromes in animals and man. II. *Brain, 88*, 585–644.

Goldman-Rakic, P. S. (1988). Topography of cognition: Parallel distributed networks in primate association cortex. *Annual Review of Neuroscience, 11*, 137–156.

Gongvatana, A., Harezlak, J., Buchthal, S., Daar, E., Schifitto, G., Campbell, T.,…Navia, B. (2013). Progressive cerebral injury in the setting of chronic HIV infection and antiretroviral therapy. *Journal of Neurovirology, 19*, 209–218.

Graus, F., & Dalmau, J. (2012). Paraneoplastic neurological syndromes. *Current Opinion in Neurology, 25*, 795–801.

Gray, F., Adle-Biassette, H., Chretien, F., Lorin de la Grandmaison, G., Force, G., & Keohane, C. (2001). Neuropathology and neurodegeneration in human immunodeficiency virus infection. Pathogenesis of HIV-induced lesions of the brain, correlations with HIV-associated disorders and modifications according to treatments. *Clinical Neuropathology, 20*, 146–155.

Greco, C. M., Berman, R. F., Martin, R. M., Tassone, F., Schwartz, P. H., Chang, A.,…Hagerman, P. J. (2006). Neuropathology of fragile X-associated tremor/ataxia syndrome (FXTAS). *Brain, 129*, 243–255.

Gregory, A., & Hayflick, S. (2013). Neurodegeneration with brain iron accumulation disorders overview. In: Pagon RA, Adam MP, Bird TD, Dolan CR, Fong CT, Smith RJH, Stephens K, editors. GeneReviews® [Internet]. Seattle (WA): University of Washington, Seattle; 1993–2014.

Griffith, J. S. (1967). Self-replication and scrapie. *Nature, 215*, 1043–1044.

Grigg-Damberger, M., & Ralls, F. (2012). Cognitive dysfunction and obstructive sleep apnea: From cradle to tomb. *Current Opinion in Pulmonary Medicine, 18*, 580–587.

Grigsby, J., Brega, A. G., Engle, K., Leehey, M. A., Hagerman, R. J., Tassone, F.,…Reynolds, A. (2008). Cognitive profile of fragile X premutation carriers with and without fragile X-associated tremor/ataxia syndrome. *Neuropsychology, 22*, 48–60.

Grois, N., Fahrner, B., Arceci, R. J., Henter, J. I., McClain, K., Lassmann, H.,…Prayer, D. (2010). Central nervous system disease in Langerhans cell histiocytosis. *Journal of Pediatrics, 156*, 873–881, 881 e1.

Grois, N., Prayer, D., Prosch, H., & Lassmann, H. (2005). Neuropathology of CNS disease in Langerhans cell histiocytosis. *Brain, 128*, 829–838.

Hagerman, R., & Hagerman, P. (2013). Advances in clinical and molecular understanding of the FMR1 premutation and fragile X-associated tremor/ataxia syndrome. *Lancet Neurology, 12*, 786–798.

Hajj-Ali, R. A., Singhal, A. B., Benseler, S., Molloy, E., & Calabrese, L. H. (2011). Primary angiitis of the CNS. *Lancet Neurology, 10*, 561–572.

Hakim, S., & Adams, R. D. (1965). The special clinical problem of symptomatic hydrocephalus with normal cerebrospinal fluid pressure. Observations on cerebrospinal fluid hydrodynamics. *Journal of Neurological Sciences, 2*, 307–327.

Halperin, J. J. (2008). Prolonged Lyme disease treatment: Enough is enough. *Neurology, 70*, 986–987.

Halperin, J. J. (2010). Nervous system Lyme disease. *Journal of the Royal College of Physicians, Edinburgh, 40*, 248–255.

Harris, M. J., Jeste, D. V., Gleghorn, A., & Sewell, D. D. (1991). New-onset psychosis in HIV-infected patients. *Journal of Clinical Psychiatry, 52*, 369–376.

Hasegawa, M., Arai, T., Akiyama, H., Nonaka, T., Mori, H., Hashimoto, T.,...Oyanagi, K. (2007). TDP-43 is deposited in the Guam parkinsonism-dementia complex brains. *Brain, 130*, 1386–1394.

Heilman, K. M., & Sypert, G. W. (1977). Korsakoff's syndrome resulting from bilateral fornix lesions. *Neurology, 27*, 490–493.

Heinrich, A., Runge, U., & Khaw, A. V. (2004). Clinicoradiologic subtypes of Marchiafava-Bignami disease. *Journal of Neurology, 251*, 1050–1059.

Heinrich, T. W., & Grahm, G. (2003). Hypothyroidism presenting as psychosis: Myxedema madness revisited. *Primary Care Companion, Journal of Clinical Psychiatry, 5*, 260–266.

Helmstaedter, C., & Elger, C. E. (2009). Chronic temporal lobe epilepsy: A neurodevelopmental or progressively dementing disease? *Brain, 132*, 2822–2830.

Henderson, R. D., Rajah, T., Nicol, A. J., & Read, S. J. (2003). Posterior leukoencephalopathy following intrathecal chemotherapy with MRA-documented vasospasm. *Neurology, 60*, 326–328.

Hillbom, M., Saloheimo, P., Fujioka, S., Wszolek, Z. K., Juvela, S., & Leone, M. A. (2013). Diagnosis and management of Marchiafava-Bignami disease: A review of CT/MRI confirmed cases. *Journal of Neurology, Neurosurgery and Psychiatry, 85*(2), 168–173.

Holle, J. U., & Gross, W. L. (2011). Neurological involvement in Wegener's granulomatosis. *Current Opinion in Rheumatology, 23*, 7–11.

Holmes, G. (1908). A form of familial degeneration of the cerebellum. *Brain, 30*, 466–488.

Hyde, T. M., Ziegler, J. C., & Weinberger, D. R. (1992). Psychiatric disturbances in metachromatic leukodystrophy. Insights into the neurobiology of psychosis. *Archives of Neurology, 49*, 401–406.

Irani, S. R., Alexander, S., Waters, P., Kleopa, K. A., Pettingill, P., Zuliani, L.,...Vincent, A. (2010). Antibodies to Kv1 potassium channel-complex proteins leucine-rich, glioma inactivated 1 protein and contactin-associated protein-2 in limbic encephalitis, Morvan's syndrome and acquired neuromyotonia. *Brain, 133*, 2734–2748.

Irani, S. R., Pettingill, P., Kleopa, K. A., Schiza, N., Waters, P., Mazia, C.,...Vincent, A. (2012). Morvan syndrome: Clinical and serological observations in 29 cases. *Annals of Neurology, 72*, 241–255.

Ironside, J. W. (1998). Neuropathological findings in new variant CJD and experimental transmission of BSE. *FEMS Immunology and Medical Microbiology, 21*, 91–95.

Ishii, K., Kanda, T., Harada, A., Miyamoto, N., Kawaguchi, T., Shimada, K.,...Mori, E. (2008). Clinical impact of the callosal angle in the diagnosis of idiopathic normal pressure hydrocephalus. *European Radiology, 18*, 2678–2683.

Ishii, N., & Nishihara, Y. (1981). Pellagra among chronic alcoholics: Clinical and pathological study of 20 necropsy cases. *Journal of Neurology, Neurosurgery and Psychiatry, 44*, 209–215.

Jackson, W. S., Borkowski, A. W., Watson, N. E., King, O. D., Faas, H., Jasanoff, A., & Lindquist, S. (2013). Profoundly different prion diseases in knock-in mice carrying single PrP codon substitutions associated with human diseases. *Proceedings of the National Academy of Science USA, 110*, 14759–14764.

Jacquemont, S., Hagerman, R. J., Leehey, M., Grigsby, J., Zhang, L., Brunberg, J. A.,...Hagerman, P. J. (2003). Fragile X premutation tremor/ataxia syndrome: Molecular, clinical, and neuroimaging correlates. *American Journal of Human Genetics, 72*, 869–878.

Jim, H. S., Phillips, K. M., Chait, S., Faul, L. A., Popa, M. A., Lee, Y. H.,...Small, B. J. (2012). Meta-analysis of cognitive functioning in breast cancer survivors previously treated with standard-dose chemotherapy. *Journal of Clinical Oncology, 30*, 3578–3587.

Jones, E. G., & Powell, T. P. (1970). An anatomical study of converging sensory pathways within the cerebral cortex of the monkey. *Brain, 93*, 793–820.

Jones, H. R., Jr., & Siekert, R. G. (1989). Neurological manifestations of infective endocarditis. Review of clinical and therapeutic challenges. *Brain, 112*(Pt 5), 1295–315.

Jongen, P. J., Ter Horst, A. T., & Brands, A. M. (2012). Cognitive impairment in multiple sclerosis. *Minerva Medicine, 103*, 73–96.

Joseph, F. G., Lammie, G. A., & Scolding, N. J. (2007). CNS lupus: A study of 41 patients. *Neurology, 69*, 644–654.

Kapas, I., Majtenyi, K., Toro, K., Keller, E., Voigtlander, T., & Kovacs, G. G. (2012). Pellagra encephalopathy as a differential diagnosis for Creutzfeldt-Jakob disease. *Metabolic Brain Disease, 27*, 231–235.

Kaufman, K. R., Zuber, N., Rueda-Lara, M. A., & Tobia, A. (2010). MELAS with recurrent complex partial seizures, nonconvulsive status epilepticus, psychosis, and behavioral disturbances: Case analysis with literature review. *Epilepsy and Behavior, 18*, 494–497.

Kayal, A. K., Goswami, M., Das, M., & Paul, B. (2011). Clinical spectrum of neurosyphilis in North East India. *Neurology India, 59*, 344–350.

Kellner, M., Sonntag, A., & Strian, F. (1990). Psychiatric sequelae of listeriosis. *British Journal of Psychiatry, 157*, 299.

Kelly, J., & Renner, A. J. (2008). Alcohol-related disorders. In T. Stern, J. Rosenbaum, M. Fava, J. Biederman, & S. Rauch (Eds.), *Massachusetts General Hospital comprehensive clinical psychiatry* (pp. 337–354). Philadelphia, PA: Mosby.

Kim, H., Schmahmann, J. S. K., Falk, W., Stern, T., & Norris, E. (1999). A neuropsychiatric presentation of mitochondrial myopathy, encephalopathy, lactic acidosis and stroke-like episodes. *Medicine and Psychiatry, 2*, 3–9.

Kishore, N., Kimchi, E., Cunningham, M., Frosch, M., & Schmahmann, J. (April 4, 2013). *A neuropsychiatric case study of early onset familial Alzheimer's Disease.* Paper presented at the Annual Meeting of the American Neuropsychiatric Association, Boston, MA.

Kitagawa, Y., Gotoh, F., Koto, A., & Okayasu, H. (1990). Stroke in systemic lupus erythematosus. *Stroke, 21*, 1533–1539.

Kleinfeld, K., Mobley, B., Hedera, P., Wegner, A., Sriram, S., & Pawate, S. (2013). Adult-onset leukoencephalopathy with neuroaxonal spheroids and pigmented glia: Report of five cases and a new mutation. *Journal of Neurology, 260*, 558–571.

Knudsen, R. (2013). Neurosyphilis: Overview of syphilis of the CNS. *Medscape.* Retrieved March 2014, from http://emedicine.medscape.com/article/1169231-overview.

Kohlschutter, A., & Eichler, F. (2011). Childhood leukodystrophies: A clinical perspective. *Expert Reviews in Neurotherapy, 11*, 1485–1496.

Kothbauer-Margreiter, I., Sturzenegger, M., Komor, J., Baumgartner, R., & Hess, C. W. (1996). Encephalopathy associated with Hashimoto thyroiditis: Diagnosis and treatment. *Journal of Neurology, 243*, 585–593.

Koziol, L. F., Budding, D., Andreasen, N., D'Arrigo, S., Bulgheroni, S., Imamizu, H.,...Yamazaki, T. (2013). Consensus paper: The cerebellum's role in movement and cognition. *Cerebellum, 13*(1), 151–177.

Kriegstein, A. R., Shungu, D. C., Millar, W. S., Armitage, B. A., Brust, J. C., Chillrud, S.,...Lynch, T. (1999). Leukoencephalopathy and raised brain lactate from heroin vapor inhalation ("chasing the dragon"). *Neurology, 53*, 1765–1773.

Kumar, N., Cohen-Gadol, A. A., Wright, R. A., Miller, G. M., Piepgras, D. G., & Ahlskog, J. E. (2006). Superficial siderosis. *Neurology, 66*, 1144–1152.

Laforce, R., Jr., Buteau, J. P., Bouchard, J. P., Rouleau, G. A., Bouchard, R. W., & Dupre, N. (2010). Cognitive impairment in ARCA-1, a newly discovered pure cerebellar ataxia syndrome. *Cerebellum, 9*, 443–453.

Lafosse, J. M., Corboy, J. R., Leehey, M. A., Seeberger, L. C., & Filley, C. M. (2007). MS vs. HD: Can white matter and subcortical gray matter pathology be distinguished neuropsychologically? *Journal of Clinical and Experimental Neuropsychology, 29*, 142–154.

Lancaster, E., & Dalmau, J. (2012). Neuronal autoantigens—pathogenesis, associated disorders and antibody testing. *Nature Reviews Neurology, 8*, 380–390.

Lancaster, E., Martinez-Hernandez, E., Titulaer, M. J., Boulos, M., Weaver, S., Antoine, J. C.,...Dalmau, J. (2011). Antibodies to metabotropic glutamate receptor 5 in the Ophelia syndrome. *Neurology, 77*, 1698–701.

Larner, A. J. (2013). Presenilin-1 mutations in Alzheimer's disease: An update on genotype-phenotype relationships. *Journal of Alzheimers Disease, 37*, 653–659.

Lasek, K., Lencer, R., Gaser, C., Hagenah, J., Walter, U., Wolters, A.,...Binkofski, F. (2006). Morphological basis for the spectrum of clinical deficits in spinocerebellar ataxia 17 (SCA17). *Brain, 129*, 2341–2352.

Lee, M. S., & Marsden, C. D. (1994). Neurological sequelae following carbon monoxide poisoning clinical course and outcome according to the clinical types and brain computed tomography scan findings. *Movement Disorders, 9*, 550–558.

Leehey, M. A., Munhoz, R. P., Lang, A. E., Brunberg, J. A., Grigsby, J., Greco, C.,...Hagerman, R. J. (2003). The fragile X premutation presenting as essential tremor. *Archives of Neurology, 60*, 117–121.

Levin, H. S., Goldstein, F. C., Norcross, K., Amparo, E. G., Guinto, F. C., Jr., & Mader, J. T. (1989). Neurobehavioral and magnetic resonance imaging findings in two cases of decompression sickness. *Aviation, Space, and Environmental Medicine, 60*, 1204–1210.

Levisohn, L., Cronin-Golomb, A., & Schmahmann, J. D. (2000). Neuropsychological consequences of cerebellar tumour resection in children: Cerebellar cognitive affective syndrome in a paediatric population. *Brain, 123*(Pt 5), 1041–1050.

Lorincz, M. T. (2010). Neurologic Wilson's disease. *Annals of the New York Academy of Sciences, 1184*, 173–187.

Lugaresi, E., Medori, R., Montagna, P., Baruzzi, A., Cortelli, P., Lugaresi, A.,...Gambetti, P. (1986). Fatal familial insomnia and dysautonomia with selective degeneration of thalamic nuclei. *New England Journal of Medicine, 315*, 997–1003.

Mangialasche, F., Solomon, A., Kareholt, I., Hooshmand, B., Cecchetti, R., Fratiglioni,

L.,...Kivipelto, M. (2013). Serum levels of vitamin E forms and risk of cognitive impairment in a Finnish cohort of older adults. *Experimental Gerontology*, 48(12), 1428–1435.

Margolin, D. H., Kousi, M., Chan, Y. M., Lim, E. T., Schmahmann, J. D., Hadjivassiliou, M.,...Seminara, S. B. (2013). Ataxia, dementia, and hypogonadotropism caused by disordered ubiquitination. *New England Journal of Medicine*, 368, 1992–2003.

Marotti, J. D., Tobias, S., Fratkin, J. D., Powers, J. M., & Rhodes, C. H. (2004). Adult onset leukodystrophy with neuroaxonal spheroids and pigmented glia: Report of a family, historical perspective, and review of the literature. *Acta Neuropathologica*, 107, 481–488.

Marshall, G. A., & Doyle, J. J. (2006). Long-term treatment of Hashimoto's encephalopathy. *Journal of Neuropsychiatry and Clinical Neuroscience*, 18, 14–20.

Mastrianni, J. (2003). Genetic prion diseases. In: Pagon RA, Adam MP, Bird TD, Dolan CR, Fong CT, Smith RJH, Stephens K, editors. GeneReviews® [Internet]. Seattle (WA): University of Washington, Seattle; 1993–2014

Matsubayashi, J., Tsuchiya, K., Matsunaga, T., & Mukai, K. (2009). Methotrexate-related leukoencephalopathy without radiation therapy: Distribution of brain lesions and pathological heterogeneity on two autopsy cases. *Neuropathology*, 29, 105–115.

Matsuda, M., Kishida, D., Kinoshita, T., Hineno, A., Shimojima, Y., Fukushima, K., & Ikeda, S. (2011). Leukoencephalopathy induced by low-dose methotrexate in a patient with rheumatoid arthritis. *Internal Medicine*, 50, 2219–2222.

Maubert, A., Hanon, C., & Metton, J. P. (2013). [Adult onset Niemann-Pick type C disease and psychosis: Literature review]. *Encephale*, 39, 315–319.

McGirr, A., Mohammed, S., Kurlan, R., & Cusimano, M. D. (2013). Clinical equipoise in idiopathic normal pressure hydrocephalus: A survey of physicians on the need for randomized controlled trials assessing the efficacy of cerebrospinal fluid diversion. *Journal of Neurological Sciences*, 333, 13–8.

McKeon, A., Frye, M. A., & Delanty, N. (2008). The alcohol withdrawal syndrome. *Journal of Neurology, Neurosurgery and Psychiatry*, 79, 854–862.

Medana, I. M., & Esiri, M. M. (2003). Axonal damage: A key predictor of outcome in human CNS diseases. *Brain*, 126, 515–530.

Meins, W., Muller-Thomsen, T., & Meier-Baumgartner, H. P. (2000). Subnormal serum vitamin B12 and behavioural and psychological symptoms in Alzheimer's disease. *International Journal of Geriatric Psychiatry*, 15, 415–418.

Melhem, E. R., Barker, P. B., Raymond, G. V., & Moser, H. W. (1999). X-linked adrenoleukodystrophy in children: Review of genetic, clinical, and MR imaging characteristics. *American Journal of Roentgenology*, 173, 1575–1581.

Melhem, E. R., Loes, D. J., Georgiades, C. S., Raymond, G. V., & Moser, H. W. (2000). X-linked adrenoleukodystrophy: The role of contrast-enhanced MR imaging in predicting disease progression. AJNR *American Journal of Neuroradiology*, 21, 839–844.

Mengel, E., Klunemann, H. H., Lourenco, C. M., Hendriksz, C. J., Sedel, F., Walterfang, M., & Kolb, S. A. (2013). Niemann-Pick disease type C symptomatology: An expert-based clinical description. *Orphanet Journal of Rare Diseases*, 8, 166.

Mesulam, M. M. (1981). A cortical network for directed attention and unilateral neglect. *Annals of Neurology*, 10, 309–325.

Minagar, A., Barnett, M. H., Benedict, R. H., Pelletier, D., Pirko, I., Sahraian, M. A.,...Zivadinov, R. (2013). The thalamus and multiple sclerosis: Modern views on pathologic, imaging, and clinical aspects. *Neurology*, 80, 210–219.

Mokri, B. (2004). Spontaneous low cerebrospinal pressure/volume headaches. *Current Neurology and Neuroscience Reports*, 4, 117–124.

Molloy, E. S., Singhal, A. B., & Calabrese, L. H. (2008). Tumour-like mass lesion: An under-recognised presentation of primary angiitis of the central nervous system. *Annals of the Rheumatic Diseases*, 67, 1732–1735.

Moser, H., Smith, K., Watkins, P., Powers, J., & Moser, A. (2000). X-linked adrenoleukodystrophy. In C. Scriver, W. S. Sly, B. Childs, A. Beaudet, D. Valle, K. Kinzler, & B. Vogelstein (Eds.), *The metabolic and molecular bases of inherited disease* (pp. 3257–3301). New York, NY: McGraw Hill.

Nanduri, V. R., Lillywhite, L., Chapman, C., Parry, L., Pritchard, J., & Vargha-Khadem, F. (2003). Cognitive outcome of long-term survivors of multisystem langerhans cell histiocytosis: A single-institution, cross-sectional study. *Journal of Clinical Oncology*, 21, 2961–2967.

Nauta, W. (1964). Some efferent connections of the prefrontal cortex in the monkey. In J. Warren & K. Akert (Eds.), *The frontal granular cortex and behavior* (pp. 397–409). New York, NY: McGraw Hill.

Navia, B. A., Jordan, B. D., & Price, R. W. (1986). The AIDS dementia complex: I. Clinical features. *Annals of Neurology*, 19, 517–24.

Offiah, C., & Hall, E. (2008). Heroin-induced leukoencephalopathy: Characterization using MRI, diffusion-weighted imaging, and MR spectroscopy. *Clinical Radiology, 63*, 146–52.

Organization, W. H. (1996). Public health issues and clinical and neurological characteristics of the new variant of Creutzfeldt-Jakob disease and other human and animal transmissible spongiform encephalopathies: Memorandum from two WHO meetings. *Bulletin of the World Health Organization, 74*, 453–463.

Orsi, L., D'Agata, F., Caroppo, P., Franco, A., Caglio, M. M., Avidano, F.,... Mortara, P. (2011). Neuropsychological picture of 33 spinocerebellar ataxia cases. *Journal of Clinical and Experimental Neuropsychology, 33*, 315–325.

Osawa, A., Maeshima, S., Kubo, K., & Itakura, T. (2006). Neuropsychological deficits associated with a tumour in the posterior corpus callosum: A report of two cases. *Brain Injury, 20*, 673–676.

Osimani, A., Berger, A., Friedman, J., Porat-Katz, B. S., & Abarbanel, J. M. (2005). Neuropsychology of vitamin B12 deficiency in elderly dementia patients and control subjects. *Journal of Geriatric Psychiatry and Neurology, 18*, 33–38.

Ozturk, A., Gurses, C., Baykan, B., Gokyigit, A., & Eraksoy, M. (2002). Subacute sclerosing panencephalitis: Clinical and magnetic resonance imaging evaluation of 36 patients. *Journal of Child Neurology, 17*, 25–29.

Palmer, M. S., Dryden, A. J., Hughes, J. T., & Collinge, J. (1991). Homozygous prion protein genotype predisposes to sporadic Creutzfeldt-Jakob disease. *Nature, 352*, 340–342.

Paloneva, J., Autti, T., & Hakola, P. (2002). Polycystic lipomembranous osteodysplasia with sclerosing leukoencephalopathy. In: Pagon RA, Adam MP, Bird TD, Dolan CR, Fong CT, Smith RJH, Stephens K, editors. GeneReviews® [Internet]. Seattle (WA): University of Washington, Seattle; 1993–2014

Pandya, D. N., & Kuypers, H. G. (1969). Cortico-cortical connections in the rhesus monkey. *Brain Research, 13*, 13–36.

Payer, M., Sottas, C., & Bonvin, C. (2010). Superficial siderosis of the central nervous system: Secondary progression despite successful surgical treatment, mimicking amyotrophic lateral sclerosis. Case report and review. *Acta Neurochirugica (Wien), 152*, 1411–1416.

Pearce, J. M. (2012). Brain disease leading to mental illness: A concept initiated by the discovery of general paralysis of the insane. *European Neurology, 67*, 272–278.

Peters, B. H., Levin, H. S., & Kelly, P. J. (1977). Neurologic and psychologic manifestations of decompression illness in divers. *Neurology, 27*, 125–127.

Petrou, P., Moscovici, S., Leker, R. R., Itshayek, E., Gomori, J. M., & Cohen, J. E. (2012). Ventriculoperitoneal shunt for intracranial hypertension in cryptococcal meningitis without hydrocephalus. *Journal of Clinical Neuroscience, 19*, 1175–1176.

Plum, F., & Posner, J. (1966). *Diagnosis of stupor and coma*. Philadelphia, PA: F.A. Davis.

Pollock, S. S., Pollock, T. M., & Harrison, M. J. (1984). Infection of the central nervous system by Listeria monocytogenes: A review of 54 adult and juvenile cases. *Quarterly Journal of Medicine, 53*, 331–340.

Poretti, A., Boltshauser, E., & Schmahmann, J. (2012). Paraneoplastic cerebellar syndromes: Neurodegeneration in Langerhans cell histiocytosis. In E. Boltshauser & J. Schmahmann (Eds.), *Cerebellar disorders in children. Clinics in developmental medicine No. 191—192* (pp. 351–357). London, UK: MacKeith Press.

Prayer, D., Grois, N., Prosch, H., Gadner, H., & Barkovich, A. J. (2004). MR imaging presentation of intracranial disease associated with Langerhans cell histiocytosis. *American Journal of Neuroradiology, 25*, 880–891.

Prosch, H., Grois, N., Wnorowski, M., Steiner, M., & Prayer, D. (2007). Long-term MR imaging course of neurodegenerative Langerhans cell histiocytosis. AJNR *American Journal of Neuroradiology, 28*, 1022–1028.

Prusiner, S. B. (1982). Novel proteinaceous infectious particles cause scrapie. *Science, 216*, 136–144.

Pyrgos, V., Seitz, A. E., Steiner, C. A., Prevots, D. R., & Williamson, P. R. (2013). Epidemiology of cryptococcal meningitis in the US: 1997–2009. *PLoS One, 8*, e56269.

Ramati, A., Rubin, L. H., Wicklund, A., Pliskin, N. H., Ammar, A. N., Fink, J. W.,... Kelley, K. M. (2009). Psychiatric morbidity following electrical injury and its effects on cognitive functioning. *General Hospital Psychiatry, 31*, 360–366.

Rao, S. M., Leo, G. J., Bernardin, L., & Unverzagt, F. (1991). Cognitive dysfunction in multiple sclerosis. I. Frequency, patterns, and prediction. *Neurology, 41*, 685–691.

Rennebohm, R., Susac, J. O., Egan, R. A., & Daroff, R. B. (2010). Susac's Syndrome—update. *Journal of Neurological Sciences, 299*, 86–91.

Rodin, G., & Ahles, T. A. (2012). Accumulating evidence for the effect of chemotherapy on cognition. *Journal of Clinical Oncology, 30*, 3568–3569.

Rodrigues, C. L., de Andrade, D. C., Livramento, J. A., Machado, L. R., Abraham, R., Massaroppe, L.,...Caramelli, P. (2012). Spectrum of cognitive impairment in neurocysticercosis: Differences according to disease phase. *Neurology, 78*, 861–866.

Rosenberg, N. L., Kleinschmidt-DeMasters, B. K., Davis, K. A., Dreisbach, J. N., Hormes, J. T., & Filley, C. M. (1988). Toluene abuse causes diffuse central nervous system white matter changes. *Annals of Neurology, 23*, 611–614.

Rudge, P., & Warrington, E. K. (1991). Selective impairment of memory and visual perception in splenial tumours. *Brain, 114*(Pt 1B), 349–360.

Sahraian, M. A., Radue, E. W., Eshaghi, A., Besliu, S., & Minagar, A. (2012). Progressive multifocal leukoencephalopathy: A review of the neuroimaging features and differential diagnosis. *European Journal of Neurology, 19*, 1060–1069.

Salkade, P. R., & Lim, T. A. (2012). Methotrexate-induced acute toxic leukoencephalopathy. *Journal of Cancer Research and Therapy, 8*, 292–296.

Savoiardo, M., Minati, L., Farina, L., De Simone, T., Aquino, D., Mea, E.,...Chiapparini, L. (2007). Spontaneous intracranial hypotension with deep brain swelling. *Brain, 130*, 1884–1893.

Schiffmann, R., & Elroy-Stein, O. (2006). Childhood ataxia with CNS hypomyelination/vanishing white matter disease—a common leukodystrophy caused by abnormal control of protein synthesis. *Molecular Genetics and Metabolism, 88*, 7–15.

Schiffmann, R., Moller, J. R., Trapp, B. D., Shih, H. H., Farrer, R. G., Katz, D. A.,...Kaneski, C. R. (1994). Childhood ataxia with diffuse central nervous system hypomyelination. *Annals of Neurology, 35*, 331–340.

Schmahmann, J. D. (1991). An emerging concept. The cerebellar contribution to higher function. *Archives of Neurology, 48*, 1178–1187.

Schmahmann, J. D. (1996). From movement to thought: Anatomic substrates of the cerebellar contribution to cognitive processing. *Human Brain Mapping, 4*, 174–198.

Schmahmann, J. D. (1997). Neurologic manifestations of late stage AIDS: Part I. *Resident and Staff Physician, 43*, 20–29.

Schmahmann, J. D. (1998). Neurologic manifestations of late stage AIDS: Part II. *Resident and Staff Physician, 44*, 45–59.

Schmahmann, J. D. (2003). Vascular syndromes of the thalamus. *Stroke, 34*, 2264–2278.

Schmahmann, J. D. (2004). Disorders of the cerebellum: Ataxia, dysmetria of thought, and the cerebellar cognitive affective syndrome. *Journal of Neuropsychiatry and Clinical Neuroscience, 16*, 367–378.

Schmahmann, J. D. (2006). Whipple disease of the central nervous system. In J. Noseworthy (Ed.), *Neurological theraputics: Principles and practice* (2nd ed., pp. 1673–16766). Oxon, UK: Informa Healthcare.

Schmahmann, J. D. (2010). The role of the cerebellum in cognition and emotion: Personal reflections since 1982 on the dysmetria of thought hypothesis, and its historical evolution from theory to therapy. *Neuropsychology Reviews, 20*, 236–260.

Schmahmann, J. D., & Pandya, D. N. (1997). The cerebrocerebellar system. *International Review of Neurobiology, 41*, 31–60.

Schmahmann, J. D., & Pandya, D. N. (2006). *Fiber pathways of the brain*. New York, NY: Oxford University Press.

Schmahmann, J. D., & Pandya, D. N. (2007). Cerebral white matter—historical evolution of facts and notions concerning the organization of the fiber pathways of the brain. *Journal of the History of Neuroscience, 16*, 237–267.

Schmahmann, J. D., & Pandya, D. N. (2008). Disconnection syndromes of basal ganglia, thalamus, and cerebrocerebellar systems. *Cortex, 44*, 1037–1066.

Schmahmann, J. D., & Sherman, J. C. (1997). Cerebellar cognitive affective syndrome. *International Review of Neurobiology, 41*, 433–440.

Schmahmann, J. D., & Sherman, J. C. (1998). The cerebellar cognitive affective syndrome. *Brain, 121*(Pt 4), 561–579.

Schmahmann, J. D., Smith, E. E., Eichler, F. S., & Filley, C. M. (2008). Cerebral white matter: Neuroanatomy, clinical neurology, and neurobehavioral correlates. *Annals of the New York Academy of Sciences, 1142*, 266–309.

Schmahmann, J. D., Weilburg, J. B., & Sherman, J. C. (2007). The neuropsychiatry of the cerebellum - insights from the clinic. *Cerebellum* 2007; 6, 254–267.

Schuelke, M. (2005). Ataxia with vitamin E deficiency. In: Pagon RA, Adam MP, Bird TD, Dolan CR, Fong CT, Smith RJH, Stephens K, editors. GeneReviews® [Internet]. Seattle (WA): University of Washington, Seattle; 1993-2014.

Schutte, C. M., Ranchhod, N., Kakaza, M., & Pillay, M. (2013). AIDS-related progressive multifocal leukoencephalopathy (PML): A retrospective study from Pretoria, South Africa. *South African Medical Journal, 103*, 399–401.

Schwarzschild, M., Rordorf, G., Bekken, K., Buonanno, F., & Schmahmann, J. D. (1997). Normal-pressure hydrocephalus with misleading features of irreversible dementias: A case report. *Journal of Geriatric Psychiatry and Neurology, 10*, 51–4.

Sciascia, S., Bertolaccini, M. L., Baldovino, S., Roccatello, D., Khamashta, M. A., & Sanna, G. (2013). Central nervous system involvement in systemic lupus erythematosus: Overview on classification criteria. *Autoimmune Reviews, 12*, 426–429.

Sellner, J., & Trinka, E. (2012). Seizures and epilepsy in herpes simplex virus encephalitis: Current concepts and future directions of pathogenesis and management. *Journal of Neurology, 259*, 2019–2030.

Seminara, S. B., Acierno, J. S., Jr., Abdulwahid, N. A., Crowley, W. F., Jr., & Margolin, D. H. (2002). Hypogonadotropic hypogonadism and cerebellar ataxia: Detailed phenotypic characterization of a large, extended kindred. *Journal of Clinical Endocrinology and Metabolism, 87*, 1607–1612.

Sepulveda-Falla, D., Glatzel, M., & Lopera, F. (2012). Phenotypic profile of early-onset familial Alzheimer's disease caused by presenilin-1 E280A mutation. *Journal of Alzheimers Disease, 32*, 1-12.

Sevin, M., Lesca, G., Baumann, N., Millat, G., Lyon-Caen, O., Vanier, M. T., & Sedel, F. (2007). The adult form of Niemann-Pick disease type C. *Brain, 130*, 120–133.

Sharma, O. P. (1997). Neurosarcoidosis: A personal perspective based on the study of 37 patients. *Chest, 112*, 220–228.

Shi, C. H., Schisler, J. C., Rubel, C. E., Tan, S., Song, B., McDonough, H.,...Xu, Y. M. (2014). Ataxia and hypogonadism caused by the loss of ubiquitin ligase activity of the U box protein CHIP. *Human Molecular Genetics, 23*(4), 1013–1024.

Shprecher, D., & Mehta, L. (2010). The syndrome of delayed post-hypoxic leukoencephalopathy. *NeuroRehabilitation, 26*, 65–72.

Shuper, A., Stark, B., Yaniv, Y., Zaizov, R., Carel, C., Sadeh, M., & Steinmetz, A. (2000). Cerebellar involvement in Langerhans' cell histiocytosis: A progressive neuropsychiatric disease. *Journal of Child Neurology, 15*, 824–826.

Sjaastad, O., & Nordvik, A. (1973). The corpus callosal angle in the diagnosis of cerebral ventricular enlargement. *Acta Neurological Scandinavica, 49*, 396–406.

Sjowall, J., Ledel, A., Ernerudh, J., Ekerfelt, C., & Forsberg, P. (2012). Doxycycline-mediated effects on persistent symptoms and systemic cytokine responses post-neuroborreliosis: A randomized, prospective, cross-over study. *BMC Infectious Disease, 12*, 186.

Smith, W. T., French, J. M., Gottsman, M., Smith, A. J., & Wakes-Miller, J. A. (1965). Cerebral complications of Whipple's disease. *Brain, 88*, 137–150.

Sokol, R. J. (1988). Vitamin E deficiency and neurologic disease. *Annual Review of Nutrition, 8*, 351–373.

Sonneville, R., Klein, I., de Broucker, T., & Wolff, M. (2009). Post-infectious encephalitis in adults: diagnosis and management. J Infect 2009; 58, 321–328.

Sproule, D. M., & Kaufmann, P. (2008). Mitochondrial encephalopathy, lactic acidosis, and strokelike episodes: Basic concepts, clinical phenotype, and therapeutic management of MELAS syndrome. *Annals of the New York Academy of Sciences, 1142*, 133–158.

Stadelmann, C., Albert, M., Wegner, C., & Bruck, W. (2008). Cortical pathology in multiple sclerosis. *Current Opinion in Neurology, 21*, 229–234.

Stefani, A., Riello, M., Rossini, F., Mariotto, S., Fenzi, F., Gambina, G.,...Monaco, S. (2013). Neurosyphilis manifesting with rapidly progressive dementia: Report of three cases. *Neurological Sciences, 34*(11), 2027–2030.

Susac, J. O. (1994). Susac's syndrome: The triad of microangiopathy of the brain and retina with hearing loss in young women. *Neurology, 44*, 591–593.

Takalo, M., Salminen, A., Soininen, H., Hiltunen, M., & Haapasalo, A. (2013). Protein aggregation and degradation mechanisms in neurodegenerative diseases. *American Journal of Neurodegenerative Diseases, 2*, 1–14.

Tan, I. L., McArthur, J. C., Clifford, D. B., Major, E. O., & Nath, A. (2011). Immune reconstitution inflammatory syndrome in natalizumab-associated PML. *Neurology, 77*, 1061–1067.

Tavano, A., Grasso, R., Gagliardi, C., Triulzi, F., Bresolin, N., Fabbro, F.,...Borgatti, R. (2007). Disorders of cognitive and affective development in cerebellar malformations. *Brain, 130*, 2646–2660.

Tedesco, A. M., Chiricozzi, F. R., Clausi, S., Lupo, M., Molinari, M., & Leggio, M. G. (2011). The cerebellar cognitive profile. *Brain, 134*(Pt 12), 3672–3686.

Terushkin, V., Stern, B. J., Judson, M. A., Hagiwara, M., Pramanik, B., Sanchez, M., & Prystowsky, S. (2010). Neurosarcoidosis: Presentations and management. *Neurologist, 16*, 2–15.

Tetzlaff, K., Friege, L., Hutzelmann, A., Reuter, M., Holl, D., & Leplow, B. (1999). Magnetic resonance signal abnormalities and neuropsychological deficits in elderly compressed-air divers. *European Neurology, 42*, 194–199.

Tian, C., Liu, D., Sun, Q. L., Chen, C., Xu, Y., Wang, H.,...Dong, X. P. (2013). Comparative analysis of gene expression profiles between cortex and thalamus in Chinese fatal familial insomnia patients. *Molecular Neurobiology, 48,* 36–48.

Todnem, K., Nyland, H., Kambestad, B. K., & Aarli, J. A. (1990). Influence of occupational diving upon the nervous system: an epidemiological study. *British Journal of Industrial Medicine, 47,* 708–714.

Toyoshima, Y., Onodera, O., Yamada, M., et al. (2012). Spinocerebellar ataxia type 17. In: Pagon RA, Adam MP, Bird TD, Dolan CR, Fong CT, Smith RJH, Stephens K, editors. GeneReviews® [Internet]. Seattle (WA): University of Washington, Seattle; 1993-2014.

Trzepacz, P. T., McCue, M., Klein, I., Levey, G. S., & Greenhouse, J. (1988). A psychiatric and neuropsychological study of patients with untreated Graves' disease. *General Hospital Psychiatry, 10,* 49–55.

Tsuji, S. (1999). DRPLA. In: Pagon RA, Adam MP, Bird TD, Dolan CR, Fong CT, Smith RJH, Stephens K, editors. GeneReviews® [Internet]. Seattle (WA): University of Washington, Seattle; 1993–2014.

Turaga, S. P., Kaul, S., Haritha Chowdary, H. A., & Praveen, P. (2012). Isolated bilateral basal ganglionic hyper intensities in early stage of subacutesclerosing panencephalitis: A case report. *Neurology India, 60,* 521-2.

Valis, M., Masopust, J., Bazant, J., Rihova, Z., Kalnicka, D., Urban, A.,...Hort, J. (2011). Cognitive changes in spinocerebellar ataxia type 2. *Neuroendocrinology Letters, 32,* 354–359.

van der Knaap, M. S., Arts, W. F., Garbern, J. Y., Hedlund, G., Winkler, F., Barbosa, C.,...van der Valk, P. (2008). Cerebellar leukoencephalopathy: Most likely histiocytosis-related. *Neurology, 71,* 1361–1367.

van der Knaap, M. S., Pronk, J. C., & Scheper, G. C. (2006). Vanishing white matter disease. *Lancet Neurology, 5,* 413–423.

van Geel, B. M., Bezman, L., Loes, D. J., Moser, H. W., & Raymond, G. V. (2001). Evolution of phenotypes in adult male patients with X-linked adrenoleukodystrophy. *Annals of Neurology, 49,* 186–194.

van Harskamp, N. J., Rudge, P., & Cipolotti, L. (2005). Does the left inferior parietal lobule contribute to multiplication facts? *Cortex, 41,* 742–752.

Vesely, S. K., George, J. N., Lammle, B., Studt, J. D., Alberio, L., El-Harake, M. A., & Raskob, G. E. (2003). ADAMTS13 activity in thrombotic thrombocytopenic purpura-hemolytic uremic syndrome: Relation to presenting features and clinical outcomes in a prospective cohort of 142 patients. *Blood, 102,* 60–68.

Victor, M., Adams, R. D., & Collins, G. H. (1971). The Wernicke-Korsakoff syndrome. A clinical and pathological study of 245 patients, 82 with post-mortem examinations. *Contemporary Neurology Series, 7,* 1–206.

Virhammar, J., Laurell, K., Cesarini, K. G., & Larsson, E. M. (2014). The callosal angle measured on MRI as a predictor of outcome in idiopathic normal-pressure hydrocephalus. *Journal of Neurosurgery, 120*(7), 178–184.

Viswanathan, A., & Greenberg, S. M. (2011). Cerebral amyloid angiopathy in the elderly. *Annals of Neurology, 70,* 871–880.

Vogel, A., Elberling, T. V., Hording, M., Dock, J., Rasmussen, A. K., Feldt-Rasmussen, U.,...Waldemar, G. (2007). Affective symptoms and cognitive functions in the acute phase of Graves' thyrotoxicosis. *Psychoneuroendocrinology, 32,* 36–43.

Walcott, B. P., Edlow, B. L., Xia, Z., Kahle, K. T., Nahed, B. V., & Schmahmann, J. D. (2012). Steroid responsive A3243G mutation MELAS: Clinical and radiographic evidence for regional hyperperfusion leading to neuronal loss. *Neurologist, 18,* 159–170.

Wang, J., Guo, Q., Zhou, P., Zhang, J., Zhao, Q., & Hong, Z. (2011). Cognitive impairment in mild general paresis of the insane: AD-like pattern. *Dementia and Geriatric Cognitive Disorders, 31,* 284–290.

Waters, F., & Bucks, R. S. (2011). Neuropsychological effects of sleep loss: implication for neuropsychologists. *Journal of the International Neuropsychology Society, 17,* 571–586.

Weaver, L. K., Valentine, K. J., & Hopkins, R. O. (2007). Carbon monoxide poisoning: Risk factors for cognitive sequelae and the role of hyperbaric oxygen. *American Journal of Respiratory Critical Care Medicine, 176,* 491-7.

Weinberger, L. M., Schmidley, J. W., Schafer, I. A., & Raghavan, S. (1994). Delayed postanoxic demyelination and arylsulfatase-A pseudodeficiency. *Neurology, 44,* 152–154.

Werder, S. F. (2010). Cobalamin deficiency, hyperhomocysteinemia, and dementia. *Neuropsychiatric Disease Treatment, 6,* 159–95.

Whatley, S., & Badminton, M. (2013). Acute intermittent porphyria. In: Pagon RA, Adam MP, Bird TD, Dolan CR, Fong CT, Smith RJH, Stephens K, editors. GeneReviews® [Internet]. Seattle (WA): University of Washington, Seattle; 1993–2014.

Wicklund, M. R., Mokri, B., Drubach, D. A., Boeve, B. F., Parisi, J. E., & Josephs, K. A. (2011). Frontotemporal brain sagging syndrome: An SIH-like presentation mimicking FTD. *Neurology, 76,* 1377–1382.

Wilson, S. (1912). Progressive lenticular degeneration: A familial nervous disease associated with cirrhosis of the liver. *Brain, 34,* 295–509.

Wnorowski, M., Prosch, H., Prayer, D., Janssen, G., Gadner, H., & Grois, N. (2008). Pattern and course of neurodegeneration in Langerhans cell histiocytosis. *Journal of Pediatrics, 153,* 127–132.

Wolters, E. C., van Wijngaarden, G. K., Stam, F. C., Rengelink, H., Lousberg, R. J., Schipper, M. E., & Verbeeten, B. (1982). Leucoencephalopathy after inhaling "heroin" pyrolysate. *Lancet, 2,* 1233–1237.

Xie, W. L., Shi, Q., Xia, S. L., Zhang, B. Y., Gong, H. S., Wang, S. B.,...Dong, X. P. (2013). Comparison of the pathologic and pathogenic features in six different regions of postmortem brains of three patients with fatal familial insomnia. *International Journal of Molecular Medicine, 31,* 81–90.

Yamashita, F., Sasaki, M., Saito, M., Mori, E., Kawaguchi, A., Kudo, K.,...Saito, K. (2013). Voxel-based morphometry of disproportionate cerebrospinal fluid space distribution for the differential diagnosis of idiopathic normal pressure hydrocephalus. *Journal of Neuroimaging,* epub ahead of print.

Yokoo, H., Nakazato, Y., Harigaya, Y., Sasaki, N., Igeta, Y., & Itoh, H. (2007). Massive myelinolytic leukoencephalopathy in a patient medicated with low-dose oral methotrexate for rheumatoid arthritis: An autopsy report. *Acta Neuropathologica, 114,* 425–430.

Yu, C. E., Bird, T. D., Bekris, L. M., Montine, T. J., Leverenz, J. B., Steinbart, E.,...Van Deerlin, V. M. (2010). The spectrum of mutations in progranulin: A collaborative study screening 545 cases of neurodegeneration. *Archives of Neurology, 67,* 161–170.

Zheng, D., Zhou, D., Zhao, Z., Liu, Z., Xiao, S., Xing, Y.,...Liu, J. (2011). The clinical presentation and imaging manifestation of psychosis and dementia in general paresis: A retrospective study of 116 cases. *Journal of Neuropsychiatry and Clinical Neuroscience, 23,* 300–307.

Zigas, V., & Gajdusek, D. C. (1957). Kuru: Clinical study of a new syndrome resembling paralysis agitans in natives of the Eastern Highlands of Australian New Guinea. *Medical Journal of Australia, 44,* 745–754.

Zuckerman, D., Seliem, R., & Hochberg, E. (2006). Intravascular lymphoma: The oncologist's "great imitator". *Oncologist, 11,* 496–502.

16

Alzheimer's Disease and Alzheimer's Dementia

Alireza Atri

Alzheimer's disease (AD) is the most common cause of neurodegenerative dementia. In the next two to three decades, with changing demographics and longevity on the rise, a worldwide pandemic of clinical AD and dementia is anticipated—that is, unless highly effective preventative or curative treatments are forthcoming. While our understanding of the scope of the AD problem and diagnostics has greatly increased in the last three decades, our understanding regarding the etiology, pathophysiology, and therapeutics in AD remains in its nascency. Similar to most chronic diseases in the elderly, AD can be managed via a multifactorial approach of nonpharmacological and pharmacological interventions that provide variable, but measurable and overall meaningful, benefits in slowing clinical decline. However, AD cannot yet be prevented, cured, or blocked from ultimately progressing to cause debilitation and death. Until highly potent therapeutic options become available, clinicians have an obligation to be knowledgeable about this common and costly condition, and they have a duty to compassionately diagnose, treat, and care for affected individuals, their loved ones, and caregivers using all options available.

When first described in 1906 by Professor Alois Alzheimer, the case of August Dieter, the index patient with early-onset AD dementia, was believed to represent a very rare condition that caused "presenile dementia." It was not until the mid-to-latter part of the 20th century that the link was made that AD greatly contributed, if not caused, most cases of "senile dementia" in older individuals. In the past two decades, there has finally been better appreciation that the AD spectrum is the most common cause of neurodegenerative dementias, that it encompasses wide age ranges and heterogeneous presentations, and that in any individual it proceeds along a lengthy clinical course that develops, progresses, and manifests insidiously over one or more decades. Brain systems that are primarily affected and are most vulnerable often become symptomatic first in AD.

The classic AD presentation (typical AD) involves initial memory difficulties attributable to dysfunction of medial temporal lobe structures, particularly the entorhinal cortex and hippocampus, and associated parietal memory processing regions. However, as the disease progresses, patients accrue additional deficits in parietal and frontal regions, thus affecting executive functions, language, visuospatial systems, personality and, ultimately, motor programming systems. Atypical presentations of AD (atypical AD) involving primarily disturbances in language, executive function and behavior, or visuospatial function are now formally recognized as part of the AD clinical syndrome.

Beyond disturbances in cognitive abilities, there is often an overlay of accumulating neuropsychiatric and behavioral symptoms and personality changes that include apathy, anxiety, depression, irritability, agitation, delusions, hallucinations, impulsivity, insensitivity, and sleep problems. Many of these, including anxiety, sleep difficulties, apathy, and irritability, may, in retrospect, be the earliest symptoms. These symptoms, along with common prominent "A" signs (amnesia, aphasia, agnosia, apathy, and anxiety; and others such as apraxia, acalculia, administrative [executive] and attentional deficits; see Chapter 19), contribute to progressive difficulties in executing activities of daily living (ADLs) and self-care, and the emergence of problem behaviors. Taken together, these eventually lead to disability and complete dependence on others.

As the population ages in the developing world, and as the percentage of elderly with dementia increases with age, the burden of care and the costs of AD will also increase (Alzheimer's-Association, 2013; Prince et al., 2013; Ziegler-Graham, Brookmeyer, Johnson, & Arrighi, 2008). In the United States, AD is the only top 10 cause of mortality that is still significantly on the rise (see Fig. 16.1; Alzheimer's-Association, 2013). Cases of AD are also projected to potentially triple in the United States over the next three to four decades (see Fig. 16.2; Hebert, Weuve, Scherr, & Evans, 2013) and to double every 20 years around the world. AD does not always cause impairment in isolation; more than have half of AD cases around the world will likely be due to mixed AD and vascular etiology (Prince et al., 2013; Saxena, 2012; Wimo & Prince, 2010).

The complex genetics of the most common form of AD dementia, the sporadic late-onset type, is not well understood, nor are the etiology or pathophysiology of AD. The leading models of AD etiology posit a central and early role of accumulation of synapto- and neurotoxic forms of the amyloid-beta protein (Aß) in inducing pathological processes involving activation of inflammatory and microglial cascades, broad ionic and neurotransmitter abnormalities, mitochondrial dysfunction, and oxidative stress. In the prevailing model, these processes are then posited to lead to hyperphosphorylation of the microtubule stabilizing protein tau and

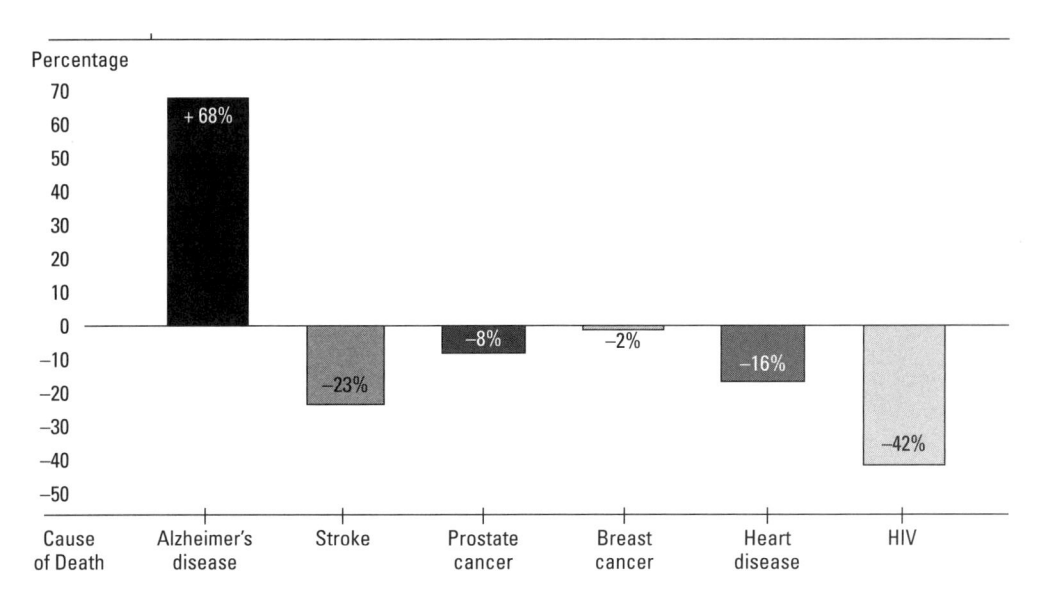

Figure 16.1 Mortality from Alzheimer's disease dementia is on the rise: percentage changes in selected causes of death (all ages) in the United States between 2000 and 2010. (Figure adapted from Alzheimer's Association Facts and Figures [Alzheimer's-Association, 2013]—data are from National Center for Health Statistics)

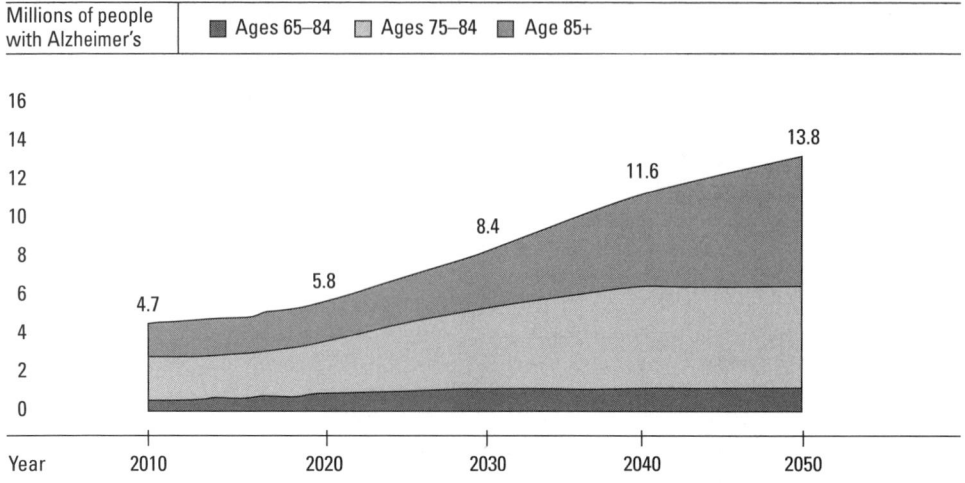

Figure 16.2 Projected numbers of individuals age 65 and over (total and by age group) in the US population anticipated to develop Alzheimer's dementia from 2010 to 2050. Projections from Hebert et al. (2013) used the US Census Bureau estimates of US population growth. Numbers, in millions of individuals, indicate middle estimates per decade, and colored area indicates different age groups (65–74; 75–84; and 85+ years of age). (Figure adapted from Alzheimer's Association Facts and Figures; Alzheimer's-Association, 2013)

formation of tangles. Tau-mediated processes are then posited to cause further synaptic and neuronal dysfunction and destruction, and, ultimately, to lead to widespread cortical dysfunction. Other emerging models posit a role of microvascular injury leading to tipping the balance in favor of accumulation of toxic Aß and subsequently a runaway cascade of synaptic and neuronal destruction. Supporting evidence for Aß accumulation playing an essential and early role in the etiology of AD mainly comes from individuals with dominantly inherited forms of AD, usually in individuals with early-onset AD, and chromosomal abnormalities that cause greater production of Aß.

While AD neuropathological changes and measures of amyloid and tau abnormalities, and neuronal destruction and dysfunction are being better understood, the diagnosis of AD remains a clinical one—no single biomarker or test provides the diagnosis. Newly revised AD clinical criteria can be reliably applied and do not require brain tissue to provide accurate diagnose. While the ancillary role of AD biomarkers in the clinical realm are being iteratively delineated, the role of obtaining a thorough and reliable history and appropriate cognitive testing remains central to establishing diagnosis in the AD clinical spectrum (see Chapters 19 and 20). Diagnosis, in some cases, can be supplemented by more experimental biomarker diagnostics. Biomarkers of AD trait and state include cerebrospinal fluid (CSF), neuroimaging (e.g., structural magnetic resonance imaging [MRI], fludeoxyglucose [FDG] and molecular positron emission tomography [PET]), and genetic tests, which are increasingly available and can be helpful to support establishing underlying pathology in selected clinical cases and in research studies (see Chapter 22). AD diagnostics have progressed not only to reliably aid in the identification of individuals at the dementia stage of AD but also to help detect high-risk individuals in potentially preclinical stages (see Chapter 18) and to assist in diagnosing early clinical stages of mild cognitive impairment (MCI) due to AD (see Chapter 17).

While a cure for AD may be far away, an individualized and multifactorial approach to AD evaluation and care that emphasizes early detection and multidisciplinary treatments can provide significant benefits to affected individuals and their caregivers. Psychoeducation and establishing a proactive and individualized care plan in the context of a strong clinician and patient–caregiver dyad therapeutic alliance lays the foundation for long-term management and care for the patient–caregiver dyad. Both pharmacologic and nonpharmacological therapies seek to minimize the effects of disabling problem symptoms, to slow clinical progression, and to mitigate care burden in AD. Currently available anti-AD medications are not disease modifying but are "disease course modifying" by slowing clinical, if not neuropathological, progression. From a clinical viewpoint, therapies aim to preserve, for longer than would be possible without intervention, cognition, independence, quality of life, and comfort. From a health economics perspective, therapies that minimize caregiver burden and delay nursing home entry translate into significant increases in productivity and savings of health care dollars (Cappell, Herrmann, Cornish, & Lanctot, 2010; Weycker et al., 2007).

Pharmacotherapy in AD first involves a thorough review of a patient's existing medications and supplements in order to eliminate redundancies and potentially inappropriate and deleterious treatments. Currently, FDA-approved anti-AD pharmacotherapies (the acetyl cholinesterase inhibitors (ChEIs) donepezil, galantamine, and rivastigmine, and the NMDA antagonist memantine) can offer meaningful benefit by potentially reducing short-term as well as long-term clinical progression of symptoms. First-line treatment for behavioral problems is nonpharmacological and involves identifying the trigger for the problem behavior. Once the trigger is identified, it is necessary to institute appropriate interventions, make environmental modifications, and then to evaluate the impact of the interventions. Finally, it is important to complete the loop by iteratively and flexibly adjusting, as necessary, or reinforcing the behavioral and environmental care plan. Use of neuroleptic medications (e.g., antipsychotics) in AD is sometimes necessary as a last resort in severe and refractory cases or in situations where safety risk is high, but it comes with a high clinical threshold and high long-term risk-benefit ratio. Persistent multifactorial treatment and care in AD can delay time to reaching costly clinical milestones: the late stages of illness when individuals require 24-hour supervision and care, and which is often, in developed countries, provided in an institutional setting. AD care in the end stages of the illness should be palliative and focus on facilitating a "good death." Clinicians can, by maintaining a proactive, positive, flexible, multifactorial, and individualized approach to compassionately caring for patient–caregiver dyads, provide meaningful care that is not only invaluable to patients, families, and caregivers on a micro level, but that is also cost-effective and beneficial to society on the macro level.

Epidemiology and Risk Factors

Alzheimer's disease and dementia are on the rise in the United States, in developed countries, and globally. As longevity trends continue to ensure that most individuals will live well into their 70s, 80s, or 90s, the prevalence of AD dementia is anticipated to rise dramatically, two- to three-fold in the coming three to four decades (see Fig. 16.2). The major risk factors of developing AD dementia (see Table 16.1) are older age (past age 65, but particularly past age 80) (see Fig. 16.2);

TABLE 16.1 Risk Factors for Alzheimer's Disease Dementia

Modifiable	Nonmodifiable
Cardiovascular and cerebrovascular risks:	Age
Diabetes	Gender (female > male)
Hypertension	Family history (particularly in first- or second-degree relative or multiple generations)
Dyslipidemia	
Metabolic syndrome	Race
Cerebral hypoperfusion	Down's syndrome
Cerebrovascular injury or stroke	ApoE-ε4 allele
Severe head trauma or traumatic brain injury	Cerebral amyloidosis—positive AD biomarker profile[*]
Low cognitive reserve (low education, intelligence, professional or social attainment/occupation)	

[*]Currently a nonmodifiable risk factor, but clinical trials with amyloid-modifying drugs are about to begin (see Chapter 18).

family history of AD or dementia in a first- or second-degree blood relative (approximately two- to six-fold relative risk [RR]); vascular risk factors (diabetes, hypertension, dyslipidemia, metabolic syndrome, smoking), altered cerebral perfusion, cerebrovascular injury and stroke; severe or repeated brain trauma; female gender; race (in the United States, African American and Hispanic race are at 1.5- to 2-fold RR compared to White Caucasians); markers of low cognitive reserve (low educational, professional, or social attainment; low intelligence); Trisomy 21 (Down syndrome), and genetic markers for higher susceptibility, most notably individuals who carry one or two ε4 alleles of the apolipoprotein-E (APOE) gene (APOE-ε4) (3-fold and 8- to 10-fold RR, respectively, compared to homozygous APOE-ε3/ε3's). Deterministic dominantly inherited AD mutations are rare and account for 1%–2% or less of AD cases, most of whom develop AD dementia before age 60. Finally, individuals who have positive biomarkers of Aß accumulation (e.g., CSF or amyloid-PET profile of the AD trait) suggesting cerebral amyloidosis are at increased risk of progressing to MCI and dementia stages of AD (see Chapters 17, 18, and 22).

Alzheimer's disease is strongly associated with increasing age beyond 65. The prevalence of AD is estimated to approximately double every 5 years from age 65 to 85 going from approximately 1%–2% at age 65 to more than 30%–50% by age 85. With the advent of greater longevity in all populations, barring development of a substantial medical breakthrough that will effectively prevent, retard, stop, or "cure" AD, countries that will experience a large demographic shift to greater numbers of elderly individuals over age 65 in the coming decades will also experience a commensurate large increase in the prevalence (number of cases) of AD. In high- and middle-income countries falling mortality for older adults, due to improvements in adult medicine and health care, are co-occurring with falling fertility rates (fewer children being born per adults) and improvements in child health, therefore causing further increased life expectancy. For example, in Japan, total life expectancy is now 86 years at birth for women and 79 years for men; those reaching the age of 60 can be expected, on average, to survive until age 88.1, and those reaching the age of 80, to survive, on average, until age 91.3 In the 34 countries that are members of the Organization of Economic Cooperation and Development (OECD), the proportion of those aged 80 years and over will increase from 4% of the total population in 2010 to 10% in 2050 (Prince et al., 2013). Between 2010 and 2050 in the United States, the percentage of people age 65 and older is expected to increase from 14% to 20% of the population (Vincent & Velkof, 2010). By 2050, the number of Americans age 85 years and older will nearly quadruple to 21 million, which will result in an additional 13 million oldest-old Americans who will be at the highest risk for developing AD (Hebert et al., 2013; Vincent & Velkof, 2010) (see Fig. 16.2).

The 2010 Alzheimer's Disease International (ADI) and the 2012 World Health Organization (WHO) World Dementia Report estimate the total number of people with dementia worldwide in 2010 at 35.6 million and project a near doubling every 20 years, to 65.7 million in 2030 and 115.4 million in 2050 (Saxena, 2012; Wimo & Prince, 2010). These reports estimate a total number of new cases of dementia each year worldwide of nearly 7.7 million, which translates into one new case of dementia every 4 seconds; the vast majority, 60%–80%, of these cases are due to AD or mixed dementia due to a combination of pathology due to AD and vascular dementia (Prince et al., 2013; Saxena, 2012; Wimo & Prince, 2010).

Estimates using data from the 2010 US Census and the Chicago Health and Aging Project (CHAP) and older AD criteria (e.g., the 1984 NINCDS-ADRDA AD criteria) place the current number of individuals with AD in the United States at 5.2 million (Hebert et al., 2013) (see Fig. 16.2). Of these 5.2 million, approximately 5 million are age 65 or older while 200,000 are younger individuals who can be classified as having early-onset AD. Current estimates are that 11% (1 in 9) of individuals age 65 and older, and 32% (1 in 3) of individuals 85 and older have AD (Hebert et al., 2013). The prevalence of all forms of dementia from population-based studies, including the Aging, Demographics, and Memory Study (ADAMS), are that 13.9% (approximately 1 in 7) of Americans age 71 and older have dementia of any kind (including AD) (Plassman et al., 2007; Wilson, Leurgans, Boyle, & Bennett, 2011). Early-onset AD currently accounts for approximately 4% of AD cases. Of the remaining 96% of AD cases who are 65 and older (late-onset AD), 13% are between age 65 and 74, 44% are between age 75 and 84, and 38% are 85 or older.

The prevalence of AD in the United States is expected to nearly triple over the next 35–40 years (Alzheimer's-Association, 2013; Hebert et al., 2013) (see Fig. 16.2); this is mainly due to the upcoming age demographic "the silver tsunami." The number and percentage of Americans who will be among the oldest-old will increase substantially in the next three decades due to a combination of increasing longevity and the baby boomer generation entering the high AD risk age category of 65 and older. Currently the 85 and older US population includes approximately 2 million individuals with AD, or 40% of all people with AD who are age 65 and older. Recent projections by Hebert and colleagues are that in year 2031, when the first wave of baby boomers reaches age 85, more than 3 million individuals age 85 and older will be affected with AD (Hebert et al., 2013). There will be a 40% increase from 2013 to 2025 in the number of Americans affected by AD; going from approximately 5.2 million now to 7.1 million in 2025 (Hebert et al., 2013). Using year 2000 and 2010 US census data, the number of people age 65 and older with AD is projected to nearly triple from approximately 5 million now to between 13.8 and 16 million individuals by 2050 (Hebert et al., 2013; Hebert, Scherr, Bienias, Bennett, & Evans, 2003).

The increasing incidence of new AD cases in the United States is also projected to continue to rise rapidly in the coming decades. While compared to 2000 (411,000 new annual AD cases), there was a 10% increase in 2010 (454,000 new annual cases) in the estimated number of new AD cases per year, projections estimate a 50% increase by 2030 (615,000 new annual cases) and a 130% increase (959,000 new annual cases) by 2050 (Hebert, Beckett, Scherr, & Evans, 2001). Future estimates that will utilize the recently updated or new AD criteria, including the AA-NIA (Alzheimer's Association-National Institute of Aging), *DSM-5* (*Diagnostic and Statistical Manual of Mental Disorders*), and IWG (International Working Group) criteria would greatly increase the incidence and prevalence of AD as they all place emphasis on early detection.

Alzheimer's disease is approximately twice more prevalent in women than men; about two thirds of Americans with AD who are age 65 and older are women. This is principally due to greater longevity in women compared to men. Recent estimates suggest that 16% of US women and 11% of US men age 71 and older are affected by AD and related dementias (Hebert et al., 2013; Seshadri et al., 1997).

Racial differences in US prevalence estimates for AD and associated dementias suggest that, proportional to their population compared to Whites, older African Americans are more than 1.5–2 times and older Hispanics are 1.4–1.5 times more likely to be affected by AD and dementias than older Whites (Gurland et al., 1999; Potter et al., 2009). In addition to genetic differences, disparities in health conditions related to cerebrovascular health, such as stroke, diabetes, hypertension, and educational and socioeconomic factors, have been especially strongly implicated as the driving factors that account for the significant differential racial prevalence proportions (Alzheimer's-Association, 2013).

The concept of "cognitive reserve" has also been implicated as a factor that can mediate the manifestation of AD dementia (Mitchell, Shaughnessy, Shirk, Yang, & Atri, 2012; Stern, 2009). Stern observed that "individual differences in how people process tasks allow some people to cope better than others with brain pathology"; Stern has defined cognitive reserve as the brain's capacity to maintain cognitive function despite neurologic damage or disease (Stern, 2009). The related concepts of brain reserve, neural reserve, and neural compensation, along with cognitive reserve, have several roots but all posit that the brain has the ability to functionally compensate for neurological damage. These concepts can help to explain early findings of discrepancies between clinical severity/cognitive performance and measures of disease burden. These observations include findings of high amyloid plaque counts in individuals who performed well on cognitive tests, presence of AD neuropathology in the absence of clinical dementia, and that 10%–40% of individuals who exceeded pathological burden for amyloid burden by PIB-PET scanning or plaque and tangle burden at autopsy showed no previous cognitive impairments (Blessed, Tomlinson, & Roth, 1968; Katzman, 1988; Rentz et al., 2010). While there is no one measure of cognitive reserve, proxies for it have been proposed that include years of education; performance on tests of intelligence, measures of verbal literacy, word reading, and vocabulary; occupational attainment; level of participation in social, mental, and leisure activities; and physiological, structural, and neuroimaging measures of brain function (e.g., brain volume, cortical thickness, neuronal count, synaptic density, activity of brain regions on functional neuroimaging). Years of education, performance on tests of estimated intelligence, and occupational attainment have all been implicated as factors that may account for differential prevalence among populations with lower versus higher levels of AD (Fratiglioni, Paillard-Borg, & Winblad, 2004; Mitchell et al., 2012; Stern et al., 1994). For example, in the Washington Heights longitudinal observational cohort study, the relative risk of developing dementia was approximately twice greater in low education as well as in low occupation groups compared groups with high levels (Stern et al., 1994).

Finally, there is a very high prevalence of an Alzheimer's-like dementia syndrome in older individuals with Trisomy 21: Down syndrome (DS). While there are no widely accepted criteria to characterize dementia in DS, about 40% of such individuals over 60 years of age have a diagnosis of dementia (Margallo-Lana et al., 2003). By age 40, virtually all individuals with DS accumulate significant AD-like brain pathology due to higher production and deposition of amyloid β as well as some neurofibrilliary tangles secondary to increased tau hyperphosphorylation (Hanney et al., 2012). The cause is believed to be due to more copies of the amyloid precursor protein (APP) gene, which is located on chromosome 21. There are over 5.8 individuals with DS worldwide, and even in the absence of a dementia diagnosis, the millions of individuals with DS over age 40 are at high risk for accelerated cognitive decline of about 11% per year (Hanney et al., 2012; Morris & Alberman, 2009).

Genetics and Etiology

The genetics and the etiology of AD are complex and incompletely understood. While degree of AD risk attributable to genetics has been estimated at 70%, many genetic variations and environmental factors likely interact to cause complex diseases such as AD. Despite great effort, only three Mendelian genetic causes of AD have been identified; all of these result in autosomal dominant familial AD (FAD), and individuals who carry the mutation have a 95% or more lifetime risk to develop the clinical manifestation of AD dementia if they live beyond the expected range for age of disease onset, which is often before age 65. These "early-onset" AD (dementia onset prior to age 65) dominantly inherited genetic mutations are due to the Amyloid Precursor Protein (APP), Presenilin 1 (PSEN1), and Presenilin 2 (PSEN2) mutations. PSEN1 mutations account for 60% of dominantly inherited AD, and APP mutations account for about 15%. PSEN2 mutations that cause AD are very rare and have only been described in 22 families (Loy, Schofield, Turner, & Kwok, 2014). However, overall, all three gene mutations only account for 1% or less of all AD cases (Loy et al., 2014).

As a complex genetic disease, there are likely many genetic variations that contribute to risk. The genetic AD susceptibility factor with the greatest risk identified to date is the apolipoprotein-E (APOE) gene. Of the three alleles of APOE (ε2, ε3, and ε4), possession of one or more ε4 alleles confers a higher risk, relative to having the ε3 allele, for accelerated Aβ deposition and manifesting the AD clinical phenotype. Possessing the ε2 allele appears to delay Aβ deposition and to be relatively protective. Meanwhile, the SorL1 gene mutation has been implicated in late-onset AD (age 65 or older); it interacts with APOE, affects APP trafficking, and gene product overexpression reduces Aβ production by decreasing APP and ß-secretase interactions (Ballard et al., 2011; Rogaeva et al., 2007; Scherzer et al., 2004).

The Amyloid Cascade Hypothesis of Alzheimer's Disease

The leading hypothesis for the etiology of AD has been the amyloid hypothesis (Hardy & Higgins, 1992; Selkoe, 1991) and remains controversial (Davies, 2000; Hyman, 2011; Zlokovic, 2011) (see Fig. 16.3). All known AD gene mutations affect Aβ metabolism to increase relative or absolute production of the Aβ$_{42}$ form of the polypeptide; this

AD genetic link to Aß has provided some of the strongest supporting arguments for the "amyloid cascade hypothesis" (Haass, Koo, Mellon, Hung, & Selkoe, 1992; Hardy & Higgins, 1992; Selkoe, 1991; Selkoe, Abraham, Podlisny, & Duffy, 1986) (see Fig. 16.3a). The original hypothesis posited that neuronal dysfunction and degeneration was a function of total Aß deposition and plaque load. The iterative evolution of this hypothesis, in various forms, posits that toxic forms of Aß oligomers play a critical and "upstream" role in the pathogenesis of AD, which subsequently causes synaptic instability, activation of inflammatory cascades, oxidative stress and mitochondrial dysfunction, tau hyperphosphorylation, synaptic and neuronal dysfunction, excitotoxicity, neurotransmitter dysregulation, and neuronal death (Hardy & Selkoe, 2002). Initially, the AD degenerative process appears to target vulnerable entorhinal, hippocampal and limbic structures, and important hubs including the posterior cingulate, precuneus, and lateral parietal association cortices, which play central roles in memory and rest-state intrinsic networks such as the default mode network (Buckner, Andrews-Hanna, & Schacter, 2008). While there is controversy regarding the amyloid hypothesis and whether amyloid is the root cause of AD, there is greater consensus that misfolded and aggregated amyloid

(A)

Amyloid cascade hypothesis

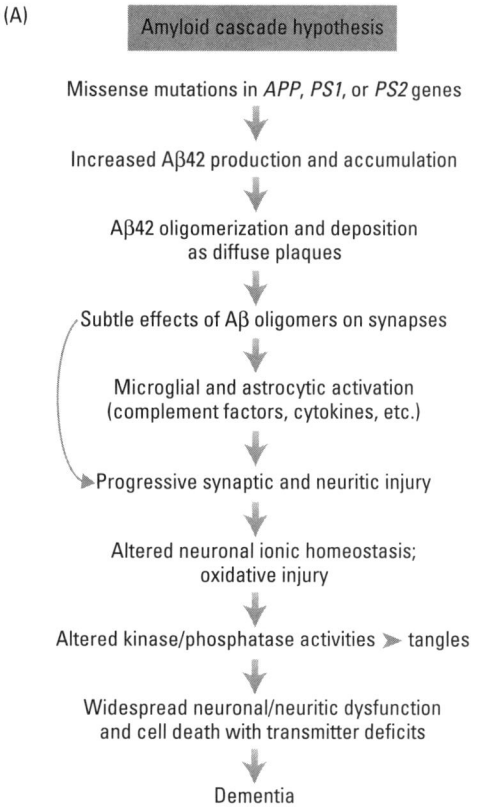

Missense mutations in *APP*, *PS1*, or *PS2* genes
↓
Increased Aβ42 production and accumulation
↓
Aβ42 oligomerization and deposition as diffuse plaques
↓
Subtle effects of Aβ oligomers on synapses
↓
Microglial and astrocytic activation (complement factors, cytokines, etc.)
↓
Progressive synaptic and neuritic injury
↓
Altered neuronal ionic homeostasis; oxidative injury
↓
Altered kinase/phosphatase activities ➤ tangles
↓
Widespread neuronal/neuritic dysfunction and cell death with transmitter deficits
↓
Dementia

Figure 16.3 Hypothesis regarding the etiology of Alzheimer's disease (AD) dementia. (*A*) The amyloid cascade hypothesis revised (Hardy and Selkoe). The leading model for AD etiology posits the sequence of pathogenic events that lead to AD dementia. Curved violet arrows indicate that Aβ oligomers directly injure synapses and neurites of brain neurons as well as activating microglia and astrocytes. The hypothesis remains controversial and several others have been proposed (Davies, 2000, Zlokovic, 2011), including (*B*) the two-hit vascular hypothesis (Zlokovic, 2011) of AD, which posits that vascular factors and injury all converge on a common final disease pathway that involves brain microvascular dysfunction and/or neuronal degeneration (hit one), which results in further neuronal injury and degeneration due to amyloid-β accumulation and tau pathology. BBB, blood–brain barrier.

(B)

[Figure: flowchart showing Vascular factors (Hypertension, diabetes, cardiac disease and/or stroke) — Hit one — branching to BBB dysfunction and Oligaemia; BBB dysfunction → Toxic accumulates; Oligaemia → App expression and processing, Capillary hypoperfusion; App expression and processing → Amyloid-β clearance, Amyloid-β production; these lead to Amyloid-β (Hit two) → p-tau; all converge on Neuronal dysfunction and injury → Cognitive decline, Neurodegeneration → Dementia]

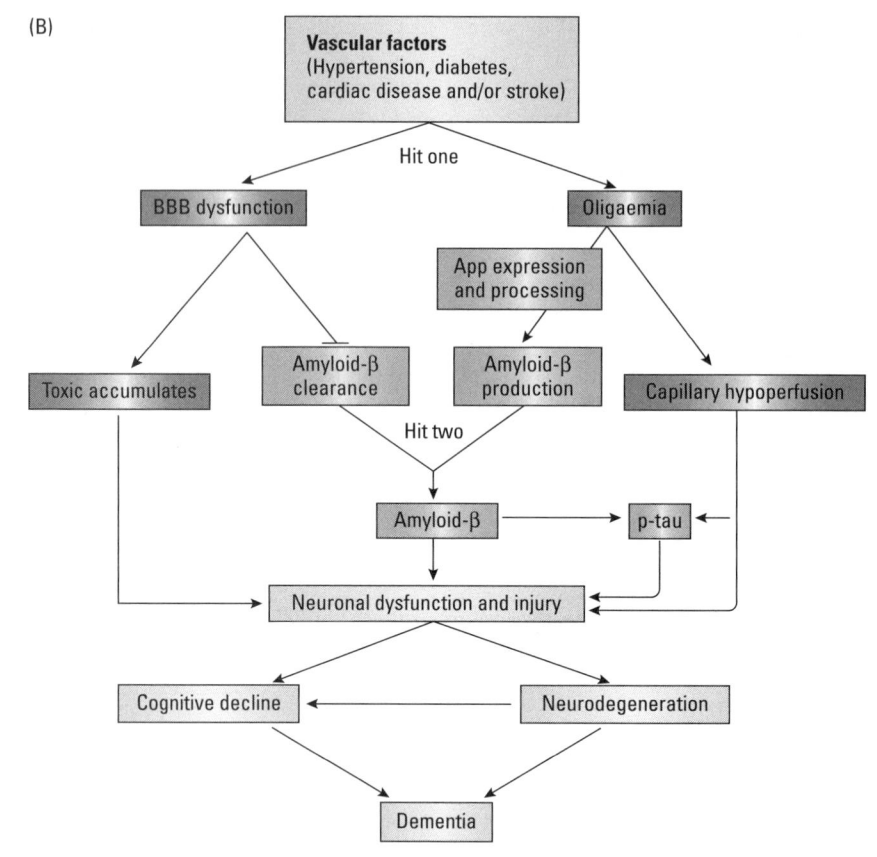

Figure 16.3 Continued

formations, whether intra- or extracellular, are associated with direct and indirect synaptotoxicity and neurotoxicity that can lead to neurodegeneration.

The Two-Stage Amyloid-Dependent and Amyloid-Independent Hypothesis of Alzheimer's Disease

While the amyloid hypothesis remains a leading hypothesis in the field, there are many other hypotheses, including those that view amyloid formation as a by-product and not a root cause of AD, and variants and reformulations to the amyloid hypothesis that have been proposed. For example, a two-stage reformulated hypothesis has been proposed (Hyman, 2011), which posits that the pathogenic process of AD may have an "amyloid-dependent" first phase, led by soluble oligomeric and fibrillar Aß accumulation, that starts a pathogenic cascade of local disruption of the neuropil, loss of dendritic spines, remodeling of neurites, and the inflammatory cascade. Over time, this process becomes increasingly decoupled from amyloid in the "amyloid-independent" second stage to cause further neurofibrillary tangle (NFT) formation, neuronal and synaptic loss, glial activation and responses in limbic and association cortices and later throughout the cortical mantle, and finally extensive neurodegeneration and the disconnection and disruption of intrinsic cognitive and behavioral networks, which ultimately leads to organ failure (Hyman, 2011). This hypothesis also serves to support the critical amyloid link found in genetics.

The Two-Hit Vascular Hypothesis of Alzheimer's Disease

Another emerging hypothesis is the two-hit vascular hypothesis for AD (Zlokovic,

2011) (see Fig. 16.3B). A significant proportion of confirmed cases of AD at autopsy in older patients contain mixed vascular pathology and small-vessel disease. There is substantial overlap in the risk factors for AD and the risk factors for cerebrovascular disease (e.g., hypertension and diabetes). Finally, cerebral ischemia, leukoaraiosis, transient ischemic attacks, and infarcts all increase the risk of AD. Taking these observations into consideration, Zlokovic proposed a model in which microvascular dysfunction ("Hit one") induces and aggravates β-amyloid accumulation ("Hit two"). In this formulation vascular factors are posited to all converge on a common final disease pathway that involves brain microvascular dysfunction and/or degeneration, as well as amyloid-β and tau pathology. "Hit one" is posited to proceed along a non-amyloid-β pathway caused by vascular risk factors and conditions that lead to blood–brain barrier dysfunction and a reduction in cerebral blood flow (oligaemia), thus initiating a cascade of events that precedes dementia. In the non-amyloid-β pathway (see the Fig. 16.3b, shown in green boxes) early neuronal dysfunction is caused by toxic accumulates and capillary hypoperfusion (Zlokovic, 2011). This vascular injury then induces "Hit Two," which proceeds along an amyloid-β pathway by reducing amyloid-β clearance at the blood–brain barrier and increasing its production from the amyloid-β precursor protein (APP), leading to amyloid-β accumulation (the amyloid-β pathway; see the figure, shown in red boxes). Increases in amyloid-β then amplify neuronal dysfunction, accelerate neurodegeneration and dementia, and contribute to disease self-propagation. Neurofibrillary tangle formation is then caused by hyperphosphorylation of tau (p-tau), which can be induced by amyloid-β accumulation and/or vascular hypoperfusion.

Deterministic Alzheimer's Disease Mutations

Multigenerational inheritance and young age of onset (<60 years of age) are the key elements that suggest a high likelihood of finding a causative mutation in one of the known AD genes. There is an 86% probability of finding a pathogenic mutation in PSEN1, APP, or PSEN2, if there are affected family members in three or more generations and the age of onset is less than 60 years. If there are two or more first-degree relatives and age of onset is less than 61 years, the probability is 68%, but this probability falls to 15% with age of onset less than 65 years, and to <1% for age of onset greater than 65 years old (Loy et al., 2014). Causative mutations are rare both in patients with onset later than 65 as well as in those with early onset but who do not have a family history. The latter can be concealed by nonpaternity and reduced penetrance confounds.

Susceptibility Alzheimer's Disease Mutations

The APOE gene is associated with relatively accelerated deposition of Aß in individuals with one or two e4 alleles and higher risk of manifesting Alzheimer's dementia. Relative to individuals with the common APOE ε3/ε3 genotype, individuals with the APOE ε2/ε2, ε3/ε4, ε4/ε4 genotypes are 0.5, 3, and 8–10 times more likely to develop Alzheimer's dementia, respectively (Corder et al., 1993; Loy et al., 2014). APOE is a major cholesterol transport protein and is the major lipoprotein in the brain; it binds Aß—different APOE isoforms have different cholesterol transport and Aß binding efficiencies—and is involved with Aß clearance, amyloid load (it is codeposited with it in neuritic plaques), and cholinergic dysfunction (Ballard et al., 2011). Other recently identified risk genes have significantly less effect than APOE in AD and include genes that increase risk for NFTs including GSK3ß (tau phosphorylation), DYRK1A (tau phosphorylation), and Tau, and genes that affect other mechanisms, which include TOMM40 (mitochondrial protein that interacts with APP), CLU (chaperone protein involved in Aß formation), and PICALM (phosphatidylinositol binding clathrin assembly protein in endosomes)—see AlzGene Database (www.alzgene.org) for regularly updated synopsis of genetic association studies (Bertram, McQueen, Mullin, Blacker, & Tanzi, 2007).

The first step in genetic assessment of AD is to obtain a thorough family history from multiple first-degree family relatives (and spouses for collateral information). Next, a detailed history should establish the dementia phenotype, including age of onset of primary and salient symptoms, progression of symptoms and signs, age of death, availability of medical records, and pathological diagnosis. When there is a high index of suspicion for a pathogenic AD, the affected individual should be offered testing, and if a known mutation is detected, then early genetic consultation should be recommended.

Clinical Features

Clinical symptoms in patients with AD do not necessarily present or progress in a uniform pattern. While certain core clinical features in "typical" (or classic) AD are remarkably consistent (e.g., early difficulty with formation of new memories and learning, apathy, mood changes, irritability, anosognosia), atypical presentations of the AD clinical syndrome are still more common in older patients than typical presentations of much less common neurodegenerative dementing conditions (e.g., FTD, CBD, MSA, PSP). This is due to (1) the high prevalence AD pathology contributing to dementia symptoms in the old (>65 years of age) and especially in the elderly population over 80 years of age where coexistent AD and vascular-ischemic pathology can additively contribute to a mixed dementia syndrome; and (2) selective vulnerability (and selective resilience) of cognitive and behavioral networks in any individual patient can trump the nature of the underlying neuropathology.

While the predominant presentation of AD is an amnestic one (typical AD) where the individual has poor recent and day-to-day memory and better memory for remote events, there can be large heterogeneity in the AD clinical phenotype; this is particularly true regarding the most prominent and initial cognitive, behavioral, and functional deficits, and the course of symptom progression and clinical decline. Recently, atypical presentations/variants of AD (atypical AD) have been formally recognized as part of AD clinical criteria; for example, the 2011 NIA-AA AD criteria recognize "nonamnestic" AD presentations that include "language," "visuospatial," and "executive dysfunction" features (McKhann et al., 2011). Yet the final common pathway of all neurodegenerative dementias converges to leave individuals who are completely dependent on caregivers and are bereft of any significant cognitive, daily living, or motor function.

Presentations of AD in the MCI phase of the illness (MCI due to AD) are reviewed in greater detail in Chapters 17, 19, and 20. Early neuropsychiatric symptoms of AD are reviewed in Chapter 21. In the earliest clinical stages a relatively isolated impairment in memory formation and inefficiency in learning is typical, and if function and behavior are not significantly affected, then the individual is likely in the transitional MCI due to AD stage of the AD clinical spectrum. While the amnestic presentation of MCI (a-MCI) due to AD is the most common, multidomain a-MCI and nonamnestic MCI can also be associated with AD pathology, the former much more than the latter. The MCI syndrome significantly increases the annual rate (incidence) of progression to the Alzheimer's dementia stage by six- to eight-fold, from approximately 1%–2% per year for individuals 65 and older to approximately 15% per year. With the advent of more recent use of biomarkers of amyloid deposition (e.g., amyloid-PET and CSF amyloid levels) and neurodegeneration (e.g., structural MRI, FDG-PET, and CSF tau and phospho-tau levels), progression rates can be further refined in individuals who have the clinical MCI phenotype and possess zero, one, or more positive AD biomarkers; the incidence rates may be two to three times higher (8% vs. 17%–22%) (Petersen et al., 2013) in those with one or more positive AD biomarkers than those who are biomarker negative.

Mild Alzheimer's Disease Versus Normal Cognitive Aging: What's Normal and What's Not

While the etiology and mechanisms that underlie AD and cognitive aging are both incompletely understood, it is more apparent that cognitive impairments and dementia in Alzheimer's disease do not represent the normal aging process but rather a disease process with its own, rather heterogeneous, clinical phenotype and spectrum.

Cognitive Aging and Changes in Cognitive Domains Across the Life Span

The phenomena of cognitive aging, and the mechanisms underlying it, are not well understood. However, converging evidence suggests that several important aspects of age-related cognitive decline begin in early adulthood, different cognitive domains decline at different rates, and individuals differ vastly in their rates of decline. Age-related declines in measures of cognitive functioning are relatively large and become evident in several different types of cognitive abilities, particularly mental processing speed, as early as one's 20s (Salthouse, 2009). Performance on measures of "fluid intelligence," such as speed of mental processing, working memory, recall and retention of verbal and visual information (learning and memory), in particular visuospatial memory, and reasoning, begin to decline in many individuals in their 20s and early 30s (Salthouse, 2009; Weintraub et al., 2013). These cognitive changes can affect creativity, abstract reasoning, and novel problem-solving abilities.

However, with increasing age, accumulation of greater experience and knowledge can allow for better performance on measures of "crystallized intelligence." These include improving or stable performance in one's 50s–70s on tests of specific procedures (e.g., acquired skills), semantic knowledge (e.g., facts about the world), and reading and vocabulary (Salthouse, 2009; Weintraub et al., 2013). These abilities still rely on successful retrieval of stored procedures and information—loss of storage is not a normal part of cognitive aging. Yet there is no consensus on the definition of "successful cognitive aging"—should this be defined as remaining free of any disease or condition that adversely affects cognition (e.g., AD, MCI, dementia) or reserved for those older individuals who cognitively perform similarly to "average" younger adults (Daffner, 2010)?

Characteristics of Alzheimer's Disease: The Symptoms and Signs

Individuals with very mild or mild AD dementia have variable but significant changes and/or mild to moderate impairments in multiple cognitive, functional, and behavioral domains. These levels and patterns of change and impairments are not part of normal cognitive aging. Normally aging persons typically retain their longstanding personalities and interests, including their levels of initiative, motivation, sociability, sensitivity to others, sympathy, affect, and behavior. However, some of the earliest signs of AD, are, in retrospect, often manifest years prior to receiving a clinical diagnosis of dementia and include changes in mood, affect, behavior and sleep patterns, and heightened anxiety; depressive symptoms, particularly apathy and withdrawal are highly prevalent in preclinical and early stages of AD (Farlow & Cummings, 2007). Progression to later stage symptoms such as impaired judgment, disorientation, and confusion; major behavioral changes such as aggression, and agitation; and neuropsychiatric symptoms such as delusions and hallucinations can go unrecognized and undertreated until AD diagnosis. Recognition of these warning signs by appropriate screening, and proper clinical evaluation is the first step of effective AD care.

The Alzheimer's Association 10 early warning signs of AD (Alzheimer's-Association, 2013) provide a practical review of the clinical manifestations of very mild to mild AD that is useful for patients, families, and caregivers, as well as for clinicians to provide psychoeducation. The AD-8 screening instrument (see Chapter 19) provides a very practical screen for changes in thinking and memory that can be a "red flag" for underlying clinical AD. The Clinical Dementia Rating Scale (CDR) also provides a useful guide for the clinical features that are salient in the different stages of AD dementia. Chapter 19 also provides a practical introduction to changes in cognitive, functional, and behavioral domains that can be seen in early AD and dementias, as well as information regarding the process and specifics of the evaluation of these domains and standard instruments that are useful in clinical practice to screen, detect, track, and stage clinically significant abnormalities (e.g., AD-8, MoCA, BDS-IMC, ACE-R, FAQ, ADL-Q, NPI, and CDR). Table 16.2 from Snowden et al. (2011) provides a good summary of the characteristic symptoms and corresponding signs elicited in the assessment of individuals with mild AD.

Memory Function

With regard to memory function, individuals with very mild or mild AD dementia

TABLE 16.2 Characteristic Symptoms and Signs of Alzheimer's Disease Dementia

Symptoms Obtained From Client History	On Assessment
Memory	
Poor recent/day to day memory	Disorientation in time and place
Better memory for remote than recent past	Impaired recall and recognition memory
Repetitive in conversation	Loses information over a delay
Mislays objects	Consistent performance
Would get lost if unaccompanied	Impaired working memory—reduced digit and word span, patent loses track of test instructions
Language	
Difficulty finding words	Conversational speech hesitant and halting, with unfinished sentence
Difficulty remembering people's names	Word retrieval difficulty
Loses train of thought in conversation	Impaired repetition, with phonemic errors
Difficulty following group conversation	Impaired sentence comprehension
Reads less	Difficulty following multistage commands
Difficulty writing, producing a signature	Problems with left/right (spatial) commands
	Reading consistent with conversational speech
	Impaired writing and spelling
Calculation	
No longer deals with bills, household accounts	Impaired mental and written arithmetic—especially subtractions involving holding and manipulating numbers, carrying across columns
Difficulty reckoning change	
Perception, Spatial Skills, Praxis	
Slow to locate and/or identify objects ("doesn't see things in front of him")	Impaired object perception for degraded stimuli/unusual Views
Difficulty remembering locations of objects ("puts things in wrong place")	Visually based errors on perceptual tasks
Disoriented in familiar environment	Slow to localize stimuli in visual field
Difficulty negotiating stairs (judging depth)	Impaired space perception
Car accidents suggesting poor spatial judgement (e.g., hitting parked car)	Loss of spatial configuration of drawings
Difficulty executing manual tasks with spatial demands (folding clothes, dressing laying table)	Spatially impaired reproduction of hand postures
	Impaired gestural praxis (spatial configuration and position in space)
Executive Skills	
Difficulty working out use of gadgets (e.g., washing machine, TV remote control)	Poor executive test performance. Patient "overloaded" by complex tasks
Difficulty organizing household affairs	
Difficulty grasping complex ideas	
Behaviour	
More irritable	Socially appropriate. Preserved social facade
More anxious	Anxious/low mood depending on insight
Less confident—takes a "backseat" in social groups	
Physical status	
Minimal physical symptoms	Few signs—mild akinesia and rigidity
Slowing—usually mid-course	Myoclonus, impaired tactile localization

Source: From Snowden et al. (2011).

show consistent difficulty with learning and remembering new information; they may partially or entirely forget important conversations, life events, dates, appointments, and obligations; misplace or lose belongings (and have difficulty retracing their steps); be highly repetitive with questions and statements (e.g., repeatedly ask for the same information, make the same statements, or tell the same stories); and increasingly need to rely on external memory aids (e.g., reminder notes, appointment books, calendars, PDAs) and others for activities they used to handle efficiently and entirely independently (e.g., recipes, hobbies, taxes, banking/finances, travel). Patients may constantly misplace or lose belongings and be unable to go back over their steps to find them again, or they may even put things in unusual places (e.g., eyeglasses in the freezer). In the moderate to severe stages of AD, progression of memory dysfunction usually results in severe memory loss and difficulty with new learning such that only highly learned or overlearned material is retained, and new information is rapidly lost, including current and historical events (usually with a retrograde gradient) and semantic knowledge. Yet patients in the moderate stages of AD may still be able to remember details of life events from many decades ago. In severe dementia no new learning and memory formation takes place and only memory fragments remain. Patients increasingly lose elementary semantic knowledge about the world, and personal and autobiographical information including relationships and names of close family members and basic details of their life become patchy or lost (e.g., whether they were married, where they went to school, and what their profession was). While this general progression is characteristic, it is important to keep in mind that individuals with AD often have both patchiness and fluctuations in cognition, function, and behavior that do not preclude islands of relative stability in some mental or daily functions and occasional moments of clarity interspersed with otherwise low function and confusion.

In contrast, patients who experience normal cognitive aging may *occasionally* have difficulty retrieving a name, appointment, or details of a conversation, but this information is not consistently lost and can typically be remembered later. This phenomenon is like a lazy Susan retrieval effect: the name or information is not readily within reach, but ultimately, as one waits long enough it comes back around and is retrieved. Cognitively healthy individuals may also occasionally misplace items but, with time, are usually able to remember and retrace their steps. By definition, this type of memory change does not consistently adversely affect daily functioning.

Executive Functions, Concentration, Judgment, Reasoning, and Insight

With regard to executive and administrative functions, reasoning, judgment, insight, and decision making, individuals with AD also experience progressive difficulties that often manifest in daily challenges in organization, planning, problem solving, social interactions, doing or completing familiar tasks at home and at work, making proper judgments and decisions, and appreciating the extent and nature of their cognitive, functional, and behavioral changes and limitations. Some individuals may experience changes in their ability to develop and follow a plan, work with numbers and money, problem solve, follow a familiar recipe, or keep track of and manage monthly bills, finances, and tax records. They may be less efficient or effective accomplishing tasks that they previously did or have great difficulty learning new tools or procedures. For example, relative to the past, they may consistently produce work of inferior quality, accomplishing their work may be more effortful and take much longer to complete, or they be unable to adequately learn a new system or procedure (e.g., writing a report, managing a budget, learning a new computer program or workflow at work). They may also have frequent difficulty with concentration, be easily distractible, and often lose their train of thought. Additionally, their ability to grasp information, manipulate, and make important connections and deductions necessary to make reasoned judgments and good decisions often deteriorates. For example, they may have poor judgment when dealing with money; give large amounts to telemarketers, strangers, or associates; make poor purchases; display major changes in their spending habits such as buying things they would not have in the past or that they do not need; and not fully appreciate that their ability to function and make decisions has changed (i.e., have anosognosia). Finally, they may be less able to modulate their affect, have poor impulse control and insight regarding their behavior, and have diminished awareness of proper grooming and hygiene.

While normal cognitive aging does not preclude *occasionally* making an error balancing the checkbook; being late with a check;

having to look up a recipe; needing greater time or help to use a new device, tool, or program; having to be reminded of details of a conversation; or sometimes losing concentration and being distracted during a task, the frequency of these occurrences is significantly greater in AD. Occasionally making a poor decision, being distractible (especially in the context of multitasking or "not being present in the moment"), or making an occasional careless mistake is normal.

Spatial and Temporal Orientation

Regarding spatial and temporal orientation, patients with AD have increased difficulty keeping track of dates, the passage of time, and geographic relations and locations. Initially this may manifest as being disoriented about the day and date, but as AD progresses into the moderate and later stages, patients can forget or be confused about the month, season, and year. In later stages, patients can have trouble understanding something if it is not happening immediately. Additionally, they become increasingly confused about their spatial location (e.g., hospital or town) and can easily forget where they are or how they got there.

In normal cognitive aging it is not uncommon to occasionally not immediately remember the date (or even day of the week) but then figure it out, or to sometimes become distracted or lose one's way, look for one's car in the parking lot, become unsure about a particular travel route, or have to ask for directions, a map, or GPS.

Visuospatial Function

Regarding visual and spatial relationships patients with AD, even in the mild stages, can have trouble understanding or interpreting visual images and spatial relationships, and navigating through space. This may include not appreciating the big picture or objects that are right in front of them, and having difficulty judging distances, colors and contrasts, and reading. For some individuals, these kinds of problems can be a predominant and presenting sign of AD (i.e., patients with the visuospatial variant of AD). This can translate into significant difficulties with work and particularly with driving.

Individuals who are undergoing normal cognitive aging can have changes in their vision related to their eyes as opposed to how their brain integrates and interprets visual images. For example, they may have shortsightedness or loss of visual clarity, due to cataracts, and low visual acuity, due to changes in the retina.

Word Finding and Language

Language difficulties in AD often present as new problems with word finding, expression, comprehension, reading, writing, repetition, naming, and understanding the meaning of words. Individuals may have trouble following or joining a conversation, frequently have long pauses in the middle of a sentence, struggle with vocabulary, and use wrong or imprecise words (e.g., call a watch a "hand clock," frequently use "thing" instead of the correct word). Over time their speech becomes increasingly inarticulate, devoid of information content, simplified, agrammatic, and short. With progression of disease they also require frequent repetition and use of simple and short sentences to affect understanding. Early on, this language problem can be mistaken for a hearing problem.

While a frequent complaint of older individuals experiencing normal cognitive aging is the inability to retrieve the right word or name, which invariably comes back later, this difficulty is of insufficient magnitude to affect consistent efficient and successful communication.

Personality, Mood, Motivation, Behavior, and Neuropsychiatric Symptoms

As detailed in Chapter 2, as well as in Chapters 19, 24, 25, and 26, the neuropsychiatric symptoms of AD and dementias, while varied, are common and can predate clinical diagnosis by years. The NPI questionnaire (see Chapter 19) provides a good instrument to detect and track neuropsychiatric symptoms in AD.

Individuals with AD can have significant changes and impairments in social interactions, mood, and affect that include being less self-motivated and more apathetic; having more anxiety and low mood; being less inhibited and more insensitive in their actions; being more irritable and easily agitated; becoming more perseverative, fixated, and compulsive; and paying less attention to grooming and hygiene. For example, individuals with early or progressing AD can show diminished initiative and greater passivity and withdrawal from activities and work. They may appear less confident and start to remove themselves from hobbies, social functions and interactions, work projects, and interests such as engaging in exercise and hobbies, and keeping up with a favorite sports team. They may show significant changes in mood, behavior, and personality, and reactions to events and stressors. For example, they may become more anxious, depressed, and fearful; be easily upset and angry at home, at work, with friends, or in places where they are out of their comfort zone or when a routine is changed; be less inhibited, appropriate, and sensitive and more judgmental in their comments and actions; become paranoid that others are stealing from them or want to hurt them; develop fixed delusions such as their spouse is having an affair; become very obsessive, compulsive, and fixated about a particular story, event, or behavior such as constantly watching a particular TV channel, talking about the same news subject, and repeating the same actions such as wiping the table or scratching; or develop hoarding habits.

Occasionally having less energy, being more tired and weary, feeling less social, wanting to stick to routine, and experiencing anxiety and fluctuations in mood in reaction to life stressors, events, and health and physiological changes is a normal part of living and cognitive aging; having major and sustained changes in personality, behavior, comportment, and social interactions is not. Such changes cannot be simply ignored in older individuals and explained as normal aging "idiosyncrasies," "eccentricity," and "quirkiness."

Neuropathology

In Alzheimer's disease, like all other dementing neurodegenerative conditions, the process that leads to the dementia stage, Alzheimer's dementia, is now believed to start decades prior to the onset of clinical symptoms. Jack et al. (2010) proposed a model of AD biomarker pathology that involves a progressive sequence of measurable biochemical, neurophysiological, and neuroanatomical alterations that can be potentially detected years prior to psychometrically and clinically noticeable deterioration in cognition, behavior, and function.

Typical AD neuropathology starts and spreads in a remarkably consistent pattern. The neuropathological hallmark of AD consists of a widespread but regionally specific pattern of intraparenchymal diffuse and neuritic ß-amyloid (Aß) plaques (cortical layers II and III) and intracytoplasmic (initially, and then extracellular) NFTs (cortical layers III and V) with synaptic and neuronal loss, and gliosis (see Fig. 6.6 in Chapter 6) (Braak, Alafuzoff, Arzberger, Kretzschmar, & Del Tredici, 2006; Hyman et al., 2012; Jellinger & Bancher, 1998; Parvizi, Van Hoesen, & Damasio, 2001). Amyloid plaques consist mostly of extracellular deposits of the 42-amino acid polypeptide Aß (Aß-42), which is cleaved via the enzymes ß–secretase and γ–secretase from the larger intermembrane amyloid precursor protein (APP). Soluble Aß-42 oligomers (2–12 or more) are considered synapto- and neurotoxic and to play an integral role in the "amyloidogenic pathway" of AD pathogenesis. Cleavage of APP by α-secretase produces shorter Aß fragments that enter a "nonamyloidogenic pathway" that is considered pathogenic. APP is an integral membrane protein that is expressed in many tissues but that is most concentrated in the neurons and synapses. The APP gene is located on Chromosome 21, and while its primary function is unknown, it has been implicated as a modulator of neural plasticity, synaptic formation, and modeling, and to play a role in memory and learning. Neurofibrillary tangles (NFTs) consist of intracellular (then extracellular) deposits of hyperphosphorylated tau protein, a microtubule-stabilizing protein.

At death, gross examination of the brain reveals that more than 90% of patients with clinical AD have substantial loss of brain weight and atrophy (with shrinkage of gyri and widening of sulci) that is more marked in the temporal (particularly the hippocampi and medial temporal lobes), frontal, and parietal lobes. There is relative sparing of primary motor and sensory cortices (less so with olfaction than in the visual cortex) in AD. Ex vacuo dilation of the ventricles and pallor of the nucleus coeruleus is also often seen. Many patients with AD also show evidence of cortical and cortico-subcortical microhemorrhages related to cerebral amyloid angiopathy-related vasculopathy and leakage (see Chapter 14; Attems, Jellinger, Thal, & van Nostrand, 2011); evidence for these types of cerebral microhemorrhages, from hemosiderin microdeposition, can be seen during life by gradient echo or susceptibility weighted MRI sequences in 15%–20% of patients with AD (Atri et al., 2005).

The hippocampal formation, entorhinal and perirhinal cortices, and their related memory networks show a selective vulnerability for the earliest micropathology in AD; the large hippocampal pyramidal neurons and entorhinal stellate neurons are particularly susceptible to NFT formation (Lace et al., 2009). Usually AD tangle pathology then spreads to homotypical association cortices, whereas heterotypical motor and visual cortices are often relatively spared until later stages of the disease.

Though not specific to AD, the cholinergic neurons of the nucleus basalis of Meynert and substantia innominata undergo either primary or retrograde degeneration, and the large cholinergic neurons of the neostriatum (caudate nucleus, putamen, nucleus accumbens) often also undergo neurofibrillary degeneration in AD. Limbic thalamic nuclei, including the anterior and dorsomedial nuclei, also appear selectively vulnerable to neurofibrillary tangles in AD and show neuronal loss. Patients with AD often also depict neurpathological changes in the amygdala and in important brainstem adrenergic (locus coeruleus) and serotonergic (dorsal and median raphe) projection nuclei. AD patients with greater extrapyramidal symptoms during life also often have tangle-related neuronal loss in the pars compacta of the substantia nigra.

The most current neuropathological criteria for AD are the "2012 National Institutes of Aging (NIA)-Alzheimer's Association (AA) guidelines for the neuropathological assessment of AD" (Hyman et al., 2012). The new 2012 guidelines/criteria are different from the previous guidelines from 1997 in several important areas; these include that a clinical diagnosis of dementia is no longer required for a neuropathological diagnosis of AD to be made, that in addition to the Braak & Braak NFT stage (Braak & Braak, 1991) and the CERAD (Consortium to Establish a Registry for Alzheimer's Disease) neuritic plaques scores, the new guidelines also incorporate the Thal Phase (Thal, Rub, Orantes, & Braak, 2002) for Aß regional accumulation. Whereas the previous guidelines offered little guidance on neuropathology related to comorbid conditions, regions to sample and stain, and reporting and clinicopathological correlation, the new criteria offer explicit recommendations and guidelines.

The CERAD classification scheme placed emphasis on neuritic plaques based on using silver stain and/or thioflavin S to determine burden in the worst areas by examination of frontal, temporal, and parietal cortex. Neuritic plaque density is reported as absent/none, sparse, moderate, or frequent. When there is evidence of any neuritic plaques, based on age category (<50, 50–75, or >75 years of age) and presence or absence of clinical dementia, a classification of definite AD, probable AD, and possible AD is made.

The Braak & Braak staging scheme (Braak & Braak, 1991), Stage I–VI, is based on silver staining techniques and assesses NFT distribution. Based on brain autopsy and clinical data from 83 individuals with and without dementia, Braak & Braak Staging assumes that AD NFT pathology is temporally acquired and progresses in a stereotyped spatiotemporal order. Stages I and II represent "transentorhinal" disease; none of the cases had clinical diagnosis of dementia. Stages III and IV represent "limbic" disease; 5/10 Stage III cases and 5/10 Stage IV cases had clinical diagnosis of dementia. Stages V and VI represent "isocortical" disease; all cases with Stage V or VI NFT pathology had a clinical diagnosis of dementia.

The Thal Phase classification of regional Aß distribution (Thal et al., 2002) utilizes antibody based methods to assess parenchymal Aß deposits (cerebral amyloid angiopathy [CAA] is excluded from this assessment) according to five progressive stages: 1–Neocortical; 2–Allocortex (hippocampal); 3–Thalamus, striatum, nucleus basalis of Meynert; 4–Brainstem; and 5–Cerebellum.

The 2012 NIA-AA guidelines state that any plaques and tangles are considered a form of "Alzheimer's disease neuropathological changes" (ADNC), report an "ABC" score ("A" for Amyloid regional distribution Thal Phase, "B" for Braak & Braak Stage NFT distribution, and "C" for CERAD neuritic amyloid plaque score) that is transformed into one of four levels, "Not," "Low," "Intermediate," or "High," to characterize the AD Neuropathological Changes (ADNC), and uses population-based observations to suggest likelihood of cognitive impairment.

Diagnosis

The first pillar in appropriate patient care is proper and timely diagnosis. The diagnosis of Alzheimer's dementia remains a clinical diagnosis. There is no one simple binary test result that provides the diagnosis. Instead, the diagnosis is made through a clinical evaluation process that ultimately conforms to established clinical criteria. Recently, three major criteria for AD dementia have been established or revised; they are the revised NIA-AA 2011 criteria (Dubois et al., 2010; McKhann et al., 2011), the International Working Group (IWG, also known as Dubois) 2010 revised New Lexicon criteria (Dubois et al., 2007, 2010), and the *DSM-5* criteria (APA, 2013). This section will review all three criteria, with a main focus on the NIA-AA 2011 criteria, and the process of the diagnostic evaluation of Alzheimer's dementia in the clinical setting.

While all three AD dementia criteria now acknowledge that the AD process occurs on a clinical continuum, for practical purposes they polychotomize the process into one or more predementia stages and a dementia stage, each with its own criteria. For example, the NIA-AA criteria provides criteria for the preclinical AD, MCI due to AD, and AD dementia stages of the Alzheimer's disease spectrum (Albert et al., 2011; McKhann et al., 2011; Sperling et al., 2011) (see Chapters 17, 18, and 22); the IWG-Dubois New Lexicon criteria provides classifications for preclinical, prodromal, and AD dementia (Dubois et al., 2010); and the *DSM-5* criteria provide minor and major neurocognitive disorder (NCD) due to AD (APA, 2013). Whereas the two former criteria opt for an integrated clinicobiological categorization of the AD spectrum where AD biomarker evidence can aid in elevating the probability of the clinical phenotype being caused by underlying AD biological and pathological changes (particularly to aid research classification of AD for clinical trials), the latter, *DSM-5* criteria, retains a purely clinical phenotype symptoms approach.

The 2010 IWG-Dubois New Lexicon Criteria

The IWG-Dubois New Lexicon criteria (see Table 16.3) establish preclinical, prodromal ("predementia"), and AD dementia stages. The preclinical stage is further subclassified into asymptomatic-at-risk state for AD (clinically normal but evidence of brain amyloidosis from PET tracer or CSF) and presymptomatic AD (clinically normal but known to carry a monogenic AD mutation for APP, PS-1, or PS-2) states. The prodromal AD stage refers to nondemented individuals with early symptomatic changes in which clinical symptoms include episodic memory loss of the hippocampal type (have free recall deficits that are not normalized with cuing) and supportive biomarker evidence from CSF or imaging for AD pathological changes. The MCI classification in the IWG-Dubois New Lexicon criteria is a term of exclusion for individuals who have measurable cognitive impairment without dementia but who deviate in the clinicobiological phenotype of prodromal AD by having memory symptoms or biomarker profiles that are not characteristic of AD (Dubois et al., 2010). AD dementia is subclassified into typical AD, atypical AD, and mixed AD (see Table 16.3).

The 2013 *DSM-5* Criteria

The recently published *DSM-5* criteria essentially replace the diagnostic term "dementia" from *DSM-IV* with "major neurocognitive disorder" (NCD), and "dementia of the Alzheimer's type" (dementia due to AD) with "major NCD due to AD." Based on the degree of cognitive symptoms and independence on ADLs, *DSM-5* distinguishes between mild NCD and major NCD. Mild NCD is defined by "modest" reported or observed cognitive decline, and cognitive

TABLE 16.3 The IWG-Dubois New Lexicon Criteria for the Alzheimer's Disease Spectrum

Panel: A new lexicon to Alzheimer's disease

Alzheimer's disease (AD)

This diagnostic label is now restricted to the clinical disorder that starts with the onset of the first specific clinical symptoms of the disease and encompasses both the predementia and dementia phases. AD thus refers to the whole spectrum of the clinical phase of the disease and is not restricted to the dementia syndrome. The diagnosis is now established in vivo and relies on a dual clinicobiological entity that requires the evidence of both specific memory changes and in-vivo markers of Alzheimer's pathology that can include the following: cerebrospinal fluid (CSF) amyloid β, total tau, and phospho-tau; retention of specific PET amyloid tracers; medial temporal lobe atrophy on magnetic resonance imaging (MRI); and/or temporal, parietal hypometabolism on fluorodeoxyglucose positron emission tomography (PET). The clinical phenotype can be typical or atypical. Additionally, two different stages might still be meaningful: a prodromal and a dementia phase.

Proldromal AD (also called "predementia stage of AD")

This term refers to the early symptomatic predementia phase of AD in which (1) clinical symptoms including episodic memory loss of the hippocampal type (characterized by a free recall deficit on testing not normalized with cueing) are present, but not sufficiently severe to affect instrumental activities of daily living and do not warrant a diagnosis of dementia; and in which (2) biomarker evidence from CSF or imaging is supportive of the presence of AD pathological changes. This phase is now included in the new definition of AD. The term of prodromal AD might disappear in the future if AD is considered to encompass both the predementia and dementia stages.

AD dementia

This term refers to the phase of AD during which cognitive symptoms are sufficiently severe to interfere with social functioning and instrumental activities of daily living, a threshold that is considered to define dementia in association with changes in episodic memory and in at least one other cognitive domain. It might still be meaningful to identify the dementia threshold for clinical trials or social/economic evaluations.

Typical AD

This term refers to the most common clinical phenotype of AD, which is characterized by an early significant and progressive episodic memory deficit that remains dominant in the later stages of the disease and is followed by or associated with other cognitive impairments (executive dysfunction, language, praxis, and complex visual processing impairments) and neuropsychiatric changes. The diagnosis is further supported by one or more in-vivo positive biomarkers of Alzheimer's pathology.

Atypical AD

This term refers to the less common and well characterized clinical phenotype of the disease that occurs with Alzheimer's pathology. This clinical syndrome includes primary progressive nonfluent aphasia, logopenic aphasia, frontal variant of AD, and posterior cortical atrophy. In the presence of one of these clinical presentations, the diagnosis of AD is supported by in-vivo evidence of amyloidosis in the brain (with retention of specific amyloid labeling radioligands) or in the CSF (with changes characteristic of Alzheimer's pathology in amyloid β, tau, and phospho-tau concentrations).

Mixed AD

This term refers to patients who fully fulfil the diagnostic criteria for typical AD and additionally present with clinical and brain imaging/biological evidence of other comorbid disorders such as cerebrovascular disease or Lewy body disease.

Preclnical states of AD (including both "asymptomatic at-risk" state for AD and "presymptomatic" AD)

These terms refer to the long asymptomatic stage between the earliest pathogenic events/brain lesions of AD and the first appearance of specific cognitive changes. Traditionally, a preclinical or asymptomatic phase was recognized postmortem by evidence of histological changes typical of Alzheimer's pathology in individuals considered as cognitively normal before death. Today, two preclinical states can be isolated in vivo:

(continued)

TABLE 16.3 Continued

- *Asymptomatic at-risk state for AD*—this state can be identified in vivo by evidence of amyloidosis in the brain (with retention of specific PET amyloid tracers) or in the CSF (with changes in amyloid ß, tau, and phospho-tau concentrations). In the absence of knowledge about the value of these biological changes to predict the further development of the disease the asymptomatic phase of AD should still be referred to as an "at-risk state for AD."
- *PresymptomaticAD*—this state applies to individuals who will develop AD. This can be ascertained only in families that are affected by rare autosomal dominant monogenic AD mutations (monogenic AD)

Alzheimer's pathology

This term refers to the underlying neurobiological changes responsible for AD that span the earliest pathogenic events in the brain and that include specific neuronal brain lesions (senile neuritic plaques and neurofibrillary tangles synaptic loss, and vascular amyloid deposits within the cerebral cortex). This term can be applied irrespective of the existence of clinical manifestation.

Mild cognitive impairment (MCI)

This term applies to individuals with measurable MCI in the absence of a significant effect on instrumental activities of daily living. This diagnostic label is applied if there is no disease to which MCI can be attributed. It remains a term of exclusion for individuals who are suspected to have but do not meet the proposed new research criteria for AD, in that they deviate from the clinicobiological phenotype of prodromal AD because they have memory symptoms that are not characteristic of AD or because they are biomarker negative.

---

impairment in one or more domains (usually a single domain) that does not interfere with "capacity for independence in daily activities" (i.e., preservation of independence on ADLs). In contrast, major NCD is defined by reported or observed cognitive decline that results in "significant" impairment in one or more (often multiple) cognitive domains that is evident or reported and that interferes with independence to the point that assistance is required with daily activities (i.e., loss of independence on ADLs). The definition of mild NCD is essentially the definition of MCI (see Chapter 17), while major NCD represents dementia. These diagnoses are precluded by the presence of delirium or primary attribution to another Axis I disorder.

The *DSM-5* still recognizes "dementia" as an acceptable alternative for the newly minted term major NCD, which the APA prefers due to a potential stigma associated with the term "dementia," which is argued to be inaccurate and stigmatizing since it can be due to any of several causes (e.g., HIV-related, alcohol-related, vascular-related) and literally means "without mind" when translated from Latin. Others have disagreed with the usefulness of the new *DSM-5* terminology, arguing that dementia is a medical term that is well established and widely used, and to change terminology from *DSM-IV* to *DSM-5* introduces unnecessary discontinuity and hardship (Tompa, 2013).

While the *DSM-IV* criteria for dementia of the Alzheimer's type required memory impairment and one or more of the following: aphasia, apraxia, agnosia, or deterioration in executive function, memory loss is not necessary for the diagnosis of major NCD. However, in order specify mild or major NCD due to AD requires "clear evidence of decline in memory and learning."

The 2011 NIA-AA Criteria

Similar to the IWG-Dubois New Lexicon criteria, the NIA-AA criteria for the AD spectrum formally characterizes asymptomatic (Sperling et al., 2011) (preclinical AD; see Chapter 18) and mildly symptomatic nondementia stages of AD (MCI due to AD; see Chapter 17) (Albert et al., 2011), incorporates the use of AD biomarkers to allow greater specificity in diagnosis, and admits nonamnestic (atypical) presentations of AD.

The original 1984 NINCDS-ADRDA criteria for Alzheimer's disease (McKhann, 1984) relied on older data and conceptualizations that AD is a clinico-pathological entity with an "all-or-none" and one-to-one coupling between the typical AD dementia phenotype and brain pathology (i.e., AD-type brain pathology and typical AD symptoms are synonymous) such that having AD pathology meant the clinical AD dementia phenotype was present and that if there was no AD dementia phenotype then no AD brain pathology was present. However, it is now established that 20%–40% of individuals age 70 and older who do not show the dementia phenotype nonetheless possess AD brain pathology at autopsy or biomarker evidence consistent with the AD cerebral amyloidosis profile (see Chapter 22). AD severity was considered binary (nondemented versus demented) as opposed to being on a continuum; the 1984 criteria did not account for cognitive impairment that did not reach the dementia threshold. The 1984 criteria also only recognized AD presenting as an amnestic disorder, defined definite AD by requiring tissue confirmation from biopsy or autopsy, and imposed strict age cutoffs for AD (40–90 years of age). The 1984 criteria were also drafted during a period when many common non-AD dementias were neither well understood nor defined (e.g., there was no definition of dementia with Lewy bodies, the FTD spectrum, or vascular dementia), there was only Pick's disease and little appreciation of mixed dementia, there was a much greater belief that reversible systemic disorder mimicking AD was common (e.g., vitamin B12 and thyroid deficiency), and the dominantly inherited monogenic causes of AD (mutations in APP, PS-1 and PS-2 genes) had not been identified. The possible AD dementia classification in the 1984 criteria included a very heterogeneous group of individuals, many of whom would now be classified as MCI (not necessarily due to AD).

The 2011 NIA-AA criteria for AD dementia update the 1984 NINCDS-ADRDA Alzheimer's disease criteria and incorporate more recent clinical, imaging, and laboratory innovations. First, an updated definition of all-cause dementia is provided utilizing core clinical criteria (see Table 16.4). The definition requires cognitive or behavioral symptoms of sufficient magnitude to interfere with usual work or daily function; evaluation of cognitive change and impairment via subjective (history from the patient and a knowledgeable informant) and objective

TABLE 16.4 2011 NIA-AA Core Clinical Criteria for All-Cause Dementia

Dementia: Cognitive or Behavioral (Neuropsychiatric) Symptoms Are Present That:
1. **Interfere with** the ability to function at work or at **usual activities**; and
2. Represent **a decline from previous levels** of functioning and performing; and
3. Are not explained by delirium or major psychiatric disorder;
4. Cognitive impairment is **detected and diagnosed** through a combination of:
   (a) **History**-taking from the *patient and a knowledgeable informant* and
   (b) An **objective cognitive assessment**, either a "bedside" *mental status examination or neuropsychological testing*. Neuropsychological testing should be performed when the routine history and bedside mental status examination cannot provide a confident diagnosis.
5. The **cognitive or behavioral impairment** involves *a minimum of two of the following domains*:
   (a) *Impaired ability to acquire and remember new information*
      Symptoms include repetitive questions or conversations, misplacing personal belongings, forgetting events or appointments, and getting lost on a familiar route.
   (b) *Impaired reasoning and handling of complex tasks, poor judgment*
      Symptoms include poor understanding of safety risks, inability to manage finances, poor decision-making ability, inability to plan complex or sequential activities.
   (c) *Impaired visuospatial abilities*
      Symptoms include inability to recognize faces or common objects or to find objects in direct view despite good acuity; inability to operate simple implements or orient clothing to the body.
   (d) *Impaired language functions* (speaking, reading, writing)
      Symptoms include difficulty thinking of common words while speaking, hesitations; speech, spelling, and writing errors.
   (e) *Changes in personality, behavior, or comportment*
      Symptoms include: uncharacteristic mood fluctuations such as agitation, impaired motivation, initiative, apathy, loss of drive, social withdrawal, decreased interest in previous activities, loss of empathy, compulsive or obsessive behaviors, and socially unacceptable behaviors.

(mental status exam or neuropsychological testing) measures; and cognitive or behavioral impairments that involve a minimum of two domains (memory; executive function, reasoning, and judgment; visuospatial function; language; personality, behavior, and comportment). Additionally, these significant changes must represent a clear decline from a previous higher baseline of performance and functioning, and they cannot be explained solely by delirium or another psychiatric illness.

The diagnosis of MCI remains a matter of "clinical judgment made by a skilled clinician" as to whether "there is significant interference in the ability to function at work or in usual daily activities," and it needs to be individualized to the patient in the context of the patient's particular circumstances and premorbid level of function and performance as appreciated through clinical interview with the patient and informant (McKhann et al., 2011).

The 2011 NIA-AA classification criteria for AD dementia proposed the following terminology for classifying individuals with dementia caused by AD: (1) probable AD dementia, (2) possible AD dementia, and (3) probable or possible AD dementia with evidence of the AD pathophysiological process. While the first two classifications are intended for use in all clinical settings, the third remains, for now, intended for research purposes. It is important to note that in order to qualify for any of these classifications, an individual must first meet criteria for dementia as delineated in Table 16.4

Probable Alzheimer's Disease Dementia

Table 16.5 delineates the core criteria for probable AD dementia. The salient inclusion criteria are as follows: (1) dementia present; (2) insidious onset over months to years; (3) history of decline/worsening; (4) initial and most prominent cognitive

TABLE 16.5　2011 NIA-AA Core Clinical Criteria for Probable Alzheimer's Disease Dementia

A diagnosis of **Probable AD dementia** can be made when the patient
1. *Meets criteria for dementia* described in Table 4, *and*
2. In addition *has the following* characteristics:
A. Insidious onset:
Symptoms have a gradual onset over months to years, not sudden over hours or days;
B. Clear-cut history of worsening of cognition by report or observation; and
C. The initial and most prominent cognitive deficits are evident on history and examination in one of the following categories:
　a. **Amnestic presentation**: It is the most common syndromic presentation of AD dementia. The deficits should include impairment in learning and recall of recently learned information. There should also be evidence of cognitive dysfunction in at least one other cognitive domain, as defined earlier in the text.
　b. **Nonamnestic presentations**:
　　(i) *Language presentation*: The most prominent deficits are in word finding, but deficits in other cognitive domains should be present.
　　(ii) *Visuospatial presentation*: The most prominent deficits are in spatial cognition, including object agnosia, impaired face recognition, simultanagnosia, and alexia. Deficits in other cognitive domains should be present.
　　(iii) *Executive dysfunction*: The most prominent deficits are impaired reasoning, judgment, and problem solving. Deficits in other cognitive domains should be present.
D. The diagnosis of probable AD dementia *should not be applied when* there is evidence of
　(a) Substantial concomitant cerebrovascular disease, defined by a history of a stroke temporally related to the onset or worsening of cognitive impairment; or the presence of multiple or extensive infarcts or severe white matter hyperintensity burden; or
　(b) Core features of Dementia with Lewy bodies other than dementia itself; or
　(c) Prominent features of behavioral variant frontotemporal dementia; or
　(d) Prominent features of semantic variant primary progressive aphasia or nonfluent/agrammatic variant primary progressive aphasia; or
　(e) Evidence for another concurrent, active neurological disease, or a nonneurological medical comorbidity or use of medication that could have a substantial effect on cognition.

deficits fall under either an amnestic (deficit in short-term and recent memory and learning) or nonamnestic (language, visuospatial, or executive dysfunction) presentation. The salient exclusion criteria are evidence for prominent features that are consistent with (1) vascular cognitive impairment/dementia (e.g., temporally related strokes; multiple infarcts; extensive leukoaraiosis); (2) DLB (see Chapter 12); (3) bvFTD (see Chapter 8); (4) semantic-variant or nonfluent/agrammatic-variant PPA (see Chapter 9); or (5) "evidence for another concurrent, active neurological disease, or a nonneurological medical comorbidity or use of medication that could have a substantial effect on cognition." By definition, all patients who previously met criteria for "probable AD" by the 1984 NINCDS–ADRDA criteria still meet the 2011 NIA-AA criteria for probable AD dementia.

Probable Alzheimer's Disease Dementia With Increased Level of Certainty

This classification (see Table 16.6) can be assigned to individuals who meet the criteria for probable AD dementia and are either clearly declining (worsening) by history and testing (probable AD dementia with evidence of documented decline) or are known to carry a causative AD mutation.

Documented cognitive decline in patients with probable AD dementia increases the certainty that the condition represents an active, evolving pathologic process, but it does not specifically increase the certainty that the process is that of AD pathophysiology. However, in carriers of a causative AD mutation (APP, PSEN1, PSEN2) who meet criteria for probable AD dementia, the certainty that the condition is caused by AD pathology is increased. Carriage of the 3/4 allele of the apolipoprotein E gene, however, is not sufficiently specific to be considered in this category.

Possible Alzheimer's Disease Dementia

A diagnosis of possible AD dementia should be made if either the individual has an *atypical course* or an *etiologically mixed presentation*.

In patients with an atypical course the core clinical criteria in terms of the nature of the cognitive deficits for AD dementia are met, but either there has been a report of sudden onset of cognitive impairment or there is insufficient historical detail or objective cognitive documentation of progressive decline.

Patients with an etiologically mixed presentation meet all core clinical criteria for AD dementia but have evidence of (a) concomitant cerebrovascular disease, defined by a history of stroke temporally related to the onset or worsening of cognitive impairment; or the presence of multiple or extensive infarcts or severe white matter hyperintensity burden; or (b) features of dementia with Lewy bodies other than the dementia itself; or (c) evidence for another neurological disease or a nonneurological medical comorbidity or medication use that could have a substantial effect on cognition. Of note, a diagnosis of "possible AD" by the 1984 NINCDS-ADRDA criteria would not necessarily meet the 2011 NIA-AA criteria for possible AD dementia. Such a patient would need to be re-evaluated.

Probable Alzheimer's Disease Dementia With Evidence of the Alzheimer's Disease Pathophysiological Process

In individuals who meet the core clinical criteria for probable AD dementia, biomarker evidence consistent with an AD profile increases the probability that the basis of the

TABLE 16.6 Probable Alzheimer's Disease Dementia With Increased Level of Certainty

In persons who meet the core clinical **criteria for Probable AD dementia**
1. **Probable AD dementia with documented decline**
Can be diagnosed when there is *evidence of progressive cognitive decline* on subsequent evaluations based on:
   (i) Information from informants, and
   (ii) Cognitive testing in the context of either formal neuropsychological evaluation or standardized mental status examinations.
2. **Probable AD dementia in a carrier of a causative AD genetic mutation**
Can be diagnosed when there is *evidence of a causative genetic mutation* (in APP, PSEN1, or PSEN2).

clinical dementia syndrome is the AD pathophysiological process (see Chapters 17, 18, and 22). Currently, the major AD biomarkers can be broadly divided into two classes based on the biology that they measure: (1) biomarkers of brain amyloid-beta (Aβ) protein deposition that include low CSF A$β_{42}$ and positive amyloid-PET imaging; and (2) biomarkers of downstream neuronal degeneration or injury that include an AD CSF profile of elevated total tau and phosphorylated tau (p-tau); an AD FDG-PET profile of decreased uptake in temporal and parietal cortices; and disproportionate atrophy on structural magnetic resonance imaging in medial, basal, and lateral temporal lobes, and medial parietal cortices.

However, due to lack of widespread standardization, availability, and longitudinal data, the use of AD biomarker tests for routine clinical diagnostic purposes is not currently recommended. Their use to enhance certainty of AD pathophysiological process has been deemed as potentially useful in three circumstances: investigational studies, clinical trials, and as *optional clinical tools* for use where available and when deemed appropriate by the clinician (McKhann et al., 2011). Based on the results of AD biomarker tests that can fall into three categories: clearly positive, clearly negative, and indeterminate.

Table 16.7 from McKhann et al. (2011) provides operational classifications (lowest, intermediate, high, uninformative) for the utility and probability that the underlying dementing process is due to AD pathophysiology.

Pathophysiologically Proven Alzheimer's Disease Dementia

The diagnosis of pathophysiologically proven AD dementia applies if the individual meets the clinical and cognitive criteria for AD dementia, and the neuropathological examination, using widely accepted criteria, demonstrates the presence of the AD pathology (Hyman & Trojanowski, 1997; Hyman et al., 2012).

Dementia Unlikely to be Due to Alzheimer's Disease

The individual does not meet clinical criteria for AD dementia *or* (1) regardless of meeting clinical criteria for probable or possible AD dementia, there is sufficient evidence for an

TABLE 16.7 Alzheimer's Disease Dementia Criteria Incorporating Biomarkers

Diagnostic Category	Biomarker Probability of AD Etiology	Aβ (PET or CSF)	Neuronal injury (CSF tau, FDG-PET, structural MRI)
Probable AD dementia			
Based on clinical criteria	Uninformative	Unavailable, conflicting, or indeterminate	Unavailable, conflicting, or indeterminate
With three levels of evidence of AD	Intermediate	Unavailable or indeterminate	Positive
	Intermediate	Positive	Unavailable or indeterminate
Pathophysiological process	High	Positive	Positive
Possible AD dementia (atypical clinical presentation)			
Based on clinical criteria	Uninformative	Unavailable, conflicting, or indeterminate	Unavailable, conflicting, or indeterminate
With evidence of AD pathophysiological process	High but does not rule out second etiology	Positive	Positive
Dementia-unlikely due to AD	Lowest	Negative	Negative

Aβ, amyloid-beta; AD, Alzheimer's disease; CSF, cerebrospinal fluid; FDG, [18]fluorocleoxyglucose; MRI, magnetic resonance imaging; PET, positron emission tomography.

Source: From McKhann et al. (2011).

alternative diagnosis such as HIV dementia, dementia of Huntington's disease, or others that rarely, if ever, overlap with AD; or (2) regardless of meeting clinical criteria for possible AD dementia, both β-amyloid and neuronal injury biomarkers consistent with AD biology are negative.

Evaluation of Alzheimer's Disease: History, Cognitive Testing, and Laboratory and Imaging Studies

In the absence of a request for an evaluation of cognitive change or dementia, clinicians need to have a high index of suspicion for cognitive, functional, or behavioral changes and dementia warning signs in older patients. Diminished cognitive capacity can seriously affect the ability of patients to manage their medications and follow medical recommendations. As detailed previously, there are no specific laboratory or imaging studies that, in isolation or combination, definitively rule-in the diagnosis of AD dementia; the AD dementia diagnoses require the presence of a clinical dementia syndrome that is consistent by history and clinical (cognitive, functional, and behavioral) profile with an AD presentation, which can be further supported by an AD biological profile, but that is not excluded by substantial evidence to support presence of another neurological, psychiatric, or medical condition that can account or contribute to the cognitive and behavioral deficits.

Unrecognized cognitive impairments affect patient health and safety, and clinicians may contribute to poor patient outcomes by violating "primum non-nocere" ("above all do no harm") when we form wrong impressions and plans based on unreliable information from a patient who may be forgetful or has unrecognized diminished cognitive capacity. In older patients with escalating decompensation of otherwise well-managed and stable chronic medical condition, such as diabetes, hypertension, congestive heart failure; new onset sleep, confusion, delirium (in the context of medical illness, medications or surgery), weight-loss, failure to thrive, anxiety, social withdrawal, apathy, depressive and behavioral symptoms (e.g., agitation, personality changes, hoarding, delusions); and symptoms of presyncope, syncope, TIA or chronic dizziness, unsteadiness, and falls that are of unclear etiology or thought to be related to medications or dehydration, subclinical cognitive impairment or dementia should be considered high in the differential diagnosis as a potential major contributing cause that warrants further investigation.

For details of history and cognitive testing, please refer to Chapter 19 on the screening clinical mental status examination and Chapter 20 on neuropsychological evaluation. For further details of studies in AD, please refer to Chapter 22.

History should be obtained from the individual as well as knowledgeable and reliable collateral informant. In addition to cognitive symptoms and dementia warning signs, history should also include an assessment of current and previous level of function and activities of daily living in the home and the community; changes in social interactions, personality, or behavior; and heightening of premorbid personality traits (e.g., hoarding—"she always had a hard time throwing things away but now her whole house is overflowing with junk"; irritability, agitation, or aggression—"he always had a short fuse and a temper, but it's much worse recently—very small things can set him off"). Qualitative and quantitative assessment of cognition, function, and behavior should be flexibly individualized with the consideration of the individual's level of education and likely intelligence, previous level of function and accomplishments, primary language, and ethnic and cultural considerations.

History of Present Illness

In obtaining history, it is important to assess both the initial presenting symptoms as well as the most salient symptoms, complaints, and problems, and how they have progressed. These questions include the following: (1) When was the last time the patient's thinking was "normal"? (2) In retrospect, what was the first major change that was noticed? (3) What is now the most prominent symptom or change? (4) What is the most bothersome symptom, problem or behavior? and (5) How have these symptoms progressed? It is important to delineate both the course (e.g., generally linear decline versus clearly stepwise decline) and the pace (e.g., very slow initially but more rapid in the last

6 months) of the progression of symptoms and problems, including any major fluctuations or full or partial recovery. Other important questions include whether there are any (1) major fluctuations in symptoms on a day-to-day (or hour-to-hour) basis; (2) unusual associated features (e.g., falls, focal weakness, tremor, myoclonus, episodes of unresponsiveness, changes in speech or handwriting, major personality changes, food cravings, or odd behaviors); and (3) temporal associations with symptoms onset or worsening (e.g., a stepwise decline after a major illness or surgery; happening mostly at night or when the patient is tired). For example, regarding the onset and pace of progression, rapid onset and deterioration (hours and days) is most consistent with an overlying encephalopathy/delirium, whereas a more subacute onset and progression (over weeks and months) may be more indicative of an overlying indolent or chronic infection, metabolic disorder, mass lesion, medication side effect, sequelae of vascular insults and infarcts, or hydrocephalus; all these may be overlying and decompensating a subclinical cognitive vulnerability in individuals with undetected cognitive impairment or dementia.

Purely neurodegenerative causes of dementia have an insidious onset and slow progression over many months and years but can be unmasked in the context of encephalopathy/delirium or other cognitive stressors.

Review of Cognitive, Functional, and Neuropsychiatric Domains

Ideally, there should be a comprehensive domain-by-domain review of cognitive systems, daily function, and neuropsychiatric symptoms and problem behaviors. Review of cognitive systems should include changes and problems with memory, orientation, language, attention, executive functions, judgment, reasoning, problem solving, visuospatial functions, and insight. Review of any changes to daily level of function should assess both instrumental ADLs (e.g., keeping appointments and checkbook; making payments and managing finances; shopping; handling money; engaging in hobbies; driving; commuting and traveling; preparing meals and cooking; using tools, electronics, and appliances; doing laundry; cleaning and housekeeping; making household repairs; and managing medications) and basic ADLs (e.g., dressing, eating, bathing, grooming, feeding, mobility, toileting, continence) that are related to changes in cognition and behaviors. A multi-domain review of the frequency and severity of any personality changes, neuropsychiatric symptoms, and problem behaviors should include false beliefs and delusions, hallucinations, apathy and indifference, anxiety, irritability and lability, dysphoria and depression, inappropriate elation or euphoria, agitation and aggression, disinhibition and impulsivity, aberrant or repetitive motor behaviors, disrupted sleep and aberrant nighttime behaviors, changes in eating habits and tastes, or aberrant oral intake. Distress in caregivers due to these changes and symptoms should also be formally quantified (see Chapters 19, 20, and 27, and the NPI questionnaire as an example of a suitable instrument) (Cummings et al., 1994).

Review of Systems

A thorough review of symptoms can be very informative regarding potential confounders and contributing causes to cognitive decompensation and unmasking of the AD clinical phenotype. It also plays an important role in excluding potential primary causes other than AD. Symptoms relating to chronic infection (e.g., Lyme disease, syphilis, HIV), malignancy, autoimmune and collagen-vascular disease (e.g., Lupus, Giant Cell Arthritis), and hormone and vitamin deficiency are particularly relevant to address. Neurological symptoms, including dysarthria, tremor, imbalance, poverty of movements, difficulty walking or shuffling gait, abnormal movements, stiffness, incoordination, numbness or dysesthesia, weakness, and dysphagia, can be helpful to alert the clinician to non-AD causes or contributing conditions (e.g., parkinsonian syndromes). It is highly recommended to always specifically ask about falls, balance, sleep, appetite, weight changes, incontinence, choking or coughing with food, and new or unusual visual problems and headaches.

Pertinent Past Medical History

This should include eliciting history regarding all potential cardiovascular and cerebrovascular risk factors such as transient ischemic attack (TIA) or stroke, hypertension, dyslipidemia, diabetes, arrhythmias, coronary artery or vascular disease, myocardial infarction, congestive heart failure, and related procedures, smoking, and snoring or obstructive sleep apnea. Other important past medical history items to be delineated are history of seizures or epilepsy, concussion or traumatic brain injury (including duration of loss of consciousness and any sequelae), meningoencephalitis, delirium/encephalopathy, immunosuppression, malignancy, hormonal disorders, thyroid disease or deficiency, vitamin deficiency (particularly vitamin B12 deficiency), severe lung disease, exposure to toxic substances (at work or environmentally), excessive alcohol use or alcoholism, substance abuse, clinical mood disorder, depression or anxiety, electroconvulsive therapy (ECT), or other neurological or psychiatric condition. It is also important to discuss developmental and school history and ask about any potential long-standing learning, attentional, or cognitive problems. For example, did the individual repeat a grade, receive extra academic support, or attend a special education program?

Medication and Supplement History

There should be special attention to medications that are included in the updated Beers Criteria that are potentially inappropriate in older individuals due to potential cognitive side effects (American Geriatric Societ [AGS], 2012). Particular attention should be paid to use of medications with strong anticholinergic effects (e.g., diphenhydramine, scopolamine, antimuscarinic agents used for urinary incontinence, antispasmodics, skeletal muscle relaxants, and tricyclic antidepressants, and some antipsychotics), benzodiazepines, sedative-hypnotics, and narcotics (see Table 16.8).

Educational, Work, and Social History

Years of formal education, educational and work history, performance, achievement, and the nature of occupation can inform the physician regarding past level of function and potential cognitive reserve, as well as serve as alerts regarding problem behaviors or cognitive and functional trends. Social history can also provide clues regarding interpersonal relationships and support networks.

Hobbies, Community Activities, and Health-Related Habits

These can inform the physician regarding past and current level of engagement, activity, and performance. Does the individual exercise regularly? What is the current level of alcohol intake (specifically quantify)? Has there been a history of past heavy drinking, alcohol problems, or drug use?

Family History

It is important to ask whether any family member (parents, siblings, children, aunts/uncles, cousins, etc.) has ever been diagnosed with (or is highly suspected to have had) Alzheimer's disease or suffered from dementia or "senility." Even if the answer is no, it is valuable to follow up by asking whether any such relative ever needed support for living when older due to changes in mental function or behavior, or whether any relative was placed in a nursing home and, if so, when and why. The ages of parents and siblings should be noted. For instance, if the patient's parents died at relatively younger ages (<65 years) of causes unrelated to dementia (e.g., cardiac, cancer), they would not have lived long enough to express the late-onset AD phenotype if they possessed the trait. Family history regarding other neurological and psychiatric diagnoses should also be sought. When a potentially affected relative is identified, the age of onset, nature and progression of symptoms, age at death, and pathological confirmation of a diagnosis should be noted.

Review of Safety and Well-Being

Are there any safety issues surrounding the patient's environment, insight, judgment, decision making, and behavior? This is an essential issue to address during the care plan; however, details of the patient's environment, daily routines, monitoring

TABLE 16.8 Medications to Avoid in Older Cognitively Impaired Individuals

Potentially Inappropriate Medications for Cognitively Impaired Older Adults (2012 Beers Criteria)

Anticholinergic		Other Mechanisms
Antihistamines • Brompheniramine • Carbinoxamine • Chlorpheniramine • Clemastine • Cyproheptadine • Dimenhydrinate • Diphenhydramine • Hydroxyzine • Loratadine • Meclizine	*Antiparkinson agents* • Benztropine • Trihexyphenidy *Skeletal muscle relaxants* • Carisoprodol • Cyclobenzaprine • Orphenadrine • Tizanidine	*Barbiturates* • Amobarbital • Butabarbital • Butalbital • Mephobarbital • Pentobarbital • Phenobarbital • Secobarbital *Nonbenzodiazepine hypnotics* • Eszopiclone • Zolpidem • Zaleplon *Chloral hydrate* *Meprobamate*
Antidepressants • Amitriptyline • Amoxapine • Clomipramine • Desipramine • Doxepin • Imipramine • Nortriptyline • Paroxetine • Protriptyline • Trimipramine	*Antipsychotics* • Chlorpromazine • Clozapine • Fluphenazine • Loxapine • Olanzapine • Perphenazine • Pimozide • Prochlorperazine • Promethazine • Thioridazine • Thiothixene • Trifluoperazine	*Benzodiazepines* *Short- and intermediate-acting:* • Alprazolam • Estazolam • Lorazepam • Oxazepam • Temazepam • Triazolam *Long-acting:* • Chlorazepate • Chlordiazepoxide • Chlordiazepoxide-amitriptyline • Clidinium-chlordiazepoxide • Clonazepam • Diazepam • Flurazepam • Quazepam
Antimuscarinics *(urinary incontinence)* • Darifenacin • Fesoterodine • Flavoxate • Oxybutynin • Solifenacin • Tolterodine • Trospium	*Antispasmodics* • Atropine products • Belladonna alkaloids • Dicyclomine • Homatropine • Hyoscyamine products • Loperamide • Propantheline • Scopolamine	

Source: Adapted from Beers Criteria (AGS, 2012).

and support systems, and access and use of machines and tools that may cause danger to self or others can be gathered during the initial evaluation. For example, it is very important to inquire about the details of driving, access to firearms, the use of the stove and power tools, and wandering.

Laboratory Studies

There are no laboratory studies that rule in the diagnosis of AD dementia—laboratory studies aid to exclude common comorbid conditions in older individuals that can contribute to cognitive impairment in susceptible individuals and can be treated. It is exceedingly rare for a hormonal or vitamin deficiency, or metabolic, infectious, autoimmune, toxic, neoplastic, or paraneoplastic condition to mimic the clinical phenotype of typical late-onset AD dementia. While many of these comorbid conditions can cause decompensation of cognitive and behavioral function in susceptible individuals with subclinical or unrecognized mild impairments or dementia, they are rarely the sole cause. A judicious and stepwise approach to screening labs that stresses more common and reversible conditions, along with prioritizing less invasive and more cost-effective tests, is suggested in evaluating individuals who present with a typical AD dementia profile. In individuals presenting with symptoms consistent with early-onset, highly atypical, or rapidly progressive dementia, a more comprehensive approach to laboratory evaluation should be pursued (also see Chapters 15 and 22), which includes assessment of spinal fluid and/or obtaining amyloid brain PET to confirm the AD profile of abnormalities (i.e., low CSF $A\beta_{42}$, high tau and phospho-tau with a amyloid-tau index [ATI] of less than 1.0; excessive and widespread binding of an amyloid PET agent in the brain) and exclusion of other less common dementing syndromes (e.g., Hashimoto's encephalopathy/SREAT).

A multitiered and individualized approach to laboratory screening in the evaluation of AD dementia is suggested here (see Table 16.9). It is reasonable to include most, if not all, Tier 1 labs to evaluate all individuals who present with dementia symptoms. These laboratory tests are widely available, low cost, and relatively high yield with respect to broadly screening for common abnormalities in older adults. For example, thyroid and vitamin B12 deficiency are common and can cause neurological, including cognitive, decompensation in susceptible individuals. Measurement of serum homocysteine levels can provide a functional/biochemical test of vitamin B12 deficiency that is inexpensive, and when elevated, and can support functional B12 deficiency even when serum B12 levels fall within the normal range; hyperhomocystenemia is also associated with vascular damage and cardio/cerebrovascular risk. Anemia, dehydration (suggested by BUN:Cr ratio of >20:1), hypo/hypernatremia, hypomagnesemia, hypercalcemia (and hypocalcemia), hypo/hyperglycemia, uremia, and hepatic dysfunction can also decompensate cognitive function. ESR and CRP can provide a very broad screen for systemic indolent or insidious inflammatory/autoimmune, infectious, and neoplastic processes (e.g., undetected lung, liver or colon cancer). Tier 2 labs are not suggested in all individuals, but they can be ordered, with a low-threshold for reason, initially or performed later based an individual's particular clinical and epidemiological profile, and findings on exam or past lab testing. For example, an individual living in an endemic area for Lyme disease who has a history of a tick bite (with or without a rash) or a patient found to have unexplained or previously undiagnosed distal symmetric neuropathy on exam (several of these labs can be then be informative depending on index of suspicion, including HgA1c, lead, Lyme, RPR, HIV, ANA, SPEP, and lipid profile).

Standard brain imaging, preferably brain MRI, should be obtained as part of the initial evaluation of dementia. Administration of a contrast agent is not routinely indicated; nor is additional Tier 3 or 4 blood tests and studies such as EEG and vascular brain imaging in most individuals with LoAD who have a typical AD profile and essentially normal elemental neurological examination and routine screening laboratories.

Biomarkers in Clinical Practice

Use of AD biomarkers is not recommended for routine use in clinical practice (Albert et al., 2011; Jack et al., 2011; McKhann et al., 2011; Sperling et al., 2011). For a review of CSF and neuroimaging biomarkers, including CSF measurements of $A\beta$, tau, and phospho-tau; FDG-PET; amyloid-PET; and structural volumetry, and their potential uses in different stages of the AD clinical spectrum, see Chapters 17, 18, and 22. In highly select situations, such as evaluation of early-onset, atypical, and/or rapidly progressive dementia, a dementia subspecialist may consider obtaining additional biomarker data to help determine etiology. Finding consistent AD biomarker patterns of abnormalities in CSF (low $A\beta_{42}$, high phospho-tau and tau with a relative amyloid-to-tau/p-tau index of <1.0), amyloid-PET (abnormal uptake of amyloid tracer), FDG-PET or SPECT (bilateral parietal and temporal hypometabolism in early/mild AD), and bi-hippocampal and cortical atrophy in other temporal and parietal regions on structural imaging (see Chapter 22) in an individual would be highly supportive that AD-related pathology may be primarily causative or contributory to his or her dementia syndrome.

TABLE 16.9 Multitiered Testing in Alzheimer's Disease (AD): A Suggested Tiered Approach to Laboratory and Ancillary Studies in the Evaluation of Alzheimer's Disease and Related Dementias

Tier	Type	What	When/Who	Why/Comments
1	Serum imaging	TSH, B12, homocysteine, CBC with differential, complete metabolic panel (including calcium, magnesium, liver function tests), ESR, CRP brain MRI without gadolinium (preferable) or noncontrast head CT	Always or often All individuals	A broad and relatively inexpensive lab screen Brain MRI (or CT). Assess for hippocampal and cortical atrophy consistent with AD; contributing infarcts, leukoaraiosis, and microhemmorhage; rule out hydrocephalus, mass lesions. Recommend most Tier 3 and 4 tests to be done by a specialist or in consultation with specialist TPO and TGA for Hashimoto's encephalopathy/ SREAT Assessment of early-onset AD should include CSF analysis for AD biomarkers (and/or brain amyloid-PET) and brain FDG-PET (or SPECT) scan to establish AD biological trait along with clinical phenotype See text above and Chapter 22 regarding role of genetic testing in dominant AD See Chapter 15 regarding comprehensive testing for rare or rapidly progressive dementia syndromes
2	Serum	Ammonia, lead, Lyme antibody, RPR, HIV, ANA, SPEP, methylmalonic acid (MMA), HgbA1c, lipid profile, folate, PT, PTT	Frequently or sometimes Individualize based on epidemiology, and profile of history, exam, or lab/studies	
3	Serum Urine CSF Imaging Other	*Thyroid peroxidase antibodies (TPO)*, antithyroglobulin antibodies (TGA)**, FTA-ABS, ACE, ANCA, viral antibody studies (hepatitis B/C, EBV, CMV) Urinalysis, urine culture, UPEP, Bence-Jones proteins *Cell count, glucose, total protein, AD CSF biomarker panel (AB-42, tau, phospho-tau) with calculation of Amyloid-Tau Index (ATI)*;* Lyme PCR; viral PCRs and cultures, VDRL, T. pallidum PCR; MR or CT angiogram of head and neck, carotid ultrasound, brain MRI with gadolinium or head CT with contrast, chest films, *brain FDG-PET (or SPECT) scan** EEG	Occasionally or sparingly Include some of these tests based on atypical clinical profile, early-onset*, or high index of clinical suspicion	
4	Serum Urine CSF Imaging Other	*AD mutation genetic panel*, APOE allele genotype**, paraneoplastic antibody panel, anti-voltage-gated potassium channel (VGKC) antibody, non-Lyme tick borne disease panel (Ehrlichiosis, Babesiosis, Anaplasmosis, Rickestsiosis, Powassan), copper and ceruloplasmin, tumor markers, rheumatological studies 24-hour urine collection for heavy metals, porphyria, and/or copper Protein 14-3-3, neuron-specific enolase (NSE), T. whipplei PCR, paraneoplastic antibody panel, anti-voltage-gated potassium channel (VGKC) antibody, cytology, flow cytommetry, other stains and cultures for infectious agents (bacterial, fungal, AFB) CT of chest/abdomen/pelvis, cerebral angiogram, *brain amyloid tracer-PET scan**, body PET scan Brain and/or meningeal vessels biopsy	Very sparingly or rarely Include based on index of suspicion in atypical cases or rapid progression	

*Consider in individuals with phenotype of early-onset AD and selected individuals with atypical AD presentation.

Cognitive Testing

Specific testing and standardized measures are discussed in detail in Chapter 19 on the mental status evaluation in clinical practice and in Chapter 20. Cognitive testing should be individually adapted with additional tests as needed and performance should be interpreted in the context of the individual's symptoms, history, demographics, and expected level of performance. As general screening instruments in AD, the MoCA and ACE-R, are both very practical, if time allows, both can be administered; if time is limited to about 10 minutes, then the MoCA is recommended. The BDS-IMC, along with the ACE-R, are both useful for tracking progression in AD dementia since they will accommodate performance across a broad range of AD stages, from mild all the way to severe; in contrast, performance on the MoCA reaches floor values in the moderate to severe stages of AD dementia.

Formal neuropsychological testing can be particularly useful (1) when the initial evaluation is borderline; (2) in patients with unusual clinical profiles; (3) to establish a comprehensive baseline, including percentile performance in each test and domain, and to detect and track longitudinal changes with good sensitivity; (4) to comprehensively clarify patterns of cognitive impairment; (5) in individuals with superior premorbid ability; (6) to help distinguish between depression and mood disorders versus dementia; (7) to help determine competency; (8) to assist in the determination of disability; (9) to delineate specific weaknesses and strengths; and (10) to provide individualized recommendations regarding effective compensatory strategies, safety, further evaluation, and care.

Management of Alzheimer's Disease Dementia

The optimal management of AD is dynamic, multifactorial, and multidisciplinary. An analogy to the legs of a stool can be made: All the legs (principles of care) are necessary to affect a functioning stool that can support the patient. Broadly speaking, the analogous important legs for AD management fall under the following categories (see Table 16.10): (1) early recognition and diagnosis of symptoms combined with a proactive care plan that is customized to the patient–caregiver dyad; (2) nonpharmacological interventions and behavioral approaches; (3) appropriate pharmacology; and (4) dynamically adjusting the care plan in a pragmatic manner according to changes in the patient–caregiver dyad's condition and resources that facilitates continued therapeutic alliance, adherence, and patient and caregiver health and safety. In this analogy, caregivers provide the glue that hold the therapeutic legs and stool together.

There is no cure for AD dementia; the current AD treatment paradigm is one of multifaceted management of symptoms and reduction of long-term clinical decline. Optimal AD management involves developing and sustaining a close therapeutic alliance within the context of caring for a patient–caregiver dyad that requires early diagnosis and multimodal care. This approach to AD management, first and foremost, involves individualized and nonpharmacological tailoring of approaches based on the patient–caregiver dyad's priorities, personal strengths, limitations, resources, and environment. A stage-appropriate pharmacological treatment plan can then be instituted based on this foundation. Long-term management of AD dementia is a dynamic process that requires proactive planning and flexibility to modify care plans according to changes in the condition and resources of the patient–caregiver dyad. Providing this multidisciplinary care provides measurable and meaningful short- and long-term benefits for patients, families, caregivers, and society.

Customizing Care to the Patient–Caregiver Dyad

Individualized tailoring of treatments and care customization should include psychoeducation; eliminating and ameliorating contributory factors (e.g., potentially harmful medications, comorbid medical conditions, treating anxiety and depression, optimizing sleep quality, simplifying routines and diminishing stress); fostering and shoring support systems; advocating for appropriate monitoring and supports to minimize health and safety risks to the patient, caregivers, and the public (e.g., monitoring or dispensing medications; home safety, driving); assisting

TABLE 16.10 Key Elements of Effective Multifactorial Management of Alzheimer's Disease: The Multilegged Approach to Effective Management of Individuals With Alzheimer's Disease Dementia Incorporates the Following Necessary Components

Individualization of Diagnosis and Care Plan
- Early detection, assessment, and staging (see Chapters 19, 20, and 22).
- Sustained targeting and tailoring of a proactive care plan to the patient and caregivers (see Chapters 19, 27, and 28).

Nonpharmacological Interventions and Behavioral Approaches
- Psychoeducation including regarding AD dementia in general and effects on cognition, function and behaviors, dementia care, expectations, "the progression and regression model of aging and dementia" (see Chapter 26).
- Behavioral approaches—both general and targeted to the patient–caregiver dyad; these include simplification of environment; establishing routines; providing a safe, calm, and consistent care environment; utilizing strategies such as interacting calmly, redirection to pleasurable activities and environment, reassurance, providing only necessary information in a manner that the patient can appreciate (i.e., in simple language and small chunks) and at the appropriate time; "benign therapeutic fibbing" and "Never saying No" to "allow the moment to pass" (see Chapter 26).
- Establishing and fostering support networks for the patient and caregivers (see Chapter 27).
- Identifying and monitoring health and safety risks for patient and others, advance planning for medical, legal, and financial decision making and needs (e.g., stove, weapon, and driving safety; falling prey to fraud or poor work or financial decision making) (see Chapter 28)
- Caring for caregivers, including caregiver support and respite care (see Chapter 27).

Appropriate Pharmacology
- Elimination of redundant and inappropriate medications—see Beers Criteria (Table 8)
- Treating underlying medical and psychiatric conditions that can exacerbate dementia symptoms (e.g., dehydration, pain, constipation, infections, electrolyte and metabolic derangements, anxiety, depression, psychosis) (see Chapters 24, 25, and 26)
- Prescription of stage-appropriate anti-AD medications; monotherapy or combination therapy with ChEI and memantine

Dynamic and Pragmatic Modifications to Sustain Alliance, Adherence, and Well-Being of Patient–Caregiver Dyad
- Flexibility to modify care plan according to important changes in the patient–caregiver dyad (see Chapter 27).
- Forging and sustaining a therapeutic alliance (see Chapter 27).
- Promoting the safety, health, and well-being of the caregivers, as well as the patient (see Chapter 27).
- Adopting a pragmatic approach to ongoing care that includes establishing and simplifying care routines where possible; modifying the environment to suit the patient–caregiver dyad; and consideration of patient and caregiver preferences, capacity, environment, and resources in devising and implementing care plans (see Chapter 26).
- Seeking, when possible, to find humor, enjoyment, and positive meaning during the dementia journey.

in identification and planning for current and future personal, psychological, medical, and legal needs; optimizing behavioral approaches and strategies to care; instituting stage-appropriate nonpharmacological interventions and pharmacological treatments; and promoting a healthy lifestyle for both the patient and caregivers. A successful long-term pharmacotherapy plan with anti-AD medications, principally involving combination treatment with a ChEI and memantine, requires sustaining a solid foundation of psychoeducation, use of behavioral care strategies, and maintaining clarity in treatment goals, expectations, and a strong therapeutic alliance between the clinician the patient–caregiver dyad.

Long-Term Treatment Expectations: Slowing Decline

The current AD treatment paradigm is to reduce progression of symptoms and disability. Despite ongoing efforts, a cure for AD dementia appears to still be far away (see Chapter 23). In contrast to the other leading medical causes of mortality in the United States, AD therapeutic research has taken place mostly for a few decades under drastically underfunded conditions. Nonpharmacological management and pharmacological therapies for AD dementia seek to minimize the disabling effects of cognitive and functional decline and emergence of problem symptoms. Alone, and particularly in combination, the only FDA-approved anti-AD pharmacotherapies, the ChEI's donepezil, galantamine, and rivastigmine, and the NMDA antagonist memantine, can reduce progression of clinical symptoms and disability. From a public health and economics perspective, therapies that minimize caregiver burden and delay nursing home entry can translate into significant benefits related to worker productivity and health care savings (Cappell et al., 2010; Weycker et al., 2007).

Nonpharmacological Interventions and Behavioral Coping Strategies

Nonpharmacological interventions and behavioral strategies should be used as the first-line option to ameliorate neuropsychiatric symptoms (e.g., agitation, apathy, delusions, disinhibition) and problem behaviors (e.g., resistance to care, caregiver shadowing, hoarding, obsessive-compulsive behaviors) in AD dementia. These problems are not only distressing to patients and caregivers but also, left untreated, their chronic effects can exact a devastating toll and lead to poor outcomes for patients and caregivers (Kales, Chen, Blow, Welsh, & Mellow, 2005; Okura et al., 2012). At least 85%–90% of patients will experience significant neuropsychiatric symptoms and problem behaviors during the course of their illness (see Chapters 24, 25, and 26).

Neuropsychiatric symptoms and problem behaviors such as resistance to care; repetitive statements and questions; caregiver shadowing and separation anxiety; irritability, agitation, and aggressiveness; argumentativeness; loss of inhibition; insensitive comments and socially inappropriate behaviors; sexualized inappropriate behaviors; using poor language and manners; utilization behavior and hoarding; inappropriate or messy urination, defecation, and cleaning; pacing and wandering; sleep-wake disturbances; paranoid delusions of theft, infidelity, and harm; spells of crying or inappropriate joviality and laughing; severe indifference and amotivation; hyperorality; poor eating or hyperphagia; repetitive motor or verbal behaviors, vocalizations, or shouting; obsessive-compulsive behaviors; hallucinations and psychosis can be variably experienced at various times, degrees, and durations in individuals with AD. Left untreated, they will lead to severe distress and negatively impact the health and well-being of patients and caregivers. Problem behaviors and neuropsychiatric symptoms (also known as noncognitive behavioral symptoms [NCBS]; behavioral and psychological symptoms of dementia [BPSD]) are associated with more rapid decline, earlier institutionalization, higher distress, worse quality of life, and greater health care utilization and costs (Kales et al., 2005; Okura et al., 2012). Treatment of BPSD using pharmacology alone has low treatment benefit effect sizes (Cohen's d of 0.2 or less) and, in some cases (e.g., antipsychotics) is associated with substantial side effects and short- and long-term risks for morbidity and mortality (see Chapters 24, 25, and 26).

Early and ongoing BPSD screening, root-cause analysis, intervention, monitoring, and care plan modification are important components of comprehensive AD dementia care; they can facilitate prevention and treatment efficacy by eliminating triggers and directing treatments to the root cause, not just at the symptoms. Adopting this kind of comprehensive approach to BPSD care decreases the likelihood of BPSD emergence, frequency, severity, and treatment failure. Unfortunately, rates of screening for BPSD in primary care are low and, even when clinically identified, individuals often receive inappropriate, ineffective, temporary, and fragmented care. However, often in a crisis, clinicians are called upon by caregivers and colleagues to acutely treat severe BPSD, including problems that are not only severely distressful but can also place the patient or others at risk of substantial harm. When identified, BPSD should be characterized, a thorough investigation of the underlying causes undertaken (root-cause analysis), and an individualized care and monitoring plan implemented.

Nonpharmacological interventions and behavioral strategies for BPSD may include a general approach such as caregiver psychoeducation and training in dementia-specific approaches to trigger avoidance, problem solving, communication, environment modification, and task simplification; patient engagement and activities; and more targeted and individually tailored approaches in which precipitating conditions of a specific behavior (triggers for a specific BPSDs) are identified, modified, and continually assessed.

Appreciating That the Disease Is Responsible, Not the Patient

Psychoeducation for caregivers should include general models to better understand the biopsychosocial substrates behind the emergence of BPSD in AD (e.g., loss of behavioral and coping reserve, compromise of "top-down" control from frontostriatal networks, regression to childhood capacities and behaviors in a progression-regression model of dementia), and strategies to better communicate, manage, and care for the patient.

It is important for the caregivers to have time to grieve and, over time, come to a resolution that their loved one has changed and is demented. It is also vital for caregivers to come to appreciate that overall "poor" and problem behaviors by the demented individual are not because the patient is being intentionally mean, ornery, or vindictive, but are due to the disease and diminished capacities. This is no one's fault—it is just part of the illness. It is also critical for caregivers to hear from clinicians that their feelings of guilt, loss, anger, and sadness are expected, normal, and are very common experiences and responses under the difficult circumstances of caregiving for a loved one with AD. Not taking the behaviors "personally" and finding a supportive environment to share these feelings is an integral part of being able to successfully cope with the long-term burdens and to find meaning in caregiving.

Facilitating the Moment to Pass

Several general behavioral strategies that can be helpful, and which leverage the fact that patients with severe memory impairment often "live in the moment," relate to helping to "keep the patient comfortable while getting her/him unstuck and allowing the moment to pass." These include utilizing strategies such as always trying to interact calmly with the patient while redirecting their attention (also known as distracting) to a pleasurable activity, and remaining reassuring. Avoidance of confrontation by not contradicting and arguing with the patient and utilizing the "never saying no" and "therapeutic fibbing" approaches can also be helpful. For example, if the patient is confused and wants to go home to see her dead spouse, not realizing at that moment that she is in her own home and that her husband has been deceased for years, it may be better to allow the moment to pass by acknowledging the request and responding in a calm and reassuring manner while redirecting her by saying something like: "I'd like to go and see dad too, let's go make an apple pie to take to him—it's his favorite, but first let's get a yummy snack and something to drink so we can have some energy to do all this; meanwhile, why don't you tell me about the first time you and dad went to the vineyard. . ." It's not always what we say to the patient, it's also how we say it—the patient will often respond to the emotional content and expression of the interaction and not always what is explicitly stated. It takes resourcefulness and emotional reserve to remain calm and be able to skillfully negotiate such interactions.

Providing Only Necessary Information in the Appropriate Way and Time: The "Presenting Small Digestible Chunks Only When Ready to Eat" Approach

It can be a difficult and lengthy process for family and caregivers to learn and adjust to the new dynamics necessary to interact and to care for the patient with dementia. Decade-long interpersonal patterns of communication, behavior, and roles will need to be adjusted as the patient with dementia progresses and has increasingly diminished capacity to remember, reason, and react. Maternal and paternal, caregiving, and familial leadership roles are reversed or changed, and the process of discussing, making, and implementing small and large daily and long-term life plans and decisions needs to be altered. Based on the patient's capacities, sometimes decisions have to be made de facto and plans implemented without communicating with the patient and allowing him or her to fully participate in the manner that had been the norm. This is a delicate balance that has to be achieved on a moving target. Doing so does not imply, and should not be interpreted as, disrespect or dishonesty. The process should be driven by appreciating the patient's diminished capacity and driven by "doing no harm"/nonmaleficence and benevolence; these trump autonomy when the patient's diminished capacity poses a significant risk of distress and harm for self and others.

Engaging in an open process of communication, planning, decision making, and implementation that relies on the patient's previous abilities to reason and appreciate consequences, have insight and foresight, to make good judgments and decisions, to relate associations and remember facts, and to correctly execute decisions and wants can be frustrating, distressing, and dangerous at times. For example, at different stages relying on the patient to be responsible or to monitor her or his own medications, investments, driving, guns, power tools, transportation, and meals, even when the patient emphatically expresses the desire for it, can be risky and lead to catastrophe (see Chapter 28).

A kind, respectful, and yet pragmatic approach to communication and shared decision making has to be adapted to the patient's capacities and may necessitate simplifying information and language, providing information piecemeal and at the appropriate time, and sometimes a degree of "maternalism and paternalism." For example, in the patient with advanced dementia who still insists on driving despite multiple attempts and conversations to bring him or her to appreciate their clearly diminished capacity and very high risk, a pragmatic approach of removing the car and allowing the moment to pass by addressing the immediate need for transportation but stating that the car is "still in the shop under repair" can allow time for adjustment by the patient and for progression of illness to serve as a solution. It is also very common for older patients with dementia to develop significant anticipatory anxiety in the face of even minor changes of routine and impending activities, travel, and appointments. This anxiety can, in many patients, serve to significantly decompensate the patient's diminished capacities and be very distressful. For example, telling some forgetful patients that they have a doctor's appointment in 2 days or that they are going to travel on the weekend can be highly distressing, even when it is a potentially pleasurable activity or appointment. The patient may experience anticipatory anxiety, or, even when the patient forgets the exact reason (e.g., appointment or travel), she or he may continue to experience underlying fear or worry that she or he may have forgotten something, is not prepared, or that something bad is going to happen. For some patients it is better to wait until the last moment to get them ready and to inform them that "we have to go out now."

An approach of providing information and requests in short and easy-to-understand phrases (i.e., "easily digestible chunks") and simple step-by-step commands, and only at the time when the individual with AD is ready and absolutely needs to know this information (i.e., "is prepared or needs to eat") can be very pragmatic and appropriate, particularly as the individual progresses to the moderate stages of AD dementia and experiences greater difficulty with receptive language, understanding, reasoning, planning, making decisions, insight, judgment, and anticipatory anxiety.

Environmental Modification, Establishing Simple Routines, and Maintaining Consistency

Modifying the patient's environment to suit the needs and capacities of the individual patient is also very important. In general, it is best to create a calm, simple, and soothing environment that feels secure and "familiar" to the patient (e.g., old pictures, a favorite comfy chair or couch, some memorabilia, soft favorite or music from their childhood or early adulthood playing), is quiet, and is not overstimulating and full of distractions (e.g., not cold, crowded, noisy, or too bright). Having the TV playing in the background all the time may not only be overstimulating but may also, at times, serve as a BPSD trigger for aggressive or inappropriately sexualized behaviors (see Chapter 25). Occasionally, patients may develop attachments and be soothed by "security objects," akin to the security blanket or a favorite stuffed animal that can provide comfort and security to young children.

Together with environmental modification comes simplification and establishing routines. For example, providing finger foods when the individual has difficulty using utensils properly; establishing a bedtime routine; providing pants with elastic waist bands without buttons or zippers, and shoes with Velcro fasteners instead of laces; allowing a patient who is apt to pace and wander to do so in an appropriately safe and enclosed space; using door locks that the individual cannot open; and disguising doors or mirrors with curtains. An environment that is too cluttered and routines that are too complex and taxing can be very stressful and fatiguing for patients with diminished capacity. Going at a reduced psychomotor pace that suits the capabilities of the patient (e.g., not talking too quickly, giving multistep commands, or rushing the patient while dressing), and allowing the patient to rest adequately between stimulating events are important factors to avoid triggering BPSD. Individuals come to rely on routine and often find comfort in an environment that is consistent. Therefore, abrupt changes in environment, caregivers, and routines, even if relatively small from an outsider's perspective, may have great potential to be very confusing, disruptive, and anxiety provoking to individuals with AD dementia.

Experiencing Humor, Meaning, and Serenity in Facing, Caregiving, and Treating Dementia

Finally, last but not least, as much as possible, trying to maintain a sense of humor, and finding meaning and experiencing some enjoyment and serenity in caregiving and facing and treating dementia can serve as high-level coping strategies that can be useful, fun, and healthy. For patients, caregivers, and clinicians, warm smiles and laughter can have powerful diffusing and therapeutic effects. Occasionally, odd and absurd statements, behaviors, and circumstances that patients and caregivers face can be, with the right perspective, fodder for a quick and hearty laugh; seen from another perspective, the same behaviors and circumstances can instead be very discouraging and depressing. When given lemons, it's okay, and therapeutic, for caregivers to sometimes make their own lemonade.

As difficult as the caregiving experience can be for many individuals, it does not have to be viewed and experienced negatively throughout; it can be a rewarding, fulfilling, and meaningful experience. To provide care for a loved one can be satisfying and purposeful in several ways. It can be viewed and experienced as an opportunity to fulfill a duty and give back; to have positive feelings about the good quality of care, love, and kindness being provided; embraced for the new dynamic and relationships being forged; and for serving as a positive role model for others in the family and community. Caregiving can also lead to experiencing higher respect from others and to greater self-actualization, self-esteem, and sense of purpose for the caregiver.

Learning to appreciate the deep meanings in the serenity prayer can be particularly useful for patients, caregivers, and clinicians alike when facing, caring, and treating dementia. The serenity prayer states: "May I be granted the serenity to accept the things I cannot change; the courage to change the things I can; and the wisdom to know the difference." Though the caregiving journey is often arduous and challenging, it can also be a positive force for finding some serenity, personal rewards, and blessings. This can come with the appreciation that one is trying to do the right thing and one's best under difficult circumstances, though no one can achieve this 100% of the time, and the acknowledgment that this work is hard, that there is no formula or optimal solution to provide care, and that one cannot restore or prevent decline in dementia, but that one can still positively affect the process of care and the experience for the patient and oneself. Peace and personal rewards for caregivers can also come with the greater sense of meaning that can be experienced by performing unheralded service, "doing good," and becoming an instrument of kindness, compassion, and care that makes a difference in the path and experiences of the patient with dementia, even if they do not alter the destruction and destination.

Pharmacological Management

Eliminating Deleterious Medications

The initial step in the pharmacologic management of AD consists of eliminating redundant and potentially deleterious medications. For example, diphenhydramine, often taken as an over-the-counter drug combination with acetaminophen for sleep and pain relief, and many medications prescribed for anxiety (e.g., benzodiazipines), urinary incontinence (e.g., those with high anticholinergic activity), and sleep are listed as medications to be avoided in the elderly. Such medications, according to the Beers Criteria, are generally contraindicated in the elderly, require close scrutiny, and can be particularly deleterious in cognitively vulnerable older persons (AGS, 2012; Rudolph et al., 2008) (see Table 16.8).

Identification and Treatment of Comorbid Conditions That Decompensate Dementia

The weakest link shows itself first; similarly, systemic conditions can affect cognitive and functional compensatory mechanisms in the brain of individuals with dementia. Treating these conditions can affect better cognition, function, and behavior in patients with AD dementia. A striking example of a common clinical scenario is an elderly individual (with or without a known diagnosis of cognitive impairment or dementia) who is brought to the emergency department for confusion, lethargy, and change in mental status and found to have a urinary tract infection (UTI) or pneumonia. In this scenario, the weakest link, the patient's cognitive reserve, has become decompensated, manifesting in worsening cognitive impairments clouded by delirium (also known as encephalopathy) (Fong et al., 2012; Rudolph et al., 2008, 2010). In many undiagnosed individuals, this is often indicative of a failed stress test that has unmasked an underlying true subclinical or undiagnosed cognitive impairment or dementia. In patients with known dementia, this is often a trigger for rapid deterioration in cognition, function, and BPSD. In many conditions, the symptoms and signs of decompensation are more subtle and chronic. Screening studies, particularly Tier 1 and Tier 2 studies discussed previously, can identify many common conditions that exacerbate dementia symptoms. These include dehydration, electrolyte and metabolic derangements, anemia, cardiac or cerebral ischemia, hypoxia, thyroid and vitamin deficiencies (e.g., vitamin B_{12} deficiency), as well as infections (e.g., urinary tract infections, pneumonia). Other conditions such as pain, for example from arthritis, constipation, hunger, thirst, and fatigue, are also very common in patients with AD dementia, and, particularly in later stages when patients cannot appropriately recognize or communicate their symptoms, can lead to BPSD, particularly anxiety, irritability, agitation, aggression, and sleep-wake disturbances. Depression, anxiety, and sleep problems should also be identified and appropriately treated. When necessary, cautious and judicious use of other, non-anti-AD medications can nonetheless significantly contribute to the comprehensive AD therapeutic plan.

Antipsychotics: Use With Extreme Caution and Only in Particular Circumstances

Another class of medications to be used with extreme caution, with ongoing monitoring, and only under strict circumstances, are antipsychotics (also known as neuroleptics) (see Chapter 24). Though antipsychotics are commonly used in an off-label manner in clinical practice in the United States, they carry an FDA black-box warning for use in dementia. Short- and long-term antipsychotic use in patients with dementia is associated with substantial risk of cognitive decline, morbidity (e.g., parkinsonism, falls, pneumonia, cardio- and cerebrovascular events), and mortality; they should be used as a last resort for severe refractory behavioral disturbances without an identifiable and treatable cause (e.g., severe aggression and agitation not due to delirium, pain, or infection) or when a serious risk of immediate harm or safety exists that cannot be otherwise ameliorated. The antipsychotic risperidone is approved in Europe by the EMA for short-term, 12-week use in dementia when there is refractory severe agitation or psychosis. Antipsychotics should optimally only be prescribed after a careful evaluation by a dementia care specialist and with the consent of caregivers; their cautious use in this manner should be limited to the lowest effective dosages for short durations. The continued use of antipsychotics requires ongoing monitoring, assessment of risk-benefit, and understanding and consent from the family regarding the goals of treatment and the potential clinical trade-offs.

Antidementia Medications: Cholinesterase Inhibitors and Memantine

Cholinesterase inhibitors (ChEIs) (donepezil, galantamine, rivastigmine) and the NMDA antagonist memantine are the only FDA-approved treatments for AD dementia; they have complementary mechanisms of action, potentially additive effects, and demonstrate good tolerability and safety profiles. A pharmacological foundation of anti-AD therapies, whether with ChEI or memantine monotherapy or, ultimately, combined together as combination therapy, most often as memantine added on to stable ChEI therapy, have demonstrated benefits in the short- and long-term to reduce decline in cognition and function, retard the emergence and impact of neuropsychiatric symptoms, and to delay nursing home placement without prolongation of time to death (Rountree et al., 2012). Viewed from the social perspective, anti-AD pharmacotherapy (donepezil, memantine, galantamine, rivastigmine) can reduce the economic burden of the illness, even in later stages of illness (Cappell et al., 2010).

Short-term responses to AD medication treatments vary greatly between individuals. Aggregate data suggests that during the initial 6–12 months of treatment, performance on measures of cognition, ADL, behavioral symptoms, or global clinical impression of change may significantly improve in a minority (10%–20%), plateau in nearly half (30%–50%), or continue to deteriorate in about a third (20%–40%) of treated patients. Some estimate higher benefits compared to placebo treatment with ChEI treatment: a four-point improvement on the ADAS-Cog (roughly equivalent to reversing six months of naturalistic decline) in 25%–30% of ChEI-treated patients compared to 15%–25% of placebo treated patients, and a seven-point improvement (roughly equivalent to reversing 12 months of naturalistic decline) in 12%–20% versus 2%–6% for ChEI- versus placebo-treated patients, respectively (Cummings, 2004). Estimates for number-needed-to-treat (NNT) in patients with AD dementia to achieve stabilization or improvement in one or more clinical domains (e.g., cognition, function, behavior, global severity) range from 5 to 9:1 for monotherapy with ChEI or memantine, and combination therapy with both (Atri, 2011; Bullock, 2006 ; Livingston & Katona, 2004). Estimates for the number-needed-to-treat (NNT) to achieve significant improvement on multiple domains simultaneously are approximately 8:1 for combination therapy in moderate to severe AD. In contrast, marked clinical worsening, defined by simultaneous significant worsening on multiple domains is also reduced by 48%–68% in patients on ChEI-memantine combination therapy compared to ChEI alone (Atri et al., 2008). There is no evidence to support that patients who do not show significant improvement or stabilization on treatment in the first few months after starting anti-AD treatment will not derive benefit from therapy in the longer run and should therefore be taken off pharmacological treatment due to presumed "nonresponse." To the contrary, discontinuation of pharmacological treatment has been shown, on aggregate, to be harmful—patients taken off or those who are impersistent in taking anti-AD medications appear to progress more rapidly than patients who continue treatments, particularly ChEIs. Therefore, clinicians should not discontinue anti-AD medications for a trial of "let's see if there is worsening" since even temporary periods of discontinuation have been associated with irreversible declines (Courtney et al., 2004; Doody et al., 2001; Farlow, Anand, Messina, Hartman, & Veach, 2000; Howard et al., 2012; Raskind, Peskind, Wessel, & Yuan, 2000).

Yet, with disease progression, patients who may initially show improvement or stability will eventually decline over years. With sustained pharmacological treatments, the care plan for individual patients should be evidence based but also customized to include patient–caregiver dyad goals, preferences, and circumstances. On aggregate, sustained treatments provide a modest expectation of overall stabilization in the short term and reduction in the rate of clinical decline in the long term. However, even a modest slowing of clinical progression provides a meaningful goal in the treatment of AD dementia. Pharmacological treatments best facilitate potentially maintaining and subsequently reducing decline in abilities and behavior when instituted appropriately early, before further abilities are lost, and when sustained until later stages of illness. In AD dementia, once an ability is lost it is very difficult to regain, and once a problem behavioral pattern is established it is hard to eliminate or suppress indefinitely. The anti-AD medications are best thought of as chronic, albeit modest, supportive crutches or "lids on boiling pots"; acute and high potency treatments and cures they are not—unfortunately, the pot will ultimately boil over in the long term. It is therefore important for clinicians to effectively communicate the practical issues associated with pharmacologic treatment that include its rationale and the expectations for treatment outcomes.

What to expect, when to start and stop pharmacological therapy, and how to monitor progression and medication side effects are all crucial questions for patients, families, caregivers, and treating clinicians to discuss openly. For clinicians, an appropriate perspective about AD outcomes and treatment expectations is especially important to guide stage-appropriate individualized care. To maximize treatment adherence and benefits, it is crucial to effectively communicate that the current treatment and disease course paradigm in AD includes progression of symptoms, long-term global decline in function, accumulation of disability, and a loss of independence in late-stage disease. In the long run, our current treatments of AD dementia mitigate decline but do not prevent it.

Cholinesterase Inhibitors

Cholinesterase inhibitors developed for the treatment of AD dementia were produced a result of rational drug design. ChEIs facilitate central cholinergic activity by reducing the physiological breakdown of ACh by the enzyme acetylcholinesterase (AChE) in the synaptic cleft. Inhibition of AChE by ChEIs thus enhances cholinergic neurotransmission.

Acetylcholine and Cholinesterase Inhibitor Mechanism of Action in Alzheimer's Disease

The central nervous system (CNS) functions of acetylcholine (ACh) include modulation of sleep, wakefulness, learning, and memory; suppression of pain at the spinal cord level; and essential roles in neural plasticity, early neural development, immunosuppression, and epilepsy (Atri, 2011). As an important modulatory neurotransmitter whose role in the neocortex includes arousal (Jones, 2005), attention (Himmelheber, Sarter, & Bruno, 2000), as well as learning and memory (Atri et al., 2004; Hasselmo, 2006), the cholinergic hypothesis regarding AD posits that patients with AD have a central ACh (cholinergic) deficit with resultant reduction in cholinergic neurotransmission. Low levels of choline acetyltransferase (ChAT), an enzyme that catalyzes the synthesis of ACh, in the brain is believed to be at least partially responsible for a decreased synthesis of ACh in cholinergic neurons affected by AD pathology. Lower levels of ACh, in, turn affect reduced cholinergic neurotransmission and hence contribute to inefficient and disordered memory and cognitive processing, and abnormal function and behavior in AD.

Through early observations that cholinergic blockade with scopolamine impairs episodic memory function (see Atri et al., 2004 for a review), and that ChEIs such as physostigmine can reverse these impairments (but have strong peripheral nervous system side effects including nausea and vomiting), centrally acting ChEIs were specifically developed as anti-AD medications to inhibit acetylcholinesterase by more selectively delaying the breakdown of ACh in cholinergic synapses in the CNS. With the introduction of tacrine in 1993, ChEIs were the first drug class approved for the treatment of AD. The current generation of anti-AD ChEIs in routine use includes donepezil, rivastigmine, and galantamine (see Table 16.11).

Pharmacokinetics and Characteristics

Although there are mechanistic and pharmacokinetic differences among the available ChEI drugs (see Table 16.11), there are no quality data to support that there are significant differences between them with respect to aggregate efficacy in AD dementia. An oral formulation of all three ChEIs is now generically available in the United States. Donpezil and rivastigmine have approved FDA-label indications in mild, moderate, and severe AD dementia; galantamine has an FDA-approved indication for mild and moderate AD. Donepezil (introduced in 1997) remains the most frequently prescribed ChEI in the United States (~70% of prescriptions). Rivastigmine

TABLE 16.11 Pharmacokinetic and Mechanistic Characteristics of the Anti-Alzheimer's Disease Dementia Cholinesterase Inhibitors

Drug	Half-life (h)	Bioavailability (%)	T_{max} (h)	Hepatic Metabolism	Absorption Affected by Food	Reversible Inhibition of AChE	Other Cholinomimetic Effects
Donepezil	60–90	100	3–5	Yes	No	Yes	--
Rivastigmine	1.5–2*	40	0.8–1.8	No	Yes	No**	BuChEI
Rivastigmine Patch	3.4*	55-65	8–12	No	No	No**	BuChEI
Galantamine	5–8	85–100	0.5–1.5	Yes	Yes	Yes	nAChR agonist
Galantamine ER	25–35	85–100	4.5–5	Yes	Yes	Yes	nAChR agonist

*Rivastigmine has plasma half-life of 2–3.4 hours but a duration of action for AChE inactivation of 9 hours.
** Rivastigmine is a "pseudo-irreversible" inhibitor of AChE and BuChE.

AChE, acetylcholinesterase; BuChEI, butyrylcholinesterase inhibitor; galantamine ER, galantamine extended-release capsules; nAChR agonist, nonpotentiating ligand of the nicotinic receptor; T_{max} = time to maximum plasma concentration.

is a "pseudo-irreversible" cholinesterase inhibitor since it forms a labile carbamoylate complex with AChE (and BuChE), inactivating the enzyme until the covalent bond is broken; the inhibitory effects of rivastigmine on CSF cholinesterase have a half-life of 9 hours. Rivastigmine is available both as an oral twice-daily preparation and, more recently, as a transdermal once-daily patch. Galantamine is both a reversible ChEI and a nonpotentiating nicotinic receptor ligand. All three drugs exhibit linear pharmacokinetics, and their time to maximum plasma concentration (t_{max}) values and elimination half-lives are prolonged in elderly patients.

Safety and Tolerability of Cholinesterase Inhibitors

With slow titration in appropriate individuals, these medications are generally tolerated well and have a safe adverse effect profile (with the exception of tacrine, which is rarely used due to reports of hepatotoxicity). While these "centrally acting" anti-AD ChEIs are mostly selective for CNS cholinesterase, the most common adverse effects—including nausea, vomiting, anorexia, flatulence, loose stools, diarrhea, salivation, and abdominal cramping—are related to peripheral cholinomimetic effects on the gastrointestinal tract. For the oral preparations, the adverse gastrointestinal effects of ChEI can be minimized by administering the drug after a meal or in combination with memantine. In general, bodily secretions can be increased—including skin, oral, and nasal. Occasionally, patients can develop mild rhinorrhea. Others can experience vivid dreams or mild insomnia; thus, doses should ideally be given after a meal in the morning. The rivastigmine transdermal patch can also cause skin irritation, redness, or rash at the site of application. For transdermal rivastigmine, adverse effects can be minimized by applying the patch to a different site each day (usually the back, upper trunk, or shoulders; applying the patch on the lower body can decrease bioavailability by 20%–30%). Overall, adverse effects may occur in 5%–20% of patients starting on ChEIs but are usually mild and transient, and often related to the dose and rate of dose escalation. These medications may also decrease heart rate and increase the risk of syncope, particularly in susceptible individuals (e.g., those with sick sinus syndrome or AV block) and with overdose. Use of these agents is contraindicated in patients with unstable or severe cardiac disease, uncontrolled epilepsy, unexplained syncope, and active peptic ulcer disease.

Efficacy and Effectiveness

In over 40 short-term randomized, placebo-controlled trials (RCTs) over 24–28 weeks investigating efficacy, and in meta-analyses of RCTs, all three ChEIs have demonstrated small to medium effect size treatment benefits at the patient-group level in terms of improving, stabilizing, or delaying decline in cognition, activities of daily living, and global status, and in ameliorating BPSD and caregiver burden (Atri, Rountree, Lopez, & Doody, 2012; Ballard et al., 2011; Birks, 2006; Cummings, 2004; Cummings, Schneider, Tariot, Kershaw, & Yuan, 2004; Cummings et al., 2006; Farlow & Cummings, 2007; Farlow et al., 2000; Greenberg et al., 2000; Howard et al., 2012; Mohs et al., 2001; Raina et al., 2008; Rockwood, 2004; Rountree et al., 2012; Tayeb, Yang, Price, & Tarazi, 2012; van de Glind et al., 2013). A majority of RCTs have been conducted in patients with MMSEs in the range of 10–26 (roughly considered equivalent by some to the range of performance in individuals with mild to moderate AD), have been of 6 months duration, and have demonstrated average MMSE treatment gains of 1.5–2 points over 6–12 months, and a 43% increase in the likelihood of remaining functionally stable at 12 months compared to placebo (Ballard et al., 2011; Mohs et al., 2001). Several RCTs and meta-analyses have demonstrated similar benefits in patients with moderate to severe AD dementia (Black et al., 2007; Bullock et al., 2005; Cappell et al., 2010; Doody et al., 2001; Farlow et al., 2011; Feldman et al., 2001; Feldman, Schmitt, & Olin, 2006; Gauthier et al., 2002; Howard et al., 2012; Winblad et al., 2006, 2009). In the few studies that have directly compared cholinesterase inhibitors to each other, no significant differences were found (Bullock et al., 2006; Wilcock et al., 2003). In longer term open-label trials, including extension trials from the original placebo-controlled, randomized studies, the cognitive benefits of the ChEIs appear to continue for at least 2–4 years (Burns, Gauthier, & Perdomo, 2007; Doody et al., 2001; Raskind, Peskind, Truyen, Kershaw, & Damaraju, 2004). Long-term prospective observation clinical cohort studies have also provided support for significant benefits of sustained ChEI treatment on ameliorating decline in cognition and function, delaying institutionalization, but not altering survival (Gillette-Guyonnet et al., 2006; Wattmo et al., 2011a; Wallin et al., 2004; Wallin et al., 2007; Wallin et al., 2011).

NMDA Antagonists (Memantine)

Memantine was the last FDA-approved treatment for AD dementia (2002) and remains the sole medication in its class. Memantine affects glutamatergic transmission; it is a low to moderate affinity N-methyl-d-aspartate (NMDA)-receptor open-channel blocker, which, in a voltage-dependent manner, modulates calcium flux through the opened channel.

Glutamate and Memantine Mechanism of Action in Alzheimer's Disease

Glutamate is the major excitatory neurotransmitter in the neocortex and plays an important role in memory and learning (Riedel, Platt, & Micheau, 2003). The glutamatergic hypothesis links cognitive decline in patients with AD to neuronal damage resulting from overactivation of NMDA receptors by glutamate (Francis, 2005). Glutamatergic transmission is disrupted in AD and the sustained low-level activation of NMDA receptors, which are pivotal in learning and memory, may result from deficiencies in glutamate reuptake by astroglial cells in the synaptic cleft, and the NMDA subtype of ionotropic glutamate receptors has been implicated (Francis, 2005; Parameshwaran, Dhanasekaran, & Suppiramaniam, 2008; Parsons, Danysz, Dekundy, & Pulte, 2013). While synaptic NMDA receptor activation may be neuroprotective, there is evidence to support that aberrant activation of extrasynaptic NMDA receptors may be neurotoxic and lead to calcium-induced excitotoxicity, neuronal amyloid-beta release, and neurodegeneration (Bordji, Becerril-Ortega, & Buisson, 2011; Parsons et al., 2013). Memantine preferentially targets extrasynaptic NMDA receptor signaling pathways. It has been further posited that due to aberrant glutamatergic exposure and stimulation in AD, synaptic signal-to-noise ratio is degraded, leading to failure or inefficient neural transmission (Francis, 2005; Parsons et al., 2013).

Physiological NMDA receptor activity is critical for normal neuronal function. However, excessive exposure to glutamate or overstimulation of its membrane receptors leads to excitotoxic neuronal injury or death. Excitotoxic neuronal cell damage is mediated in part by overactivation of NMDA-type receptors, which results in excessive Ca(2+) influx through the receptor-associated ion channel and subsequent free radical formation (Lipton, 2007). Thus, potential neuroprotective agents that excessively block NMDA receptor activity will likely produce unacceptable clinical and cognitive side effects (e.g., hallucinations with phencyclidine). However, memantine, through its action as an uncompetitive, low-to-moderate affinity, open-channel blocker may preferentially block excessive NMDA receptor activity without disrupting normal activity (Lipton, 2007). Entering the receptor-associated ion channel preferentially when it is excessively open, and with a fast off-rate, memantine does not substantially accumulate in the channel to interfere with subsequent normal synaptic transmission (Lipton, 2007).

Pharmacokinetics and Characteristics

Memantine is available in immediate-release twice daily (expected to be available generically in the United States by mid-2014) and extended-release once daily (recently available in the United States) preparations. The pharmacokinetic profiles and characteristics of these formulations are reviewed in Table 16.12 Memantine is mostly renally cleared and does not affect the hepatic CYP450 enzyme system.

Safety and Tolerability of Memantine

Titrated appropriately, memantine has a highly favorable safety and tolerability profile. Mild and transient treatment-emergent side effects include confusion, dizziness, constipation, headache, and somnolence; these may be encountered during, or soon after, titration to the maximum total daily dose of 10 mg twice daily for immediate-release memantine or 28 mg once daily for memantine extended release. In patients with severe renal insufficiency (creatinine clearance <30 mL/min) a dose adjustment to 5 mg twice daily for immediate-release memantine and 14 mg daily for memantine extended release is recommended. Memantine can be taken with or without food, does not produce significant changes in heart rate or blood pressure, and does not have significant interactions with other medications, including the ChEIs. Due to its mechanism of action, however, coadministration with other medications that have antiglutamatergic effects (e.g., amantadine, dextromethorphan) should be approached with caution.

TABLE 16.12 Pharmacokinetic Characteristics and Effects of the Anti-Alzheimer's Disease Dementia Voltage-Dependent, Low-Affinity, Open-Channel NMDA Blockers

Drug	Half-life (h)	Bioavailability (%)	T_{max} (h)	Hepatic Metabolism	Renal Excretion	Absorption Affected by Food	Effects on Other Receptors	Other Notes
Memantine	60–80	95–100	9–12	Little (<10%)*	Yes**	No	HT_3 antagonist	10 mg twice daily max dose (20 mg total daily max)#
Memantine extended release	60–80	95–100	18–25+	Little (<10%)*	Yes**	Yes+	HT_3 antagonist	28 mg once daily max dose#

*Memantine does not significantly inhibit the CYP450 hepatic enzyme system

**Renal excretion is the main factor for memantine elimination—maximum dosages are halved in individuals with CrCl<30.

+Memantine extended release absorption is slower after food than on an empty stomach; peak plasma concentrations are achieved 18 hours on an empty stomach and 25 hours after food.

#Memantine extended release affects a slower release compared to memantine and a potentially higher target dose (compared with twice-daily 10-mg dosing of immediate-release memantine it achieved a 48% higher steady-state maximum plasma concentration (Cmax) and 33% higher area under the plasma concentration– time curve from time 0 to 24 hours (AUC0–24))

T_{max} = time to maximum plasma concentration.

Efficacy and Effectiveness

Memantine is FDA-approved for the treatment of moderate to severe AD dementia, as monotherapy or in combination with a ChEI (often added on to existing ChEI treatment). In moderate and severe stage AD dementia, the short-term efficacy of memantine monotherapy over treatment with placebo has been demonstrated in several RCTs of 12–50 weeks duration and supported by meta-analyses; these treatment benefits include improvement, stabilization or reduced decline in the domains of cognition, function (ADLs), and global status, and by amelioration of BPSD and caregiver burden (Atri et al., 2008; Bullock, 2006; Doody, Wirth, Schmitt, & Mobius, 2004; Grossberg et al., 2009; Howard et al., 2012; Livingston & Katona, 2004; McShane, Areosa Sastre, & Minakaran, 2006; Puangthong & Hsiung, 2009; Reisberg et al., 2003; Schmitt, van Dyck, Wichems, & Olin, 2006; van Dyck, Tariot, Meyers, & Malca Resnick, 2007; Weycker et al., 2007; Wilcock, Ballard, Cooper, & Loft, 2008; Wilkinson & Andersen, 2007; Wimo, Winblad, Stoffler, Wirth, & Mobius, 2003; Winblad, Jones, Wirth, Stoffler, & Mobius, 2007; Winblad & Poritis, 1999). Short-term (6 months or less) memantine treatment effect sizes are small to medium in size and clinically significant at the moderate to severe stages of AD (Livingston & Katona, 2004; Wilkinson et al., 2009; Winblad et al., 2007). However, effect sizes associated with memantine treatment may be smaller and not readily detectable in mild AD, particularly over short durations of treatment (Atri et al., 2008; Bakchine & Loft, 2008; McShane et al., 2006; Peskind et al., 2006; Porsteinsson et al., 2008; Raina et al., 2008). Yet the practice of off-label prescription of memantine, most often in combination with a ChEI, in patients with mild AD is common, particularly in patients who are younger or may have faster progression, and has been criticized as unsupported by some (Schneider, Dagerman, Higgins, & McShane, 2011; Schneider, Insel, & Weiner, 2011). Nonetheless, longer term prospective observational clinical patient cohort studies have reported reduced clinical decline in patients with AD who are treated at any stage of the illness (Atri et al., 2008; Chou et al., 2009; Gillette-Guyonnet et al., 2011; Lopez et al., 2009; Rountree et al.; Vellas et al., 2012).

Add-on Combination Therapy With Acetyl Cholinesterase Inhibitors and Memantine

Several types and grades of clinical data, including those from short-term (6–12 months) RCTs (Level I evidence), longer term (12–36 months) open-label extensions to RCTs (Level II/III evidence), and from long-term (2 to 5-plus years) observational prospective clinical cohort effectiveness studies (Level II evidence) support the safety and benefits of anti-AD treatments in combination—most frequently as memantine added on to a stable regimen of background ChEI treatment (Atri et al., 2008; Chou et al., 2009; Gillette-Guyonnet et al., 2011; Lopez et al., 2009; Rountree et al., 2009; Vellas et al., 2012). Systematic reviews and meta-analysis also provide Level II grade evidence for the benefits of ChEI-memantine add-on combination treatment in AD dementia (Atri et al., 2011; Molinuevo, Gauthier, & Molinuevo, 2013; Raina et al., 2008; Rountree et al., 2013; Patel & Grossberg, 2011).

Mechanism of Action, Preclinical Data, and Rationale for Combination Therapy

Cholinergic and glutamatergic brain pathways are highly structurally and functionally linked (Francis, 2005). Glutamatergic cortical and hippocampal neurons receive widespread cholinergic inputs, and this, along with cholinergic suppression of excitatory feedback, allows ACh to set up the neural dynamics to enhance encoding of new information and to diminish proactive interference from previously learned information (Atri et al., 2004; Francis, 2005; Hasselmo, 2006). Conversely, glutamatergic inputs to cholinergic projection neurons can facilitate increased firing and ACh release, while ACh serves as a key modulator in glutamatergic, hippocampal, and cortical memory networks (Parsons et al., 2013).

Parsons and colleagues have proposed the "three-neuron model" to explain the higher efficacy of combination treatment compared to monotherapy with either ChEI or memantine alone (Parsons et al., 2013) (see Fig. 16.4). According to this model, since memantine and the ChEIs intervene at separate points of the disrupted signaling cascades in AD, memantine, acting at the NMDA receptor, and ChEIs, by delaying breakdown of ACh at cholinergic synapses, together act to better facilitate LTP and successful memory processing. As seen in Figure 16.4, memantine is posited to lower the pathologically increased tonic level of excitation of the glutamatergic synapse at rest (neuron 2—see Fig. 16. 4). A dual impact is hypothesized from this: (1) reduction of the "background noise," so that incoming physiological signals can be better distinguished; and (2) reduction of the constant pathological influx of Ca^{2+}, thereby reducing the likelihood of the neuron from being stimulated in a way that would cause dysfunction, synaptotoxicity, and, ultimately, cell death (neuron 2). In this model, combination treatment reduces the overall tonic activation of NMDA receptors, which delays neurodegeneration of cholinergic neurons bearing NMDA receptors and thus facilitates synaptic NMDA receptor activation. Supplementing this effect, the ChEIs are posited to amplify (i.e., bring toward normal) the AD pathologically weakened signal from cholinergic neurons by delaying ACh breakdown at cholinergic nerve endings such that neurotransmission (to neuron 3) is preserved by the improved signal detected against the lowered background noise (Fig. 16.4). Together, these effects are posited to help maintain glutamatergic/cholinergic signaling cascades and to consequently facilitate LTP and memory processing (Parsons et al., 2013).

Not only do ChEIs and memantine work via different mechanisms, thus providing a dual pharmacologic strategy, but in vitro and animal data suggest that the combination of a ChEI and memantine may, under certain conditions, act potentially synergistically to increase release of hippocampal ACh (Ihalainen et al., 2011). In preclinical animal models, both ChEIs and memantine have been observed to improve memory performance (Wise & Lichtman, 2007; Yamada et al., 2005). As they work via potentially complementary mechanisms and data support benefits of these drugs in improving memory performance in animal models, the use of ChEI and memantine combination therapy is supported by a sound scientific basis and rationale.

Efficacy in Short-Term Randomized, Double-Blind, Placebo-Controlled Trials

Three 24-week, randomized, double-blind, placebo-controlled trials (RCTs) have investigated the efficacy and safety of memantine 20–28 mg/day in combination with a ChEI (see Table 16.13) (Tariot et al., 2004; Porsteinsson et al., 2008). Two of these trials were conducted with patients in the moderate to severe range of AD severity and were successful in demonstrating efficacy on multiple prespecified outcome measures at study endpoint (Tariot et al., 2004). Another study conducted in patients in the mild to moderate AD severity range failed to demonstrate statistically significant results on prespecified outcomes and is considered an underpowered and indeterminate study by some (Atri et al., 2013; Porsteinsson et al., 2008). All three studies demonstrated overall good tolerability and safety for combination treatment compared to chronic baseline ChEI monotherapy.

The first RCT of anti-AD combination treatment assessed the efficacy of administration of memantine (10 mg twice daily) versus placebo to patients with moderate to severe AD (MMSE 5–14; n = 404) receiving stable donepezil therapy (Tariot et al., 2004). Relative to placebo, memantine produced significant benefits in all primary and secondary outcome measures and all four key symptom domains of AD—cognition, function, behavior, and global status (Tariot et al., 2004). Notably, the average score on the primary outcome measure of cognition, the Severe Impairment Battery (SIB), was 0.9 points better at the 24-week study endpoint than at baseline with ChEI-memantine treatment. In contrast, with donepezil-placebo treatment SIB scores worsened by 2.5 points in the same interval. Combination treatment effect sizes on cognition (SIB) and global severity (CIBIC-plus) were 0.4 and 0.24, respectively. Several post-hoc analyses of this data have identified specific significant benefits of memantine add-on treatment relative to chronic donepezil monotherapy; these include the following (1) decreases in

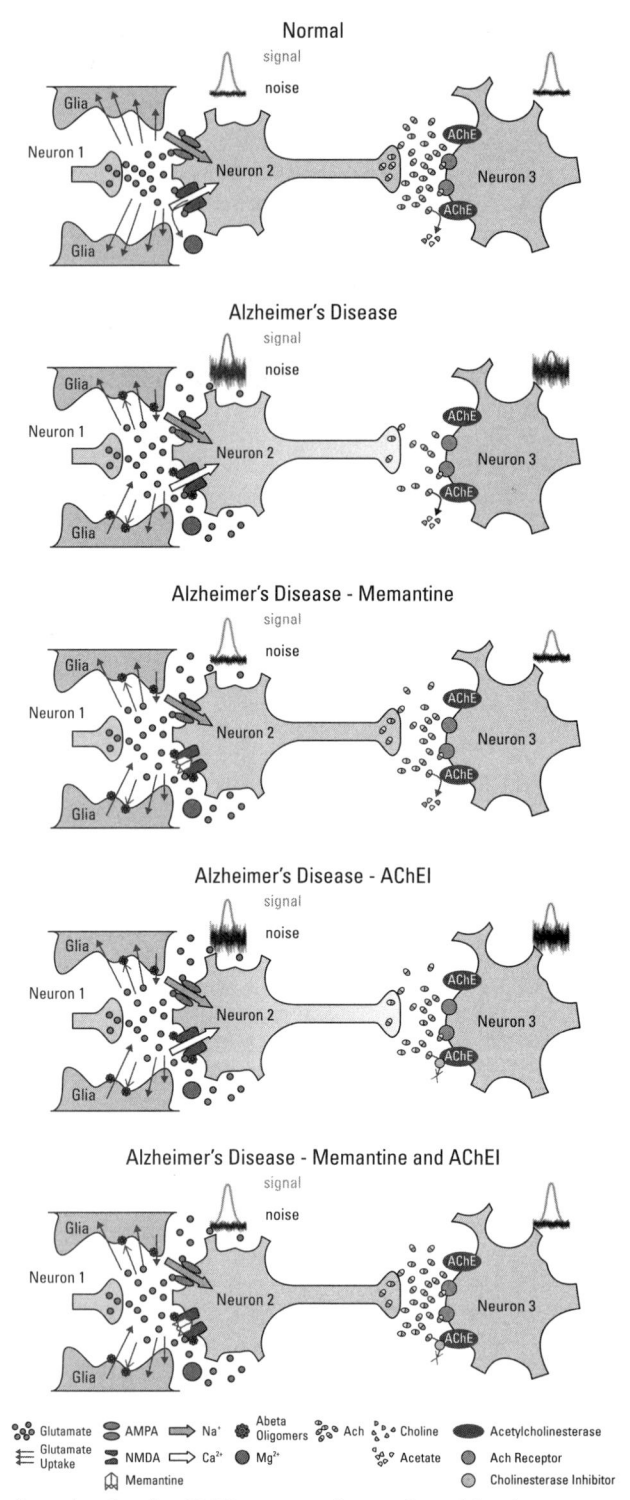

Figure 16.4 Mechanism of action for ChEIs, memantine, and combination treatment with both in Alzheimer's disease (AD) (from the Parsons et al. "three-neuron model" for the action of memantine and the AChEIs in AD; Parsons et al., 2013).

TABLE 16.13 Level I and Level II Evidence Grade Controlled Clinical Efficacy and Effectiveness Studies of and Memantine Add-on Combination Therapy

Study	Design	No. of Patients	Duration or Mean Follow-up	AD Stage	Study Goal	Primary End Points	Results	Evidence Level
Tariot et al. (2004)	RCT—efficacy trial	404	24 weeks	Moderate–severe	Safety and efficacy of adding 10 mg twice daily memantine immed iate-release to stable background donepezil treatment	Cognition: SIB Function: ADCS-ADL$_{19}$ Safety & tolerability: TEAE	Significantly Better outcome with addition of memantine vs. placebo in all primary endpoints; good safety profile and well tolerated	Class I
Porsteinsson et al. (2008)	RCT—efficacy trial	433	24 weeks	Mild–moderate	Safety & efficacy of adding 20 mg once daily memantine immediate-release to stable background ChEI treatment (donepezil, rivastigmine, or galantamine)	Cognition: ADAS-cog Global Change: CIBIC-Plus Safety & tolerability: TEAE	No statistical treatment differences on primary endpoints; underpowered study*; good safety profile and well tolerated	Class II
Grossberg et al. (2013)	RCT—efficacy trial	677	24 weeks	Moderate–severe	Safety and efficacy of adding 28 mg once daily memantine extended-release to stable background ChEI treatment (donepezil, rivastigmine, or galantamine)	Cognition: SIB Function: ADCS-ADL$_{19}$ Behavior: NPI Global Change: CIBIC-Plus Fluency: VFT Safety and tolerability: TEAE	Significantly Better outcome with addition of memantine vs. placebo in all primary endpoints (SIB and CIBIC-Plus), and secondary endpoints of NPI and VFT, but not ADLs. Good safety profile and well tolerated	Class I
Howard et al. (2012)	RCT—effectiveness trial	295	52 weeks	Moderate–severe	Comparative effectiveness of discontinuing background donepezil and adding placebo or memantine, or continuing donepezil and adding placebo or memantine	Cognition: SMMSE Function: BALDS Behavior: NPI QOL: DEMQOL-proxy Caregiver health: GHQ-12	Significantly better outcomes on SMMSE, BALDS, and NPI at 52 week endpoint for all treatment groups compared to discontinuation of donepezil and starting placebo; overall, treatment groups undifferentiated at 52-weeks	Class II (due to >72% attrition and inadequate power

(continued)

TABLE 16.13 Continued

Study	Design	No. of Patients	Duration or Mean Follow-up	AD Stage	Study Goal	Primary End Points	Results	Evidence Level
Atri et al. (2008)	CLOC—effectiveness cohort study	382	Mean 2.5 years	Mild, moderate, and severe	Long-term clinical effectiveness of combination therapy (CT) vs. ChEI alone vs. standard care without ChEI or memantine	Cognition: BDS Function: ADL	Significantly slower trajectory of cognitive and functional decline for CT; slower decline in cognition for ChEI than standard care; effect sizes increase with time on CT	Class II
Lopez et al. (2009)	CLOC—effectiveness cohort study	943	Mean 5.2 years	Mild, moderate, and severe	Effects of combination therapy vs. ChEI alone vs. standard care without ChEI or memantine on time to death or nursing home admission	Time to nursing home admission or death	Longer time to nursing home admission for CT over ChEIs alone, and for ChEIs vs. standard care. No differences in time to death.	Class II
Rountree et al. (2009)	CLOC—effectiveness cohort study	641	Mean 3.0 years	Mild, moderate, and severe	Clinical effectiveness of persistence of anti-AD therapies with ChEI, memantine, and CT	Cognition: ADAS-cog, MMSE, BPMSE Function: PSMS & IADL Severity: CDR-sb	Treatment persistence associated with significant benefits in outcomes (slower decline) in all domains; treatment benefits are cumulative	Class II
Gillette-Guyonnet et al. (2012)	CLOC—effectiveness cohort study	686	Mean 2.6 years	Mild, moderate, and severe	Delineation and comparison of rates of deterioration on clinical measures between ChEI and/or memantine treated and untreated (historical) cohorts	Cognition: ADAS-cog, MMSE, Function: ADL Behavior: NPI Severity: CDR-sb	Significantly lower rates of deterioration on MMSE and ADAS-cog in treated AD patients compared to untreated patients in the Pre-ChEI era. No Pre-ChEI vs. post-ChEI/memantine era comparative data for ADL, NPI, and CDR	Class II

*Numerically favorable results observed for CT at an effect size (0.12) that was lower than the effect size estimate (0.325) the study was powered for to detect a statistically significant difference.

ADAS-cog, AD Assessment Scale-cognitive subscale; ADCS-ADL$_{19}$, modified 19-item AD Cooperative Study–Activities of Daily Living Inventory; ADL, Weintraub Activities of Daily Living Scale; BALDS, Bristol Activities of Daily Living scale; BDS, Blessed Dementia Scale; BPMSE, Baylor Profound Mental Status Examination; ChEI, cholinesterase inhibitor; CIBIC-Plus, Interview-Based Impression of Change Plus Caregiver Input; CLOC, controlled long-term observational prospective clinical cohort; CT, combination therapy (ChEI plus memantine); DEMQOL-proxy, Health-related Quality of Life; GHQ-12, General Health Questionnaire 12-item; IADL, instrumental activities of daily living; MMSE, Mini-Mental State Examination; NPI, Neuropsychiatric Inventory; PSMS, Physical Self-Maintenance Scale; RCT, randomized clinical trial; SIB, Severe Impairment Battery; SMMSE, standardized MMSECDR-sb, Clinical Dementia Rating-Sum of Boxes; TEAE, Treatment Emergent Adverse Event reporting; VFT, semantic verbal fluency test.

frequency, severity, and duration of existing neuropsychiatric and behavioral symptoms, in addition to a reduction in the emergence of these symptoms; (2) lowering of caregiver distress and burden; (3) improved daily functioning in ADLs that require greater connectedness/autonomy and higher level functions; and (4) better cognitive performance related to memory, language, and praxis (Cummings et al., 2006; Feldman et al., 2006; Schmitt et al., 2006).

The second 24-week RCT assessed the efficacy of administration of memantine (20 mg once daily) versus placebo to patients with mild to moderate AD (MMSE 10–22; n = 433) taking a stable dose of any approved ChEI therapy (donepezil, rivastigmine, galantamine) (Porsteinsson et al., 2008) and failed to meet a priori outcome endpoints in cognition and daily functioning. There were no significant differences observed in tolerability and safety between the memantine and placebo groups. There were also no clinically significant differences between treatment groups in laboratory tests, vital signs measurements, or electrocardiogram parameters. A greater proportion of participants in the memantine group (9.7%) than in the placebo group (5.0%) demonstrated a significant weight increase (at least 7% over the baseline value), which may be a clinically important beneficial "side effect" in this often frail elderly population—a population that is highly susceptible to anorexia and weight loss due to potential side effects from ChEIs and from low caloric intake due to forgetfulness, depression, and apathy.

Other than dementia stage (as gauged by MMSE inclusion criteria: 3–14 versus 10–22), the major inclusion and design differences between these first two RCTs were that the Porsteinsson et al. (2008) study (MMSE 10-22) allowed use of any ChEI (not just donepezil) and had a once daily dosing regimen using immediate-release memantine (as opposed to a twice daily dosing in the Tariot et al., 2004, study). The observed effect size of 0.118 on the ADAS-cog cognitive outcome, which was numerically in a favor of ChEI-memantine add-on combination treatment but was not statistically significant (p = 0.18), was a much lower value than was used a priori (effect size of 0.325) to power the study for an adequate sample size to be able to reliably detect a possible treatment effect. This suggests that the Porsteinsson et al. study in mild to moderate subjects was underpowered to be able to detect a potentially statistically significant benefit of combination therapy in this population, and that, along with increased severity range-, ChEI type- and dose-related heterogeneities, may have contributed to the observed null results. This hypothesis was tested in a recent post-hoc meta-analysis that included this data. This study reported significant results with effect size estimates in the 0.21–0.36 range for multiple domains (cognition, function, global status) in favor of stable donepezil-memantine add-on combination therapy in patients in the moderate range of severity (MMSE 10-19) (Atri et al., 2013). Long-term effectiveness studies in clinical cohorts of patients with AD dementia support beneficial combination treatment effects for at least 2 years; these benefits were not limited to patients with moderate or severe stage dementia but were statistically observed in the later years of treatment (Atri, Shaughnessy, Locascio, & Growdon, 2008). For example, Atri et al. observed that in mild AD, cognitive and functional effects of combination therapy over ChEI monotherapy have small effect sizes (0.10–0.21 range) within the first year of treatment (Atri et al., 2008) but manifest larger benefits (effect sizes in the 0.34–0.73 range) as treatment continues over 4 years.

Unless similar studies in mild AD are powered accordingly (and/or are appropriately extended to multiple years), they may not be able to adequately address whether an actual treatment benefit has been missed due to inadequate design (an indeterminate study) or that it simply does not exist. Statistically failing to observe an effect (i.e., to reject the null hypothesis) is not the same as confirming that a significant effect does not exist (i.e., to confirm the null hypothesis of equivalence)—absence of evidence is not evidence of absence. This is an important caveat for the interpretation of studies with design or execution limitations that produce potential bias (e.g., disproportional and nonrandom missing data between comparison groups), unplanned variability, and results that fail to meet a priori criteria to detect a difference in outcomes at the desired significance level. Also, results from studies that fail to reject the null hypothesis cannot be interpreted as having demonstrated "equivalence" of treatments. To show this, an appropriate equivalence analysis must be designed that specifies the parameters for treatments being deemed equivalent (e.g., less than a +/− 0.5 point difference in drug-placebo performance on the MMSE at 24 weeks).

The third and final short-term RCT was a recently published study by Grossberg et al. (2013) that also demonstrated multidomain superiority of ChEI-memantine add-on combination treatment compared to chronic ChEI-placebo add-on treatment in 661 subjects with AD in the moderate to severe range (MMSE 3–14; Grossberg et al., 2013). This study was novel in that it utilized a once-daily memantine extended-release preparation at a higher dose of 28 mg daily. It also allowed baseline ChEI treatment with any oral ChEI preparation (donepezil, rivastigmine, galantamine). Significant combination treatment benefits were observed at the 24-week study endpoint on primary and secondary outcome measures in the domains of cognition, global status, neuropsychiatric symptoms and behaviors, and verbal fluency (p <.01 for all). Activities of daily living showed statistical trends in favor of combination treatment at weeks 18 (p = .068) and 24 (p = .155). The combination treatment again showed an expected and good profile of overall tolerability and safety.

Longer Term Randomized Controlled Trials, Open-Label Extensions, and Naturalistic Observational Clinical Cohort Studies

The preponderance of evidence from longer term clinical studies also supports that the benefits of anti-AD medications, particularly in combination, are sustained for 1 or more years when treatment is continued (see Table 16.13). Multiple, open-label extension studies of short-term RCTs have reported sustained benefits for persistent treatment with ChEIs (3–5 years) (Doody et al., 2001; Lyketsos, Reichman, Kershaw, & Zhu, 2004; Raskind et al., 2004; Rogers, Doody, Pratt, & Ieni, 2000) and memantine (52 weeks) (Reisberg et al., 2006). Longer RCTs and long-term observational clinical cohort studies also support effectiveness of ChEI, memantine, and combination therapy (Atri et al., 2008; Howard et al., 2012; Lopez et al., 2009) (for reviews see Atri et al., 2012; Rountree et al., 2012).

The DOMINO-AD 52-week RTC in patients with moderate to severe AD (MMSE 5–13) in the United Kingdom treated in the community was a recently reported effectiveness study (Howard et al., 2012). Despite its significant methodological limitations, which included high and imbalanced attrition (72% overall; attrition was significantly less in patients on 2 vs. 1 vs. no anti-AD medications) and inadequate power and analysis to demonstrate potential equivalence of treatments at 52 weeks, it nonetheless provided further evidence to support that, compared to discontinuation of donepezil, the continuation of donepezil, and the starting of memantine treatment despite discontinuation of donepezil, provided significant benefits on cognition, function, and behavior (Atri et al., 2013; Howard et al., 2012; Shaw, 2012). The addition of memantine to donepezil to achieve combination therapy was again well tolerated (significantly fewer patients withdrew who were on combination treatment) and no less effective, while discontinuation of donepezil was clearly detrimental to cognition and function (Atri et al., 2013; Howard et al., 2012; Shaw, 2012).

Long-term observational clinical cohort studies performed in naturalistic settings with prospectively collected data show similar patterns to RCTs. They provide supportive Level II grade and more generalizable evidence to patients treated in clinical practice that combination treatment is more effective than monotherapy, and that monotherapy is better than no antidementia medication treatment (Atri et al., 2008, 2012; Gauthier & Molinuevo, 2013; Lopez et al., 2009; Rountree et al., 2009). In patient cohorts, long-term ChEI-memantine combination therapy significantly reduced cognitive and functional decline (see Fig. 16.5), and delayed time to nursing home admission, compared to ChEI monotherapy and to standard care without a ChEI or memantine (Atri et al., 2008; Gillette-Guyonnet et al., 2011; Lopez et al., 2009; Rountree et al., 2009). Furthermore, the benefits of combination therapy accumulate with time on treatment and are sustained for years (Atri et al., 2008; Rountree et al., 2009). Benefits of anti-AD medications significantly

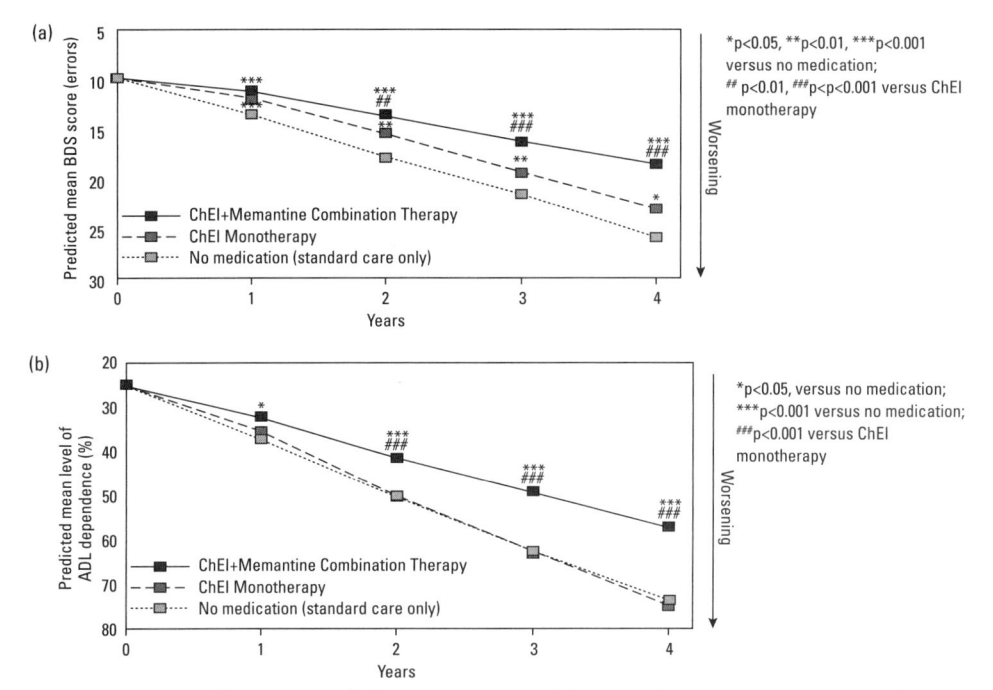

Figure 16.5 Clinical effectiveness of ChEI-memantine add-on combination treatment to reduce long-term progression of cognitive and functional decline in Alzheimer's disease (AD) dementia. (A) Estimated trajectory of cognitive decline over 4 years for groups of patients with AD dementia starting with 10 errors on the BDS (~MMSE 22) is lowest in the combination treatment group. (B) Estimated trajectory of functional decline over 4 years for groups of patients with AD starting with 25% dependence on the Weintraub ADL scale is lowest in the combination treatment group. Similar graphs (not shown) demonstrate significant benefits of combination treatment to reduce clinical progression in groups of patients with very mild and with severe AD dementia (Atri et al., 2008).

increased with treatment persistence in several symptom domains (cognition, function, global severity) and in all stages of AD (Rountree et al., 2009). Gillette-Guyonnet et al. (2011) also reported slower decline of cognition associated with anti-AD medication use in France.

Delaying Major Clinical Milestones: Nursing Home Placement and Death

There is evidence that ChEI and memantine, especially in combination, delay clinically relevant endpoints, particularly nursing home placement. Several studies support delayed nursing home placement in patients treated with ChEIs (Lopez et al., 2005, 2009; Wallin et al., 2011), memantine (Wimo et al., 2003), and combination therapy (Lopez et al., 2009). In two separate cohort analyses totaling more than 932 patients with AD dementia (mean MMSE 18.8 at baseline study entry) followed annually for a mean duration of 5.2 years, those patients taking combination therapy were three to seven times less likely to be placed in a nursing home than patients receiving ChEI monotherapy. The same study found no association with anti-AD medication use and time to death; similar results were reported by Rountree and colleagues, who also concluded that anti-AD medications do not prolong survival (Rountree et al., 2012), and by Wallin and colleagues, who reported early response to chronic ChEI treatment was associated with delayed institutionalization but not with increased survival (Wallin et al., 2011). These data infer that anti-AD treatments with ChEIs and memantine, alone or in combination, may cause an expansion of the mid- to late-stages of AD-related disability, thus to effectively delay end-stage disability and to produce a contraction of the end/terminal stages of AD without prolonging life in the profound and end stages of AD.

Reduction of Caregiving Time and Health Care Costs

Data also support the pharmacoeconomic and direct benefits of AD therapies on reducing costs and in beneficially affecting quality of life, particularly for patient caregivers. Caregivers of patients enrolled in a 24-week RCT who received memantine (Reisberg et al., 2003) spent an average of 52 hours fewer per month on caregiving tasks than caregivers of patients in the placebo group ($p = .02$) (Wimo et al., 2003). A reduction of 52 hours per month equates to saving caregivers, on average, 1.7 hours per day—a clinically and financially meaningful outcome. Wimo et al. also reported a treatment advantage in terms of patients remaining in residential status longer and delaying time to institutionalization (Wimo et al., 2003). Originally the United Kingdom's National Institute for Health and Care Excellence (NICE) recommended, on the basis of perceived cost-effectiveness and highly flawed data and interpretations from the AD-2000 study (Courtney et al., 2004), to reserve donepezil treatment only for patients with moderate-stage dementia (MMSE10-20). However, more recent data demonstrated clear cost benefits in terms of reducing both direct patient care costs and unpaid caregiver time in the UK health care system (Getsios, Blume, Ishak, & Maclaine, 2010), and the indication for treatment was expanded to all stages of AD dementia. Donepezil prescribed in routine clinical practice was demonstrated in a case-control study in patients with predominantly mild to moderate AD to be associated with reduced health care costs to a Medicare managed care plan (Lu, Hill, & Fillit, 2005). Similarly, when adding memantine to stable doses of donepezil for patients with moderate to severe AD, cost reduction in terms of formal and informal care outweighed the additional cost of memantine itself (Weycker et al., 2007). Reductions in cost benefits are not surprising when considering that each month of delay in nursing home placement can save up to $2,029 in direct health care and supportive care costs (Stefanacci, 2007).

Effects on Domains of Cognition

Patients with MMSEs in the 3-15 range (moderate to severe AD dementia) who were on combination treatment demonstrated significant benefits over ChEI monotherapy on the SIB in two large 24-week RCTs (Grossberg et al., 2013; Tariot et al., 2004). A post-hoc analysis reported particularly beneficial combination treatment effects in the domains of memory, language, and praxis (Schmitt et al., 2006). A recent meta-analysis of 24-week RCTs that included 510 subjects reported benefits on cognitive measures (ADAS-cog and SIB) with effect sizes ranging from 0.28 to 0.36 in patients with MMSEs from 3 to 19 (Atri et al., 2013). A 12-week RCT with memantine mono- or ChEI combination-therapy reported treatment benefits on functional communication, as recognized by caregivers (Saxton et al., 2012). In the DOMINO-AD RCT, treatment benefits of donepezil and memantine, alone or in combination, were also evident throughout 52 weeks on the MMSE (Howard et al., 2012). Benefits on cognition have also been reported from observational prospective clinical cohort effectiveness studies. Patients on ChEI-memantine combination therapy, as compared to a ChEI alone, accumulated significantly fewer errors on the Attention-Memory-Concentration subscale of the Blessed Dementia Scale (BDS) over several years (Atri et al., 2008) (see Fig. 16.5a). Lower rates of cognitive decline on the MMSE, equating to about one point less decline per year, and the ADAS-cog, equating to about 4.5–6.5 less errors per year, have also been reported by Rountree and colleagues and Gillette-Guyonnet and colleagues to be associated with anti-AD medication persistence and use (Gillette-Guyonnet et al., 2011; Rountree et al., 2009).

Effects on Daily Function

In the 24-week Tariot et al. RCT (MMSE 3–14), caregivers rated patients who received combination therapy as being significantly more independent and higher functioning on ADLs than those on donepezil alone (Tariot et al., 2004). The recent meta-analysis by Atri et al. showed a similar pattern in ADLs in favor of combination treatment over ChEI alone with a treatment effect size of 0.21 in patients with both moderate AD and more severe AD (MMSE ranges of 5–19) (Atri et al., 2013). Long-term observational prospective clinical cohort studies have also reported similar results. Patients on ChEI-memantine combination therapy as compared to a ChEI alone also retained more independence on ADLs over several years with effect sizes of 0.23 at year one, 0.46 at year two, 0.62 at year three, and 0.73 by year four of combination treatment (Atri et al., 2008) (see Fig. 16.5b). Similarly, Rountree et al. also reported slower decline on daily function as measured by the Physical Self-Maintenance scale (PSMS), and Independent Activities of Daily Living scale (IADL) for patients with more persistent treatment with anti-AD medications (Rountree et al., 2009).

Effects on Domains of Neuropsychiatric Symptoms and Behavior

The benefits of monotherapy with a ChEI or memantine on ameliorating BPSD may be complementary (see Fig. 16.6). Compared to 24-week treatment with placebo, donepezil monotherapy was associated with significant behavioral benefits in the NPI subdomains of depression/dysphoria, anxiety and apathy (Feldman, Van Baelen, Kavanagh, & Torfs, 2005) (Fig. 16.6a), while memantine monotherapy was associated with benefits in the subdomains of delusions, agitation/aggression, and irritability/lability (Gauthier, Loft, & Cummings, 2008) (Fig. 16.6b). The benefits of combination treatment on BPSD appear to be superior to monotherapy with a ChEI donepezil (Cummings et al., 2006). Cummings et al. analyzed data from the Tariot et al.'s 24-week RCT and observed that memantine added on to chronic background donepezil treatment was associated with significantly reduced agitation, irritability, and appetite/eating changes compared to adding placebo to chronic background treatment with donepezil (Cummings et al., 2006). In patients receiving donepezil-memantine combination treatment, caregivers also reported significantly less distress related to agitation and aggression, nighttime behavior, and eating changes, and there was greater delay and reduction in the emergence of new agitation and aggression, irritability, and nighttime behaviors compared to patients on donepezil-placebo (Cummings et al., 2006). Beneficial treatment effects on the NPI were also reported for donepezil-memantine add-on combination in the 52-week DOMINO-AD RCT. Memantine add-on combination treatment was associated with a significantly smaller worsening of NPI scores, and with a benefit that was equivalent to 83% of the 12-month deterioration (4.8 NPI points) observed in the group of patients who discontinued donepezil and received placebo (Howard et al., 2012).

Safety and Tolerability of ChEI-Memantine Add-on Combination Treatment

Several studies have reported on safety and tolerability of combination therapy; overall, there is a good profile for both. Addition of memantine to stable doses of ChEIs does not correspond to significant overall increases in adverse events (AEs). The rates of discontinuation due to AEs for ChEIs and memantine combination treatment are low, between 5% and 10%, and not generally significantly different from placebo (Choi et al., 2011; Grossberg et al., 2013; Porsteinsson et al., 2008; Reisberg et al., 2003; Tariot et al., 2004). Among ChEIs, the highest reports of AEs are due to nausea, vomiting, and diarrhea, and appear to be higher for patients taking oral rivastigmine; this is much less of an issue with the rivastigmine patch. The rates for donepezil are approximately 5% for those taking 10 mg daily and ≤12% for those taking 23 mg daily (Farlow et al., 2011). Meanwhile, memantine monotherapy is not associated with a significant increase in AEs compared to treatment with placebo (Reisberg et al., 2003).

In Tariot et al., significantly fewer patients on donepezil-memantine (10 mg twice daily memantine immediate release) combination treatment, compared to donepezil-placebo, discontinued the study due to AEs (Tariot et al., 2004). Reports of transient and mild or moderate confusion were higher (7.9% vs. 2.0%), but reported AEs for agitation (9.4% vs. 11.9%), diarrhea (4.5% vs. 8.5%), and fecal incontinence (2.0% vs. 5.0%) were lower in the combination group. In Porsteinsson et al.'s study, overall AE reports were no different between ChEI-memantine (20 mg once daily immedeiate-release) and ChEI-placebo (Porsteinsson et al., 2008). In the recently published study with the

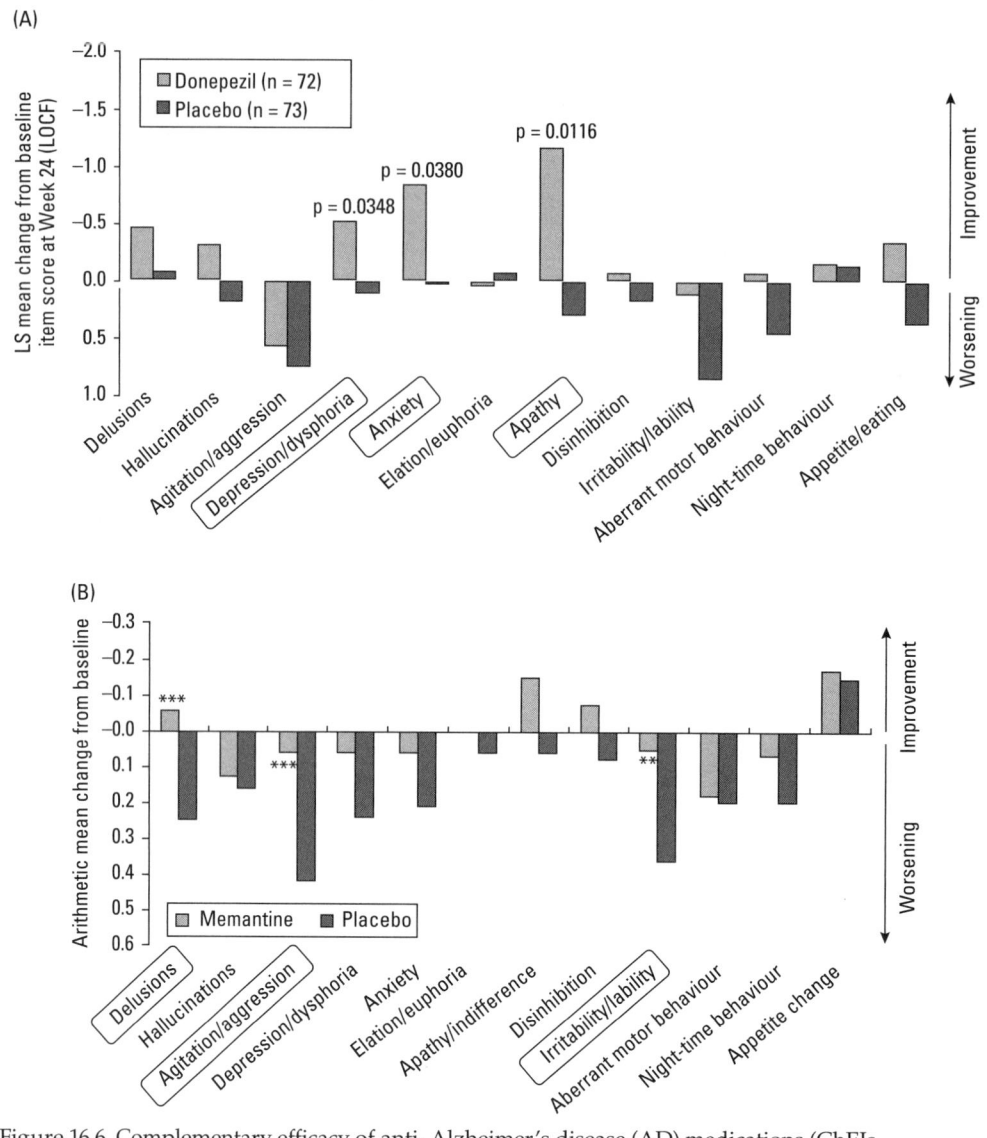

Figure 16.6 Complementary efficacy of anti-Alzheimer's disease (AD) medications (ChEIs, memantine) on amelioration of behavioral and psychological symptoms of dementia (BPSD) as measured by NPI domains in AD dementia. (A) Donepezil, compared to placebo, treatment was associated with significant behavioral benefits over 24 weeks in the NPI subdomains of depression/dysphoria, anxiety, and apathy (Feldman et al., 2005); and (B) memantine, compared to placebo, treatment was associated with significant behavioral benefits over 24 weeks in the NPI subdomains of delusions, agitation/aggression, and irritability/lability (Gauthier et al., 2008).

higher dose of 28 mg once daily memantine extended release, AEs with a frequency of at least 5.0% that were more prevalent in the ChEI-memantine extended-release group than the ChEI-placebo group were diarrhea (5.0% vs. 3.9%) and headache (5.6 vs. 5.1%) (Grossberg et al., 2013). In a meta-analysis of 520 subjects, adding memantine 20 mg daily to background donepezil 10 mg daily did not result in an AE profile that was significantly different compared to donepezil and placebo (see Table 16.14); there were also approximately half as many reports of agitation as an AE in donepezil-memantine combination treatment compared to donepezil-placebo (Atri et al., 2013).

TABLE 16.14 Comparison of Adverse Events With an Incidence ≥5% Between Alzheimer's Disease Treatment Groups

Adverse Event	Moderate and Severe AD MMSE<20 (5–19)[a]		Moderate ADMMSE 10–19[b]	
	Memantine Added to Donepezil ($n = 269$)	Placebo Added to Donepezil ($n = 251$)	Memantine Added to Donepezil ($n = 190$)	Placebo Added to Donepezil ($n = 185$)
Patients with AEs	206 (76.6)	186 (74.1)	144 (75.8)	136 (73.5)
Dizziness	20 (7.4)	19 (7.6)	17 (8.9)	16 (8.6)
Agitation	17 (6.3)*	29 (11.6)	9 (4.7)*	19 (10.3)
Confusional state	15 (5.6)	6 (2.4)	–	–
Diarrhea	14 (5.2)	21 (8.4)	12 (6.3)	14 (7.6)
Nasopharyngitis	14 (5.2)	6 (2.4)	–	–
Falls	11 (4.1)	15 (6.0)	10 (5.3)	11 (5.9)
Urinary tract infection	–	–	10 (5.3)	8 (4.3)
Depression	–	–	6 (3.2)	11 (5.9)

Note: Incidence of AEs over 24 weeks was similar between the patients treated with memantine added to donepezil versus placebo added to donepezil (Atri et al., 2013).

Data are number (%).

[a]Moderate to severe AD (MMSE 5–19 at baseline), receiving donepezil (10 mg/day).
[b]Moderate AD (MMSE 10–19 at baseline), receiving donepezil (10 mg/day).
*$p < .05$ versus placebo added to donepezil.
APT, all patients treated; AD, Alzheimer's disease; AE, adverse event. "–" denotes AEs with an incidence <5% in both treatment groups in the respective severity subgroup.

Evidence-Based Medication Therapeutics by Stage of Alzheimer's Disease

In the United States, the ChEIs donepezil and rivastigmine are FDA approved for use in mild, moderate, and severe AD dementia, while memantine is FDA approved for use in moderate and severe AD dementia. There is, however, support in the literature, with differential grades/levels of evidence and treatment effect sizes, for use of anti-AD medications at different stages of AD. Overall, it appears that the grade of evidence is higher and the effect sizes are bigger for use of ChEI monotherapy in mild and moderate AD dementia than in severe AD dementia; the grade of evidence and effect sizes then drop in very mild AD dementia and are lowest for MCI (i.e., mild and moderate > severe > very mild > very severe and MCI). For memantine monotherapy the overall gradient of evidence and effect sizes are as follows according to AD dementia stage: moderate-to-severe and severe > moderate > very severe >>> mild; none in MCI. Finally, for combination treatment with memantine added on to baseline/chronic ChEI, the overall gradient of evidence and effect sizes are as follows according to AD dementia stage: moderate-to-severe and severe > moderate >> mild and very severe >> very mild and in MCI; the latter are from subsets of patients in long-term observational cohorts. Some of this evidence is reviewed according to stage of disease severity. Overall, regardless of severity stage, higher persistence, dose (approved dosages), and duration of treatments are associated with better outcomes over slowing clinical decline.

Mild Cognitive Impairment: Very Early/Mild Alzheimer's Disease

Randomized, placebo-controlled trials of ChEI treatment in MCI have shown mixed results; while some studies suggest treatment-related preserved cognitive functions (but no effects for other outcome measures) (Salloway et al., 2004), other data support that ChEI treatment (donepezil) delays time to dementia diagnosis by up to 2–3 years in those who carry one or more APOE ε4 alleles (Petersen et al., 2005) or in those who show symptoms of depression (Lu et al., 2009). Petersen et al. found that "the observed relative reduction in the risk of progression to Alzheimer's disease of 58% at one year and 36% at two years in the entire cohort is likely to be clinically significant."

However, systematic reviews of RCTs have yet to demonstrate clear efficacy for all MCI groups (Raschetti, Albanese, Vanacore, & Maggini, 2007).

Heterogeneity of underlying pathology leading to MCI in different subjects in past RCTs, including non-AD pathology, may confound results and obscure potential efficacy; for this reason, more recent and future RCTs investigating MCI due to AD are starting to employ AD biomarker inclusion criteria (e.g., AD CSF profile, evidence of amyloid-PET positivity) along with biomarkers of neuronal injury (e.g., CSF tau profile, FDG-PET hypometabolism pattern, structural MRI atrophy pattern) to ensure a diagnosis of "High Likelihood MCI due to AD" according to the new NIA-AA criteria (Albert et al., 2011).

While there are potential signals of benefit observed in RCT and clinical effectiveness studies with observational cohorts that there may be long-term clinical treatment benefits even in early disease and with sustained use of antidementia medications (Atri et al., 2008; Petersen et al., 2005; Rountree et al., 2009), the strength of evidence does not provide support for a clear recommendation for or against the use of donepezil or other antidementia medications (memantine and combination treatment) in persons with MCI. The general good safety and tolerability profile of these medications, along with signals of potential efficacy and effectiveness and the generic availability of most of these medications, could prompt a discussion between the clinician and the patient about this possibility.

Mild Stage

Level I grade evidence for the efficacy of ChEI monotherapy in mild AD has been established by multiple RCTs for benefits in the domains of cognition, function, global status, and behavior. The ChEI treatment effect sizes for cognition in short-term RCTs appear to be small (Cohen's d: 0.2–0.3 range) but larger than treatment effects on functional measures. There is no Level I grade evidence to support short-term efficacy of memantine monotherapy or combination treatment in mild AD (Schneider et al., 2011).

Level II grade evidence exists for short- and long-term effectiveness of ChEI monotherapy, memantine monotherapy, and memantine add-on combination treatment with a ChEI. Level II grade evidence from clinical effectiveness studies in observational cohorts have supported that long-term clinical treatment benefits are not limited to moderate and later stages of the disease but may be observed in early/mild stages of AD, increased with sustained use and time on treatment, and that rates of cognitive and functional decline are lower now in cohorts treated with antidementia medications than in untreated control or historical cohorts (Atri et al., 2008; Gillette-Guyonnet et al., 2011; Lopez et al., 2009; Rountree et al., 2009; Vellas et al., 2012; Wallin et al., 2011; Wattmo et al., 2011).

For those RCTs that have specifically limited enrollment to those in the mild to moderate stages of AD, the ChEIs have demonstrated significant, if modest, benefits in terms of cognitive and global decline versus placebo (Takeda et al., 2006; Whitehead et al., 2004). Even in those patients who decline substantially while on a ChEI, evidence suggests that the magnitude of decline may be significantly less for patients who are treated than those on placebo (Wilkinson et al., 2009).

Moderate Stage

There is Level I and II support for monotherapy with ChEI and memantine, and combination treatment in the moderate stages of AD dementia (Atri et al., 2008; Feldman et al., 2001; Howard et al., 2012; McShane et al., 2006; Reisberg et al., 2003; Rountree et al., 2009; Tariot et al., 2004). Atri, Molinuevo, and colleagues assessed, by meta-analysis of short-term efficacy RCTs, the benefits of combination treatment with memantine added to baseline donepezil and observed that treatment benefits with effect sizes in the range of 0.2–0.3 were evident in moderate, as well as moderate to severe, stage AD in the domains of cognition, daily function, and global status (Atri et al., 2013).

Moderate to Severe, and Severe Stages

Level I grade evidence from short-term RCTs supports anti-AD medication treatment, in monotherapy or combination therapy, in the moderate to severe and severe stages of AD (Feldman et al., 2001; McShane et al., 2006; Reisberg et al., 2003; Tariot et al., 2004; van Dyck et al., 2007; van de Glind et al., 2013).

Tariot and colleagues' 24-week RCT (Tariot et al., 2004) demonstrated that the combination of memantine added to long-term stable donepezil therapy has beneficial effects on cognition, ADLs, and global function at these stages of AD. Grossberg and colleagues recently reported treatment benefits of memantine add-on combination treatment with any baseline ChEI in multiple domains (Grossberg et al., 2013). Level II grade evidence from multiple studies supports the long-term benefits of antidementia medication treatments in multiple domains (Atri et al., 2008; Gillette-Guyonnet et al., 2011; Howard et al., 2012; Lopez et al., 2009; Rountree et al., 2009; Vellas et al., 2012; Wallin et al., 2011; Wattmo et al., 2011).

Very Severe (Nursing Home) Stage

Treatment benefits of ChEI therapy, even when initiated in individuals in nursing homes with very severe stage dementia, have been demonstrated in RCTs to be of benefit in the domains of cognition, function/ADLs (Winblad et al., 2006), and global function (Black et al., 2007). Similarly, an RCT by Winblad and colleagues (Winblad & Poritis, 1999) reported that initiation of memantine in late-stage nursing home patients with dementia (AD dementia, vascular dementia, or mixed dementia from both) was associated with significant functional improvement and reduction of care dependence.

Persistence, Dose, and Duration of Treatment Are Associated With Better Outcomes

There is evidence that persistence in antidementia therapy—either ChEI monotherapy or combotherapy—results in better cognitive, functional, and disease severity outcomes, even in those with advanced dementia (Atri et al., 2008; Rountree et al., 2009). Higher doses of ChEI (up to the recommended maximums), have been shown to correlate with better long-term cognitive, functional, and global outcomes over 3 years of follow-up (Wallin et al., 2011; Wattmo et al., 2011). Rountree and colleagues calculated that high persistence in adherence to antidementia medication regimens is of 1 point/year benefit in reducing decline in MMSE score, and their data suggest that incremental benefits associated with greater cumulative antidementia treatment may be equivalent to expanding the span of the early and mid-stages of the illness up to 56% or more (Rountree et al., 2009).

Best Practices and Recommendations

The evidence supporting use of ChEIs and memantine reviewed supports, with Level I evidence, initiating a ChEI in the mild stages of AD and adding memantine at the moderate stage. For those not diagnosed until the moderate to severe stages, either a ChEI or memantine can be initiated. Data further support the added benefits of achieving ChEI-memantine add-on combination therapy in moderate and later stages of AD dementia. Level II evidence or equivocal Level I data suggest that treatment with ChEI may also be significantly beneficial in very mild stage AD or for particular subgroups of patients with MCI due to AD (i.e., carriers of APOE-e4 allele; Petersen et al., 2005; those with depression or depressive symptoms; Lu et al., 2005). Such off-FDA label pharmacotherapy is not sufficiently supported by Level I evidence to warrant an unequivocal recommendation for blanket use in all patients. However, available benefit, risk (tolerability and safety) and cost data, individual clinical circumstances, and patient–caregiver dyad preferences warrant prompting a discussion between clinicians, patients, and caregivers about this possibility.

In practice, patients are treated differently depending on their geographic location and what kind of clinician evaluates them (Iliffe, 2007; Vellas et al., 2012). While treatment rates with one or more antidementia medications are on the rise in the United States and elsewhere (Gillette-Guyonnet et al., 2011; Vellas et al., 2012), regrettably, a significant percentage of patients remain untreated with medications at any given stage of AD dementia, and too many patients who are prescribed stop medications within 1–2 years (Alzheimer's-Association, 2013; Sun, Lai, Lu, & Chen, 2008). In the United States, patients are more likely to receive a ChEI and/or memantine when seen in a specialized dementia clinic than if seen in a mental health setting (Rattinger, Mullins, Zuckerman, Onukwugha, & Delisle, 2010). Among US neurologists, most routinely prescribe ChEIs for mild to moderate AD and add memantine later, but some, at least at times, also prescribe

ChEIs in MCI and, less often, memantine for individuals with MCI or mild AD (Roberts, Karlawish, Uhlmann, Petersen, & Green, 2010). Among academic Alzheimer's disease research centers, for those patients followed from early disease stages for 6 years, the dominant practice pattern was to initiate ChEIs in the mild to moderate stages and memantine in the moderate to severe stage (Schneider et al., 2011). A similar pattern was observed in France: Over 90% of patients were treated with anti-AD medications, with a ChEI usually started first and then memantine added in the moderate stages (Gillette-Guyonnet et al., 2011).

Vitamins, Medical Foods, and Supplements

Supplements, including vitamin E, fish oil, and vitamin C, may benefit some patients with AD, although controversy surrounds their efficacy and potential risks.

Vitamin E

Unless contraindicated due to bleeding diatheses, coronary artery disease, or another comorbidity, vitamin E (α-tocopherol 1,000 international units twice daily) may be considered. In a randomized, double-blind, placebo-controlled study of moderately severe AD (n = 341), patients received selegiline, vitamin E, both, or placebo and were followed for 2 years (Sano et al., 1997). The primary outcomes were time to severe dementia, loss of ability to perform ADLs, institutionalization, or death. All active treatment groups had significant delays in the time to primary outcome compared with placebo. A meta-analysis suggested that low-dose vitamin E supplementation (up to 150 IU daily) is associated with less all-cause mortality but that high-dose vitamin E may be associated with a very small increase in relative risk (RR) of mortality (approximately 1.05). However, the subgroup of patients with AD included in this study was observed to have a lower relative risk of mortality associated with high-dose vitamin E supplementation. A large longitudinal observational clinical cohort study also supports that high-dose vitamin E supplementation is not associated with death in patients with AD (Pavlik, Doody, Rountree, & Darby, 2009). Finally, a recently published randomized, double-blind, placebo-controlled trial performed in a U.S. veterans with mild to moderate AD who were already taking a cholinesterase-inhibitor further supported the benefits of high-dose vitamin E (α-tocopherol 1,000 international units twice daily) treatment on slowing functional decline (Dysken et al., 2014). In this multiyear study, decline in activities of daily living was 19% per year slower in the group of subjects who received vitamin E in addition to their background cholinesterase-inhibitor treatment, than in the group of subjects who received placebo in addition to their background cholinesterase-inhibitor. Furthermore, all-cause mortality and safety analyses did not suggest increased risks, compared to placebo, of vitamin E supplementation (Dysken et al., 2014).

Medical Foods

Souvenaid®, a prescription nutritional supplement (also known as medical food), containing Fortasyn® Connect includes precursors (uridine monophosphate; choline; phospholipids; eicosopentaenoic acid; docosahexaenoic acid) and cofactors (vitamins E, C, B12, and B6; folic acid; selenium), which are posited to support synapse synthesis and the formation of neuronal membranes in individuals with AD. Short-term (12- to 24-week) efficacy data have been conflicting and generally do not support significant benefits of Souvenaid® in patients with AD who are being treated with anti-AD medications. Potential signals of very modest benefit were reported in two short-term 12- to 24-week studies in drug-naïve patients with mild AD dementia (N's = 225–259 subjects; mean MMSE 24-25) (Scheltens et al., 2010; Scheltens et al., 2012). However, a very recently reported 24-week study of Souvenaid® added onto baseline anti-AD medications did not show any benefit of slowing cognitive decline in individuals treated for mild-to-moderate AD (Shah et al., 2013). In 527 individuals with mild to moderate AD (mean MMSE score 19.5; SD = 3.1, range 14–24), taking anti-AD medications who were randomized 1:1 to daily, 125 mL (125 kcal) oral intake of the active product (Souvenaid®) or an iso-caloric control, at the 24-week study endpoint, there were no significant differences between treatment groups on the primary outcome of cognition as assessed by the 11-item ADAS-cog subscale

(Shah et al., 2013). In this study, Souvenaid® was, however, well tolerated in combination with standard care anti-AD medications.

Other Vitamins and Supplements

Unfortunately, large RCTs have, thus far, failed to support any significant benefit from ginkgo biloba, high-dose vitamin B_{12}/folic acid combinations, omega-3 fatty acid/fish oil components/preparations, nonsteroidal anti-inflammatory drugs, and statin medications at the dementia stage of AD (Ballard et al., 2011; Tayeb et al., 2012). While epidemiological and Level III/IV grade evidence has suggested potential benefits associated with individuals who take these supplements, all efficacy RCTs in individuals with AD dementia have failed to show benefit.

Practical Implementation of Pharmacotherapy

Unless contraindicated due to conditions, including unstable cardiac arrhythmias, uncontrolled seizures, active peptic ulcer disease and gastrointestinal bleeding, and unexplained syncope, ChEI therapy should be initiated and slowly titrated over months to a maximal clinical or tolerated dose following diagnosis of AD dementia (see Table 16.15). For patients with moderate to severe AD, memantine can be initiated once patients have received stable ChEI therapy for several months without adverse effects (Table 16.15). Memantine monotherapy can be initiated on-label in the United States if the patient has moderate or later stage AD; conversely, a ChEI can be added after several months of stable memantine therapy. The latter may be a particularly useful strategy in patients who are very sensitive to or experience gastrointestinal side effects with ChEIs. In the event of marked AEs, trying a very low and slow titration (e.g., starting donepezil 2.5 mg daily after breakfast; increasing it to 5 mg daily if no side effects emerge within 6 weeks) may be helpful. In highly refractory situations, switching to another ChEI at a low dose can also be tried.

TABLE 16.15 Recommended Dosing for Anti-Alzheimer's Disease Medications

Drug	Dose
Donepezil	Starting dose: 5 mg/day; can be increased to 10 mg/day after 4–6 weeks. Before starting donepezil 23 mg/day, patients should be on donepezil 10 mg/day for at least 3 months.
Rivastigmine	Oral: Starting dose: 1.5 mg twice daily. If well tolerated, the dose may be increased to 3 mg twice daily after 2 weeks. Subsequent increases to 4.5 and 6 mg twice daily should be attempted after 2-week minimums at previous dose. Maximum dose: 6 mg twice daily. Patch: Starting dose: one 4.6 mg patch once daily for a period of 24 hours Maintenance dose: one 9.5 mg or 13.3 mg patch once daily for a period of 24 hours. Before initiating a maintenance dose, patients should undergo a minimum of 4 weeks of treatment at the initial dose (or at the lower patch dose of 9.5 mg) with good tolerability.
Galantamine	Extended-release: Start at 8 mg once daily for 4 weeks; increase to 16 mg once daily for 4weeks; increase to 24 mg once daily. Generic: Start at 4 mg twice daily for 4 weeks; increase to 8 mg twice daily for 4 weeks; increase to 12 mg twice daily.
Memantine	Immediate-release: Starting dose: 5 mg once daily; increase dose in 5-mg increments to a maximum of 20 mg daily (divided doses taken twice daily) with a minimum of 1week between dose increases. The maximum recommended dose in severe renal impairment is 5 mg twice daily. Extended-release: For patients new to memantine, the recommended starting dose of memantine extended release is 7 mg once daily, and the recommended target dose is 28 mg once daily. The dose should be increased in 7 mg increments every seventh day. The minimum recommended interval between dose increases is 1 week, and only if the previous dose has been well tolerated. The maximum recommended dose in severe renal impairment is 14 mg once daily.

All patients should have their vascular risk factors managed diligently. This includes, in at-risk individuals, optimization of lipids (preferably with a statin), blood pressure, and serum glucose, and, if not contraindicated, use of daily enteric-coated baby aspirin (81 mg). There should be screening and ongoing monitoring for anxiety and clinical depression, and when present these should be treated with a trial of an antidepressant—preferably with a selective serotonin reuptake inhibitor with low anticholinergic load and a favorable geriatric profile (e.g., citalopram, sertraline). Sleep and nutrition should be optimized, and any deficiencies (e.g., thyroid, vitamin B_{12}) and systemic conditions that can decompensate mental functions should be treated (e.g., UTI, dehydration, hyponnatremia). Promotion of good health habits, including exercise, nutrition, stress management, adequate sleep, and social and mental engagement, should be actively promoted.

In general, benzodiazepines (e.g., lorazepam used for anxiety or as a sedative-hypnotic) and medications with high anticholinergic activity, for example, those used in the treatment of urinary incontinence, allergies (antihistamines), pain or sleep disorders (e.g., tricyclic antidepressants, diphenhydramine), should be avoided (see Table 16.8). Antipsychotics should be used with great caution and only under specific circumstances (see Chapter 24 and below). Along with psychosocial interventions, a trial of low-dose citalopram (starting low at 10 mg nightly, and increasing after 4-6 weeks, if response is insufficient, to preferably no higher than 20 mg nightly) can be considered in individuals with significant agitation (see below). Stimulants are seldom indicated except for a trial in patients with severe and refractory daytime somnolence or apathy, in which case low-dose modafinil may be tried. However, all stimulants may lower threshold for causing irritability, agitation, aggression, and dysphoria, particularly in individuals who are susceptible. Additionally, one can avoid the common syndrome of "chasing one's tail," which includes prescribing medications that exacerbate a seemingly "separate" condition for which another medication is being prescribed for as treatment. For example, it is not uncommon to come across patients who are treated with increasing numbers and dosages of medications that are activating (e.g., stimulants) and who are also being treated with large dosages of sedative/hypnotics at night in order to induce sleep.

Antipsychotics for Treatment of Severe and Refractory Agitation, Aggression, and Psychosis

Severe agitation, aggression, and psychosis are prevalent BPSDs in advancing AD that can respond to atypical antipsychotics. However, the use of antipsychotics for BPSD in AD dementia is off-label in the United States, and the prescribing information carries a FDA black box warning. Clinicians should resist starting antipsychotics in patients with dementia and only do so when strict conditions have been met, including a careful consideration of risks, benefits, side effects, and alternatives. As antipsychotics can have detrimental effects on cognition, function, and patient safety, they should generally be reserved for a trial in selected patients who are on a multidisciplinary behavioral plan, already on stable background combination therapy, and are under the supervision of a dementia specialist; or when there is an immediate or impending high risk to the safety or well-being of the patient or others.

In the absence of a great immediate or impending safety risk, an alternative pharmacological approach that can be considered is a trial treatment with low-dose citalopram. A very recently published study, the CitAD trial, reported that among AD patients with clinically significant agitation who were receiving psychosocial intervention, the addition of citalopram (started at 10 mg daily and titrated, based on response and tolerability, to 30 mg daily over three weeks) compared with placebo significantly reduced agitation and caregiver distress (Porsteinsson et al., 2014). However, it is cautioned that potential worsening of cognitive functions and emergence of cardiac adverse effects (e.g., prolongation of QT interval) could limit the practical application of citalopram at dosages as high as 30 mg per day. For a more detailed discussion of approaches to treating agitation, aggression and psychosis, see Chapter 24.

When to Start and Stop Anti-Alzheimer's Disease Medications

The questions of when to start and when to stop AD medications are of utmost importance to clinicians, patients, and families. While there is no clear consensus on either front, the question of when to start anti-AD medications appears to be the simpler one to address as there are FDA indications for each drug class. Yet this presupposes that the clinician is adept at appropriately staging dementia severity in all individuals with AD, and that individuals in other stages may not benefit from treatment. As the first caveat, there is no single measure of cognition, function, or behavior that can, in isolation, characterize AD dementia stage in every patient. Staging disease severity should also consider changes from premorbid levels and the impact of the illness on family and caregivers; it requires a multidimensional picture of an individual and depends on a variety of subjective factors. Per US FDA prescribing information, clinicians may start a ChEI in mild, moderate, or severe AD, and memantine in moderate or severe AD. Patients in the moderate stages can be started with a ChEI or memantine, and, ultimately, the complementary agent should be added to achieve combination therapy. As reviewed previously, there are data with lower grades of evidence to support potential benefits of antidementia medication in other stages of AD. Therefore, based on the patient–caregiver dyad preferences and clinician comfort and expertise, an individualized discussion may be prompted regarding the pros and cons, cost and uncertainties of potential off-label prescription of anti-AD medications.

There are no appropriate studies to guide when anti-AD medications should be withdrawn in AD dementia. In addition to other stages, memantine and the ChEIs donepezil and rivastigmine have FDA indications in severe AD—studies support their treatment benefits even in late stages of dementia when patients may require nursing home level of care. It is important for clinicians, caregivers, and families to appreciate that the practical benefits of anti-AD medications in very severe/late-stage AD are no longer aimed at reducing decline in memory and other higher level cognitive functions; these functions are no longer viable. Anti-AD medications can be maintained in late-stage AD with a goal to support basic psychomotor processes; praxis; functional communication; behavioral responses required to assist caregivers to deliver basic care involving feeding, dressing, grooming, and bathing; and the elementary processes of movement, turning, sitting, standing, chewing, and swallowing. The benefits may also extend to reducing antipsychotic usage.

In the end/terminal stages of AD when personhood has disintegrated, and when there is no meaningful communication or interaction, patients should only receive care (pharmacological or otherwise) that is directed to provide palliation and comfort. There is no economic, moral, scientific, or ethical reason for other medications, including anti-AD medications, statins, or for performance of intrusive evaluations and interventions. The health care team must focus on providing an environment that promotes a "good death"; one that fosters, supports, and safeguards the dignity and integrity of the patient's lifelong wishes regarding his or her dying process and also provides the necessary care, consideration, and comfort to the patient's loved ones to prepare and assist them in this process.

Practical Tips for Other Therapeutic Challenges: Sleep-Wake Disturbances, Wandering, Eating Issues, and Incontinence

These challenges posed to caregivers and patients are myriad and often incompletely respond or are suboptimally addressed only by drug interventions (see Chapters 24, 25, and 26 for further discussion and recommendations regarding approaches to common BPSD). Many of these conditions are also incompletely studied and clinical recommendations regarding them often fall in the realm of "evidenced-based opinion" as opposed to being fully supported by evidence-based medicine.

Sleep-Wake Dysregulation

Abnormal or distorted sleep-wake patterns are very common in AD dementia, and they often become worse as the illness progresses. This can lead to significant additional strains on caregivers, such as when patients are awake or wander at night, wake up too early, or sleep most of the day. Patients with significant apathy who experience inactivity during the day and who are not kept engaged may sit around and regularly fall asleep several times during the day. This can produce fragmented and poor quality sleep and lead to a vicious cycle of sleeping/napping several times during the day and difficulty sleeping or awakening during the night or very early morning. A review of systems for obstructive sleep apnea (OSA) should be undertaken, and, if positive, appropriate evaluation and treatment of OSA should be sought, particularly early in the course of dementia. Additionally, in some individuals ChEIs, especially if given at night, can adversely affect sleep by being overly activating, delaying sleep onset, producing very vivid dreams, or affecting low quality sleep.

First-line treatment is nonpharmacological and involves common sleep hygiene strategies. These include keeping the individual awake and physically, socially, and mentally active during the day; avoiding caffeine in the afternoon and nicotine in the evening; limiting naps to at most one 1–1.5 hour scheduled nap in the early afternoon; limiting stimulating activities, exercise, and big meals in the later evening or before bedtime; ensuring that a strict sleep and wake schedule is kept and that the individual is out of bed and dressed in the morning; and ensuring the bedroom is quiet, dark, cool, devoid of TV and other distractions. In refractory situations, melatonin can be tried. In severely refractory cases, pharmacological treatment can include trials of low-dose trazodone (25–50 mg to start; increased to 100 mg at bedtime as needed); zolpidem; or quetiapine or mirtazipine, particularly if these are being considered for pharmacological treatment of coexisting severe refractory agitation, aggression, or psychosis (quetiapine), or anxiety and depression (mirtazipine).

Wandering

A particularly disturbing and dangerous behavioral symptom in individuals with AD dementia is wandering, particularly when it occurs at night or when the patient strays outside in unhospitable conditions. The underlying etiology of wandering should be sought and treated, and it can include anxiety, confusion, lack of physical and social activity, and side effects from medications (e.g., antipsychotics). Medications are unlikely to be of benefit to safely suppress wandering—the individual can become oversedated and then be at higher risk of aspiration and falls. Providing the individual with plenty of engagement and activity (including exercise during the day) and a safe environment to roam (e.g., a fenced back yard, corridors without access to the outside) is key. The use of door locks and alarms that the patient cannot disengage, and disguising routes of entry and egress can also be helpful. Finally, the patient who has a tendency to wander should be provided with a medical identification bracelet and can be registered in a safety program (e.g., the Alzheimer's Association Safe Return program).

Abnormal Eating Behaviors and Eating-Related Problems

Individuals with AD dementia can experience a variety of eating changes and problems that can include overeating, undereating, and abnormal eating behaviors (Ikeda, Brown, Holland, Fukuhara, & Hodges, 2002). Food tastes and preferences can change along with an individual's interest, mood, motivation, energy, appetite, and self-restraint. Changes in an individual's senses of taste and smell are common, and so is a particular craving for sweets. In some individuals with AD or mixed AD dementia, especially in those with particular frontal syndromes, hyperorality, poor impulse control, compulsions, and memory problems can synergize to manifest in binging or overeating (or drinking), and eating and tasting things that inappropriate, inedible, or dangerous. In others, lack of appetite, interest, and activity, and forgetfulness can lead to undereating that results in medically significant dehydration, malnutrition, and frailty.

As always, a root cause analysis should include investigation of potential biopsychosocial causes, particularly medical and medication-relation causes, including thyroid, diabetes and other endocrine abnormalities. Commonly prescribed medications such as antipsychotics (particularly quetiapine), antidepressants (tricyclic antidepressants, SSRIs, mirtazipine), and antiepileptics (valproic acid, gabapentin) can increase appetite and weight gain. Stimulants can have the opposite effect. Behavioral interventions and strategies usually provide the most effective approach. In binge-, compulsive-, and overeaters regulating access to food, drink, and objects provides the most effective strategy. In some cases, cabinets and refrigerators have to be locked, and in other cases, the particular food or drink that is being compulsively consumed has to be rationed and brought into the house in limited quantities. Compulsive eating in some individuals may respond to a trial of SSRI or carbamazepine.

For individuals who are undereating, practical approaches such as providing favorite foods (particularly from childhood); high caloric foods, drinks, and nutritional supplements; eating with the individual (social eating); providing small portions on a large plate and then replenishing it when the portion is eaten; allowing more time for individuals to eat; and serving meals in an environment that is peaceful, uncluttered, and devoid of distractions (e.g., is quiet but has peaceful music in the background) may be effective. In more advanced stage patients, providing supervision at mealtime and finger foods; and ensuring that dental and denture problems and chewing and choking difficulties do not exist can also be helpful. For individuals who are inactive, increasing their activity and facilitating exercise is recommended. If a comorbid condition such as depression or severe agitation is also being treated, then switching to a medication in the same class that also increases appetite, such as mirtazipine or quetiapine, may be tried. Appetite stimulants, such as megestrol and dronabinol, can be tried as a last resort.

Incontinence

Urinary and, particularly, fecal incontinence are very challenging for patients and caregivers. When a medical assessment and medication review eliminates other contributing causes such as a urinary tract infection, prostatic hypetrophy, or a poorly scheduled diuretic dose, then behavioral and environmental strategies are the recommended approach to management of incontinence. These include optimizing the timing of food and fluid intake and coordinating and scheduling bathroom visits with meals, travel, and sleep (e.g., reminding or taking the individuals to the bathroom immediately after meals, then an hour later; before naps; and before travel; limiting fluid intake in the evening, particularly fluids such as caffeinated tea, coffee, and sodas that can act as a diuretic); wearing adult diapers; wearing clothes that are easy to quickly remove (and to clean); facilitating easy access to the bathroom (e.g., clear path and lighting); providing a urinal or bedside commode; using bed or floor pads that are absorbent and easy to clean; and using special incontinence bed sheets (rubber-like). Pelvic floor (Kegel) exercises can be taught and may be of benefit to women and men with urge and stress incontinence or urinary leakage who have sufficient cognitive function. Identifying patterns, clues, and triggers for incontinence can also be helpful. For example, if urinary incontinence occurs at night, one can limit fluid and caffeinated product intake in the later evening, switch a diuretic dose to earlier in the day, and ensure that the individual is not oversedated due to medications or supplements. Unfortunately, common medications prescribed for urinary incontinence in the elderly all have anticholinergic properties (see Table 16.8), effectively counteract ChEIs, and can cause increased confusion in individuals with dementia. In individuals in whom prostatic hypertrophy can contribute to their urinary problems, a trial of low-dose tamsulosin by be tried.

The Therapeutic Glue: The Caregivers, and Caring for Them

Caregivers are the glue in the clinician and patient–caregiver dyad therapeutic relationship. They are "where the rubber meets the road"—no plans for therapeutics and care, no matter how detailed and optimized in theory, can be realized without the caregivers. The importance of forging and maintaining a therapeutic alliance with caregivers in order to provide the best care to the patient–caregiver dyad cannot be understated. The complex biopsychosocial and cultural factors that influence patient care and their effects on caregiver well-being and participation are reviewed in Chapter 27. Caregivers require psychoeducation, support, and care—this can provide meaningful benefits to both patient and caregivers.

The Medication Drift Syndrome

The syndrome of chasing one's tail frequently arises from another syndrome: the medication drift of "subtraction by addition." Many elderly individuals unnecessarily suffer from this syndrome by gradually accumulating, without professional review or discontinuation when appropriate, numerous medications prescribed by a multitude of clinicians and specialists for various and seemingly separate, but in reality related, conditions. Often, medications prescribed for different conditions can have additive effects (e.g., anticholinergic load) to produce deleterious outcomes (e.g., confusion, orthostasis, falls). In some cases the medications are prescribed for complementary or opposite conditions, such as excessive daytime sleep or lethargy versus inability to initiate or maintain asleep at night (e.g., stimulants versus sedative-hypnotics), and produce effects that are counteractive (e.g., anticholinergics prescribed for urinary incontinence and ChEIs prescribed for AD). A good example of this was reported by Tsao and Heilman in the case of an elderly woman who began to experience cognitive and memory problems and hallucinations soon after being prescribed tolterodine, an anticholinergic agent used in the treatment of urinary incontinence (Tsao & Heilman, 2003). Her primary care physician, suspecting that the cognitive and neuropsychiatric symptoms were due to dementia, then prescribed the ChEI donepezil, which resulted in improvement of her memory problems and resolution of her hallucinations. Later, when the patient discontinued the tolterodine, her memory and cognitive improved further. However, upon subsequently reintroducing the tolterodine, her memory and cognitive problems re-emerged, and they did not resolve until this medication was finally discontinued. While this particular patient effectively failed the "anticholinergic stress test" of tolterodine and appeared to be demented, and potentially may have been particularly susceptible due to a subclinical stage of AD or another neurodegenerative dementia, she was, however, not demented at the time, and her symptoms were due to iatrogenesis.

Clinicians should, therefore, adopt a broad and integrative perspective regarding medical conditions and cognitive health to periodically review all medications and supplements and to safely eliminate potentially cognitively deleterious and redundant medications. Medications that appear on Beers Criteria (AGS, 2012) should be particularly avoided and substituted when possible (see Table 16.8). This type of "addition by subtraction" can be a powerful clinical approach to regain seemingly lost cognition and function in individuals with AD dementia, and it should be undertaken periodically, even before anti-AD medications are prescribed.

Recommendations

Evidence- and experience-based opinion supports the following: (1) AD dementia treatments should be individualized based upon an open discussion with the patient and caregivers regarding the prognosis, goals, and expectations of therapy; (2) all discussions should involve clarifying goals and expectations of treatments, make clear which treatments are on-label or off-label, and include an honest assessment of current and future potential benefits, risks, side effects, costs, alternatives, and uncertainties; (3) elimination of redundant and potentially inappropriate medications; (4) initiation and maintenance of anti-AD medications: Level I evidence supports short-term benefits of ChEI-memantine add-on combination therapy in moderate and severe AD, and long-term Level II evidence support that for any individual, irrespective of AD stage, sustained combination therapy may potentially best provide the greatest likelihood of slowing long-term clinical decline; (5) first-line treatment of BPSD involves psychoeducation and behavioral and environmental interventions; the prescription of atypical antipsychotics for BPSD should be reserved for a trial in selected highly refractory patients who are on a multidisciplinary behavioral plan, are already on stable background combination therapy, and are under the supervision of a dementia specialist; or when there is an immediate or impending high risk to the safety or well-being of the patient or others; and (6) maintaining an open-minded, proactive, positive, and flexible individualized approach to compassionately caring for individuals and caregivers that utilizes "thinking and caring on the margin," which is realistic but does not take away hope, and that establishes a strong therapeutic alliance that is holistic and pragmatic and involves psychoeducation; behavioral and environmental approaches to care; planning for current and future care needs; and promoting vascular and general health, psychosocial well-being, safety, and quality of life; and (7) care in the end stages of the illness should be palliative and focus on facilitating a "good death."

References

Albert, M. S., DeKosky, S. T., Dickson, D., Dubois, B., Feldman, H. H., Fox, N. C.,...Phelps, C. H. (2011). The diagnosis of mild cognitive impairment due to Alzheimer's disease: Recommendations from the National Institute on Aging-Alzheimer's Association workgroups on diagnostic guidelines for Alzheimer's disease. *Alzheimers and Dementia,* 7(3), 270–279.

Alzheimer's-Association. (2013). 2013 Alzheimer's disease facts and figures. *Alzheimers and Dementia,* 9(2), 208–245.

American Geriatric Society (AGS). (2012). American Geriatrics Society updated Beers Criteria for potentially inappropriate medication use in older adults. *Journal of the American Geriatrics Society,* 60(4), 616–631.

American Psychiatric Association (APA). *Diagnostic and statistical manual of mental disorders* (5th ed.). Washington, DC: American Psychiatric Publishing.

Atri, A. (2011). Effective pharmacological management of Alzheimer's disease. *American Journal of Managed Care,* 17(Suppl 13), S346–S355.

Atri, A., Locascio, J. J., Lin, J. M., Yap, L., Dickerson, B. C., Grodstein, F.,...Greenberg, S. M. (2005). Prevalence and effects of lobar microhemorrhages in early-stage dementia. *Neurodegener Dis.* (6):305–312.

Atri, A., Molinuevo, J., Lemming, O., Wirth, Y., Pulte, I., & Wilkinson, D. (2013). Memantine in patients with Alzheimer's disease receiving donepezil: New analyses of efficacy and safety for combination therapy. *Alzheimers Research and Therapy,* 5(1), 6.

Atri, A., Rountree, S., Lopez, O., & Doody, R. (2012). Validity, significance, strengths, limitations, and evidentiary value of real-world clinical data for combination therapy in Alzheimer's disease: comparison of efficacy and effectiveness studies. *Neurodegenerative Diseases,* 10(1–4), 170–174.

Atri, A., Shaughnessy, L. W., Locascio, J. J., & Growdon, J. H. (2008). Long-term course and effectiveness of combination therapy in Alzheimer disease. *Alzheimer Disease and Associated Disorders,* 22(3), 209–221.

Atri, A., Sherman, S., Norman, K. A., Kirchhoff, B. A., Nicolas, M. M., Greicius, M. D.,...Stern, C. E. (2004). Blockade of central cholinergic receptors impairs new learning and increases proactive interference in a word paired-associate memory task. *Behavioral Neuroscience,* 118(1), 223–236.

Atri, A., Chang, M. S. & Strichartz, G. R. (2011). Cholinergic pharmacology. In D. Golan, A. Tashjian, E. Armstrong, & A. W. Armstrong (Eds.), *Principles of pharmacology: The pathophysiological basis for drug therapy* (3rd ed., pp. 125–148. Philadelphia, PA: Lippencott & Williams.

Attems, J., Jellinger, K., Thal, D. R., & van Nostrand, W. (2011). Review: Sporadic cerebral amyloid angiopathy. *Neuropathology and Applied Neurobiology,* 37, 75–93.

Bakchine, S., & Loft, H. (2008). Memantine treatment in patients with mild to moderate Alzheimer's disease: Results of a randomised, double-blind, placebo-controlled 6-month study. *Journal of Alzheimers Disease,* 13(1), 97–107.

Ballard, C., Gauthier, S., Corbett, A., Brayne, C., Aarsland, D., & Jones, E. (2011). Alzheimer's disease. *Lancet,* 377(9770), 1019–1031.

Bertram, L., McQueen, M. B., Mullin, K., Blacker, D., & Tanzi, R. E. (2007). Systematic meta-analyses of Alzheimer disease genetic association studies: The AlzGene database. *Nature Genetics,* 39(1), 17–23.

Birks, J. (2006). Cholinesterase inhibitors for Alzheimer's disease. *Cochrane Database of Systematic Reviews,* (1), CD005593.

Black, S. E., Doody, R., Li, H., McRae, T., Jambor, K. M., Xu, Y.,...Richardson, S. (2007). Donepezil preserves cognition and global function in patients with severe Alzheimer disease. *Neurology,* 69(5), 459–469.

Blessed, G., Tomlinson, B. E., & Roth, M. (1968). The association between quantitative measures of dementia and of senile change in the cerebral grey matter of elderly subjects. *British Journal of Psychiatry,* 114, 797–811.

Bordji, K., Becerril-Ortega, J., & Buisson, A. (2011). Synapses, NMDA receptor activity and neuronal abeta production in Alzheimer's disease. *Reviews in the Neurosciences,* 22(3), 285–294.

Braak, H., Alafuzoff, I., Arzberger, T., Kretzschmar, H., & Del Tredici, K. (2006). Staging of Alzheimer disease-associated neurofibrillary pathology using paraffin sections and immunocytochemistry. *Acta Neuropathologica,* 112, 389–404.

Braak, H., & Braak, E. (1991). Neuropathological stageing of Alzheimer-related changes. *Acta Neuropathologica,* 82(4), 239–259.

Buckner, R. L., Andrews-Hanna, J. R., & Schacter, D. L. (2008). The brain's default network: Anatomy, function, and relevance to disease. *Annals of the New York Academy of Sciences*, *1124*, 1–38.

Bullock, R., Bergman, H., Touchon, J., Gambina, G., He, Y., Nagel, J.,...Lane, R. (2006). Effect of age on response to rivastigmine or donepezil in patients with Alzheimer's disease. *Current Medical Research and Opinion*, *22*(3), 483–494.

Bullock, R. (2006). Efficacy and safety of memantine in moderate-to-severe Alzheimer disease: The evidence to date. *Alzheimer Disease and Associated Disorders*, *20*(1), 23–29.

Bullock, R., Touchon, J., Bergman, H., Gambina, G., He, Y., Rapatz, G.,...Lane, R. (2005). Rivastigmine and donepezil treatment in moderate to moderately-severe Alzheimer's disease over a 2-year period. *Current Medical Research and Opinion*, *21*(8), 1317–1327.

Burns, A., Gauthier, S., & Perdomo, C. (2007). Efficacy and safety of donepezil over 3 years: An open-label, multicentre study in patients with Alzheimer's disease. *International Journal of Geriatric Psychiatry*, *22*(8), 806–812.

Cappell, J., Herrmann, N., Cornish, S., & Lanctot, K. L. (2010). The pharmacoeconomics of cognitive enhancers in moderate to severe Alzheimer's disease. *CNS Drugs*, *24*(11), 909–927.

Choi, S. H., Park, K. W., Na, D. L., Han, H. J., Kim, E. J., Shim, Y. S., & Lee, J. H. (2011). Tolerability and efficacy of memantine add-on therapy to rivastigmine transdermal patches in mild to moderate Alzheimer's disease: A multicenter, randomized, open-label, parallel-group study. *Current Medical Research and Opinion*, *27*(7), 1375–1383.

Chou, Y. Y., Lepore, N., Avedissian, C., Madsen, S. K., Parikshak, N., Hua, X.,...Thompson, P. M. (2009). Mapping correlations between ventricular expansion and CSF amyloid and tau biomarkers in 240 subjects with Alzheimer's disease, mild cognitive impairment and elderly controls. *NeuroImage*, *46*(2), 394–410.

Corder, E. H., Saunders, A. M., Strittmatter, W. J., Schmechel, D. E., Gaskell, P. C., Small, G. W.,...Pericak-Vance, M. A. (1993). Gene dose of apolipoprotein E type 4 allele and the risk of Alzheimer's disease in late onset families. *Science*, *261*(5123), 921–923.

Courtney, C., Farrell, D., Gray, R., Hills, R., Lynch, L., Sellwood, E.,...Bentham, P. (2004). Long-term donepezil treatment in 565 patients with Alzheimer's disease (AD2000), randomised double-blind trial. *Lancet*, *363*(9427), 2105–2115.

Cummings, J. L. (2004). Alzheimer's disease. *New England Journal of Medicine*, *351*(1), 56–67.

Cummings, J. L., McRae, T., & Zhang, R. (2006). Effects of donepezil on neuropsychiatric symptoms in patients with dementia and severe behavioral disorders. *American Journal of Geriatric Psychiatry*, *14*(7), 605–612.

Cummings, J. L., Mega, M., Gray, K., Rosenberg-Thompson, S., Carusi, D. A., & Gornbein, J. (1994). The Neuropsychiatric Inventory: Comprehensive assessment of psychopathology in dementia. *Neurology*, *44*(12), 2308–2314.

Cummings, J. L., Schneider, E., Tariot, P. N., & Graham, S. M. (2006). Behavioral effects of memantine in Alzheimer disease patients receiving donepezil treatment. *Neurology*, *67*(1), 57–63.

Cummings, J. L., Schneider, L., Tariot, P. N., Kershaw, P. R., & Yuan, W. (2004). Reduction of behavioral disturbances and caregiver distress by galantamine in patients with Alzheimer's disease. *American Journal of Psychiatry*, *161*(3), 532–538.

Daffner, K. R. (2010). Promoting successful cognitive aging: A comprehensive review. *Journal of Alzheimers Disease*, *19*(4), 1101–1122.

Davies, P. (2000). A very incomplete comprehensive theory of Alzheimer's disease. *Annals of the New York Academy of Sciences*, *924*, 8–16.

Doody, R., Geldmacher, D., Gordon, B., Perdomo, C., & Pratt, R. (2001). Open-label, multicenter, phase 3 extension study of the safety and efficacy of donepezil in patients with Alzheimer disease. *Archives of Neurology*, *58*(3), 427–433.

Doody, R., Wirth, Y., Schmitt, F., & Mobius, H. J. (2004). Specific functional effects of memantine treatment in patients with moderate to severe Alzheimer's disease. *Dementia and Geriatric Cognitive Disorders*, *18*(2), 227–232.

Doody, R. S., Dunn, J. K., Clark, C. M., Farlow, M., Foster, N. L., Liao, T.,...Massman, P. (2001). Chronic donepezil treatment is associated with slowed cognitive decline in Alzheimer's disease. *Dementia and Geriatric Cognitive Disorders*, *12*(4), 295–300.

Doody, R. S., Geldmacher, D. S., Gordon, B., Perdomo, C. A., & Pratt, R. D. (2001). Open-label, multicenter, phase 3 extension study of the safety and efficacy of donepezil in patients with Alzheimer disease. *Archives of Neurology*, *58*(3), 427–433.

Dubois, B., Feldman, H., Jacova, C., DeKosky, S., Barberger-Gateau, P., Cummings, J.,...Scheltens, P. (2007). Research criteria for the diagnosis of Alzheimer's disease: Revising the NINCDS-ADRDA criteria. *Lancet Neurology*, *6*(8), 734–746.

Dubois, B., Feldman, H. H., Jacova, C., Cummings, J. L., Dekosky, S. T., Barberger-Gateau, P.,...Scheltens, P. (2010).

Revising the definition of Alzheimer's disease: A new lexicon. *Lancet Neurology*, *9*(11), 1118–1127.

Dysken, M. W., Sano, M., Asthana, S., Vertrees, J. E., Pallaki, M., Llorente, M.,...Guarino, P. D. (2014). Effect of Vitamin E and Memantine on Functional Decline in Alzheimer Disease. *JAMA*. *311*(1), 33–44.

Farlow, M., Anand, R., Messina, J., Jr., Hartman, R., & Veach, J. (2000). A 52-week study of the efficacy of rivastigmine in patients with mild to moderately severe Alzheimer's disease. *European Neurology*, *44*(4), 236–241.

Farlow, M. R., & Cummings, J. L. (2007). Effective pharmacologic management of Alzheimer's disease. *American Journal of Medicine*, *120*(5), 388–397.

Farlow, M., Veloso, F., Moline, M., Yardley, J., Brand-Schieber, E., Bibbiani, F.,...Satlin, A. (2011). Safety and tolerability of donepezil 23 mg in moderate to severe Alzheimer's disease. *BMC Neurology*, *11*, 57.

Feldman, H., Gauthier, S., Hecker, J., Vellas, B., Subbiah, P., & Whalen, E. (2001). A 24-week, randomized, double-blind study of donepezil in moderate to severe Alzheimer's disease. *Neurology*, *57*, 613–620.

Feldman, H., Schmitt, F., & Olin, J. (2006). Activities of daily living in moderate-to-severe Alzheimer disease: An analysis of the treatment effects of memantine in patients receiving stable donepezil treatment. *Alzheimer Disease and Associated Disorders*, *20*, 263–268.

Feldman, H. H., Van Baelen, B., Kavanagh, S. M., & Torfs, K. E. (2005). Cognition, function, and caregiving time patterns in patients with mild-to-moderate Alzheimer disease: A 12-month analysis. *Alzheimer Disease and Associated Disorders*, *19*(1), 29–36.

Fong, T. G., Jones, R. N., Marcantonio, E. R., Tommet, D., Gross, A. L., Habtemariam, D.,...Inouye, S. K. (2012). Adverse outcomes after hospitalization and delirium in persons with Alzheimer disease. *Annals of Internal Medicine*, *156*(12), 848–856, W296.

Francis, P. T. (2005). The interplay of neurotransmitters in Alzheimer's disease. *CNS Spectrums*, *10*(11 Suppl 18), 6–9.

Fratiglioni, L., Paillard-Borg, S., & Winblad, B. (2004). An active and socially integrated lifestyle in late life might protect against dementia. *Lancet Neurology*, *3*(6), 343–353.

Gauthier, S., Feldman, H., Hecker, J., Vellas, B., Ames, D., Subbiah, P.,...Emir, B. (2002). Efficacy of donepezil on behavioral symptoms in patients with moderate to severe Alzheimer's disease. *International Psychogeriatrics*, *14*(4), 389–404.

Gauthier, S., Loft, H., & Cummings, J. (2008). Improvement in behavioural symptoms in patients with moderate to severe Alzheimer's disease by memantine: A pooled data analysis. *International Journal of Geriatric Psychiatry* 2008 May;*23*(5), 537–545.

Gauthier, S., & Molinuevo, J. L. (2013). Benefits of combined cholinesterase inhibitor and memantine treatment in moderate-severe Alzheimer's disease. *Alzheimers and Dementia*, *9*(3), 326–331.

Getsios, D., Blume, S., Ishak, K. J., & Maclaine, G. D. (2010). Cost effectiveness of donepezil in the treatment of mild to moderate Alzheimer's disease: A UK evaluation using discrete-event simulation. *PharmacoEconomics*, *28*(5), 411–427.

Gillette-Guyonnet, S., Andrieu, S., Cortes, F., Nourhashemi, F., Cantet, C., Ousset, P. J.,...Vellas, B. (2006). Outcome of Alzheimer's disease: potential impact of cholinesterase inhibitors. *Journals of Gerontology Series A, Biological Sciences and Medical Sciences*, *61*(5), 516–520.

Gillette-Guyonnet, S., Andrieu, S., Nourhashemi, F., Gardette, V., Coley, N., Cantet, C.,...Vellas, B. (2011). Long-term progression of Alzheimer's disease in patients under antidementia drugs. *Alzheimers and Dementia*, *7*, 579–92.

Greenberg, S. M., Tennis, M. K., Brown, L. B., Gomez-Isla, T., Hayden, D. L., Schoenfeld, D. A.,...Growdon, J. H. (2000). Donepezil therapy in clinical practice: A randomized crossover study. *Archives of Neurology*, *57*(1), 94–99.

Grossberg, G. T., Manes, F., Allegri, R. F., Gutierrez-Robledo, L. M., Gloger, S., Xie, L.,...Graham, S. M. (2013). The safety, tolerability, and efficacy of once-daily memantine (28 mg): A multinational, randomized, double-blind, placebo-controlled trial in patients with moderate-to-severe Alzheimer's disease taking cholinesterase inhibitors. *CNS Drugs*, *27*(6), 469–478.

Grossberg, G. T., Pejovic, V., Miller, M. L., & Graham, S. M. (2009). Memantine therapy of behavioral symptoms in community-dwelling patients with moderate to severe Alzheimer's disease. *Dementia and Geriatric Cognitive Disorders*, *27*(2), 164–172.

Gurland, B. J., Wilder, D. E., Lantigua, R., Stern, Y., Chen, J., Killeffer, E. H., & Mayeux, R. (1999). Rates of dementia in three ethnoracial groups. *International Journal of Geriatric Psychiatry*, *14*(6), 481–493.

Haass, C., Koo, E. H., Mellon, A., Hung, A. Y., & Selkoe, D. J. (1992). Targeting of cell-surface beta-amyloid precursor protein to lysosomes: Alternative processing

into amyloid-bearing fragments. *Nature, 357*(6378), 500–503.
Hanney, M., Prasher, V., Williams, N., Jones, E. L., Aarsland, D., Corbett, A.,...Ballard, C. (2012). Memantine for dementia in adults older than 40 years with Down's syndrome (MEADOWS): A randomised, double-blind, placebo-controlled trial. *Lancet, 379*(9815), 528–536.
Hardy, J., & Selkoe, D. J. (2002). The amyloid hypothesis of Alzheimer's disease: Progress and problems on the road to therapeutics. *Science, 297*(5580), 353–356.
Hardy, J. A., & Higgins, G. A. (1992). Alzheimer's disease: The amyloid cascade hypothesis. *Science, 256*(5054), 184–185.
Hasselmo, M. E. (2006). The role of acetylcholine in learning and memory. *Current Opinion in Neurobiology, 16*(6), 710–715.
Hebert, L., Beckett, L., Scherr, P., & Evans, D. (2001). Annual incidence of Alzheimer disease in the United States projected to the years 2000 through 2050. *Alzheimer Disease and Associated Disorders, 15*(4), 169.
Hebert, L. E., Scherr, P. A., Bienias, J. L., Bennett, D. A., & Evans, D. A. (2003). Alzheimer disease in the US population: Prevalence estimates using the 2000 census. *Archives of Neurology, 60*(8), 1119–1122.
Hebert, L. E., Weuve, J., Scherr, P. A., & Evans, D. A. (2013). Alzheimer disease in the United States (2010–2050) estimated using the 2010 census. *Neurology, 80*(19), 1778–1783.
Himmelheber, A. M., Sarter, M., & Bruno, J. P. (2000). Increases in cortical acetylcholine release during sustained attention performance in rats. *Brain Research Cognitive Brain Research, 9*(3), 313–325.
Howard, R., McShane, R., Lindesay, J., Ritchie, C., Baldwin, A., Barber, R.,...Phillips, P. (2012). Donepezil and memantine for moderate-to-severe Alzheimer's disease. *New England Journal of Medicine, 366*(10), 893–903.
Hyman, B. T. (2011). Amyloid-dependent and amyloid-independent stages of Alzheimer disease. *Archives of Neurology, 68*(8), 1062–1064.
Hyman, B. T., Phelps, C. H., Beach, T. G., Bigio, E. H., Cairns, N. J., Carrillo, M. C.,...Montine, T. J. (2012). National Institute on Aging-Alzheimer's Association guidelines for the neuropathologic assessment of Alzheimer's disease. *Alzheimers and Dementia, 8*(1), 1–13.
Hyman, B. T., & Trojanowski, J. Q. (1997). Consensus recommendations for the postmortem diagnosis of Alzheimer disease from the National Institute on Aging and the Reagan Institute Working Group on diagnostic criteria for the neuropathological assessment of Alzheimer disease. *Journal of Neuropahtology and Experimental Neurology, 56*(10), 1095–1097.
Ihalainen, J., Sarajarvi, T., Rasmusson, D., Kemppainen, S., Keski-Rahkonen, P., Lehtonen, M.,...Tanila, H. (2011). Effects of memantine and donepezil on cortical and hippocampal acetylcholine levels and object recognition memory in rats. *Neuropharmacology, 61*(5-6), 891–899.
Ikeda, M., Brown, J., Holland, A. J., Fukuhara, R., & Hodges, J. R. (2002). Changes in appetite, food preference, and eating habits in frontotemporal dementia and Alzheimer's disease. *Journal of Neurology, Neurosurgery and Psychiatry, 73*(4), 371–376.
Iliffe, S. (2007). The National Institute for Health and Clinical Excellence (NICE) and drug treatment for Alzheimer's disease. *CNS Drugs, 21*(3), 177–184.
Jack, C. R., Albert, M. S., Knopman, D. S., McKhann, G. M., Sperling, R. A., Carillo, M.,...Phelps, C. H. (2011). Introduction to the recommendations from the National Institute on Aging-Alzheimer's Association workgroups on diagnostic guidelines for Alzheimer's disease. *Alzheimers and Dementia, 7*(3), 257–262.
Jack, C. R., Knopman, D., Jagust, W., Shaw, L. M., Aisen, P. S., Weiner, M.,...Trojanowski, J. Q. (2010). Hypothetical model of dynamic biomarkers of the Alzheimer's pathological cascade. *Lancet, 9*(1), 119–128.
Jellinger, K. A., & Bancher, C. (1998). Neuropathology of Alzheimer's disease: A critical update. *Journal of Neural Transmission, 54*, 77–95.
Jones, B. E. (2005). From waking to sleeping: Neuronal and chemical substrates. *Trends in Pharmacological Sciences, 26*(11), 578–586.
Kales, H. C., Chen, P., Blow, F. C., Welsh, D. E., & Mellow, A. M. (2005). Rates of clinical depression diagnosis, functional impairment, and nursing home placement in coexisting dementia and depression. *American Journal of Geriatric Psychiatry, 13*(6), 441–449.
Katzman, R., Terry, R., DeTeresa, R., Brown, T., Davis, P., Fuld, P.,...Peck, A. (1988). Clinical, pathological, and neurochemical changes in dementia: A subgroup with preserved mental status and numerous neocortical plaques. *Annals of Neurology, 23*, 138–144.
Lace, G., Savva, G. M., Forster, G., de Silva, R., Brayne, C., Matthews, F. E.,...Wharton, S. B. (2009). Hippocampal tau pathology is related to neuroanatomical connections: An ageing population-based study. *Brain, 132*, 1324–1334.
Lipton, S. A. (2007). Pathologically-activated therapeutics for neuroprotection: Mechanism

of NMDA receptor block by memantine and S-nitrosylation. *Current Drug Targets*, 8(5), 621–632.

Livingston, G., & Katona, C. (2004). The place of memantine in the treatment of Alzheimer's disease: A number needed to treat analysis. *International Journal of Geriatric Psychiatry*, 19(10), 919–925.

Lopez, O. L., Becker, J. T., Saxton, J., Sweet, R. A., Klunk, W., & DeKosky, S. T. (2005). Alteration of a clinically meaningful outcome in the natural history of Alzheimer's disease by cholinesterase inhibition. *Journal of the American Geriatrics Society*, 53(1), 83–87.

Lopez, O. L., Becker, J., Wahed, A., Saxton, J., Sweet, R., Wolk, D.,...Dekosky, S. T. (2009a). Long-term effects of the concomitant use of memantine with cholinesterase inhibition in Alzheimer disease. *Journal of Neurology, Neurosurgery and Psychiatry*, 80, 600–607.

Lopez, O. L., Becker, J. T., Whahed, A., Saxton, J. A., Sweet, R. D., Wolk, D.,...Dekosky, S. T. (2009b). Memantine augments the effects of cholinesterase inhibition in the treatment of Alzheimer's disease. *Journal of Neurology, Neurosurgery and Psychiatry.* doi:10.1136/jnnp.2008.158964

Loy, C. T., Schofield, P. R., Turner, A. M., & Kwok, J. B. (2014). Genetics of dementia. *Lancet*, 383(9919), 828–840.

Lu, P. H., Edland, S. D., Teng, E., Tingus, K., Petersen, R. C., & Cummings, J. L. (2009). Donepezil delays progression to AD in MCI subjects with depressive symptoms. *Neurology*, 72(24), 2115–2121.

Lu, S., Hill, J., & Fillit, H. (2005). Impact of donepezil use in routine clinical practice on health care costs in patients with Alzheimer's disease and related dementias enrolled in a large medicare managed care plan: A case-control study. *American Journal of Geriatric Pharmacotherapy*, 3(2), 92–102.

Lyketsos, C. G., Reichman, W. E., Kershaw, P., & Zhu, Y. (2004). Long-term outcomes of galantamine treatment in patients with Alzheimer disease. *American Journal of Geriatric Psychiatry*, 12(5), 473–482.

Margallo-Lana, M. L., Ballard, C., Morris, C., Kay, D., Tyrer, S., & Moore, B. (2003). Cognitive decline in Down syndrome. *Archives of Neurology*, 60(7), 1024; author reply.

McKhann, G., Drachman, D., Folstein, M., Katzman, R., Price, D., & Stadlan, E. M. (1984). Clinical diagnosis of Alzheimer's disease: Report of the NINCDS-ADRDA Work Group under the auspices of Department of Health and Human Services Task Force on Alzheimer's Disease. *Neurology*, 34, 939–944.

McKhann, G. M., Knopman, D. S., Chertkow, H., Hyman, B. T., Jack, C. R., Jr., Kawas, C. H.,...Phelps, C. H. (2011). The diagnosis of dementia due to Alzheimer's disease: Recommendations from the National Institute on Aging-Alzheimer's Association workgroups on diagnostic guidelines for Alzheimer's disease. *Alzheimers and Dementia*, 7(3), 263–269.

McShane, R., Areosa Sastre, A., & Minakaran, N. (2006). Memantine for dementia. *Cochrane Database of Systematic Reviews*, (2), CD003154.

Mitchell, M. B., Shaughnessy, L. W., Shirk, S. D., Yang, F. M., & Atri, A. (2012). Neuropsychological test performance and cognitive reserve in healthy aging and the Alzheimer's disease spectrum: A theoretically driven factor analysis. *Journal of the International Neuropsychological Society*, 18, 1071–1080.

Mohs, R. C., Doody, R. S., Morris, J. C., Ieni, J. R., Rogers, S. L., Perdomo, C. A., & Pratt, R. D. (2001). A 1-year, placebo-controlled preservation of function survival study of donepezil in AD patients. *Neurology*, 57(3), 481–488.

Morris, J. K., & Alberman, E. (2009). Trends in Down's syndrome live births and antenatal diagnoses in England and Wales from 1989 to 2008: Analysis of data from the National Down Syndrome Cytogenetic Register. *British Medical Journal*, 339, b3794.

Okura, T., Plassman, B. L., Steffens, D. C., Llewellyn, D. J., Potter, G. G., & Langa, K. M. (2012). Neuropsychiatric symptoms and the risk of institutionalization and death: The aging, demographics, and memory study. *Journal of the American Geriatrics Society*, 59(3), 473–481.

Parameshwaran, K., Dhanasekaran, M., & Suppiramaniam, V. (2008). Amyloid beta peptides and glutamatergic synaptic dysregulation. *Experimental Neurology*, 210(1), 7–13.

Parsons, C. G., Danysz, W., Dekundy, A., & Pulte, I. (2013). Memantine and cholinesterase inhibitors: Complementary mechanisms in the treatment of Alzheimer's disease. *Neurotoxicity Research*, 24(3), 358–369.

Parvizi, J., Van Hoesen, G. W., & Damasio, A. (2001). The selective vulnerability of brainstem nuclei to Alzheimer's disease. *Annals of Neurology*, 49, 53–66.

Patel, L., & Grossberg, G. (2011). Combination therapy for Alzheimer's disease. *Drugs and Aging*, 28, 539–546.

Pavlik, V. N., Doody, R. S., Rountree, S. D., & Darby, E. J. (2009). Vitamin E use is associated with improved survival in an Alzheimer's disease cohort. *Dementia and Geriatric Cognitive Disorders*, 28(6), 536–540.

Peskind, E. R., Potkin, S. G., Pomara, N., Ott, B. R., Graham, S. M., Olin, J. T., & McDonald, S. (2006). Memantine treatment in mild to moderate Alzheimer disease: A 24-week randomized, controlled trial. *American Journal of Geriatric Psychiatry*, 14(8), 704–715.

Petersen, R. C., Aisen, P., Boeve, B. F., Geda, Y. E., Ivnik, R. J., Knopman, D. S.,...Jack, C. R., Jr. (2013). Criteria for mild cognitive impairment due to Alzheimer's disease in the community. *Annals of Neurology*. doi: 10.1002/ana.23931.

Petersen, R. C., Thomas, R. G., Grundman, M., Bennett, D., Doody, R., Ferris, S.,...Thal, L. J. (2005). Vitamin E and donepezil for the treatment of mild cognitive impairment. *New England Journal of Medicine*, 352(23), 2379–2388.

Plassman, B. L., Langa, K. M., Fisher, G. G., Heeringa, S. G., Weir, D. R., Ofstedal, M. B.,...Wallace, R. B. (2007). Prevalence of dementia in the United States: The aging, demographics, and memory study. *Neuroepidemiology*, 29(1-2), 125–132.

Porsteinsson, A. P., Grossberg, G. T., Mintzer, J., & Olin, J. T. (2008). Memantine treatment in patients with mild to moderate Alzheimer's disease already receiving a cholinesterase inhibitor: A randomized, double-blind, placebo-controlled trial. *Current Alzheimer Research*, 5(1), 83–89.

Porsteinsson, A. P., Drye, L. T., Pollock, B. G., Devanand, D. P., Frangakis, C., Ismail, Z.,...Lyketsos, C. G.; CitAD Research Group (2014). Effect of citalopram on agitation in Alzheimer disease: the CitAD randomized clinical trial. *JAMA.* 311(7), 682–691.

Potter, G. G., Plassman, B. L., Burke, J. R., Kabeto, M. U., Langa, K. M., Llewellyn, D. J.,...Steffens, D. C. (2009). Cognitive performance and informant reports in the diagnosis of cognitive impairment and dementia in African Americans and whites. *Alzheimers and Dementia*, 5(6), 445–453.

Prince, M., Prina, M., & Guerchet, M. (2013). The World Alzheimer Report 2013. Journey of caring: An analysis of long-term care for dementia. *Alzheimer's Disease International*. Retrieved March 2014, from http://www.alz.co.uk/research/WorldAlzheimerReport2013.pdf.

Puangthong, U., & Hsiung, G. Y. (2009). Critical appraisal of the long-term impact of memantine in treatment of moderate to severe Alzheimer's disease. *Neuropsychiatric Disease and Treatment*, 5, 553–561.

Raina, P., Santaguida, P., Ismaila, A., Patterson, C., Cowan, D., Levine, M.,...Oremus, M. (2008). Effectiveness of cholinesterase inhibitors and memantine for treating dementia: Evidence review for a clinical practice guideline. *Annals of Internal Medicine*, 148(5), 379–397.

Raschetti, R., Albanese, E., Vanacore, N., & Maggini, M. (2007). Cholinesterase inhibitors in mild cognitive impairment: A systematic review of randomised trials. *PLoS Medicine*, 4(11), e338.

Raskind, M. A., Peskind, E. R., Truyen, L., Kershaw, P., & Damaraju, C. V. (2004). The cognitive benefits of galantamine are sustained for at least 36 months: A long-term extension trial. *Archives of Neurology*, 61(2), 252–256.

Raskind, M. A., Peskind, E. R., Wessel, T., & Yuan, W. (2000). Galantamine in AD: A 6-month randomized, placebo-controlled trial with a 6-month extension. The Galantamine USA-1 Study Group. *Neurology*, 54, 2261–2268.

Rattinger, G. B., Mullins, C. D., Zuckerman, I. H., Onukwugha, E., & Delisle, S. (2010). Clinic visits and prescribing patterns among Veterans Affairs Maryland Health Care System dementia patients. *Journal of Nutrition, Health and Aging*, 14(8), 677–683.

Reisberg, B., Doody, R., Stoffler, A., Schmitt, F., Ferris, S., & Mobius, H. J. (2003). Memantine in moderate-to-severe Alzheimer's disease. *New England Journal of Medicine*, 348(14), 1333–1341.

Reisberg, B., Doody, R., Stoffler, A., Schmitt, F., Ferris, S., & Mobius, H. J. (2006). A 24-week open-label extension study of memantine in moderate to severe Alzheimer disease. *Archives of Neurology*, 63(1), 49–54.

Rentz, D. M., Locascio, J. J., Becker, J. A., Moran, E. K., Eng, E., Buckner, R. L.,...Johnson, K. A. (2010). Cognition, reserve, and amyloid deposition in normal aging. *Annals of Neurology*, 67(3), 353–364.

Riedel, G., Platt, B., & Micheau, J. (2003). Glutamate receptor function in learning and memory. *Behavioural Brain Research*, 140(1-2), 1–47.

Roberts, J. S., Karlawish, J. H., Uhlmann, W. R., Petersen, R. C., & Green, R. C. (2010). Mild cognitive impairment in clinical care: A survey of American Academy of Neurology members. *Neurology*, 75(5), 425–431.

Rockwood, K. (2004). Size of the treatment effect on cognition of cholinesterase inhibition in Alzheimer's disease. *Journal of Neurology, Neurosurgery and Psychiatry*, 75(5), 677–685.

Rogaeva, E., Meng, Y., Lee, J. H., Gu, Y., Kawarai, T., Zou, F.,...St George-Hyslop, P. (2007). The neuronal sortilin-related receptor SORL1 is genetically associated with Alzheimer disease. *Nature Genetics*, 39(2), 168–177.

Rogers, S., Doody, R., Pratt, R., & Ieni, J. (2000). Long-term efficacy and safety of donepezil in the treatment of Alzheimer's disease: Final analysis of a US multicentre open-label study. *European Neuropsychopharmacology*, 10(3), 195–203.

Rountree, S., Chan, W., Pavlik, V., Darby, E., & Doody, R. (2012). Factors that influence survival in a probable Alzheimer disease cohort. *Alzheimers Research and Therapy*, 4(3), 16.

Rountree, S. D., Atri, A., Lopez, O. L., & Doody, R. S. Effectiveness of antidementia drugs in delaying Alzheimer disease progression. *Alzheimers and Dementia*, 9(3), 338–345.

Rountree, S. D., Chan, W., Pavlik, V. N., Darby, E. J., Siddiqui, S., & Doody, R. S. (2009). Persistent treatment with cholinesterase inhibitors and/or memantine slows clinical progression of Alzheimer disease. *Alzheimers Research and Therapy*, 1(2), 7.

Rudolph, J. L., Inouye, S. K., Jones, R. N., Yang, F. M., Fong, T. G., Levkoff, S. E., & Marcantonio, E. R. (2010). Delirium: An independent predictor of functional decline after cardiac surgery. *Journal of the American Geriatrics Society*, 58(4), 643–649.

Rudolph, J. L., Marcantonio, E. R., Culley, D. J., Silverstein, J. H., Rasmussen, L. S., Crosby, G. J.,...Inouye, S. K. (2008). Delirium is associated with early postoperative cognitive dysfunction. *Anaesthesia*, 63(9), 941–947.

Rudolph, J. L., Salow, M. J., Angelini, M. C., & McGlinchey, R. E. (2008). The anticholinergic risk scale and anticholinergic adverse effects in older persons. *Archives of Internal Medicine*, 168(5), 508–513.

Salloway, S., Ferris, S., Kluger, A., Goldman, R., Griesing, T., Kumar, D., & Richardson, S. (2004). Efficacy of donepezil in mild cognitive impairment: A randomized placebo-controlled trial. *Neurology*, 63(4), 651–657.

Salthouse, T. A. (2009). When does age-related cognitive decline begin? *Neurobiology of Aging*, 30(4), 507–514.

Sano, M., Ernesto, C., Thomas, R. G., Klauber, M. R., Schafer, K., Grundman, M.,...Thal, L. J. (1997). A controlled trial of selegiline, alpha-tocopherol, or both as treatment for Alzheimer's disease. The Alzheimer's Disease Cooperative Study. *New England Journal of Medicine*, 336(17), 1216–1222.

Saxena, S. (2012). *Dementia world report: A public health priority*. Geneva, Switzerland: World Health Organization.

Saxton, J., Hofbauer, R. K., Woodward, M., Gilchrist, N. L., Potocnik, F., Hsu, H. A.,...Perhach, J. L. (2012). Memantine and functional communication in Alzheimer's disease: Results of a 12-week, international, randomized clinical trial. *Journal of Alzheimers Disease*, 28(1), 109–118.

Scheltens, P., Kamphuis, P. J., Verhey, F. R., Olde Rikkert, M. G., Wurtman, R. J., Wilkinson, D.,...Kurz, A. (2010). Efficacy of a medical food in mild Alzheimer's disease: A randomized, controlled trial. *Alzheimers and Dementia*, 6(1), 1–10 e1.

Scheltens, P., Twisk, J. W., Blesa, R., Scarpini, E., von Arnim, C. A., Bongers, A.,...Kamphuis, P. J. (2012). Efficacy of Souvenaid in mild Alzheimer's disease: Results from a randomized, controlled trial. *Journal of Alzheimers Disease*, 31(1), 225–236.

Scherzer, C. R., Offe, K., Gearing, M., Rees, H. D., Fang, G., Heilman, C. J.,...Lah, J. J. (2004). Loss of apolipoprotein E receptor LR11 in Alzheimer disease. *Archives of Neurology*, 61(8), 1200–1205.

Schmitt, F. A., van Dyck, C. H., Wichems, C. H., & Olin, J. T. (2006). Cognitive response to memantine in moderate to severe Alzheimer disease patients already receiving donepezil: An exploratory reanalysis. *Alzheimer Disease and Associated Disorders*, 20(4), 255–262.

Schneider, L. S., Dagerman, K. S., Higgins, J. P., & McShane, R. (2011). Lack of evidence for the efficacy of memantine in mild Alzheimer disease. *Archives of Neurology*, 68(8), 991–998.

Schneider, L. S., Insel, P. S., & Weiner, M. W. (2011). Treatment with cholinesterase inhibitors and memantine of patients in the Alzheimer's Disease Neuroimaging Initiative. *Archives of Neurology*, 68(1), 58–66.

Selkoe, D. J. (1991). Amyloid protein and Alzheimer's disease. *Scientific American*, 265(5), 68–71, 4–6, 8.

Selkoe, D. J., Abraham, C. R., Podlisny, M. B., & Duffy, L. K. (1986). Isolation of low-molecular-weight proteins from amyloid plaque fibers in Alzheimer's disease. *Journal of Neurochemistry*, 46(6), 1820–1834.

Seshadri, S., Wolf, P. A., Beiser, A., Au, R., McNulty, K., White, R., & D'Agostino, R. B. (1997). Lifetime risk of dementia and Alzheimer's disease. The impact of mortality on risk estimates in the Framingham Study. *Neurology*, 49(6), 1498–1504.

Shah, R. C., Kamphuis, P. J., Leurgans, S., Swinkels, S. H., Sadowsky, C. H., Bongers, A.,...Bennett, D. A. (2013). The S-Connect study: Results from a randomized, controlled trial of Souvenaid in mild-to-moderate Alzheimer's disease. *Alzheimers Research and Therapy*, 5(6), 59.

Shaw, G. (2012). Two drugs are not better than one for treating moderate to severe Alzheimer disease, British investigators report: Why some US neurologists don't agree. *Neurology Today*, 12, 12–13.

Snowden, J. S., Thompson, J. C., Stopford, C. L., Richardson, A. M., Gerhard, A., Neary, D., & Mann, D. M. (2011). The clinical diagnosis of early-onset dementias: diagnostic accuracy and clinicopathological relationships. *Brain*, 134(Pt 9), 2478–2492.

Sperling, R. A., Aisen, P. S., Beckett, L. A., Bennett, D. A., Craft, S., Fagan,

A. M., ... Phelps, C. H. (2011). Toward defining the preclinical stages of Alzheimer's disease: Recommendations from the National Institute on Aging-Alzheimer's Association workgroups on diagnostic guidelines for Alzheimer's disease. *Alzheimers and Dementia, 7*(3), 280–292.

Stefanacci, R. G. (2007). Current implications for the managed care of dementia. *American Journal of Managed Care, 13*(Suppl 8), S203–S205; discussion S6–S7.

Stern, Y. (2009). Cognitive reserve. *Neuropsychologia, 47*, 2015–2028.

Stern, Y., Gurland, B., Tatemichi, T. K., Tang, M. X., Wilder, D., & Mayeux, R. (1994). Influence of education and occupation on the incidence of Alzheimer's disease. *Journal of the American Medical Association, 271*(13), 1004–1010.

Sun, Y., Lai, M. S., Lu, C. J., & Chen, R. C. (2008). How long can patients with mild or moderate Alzheimer's dementia maintain both the cognition and the therapy of cholinesterase inhibitors: A national population-based study. *European Journal of Neurology, 15*(3), 278–283.

Takeda, A., Loveman, E., Clegg, A., Kirby, J., Picot, J., Payne, E., & Green, C. (2006). A systematic review of the clinical effectiveness of donepezil, rivastigmine and galantamine on cognition, quality of life and adverse events in Alzheimer's disease. *International Journal of Geriatric Psychiatry, 21*(1), 17–28.

Tariot, P. N., Farlow, M. R., Grossberg, G. T., Graham, S. M., McDonald, S., & Gergel, I. (2004). Memantine treatment in patients with moderate to severe Alzheimer disease already receiving donepezil: a randomized controlled trial. *Journal of the American Medical Association, 291*(3), 317–324.

Tayeb, H., Yang, H., Price, B., & Tarazi, F. (2012). Pharmacotherapies for Alzheimer's disease: Beyond cholinesterase inhibitors. *Pharmacology and Therapeutics, 134*, 8–25.

Thal, D. R., Rub, U., Orantes, M., & Braak, H. (2002). Phases of A beta-deposition in the human brain and its relevance for the development of AD. *Neurology* 2002 Jun 25;*58*(12), 1791–1800.

Tompa, R. (Ed.) (2013). DSM-5: Debated? Yes. Important for AD diagnosis? Maybe not. June 13, Alzheimer Research Forum.

Tsao, J. W., & Heilman, K. M. (2003). Transient memory impairment and hallucinations associated with tolterodine use. *New England Journal of Medicine, 349*(23), 2274–2275.

van de Glind, E. M., van Enst, W. A., van Munster, B. C., Olde Rikkert, M. G., Scheltens, P., Scholten, R. J., & Hooft, L. (2013). Pharmacological treatment of dementia: A scoping review of systematic reviews. *Dementia and Geriatric Cognitive Disorders, 36*(3-4), 211–228.

van Dyck, C. H., Tariot, P. N., Meyers, B., & Malca Resnick, E. (2007). A 24-week randomized, controlled trial of memantine in patients with moderate-to-severe Alzheimer disease. *Alzheimer Disease and Associated Disorders, 21*(2), 136–143.

Vellas, B., Hausner, L., Frolich, L., Cantet, C., Gardette, V., Reynish, E., ... Andrieu, S. (2012). Progression of Alzheimer disease in Europe: Data from the European ICTUS study. *Current Alzheimer Research, 9*(8), 902–912.

Vincent, G., & Velkof, V. (2010). *The next four decades: The older population in the United States: 2010 to 2050.* Washington, DC: US Census Bureau.

Wallin, A., Andreasen, N., Eriksson, S., Batsman, S., Nasman, B., Ekdahl, A., ... Minthon, L. (2007). Donepezil in Alzheimer's disease: What to expect after 3 years of treatment in a routine clinical setting. *Dementia and Geriatric Cognitive Disorders, 23*, 150–160.

Wallin, A., Gustafson, L., Sjogren, M., Wattmo, C., & Minthon, L. (2004). Five-year outcome of cholinergic treatment of Alzheimer's disease: Early response predicts prolonged time until nursing home placement, but does not alter life expectancy. *Dementia and Geriatric Cognitive Disorders* 2004; *18*(2), 197–206.

Wallin, A. K., Wattmo, C., & Minthon, L. (2011). Galantamine treatment in Alzheimer's disease: response and long-term outcome in a routine clinical setting. *Neuropsychiatric Disease and Treatment, 7*, 565–576.

Wattmo, C., Wallin, A. K., Londos, E., & Minthon, L. (2011a). Long-term outcome and prediction models of activities of daily living in Alzheimer disease with cholinesterase inhibitor treatment. *Alzheimer Disease and Associated Disorders, 25*(1), 63–72.

Wattmo, C., Wallin, A. K., Londos, E., & Minthon L. (2011b). Predictors of long-term cognitive outcome in Alzheimer's disease. *Alzheimers Research and Therapy, 3*(4), 23.

Weintraub, S., Dikmen, S. S., Heaton, R. K., Tulsky, D. S., Zelazo, P. D., Bauer, P. J., ... Gershon, R. C. (2013). Cognition assessment using the NIH Toolbox. *Neurology, 80*(11 Suppl 3), S54–S64.

Weycker, D., Taneja, C., Edelsberg, J., Erder, M. H., Schmitt, F. A., Setyawan, J., & Oster, G. (2007). Cost-effectiveness of memantine in moderate-to-severe Alzheimer's disease patients receiving donepezil. *Current Medical Research and Opinion, 23*(5), 1187–1197.

Whitehead, A., Perdomo, C., Pratt, R. D., Birks, J., Wilcock, G. K., & Evans, J. G. (2004). Donepezil for the symptomatic treatment of patients with mild to moderate Alzheimer's disease: A meta-analysis of individual patient data from randomised controlled trials. *International Journal of Geriatric Psychiatry, 19*(7), 624–633.

Wilcock, G., Ballard, C., Cooper, J., & Loft, H. (2008). Memantine for agitation/aggression and psychosis in moderately severe to severe Alzheimer's disease: A pooled analysis of 3 studies. *Journal of Clinical Psychiatry, 69*, 341–348.

Wilcock, G., Howe, I., Coles, H., Lilienfeld, S., Truyen, L., Zhu, Y.,…Kershaw, P. (2003). A long-term comparison of galantamine and donepezil in the treatment of Alzheimer's disease. *Drugs and Aging, 20*(10), 777–789.

Wilkinson, D., & Andersen, H. (2007). Analysis of the effect of memantine in reducing the worsening of clinical symptoms in patients with moderate to severe Alzheimer's disease. *Dementia and Geriatric Cognitive Disorders, 24*, 138–145.

Wilkinson, D., Schindler, R., Schwam, E., Waldemar, G., Jones, R. W., Gauthier, S.,…Feldman, H. H. (2009). Effectiveness of donepezil in reducing clinical worsening in patients with mild-to-moderate alzheimer's disease. *Dementia and Geriatric Cognitive Disorders, 28*(3), 244–251.

Wilson, R. S., Leurgans, S. E., Boyle, P. A., & Bennett, D. A. (2011). Cognitive decline in prodromal Alzheimer disease and mild cognitive impairment. *Archives of Neurology* 2011 Mar;*68*(3), 351–356.

Wimo, A., & Prince, M. (2010). The World Alzheimer Report 2010: The global impact of dementia. *Alzheimer's Disease International*. Retrieved March 2014, from http://www.alz.org/documents/national/world_alzheimer_report_2010.pdf.

Wimo, A., Winblad, B., Stoffler, A., Wirth, Y., & Mobius, H. J. (2003). Resource utilisation and cost analysis of memantine in patients with moderate to severe Alzheimer's disease. *PharmacoEconomics, 21*(5), 327–340.

Winblad, B., Black, S., Homma, A., Schwam, E., Moline, M., Xu, Y.,…Albert, K. (2009). Donepezil treatment in severe Alzheimer's disease: A pooled analysis of three clinical trials. *Current Medical Research and Opinion, 25*, 2577–2587.

Winblad, B., Jones, R., Wirth, Y., Stoffler, A., & Mobius, H. (2007). Memantine in moderate to severe Alzheimer's disease: A meta-analysis of randomised clinical trials. *Dementia and Geriatric Cognitive Disorders, 24*, 20–27.

Winblad, B., Kilander, L., Eriksson, S., Minthon, L., Batsman, S., Wetterholm, A. L.,…Haglund, A. (2006). Donepezil in patients with severe Alzheimer's disease: Double-blind, parallel-group, placebo-controlled study. *Lancet, 367*(9516), 1057–1065.

Winblad, B., & Poritis, N. (1999). Memantine in severe dementia: Results of the 9M-Best Study (Benefit and efficacy in severely demented patients during treatment with memantine). *International Journal of Geriatric Psychiatry, 14*(2), 135–146.

Wise, L. E., & Lichtman, A. H. (2007). The uncompetitive N-methyl-D-aspartate (NMDA) receptor antagonist memantine prolongs spatial memory in a rat delayed radial-arm maze memory task. *European Journal of Pharmacology, 575*(1-3), 98–102.

Yamada, K., Takayanagi, M., Kamei, H., Nagai, T., Dohniwa, M., Kobayashi, K.,…Nabeshima, T. (2005). Effects of memantine and donepezil on amyloid beta-induced memory impairment in a delayed-matching to position task in rats. *Behavioural Brain Research, 162*(2), 191–199.

Ziegler-Graham, K., Brookmeyer, R., Johnson, E., & Arrighi, H. M. (2008). Worldwide variation in the doubling time of Alzheimer's disease incidence rates. *Alzheimers and Dementia, 4*(5), 316–323.

Zlokovic, B. V. (2011). Neurovascular pathways to neurodegeneration in Alzheimer's disease and other disorders. *Nature Reviews Neuroscience, 12*(12), 723–738.

17

Mild Cognitive Impairment

Meredith Wicklund and Ronald C. Petersen

The field of aging and dementia is moving toward an earlier identification of symptomatic subjects with the intent to identify individuals as soon as possible in the pathophysiologic process of disorders such as Alzheimer's disease (AD), and a great deal of effort is being expended toward detecting individuals early in the symptomatic disease process (Petersen et al., 1999). With the recent publication of sets of criteria for individuals along the AD spectrum, dementia is the most advanced stage while mild cognitive impairment (MCI) constitutes the earliest manifestation of clinical symptoms. In addition to dementia and MCI, a preclinical stage was also proposed as being useful for identifying individuals with the biological predisposition to AD but being clinically asymptomatic (Jack et al., 2012; Knopman et al., 2012; Sperling et al., 2011).

Brief History of the Mild Cognitive Impairment Construct

The construct of MCI has risen and become popular over the past 15 years (Petersen et al., 2009). Initially, investigators at New York University used the term "MCI" to characterize individuals whom they designated as being at Stage 3 on the Global Deterioration Scale (Reisberg et al., 1988). The construct was limited to individuals with that particular degree of severity on the scale, but the clinical criteria were not clearly delineated.

In 1999, investigators at the Mayo Clinic published criteria for memory-impaired individuals who did not meet criteria for dementia and called them MCI. These criteria are shown in Table 17.1 and became heavily investigated in the field to determine their validity. The criteria emphasized a change in memory function for individuals from their prior level of performance, and yet other cognitive domains such as language, attention, executive function, and visuospatial skills were preserved. Functionally, the individuals were essentially normal without the degree of loss of social or occupational function consistent with dementia. These subjects were followed longitudinally and were shown to have an increased risk of developing subsequent dementia.

In 2003, an international conference was held in Stockholm to expand the construct of MCI and determine its relevance for the field (Petersen, 2004; Winblad et al., 2004). At that time, MCI was divided into two subclasses, amnestic MCI (aMCI) and non-amnestic MCI (naMCI). The aMCI subtype essentially conformed to the 1999 criteria cited and characterized a set of individuals

TABLE 17.1 Criteria for Amnestic Mild Cognitive Impairment—1999

1. Cognitive concern
2. Objective impairment in memory
3. Relative preservation of nonmemory cognitive functions
4. Preservation of activities of daily living
5. Not demented

who had a primary memory impairment with relative preservation of other cognitive domains and function. Technically, these individuals could also be slightly impaired in other cognitive domains such as executive function, and as such, the constructs of aMCI single domain (memory only) and multidomain (memory plus one or more other cognitive domains) were established. However, if the individual was judged to be between normal cognition and dementia but not have significant memory impairment, the naMCI label was given with the additional qualifiers of single and multiple domains. Over the ensuing years, these entities were investigated quite extensively, and general support for the entity was achieved, but notable concerns were also raised. These criteria were also used for several epidemiologic explorations (Busse, Hensel, Guhne, Angermeyer, & Riedel-Heller, 2006; Di Carlo et al., 2007; Manly et al., 2008).

Epidemiology of Mild Cognitive Impairment

Numerous epidemiologic studies have been conducted internationally to determine the frequency of MCI (Ganguli, Dodge, Shen, & DeKosky, 2004; Lopez et al., 2003; Ritchie, Artero, & Touchon, 2001; Unverzagt et al., 2001; Larrieu et al., 2002). In general, the prevalence figures have varied from 3% to 30% in the literature with most studies coalescing around 15% (Ganguli et al., 2004; Lopez et al., 2003; Petersen et al., 2010). Numerous methodologic issues contributed to the variable prevalence rates reported in the literature, including the nature of the underlying population, the specific implementation of the criteria for MCI, and whether the studies were performed retrospectively or prospectively. In recent years, prospective studies employing MCI criteria at the outset have tended to report results in the 10%–20% range, and these figures are generally accepted (Manly et al., 2008).

Incidence studies for the conversion from normal cognition to MCI have only recently been reported and characterize subjects who have been tracked from being clinically normal to newly diagnosed with MCI (Larrieu et al., 2002; Roberts et al., 2012). Again, there is a great deal of variability in this literature, but the majority of the studies have indicated an annual incidence rate of from 3% to 10% per year (Roberts et al., 2012). As such, the incidence rates are significant and have implications for aging societies around the world.

Clinical Characterization

Clinical Vignette

Part 1

A 68-year-old businesswoman with a master's degree began noting increasing forgetfulness for recent events. She had been having some problems coming up with the names of acquaintances with whom she had not had contact for several months, but perhaps more bothersome to her was the fact that she was occasionally missing appointments. She was quite meticulous about her daily calendar but now was overlooking important appointments, which was uncharacteristic of her. When her husband was questioned about this, he indicated that he had noticed the same behaviors in her but was not concerned about them. They both noted that she continued to run her business quite well without any problems, and those around her who had been working closely with her had not noticed a change. On a personal level, she still handled her own finances, was driving, and showed no signs of depression or anxiety. She came for a clinical evaluation, and the history, in addition to the above, revealed that her maternal grandmother had developed dementia in her late 70s, but otherwise, there was no other dramatic history for cognitive impairment. She was on medications for hyperlipidemia and a calcium supplement. Her clinical assessment revealed a Mini-Mental State Exam score of 28, and the remainder of the neurologic examination was normal.

At this point, do you reassure her that she is manifesting signs of aging but nothing more worrisome, or do you pursue it further?

The clinician wanted to obtain neuropsychological testing to get a more complete picture of the woman's cognitive profile. The testing revealed summary scores in the area of executive function and attention at the 60th percentile for her age and education. Comparable measures on language (70th percentile) and visuospatial skills (65th percentile) were above what would be expected. Her memory profile, however, including several measures of delayed verbal and nonverbal recall indicated performance at the 40th percentile. As such, this clinical profile corroborated her and her husband's concern and raised a suspicion of amnestic mild cognitive impairment.

What Does the Clinician Do at This Point?

Figure 17.1 depicts the general evaluation scheme for an individual suspected of having MCI (Petersen, 2004). Typically, a patient will present to a clinician with a concern about a new memory problem, and the clinician's obligation is to determine whether this is a manifestation of aging or may represent the earliest stages of a pathologic condition. As is indicated in Figure 17.1, the clinician should start with the history, preferably from the patient and someone who knows the patient well, and examination in the office. This can involve a mental status exam such as the Mini-Mental State Exam (Folstein, Folstein, & McHugh, 1975), the Short Test of Mental Status (Kokmen, Naessens, & Offord, 1987), or the Montreal Cognitive Assessment (Nasreddine et al., 2005), among others, but it should be augmented by additional tools to determine the presence and extent of cognitive impairments since the global screening instruments may be insensitive, particularly in individuals with a high level of educational or occupational attainment (Lonie, Tierney, & Ebmeier, 2009). Neuropsychological testing can be quite useful in this regard since it will provide a more thorough characterization of cognitive function in multiple domains as well as the degree of impairment if one exists (Petersen et al., 2010). Preferably, neuropsychological testing should be used in the setting of appropriate normative data for the patient's age, education, and ethnicity. Often in the clinical setting, the individual is seen at one time point and a diagnosis needs to be made. However, if longitudinal data are available, they can be very helpful in assessing change for a given individual with respect to his or her own baseline. The criteria for MCI require the clinician to assess whether or not there has been a change in cognitive function over time. Again, if serial data exist, they can be quite helpful; but often, the clinician has to infer this from the history provided by the patient and someone who knows the patient well. The history of a change coupled with appropriate neuropsychological data can be very useful for the clinician to determine whether there has been a substantive cognitive change.

If the clinician determines that the patient has experienced a change in cognition, and yet

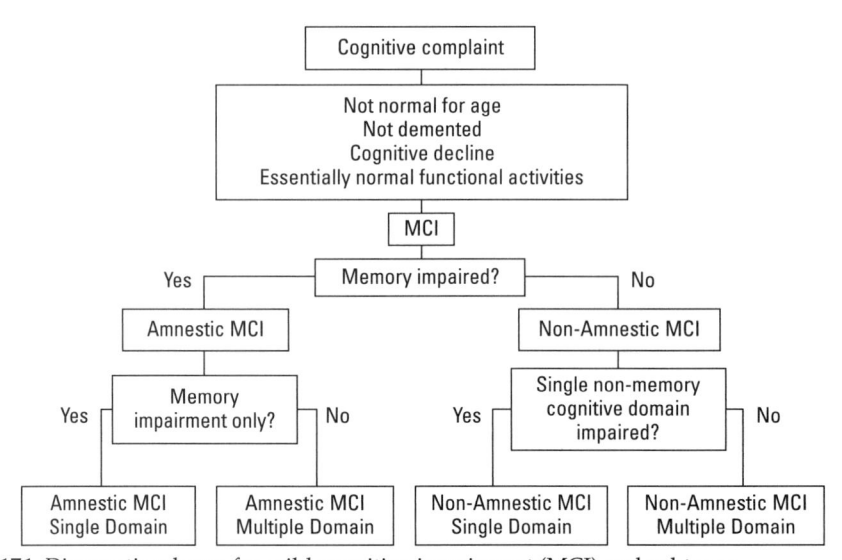

Figure 17.1 Diagnostic scheme for mild cognitive impairment (MCI) and subtypes.

MCI Subtypes

		Etiology			
		Degen-erstive	Vascular	Psychiatric	Medical conditions
Amnestic MCI	Single domain	AD		Depr	
	Multiple domain	AD	VaD	Depr	
Non-amnestic MCI	Single domain	FTD			
	Multiple domain	DLB	VaD		

(Clinical classification on vertical axis)

Figure 17.2 Clinical classification and etiology in mild cognitive impairment (MCI). AD, Alzheimer's disease; FTD, frontotemporal dementia; LBD, dementia with Lewy bodies; VaD, vascular dementia.

general function is well preserved, the diagnosis of MCI can be entertained. The next task for the clinician is to determine the cause of the clinical syndrome. Difficulties in investigating MCI have arisen due to issues in terminology. Since the bulk of the literature on MCI has arisen in the setting of AD, some individuals assume that MCI means "early AD." However, as is evident from Figure 17.1, MCI is a clinical syndrome, and there may be multiple etiologies. As is shown in Figure 17.2, while degenerative diseases are common causes of MCI, especially in older patients, there can be other etiologies. For example, vascular insults can produce cognitive impairment in various domains, and this has typically been referred to in the literature as vascular cognitive impairment (Hachinski et al., 2006; Petersen et al., 2009). In addition, MCI can arise in the setting of certain psychiatric illnesses such as depression and anxiety as well as in the setting of medical comorbidities such as diabetes, heart failure, and chronic obstructive pulmonary disease. As such, it is incumbent upon the clinician to investigate other possible causes of MCI or contributing factors to MCI even in the setting of a degenerative disease.

Mild cognitive impairment can also arise as a prodromal state of other dementing disorders in addition to AD. There can be prodromal states to frontotemporal lobar degeneration (FTLD) and dementia with Lewy bodies (DLB). In FTLD, the presenting clinical picture may involve behavioral abnormalities prior to actual cognitive impairment. Similarly, in DLB, some of the presenting clinical features may constitute sleep disorders, parkinsonism, or behavioral disturbances, and these may be the hallmarks of prodromal DLB (Molano et al., 2009).

Recently, MCI has been described in the setting of Parkinson's disease, and the condition known as PD-MCI has been described (Litvan et al., 2012). In this situation, patients must first have the diagnosis of Parkinson's disease, and then criteria for PD-MCI, to characterize impaired cognitive function in these individuals prior to the development of Parkinson's disease dementia, have been published (Emre et al., 2007).

It is important to determine the etiology of the MCI syndrome since it may be possible to reverse or at least slow the course of some of these conditions; if this is possible, the MCI syndrome can improve. This has also led to some misunderstanding in the literature since, when MCI is viewed as prodromal AD, generally, this is not believed to be reversible. However, when MCI is due to other conditions, such as depression or medical comorbidities, when the underlying conditions are treated, the MCI syndrome may improve. This has led to criticism in the literature that the MCI construct is unstable when, in fact, one would expect an improvement in the symptoms if the underlying cause is potentially reversible.

Predictors of Progression

Over the past decade, a great deal of literature has accumulated regarding the ability to predict which MCI patients will progress to dementia more rapidly than others. Table 17.2 outlines several of these predictors, and additional data are accumulating at a rapid pace. In general, the greater the clinical severity of the MCI at the time of diagnosis tends to predict a more rapid progression (Dickerson, Sperling, Hyman, Albert, & Blacker, 2007; Visser et al., 1999). That is, individuals who have more severe memory impairment or have memory impairment plus the involvement of other cognitive domains (multidomain aMCI) tend to progress to the dementia stage more rapidly than those with less severe impairment. In many respects, this represents a further progression of the underlying pathology, usually degeneration, and constitutes more extensive pathological involvement.

TABLE 17.2 Possible Predictors of Progression in Mild Cognitive Impairment

1. Severity of clinical impairment
2. Apolipoprotein E4 carrier
3. MRI: Atrophy of medial temporal lobe structures
4. FDG PET: Evidence of parietotemporal hypometabolism
5. Amyloid imaging: Positive for the presence of amyloid
6. Cerebrospinal fluid: Lower Abeta 42 and elevated tau
7. Positive family history for dementia

Magnetic Resonance Imaging

There has been more literature generated on the utility of MRI in predicting progression to dementia than most of the other biomarkers (Apostolova et al., 2006; Jack et al., 2008, 2010), particularly hippocampal atrophy (Fig. 17.3). Jack and colleagues documented the utility of hippocampal atrophy at predicting rates of progression in MCI over a decade ago (Jack et al., 1999). In general, more sophisticated MRI measures have evolved in recent years, including other volumetric measurements such as ventricular volume and whole-brain atrophy, entorhinal atrophy (Dickerson et al., 2001), as well as cortical thinning (Bakkour, Morris, & Dickerson, 2009) and functional MRI studies of the medial temporal lobe (Dickerson et al., 2005). While some of these measures may vary in a given study, in general, the greater the degree of hippocampal atrophy, whole-brain atrophy, ventricular dilatation, and cortical thinning are present, the progression rate is accelerated

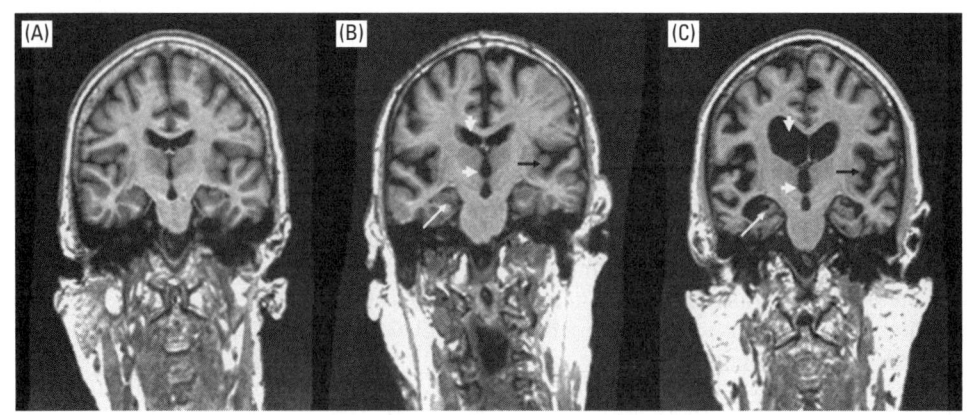

Figure 17.3 Magnetic resonance imaging (MRI) in mild cognitive impairment (MCI). Coronal T1 MP RAGE sections through the hippocampus in a cognitively normal individual (A) and individuals with MCI (B) and dementia (C). The presence of hippocampal atrophy (long white arrows), ventricular dilation (short white arrows), and cortical thinning (black arrows) with widening of the sulci in MCI predicts conversion to dementia. These structural brain changes are first subtly noted in the MCI stage (B) and rapidly increase through the dementia stage (C), when they become quite prominent.

(Bakkour et al., 2009). The Alzheimer's Disease Neuroimaging Initiative (ADNI) has been a hallmark study designed to evaluate the utility of a variety of imaging and fluid biomarkers with respect to their ability to predict progression in MCI (Landau et al., 2010). Numerous studies have documented that many of these individual quantitative measures are quite useful at predicting progression and, when used in the setting of a clinical trial, can reduce the number of subjects needed to document a change in performance (Landau et al., 2010).

The data indicate that certain measures are more indicative of progression at various stages in the evolutionary process of degeneration in the AD spectrum, and these have proven to be quite useful. While quantitative measures may not be available in most clinical situations, the efficacy of visual rating of hippocampal atrophy can be useful (van de Pol et al., 2007). There are several scales that have been introduced to allow the clinician to assess medial temporal lobe atrophy in the office, and for the practicing clinician, they can be quite useful. However, automated volumetric MRI measurements have also become available through programs like FreeSurfer (Fischl et al., 2002), and these are becoming more widely available for use in clinical practice. The field is sufficiently advanced that standardized measurements are being established and will likely become available to the clinician. It is anticipated that volumetric MRI measurements of the brain may be used in a fashion similar to bone density measures used to assess osteoporosis (Jack et al., 2011).

Positron Emission Tomography

The application of positron emission tomography (PET) imaging to degenerative dementias has increased dramatically in recent years. Fluorodeoxyglucose (FDG) has been available for many decades to evaluate metabolic activity in the brain. Certain patterns that have been characteristic of an AD-like process have been known for years and generally involve hypometabolism in the temporal and parietal regions (Fig. 17.4). This pattern is in distinction to that seen in frontotemporal lobar degeneration where hyperperfusion is most prominent in the anterior frontal and temporal lobes. The Center for Medicare and Medicaid Services (CMS) has approved coverage for the FDG distinction between frontotemporal lobar degeneration and AD, and consequently, this has been a useful technique for that clinical distinction. Early work had indicated that individuals with an apolipoprotein

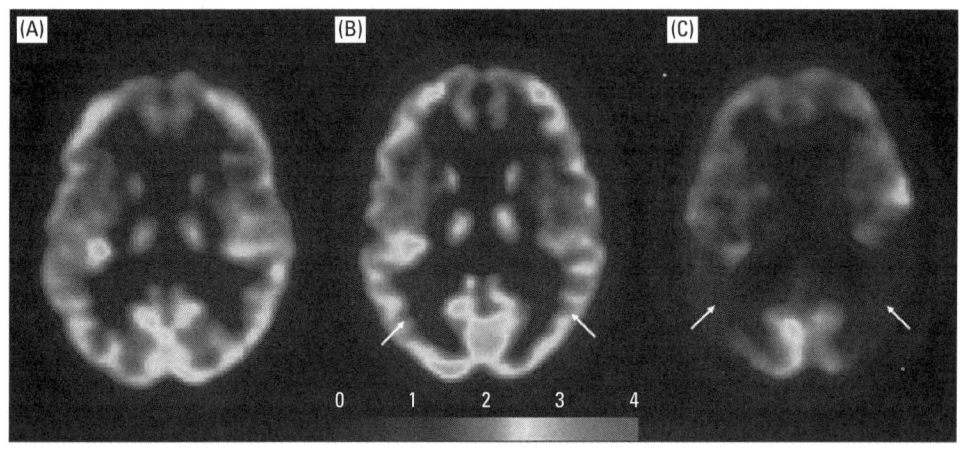

Figure 17.4 Fludeoxyglucose positron emission tomography (FDG-PET) in mild cognitive impairment (MCI). Axial section of FDG-PET scans in a cognitively normal individual (A) and individuals with MCI (B) and dementia (C). Red indicates the greatest areas of metabolism, while blue and black are the least. FDG-PET hypometabolism is a marker of neuronal injury and dysfunction. Bilateral temporoparietal hypometabolism is noted in MCI (B, white arrows) and even more so in dementia (C, white arrows) due to Alzheimer's disease and is indicative of an increased rate of progression from MCI to dementia. (See color plate section)

E4 carrier status had a hypometabolic pattern on FDG-PET prior to the demonstration of any clinical symptoms (Reiman et al., 1996). This pattern was most prominent in apolipoprotein E4 homozygotes but also has been seen in heterozygotes, raising the question of evidence for the pathophysiologic process leading to the dementia of AD many years before symptoms appear (Reiman et al., 2001). More recently, there have been several studies documenting the utility of the temporoparietal hypometabolism pattern in MCI as being indicative of increased rate of progression to dementia (Chetelat et al., 2003). The ADNI has generated data in support of this position, as well, and FDG-PET has been compared to other indices of progression from MCI (Landau et al., 2010).

More recently, the utility of amyloid imaging in characterizing patients who have MCI has become apparent (Engler et al., 2006). Amyloid imaging was introduced around 2004, using the carbon 11 Pittsburgh compound B (PiB) (Klunk et al., 2004). A great deal of data have been generated over the past several years, suggesting the utility of a positive amyloid imaging scan in predicting the progression from MCI to dementia due to AD (Wolk et al., 2009). Again, ADNI has been at the forefront of these studies and has shown that individuals with the clinical symptoms of MCI and having a positive amyloid imaging scan progress to the dementia stage much more rapidly than MCI subjects with a negative amyloid imaging scan (Jack et al., 2010, Landau et al., 2012) (Fig. 17.5). While these data are convincing, precise prediction models have not been generated as of yet. There still can be a considerable time lag for individuals with positive amyloid imaging scans with respect to their progression from the MCI to the dementia stage of AD, and more research needs to be done to clarify this progression pattern.

Cerebrospinal Fluid

In recent years, a great deal of data regarding the utility of cerebrospinal fluid (CSF) in characterizing the underlying AD pathophysiology has emerged. In particular, with respect to MCI, numerous studies have documented that individuals with the AD

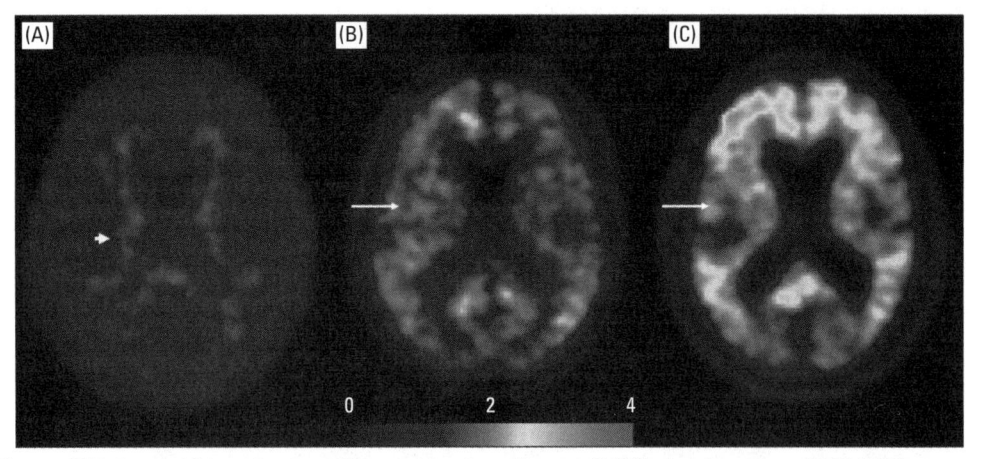

Figure 17.5 Amyloid imaging in mild cognitive impairment (MCI). Axial section of PiB-PET scans in a cognitively normal individual (*A*) and individuals with MCI (*B*) and dementia (*C*). PiB is a positron emission tomography (PET) tracer useful for detecting amyloid deposition in the brain. Brain areas where amyloid is absent appear blue; brain areas with the greatest tracer uptake appear red, while areas with less tracer uptake appear green or yellow. Amyloid deposition of the white matter, but not gray matter, is seen in cognitively normal individuals, creating a clear contrast in radioactivity between gray and white matter (*A*, short arrow). When amyloid is deposited in the cortices, as occurs in MCI (*B*, long arrow) and dementia (*C*, long arrow) due to Alzheimer's disease, diffuse reduction or loss of the normal gray-white contrast is noted. Amyloid deposition occurs early in the pathological cascade and before development of symptoms, creating relatively similar distribution and concentration of deposition between the MCI and dementia subjects. (See color plate section)

pathophysiologic fingerprint (i.e., low amyloid beta 42 levels and elevated total tau or phospho-tau levels) predict a more rapid progression (Shaw et al., 2009). A great deal of this work has been done in Europe, and there are several review studies indicating that combining samples from several medical centers have demonstrated that the low Abeta 42 and elevated tau or p-tau ratios can also be quite suggestive (Hansson et al., 2006). Investigators from ADNI have also demonstrated the utility of CSF in predicting progression from MCI to dementia (Shaw et al., 2009). While these data have been intriguing and likely to be quite useful in assisting clinicians, there has been a great deal of difficulty encountered in standardizing CSF assays around the world (Mattsson et al., 2009). Currently, there is an international standardization exercise under way sponsored by the Alzheimer's Association to bring multiple laboratories together to standardize the methodology for CSF collection and the assays themselves. While this work is progressing, there is currently not a standard cutoff threshold for CSF measures, and this presents a problem for the practicing clinician. Nevertheless, CSF is likely to be very useful in characterizing the underlying pathophysiologic nature of clinical symptoms found in MCI.

Theoretical Foundation for Biomarkers

A great deal of work has been completed and is undergoing regarding the establishment of the utility of the variety of fluid and biomarkers in characterizing the AD pathophysiologic process. Jack and colleagues presented convincing data in a very influential paper in 2010, setting forth the hypothetical sequence of events that occurs as the AD process unfolds (Jack et al., 2010). As is seen in Figure 17.6, the initiating process in the AD cascade involves the deposition of amyloid in the brain typically during the asymptomatic stage. The precise timing of this relative to the subsequent presentation of clinical symptoms is not known, and the shape of the deposition curve needs to be elucidated,

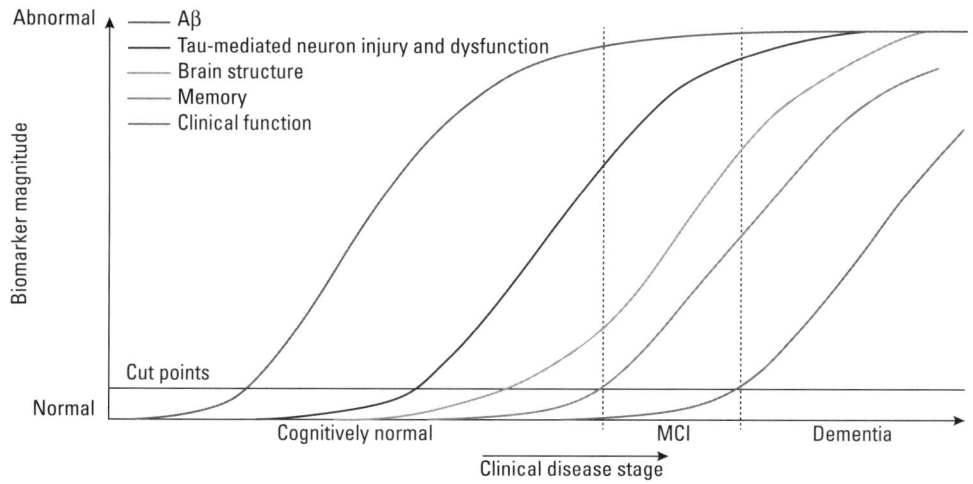

Figure 17.6 The evolution of biomarkers in the Alzheimer's pathological cascade. With the early deposition of amyloid in the pathological cascade, corresponding biomarkers (low cerebrospinal fluid [CSF], Aβ declines, and positive amyloid imaging) are detected before the development of clinical symptoms. Following this, there is a sequence of events characterizing neurodegeneration where evidence of brain dysfunction can be measured through CSF tau levels or fludeoxyglucose positron emission tomography (FDG-PET). As memory and clinical function decline, structural changes of the brain are noted on magnetic resonance imaging (MRI). MCI, mild cognitive impairment. (Reprinted from *The Lancet Neurology*, Vol. number 9, Clifford R Jack, David S Knopman, William J Jagust, Leslie M Shaw, Paul S Aisen, Michael W Weiner, Ronald C Petersen, John Q Trojanowski. Hypothetical model of dynamic biomarkers of the Alzheimer's pathological cascade, pages 119–128. Copyright (2010), with permission from Elsevier) (See color plate section)

but the construct of the initiating event being amyloid deposition is well documented (Hardy & Selkoe, 2002). Following the deposition of amyloid, there is a sequence of events characterizing neurodegeneration. One of the early events may be the development of an abnormal pattern of glucose metabolism on FDG-PET scanning. There is some evidence that this may occur quite early in the pathophysiologic process but at present is being characterized as occurring after the deposition of amyloid. Another event that occurs to index neurodegeneration is depicted by the abnormal processing of the tau protein (Buerger et al., 2006). In general, when tau becomes hyperphosphorylated, it reflects underlying neurodegeneration, and this can be an early event in the neurodegeneration process. The model then indicates that, after these events have occurred, one is likely to see structural changes on magnetic resonance imaging (MRI) such as hippocampal atrophy, whole-brain atrophy, ventricular dilatation, and cortical thinning (Dickerson et al., 2009; Fox, Warrington, & Rossor, 1999; Jack et al., 2004; Kaye et al., 1997). As such, quantitative measures of MRI can be very useful but are likely most dynamic during the symptomatic stage of the process such as that seen during MCI. As is depicted in Figure 17.2, it is only after these events take place that clinical symptoms evolve. Typically, memory impairment is the first hallmark characterized during the MCI stage, and as that progresses and other cognitive domains become impaired and daily function is compromised, then one crosses the threshold for dementia.

This model, which was recently revised (Jack et al., 2013), has proved to be extremely useful for the field of aging and dementia at characterizing putative pathologic processes and their consequences. However, as indicated previously, the precise temporal ordering of these events, the shapes of the curves, and the thresholds for normal and abnormal on each of these markers are largely unknown. A wealth of research is being done to elucidate these processes further, but the specific calibration of the various biomarkers remains to be done. However, this basic formulation of pathological events provides the backdrop for the use of individual biomarkers in characterizing individuals across the AD spectrum. As will be discussed later in the chapter, this model also serves as the framework for the revised criteria for the AD spectrum.

New Criteria for the Alzheimer's Disease Spectrum

In 2011, the National Institute on Aging and the Alzheimer's Association published the results of several expert groups who had been working on a revision of the criteria for Alzheimer's disease (Jack et al., 2011). The previously published criteria from 1984 were updated and expanded to reflect all of the activity in the field over the intervening two and a half decades. There were two major changes to the overall conceptualization of the criteria. First, the notion of Alzheimer's disease being a clinical-pathologic entity was discarded. Since the clinical spectrum can vary according to disease severity, it was believed that the clinical aspects of the disease should be characterized from the most severe state being dementia back through the intermediate state of MCI and ultimately to a preclinical state, which is the point at which individuals are clinically normal but may harbor the underlying pathophysiological characteristics of Alzheimer's disease. Correspondingly, there is a pathological spectrum for Alzheimer's disease stretching backward from the most severe stage of well-established neuritic plaques and neurofibrillary tangles to stages of much lesser pathophysiology, yet believed to be on the pathology spectrum. Secondly, as indicated previously, the disease was now being characterized as a full spectrum and not just at the dementia stage. Relevant to our current discussion, the MCI stage is now called "MCI due to AD." This stage is meant to reflect the fact that a person may be minimally symptomatic, demonstrating a mild episodic memory deficit, but has underlying features of Alzheimer's disease pathophysiology.

To implement this thinking in the criteria, biomarkers become an essential component. As mentioned previously, the theoretical model characterizing the evolution of Alzheimer's disease pathophysiology and clinical symptoms was outlined by Jack and colleagues (Jack et al., 2010). This model implies that the deposition of amyloid was the initiating event followed by neurodegeneration and

TABLE 17.3 Use of Biomarkers to Enhance Diagnostic Certainty in Mild Cognitive Impairment (MCI)

Diagnostic Category	Biomarker Probability of AD Etiology	Aβ (PET or CSF)	Neuronal Injury (tau, FDG, sMRI)
MCI	Uninformative	Conflicting/indeterminant Untested	
MCI due to AD – intermediate likelihood	Intermediate Intermediate	Positive Untested	Untested Positive
MCI due to AD – high likelihood	Highest	Positive	Positive
MCI—unlikely due to AD	Lowest	Negative	Negative

AD, Alzheimer's disease; CSF, cerebrospinal fluid; PET, positron emission tomography.

then clinical manifestations. With this model in mind, the MCI-due-to-AD stage is characterized as a state in which the subjects have minimal clinical symptoms, usually mild memory impairment, but are otherwise functioning reasonably normal. The subjects may have some inefficiency in conducting their daily activities but are able to do them without any assistance. The subjects may have a memory impairment (aMCI) or, less commonly, mild impairments in nonmemory cognitive domains (naMCI). However, the new criteria for MCI due to AD do not distinguish between aMCI and naMCI, but this remains an area of investigation.

To enhance the clinician's suspicion that the clinical syndrome of MCI is due to Alzheimer's disease, biomarkers must be invoked. As is shown in Table 17.3, the first level of certainty is reflected in just the clinical syndrome alone. That is, in addition to the MCI diagnostic criteria being fulfilled, the clinician does not have any information regarding the underlying biomarker status for a given person. The next level of certainty, which is called intermediate, is higher with respect to the likelihood of the clinical syndrome being due to underlying Alzheimer's disease, and this can be achieved by either having evidence for amyloid deposition, via amyloid PET or CSF Abeta, or evidence for neurodegeneration, as indicated by an abnormal FDG-PET scan, CSF tau levels, or atrophy on MRI. The criteria do not weight one set of biological markers as being more important than the other at this point in time due to insufficient data. However, as the field evolves, it is likely that these biomarkers will be rank ordered. Finally, the highest level of certainty that the MCI syndrome is due to underlying Alzheimer's disease pathophysiology is achieved when the clinical syndrome is present and is accompanied by evidence for amyloid deposition and neurodegeneration. For completeness, a low level of certainty is also demonstrated when the clinical syndrome is present and biomarkers are available, but they are negative for underlying Alzheimer's disease pathophysiology.

Clinical Vignette

Part 2

Resumption of Evaluation of Clinical Case

Due to the concern about possible aMCI, the clinician decided to obtain additional measures. An MRI scan was performed, which showed only slight atrophy in the medial temporal lobe, most notably in the hippocampal formations, but was judged to be within normal limits for age. A functional imaging test involving FDG-PET also was equivocal. There was a suggestion of temporoparietal hypometabolism on the left, but it was of insufficient severity to be judged as abnormal. However, an amyloid imaging study was performed, and this was positive. The patient was entered into a research protocol, and a lumbar puncture was performed, and the cerebrospinal fluid measure for Abeta 42 was low, and the indices for total tau and p-tau were elevated.

Conclusion

It appears that this woman had a gradual onset of a memory difficulty which by evaluation was judged to be beyond what one would expect for age. The neuropsychological testing profile confirmed her suspicions of a decrement in memory, and by history, one can infer that this is a change in performance for her. As such, the diagnosis of aMCI was established, but the etiology was uncertain. Since the woman was relatively young, additional imaging studies were performed, and the structural imaging MRI and functional imaging FDG-PET scan were equivocal. However, the more definitive molecular neuroimaging measures, as determined by amyloid PET imaging and CSF, did, in fact, indicate that she had the presence of amyloid in the brain, and the suspicion is that this is now MCI due to AD with a high likelihood, according to the new criteria.

At this point, these criteria are for research purposes, and a great deal of additional data needs to be developed. In particular, as mentioned previously, we need to determine whether markers for amyloid deposition carry more weight than those of neurodegeneration with respect to Alzheimer's disease pathophysiology specificity. One would suspect that this is the case given that amyloid is a sine qua non for the diagnosis of Alzheimer's disease pathophysiologically. That is, one must have evidence of amyloid deposition in the brain to make the pathophysiologic diagnosis of Alzheimer's disease, and hence, a biomarker reflecting that pathologic characteristic would be quite reasonable.

There is also a variable degree of specificity of the biomarkers. As indicated, the amyloid biomarkers reflect underlying amyloid pathology, as has been demonstrated in amyloid PET pathology correlations, whereas biomarker measures of neurodegeneration are relatively nonspecific. One can see atrophy on an MRI from a variety of pathologic entities, including neurodegeneration, vascular disease, or combinations of them (Barber, Ballard, McKeith, Gholkar, & O'Brien, 2000, O'Brien et al., 2001). Similarly, CSF tau can be elevated in a variety of neurologic conditions, such as stroke, traumatic brain injury, or Creutzfeldt-Jakob disease (Hesse et al., 2001; Ost et al., 2006; Otto et al., 2002). In addition, research needs to be done to characterize the outcome of subjects whose biomarkers do not agree. That is, how does one classify an individual who may have evidence for amyloid deposition but no degeneration? What about the subject who has evidence for neurodegeneration but is amyloid negative?

These data are beginning to emerge, and their implication for the application of the new criteria remains to be determined.

Diagnostic and Statistical Manual for Mental Disorders, Fifth Edition

In conjunction with the National Institute on Aging/Alzheimer's Association criteria for the Alzheimer's disease spectrum, the *Diagnostic and Statistical Manual for Mental Disorders (fifth ed.) (DSM-5)* was recently finalized and published (Ganguli et al., 2011). The construct of MCI is included in the section dealing with neurocognitive disorders. This area of neurocognitive disorders is labeled "minor neurocognitive disorders" and essentially captures the clinical criteria of MCI, as discussed here. The construct of neurocognitive disorders for *DSM-5* is broader than just Alzheimer's disease, and consequently, the criteria must be more flexible to encompass other disorders such as frontotemporal lobar degeneration, dementia with Lewy bodies, Parkinson's disease—mild cognitive impairment, vascular cognitive impairment, HIV, AIDS, neurocognitive disorders, and traumatic brain injury. Nevertheless, the construct of a predementia clinical state has officially been recognized in *DSM-5*, and this will coincide with MCI due to Alzheimer's disease, as discussed previously.

Clinical Acceptance

In summary, the construct of MCI has been intensely investigated over the past 10 to 15 years. While there is not complete agreement on the clinical characterization, it has been adopted in clinical practice. A study published in *Neurology* reflecting the opinions of practicing neurologists with respect to the construct of MCI was quite illuminating (Roberts, Karlawish, Uhlmann, Petersen, & Green, 2010). This study indicated that most practicing neurologists see patients with this intermediate degree of cognitive impairment and prefer to use the term MCI to other nomenclatures. The neurologists indicated that MCI is a useful term for them, and in spite of the challenges of making the diagnosis at times, they find it quite useful. They prefer to use MCI rather than other terms such as prodromal Alzheimer's disease because there is uncertainty at the MCI stage as to the outcome of the patients, and clinicians are reluctant to mislabel someone with an Alzheimer's disease type of label because of the disservice that would be done to the patient. As such, they would prefer to use the term "MCI" since it does reflect a probabilistic progression to dementia due to Alzheimer's disease but not a definitive state. This more accurately characterizes the clinical condition, and as such, most clinicians are quite comfortable using it.

Treatment of Mild Cognitive Impairment

Currently, there are no FDA-approved treatments for MCI. There have been numerous clinical trials conducted over the past several years, largely involving established therapies for Alzheimer's disease, and virtually all of these have been unsuccessful (Petersen, 2011). One trial sponsored by the Alzheimer's Disease Cooperative Study through the National Institute on Aging in conjunction with Pfizer, Inc., evaluated high-dose vitamin E (2000 IU) and donepezil for the treatment of MCI with the clinical endpoint being conversion to dementia (Petersen et al., 2005). This study was designed as a 36-month trial and, as such, was unsuccessful at demonstrating the utility of either of these treatments over that timeframe. However, a prespecified analysis indicated that donepezil was efficacious at reducing the rate at which subjects progress to dementia over the first 12 months of the study and for up to 24 months in subjects who were Apolipoprotein ε4 carriers. However, as indicated previously, all of the treatment curves converged at 36 months. Vitamin E was not demonstrated to be of any value throughout the treatment. A subsequent trial of donepezil alone for 18 months, however, failed to replicate the ADCS finding (Doody et al., 2009).

Additional studies using galantamine and rivastigmine were not successful (Feldman et al., 2007; Winblad et al., 2008). These studies were plagued by a relatively low progression rate from MCI to dementia, and consequently, the power analyses were inaccurate. In particular, the rivastigmine trial was planned for 2 years but had to be extended to 3–4 years, and this extension resulted in a significant number of discontinued subjects. As such, that and several other factors contributed to a null finding. The galantamine trials were suggestive of therapeutic effect, but again, no statistical effect was found after 2 years of treatment (Winblad et al., 2008). Interestingly, a study with rofecoxib failed to demonstrate a beneficial effect, and there was even a suggestion of more rapid progression in the rofecoxib-treated group; however, the cognitive data did not support that conclusion (Thal et al., 2005).

Several studies evaluating lifestyle modifications and nonpharmacologic treatments have been suggestive of a benefit (Jean, Bergeron, Thivierge, & Simard, 2010). Aerobic exercise appears to be effective a reducing the rate at which subjects may progress in degree of cognitive impairment in aging, and numerous other studies are currently under way (Lautenschlager et al., 2008). At present, many clinicians recommend subjects engage in physical exercise, stay intellectually engaged, and maintain their social networks. From a dietary and supplement perspective, there is no evidence of any particular diets or compounds that can be used to prevent cognitive impairment.

Conclusion

The field of aging and dementia is progressing rapidly with regard to clinical characterization of persons at earlier stages of cognitive impairment. The construct of MCI has been useful as a heuristic and, clinically, to encourage research on this stage of impairment and also allow clinicians a category to use in characterizing subjects who are not normal but do not meet criteria for dementia. Ultimately, as biomarkers evolve, these types of arbitrary clinical distinctions may not be necessary, and the field will move to a more biological characterization of subjects underlying pathophysiologic spectra. However, prior to that stage of development, the clinical labels such as MCI are useful and facilitate communication with patients and promote research.

References

Apostolova, L. G., Dutton, R. A., Dinov, I. D., Hayashi, K. M., Toga, A. W., Cummings, J. L., & Thompson, P. M. (2006). Conversion of mild cognitive impairment to Alzheimer disease predicted by hippocampal atrophy maps. *Archives of Neurology, 63*(5), 693–699.

Bakkour, A., Morris, J. C., & Dickerson, B. C. (2009). The cortical signature of prodromal AD: Regional thinning predicts mild AD dementia. *Neurology, 72*(12), 1048–1055.

Barber, R., Ballard, C., McKeith, I. G., Gholkar, A., & O'Brien, J. T. (2000). MRI volumetric study of dementia with Lewy bodies. *Neurology, 54*(6), 1304–1309.

Buerger, K., Ewers, M., Pirttila, T., Zinkowski, R., Alafuzoff, I., Teipel, S. J.,...Hample, H. (2006). CSF phosphorylated tau protein correlates with neocortical neurofibrillary pathology in Alzheimer's disease. *Brain, 129*(Pt 11), 3035–3041.

Busse, A., Hensel, A., Guhne, U., Angermeyer, M. C., & Riedel-Heller, S. G. (2006). Mild cognitive impairment: Long-term course of four clinical subtypes. *Neurology, 67*(12), 2176–2185.

Chetelat, G., Desgranges, B., de la Sayette, V., Viader, F., Eustache, F., & Baron, J. C. (2003). Mild cognitive impairment: Can FDG-PET predict who is to rapidly convert to Alzheimer's disease? *Neurology, 60*(8), 1374–1377.

Di Carlo, A., Lamassa, M., Baldereschi, M., Inzitari, M., Scafato, E., Farchi, G., & Inzitari, D. (2007). CIND and MCI in the Italian elderly: Frequency, vascular risk factors, progression to dementia. *Neurology, 68*(22), 1909–1916.

Dickerson, B. C., Feczko, E., Augustinack, J. C., Pacheco, J., Morris, J. C., Fischl, B., & Buckner, R. L. (2009). Differential effects of aging and Alzheimer's disease on medial temporal lobe cortical thickness and surface area. *Neurobiology of Aging, 30*(3), 432–440.

Dickerson, B. C., Goncharova, I., Sullivan, M. P., Forchetti, C., Wilson, R. S., Bennett, D. A.,...deToledo-Morrell, L. (2001). MRI-derived entorhinal and hippocampal atrophy in incipient and very mild Alzheimer's disease. *Neurobiology of Aging, 22*(5), 747–754.

Dickerson, B. C., Salat, D. H., Greve, D. N., Chua, E. F., Rand-Giovannetti, E., Rentz, D. M.,...Sperling, R. A. (2005). Increased hippocampal activation in mild cognitive impairment compared to normal aging and AD. *Neurology, 65*(3), 404–411.

Dickerson, B. C., Sperling, R. A., Hyman, B. T., Albert, M. S., & Blacker, D. (2007). Clinical prediction of Alzheimer disease dementia across the spectrum of mild cognitive impairment. *Archives of General Psychiatry, 64*(12), 1443–1450.

Doody, R. S., Ferris, S. H., Salloway, S., Sun, Y., Goldman, R., Watkins, W. E.,...Murthy, A. K. (2009). Donepezil treatment of patients with MCI: A 48-week randomized, placebo-controlled trial. *Neurology, 72*(18), 1555–1561.

Emre, M., Aarsland, D., Brown, R., Burn, D. J., Duyckaerts, C., Mizuno, Y.,...Dubois, B. (2007). Clinical diagnostic criteria for dementia associated with Parkinson's disease. *Movement Disorders, 22*(12), 1689–1707; quiz 837.

Engler, H., Forsberg, A., Almkvist, O., Blomquist, G., Larsson, E., Savitcheva, I.,...Nordberg, A. (2006). Two-year follow-up of amyloid deposition in patients with Alzheimer's disease. *Brain, 129*, 2856–2866.

Feldman, H. H., Ferris, S., Winblad, B., Sfikas, N., Mancione, L., He, Y.,...Lane, R. Effect of rivastigmine on delay to diagnosis of Alzheimer's disease from mild cognitive impairment: The InDDEx study. *Lancet Neurology, 6*(6), 501–512.

Fischl, B., Salat, D. H., Busa, E., Albert, M., Dieterich, M., Haselgrove, C.,...Dale, A. M. (2002). Whole brain segmentation: Automated labeling of neuroanatomical structures in the human brain. *Neuron, 33*(3), 341–355.

Fox, N. C., Warrington, E. K., & Rossor, M. N. (1999). Serial magnetic resonance imaging of cerebral atrophy in preclinical Alzheimer's disease. *Lancet, 353*(9170), 2125.

Folstein, M. F., Folstein, S. E., & McHugh, P. R. (1975). "Mini-mental state." A practical method for grading the cognitive state of patients for the clinician. *Journal of Psychiatric Research, 12*(3), 189–198.

Ganguli, M., Blacker, D., Blazer, D. G., Grant, I., Jeste, D. V., Paulsen, J. S.,...Sachdev, P. S. (2011). Classification of neurocognitive disorders in DSM-5: A work in progress. *American Journal of Geriatric Psychiatry, 19*(3), 205–210.

Ganguli, M., Dodge, H. H., Shen, C., & DeKosky, S. T. (2004). Mild cognitive impairment, amnestic type: An epidemiologic study. *Neurology, 63*, 115–121.

Hachinski, V., Iadecola, C., Petersen, R. C., Breteler, M. M., Nyenhuis, D. L., Black, S. E.,...Leblanc, G. G. (2006). National Institute of Neurological Disorders and Stroke-Canadian Stroke Network vascular cognitive impairment harmonization standards. *Stroke, 37*(9), 2220–2241.

Hansson, O., Zetterberg, H., Buchhave, P., Londos, E., Blennow, K., & Minthon, L. (2006). Association between CSF biomarkers and incipient Alzheimer's disease in patients with mild cognitive impairment: A follow-up study. *Lancet Neurology, 5*, 228–234.

Hardy, J., & Selkoe, D. J. (2002). The amyloid hypothesis of Alzheimer's disease: Progress and problems on the road to therapeutics. *Science, 297*(5580), 353–356.

Hesse, C., Rosengren, L., Andreasen, N., Davidsson, P., Vanderstichele, H., Vanmechelen, E., & Blennow, K. (2001). Transient increase in total tau but not phospho-tau in human cerebrospinal fluid after acute stroke. *Neuroscience Letters, 297*(3), 187–190.

Jack, C., Barkhof, F., Bernstein, M., Cantillon, M., Cole, P., DeCarli, C.,...Foster, N. L. (2011). Steps to standardization and validation of hippocampal volumetry as a biomarker in clinical trials and diagnostic criteria for Alzheimer's disease. *Alzheimer Dementia, 7*(4), 474–485.

Jack, C., Knopman, D., Jagust, W., Shaw, L. M., Aisen, P. S., Weiner, M.,...Trojanowski, J. Q. (2010). Hypothetical model of dynamic biomarkers of the Alzheimer's pathological cascade. *Lancet, 9*(1), 119–128.

Jack, C. R., Albert, M. S., Knopman, D. S., McKhann, G. M., Sperling, R. A., Carillo, M.,...Phelps, C. H. (2011). Introduction to the recommendations from the National Institute on Aging-Alzheimer's Association workgroups on diagnostic guidelines for Alzheimer's disease. *Alzheimers Dementia, 7*(3), 257–262.

Jack, C. R., Knopman, D. S., Jagust, W. J., Petersen, R. C., Weiner, M. W., Aisen, P. S.,...Trojanowski, J. Q. (2013). Tracking pathophysiological processes in Alzheimer's disease: an updated hypothetical model of dynamic biomarkers. *Lancet Neurology, 12*(2), 207–216.

Jack, C. R., Knopman, D. S., Weigand, S. D., Wiste, H. J., Vemuri, P., Lowe, V.,...Petersen, R. C. (2012). An operational approach to NIA-AA crtiteria for preclinical Alzheimer's disease. *Annals of Neurology, 71*(6), 765–775.

Jack, C. R., Petersen, R. C., Xu, Y. C., O'Brien, P. C., Smith, G. E., Ivnik, R. J.,...Kokmen, E. (1999). Prediction of AD with MRI-based hippocampal volume in mild cognitive impairment. *Neurology, 52*(7), 1397–1403.

Jack, C. R., Shiung, M. M., Gunter, J. L., O'Brien, P. C., Weigand, S. D., Knopman, D. S.,...Petersen, R. C. (2004). Comparison of different MRI brain atrophy rate measures with clinical disease progression in AD. *Neurology, 62*(4), 591–600.

Jack, C. R., Weigand, S. D., Shiung, M. M., Przybelski, S. A., O'Brien, P. C., Gunter, J. L.,...Petersen, R. C. (2008). Atrophy rates accelerate in amnestic mild cognitive impairment. *Neurology, 70*(19 Pt 2), 1740–1752.

Jack, C. R., Wiste, H. J., Vemuri, P., Weigand, S. D., Senjem, M. L., Zeng, G.,...Knopman, D. S. (2010). Brain beta-amyloid measures and magnetic resonance imaging atrophy both predict time-to-progression from mild cognitive impairment to Alzheimer's disease. *Brain, 133*(11), 3336–3348.

Jean, L., Bergeron, M. E., Thivierge, S., & Simard, M. (2010). Cognitive intervention programs for individuals with mild cognitive impairment: Systematic review of the literature. *American Journal of Geriatric Psychiatry, 18*(4), 281–296.

Kaye, J. A., Swihart, T., Howieson, D., Dame, A., Moore, M. M., Karnos, T.,...Sexton, G. (1997). Volume loss of the hippocampus and temporal lobe in healthy elderly persons destined to develop dementia. *Neurology, 48*, 1297–1304.

Klunk, W. E., Engler, H., Nordberg, A., Wang, Y., Blomqvist, G., Holt, D. P.,...Långström, B. (2004). Imaging brain amyloid in Alzheimer's disease with Pittsburgh Compound-B. *Annals of Neurology, 55*(3), 306–319.

Knopman, D. S., Jack, C. R., Jr., Wiste, H. J., Weigand, S. D., Vemuri, P., Lowe, V.,...Petersen, R. C. (2012). Short-term clinical outcomes for stages of NIA-AA preclinical Alzheimer disease. *Neurology, 78*(20), 1576–1582.

Kokmen, E., Naessens, J. M., & Offord, K. P. (1987). A short test of mental status: Description and preliminary results. *Mayo Clinic Proceedings, 62*(4), 281–288.

Landau, S. M., Harvey, D., Madison, C. M., Reiman, E. M., Foster, N. L., Aisen, P. S.,...Jagust, W. J. (2010). Comparing predictors of conversion and decline in mild cognitive impairment. *Neurology, 75*(3), 230–238.

Landau, S. M., Mintun, M. A., Joshi, A. D., Koeppe, R. A., Petersen, R. C., Aisen, P. S.,...Jagust, W. J. (2012). Amyloid deposition, hypometabolism, and longitutdinal cognitive decline. *Annals of Neurology, 72*(4), 578–586.

Larrieu, S., Letenneur, L., Orgogozo, J. M., Fabrigoule, C., Amieva, H., Le Carret, N.,...Dartigues, J. F. (2002). Incidence and outcome of mild cognitive impairment in a population-based prospective cohort. *Neurology, 59*(10), 1594–1599.

Lautenschlager, N. T., Cox, K. L., Flicker, L., Foster, J. K., van Bockxmeer, F. M., Xiao, J.,...Almedia, O. P. (2008). Effect of physical activity on cognitive function in older adults at risk for Alzheimer disease: A randomized trial. *Journal of the American Medical Association, 300*(9), 1027–1037.

Litvan, I., Goldman, J. G., Troster, A. I., Schmand, B. A., Weintraub, D., Petersen, R. C.,...Emre, M. (2012). Diagnostic criteria for mild cognitive impairment in Parkinson's disease: Movement Disorder Society Task Force guidelines. *Movement Disorders, 27*(3), 349–356.

Lonie, J. A., Tierney, K. M., & Ebmeier, K. P. (2009). Screening for mild cognitive impairment: A systematic review. *International Journal of Geriatric Psychiatry, 24*(9), 902–915.

Lopez, O. L., Jagust, W. J., DeKosky, S. T., Becker, J. T., Fitzpatrick, A., Dulberg, C.,...Kuller, J. H. (2003). Prevalence and classification of mild cognitive impairment in the Cardiovascular Health Study Cognition Study: Part 1. *Archives of Neurology, 60*(10), 1385–1389.

Manly, J. J., Tang, M. X., Schupf, N., Stern, Y., Vonsattel, J. P., & Mayeux, R. (2008). Frequency and course of mild cognitive impairment in a multiethnic community. *Annals of Neurology, 63*(4), 494–506.

Mattsson, N., Zetterberg, H., Hansson, O., Andreasen, N., Parnetti, L., Jonsson, M.,...Blennow, K. (2009). CSF biomarkers and incipient Alzheimer disease in patients with mild cognitive impairment. *Journal of the American Medical Association, 302*(4), 385–393.

Molano, J., Boeve, B., Ferman, T., Smith, G., Parisi, J., Dickson, D.,...Petersen, R. (2009). Mild cognitive impairment associated with limbic and neocortical lewy body disease: A clinicopathological study. *Brain, 133*, 540–556.

Nasreddine, Z. S., Phillips, N. A., Bedirian, V., Charbonneau, S., Whitehead, V., Collin, I.,...Chertkow, H. (2005). The Montreal Cognitive Assessment (MoCA): A brief screening tool for mild cognitive impairment. *Journal of the American Geriatric Society, 53*, 695–699.

O'Brien, J. T., Paling, S., Barber, R., Williams, E. D., Ballard, C., McKeith, I. G.,...Fox, N. C. (2001). Progressive brain atrophy on serial MRI in dementia with Lewy bodies, AD, and vascular dementia. *Neurology, 56*(10), 1386–1388.

Ost, M., Nylen, K., Csajbok, L., Ohrfelt, A. O., Tullberg, M., Wikkelso, C.,...Nellgård, B. (2006). Initial CSF total tau correlates with 1-year outcome in patients with traumatic brain injury. *Neurology, 67*(9), 1600–1604.

Otto, M., Wiltfang, J., Cepek, L., Neumann, M., Mollenhauer, B., Steinacker, P.,...Poser, S. (2002). Tau protein and 14-3-3 protein in the differential diagnosis of Creutzfeldt–Jakob disease. *Neurology, 58*(2), 192–197.

Petersen, R., Knopman, D., Boeve, B., Geda, Y., Ivnik, R., Smith, G., & Jack, C. R., Jr. (2009). Mild cognitive impairment: Ten years later. *Archives of Neurology, 66*(22), 1447–1455.

Petersen, R. C. (2004). Mild cognitive impairment as a diagnostic entity. *Journal of Internal Medicine, 256*(3), 183–194.

Petersen, R. C. (2011). Clinical practice. Mild cognitive impairment. *New England Journal of Medicine, 364*(23), 2227–2234.

Petersen, R. C., Aisen, P. S., Beckett, L. A., Donohue, M. C., Gamst, A. C., Harvey, D. J.,...Weiner, M. W. (2010). Alzheimer's Disease Neuroimaging Initiative (ADNI): Clinical characterization. *Neurology, 74*(3), 201–209.

Petersen, R. C., Roberts, R. O., Knopman, D. S., Geda, Y. E., Cha, R. H., Pankratz, V. S.,...Rocca, W. A. (2010). Prevalence of mild cognitive impairment is higher in men. The Mayo Clinic Study of Aging. *Neurology, 75*(10), 889–897.

Petersen, R. C., Smith, G. E., Waring, S. C., Ivnik, R. J., Tangalos, E. G., & Kokmen, E. (1999). Mild cognitive impairment: Clinical characterization and outcome. *Archives of Neurology, 56*, 303–308.

Petersen, R. C., Thomas, R. G., Grundman, M., Bennett, D., Doody, R., Ferris, S.,...Thal, L. J. (2005). Donepezil and vitamin E in the treatment of mild cognitive impairment. *New England Journal of Medicine, 352*, 2379–2388.

Reiman, E. M., Caselli, R. J., Chen, K., Alexander, G. E., Bandy, D., & Frost, J. (2001). Declining brain activity in cognitively normal apolipoprotein E epsilon 4 heterozygotes: A foundation for using positron emission tomography to efficiently test treatments to prevent Alzheimer's disease. *Proceedings of the National Academy of Sciences USA, 98*(6), 3334–3339.

Reiman, E. M., Caselli, R. J., Lang, S., Yun, M. S., Chen, K., Bandy, D.,...Greicius, M. D. (1996). Preclinical evidence of Alzheimer's disease in persons homozygous for the E4 allele for apolipoprotein E. *New England Journal of Medicine, 334*, 752–758.

Reisberg, B., Ferris, S., & de Leon, M. J. (1988). Stage-specific behavioral, cognitive, and in vivo changes in community residing subjects with age-associated memory impairment and primary degenerative dementia of the Alzheimer type. *Drug Development Research, 15*(2-3), 101–114.

Ritchie, K., Artero, S., & Touchon, J. (2001). Classification criteria for mild cognitive impairment: A population-based validation study. *Neurology, 56*, 37–42.

Roberts, J. S., Karlawish, J. H., Uhlmann, W. R., Petersen, R. C., & Green, R. C. (2010). Mild cognitive impairment in clinical care: A survey of American Academy of Neurology members. *Neurology, 75*(5), 425–431.

Roberts, R. O., Geda, Y. E., Knopman, D. S., Cha, R. H., Pankratz, V. S., Boeve, B. F.,...Petersen, R. C. (2012). The incidence of MCI differs by subtype and is higher in men: The Mayo Clinic Study of Aging. *Neurology, 78*(5), 342–351.

Shaw, L. M., Vanderstichele, H., Knapik-Czajka, M., Clark, C. M., Aisen, P. S.,

Petersen, R. C., ...Trojanowski, J. Q. (2009). Cerebrospinal fluid biomarker signature in Alzheimer's disease neuroimaging initiative subjects. *Annals of Neurology, 65*(4), 403–413.

Sperling, R. A., Aisen, P. S., Beckett, L. A., Bennett, D. A., Craft, S., Fagan, A. M.,...Phelps, C. H. (2011). Toward defining the preclinical stages of Alzheimer's disease: Recommendations from the National Institute on Aging-Alzheimer's Assocation workgroups on diagnostic guidelines for Alzheimer's disease. Alzheimers Dementia, 7(3), 280–292.

Thal, L. J., Ferris, S. H., Kirby, L., Block, G. A., Lines, C. R., Yuen, E.,...Reines, S. A. (2005). A randomized, double-blind, study of rofecoxib in patients with mild cognitive impairment. *Neuropsychopharmacology, 30,* 1204–1215.

Unverzagt, F. W., Gao, S., Baiyewu, O., Ogunniyyi, A. O., Gureje, O., Perkins, A.,...Hendrie, H. C. (2001). Prevalence of cognitive impairment: Data from the Indianapolis Study of Health and Aging. *Neurology, 57*(9), 1655–1662.

van de Pol, L. A., van der Flier, W. M., Korf, E. S., Fox, N. C., Barkhof, F., & Scheltens, P. (2007). Baseline predictors of rates of hippocampal atrophy in mild cognitive impairment. *Neurology, 69*(15), 1491–1497.

Visser, P. J., Scheltens, P., Verhey, F. R., Schmand, B., Launer, L. J., Jolles, J., & Jonker, C. (1999). Medial temporal lobe atrophy and memory dysfunction as predictors for dementia in subjects with mild cognitive impairment. *Journal of Neurology, 246*(6), 477–485.

Winblad, B., Gauthier, S., Scinto, L., Feldman, H., Wilcock, G. K., Truyen, L.,...Nye, J. S. (2008). Safety and efficacy of galantamine in subjects with mild cognitive impairment. *Neurology, 70*(22), 2024–2035.

Winblad, B., Palmer, K., Kivipelto, M., Jelic, V., Fratiglioni, L., Wahlund, L-O.,...Petersen, R. C. (2004). Mild cognitive impairment—beyond controversies, towards a consensus. *Journal of Internal Medicine, 256,* 240–246.

Wolk, D., Price, J., Saxton, J., Snitz, B., James, J., Lopez, O.,...De-Kosky, S. T. (2009). Amyloid imaging in mild cognitive impairment subtypes. *Annals of Neurology, 65*(5), 557–568.

18

Preclinical Alzheimer's Disease

Reisa A. Sperling

In 2010, more than a quarter of a century after the original clinical criteria for Alzheimer's disease (AD) were published (McKhann et al., 1984), the National Institute on Aging and the Alzheimer's Association convened three working groups to develop recommendations for updated diagnostic criteria for AD. One of the workgroups was charged with exploring the border zone between "normal aging" and the earliest stages of AD. After much discussion and debate, this workgroup suggested the term "preclinical AD" to connote the stage when the pathophysiological process of AD has begun in the brain but clinically evident symptoms of AD are not yet clearly manifest.

Converging evidence from studies of clinically normal elders and genetic at-risk cohorts strongly suggests that the AD pathophysiological process begins years, perhaps decades, prior to the diagnosis of clinical dementia. Recent advances in neuroimaging, cerebrospinal fluid (CSF) assays, and other biomarkers now allow the in vivo detection of AD pathology. As data began to accumulate from large cohorts of cognitively normal older individuals and asymptomatic autosomal dominant mutation carriers, it became clear that a substantial proportion of these individuals harbored biomarker or imaging evidence of amyloid-β (Aβ) accumulation.

Moreover, the presence of Aβ markers in these asymptomatic individuals was often associated with functional and structural brain alterations, consistent with the patterns of abnormality seen in patients with mild cognitive impairment (MCI) and dementia due to AD. In addition, longitudinal studies suggest that are very subtle alterations in cognition and behavior that are detectable in these "normal" individuals years prior to meeting criteria for MCI and AD dementia. Thus, it is increasingly evident that AD represents a disease continuum, beginning with a preclinical phase that may gradually progress toward the earliest symptomatic stages of AD, through MCI due to AD and ultimately to AD dementia.

It is also clear, however, that some clinically normal older individuals with biomarker evidence of AD may not become symptomatic during their lifetime. The moniker "preclinical AD" does not suppose that all individuals with evidence of preclinical AD will progress to AD dementia—merely that the pathophysiological process of AD is present prior to clinically evident symptoms of AD. Currently, there are insufficient data to predict the likelihood of clinical decline on an individual basis. Thus, the workgroup recommendations for defining the preclinical stages of AD are intended only for research purposes and have no clinical utility at this point.

Redefining the Earliest Stages of Alzheimer's Disease

To facilitate the possibility of presymptomatic treatment of AD in the future, the NIA-AA workgroup felt it was important to define AD as including the underlying pathophysiological disease process, as opposed to having "AD" connote only the clinical stages of the disease as suggested by other criteria (Dubois et al., 2010). In particular, emerging evidence from both genetic at-risk and aging cohorts suggests that there may be a time lag of a decade or more between the beginning of the pathological cascade of AD and the onset of clinically evident impairment. The extent to which biomarkers of AD predict a cognitively normal individual's subsequent clinical course remain to be elucidated, and it is likely that some of individuals with biomarker evidence of AD will never manifest clinical symptoms in their lifetime. Thus, it is critical to determine the factors that best predict the emergence of clinical impairment and progression to eventual AD dementia, and to identify individuals most likely to benefit from early intervention.

Although the concept of a "preclinical" stage of AD has been somewhat controversial, this notion should not be too foreign, as medical professionals readily acknowledge that cancer can be detected at the stage of "carcinoma in situ" and that hypercholesterolemia and atherosclerosis can result in narrowing of coronary arteries that is detectable prior to myocardial infarction. In most areas of medicine, symptoms are not required to diagnose human disease. Type II diabetes, hypertension, renal insufficiency, and osteoporosis are primarily detected through laboratory tests (i.e., biomarkers), and effective treatment can prevent the emergence of symptoms. The field of AD has not yet firmly established the link between the appearance of any specific biomarker in asymptomatic individuals and the subsequent emergence of clinical symptomatology; however, accumulating data suggest that we will someday be able to utilize a combination of biomarkers, genetics, and sensitive neuropsychological measures to identify individuals at high risk for cognitive decline

It is likely that even the preclinical stage of AD represents a continuum from completely asymptomatic individuals with biomarker evidence of AD to biomarker positive individuals who are already demonstrating very subtle decline but whom do not yet meeting standardized criteria for MCI (see Fig. 18.1). It is for this reason that the NIA-AA workgroup chose the term "preclinical AD" rather than asymptomatic or presymptomatic, as it is clear that there is evidence of decline from baseline and very subtle symptoms that are detectable prior to the stage of MCI or prodromal AD. The continuum of preclinical AD also encompasses: (1) individuals who carry one or more apolipoprotein E (*APOE*) ε4 alleles who are known to have an increased risk of developing AD dementia, at the point they are biomarker positive, and (2) carriers of autosomal dominant mutations, who are in the presymptomatic biomarker positive stage of their illness, and who will almost certainly manifest clinical symptoms and progress to dementia.

Models of the Pathophysiological Sequence of Alzheimer's Disease

The majority of biological models of AD continue to suggest that abnormal accumulation of $A\beta_{42}$ is an early event in the pathophysiologic cascade. All of the known autosomal dominant, early-onset forms of AD are thought to be due, at least in part, to alterations in amyloid precursor protein (APP) production or enzymatic cleavage (presenilin 1 and 2). Similarly, trisomy-21 invariably results in AD pathology in individuals who have three intact copies of the *APP* coding region located on chromosome 21. Finally, apolipoprotein E (*APOE*), the major genetic risk factor for late-onset AD, has been implicated in amyloid trafficking and plaque clearance. Both autopsy and biomarker studies suggest that $A\beta_{42}$ accumulation increases with advanced aging, the greatest risk factor for developing AD. There remains significant debate in the field as to whether abnormal processing or clearance of $A\beta_{42}$ is actually an etiologic event in sporadic, late-onset AD (Mawuenyega et al., 2010), and some investigators have suggested that sequestration

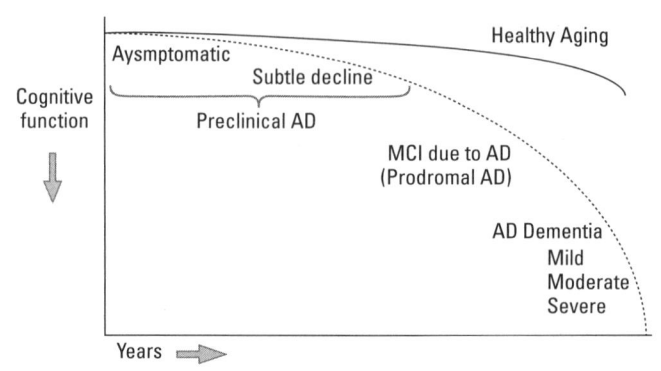

Figure 18.1 The continuum of Alzheimer's disease (AD). The stage of preclinical AD precedes mild cognitive impairment (MCI) and encompasses the spectrum of asymptomatic biomarker-positive older individuals at risk for progression to MCI due to AD and AD dementia, as well as biomarker-positive individuals who have demonstrated subtle decline from their own baseline that exceeds that expected in typical aging but would not yet meet criteria for MCI. Preclinical AD also encompasses individuals at genetic risk for AD, both presymptomatic autosomal dominant mutation carriers and asymptomatic *APOE* ε4 carriers at the point they begin to demonstrate abnormalities on AD biomarkers.

of Aβ into fibrillar forms may even serve as a protective mechanism (Lee et al., 2004; Shankar et al., 2008).

It is also clear that intracellular hyperphosphorylated forms of tau, synaptic, and neuronal loss invariably occur in AD. Thus far, markers of synaptic and neuronal injury appear to correlate better than Aβ plaque burden with clinical status. Although overproduction of Aβ due to autosomal dominant mutations appear to result in "downstream" neuronal pathology (Bateman et al., 2012), it remains to be proven whether Aβ accumulation is sufficient to incite the downstream pathological cascade of AD in late-onset AD. Furthermore, it is not yet clear whether the associated neurodegenerative processes are related to direct synaptic toxicity from oligomeric forms of Aβ, disruption of axonal trajectories from fibrillar forms of Aβ, or a "second hit" (another X factor) that leads to synaptic dysfunction, neurofibrillary tangle formation, neurodegeneration, and ultimately neuronal loss.

Biomarker Model of the Preclinical Stage of Alzheimer's Disease

Jack and colleagues proposed a hypothetical model in which the most widely validated biomarkers of AD become increasingly abnormal in an ordered manner (Jack et al., 2010; see Fig. 18.2). Figure 18.2 was adapted from the original graph proposed by Jack (Jack et al., 2010), which has recently been revised, to expand the preclinical phase. This biomarker model parallels the hypothetical pathophysiological sequence of AD and is particularly relevant to tracking the preclinical stages of AD. Biomarkers of brain Aβ amyloidosis are reductions in CSF Aβ$_{42}$ and increased amyloid positron emission tomography (PET) tracer retention. Elevated CSF tau is thought to be a biomarker of neuronal injury but is not specific to AD, whereas increased CSF phospho-tau may reflect ongoing injury and make be somewhat more specific. Decreased fludeoxyglucose (FDG) uptake on PET in a characteristic temporal-parietal pattern is thought to reflect AD-related synaptic dysfunction. More recently, resting state or "task-free" functional connectivity magnetic resonance imaging (MRI) has also demonstrated a similar pattern of dysfunction in early AD. Note that biomarkers of synaptic dysfunction may demonstrate abnormalities very early, particularly in apolipoprotein E (*APOE*) ε4 allele and autosomal dominant mutation carriers, who may manifest functional abnormalities prior to detectable Aβ deposition (Filippini et al., 2009; Reiman et al., 2004, 2012; Sheline et al., 2010). Brain atrophy on structural MRI in a characteristic pattern involving medial temporal regions and thinning of temporo-parietal cortices

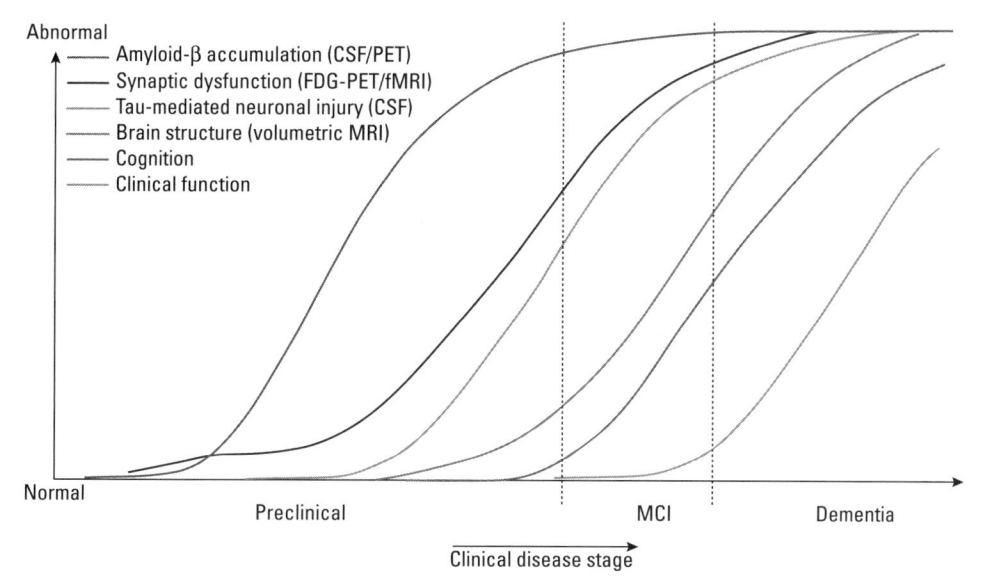

Figure 18.2 Hypothetical model of dynamic biomarkers of Alzheimer's disease (AD) expanded to explicate the preclinical phase: Aβ accumulation detected by cerebrospinal fluid (CSF) Aβ$_{42}$ assays or positron emission tomography (PET) amyloid imaging. Synaptic dysfunction evidenced by fludeoxyglucose (FDG)-PET or functional magnetic resonance imaging (MRI), with a dashed line to indicate that synaptic dysfunction may be detectable in carriers of the ε4 allele of the apolipoprotein E gene (*APOE*) prior to detectable Aβ deposition. Neuronal injury evidenced by CSF tau or phospho-tau. Brain structure by structural MRI. Biomarkers change from maximally normal to maximally abnormal (y axis) as a function of disease stage (x axis). The temporal trajectory of two key indicators used to stage the disease clinically, cognition and clinical function, are also illustrated. MCI, mild cognitive impairment. (Figure adapted with permission from Cliff Jack [Jack et al., 2010]) (See color plate section)

are later biomarkers of AD-related neurodegeneration that may also become subtly abnormal even before clinical symptoms are evident.

The temporal lag between the earliest positivity on AD biomarkers and the emergence of clinical symptoms also may be altered by factors such as brain or cognitive reserve (Stern, 2009). The concept of reserve was originally invoked to account for the observation that the extent of AD histopathologic changes at autopsy was not tightly correlated with the degree of clinical impairment. Reserve can be conceptualized as the ability to tolerate higher levels of brain injury without exhibiting clinical symptoms. "Cognitive reserve" is thought to represent the ability to engage alternate brain networks or cognitive strategies to cope with the effects of encroaching pathology, whereas "brain reserve" refers to the capacity of the brain to withstand pathologic insult, perhaps due to greater synaptic density or larger number of healthy neurons, such that sufficient neural substrate remains to support normal function. It is not clear, however, that the data support a clear demarcation between these two concepts, as many factors, such as higher socioeconomic status or engagement in cognitively stimulating activities, may contribute to both types of reserve. Recent studies suggest that high reserve may primarily influence the capability of individuals to tolerate occult AD pathology without evidence of subtle cognitive signs (Rentz et al., 2010; Roe et al., 2008), but it may be associated with rapid decline once the "tipping point" is reached and compensatory mechanisms begin to fail (Fotenos, Mintun, Snyder, Morris, & Buckner, 2008; Wilson et al., 2010).

Epidemiological studies suggest there are factors that may significantly modulate the clinical expression of AD pathology, although evidence that these factors alter the underlying pathophysiologic process itself is less clear. Large cohort studies have implicated multiple health factors that may increase the risk for developing cognitive decline and dementia thought to be due to AD (Yaffe et al., 2009). In particular, vascular risk factors such as hypertension, hypercholesterolemia, and diabetes have been associated with an increased risk of dementia, and they may contribute directly to the impact of AD pathology on the aging brain (Arvanitakis, Wilson, Bienias, Evans, & Bennett, 2004; Craft, 2009). On the positive side, there is some evidence that engagement in specific activities, including cognitive, physical, leisure, and social activity, may be associated with decreased risk of AD pathology (Landau et al., 2012; Vidoni et al., 2012), and also progression toward MCI and AD dementia (Wilson, Scherr, Schneider, Tang, & Bennett, 2007).

Biomarker Evidence Linking Alzheimer's Disease Pathology to Early Symptomatology

Several multicenter biomarker initiatives, including the Alzheimer's Disease Neuroimaging Initiative (ADNI), and the Australian Imaging, Biomarker & Lifestyle Flagship Study of Ageing (AIBL), as well as longitudinal biomarker studies in preclinical AD populations at several academic centers, including Harvard, Washington University, and the Mayo Clinic, are ongoing. Many of the recent studies have focused on markers of Aβ, using either CSF assays of Aβ42 or PET amyloid imaging with radioactive tracers that bind to fibrillar forms of Aβ. Both CSF and PET amyloid imaging studies suggest that a substantial proportion of clinically normal older individuals demonstrate evidence of Aβ accumulation (De Meyer et al., 2011; Gomperts et al., 2008; Jack et al., 2008; Mintun et al., 2006; Montine et al., 2011; Rowe et al., 2006). The exact proportion of "amyloid-positive" normal individuals is dependent on the age and genetic background of the cohort, but it ranges from approximately 20%–40% and is very consonant with large postmortem series (Arriagada, Marzloff, & Hyman, 1992; Morris et al., 1996, Bennett et al., 2006). Interestingly, the percentage of "amyloid-positive" normal individuals at autopsy detected at a given age closely parallels the percentage of individuals diagnosed with AD dementia a decade later (Rowe et al., 2010). Similarly, genetic at-risk cohorts demonstrate evidence of Aβ accumulation many years prior to detectable cognitive impairment (Bateman et al., 2012; Klunk et al., 2007; Moonis et al., 2005; Reiman et al., 2009; Ringman et al., 2008). Both autosomal dominant cohorts and *APOE* ε4 carrier data suggest that synaptic function markers may be abnormal prior to detectable Aβ deposition on PET amyloid imaging or the drop in CSF Aβ levels, supporting the hypothesis that soluble forms of Aβ may be responsible for synaptic toxicity.

Multiple groups have reported that cognitively normal older individuals with low CSF Aβ$_{1-42}$ or high PET amyloid tracer retention demonstrate disruption of functional networks during cognitive tasks or altered connectivity at rest (Hedden et al., 2009; Kennedy et al., 2012; Mormino et al., 2011; Sheline et al., 2009; Sperling et al., 2009). In addition, Aβ-"positive" clinically normal older adults demonstrate decreased brain volume at baseline (Becker et al., 2011; Desikan et al., 2010; Dickerson et al., 2009; Fjell et al., 2010; Oh et al.,) consistent with the patterns seen in AD dementia, and increased rates of atrophy (Chetelat et al., 2012; Sabuncu et al., 2011; Schott, Bartlett, Fox, & Barnes, 2010). There have been variable reports in the literature thus far as to whether Aβ positive individuals demonstrate lower neuropsychological test scores cross-sectionally at the time of biomarker acquisition (Aizenstein et al., 2008; Hedden et al., 2012; Mormino et al., 2009; Pike et al., 2007; Rentz et al., 2010; Sperling, Karlawish, & Johnson, 2013), which may represent heterogeneity in where these individuals fall on the preclinical continuum, the cognitive measures evaluated, and the degree of cognitive reserve in the cohorts. Interestingly, two recent reports also link PET evidence of Aβ to increased subjective cognitive concerns, particularly with self-report of increasing memory difficulty in everyday life (Amariglio et al., 2012; Perrotin, Mormino, Madison, Hayenga, & Jagust, 2012). Several longitudinal studies have now reported that Aβ positivity in clinically normal older individuals an increased risk of cognitive decline and progression to dementia (Chételat et al., 2011; Doraiswamy et al., 2012; Fagan et al., 2007; Knopman et al., 2012; Li et al., 2007; Lim et al., 2013; Morris et al., 2009; Resnick et al.,

2010; Storandt, Mintun, Head, & Morris, 2009; Villemagne et al., 2008). Additional longitudinal studies are clearly needed to confirm these findings and to elucidate the combination of factors or biomarkers that best predict likelihood and rate of decline, and to better understand individual differences in risk for decline.

In addition to the aforementioned longitudinal studies in older at-risk populations, researchers continue to investigate the biomarker changes associated with genetic risk for AD. To date, the best established genetic risk factors for AD include common allelic variants of *APOE*, the major late-onset AD susceptibility gene, uncommon early-onset AD-causing mutations in the presenilin 1 (*PSEN1*), presenilin 2 (*PSEN2*), and amyloid precursor protein (*APP*) genes, and Trisomy 21 (Down syndrome). Biomarker studies in presymptomatic carriers of autosomal dominant mutations have revealed evidence of Aβ accumulation on CSF and PET amyloid imaging more than 20 years prior to the expected age of dementia onset in their families, as well as FDG-PET hypometabolism, functional MRI abnormalities, and brain atrophy that may also precede symptoms by more than a decade (Bateman et al., 2012; Reiman et al., 2012).

A Conceptual Framework for Staging Preclinical Alzheimer's Disease

Based on the available data in 2010 and the biomarker framework utilized by the MCI and AD dementia workgroups, the NIA-AA preclinical workgroup proposed a three-stage model for preclinical AD to characterize individuals at increasing risk of progression toward MCI and dementia (Sperling, Jack, & Aisen, 2011). Table 18.1 summarizes the categorization of biomarkers across the stages of preclinical AD. Stage 1 is characterized as asymptomatic cerebral amyloidosis; Stage 2 is amyloidosis plus neurodegeneration; and Stage 3 is amyloidosis, neurodegeneration, and evidence of very subtle change in cognition, including subjective cognitive concern, or behavior that is insufficient to be diagnosed with MCI. Cliff Jack and colleagues from the Mayo Clinic added two additional categories that may be useful in capturing the full spectrum of the clinically normal populations: (1) Stage 0 to connote older individuals without any biomarker evidence of AD pathology and (2) Suspected non-Alzheimer's pathology (SNAP) to categorize individuals who do not have biomarker evidence of amyloid pathology but who demonstrate abnormalities on markers of neuronal injury or subtle cognitive abnormalities (Jack et al., 2012). Additional work is required to determine the utility of such a staging framework; however, initial results suggest that individuals in preclinical Stage 2 or 3 are indeed at increased risk of progression to MCI and AD dementia (Knopman et al., 2012).

The definitive studies to determine whether the majority of asymptomatic individuals with Aβ accumulation are indeed destined to develop AD dementia, and to elucidate the biomarker and/or cognitive endophenotype that is most predictive of cognitive decline will likely take more than a decade to fully accomplish. Even if all of the postulates mentioned previously prove to be correct, a number of challenges remain

TABLE 18.1 Staging Categories for Preclinical Alzheimer's Disease Research

Stage	Description	Markers of Aβ Accumulation (PET or CSF)	Markers of Neuronal Injury (CSF tau, FDG, MRI)	Evidence of Subtle Cognitive Change
Stage 1	Asymptomatic cerebral amyloidosis	Positive	Negative	Negative
Stage 2	Asymptomatic amyloidosis + "downstream" neurodegeneration	Positive	Positive	Negative
Stage 3	Amyloidosis + neuronal injury + subtle cognitive decline	Positive	Positive	Positive

Source: From Sperling et al. (2011).

before these research recommendations can be translated into clinical practice (Sperling et al., 2013). The ethical and practical implications of future implementation of making a "diagnosis" of AD at a preclinical stage need to be carefully studied before any of these diagnostic tests are offered to clinically normal older individuals. In particular, the poignant question of "Why would individuals want to know they have AD a decade before they might develop symptoms, if there is nothing they can do about it?" needs to be carefully considered well before any results from research is translated into clinical practice. There may be important reasons, including social and financial planning, that some individuals would want to know their likelihood of developing AD dementia within the next decade, even in the absence of an available disease-modifying therapy. It is our hope, however, that the advances in preclinical detection of AD will enable earlier, more effective treatment, just as nearly all of therapeutic gains in cancer, cardiovascular disease, osteoporosis, and diabetes involve treatment before significant clinical symptoms are present.

Why Would We Want to Detect Alzheimer's Disease a Decade Before Dementia?

The long preclinical phase of AD provides a critical opportunity for potential intervention with disease-modifying therapy, if we are able to elucidate the link between the presence of AD biomarkers in asymptomatic individuals and the emergence of the clinical syndrome. As our population ages, with 10,000 baby boomers turning age 65 every day in the United States and entering the age of increased risk for AD, early detection and intervention is increasingly imperative. Recent analyses by the Alzheimer's Association suggest that a hypothetical intervention that delayed the onset of AD dementia by just 5 years would result in a 57% reduction in the number of AD dementia patients and reduce the projected Medicare costs of AD from $627 to $344 billion (http://www.alz.org/alzheimers_disease_trajectory.asp). These models suggest that a screening instrument for the presence of AD pathology (with 90% sensitivity and specificity), and a treatment that slows progression by 50%, would reduce the lifetime risk for AD dementia for a 65-year-old from 10.5% to 5.7%.

The recognition that the pathophysiological process of AD is already well under way prior to the stage of clinically evident symptoms has already spurred plans for very early intervention trials. These studies might be thought of as "secondary prevention" to delay the onset of the clinical syndrome in individuals in whom the brain disease has already begun. The Alzheimer's Prevention Initiative (API) (Reiman et al., 2011) and Dominantly Inherited Alzheimer Network (DIAN) (Bateman et al., 2012) clinical trials will enroll asymptomatic individuals from families with autosomal dominant mutations with two monoclonal antibodies against Aβ (solanezumab and gantanerumab). The "A4" Anti-Amyloid Treatment of Asymptomatic Alzheimer's disease trial will enroll clinically normal older individuals with evidence of amyloid pathology on PET amyloid imaging and treat with a monoclonal antibody against Aβ (solanezumab) for 3 years in a placebo-controlled trial. Additional anti-amyloid trials in preclinical AD populations are currently in the planning stages. The results from these studies will provide important information regarding the role of amyloid in early cognitive decline in AD.

The success of these prevention trials, however, does not require that amyloid is "the" cause of AD, merely that amyloid is "a" critical factor in the pathway that can be treated at the right stage of AD. A useful analogy may be cholesterol lowering in cardiac disease. Many individuals with high cholesterol never experience a myocardial infarction (MI), but lowering cholesterol at the population level has substantially decreased cardiac morbidity and mortality over the past decade. The relationship between cholesterol and cardiac disease took many years to establish, requiring both large natural history studies, such as the Framingham study, and multiple prevention trials in familial hypercholesterolemia, individuals with early symptoms of ischemic hear disease, and ultimately in healthy individuals at high risk for coronary heart disease. Lowering cholesterol may be very helpful in reducing an individual's risk prior to any cardiac symptoms, and even after a single MI, but is unlikely to improve cardiac function at the end stage of ischemic heart failure. Similarly, it is likely that we may need to intervene with anti-amyloid therapies at a much earlier stage of AD to maximally impact the clinical course of the disease (Sperling et al., 2011). Studies with transgenic mouse models strongly suggest that Aβ-modifying therapies may have limited impact once neuronal degeneration has begun (Oddo, Billings, Kesslak, Cribbs, & LaFerla, 2004). Disappointing results from Phase 3 studies of anti-Aβ monoclonal antibodies at the stage of dementia, despite evidence of biological activity, also support the need for earlier intervention. Although secondary prevention trials at the stage of preclinical AD will be long, expensive, and challenging to execute, the potential public health impact is tremendous.

Acknowledgments

The author wishes to acknowledge the invaluable contributions of the NIA-AA Workgroup on Preclinical Alzheimer's disease.

References

Aizenstein, H. J., Nebes, R. D., Saxton, J. A., Price, J. C., Mathis, C. A., Tsopelas, N. D.,... Klunk, W. E (2008). Frequent amyloid deposition without significant cognitive impairment among the elderly. *Archives of Neurology*, 65(11), 1509–1517.

Amariglio, R. E., Becker, J. A., Carmasin, J., Wadsworth, L. P., Lorius, N., Sullivan, C.,...Rentz, D. M. (2012). Subjective cognitive complaints and amyloid burden in cognitively normal older individuals. *Neuropsychologia*, 50(12), 2880–2886.

Arriagada, P. V., Marzloff, K., & Hyman, B. T. (1992). Distribution of Alzheimer-type pathologic changes in nondemented elderly individuals matches the pattern in Alzheimer's disease. *Neurology* 1992;42(9), 1681–1688.

Arvanitakis, Z., Wilson, R. S., Bienias, J. L., Evans, D. A., & Bennett, D. A. (2004). Diabetes mellitus and risk of Alzheimer disease and decline in cognitive function. *Archives of Neurology*, 61(5), 661–666.

Bateman, R. J., Xiong, C., Benzinger, T. L., Fagan, A. M., Goate, A., Fox, N. C.,...Morris, J. C. (2012). Clinical and biomarker changes in dominantly inherited Alzheimer's disease. *New England Journal of Medicine*, 367(9), 795–804.

Becker, J. A., Hedden, T., Carmasin, J., Maye, J., Rentz, D. M., Putcha, D.,...Johnson, K. A. (2011). Amyloid-beta associated cortical thinning in clinically normal elderly. *Annals of Neurology*, 69(6), 1032–1042.

Bennett, D., Schneider, J., Arvanitakis, Z., Kelly, J., Aggarwal, N., Shah, R., & Wilson, R. S. (2006). Neuropathology of older persons without cognitive impairment from two community-based studies. *Neurology*, 66, 1837–1844.

Chételat, G., Villemagne, V. L., Pike, K., Ellis, K., Bourgeat, P., Jones, G.,...Rowe, C. C. (2011). Independent contribution of temporal b-Amyloid deposition to memory decline in non-demented elderly. *Brain*, 134(Pt 3), 798–807.

Chetelat, G., Villemagne, V. L., Villain, N., Jones, G., Ellis, K. A., Ames, D.,...Rowe, C. C. (2012). Accelerated cortical atrophy in cognitively normal elderly with high beta-amyloid deposition. *Neurology*, 78(7), 477–484.

Craft, S. (2009). The role of metabolic disorders in Alzheimer disease and vascular dementia: Two roads converged. *Archives of Neurology*, 66(3), 300–305.

De Meyer, G., Shapiro, F., Vanderstichele, H., Vanmechelen, E., Engelborghs, S., De Deyn, P. P.,...Trojanowski, J. Q. (2011). Diagnosis-independent Alzheimer disease biomarker signature in cognitively normal elderly people. *Archives of Neurology*, 67(8), 949–956.

Desikan, R. S., Sabuncu, M. R., Schmansky, N. J., Reuter, M., Cabral, H. J., Hess, C. P.,...Fischl, B. (2010). Selective disruption of the cerebral neocortex in Alzheimer's disease. *PLoS One*, 5(9), e12853.

Dickerson, B. C., Bakkour, A., Salat, D. H., Feczko, E., Pacheco, J., Greve, D. N.,...Buckner, R. L. (2009). The cortical signature of Alzheimer's disease: Regionally specific cortical thinning relates to symptom severity in very mild to mild AD dementia and is detectable in asymptomatic amyloid-positive individuals. *Cereb Cortex*, 19(3), 497–510.

Doraiswamy PM, Sperling RA, Coleman RE, Johnson KA, Reiman EM, Davis MD,...Pontecorvo, M. J. (2012). Amyloid-beta assessed by florbetapir F 18 PET and 18-month cognitive decline: A multicenter study. *Neurology*, 79(16), 1636–1644.

Dubois, B., Feldman, H. H., Jacova, C., Cummings, J. L., Dekosky, S. T., Barberger-Gateau, P.,...Scheltens, P. (2010). Revising the definition of Alzheimer's disease: A new lexicon. *Lancet Neurology*, 9(11), 1118–1127.

Fagan, A. M., Roe, C. M., Xiong, C., Mintun, M. A., Morris, J. C., & Holtzman, D. M. (2007). Cerebrospinal fluid tau/beta-amyloid(42) ratio as a prediction of cognitive decline in nondemented older adults. *Archives of Neurology*, 64(3), 343–349.

Filippini, N., MacIntosh, B. J., Hough, M. G., Goodwin, G. M., Frisoni, G. B., Smith, S. M.,...Mackay, C. E. (2009). Distinct patterns of brain activity in young carriers of the APOE-epsilon4 allele. *Proceedings of the National Academy of Science USA, 106*(17), 7209–7214.

Fjell, A. M., Walhovd, K. B., Fennema-Notestine, C., McEvoy, L. K., Hagler, D. J., Holland, D.,...Dale, A. M. (2010). Brain atrophy in healthy aging is related to CSF levels of Abeta1-42. *Cerebral Cortex, 20*(9), 2069–2079.

Fotenos, A. F., Mintun, M. A., Snyder, A. Z., Morris, J. C., & Buckner, R. L. (2008). Brain volume decline in aging: Evidence for a relation between socioeconomic status, preclinical Alzheimer disease, and reserve. *Archives of Neurology, 65*(1), 113–120.

Gomperts, S. N., Rentz, D. M., Moran, E., Becker, J. A., Locascio, J. J., Klunk, W. E.,...Johnson, K. A. (2008). Imaging amyloid deposition in Lewy body diseases. *Neurology, 71*(12), 903–910.

Hedden, T., Mormino, E. C., Amariglio, R. E., Younger, A. P., Schultz, A. P., Becker, J. A.,...Rentz, D. M. (2012). Cognitive profile of amyloid burden and white matter hyperintensities in cognitively normal older adults. *Journal of Neuroscience, 32*(46), 16233–16242.

Hedden, T., Van Dijk, K. R., Becker, J. A., Mehta, A., Sperling, R. A., Johnson, K. A., & Buckner, R. L. (2009). Disruption of functional connectivity in clinically normal older adults harboring amyloid burden. *Journal of Neuroscience, 29*(40), 12686–12694.

Jack, C. R., Jr., Knopman, D. S., Jagust, W. J., Shaw, L. M., Aisen, P. S., Weiner, M. W.,...Trojanowski, J. Q. (2010). Hypothetical model of dynamic biomarkers of the Alzheimer's pathological cascade. *Lancet Neurology, 9*(1), 119–128.

Jack, C. R., Jr., Knopman, D. S., Weigand, S. D., Wiste, H. J., Vemuri, P., Lowe, V.,...Petersen, R. C. (2012). An operational approach to National Institute on Aging-Alzheimer's Association criteria for preclinical Alzheimer disease. *Annals of Neurology, 71*(6), 765–775.

Jack, C. R., Jr., Lowe, V. J., Senjem, M. L., Weigand, S. D., Kemp, B. J., Shiung, M. M.,...Petersen, R. C. (2008). 11C PiB and structural MRI provide complementary information in imaging of Alzheimer's disease and amnestic mild cognitive impairment. *Brain, 131*(Pt 3), 665–680.

Kennedy, K. M., Rodrigue, K. M., Devous, M. D., Sr., Hebrank, A. C., Bischof, G. N., & Park, D. C. (2012). Effects of beta-amyloid accumulation on neural function during encoding across the adult lifespan. *Neuroimage, 62*(1), 1–8.

Klunk, W. E., Price, J. C., Mathis, C. A., Tsopelas, N. D., Lopresti, B. J., Ziolko, S. K.,...DeKosky, S. T. (2007). Amyloid deposition begins in the striatum of presenilin-1 mutation carriers from two unrelated pedigrees. *Journal of Neuroscience, 27*(23), 6174–6184.

Knopman, D. S., Jack, C. R., Jr., Wiste, H. J., Weigand, S. D., Vemuri, P., Lowe, V.,...Petersen, R. C. (2012). Short-term clinical outcomes for stages of NIA-AA preclinical Alzheimer disease. *Neurology, 78*(20), 1576–1582.

Landau, S. M., Marks, S. M., Mormino, E. C., Rabinovici, G. D., Oh, H., O'Neil, J. P.,...Jagust, W. J. (2012). Association of lifetime cognitive engagement and low beta-amyloid deposition. *Archives of Neurology, 69*(5), 623–629.

Lee, H. G., Casadesus, G., Zhu, X., Takeda, A., Perry, G., & Smith, M. A. (2004). Challenging the amyloid cascade hypothesis: Senile plaques and amyloid-beta as protective adaptations to Alzheimer disease. *Annals of the New York Academy of Sciences, 1019*, 1–4.

Li, G., Sokal, I., Quinn, J. F., Leverenz, J. B., Brodey, M., Schellenberg, G. D.,...Montine, T. J. (2007). CSF tau/Abeta42 ratio for increased risk of mild cognitive impairment: A follow-up study. *Neurology, 69*(7), 631–639.

Lim, Y. Y., Pietrzak, R. H., Ellis, K. A., Jaeger, J., Harrington, K., Ashwood, T.,...Maruff, P. (2013). Rapid decline in episodic memory in healthy older adults with high amyloid-beta. *Journal of Alzheimers Disease, 33*(3), 675–679.

Mawuenyega, K. G., Sigurdson, W., Ovod, V., Munsell, L., Kasten, T., Morris, J. C.,...Bateman, R. J. (2010). Decreased clearance of CNS beta-amyloid in Alzheimer's disease. *Science, 330*(6012), 1774.

McKhann, G., Drachman, D., Folstein, M., Katzman, R., Price, D., & Stadlan, E. M. (1984). Clinical diagnosis of Alzheimer's disease: Report of the NINCDS-ADRDA Work Group under the auspices of Department of Health and Human Services Task Force on Alzheimer's Disease. *Neurology, 34*(7), 939–944.

Mintun, M. A., Larossa, G. N., Sheline, Y. I., Dence, C. S., Lee, S. Y., Mach, R. H.,...Morris, J. C. (2006). [11C]PIB in a nondemented population: Potential antecedent marker of Alzheimer disease. *Neurology, 67*(3), 446–452.

Montine, T. J., Peskind, E. R., Quinn, J. F., Wilson, A. M., Montine, K. S., & Galasko, D. (2011). Increased cerebrospinal fluid F(2)-isoprostanes are associated with aging and latent Alzheimer's disease as identified by biomarkers. *Neuromolecular Medicine, 13*(1), 37–43.

Moonis, M., Swearer, J. M., Dayaw, M. P., St George-Hyslop, P., Rogaeva, E., Kawarai, T.,...Pollen, D. A. (2005). Familial Alzheimer disease: Decreases in CSF Abeta42 levels precede cognitive decline. *Neurology, 65*(2), 323–325.

Mormino, E. C., Kluth, J. T., Madison, C. M., Rabinovici, G. D., Baker, S. L., Miller, B. L., (2009). Episodic memory loss is related to hippocampal-mediated {beta}-amyloid deposition in elderly subjects. *Brain, 132*(5), 1310–1323.

Mormino, E. C., Smiljic, A., Hayenga, A. O., Onami, S. H., Greicius, M. D., Rabinovici, G. D.,...Jagust, W. J. (2011). Relationships between beta-amyloid and functional connectivity in different components of the default mode network in aging. *Cerebral Cortex, 21*(10), 2399–2407.

Morris, J. C., Roe, C. M., Grant, E. A., Head, D., Storandt, M., Goate, A. M.,...Mintun, M. A. (2009). Pittsburgh Compound B imaging and prediction of progression from cognitive normality to symptomatic Alzheimer disease. *Archives of Neurology, 66*(12), 1469–1475.

Morris, J. C., Storandt, M., McKeel, D. W., Jr., Rubin, E. H., Price, J. L., Grant, E. A., & Berg, L. (1996). Cerebral amyloid deposition and diffuse plaques in "normal" aging: Evidence for presymptomatic and very mild Alzheimer's disease. *Neurology, 46*(3), 707–719.

Oddo, S., Billings, L., Kesslak, J. P., Cribbs, D. H., & LaFerla, F. M. (2004). Abeta immunotherapy leads to clearance of early, but not late, hyperphosphorylated tau aggregates via the proteasome. *Neuron, 43*(3), 321–332.

Oh, H., Mormino, E. C., Madison, C., Hayenga, A., Smiljic, A., & Jagust, W. J. beta-Amyloid affects frontal and posterior brain networks in normal aging. *Neuroimage, 54*(3), 1887–1895.

Perrotin, A., Mormino, E. C., Madison, C. M., Hayenga, A. O., & Jagust, W. J. (2012). Subjective cognition and amyloid deposition imaging: A Pittsburgh compound B positron emission tomography study in normal elderly individuals. *Archives of Neurology, 69*(2), 223–229.

Pike, K. E., Savage, G., Villemagne, V. L., Ng, S., Moss, S. A., Maruff, P.,...Rowe, C. C. (2007). Beta-amyloid imaging and memory in non-demented individuals: Evidence for preclinical Alzheimer's disease. *Brain, 130*(Pt 11), 2837–2844.

Reiman, E. M., Chen, K., Alexander, G. E., Caselli, R. J., Bandy, D., Osborne, D.,...Hardy, J. (2004). Functional brain abnormalities in young adults at genetic risk for late-onset Alzheimer's dementia. *Proceedings of the National Academy of Science USA, 101*(1), 284–289.

Reiman, E. M., Chen, K., Liu, X., Bandy, D., Yu, M., Lee, W.,...Caselli, R. J. (2009). Fibrillar amyloid-beta burden in cognitively normal people at 3 levels of genetic risk for Alzheimer's disease. *Proceedings of the National Academy of Science USA, 106*(16), 6820–6825.

Reiman, E. M., Langbaum, J. B., Fleisher, A. S., Caselli, R. J., Chen, K., Ayutyanont, N.,...Tariot, P. N. (2011). Alzheimer's Prevention Initiative: A plan to accelerate the evaluation of presymptomatic treatments. *Journal of Alzheimers Disease, 26*(Suppl 3), 321–329.

Reiman, E. M., Quiroz, Y. T., Fleisher, A. S., Chen, K., Velez-Pardo, C., Jimenez-Del-Rio, M.,...Lopera, F. (2012). Brain imaging and fluid biomarker analysis in young adults at genetic risk for autosomal dominant Alzheimer's disease in the presenilin 1 E280A kindred: A case-control study. *Lancet Neurology, 11*(12), 1048–1056.

Rentz, D. M., Locascio, J. J., Becker, J. A., Moran, E. K., Eng, E., Buckner, R. L.,...Johnson, K. A. (2010). Cognition, reserve, and amyloid deposition in normal aging. *Annals of Neurology, 67*(3), 353–364.

Resnick, S. M., Sojkova, J., Zhou, Y., An, Y., Ye, W., Holt, D. P.,...Wong, D. F. (2010). Longitudinal cognitive decline is associated with fibrillar amyloid-beta measured by [11C]PiB. *Neurology, 74*(10), 807–815.

Ringman, J. M., Younkin, S. G., Pratico, D., Seltzer, W., Cole, G. M., Geschwind, D. H.,...Cummings, J. L. (2008). Biochemical markers in persons with preclinical familial Alzheimer disease. *Neurology, 71*(2), 85–92.

Roe, C. M., Mintun, M. A., D'Angelo, G., Xiong, C., Grant, E. A., & Morris, J. C. (2008). Alzheimer disease and cognitive reserve: Variation of education effect with carbon 11-labeled Pittsburgh Compound B uptake. *Archives of Neurology, 65*(11), 1467–1471.

Rowe, C. C., Ellis, K. A., Rimajova, M., Bourgeat, P., Pike, K. E., Jones, G.,...Villemagne, V. L. (2010). Amyloid imaging results from the Australian Imaging, Biomarkers and Lifestyle (AIBL) study of aging. *Neurobiology of Aging, 31*(8), 1275–1283.

Rowe, C. C., Ng, S., Gong, S. J., Ackermann, W., Pike, K., Savage, G., (2006). *C-11 PIB PET amyloid imaging in ageing and dementia.* Presentation at the Alzheimer Imaging Consortium, International Conference on Alzheimer's Disease, Madrid, Spain.

Sabuncu, M. R., Desikan, R. S., Sepulcre, J., Yeo, B. T., Liu, H., Schmansky, N. J.,...Fischl, B. (2011). The dynamics of cortical and hippocampal atrophy in Alzheimer disease. *Archives of Neurology, 68*(8), 1040–1048.

Schott, J. M., Bartlett, J. W., Fox, N. C., & Barnes, J. (2010). Increased brain atrophy rates in cognitively normal older adults with low cerebrospinal fluid Abeta1-42. *Annals of Neurology, 68*(6), 825–834.

Shankar, G. M., Li, S., Mehta, T. H., Garcia-Munoz, A., Shepardson, N. E., Smith, I., ... Selkoe, D. J. (2008). Amyloid-beta protein dimers isolated directly from Alzheimer's brains impair synaptic plasticity and memory. *Nature Medicine, 14*(8), 837–842.

Sheline, Y. I., Morris, J. C., Snyder, A. Z., Price, J. L., Yan, Z., D'Angelo, G., ... Mintun, M. A. (2010). APOE4 allele disrupts resting state fMRI connectivity in the absence of amyloid plaques or decreased CSF Abeta42. *Journal of Neuroscience, 30*(50), 17035–17040.

Sheline, Y. I., Raichle, M. E., Snyder, A. Z., Morris, J. C., Head, D., Wang, S., & Mintun, M. A. (2009). Amyloid plaques disrupt resting state default mode network connectivity in cognitively normal elderly. *Biological Psychiatry, 67*(6), 584–587.

Sperling, R. A., Aisen, P. S., Beckett, L. A., Bennett, D. A., Craft, S., Fagan, A. M., ... Phelps, C. H. (2011). Toward defining the preclinical stages of Alzheimer's disease: Recommendations from the National Institute on Aging-Alzheimer's Association workgroups on diagnostic guidelines for Alzheimer's disease. *Alzheimers Dementia, 7*(3), 280–292.

Sperling, R. A., Jack, C. R., Jr., & Aisen, P. S. (2011). Testing the right target and right drug at the right stage. *Science Translational Medicine, 3*(111), 111cm33.

Sperling, R. A., Johnson, K. A., Doraiswamy, P. M., Reiman, E. M., Fleisher, A. S., Sabbagh, M. N., ... Pontecorvo, M. J. (2013). Amyloid deposition detected with florbetapir F 18 ((18)F-AV-45) is related to lower episodic memory performance in clinically normal older individuals. *Neurobiology of Aging, 34*(3), 822–831.

Sperling, R. A., Karlawish, J., & Johnson, K. A. (2013). Preclinical Alzheimer disease-the challenges ahead. *Nature Reviews Neurology, 9*(1), 54–58.

Sperling, R. A., Laviolette, P. S., O'Keefe, K., O'Brien, J., Rentz, D. M., Pihlajamaki, M., ... Johnson, K. A. (2009). Amyloid deposition is associated with impaired default network function in older persons without dementia. *Neuron, 63*(2), 178–188.

Stern, Y. (2009). Cognitive reserve. *Neuropsychologia, 47*(10), 2015–2028.

Storandt, M., Mintun, M. A., Head, D., & Morris, J. C. (2009). Cognitive decline and brain volume loss as signatures of cerebral amyloid-beta peptide deposition identified with Pittsburgh compound B: Cognitive decline associated with Abeta deposition. *Archives of Neurology, 66*(12), 1476–1481.

Vidoni, E. D., Van Sciver, A., Johnson, D. K., He, J., Honea, R., Haines, B., ... Burns, J. M. (2012). A community-based approach to trials of aerobic exercise in aging and Alzheimer's disease. *Contemporary Clinical Trials, 33*(6), 1105–1116.

Villemagne, V. L., Pike, K. E., Darby, D., Maruff, P., Savage, G., Ng, S., ... Rowe, C. C. (2008). Abeta deposits in older non-demented individuals with cognitive decline are indicative of preclinical Alzheimer's disease. *Neuropsychologia, 46*(6), 1688–1697.

Wilson, R. S., Barnes, L. L., Aggarwal, N. T., Boyle, P. A., Hebert, L. E., Mendes de Leon, C. F., & Evans, D. A. (2010). Cognitive activity and the cognitive morbidity of Alzheimer disease. *Neurology, 75*(11), 990–996.

Wilson, R. S., Scherr, P. A., Schneider, J. A., Tang, Y., & Bennett, D. A. (2007). Relation of cognitive activity to risk of developing Alzheimer disease. *Neurology, 69*(20), 1911–1920.

Yaffe, K., Fiocco, A. J., Lindquist, K., Vittinghoff, E., Simonsick, E. M., Newman, A. B., ... Harris, T. B. (2009). Predictors of maintaining cognitive function in older adults: The Health ABC study. *Neurology, 72*(23), 2029–2035.

Part III

Assessment, Diagnosis, and Comprehensive Treatment: From Principles to Practice

19

Dementia Screening and Mental Status Examination in Clinical Practice

Meghan B. Mitchell and Alireza Atri

The mental status examination is a critical first step in identifying individuals with potential cognitive problems in primary care, specialty clinic, and other outpatient settings. It is additionally an invaluable tool for tracking changes in a patient's overall level of cognitive function in an inpatient setting or after a clinical dementia diagnosis has been established. It is frequently a mental status examination that provides a first indication that a patient may be in the early stages of dementia. Frequently, it is also a change in mental status noted in an inpatient setting that can alert clinicians that an acute and systemic change in a patient's health has led to a potentially reversible cognitive, functional, or behavioral problem such as delirium (Rudolph et al., 2008). This chapter provides a review of approaches to the mental status examination that includes comparison of standardized instruments and measures to detect cognitive impairment and dementia in the office or hospital setting, as well as additional observations and tests that can complement standardized measures in the screening mental status evaluation.

While there are many approaches to conducting the mental status examination, clinicians typically include their own qualitative evaluation of different aspects of a patient's level of awareness and cognitive function, in addition to one of several standardized measures that provide a brief assessment of multiple domains of cognitive function. These measures are typically summarized in one global summary score, and cutoff scores can be applied to optimally maximize the sensitivity of the measure at detecting impairment. As such, these tools can be thought of as screening tools that identify cases for which a referral can be made for more extensive evaluation of cognitive function by a neuropsychologist or other subspecialized clinician.

Typically the goal of a mental status examination is to provide a brief assessment of multiple aspects of the patients behavioral, psychological, daily, and cognitive functioning. This typically includes consideration of the patient's appearance, ability to carry out activities of daily living, mood and insight, level of arousal and orientation, and multiple aspects of cognitive function, including processing speed; psychomotor function; attention; and executive, language, visuospatial, and memory functions. The examination should ideally be applied using a flexible approach, in which the clinician adapts to the presentation of each patient. For example, if it becomes clear upon initial introductions that a patient is extremely disinhibited (e.g., making inappropriate sexual comments), a mental status examination with more elaborate assessment of executive and frontal lobe functioning would be warranted, whereas memory function might be more of a focus if the patient has trouble recalling details of her recent personal history. Before and while meeting with a patient, consider the following questions to form a hypothesis and appropriate plan of action:

- What is the purpose of this examination?
- What is the primary presenting symptom, complaint, or problem?
- What is/has been the most salient symptom, complaint, or problem?
- What is the pace of progression of symptoms or problems?
- Are there any unusual associated features or temporal associations?
- What diagnoses may be considered in this case?
- What particular aspects of cognition or psychological function may be affected?
- How should the testing and interpretation of the results be adjusted to the patient's level of education, intelligence, and estimated previous intellectual and functional capacities?
- Are there cultural, ethnic, or primary language considerations that should be made while testing and interpreting the results?

In the context of performing mental status examinations where dementia diagnosis is at the forefront of the differential diagnosis, appropriate consideration of the base rates of different forms of dementia is warranted. Specifically, as Alzheimer's dementia is the most common form of dementia (Hebert, Weuve, Scherr, & Evans, 2013), and changes in memory function tend to be the first clinically observable signs in the Alzheimer's disease (AD) spectrum (Albert et al., 2011; Mckhann et al., 2011; Petersen et al., 1999; Sperling et al., 2011), evaluation of memory is almost always an essential aspect, if not the central focus, of a mental status examination in this context. Despite this point related to prior probability, this primary focus on memory function should be flexibly shifted to other cognitive domains if the presenting symptoms differ (e.g., if a patient presents with language or visuospatial symptoms).

Qualitative Evaluation by Domain

Many behaviors can be informally assessed through careful behavioral observations of the patient. While some clinicians prefer to do this assessment in an unstructured format, others benefit from having the structure of a checklist, outline, or standardized tool for answering basic questions about the patient's presentation. We will first provide an overview of the domains that are typically assessed in a mental status examination and provide examples of observations or tasks that illustrate or assess each. Next, we will review some of the most common and empirically supported standardized tools for the brief evaluation of mental status. Whenever possible, we recommend use of a standardized tool in addition to informal observations.

Appearance and Indicators of Functional Status

Basic observations regarding the patient's physical characteristics, such as the patient's sex, age, race, dress, posture, hygiene, grooming, and social interactions are essential to consider and describe in the office report. "Functional status" is a term used to describe one's ability to carry out basic activities of daily living (BADLs; e.g., dressing, bathing) and instrumental activities of daily living (IADLs; e.g., grocery shopping, financial management) (Lawton & Brody, 1969; Njegovan, Hing, Mitchell, & Molnar, 2001; Weintraub, 1986). While not always a standard component of a mental status exam with all patient populations, assessment of functional status is an essential aspect of dementia diagnosis (Mckhann et al., 2011) and is thus an essential component of the mental status examination with geriatric patients. Regardless of the consideration of a dementia diagnosis, it is important to assess functional status of older adults, as impairment in daily functioning puts patients at risk for many detrimental outcomes, such as car accidents (O'Connor, Kapust, & Hollis, 2008); falls (Lakhan, Jones, Wilson, & Gray,

2012); medication noncompliance (Edelberg, Shallenberger, Hausdorff, & Wei, 2000; Edelberg, Shallenberger, & Wei, 1999); and fraud, abuse, and poor decisions; or undue influence related to finances, health, sexual consent, legal contracts, and living situation (Edelstein et al., 2008). While several standardized measures of daily function will be summarized later in the chapter, there are many signs of impaired daily function that are directly observable and evident within the first few minutes of meeting with a patient. Any subtle or obvious suggestion of a problem with self-care is clinically relevant, should be noted, and can be explored further with questions regarding specific activities of daily living. For older adults who require assistance for activities, it is important to determine whether their limitations are attributable to physical versus cognitive limitations. For example, if a patient has exhibited a recent change in the ability to dress herself, clarification is needed to determine whether she has experienced a physical change or injury (e.g., increased arthritis symptoms), or whether she has instead experienced a cognitive change (e.g., forgetting to get dressed or lacking the volition to initiate getting dressed). Functional impairments that are clearly attributable to a cognitive change would be consistent with those seen in dementia, while any functional change is of course clinically relevant and warrants further evaluation to ensure safety (e.g., consideration of a referral to physical or occupational therapy to provide modifications to the home).

Mood and Psychological Functioning

Informal evaluation of mood and psychological functioning includes observing the patient's affect. Overt signs of depression or dysphoria include tearfulness, verbal expression of feeling hopeless or in extreme cases suicidal, and can also be expressed by overt emotional outbursts of anger or irritability. Another important aspect of mood that can go undetected is apathy or emotional withdrawal. In evaluating psychological functioning in older adults, it is important to determine the onset and duration of mood symptoms. Specifically, does the patient have a lifelong history of psychiatric problems (e.g., depression, anxiety), or is the current change in mood or behavior the patient's first experience of significant psychiatric difficulties? If the latter is the case, consideration of dementia as the potential cause of the change should be considered. While it is possible for depression or other psychiatric problems to emerge in later life, it is more likely for psychiatric changes in older adults with no prior history of such problems to be driven by an underlying neurodegenerative process (Barnes et al., 2012; Boustani, Peterson, Hanson, Harris, & Lohr, 2003; Jost & Grossberg, 1996). Other aspects of psychological functioning that are directly observable are overt signs of psychosis (e.g., hallucinations, delusions, paranoia), which can emerge in the context of delirium but can also be present in advancing dementia, and as a prominent earlier feature in dementia with Lewy bodies. Such signs can be observed in patients who appear to be responding to internal stimulus (e.g., talking or laughing to themselves), who express delusional thoughts or beliefs during conversation (e.g., people are coming in the house and taking all my things; my wife is having an affair; my wife is not my wife but an imposter), or who have grossly disorganized speech (e.g., circumlocutory, tangential). Disinhibition; compulsive behaviors; perseveration; utilization behavior; and insensitive, inappropriate, and odd behaviors can also be directly observed and are cardinal symptoms of frontal systems dysfunction that can be featured prominently in vascular-ischemic cognitive impairment or dementia, traumatic brain injury/chronic traumatic encephalopathy, and particularly in behavioral-variant frontotemporal dementia (bv-FTD; Hardy, Momeni, & Traynor, 2006; Rascovsky et al., 2011; Slachevsky et al., 2011).

Arousal and Orientation

General level of arousal and alertness can be assessed through passive observation of the patient, and in cases where extremely diminished arousal or fluctuations in arousal are present, a thorough and active assessment of level of consciousness may be necessary; verbal, nonverbal, and motor responses are assessed to determine what level of stimulation is required to elicit different levels of response from the patient. As a clinician, it is important to keep in mind that the same word may represent different meanings between individuals; for example, "sleepy" can elicit a different mental picture to the reader, ranging from awake and relatively alert to nearly comatose. It is therefore better to describe the patient's spontaneous engagement and responses to the examiner's commands and stimuli (e.g., "The patient had his eyes closed without spontaneous movements, was breathing loudly, and did not open his eyes to loud voice command or to gentle tactile stimuli, including tickling of his feet and shaking of his fingers and hands. He partially opened both eyes for less than 5 seconds and grunted to vigorous sternal rub while also reaching with his left hand to localize by grabbing my hand on his sternum"). If the patient appears to have low arousal and alertness, consideration of current medications, assessment of sleep quality, and questioning the patient and a reliable informant about specifics regarding the energy and activity level of the patient during the day (and night) can help to determine whether the sedation represents a change in the patient's typical level of functioning.

Assessment of orientation can be more formally assessed by asking the examinee to provide levels of details about her or his knowledge regarding current location (spatial orientation; e.g., state, town, name of location/hospital/clinic, address, building, floor), aspects of time (temporal orientation; e.g., year, season, month, date, day, time of day, estimate of exact time), persons (orientation to person; e.g., people present at evaluation; name(s) of clinician, person(s) accompanying the patient, the patient her/himself), and situation (orientation to context; e.g., medical/neurological/psychiatric evaluation of patient for cognitive change or problems by the clinician). While some of these questions may have limited utility in detecting subtle signs of early dementia, they can provide useful information for staging and tracking patients who are in the middle to late stages of dementia or have mild dementia but have a relatively greater disorientation, impairment in forming new memories, or lack of insight and awareness into their cognitive problems. Assessment of arousal and orientation may also provide the clinician with an indication that an acute or subacute change or fluctuation in mental status is due to an acute or gradually progressing underlying medical complication that is causing mental decompensation that may manifest as confusion and delirium. Fluctuations in arousal or orientation are often a prominent feature in the early stages of dementia with Lewy bodies (DLB) (see Chapter 2 for a review), but they can also be seen in some patients with mild or moderate vascular-ischemic dementia and cerebral amyloid angiopathy.

Attention, Working Memory, Processing Speed, and Psychomotor Function

Attention, working memory, and processing speed are interrelated concepts that are represented diffusely in the brain and tend to show a gradual decline in normal aging (Robitaille et al., 2013; Salthouse, 2010). As they have diffuse neuroanatomical substrates, impairments in these aspects of cognition can be due to many underlying causes.

Attention was famously described in 1890 by the father of American psychology, William James, in *The Principles of Psychology* as follows: "Every one knows what attention is. It is the taking possession by the mind, in clear and vivid form, of one out of what seem several simultaneously possible objects or trains of thought. Focalization, concentration of consciousness are of its essence. It implies withdrawal from some things in order to deal effectively with others, and is a condition which has a real opposite in the confused, dazed, scatterbrained state which in French is called *distraction*, and *Zerstreutheit* in German" (James, 1890, pp. 403–404). Informally, elements of the patient's attention can be observed by how attentive she is to the examiner, conversation, and instructions; how distractible she is; and whether she has difficulty maintaining focus or loses her train of thought and is impersistent during conversations, actions, tasks, or instructions. Evaluation of attention is typically covered by items on formal mental status exams that involve asking the patient to repeat a string of numbers in forward and backward order. Other commonly used tasks include asking a patient to recite the days of the week or months of the year in forward and reverse order, to count or spell words in forward and reverse order (e.g., counting back from 20 to 1; spelling "world" or "sailor" forward and backward), to repeatedly do fixed subtractions from starting number (e.g., subtracting 7's starting from 100, subtracting 3's starting at 20), or to rearrange a sequence according to a certain rule (e.g., reordering the alphanumeric sequence: "8, A, 3, L, 6, I" presented at one number/letter per second into ascending alphabetic and numerical order as "A, I, L, 3, 6, 8"). These tasks all have the common component of asking a patient to attend to a verbal instruction set and to mentally "hold" and manipulate a set of information to provide accurate responses.

Many patients with mild Alzheimer's dementia can display relatively preserved attention but may show subtle deficits in speed or psychomotor function. In dementias that have more subcortical or diffuse white matter involvement, such as Parkinsonian dementias or vascular dementia, more notable difficulties with speed and motor function are often evident (Cherrier et al., 1997; O'Brien et al., 2002). At the outset of any clinical office visit, motor function can be assessed by informally observing the patient's gait, posture, stability, facial movements (e.g., blink rate), and the speed of performing basic motor functions and overall movements (e.g., rising from sitting to standing). Processing speed can also be informally observed by the patient's response latency to questioning during the interview.

Executive Function

"Executive function," a term often used to refer to the cognitive tasks primarily controlled by the frontal lobes or frontal systems of the brain, includes cognitive abilities such as planning, organization, inhibition, shifting from one task to another, fluency, and abstract reasoning (Stuss & Alexander, 2000). Informal assessment of executive functions can be obtained by observing for signs of disinhibition, such as frequently interrupting or making socially inappropriate comments. Patients with executive dysfunction also commonly have difficulty shifting from one task to another; this can be observed during interview if the patient exhibits difficulty when the topic of conversation or task changes, is perseverative, or has poor mental flexibility. Formal assessment of elements of executive function can be done by asking the patient to alternate between reciting or drawing lines on a piece of paper between two sequences (e.g., alternating between counting by 7s and reciting the months of the year; alternating between stating the letters of the alphabet starting at A and ending at Z and counting numbers from 1 to 26; alternate between connecting numbers and letters on a page as in the trails B test (Reitan & Wolfson, 1985). There are a diverse array of formal and informal measures of many aspects of executive function that have been developed; some provide qualitative information regarding a patient's approach to problem solving, and some have systematic scoring criteria for objective quantification of performance. Several commonly used screening measures include items specifically designed to assess executive function (e.g., MoCA, ACE-R), while there are also domain-specific screening measures, such as the Clock Drawing Test (see later for a review of several variants on this task). Importantly, the Mini Mental State Examination provides very limited assessment of executive functioning through spelling of the word "world" backward. Other bedside tasks to assess executive function include performance of Luria-type motor programming sequences to test ordering, set-maintenance/shifting, and perseveration, and the visual pattern completion test. For example, Weiner and colleagues (2011) devised a more difficult Luria-type task by modifying the original Luria three-step sequence task of "fist-cut-slap" by asking the patient to first mimic the examiner and then to perform several cycles of a hand motor sequence of "cut, fist, slap" (Weiner, Hynan, Rossetti, & Falkowski, 2011) with the knuckles pointing down during the formation of a fist (see Fig. 19.1). An example of the visual pattern completion task involves asking the patient to extend an alternating pattern of connected open-square and triangular shapes (i.e., "ramparts"; see Fig. 19.2).

Another aspect of executive functioning is the ability to generate responses, either verbally or nonverbally. Verbal fluency is discussed later in the language section, but the executive component of these types of tasks is that they require the examinee to generate novel responses according to a set of rules (e.g., to say or write words following

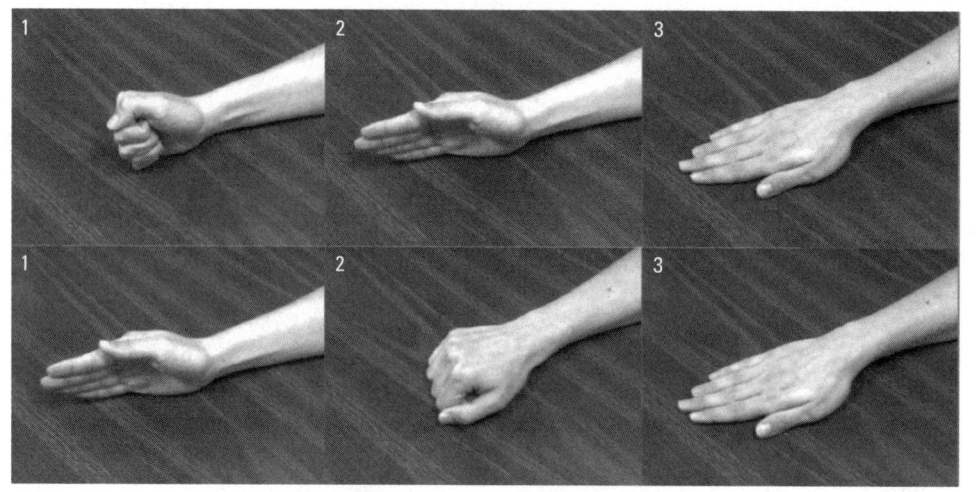

Figure 19.1 Demonstration of the original Luria motor sequencing test (top) and the modified, slightly more challenging motor sequence (bottom) used by Weiner et al. (2011).

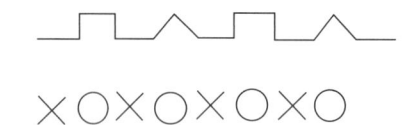

Figure 19.2 Examples of graphomotor sequences that can be started by the examiner and completed by the patient.

a rule set; to create designs by connecting dots according to a rule set). Difficulties with executive function are reflected on these tasks by a reduction or inability to generate responses, difficulties maintaining cognitive set (e.g., when instructed to say as many "A" words as she can, a patient says a word beginning with another letter), and perseverative errors (i.e., repeating previously stated responses).

Language

Evaluation of the patient's speech and language includes noting gross signs of the motoric aspects of speech (e.g., dysarthria, and speech rhythm, prosody, and volume) as well as multiple aspects of language function, which can broadly be conceptualized as receptive language abilities (i.e., the ability to process and understand written or spoken language) and expressive abilities (i.e., the ability to express oneself in verbal or written language). An important distinction to make is whether a patient has a motor speech disorder (e.g., dysarthria) or aphasia, is a disorder of communication. General elements of the language exam include fluency, comprehension, reading, writing, repeating, and naming. While a fine-grained analysis of language function would not be possible or appropriate in a screening mental status examination format, a gross evaluation of expressive abilities can be obtained, for example, by noting the patient's ability to verbally express herself in conversation and to state an understanding of the purpose of the current office visit (unless there is an underlying lack of awareness of deficits).

Brief informal evaluation of naming ability can be assessed by asking the patient to name a few objects starting with items that are higher frequency words (e.g., glasses, thumb) and progressing to lower frequency words (e.g., the lens of a pair of glasses, fingernail, cuticle, lapel). Comprehension can be assessed by asking a question that requires processing of sentences with complex grammatical constructions (e.g., "If a lion is eaten by a tiger, which animal is still alive?") or the performance of a multistep command, preferably across midline (e.g., "Please take your left thumb, touch your right ear, and then point to the door"). It is important to keep in mind that longer verbal statements such as these draw on not only language abilities but also working memory abilities, so if a patient fails to perform such a task, further testing is warranted to better define the nature of the performance deficit. Reading and writing can be assessed directly by asking the patient to read a paragraph and to write a complete sentence (which should include a subject and a verb). Repetition is tested using medium to long phrases or sentences (e.g., "The naughty boys always chased the innocent girls during recess" or "The Patriots scored two touchdowns in the fourth quarter to beat the Bears"). Fluency can be assessed by noting the fluidity, speed, and ease with which a patient expresses him or herself in conversation—long pauses or word-finding hesitations or word substitutions may be indicative of a nonfluent or dysnomic language disorder (assuming psychomotor processing is not also generally affected to the same degree).

Verbal fluency is an aspect of language abilities that is conceptualized to fall under both the domain of executive and language function. Formal evaluation of verbal fluency is included on several of the standardized measures summarized later (e.g., SLUMS, MoCA, ACE-R) and is typically assessed by asking the patient to say as many words as she can think of that begin with a certain letter (letter or phonemic fluency task) or that belong to a certain semantic category (e.g., animals, vegetables, tools; semantic category task). The pattern of verbal fluency deficits can also be informative. For example, in early AD the pattern of language dysfunction is often a verbal fluency profile of worse performance on semantic than letter fluency tasks, likely reflecting temporal cortical dysfunction. In contrast, early-stage patients with vascular cognitive impairment (VCI) or other disorders that prominently affect frontoparietal language systems (e.g., agrammatic or logopenic variants of primary progressive aphasia) often show profiles of impaired word finding and naming (but improved naming when provided with hints or cues), and worse performance on letter fluency than semantic category fluency. If language difficulty is the primary symptom, a more detailed language assessment is essential, usually performed by a specialist. A patient whose most salient symptom involves language may be presenting with primary progressive aphasia (see Chapter 9) or another variant of frontotemporal dementia (see Chapter 2).

Visuospatial Function

Visuospatial function involves the abilities to identify, integrate, and analyze space, and visual form, details, structure, and spatial relations in several (usually two or three) dimensions. Visuospatial skills include spatial navigation; perception of distance, depth, movement, and visual relations; visuospatial construction; and mental imagery. Gross visuospatial dysfunction can be observed by evidence that the patient has trouble navigating through space (e.g., observed to frequently bump into things). Importantly, intact visuospatial functioning is essential for driving (Reger et al., 2004), and given the safety implications, detailed questioning of patients and their caregivers regarding recent changes in driving ability is essential. Common difficulties with driving that emerge in early dementia that reflect difficulties with visuospatial function include minor accidents due to misjudging the location of surrounding objects (e.g., hitting adjacent cars while parking).

Brief assessments of visuospatial abilities are included in all of the standardized mental status examination tools discussed later. In the event a standardized tool is not used, a basic screen for visuospatial problems may include instructing the patient to copy predrawn shapes on a page, starting with simple shapes (e.g., a square, pentagon) and progressing to more complex shapes (e.g., a cube, intersecting pentagons), building shapes with triangles or blocks, and drawing a clock. Simple visual perception can be tested by asking the patient to count the number of irregularly spaced dots on a card without using any fingers to point or count. More complex visual perception, attention, and integration can be tested by showing the patient a picture and asking him to describe what he sees (e.g., using the "Boston Cookie Theft Picture," from the Boston Diagnostic Aphasia Examination, where a line drawing picture portrays a complex scene). Visuospatial construction can also be tested by asking the patient to imitate the construction of different interlocking finger patterns made by the examiner. Navigation can be tested by asking the patient to recount a familiar route that can be verified by a reliable informant (e.g., "Turn by turn, can you tell me how you get from your house to the grocery store?") or the route the patient traveled to come to the office visit; the latter task also makes demands on episodic memory function. Mental visualization may also be tested by asking the patient to perform mental rotations, spatial navigation, or by the clock visualization and projection (CVP) task. During this multimodal screening task, which also requires good attention, comprehension, and working memory, the patient is asked to close her eyes and to visualize a clock face; the patient is then instructed to "imagine the short-hand of the clock is pointing to three and the long-hand is pointing to five. What time will the clock show in half-an-hour?" It is possible, however, to use alternative strategies, such as using semantic knowledge and working memory without utilizing mental imagery, to solve the CVP task.

Visuospatial function can be impaired early in several conditions, including dementia with Lewy bodies, vascular cognitive impairment, corticobasal syndrome, or the posterior cortical atrophy syndrome. A patient who reports abnormalities in perception, such as detailed visual hallucinations or subtle perceptual distortions, should be referred for further subspecialty evaluation. Visual hallucinations can also be due to a medication side effect in susceptible individuals, such as in patients with Parkinson's disease prescribed dopamine-enhancing medications.

Memory Function

Memory is the capacity to store, retain, and recall information and experiences (see Chapter 1 for review of memory systems). The aspect of cognition most affected by Alzheimer's disease in its earliest stages is episodic memory, and the difficulty lies with the formation of new memories. This can often translate to a patient with early Alzheimer's disease who may have an excellent memory for information learned and events that occurred in their remote past (e.g., many lines of poetry, autobiographical information such as where she went to grade school) but may have less ability to learn new information or form detailed memories for more recent events (e.g., names of new coworkers, details of current events, what restaurant she went to last week, what meal she ate last night).

Assessment of recent episodic memory can be evaluated informally while interviewing the patient by asking questions about recent events in the news. Ideally, this is done after obtaining some information about the patient's interests (e.g., a particular sports team; a current political issue) and asking questions specific to those interests (e.g., details and the score of the last game he watched) that can be verified. Alternatively, if a family member is available to provide the clinician with details about a recent family event, the clinician can ask questions about the patient's recent personal history. If such information is not readily available, one can assess nonpersonal semantic memory by asking the patient to name, for example, the current president (prime minister or monarch), vice president, state governor or senator, the mayor of the patient's town, the name of the US President who was assassinated in the 1960s (and what city he was in), or naming the US Presidents in reverse temporal order starting with the current president. Often the last type of memory to be affected is personal or autobiographic memory such as the patient's current age, date and place of birth, her profession and names and places of past major employment, names of schools attended, and names of family members.

All of the cognitive screening tools discussed later provide objective assessment of memory and include tasks on which the patient is asked to learn and recall (or recognize), after a delay in which the patient is mentally engaged and not allowed to rehearse the presented materials, a verbally presented word list or story, or to redraw a previously copied figure. When expressive language function can significantly interfere with verbal recall during memory testing, other alternatives to redrawing previously copied figures include testing recognition memory through presenting lists of words, patterns, or pictures, or to hide objects in particular locations in the exam room and ask the patient to remember and later show you their locations.

It is important to always assess that the patient has been able to immediately register or encode the material, as well as to ensure that the patient's hearing is intact, by asking the patient to first repeat the presented items (at least once, and preferably twice or more when a greater learning load is being demanded). If the patient is unable to adequately register this material (e.g., because of an attentional, learning, or severe hearing problem) then subsequent assessment of memory storage capacity may not be completely made. After a delay, ideally of at least 5 minutes, when the patient has been mentally engaged with other tasks that do not require substantial learning and remembering of material that can interfere with this material/information, the patient is asked to recall the specific information he was asked to remember. Any items the patient cannot recall can be first cued by category (e.g., a category cue of "building" for the learned item of "church") and then by multiple-choice recognition (e.g., "Was it school, church, hospital, or train station?"). The hallmark of patients with early to mid-stage Alzheimer's dementia is a relatively preserved ability to immediately register new information but significant "storage loss" for this information when tested after an adequate delay that is not substantially amenable to cues or recognition by multiple/forced-choice testing.

Specialized Mental Functions and Multimodal Cognitive Operations

While not necessary to evaluate these functions during all screening MSEs in the primary care setting, some tests of specialized cognitive functions can be included in certain primary care situations and should be often included in screening MSEs by subspecialists. These include assessment of calculations, reasoning and problem solving, abstraction, agnosia, neglect, praxis (see Chapter 1), insight, and judgment (see Table 19.1).

Complexity of calculations should be adjusted to the patient's level of education or highest function. This can range from simple arithmetic (e.g., "What is 9 plus 14?") to calculations involving money (e.g., "How many nickels are there in 65 cents?"), to making change (e.g., "If you bought something that cost $3.73 and you paid with a $5 bill, how much change should you receive back?), to calculating more complex bills involving percentages (e.g., "If you went to a restaurant and the bill came to $120, how much total money would you leave if you wanted to also include a 15% tip?"), and to solving more complex word problems.

Simple reasoning and problem solving can be tested in a variety of ways, including asking the patient to address a simple life scenario such as "What would you do if you found a stamped and addressed envelope on the street?" or "You find water pouring out from a cracked pipe in your bathroom; what do you do?"

Abstraction can be assessed by asking for the meaning of common proverbs as well as asking the patient to delineate the similarity (e.g., "In the most general sense, how are bicycle and train similar?") and difference between two things (e.g., "What is the difference between a lie and a mistake?").

Agnosia, derived from *a-gnosis* or "non-knowledge," is the loss of ability to recognize objects, persons, sounds, shapes, or smells while the specific sense is not defective. Anosognosia is the lack of awareness of or denial of the existence of a deficit or handicap (Greek: *nosos* or "disease" and *gnosis* or "knowledge") and is a common (but not necessary), and relatively early, feature of several dementias, particularly AD and bvFTD. It is important to gauge anosognosia, and the patient's overall insight, for several reasons, including to advise the caregivers about the best approaches to the patient's care and safety considerations (including driving, guns, cooking). Anosognosia can be assessed by comparing actual facts to the patient's insight, perception, and understanding of her condition (deficits, disabilities, and behaviors, and their impact on others), current station in life, and the reason and context of the medical evaluation. Patients with simultanagnosia can recognize objects or details in their visual field, but only one at a time. They cannot make out the scene they belong to or make out a whole image out of the details—they literally cannot see the forest for the trees. Simultanagnosia can be tested using scenes (e.g., The Cookie Theft Picture) or asking the patient to identify specific targets of various sizes such as letters, numbers, or shapes on a page—affected patients may be able to identify smaller individual targets but not larger ones (e.g., the patient can circle all small "A"s on a page with an array of small and large letters, but not the very large "A"s) or ones that are produced by smaller shapes (see Fig. 19.3).

Hemispatial neglect (also known as unilateral neglect, spatial neglect, or neglect

TABLE 19.1 Summary of Cognitive Domains and Examples of Their Informal Assessment in an Office Visit

Domain *Subcomponent*	Instruct the patient to...
Orientation	State his or her name; name family members present
Person	Name the state, county, town, hospital building, floor
Place	State the year, month, date, day, time of day
Time	
Attention	Recite the days of week or months of year in forward, then reverse order
	Spell a word (e.g., WORLD) in forward, then reverse order
	Recite a string of numbers (presented at a rate of a number per second, starting with a shorter string and increasing string length by one number each time; e.g., "2-7...5-8-6....6-9-3-4...")
Working memory	Recite a string of numbers using the same method as above, but instructing the patient to recite the numbers in reverse order of what you say (e.g., "If I say 7-8-3, you would say 3-8-7")
	Recite a string of numbers using the same method as above, but instructing the patient to recite the numbers in numeric order, starting with the lowest number (e.g., "If I say 7-2-5, you would say 2-5-7")
Processing speed	Note the response latency and overall speed of verbal response on attention measures above (e.g., counting in forward and reverse order)
Executive	
Sequencing	Imitate hand movements in a sequence demonstrated by the examiner (see Fig. 19.1)
	Continue a sequenced drawing that is started by the examiner (e.g., XOXO; ramparts)
Set switching	Alternate between counting and reciting the alphabet (e.g., "I want you to switch between counting in numeric order and reciting the alphabet, like this: 1-A-2-B-3... now you try it")
	Alternate between counting by 6s and reciting the days of the week (e.g., "I want you to alternate between counting by 6s and reciting the days of the week in order, like this: 0-Sunday, 6-Monday, 12... now you try it")
Fluency	Recite as many words as possible in 1 minute that start with a given letter (e.g., "C") or a given semantic category (e.g., "grocery store items")
Language	Name several objects in the room, starting with high-frequency items (pen, pencil, watch, ruler, glasses) and moving to low-frequency items (glasses lens, watch clasp, tip of pencil).
	Follow a multistep verbal command (e.g., "Touch your left ear with your right index finger, then touch your nose").
	Follow a written command (e.g., "Close your eyes").
	Answer a complex question (e.g., "If a lion and a tiger fight and the tiger eats the lion, which animal is still alive?")
Visuospatial	Copy a simple shape (e.g., a square), then a more complex shape (e.g., a cube)
	Draw a mark where they think the middle of a provided line is.
Memory	Repeat a list of words immediately, and again after 10 minutes
	At the beginning of the visit, tell the patient you will be hiding three objects in the room (e.g., watch, pencil, ruler). Then show the patient where you are hiding them, and ask the patient to try to remember the items and their location. At the end of the visit, ask the patient to name the objects and to show (or tell) you where they are located.
Specialized mental functions/multimodal operations	
Calculations	Perform mental arithmetic (e.g., "What is 28 minus 17?")
	Make change (e.g., "Of you bought something for $3.73 and paid with a 5 dollar bill, how much change should you get?")
Reasoning/ problem solving	Provide solutions to everyday problems (e.g., "What should you do if you are in a movie theatre and you smell smoke)
Abstraction	Identify the similarities between words (e.g., "In what way are a banana and an orange alike?")

(continued)

TABLE 19.1 Continued

Domain *Subcomponent*	Instruct the patient to...
Anosognosia	Describe his or her understanding of the reasons why a given safety measure has been taken or restriction has been made (e.g., if the patient's driver's license has been revoked) and compare his or her provided reasons to known facts (e.g., the patient has a recent history of several minor car accidents).
Simultanagnosia	Describe a complex scene (e.g., the Boston Cookie Theft picture) or identify a large object that is made up of smaller shapes (e.g., an A made on a page with small A's)
Neglect	Bisect a line drawn on a page
Apraxia	Show you how he or she would cut with scissors; sweep with a broom; strike a match

syndrome) is broadly defined when a deficit in attention to the opposite side of space is observed. When florid, it will be symptom described by the informant, which can be observed during the examination by noticing that the patient has not shaved, applied makeup, or brushed the hair on the left side of her body. When more subtle, it can be assessed by asking the patient to bisect a horizontal line, cross out a target letter on a page of randomly placed letters, copy a geometric figure, describe the examination room, or a picture presented to her (see Fig. 19.4 for an example task). When the primary modality is intact, extinction to double-sided stimulation in any modality (e.g., visual, tactile) can also indicate neglect (e.g., with eyes closed the patient indicates the light touch by the examiner on the left and right side of his body when touched in sequence, but not when touched at the same time—in left-sided neglect he would only indicate being touched on his right side though he is touched simultaneously on the right and left). While the sequelae of large right middle cerebral artery stroke is the most common cause of hemispatial neglect, traumatic brain injury, brain tumors, and neurodegenerative conditions such as corticobasal degeneration (CBD) and Creutzfeldt-Jakob disease may also cause this condition.

Apraxia can be broadly defined as the loss of the ability to execute or carry out learned purposeful movements, despite having the desire and the physical ability to perform the movements (see Chapter 1). Ideomotor praxis, the ability to correctly form the necessary postures and movements to perform a task using a tool, can be tested by asking the patient to pretend by showing you how

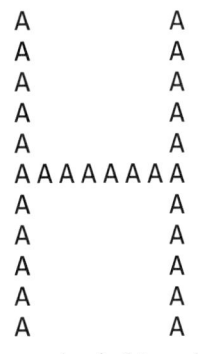

```
A           A
A           A
A           A
A           A
A           A
A A A A A A A A
A           A
A           A
A           A
A           A
A           A
```

Figure 19.3 A sample of a hierarchical figure in which the smaller letters make up a larger letter. In patients with simultagnosia (seen in Balint's syndrome), there would be difficulty in seeing the larger letter (H) below.

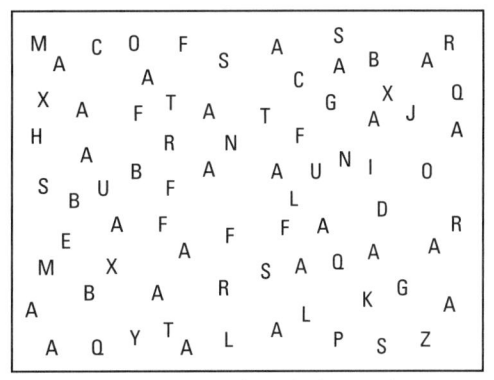

Figure 19.4 Example of a task that evaluates visual field perception and hemifield attention. The patient can be shown such an array of letters or objects on a page and be instructed to cross out all of the "As" on the page. People with visual neglect (typically left) will have a high rate of omissions on the left side of the page. Similarly, when asked to bisect a line by marking the center of the line, patients with neglect will mark the line to the right of center.

she would "scramble an egg with a fork" (a transitive task) or by asking her to show you how she would salute (a nontransitive task). Ideational praxis, the ability to correctly temporally sequence independent actions/task components to perform a goal, can be tested by asking the patient to verbalize, step by step, how she would make a sandwich.

An overall general estimate of the patient's insight and judgment can be made after obtaining a complete history (from patient and informant), performing the assessment discussed previously, and gauging the patient's understanding, response, and receptiveness to the clinical impression and recommendations made by the clinician.

Review of Common Standardized Mental Status Examination Tools

Functional Status and Dementia Symptom Questionnaires

Functional status instruments are meant to capture the degree to which cognitive and/or behavioral symptoms interfere with a patient's independence in daily functioning. It is critical for the clinician to gauge functional status in order to develop an overall assessment of the patient's clinical status (i.e., mild cognitive impairment vs. dementia). Dementia symptom questionnaires are meant to capture the types and severity of behavioral symptoms, many of which are not yet possible to measure using psychometric tests. All of these instruments can be sent (or can be adapted to be sent) to the informant in advance or filled out in the waiting room, and then reviewed with the clinician to increase efficiency in a practice setting.

Functional Assessment Questionnaire

The Functional Assessment Questionnaire (FAQ) is a 10-item questionnaire assessing instrumental activities of daily living (IADLs) administered by a clinician to a reliable informant (e.g., caregiver or spouse) regarding the patient's ability to carry out complex daily tasks independently (Pfeffer, Kurosaki, Harrah, Chance, & Filos, 1982). Ten different items assess instrumental tasks of daily living such as managing finances, shopping, food preparation, managing appointments, and traveling independently. Each item on the FAQ is rated on a scale of 0–3, with a rating of 0 indicating complete independence and a score of 3 indicating complete reliance on caregivers. The FAQ is helpful as a screening tool, as any score greater than 0 would indicate some level of functional impairment and would thus represent a red flag for further evaluation of dementia. As suggested by the Alzheimer's Association recommendations for primary care clinicians conducting the Medicare Annual Wellness Visit (Cordell et al., 2013), a questionnaire such as the FAQ to screen for functional impairment should be used in conjunction with a screening tool for cognitive function, such as those described later. This recommendation is made because subtle changes in cognition often predate overt problems with daily function (Petersen et al., 1999).

AD8

The AD8 is an eight-item questionnaire assessing changes in cognition or daily function that are attributable to problems with thinking or memory (Galvin et al., 2005). Each item on the AD8 is rated dichotomously with a Yes/No answer indicating whether there has been a change from a previous level of function for the patient. The important factor is to indicate whether there has been a change and not to attribute cause or reasons for the change. The measure is ideally administered by a clinician in an interview with a reliable informant, but it can also be completed by the informant or patient independently if the situation necessitates.

The AD8 was developed by the creators of the Clinical Dementia Rating scale (CDR) (Morris, 1993), by independently administering the CDR and a separate 52-item informant questionnaire regarding aspects of cognitive and daily function to informants of participants enrolled in the Washington University Alzheimer's Disease Research Center. The initial 52-item questionnaire was analyzed in a subset of participants with CDR scores of 0.5, indicating questionable or very mild dementia (n = 103), to identify the optimal subset of 10 of the 52 items that were the strongest predictor of CDR sum of boxes (CDR-sb) in this group. Using these 10 items, an eight-item questionnaire was developed and then validated in a separate sample of participants and found to have a sensitivity of .74 (ROC AUC = .83) when using a cutoff of AD8 ≥ 2 to distinguish between nondemented participants (CDR = 0, n = 112) and participants with questionable or very mild dementia (CDR = 0.5, n = 68), while sensitivity improved to .85 (receiver operating characteristic area under the curve, ROC AUC = .90) when using the same cutoff to distinguish between the nondemented group and participants at all levels of dementia (CDR ≥ 0.5, n = 124). Replication studies have further supported the validity and reliability of the AD8. In 225 patient–caregiver dyads, the AD8 was found to have very good interrater reliability (intraclass correlation coefficient = 0.80, 95% CI 0.55 to 0.92) and a ROC AUC of 0.92 (95% CI 0.88 to 0.95) that suggests excellent discrimination between nondemented individuals and those with cognitive impairment regardless of etiology (Galvin, Roe, Xiong, & Morris, 2006). The AD8 is estimated to only take 3 minutes to complete and can be used alone or in conjunction with a brief cognitive screening tool, as is recommended by the measure's authors. Finally, the AD8 is freely available for general clinical use at: http://alzheimer.wustl.edu/About_Us/PDFs/AD8form2005.pdf.

General Practitioner Assessment of Cognition Informant Interview

The General Practitioner Assessment of Cognition (GPCOG) is a dementia screening tool that includes both a brief informant interview (GPCOG Informant Interview; Brodaty et al., 2002), discussed here, and a brief cognitive screening test for the patient (GPCOG Patient Examination), discussed in the cognitive screening tool section discussed later. The informant interview consists of six questions, rated dichotomously regarding the patient's current cognitive or daily function relative to his level of function a few years prior (e.g., "Does the patient have more trouble remembering things that have happened recently?"). Each item with a "yes" response is given a score of 1, and a total score ≥ 4 is recommended as the cutoff for impairment.

In the original validation study for the GPCOG (Brodaty et al., 2002), both informant and patient sections were administered to 283 older adults and divided into a nondemented group (n = 151) and a group with possible or probable dementia (n = 132). Using the cutoff of ≥ 4 on the GPCOG Informant Interview had a sensitivity of .89 (ROC AUC = .84), and when combined with the cognitive testing portion (GPCOG Patient Examination discussed later), the total scale had a sensitivity of 0.82 (ROC AUC = .91). These sensitivities were significantly higher than the Abbreviated Mental Test (AMT; Hodkinson, 2012; sensitivity = .42; ROC AUC = .78) and were higher (although not significantly higher) than the MMSE (sensitivity = .81, ROC AUC = .85).

A benefit of the GPCOG is that it integrates both objective cognitive testing and caregiver report into one comprehensive summary score, and also allows the clinician to choose to administer either or both sections based on the clinical situation at hand. Furthermore, in the initial validation paper of the GPCOG, both individual components had higher specificity values compared to the MMSE, providing support for potentially using one of these subtests in lieu of the MMSE. However, as is the case with the MMSE, the sensitivity to detect decline in the earlier stage of mild cognitive impairment (MCI) has not been established. The Informant Interview portion of the GPCOG is extremely brief, taking approximately 1–3 minutes to administer.

Relevant Outcome Scale for Alzheimer's Disease

The Relevant Outcome Scale for Alzheimer's Disease (ROSA) is a 16-item, clinician-administered questionnaire that is ideally administered to a patient caregiver, although it can be administered to the patient in early stages of dementia. As opposed to the other measures mentioned in this section, which were primarily developed to detect the first signs of dementia, the ROSA was designed to track the progression of symptoms of dementia over time, and thus includes items that are largely inapplicable to many patients in the earliest stages of AD (e.g., experiencing delusions or becoming disoriented). However, the ROSA does include several items relevant to early-stage AD (e.g., difficulties remembering details of recent events), and the rating of each item on the ROSA is on a scale of 0–10, with 0 indicating the most difficulty and 10 indicating no difficulty. Thus, the ROSA offers the benefit of a wider range of scores on each item and can thus potentially be used as a more sensitive measure of very early changes in cognitive or daily function. However, administration time for the ROSA is estimated to be approximately 13–15 minutes and requires a clinician to administer (versus measures such as the AD8, which could be completed by the reporter in the waiting room), which may make it less attractive for use in the busy primary care settings.

Brief Measures of Psychological Function

Geriatric Depression Scale, Short Form

The Geriatric Depression Scale, Short Form (GDS-SF) is a 15-item, yes/no symptom checklist containing 15 of the 30 items from the original, longer version of the geriatric depression scale (Sheikh & Yesavage, 1986; Yesavage et al., 1983). The GDS and its short form were developed specifically for older adults; this is in contrast to most other self-report inventories of depression that were developed and validated in younger samples and include depression symptoms less prevalent in older adults. Furthermore, the wording and complexity of items on depression inventories designed with younger patients in mind may also be difficult for older adults with cognitive impairments to complete accurately. For example, the Beck Depression Inventory (Beck, Ward, Mendelson, Mock, & Erbaugh, 1961) requires the patient to choose from four multiple-choice responses to question items that often have complex wording. A cutoff score of >5 on the GDS-SF is recommended for further clinical evaluation of depression by the scale's authors. The GDS is solely designed to screen for depression and should be used in conjunction with a cognitive or dementia screening tool in the context of mental status exams with older adults. Both forms of the GDS are freely available for clinical use at the author's Web site: http://www.stanford.edu/~yesavage/GDS.html

Neuropsychiatric Inventory Questionnaire

The Neuropsychiatric Inventory Questionnaire (NPI-Q) is a 13-item clinician-administered questionnaire that is conducted with an informant (Kaufer et al., 2000). The questionnaire is an abbreviated form of the Neuropsychiatric Inventory (NPI), both of which were designed to grade the presence and severity of psychiatric and behavioral problems often seen in dementia (e.g., agitation, irritability, disinhibition, delusions). Similar to other noncognitive screening instruments for dementia detection, the NPI-Q is intended to be used in conjunction with complementary measures of cognitive and daily functioning, and it may be more useful in tracking noncognitive behavioral problem symptoms in established dementia cases versus screening for the presence of dementia in general clinical practice. However, when there is concern on interview with a patient regarding a recent change in behavior, the NPI-Q is extremely helpful in operationalizing each of the most common behavioral disturbances seen in older adults with dementia. Furthermore, several forms of dementia include early behavioral disturbances as hallmark symptoms (e.g., the behavioral variant of frontotemporal dementia; dementia with Lewy bodies; vascular cognitive impairment/dementia).

Cognitive Test Instruments and Screening Tools

The following is a review of the most widely used and extensively studied standardized mental status tests in the context of dementia evaluations. Which tool is chosen by a given clinician in any given context can be determined by practical (e.g., time) and clinical considerations (e.g., does the patient have a high level of education and previous function), clinical experience with the measures, and consideration of the empirical support for each instrument (as reviewed later). We recommend an approach that individualizes the evaluation by integrating the qualitative aspects of the mental status examination discussed previously with administration of at least one standardized screening tool with which the clinician has acquired appropriate training and supervision in administering and interpreting. For clinicians who are not familiar or comfortable using standardized measures, we have provided information discussed later on how to obtain the measures and resources on receiving training in their administration.

It is important to note that most screening tools are purposely designed to be sensitive to *many* types of cognitive impairment and should not be used as standalone measures to attribute cause and diagnose dementia. An ideal screening tool for dementia would correctly classify all patients with dementia as having dementia (i.e., 100% sensitivity) and all those without as "normal" (i.e., 100% specificity). Of course, such a perfect screening test does not yet exist, sensitivity and specificity trade-offs have to be considered for all tests, and there are multiple factors, such as education level, cultural and language barriers, and premorbid level of cognitive function that influence performance on even the most basic screens of cognitive function (Crum, Anthony, Bassett, & Folstein, 1993). The threshold for a score on a screening tool to be flagged as "abnormal" is typically determined by choosing a cutoff score that minimizes the change of a false negative (i.e., sensitivity: incorrectly classifying a dementia patient as not demented), the idea being that it would be less desirable to miss a diagnosis of dementia than to have a false alarm (i.e., incorrectly classifying a nondemented individual as demented). Thus, the screening should be framed to the patient as part of a procedure ("answering some questions") that can help to determine whether further evaluation may be helpful, and performance should never be presented or interpreted as a definitive "pass" or "fail" on a "test."

With these points in mind, the following review considers the main aspects of test comparison for the clinician to consider: (1) test length; (2) ease of obtaining test materials and appropriate training; (3) complexity of administration and scoring procedures; and (4) evidence of a test's sensitivity to detect mild cognitive impairment (versus more advanced stages of dementia). Aspects of screening tests that we regard with less emphasis in this review include the availability of alternate test forms for serial evaluations, development and availability of translated versions for international clinical or research use, and evidence for a test's specificity (i.e., the ability of a test to distinguish between different forms of cognitive impairment or diagnostic groups, including false positives in nondemented individuals). While all of the following are considered brief screening measures, they are presented in order of estimated administration time from the shortest to longest (see Table 19.2).

Clock Drawing Test and Its Variants

The Clock Drawing Test (CDT) has the benefit of being an extremely short measure (approximately 1 minute) that taps multiple cognitive abilities, including visuospatial, memory, and executive functions. While the brevity and complexity of the task make it a very good screening tool, it is important to note that the sensitivity of the test comes at a cost to specificity; there are many underlying cognitive problems that can lead to impaired clock drawing, and the CDT does not test learning and remembering of new information (including episodic memory), thus underscoring the importance of viewing this task as a limited screening tool when used in isolation.

In the most common variant of this task, the patient is given a blank sheet of paper and given the verbal instructions to "Draw the face of a clock, place all of the numbers on the clock face, and set the hands to ten after eleven." There has been an entire literature on this task and its variants (Cahn-Weiner et al., 1999; Royall, Cordes, & Polk, 1998), and there have been many different proposed scoring criteria (Libon, Swenson, Barnoski, & Sands, 1993; Storey, Rowland, Basic, & Conforti, 2001; Sunderland et al., 1989) and "classic" signs of impairment that are exhibited on the task. To highlight a few of the main considerations that a clinician should look for in this task, there are several types of errors reflecting different cognitive problems, including graphomotor difficulties, perseverative errors, stimulus-bound responses, errors in conceptualization, and problems with planning and spatial organization (Eknoyan, Hurley, & Taber, 2012). Graphomotor problems (e.g., imprecise lines, distorted or illegible numbers, micrographia) reflect underlying problems with motor functioning and are more common in subcortical dementias (e.g., Parkinson's disease, vascular dementia) than in early stages of Alzheimer's disease (Kitabayashi et al., 2001; Rouleau, Salmon, Butters, Kennedy, & Mcguire, 1992). Planning ability can be assessed by observing the approach the examinee takes to drawing the clock, with a planful approach being characterized by "anchoring," or first placing the numbers 12, 3, 6, and 9 on the clock face, and then filling in the other numbers appropriately. A classic example of a poorly

TABLE 19.2 Brief Screening Tools for Cognitive Impairment in Older Adults

Measure	Time (~min.)	Score Range	Suggested Cutoff	Strengths	Weaknesses
Clock Drawing	1		Varies by scoring system	Very brief; taps multiple cognitive functions in a single task	Low specificity; many scoring systems
Mini-Cog	2–4	0–3	See decision rules in text	Simple scoring algorithm	Limited evidence for sensitivity to MCI
Memory Impairment Screen (MIS)	4	0–8	See decision rules in text	Better sensitivity than three-word recall from MMSE	Only assesses memory
General Practitioner Assessment of Cognition (GPCOG) Patient Version	2–5	0–9	≥ 7 indicates impairment	Has accompanying informant interview questions	Limited evidence for sensitivity to MCI
St. Louis University Mental Status (SLUMS) examination	7	0–30	Varies by education level: ≤ 26 for those with 12+ years ≤ 24 for those with <12	Evidence for sensitivity to predementia cognitive impairment	Largely studied in VA clinical settings
7-minute Screen (7MS)	7–12		Requires use of scoring calculator available at memorydoc.org	Multidomain tool	Original validation study had small sample size; Limited evidence for sensitivity to MCI
Mini Mental State Examination (MMSE)	7–10	0–30	<24 indicates impairment, but use of available normative data recommended (Crum et al., 1993)	Widely known, allowing for ease of communication among clinicians	Limited evidence for sensitivity to MCI
The Modified Mini Mental Sate Examination (3MS)	10	0–100	<77 generally indicates impairment, but use of available normative data recommended (Tombaugh et al., 1996)	Generates MMSE and 3MS score from a single administration; verbal fluency item improves sensitivity of original MMSE	Limited evidence for sensitivity to MCI
Blessed Dementia Scale Information-Memory-Concentration (BDS-IMC)	10	0–37	>3 errors generally indicates impairment 4–10 errors: suggests mild AD 11–16 errors: suggests moderate AD 17–37 errors: suggests advanced AD	Ideal for tracking global impairment in established dementia cases	Limited evidence for sensitivity to MCI
6-Item Impairment Test (6CIT)	4–6	0–16	>7 errors indicates impairment	Superior sensitivity to MMSE with shorter administration time	Limited sensitivity to MCI

(continued)

TABLE 19.2 Continued

Measure	Time (~min.)	Score Range	Suggested Cutoff	Strengths	Weaknesses
Montreal Cognitive Assessment (MoCA)	10–12	0–30	<26 indicates impairment	Superior sensitivity to MMSE	Empirical support for its use as a screening tool for MCI
Addenbrooke's Cognitive Examination, Revised (ACE-R)	12–20	0–100	<83 indicates impairment	Global and domain-specific scores are generated	Lengthier than most screening measures

MCI, mild cognitive impairment.

planned clock draw would be one in which the numbers are drawn in numeric order and poorly spaced, such that the examinee runs out of room for the last few numbers on the clock.

Several different scoring criteria have been proposed for the CDT, ranging from dichotomous scoring for normal versus abnormal performance, to detailed scoring of each aspect of the clock drawing. Generally, scoring systems include consideration for the general shape or contour of the clock face (i.e., specifying that the clock face is approximately circular in shape), accurate placement and sequencing of the numbers on the clock face (i.e., all numbers present and spaced approximately evenly around the entire inner circle of the clock face), and accurate placement of clock hands (i.e., pointing to the correct numbers with a clear differentiation in the lengths of the hour and minute clock hands). Overall, the CDT, when scored on 10-point scale, has been found to have good interrater reliability and sensitivity in distinguishing patients with mild AD from cognitively normal older individuals (Nair et al., 2010).

Mini-Cog

The Mini-Cog consists of a combination of a clock drawing task and a three-item word list recall (Borson, Scanlan, Brush, Vitaliano, & Dokmak, 2000). Scoring for the Mini-Cog consists of numbered scores for each item as well as a scoring algorithm to classify examinees as demented or nondemented. The clock drawing test (CDT) for the Mini-Cog is scored on a scale of 0–3 with 0 indicating no impairment and 3 indicating severe impairment according to the Consortium to Establish a Registry for Alzheimer's Disease (CERAD) scoring criteria (Morris et al., 1989). These scores were reduced to a dichotomous scale (0 = normal, 1–3 = abnormal) to evaluate the Mini-Cog's diagnostic accuracy (Borson et al., 2000). Words recalled (after a filled delay during which the CDT is completed) are scored on a scale of 0–3. The scoring algorithm specifies that one would arrive at a dementia classification in one of two ways: (1) 3-Item Recall = 0, or (2) 3-Item Recall = 1–2 and CDT is abnormal. Conversely, a nondemented classification would be given if 3-Item recall = 3, or if 3-Item recall = 1–2 and CDT is normal. The Mini-Cog has been reported to have higher sensitivity than the Mini Mental State Exam (MMSE;.99 versus.91) when distinguishing between older adults with normal cognition ($n = 120$) versus those with dementia ($n = 129$). The Mini-Cog has the added benefit over the MMSE of having a shorter administration time (approximately 3 versus 10 minutes). However, in contrast to some of the tools listed later (e.g., the MoCA and ACE-R), the diagnostic accuracy of the Mini-Cog has not been well characterized in distinguishing between normal aging and MCI.

Memory Impairment Screen

The Memory Impairment Screen (MIS; Buschke et al., 1999) is a screening tool designed to detect memory impairment at the exclusion of any other cognitive difficulties and is thus designed to better detect AD dementia compared to other forms of dementia. The MIS is estimated to take approximately 4 minutes to administer and consists of a 4-item learning and memory task during which the examinee is presented with a page and asked to read the four printed words on the page. Next, the examinee is asked to state the word on the page associated with a given semantic category (e.g., the examiner says, "Which word is a type of fruit?" to which the examinee would respond, "Orange"). After these semantic associations are made for all words, the examinee engages in a different mentally occupying task for 2–3 minutes and is then asked to freely recall the four words. The examiner provides semantic cues for those items not freely recalled, and the total score on the MIS is represented by doubling the number of items freely recalled and adding that number to the number of items recalled with semantic cueing (MIS = (free recall X 2) + cued recall), generating a summary score ranging from 0 to 8 with higher scores indicating better performance. The MIS has been compared to the 3-word recall from the MMSE and found to have higher sensitivity than the 3-word recall MMSE item at detecting dementia (sensitivities = .86 and .65, respectively). Limitations of the MIS include that it only assesses memory function and has not been demonstrated to be sensitive to detecting MCI.

General Practitioner Assessment of Cognition, Patient Version

The General Practitioner Assessment of Cognition (GPCOG; Brodaty et al., 2002) Patient Examination is one of two subtests that comprise the GPCOG and includes six clinician-administered items assessing memory (recall of a previously repeated name and address), orientation (to exact date), information (ability to provide examiner with a news item occurring in the last week), and executive, and visuospatial function (clock drawing test). Scores on the GPCOG range from 0 to 9 with higher scores indicating more impairment. In the original validation study for the GPCOG (Brodaty et al., 2002), both informant and patient sections were administered to 283 older adults who were divided into a nondemented group (n = 151) and a group with possible or probable dementia (n = 132).

Using the cutoff of ≥ 7 on the GPCOG Patient Examination, the measure had a sensitivity of .82 (ROC AUC = .86), while the total scale had a sensitivity of 0.82 (ROC AUC = .91), both of which were higher than the sensitivities observed for the AMT or MMSE. An advantage of the GPCOG is short time of administration as it is estimated to take approximately 2–5 minutes to administer. The main limitation of the GPCOG Patient Examination is that there is limited evidence of its sensitivity to distinguish between older adults with normal versus mildly impaired cognitive function. The GPCOG is freely available in multiple languages for general clinical use on the author's Web site: http://www.gpcog.com.au

St. Louis University Mental Status Examination

The St. Louis University Mental Status (SLUMS; Tariq, Tumosa, Chibnall, Perry, & Morley, 2006) is a screening tool that has been largely studied in a VA geriatric clinic setting that takes approximately 7 minutes to administer. Similar to the MMSE and MoCA, SLUMS scores range from 0 to 30, with higher scores indicating better performance. As is the case with the MoCA, the SLUMS provides normative score ranges for older adults at two education levels (12+ years versus less than 12 years), and three different levels of cognitive impairment (normal, mild neurocognitive disorder or "MNCD," and dementia). Also similar to the MoCA, the SLUMS includes items that assess a broader range of cognitive domains compared to other screening measures, including items to assess orientation, memory, attention, and executive function. Items for each of these domains are also more difficult than the comparable items on the MMSE (e.g., the SLUMS, like the MoCA, as a five-word list learning task as opposed to the MMSE's three-word item).

In the original validation study (Tariq et al., 2006), sensitivity of the SLUMS to detect mild neurocognitive disorder (MCND) and dementia were compared with the MMSE in a sample of older veterans (n = 702), who were classified into three groups: normal cognition (n = 440), MCND (n = 180), and dementia (n = 82). Using different cutoff scores for those with <12 versus 12+ years of education, the SLUMS was consistently more sensitive than the MMSE at detecting MCND from normal cognition. Specifically, in the

<12-year education group, using the optimal SLUMS cutoff score of 23.5, sensitivity was .92 (ROC AUC = .93), while the optimal cutoff for the MMSE was 28.5 with a sensitivity of .60 (ROC AUC = .67). Similarly, in the 12+ year education group, using a SLUMS cutoff score of 25.5, sensitivity was .95 (ROC AUC = .94), while the optimal cutoff for the MMSE was 29.5 with a sensitivity of .75 (ROC AUC = .64). Both SLUMS and MMSE did an acceptable job at detecting dementia from normal cognition across education groups, although the sensitivity and ROC AUC values for the SLUMS in these analyses were consistently higher than the MMSE. Detailed information on all recommended cutoff scores for each diagnostic distinction and education level can be found in the original SLUMS validation paper (Tariq et al., 2006).

The SLUMS shows clear superiority to the MMSE at detecting mild neurocognitive disorder, but more research is needed on the sensitivity of the SLUMS to detect MCI. The diagnosis of MCND is based on a set of suggested research criteria set forth in the *Diagnostic and Statistical Manual of Mental Disorders*, 4th edition (*DSM-IV*, American Psychiatric Association, 2000), which essentially defines MCND as impaired function in two or more cognitive domains that cause impaired daily function for at least 2 weeks and is accompanied by medical evidence (e.g., neurologic exam or imaging) thought to be related to the cognitive change. Essentially, the main difference between the criteria for MCND and frank dementia in the DSM-IV definition is the description of the cognitive symptoms in dementia gradually worsening over time. Thus, MCND as a diagnostic entity is much closer on the continuum to the diagnosis of dementia than the diagnosis MCI, as it includes individuals with two domains of impaired cognition with associated functional impairment. While the SLUMS holds promise as a dementia screening instrument, it needs further validation at detecting subtle cognitive problems in patients with MCI and validation in nonveteran patient populations. The SLUMS is freely available for general clinical use at http://aging.slu.edu

7-Minute Screen

The 7-Minute Screen (7MS; Solomon et al., 1998) was developed to provide a rapid assessment capable of distinguishing between cognitively healthy older adults and those with AD. The measure is comprised of four previously developed tests, each with slight modifications, including a modified version of the Free and Cued Selective Reminding Test (Grober & Buschke, 1987), a 60-second trial of semantic verbal fluency (animal naming), the Benton Temporal Orientation Test (Benton, Sivan, Hamsher, Varney, & Spreen, 1994), and a variant of the clock drawing test (with instructions to set the hands to "seven to four" and use of a 7-point scoring system originally developed by Freedman and colleagues (Freedman et al., 1994).

The original validation study for the 7MS compared performance in 60 community-dwelling older adults to a demographically comparable clinical sample of older adults with probable AD diagnoses. It reported the 7MS to have extremely high sensitivity in the overall sample (1.0), and when repeatedly testing sensitivity on 1,000 random samples of 30 AD and 30 control subjects, sensitivity was found to have an average value of .92. Strengths of the 7MS include its relative brevity, while still providing a more detailed assessment of memory function than most screening measures, and its high sensitivity. Limitations of the 7MS include the small sample size with which it was developed and validated, and its administration and scoring, which require slightly more training than some of the more widely used measures. Finally, the 7MS has not been well studied in distinguishing between groups of older adults with normal cognition versus patients with MCI.

Mini Mental State Examination

Historically, the Mini Mental State Examination (MMSE; Folstein, Robins, & Helzer, 1983) has been the most widely used and recognized of standardized mental status measures, which greatly increases the ease of communication among clinicians regarding scores and specific test items. The test takes approximately 10 minutes to administer and generates a summary score ranging from 0 to 30, including items assessing orientation to time and place (10 points), repetition of three words (3 points), attention and mental control (5 points), recall of three words following a 3-minute delay (3 points), language abilities (8 points), and visuoconstruction (1 point). The original validation study for the MMSE suggested use of a cutoff score of 24 (Folstein, Folstein, & Mchugh, 1975), but sensitivity of the MMSE using cutoff scores alone has been shown to be highly dependent on the sample with which its accuracy is tested. Specifically, as a broad-based screening measure in a general population, the MMSE has limited utility in providing distinctions between older adults with normal cognition versus MCI (Lonie, Tierney, & Ebmeier, 2009), while it generally distinguishes older adults with normal cognition from those with more advanced stages of dementia (Folstein et al., 1975).

Despite its limitations, the MMSE is still often considered a corner stone standardized test to include in dementia clinical trials; this is likely a function of its long history of use (first published in 1975), and its wide use in clinical and research settings to detect and track cognitive impairment (Cullen, O'neill, Evans, Coen, & Lawlor, 2007; Tangalos et al., 1996), in epidemiologic studies (Crum et al., 1993), in clinical trials as a tool for operationalizing inclusion/exclusion criteria based on level of cognitive impairment (Raskind, Peskind, Wessel, & Yuan, 2000), and as a cognitive outcome measure to track response to treatment (Wallin, Wattmo, & Minthon, 2011). Given its ubiquity, it is frequently used as a reference for comparison for newer mental status exams and cognitive screening measures and has generally been shown to stand the test of time as a tool for detecting and tracking moderate to severe levels of cognitive impairment. However, the MMSE does not perform as well as several newer screening tools (e.g., the Montreal Cognitive Assessment) at detecting the more subtle changes in cognitive function seen in MCI (Freitas, Simoes, Alves, & Santana, 2013; Nasreddine et al., 2005). Additionally, using traditional cutoffs, the MMSE has been particularly criticized for having low sensitivity to detect cognitive impairment and dementia in individuals with high education or intelligence (Alves, Simoes, Martins, Freitas, & Santana, 2013; Christensen & Jorm, 1992). As is reflected in the reviews of these other screening tools, there are several alternatives to the MMSE that have higher sensitivity for this diagnostic distinction. A final limitation of the MMSE is that it is not free but copyrighted; it can be purchased for general clinical use at http://www.minimental.com

The Modified Mini-Mental State Examination

The Modified Mini-Mental State Examination (3MS; Teng & Chui, 1987) is a modification of the MMSE that was developed upon on the concept that adding a few additional items to the original MMSE and changing the scoring to create a broader range of scores (0–30 versus 0–100) would increase the sensitivity of the screening tool while still allowing for the provision of an original MMSE score. The benefit of this approach is that the full 3MS expands on the original, while still allowing clinicians familiar with the original MMSE to reference the 0–100 scale performance to a 0–30 MMSE score. The original paper presenting the 3MS (Teng & Chui, 1987) offers a full description of the changes in scoring from the original MMSE to the 3MS and includes side-by-side administration and scoring protocols for both the 3MS and MMSE. Briefly, the 3MS includes additional items assessing orientation (year, month, day, town, and state of birth), more unusual words for the 3-item registration and recall, standardized semantic and multiple-choice cueing for 3-item recall, finer gradation of scoring for existing MMSE items (e.g., a 10-point scoring system for overlapping pentagon copy versus the dichotomous 0 vs. 1 scoring on the original MMSE), additional naming items, a brief (30-second) test of semantic verbal fluency, several word similarity items, and a second 3-word recall trial at the end of the test, allowing for additional memory testing.

In a study comparing sensitivity of the 3MS to MMSE in a sample of cognitively healthy older adults ($n = 406$) versus those with Alzheimer's disease ($n = 119$), Tombaugh and colleagues (1996) found that the 3MS was more sensitive than the MMSE overall (.926 versus .905), and that this difference was more pronounced in a subsample of individuals with lower (0–8 years) education (.901 versus .848). While these differences in sensitivity were not statistically significant, the authors suggest that the addition of a verbal fluency test to the MMSE would increase its sensitivity (Tombaugh, Mcdowell, Kristjansson, & Hubley, 1996).

Blessed Dementia Scale Information-Memory-Concentration

The Blessed Dementia Scale Information-Memory-Concentration (BDS-IMC; Blessed, Tomlinson, & Roth, 1968) was originally designed to track cognitive impairment in patients with established dementia diagnoses and thus contains a number of test items that have ceiling effects in less impaired patients and may be less sensitive at detecting early, subtle signs of cognitive impairment seen in MCI. While the BDS is heavily weighted toward a continuum of memory and orientation items of easy to moderate difficulty, it also includes several items that assess working memory and executive function (e.g., reciting the months of the year in reverse order; counting backward from 20 to 1). The BDS is scored on a scale of 0–37, with higher scores indicating more errors and more cognitive impairment. The generally accepted cutoff score for dementia-level cognitive impairment on the BDS is >3 errors, and nonadjusted (e.g., for age, education, premorbid IQ) error score ranges for mild, moderate, and severe impairments in patients with AD are reported as 4–10, 11–16, and 17–37 errors, respectively (Locascio, Growdon, & Corkin, 1995). While neuropsychological testing plays an important role in detecting, verifying, and delineating patterns of cognitive dysfunction in AD, the BDS, due to its range, has been shown to be superior to cognitive test domains in staging and tracking dementia severity in patients with AD.

The BDS-IMC has been adapted to create a shorter, 6-item version that is more amenable for use as a screening tool; this was originally named the 6-Item Cognitive Impairment Test (6CIT) (Katzman et al., 1983) but has also been referred to in the literature as the 6-Item or Short Orientation-Memory-Concentration Test (6OMCT), or the Short Blessed Test (SBT) (Brooke & Bullock, 1999). Scoring from the original BDS-IMC was modified in the 6CIT to include a broader range of scores and to weight some items more than others to yield a total score range of 0–16, with higher scores indicating more impairment. The 6CIT has demonstrated a strong correlation to MMSE ($r = .91$) in a sample of 287 older adults ranging from normal cognitive function to severe dementia (Brooke & Bullock, 1999). Using a cutoff score of 8 or more on the 6CIT, it was shown in the same study to have superior sensitivity to the MMSE (using a cutoff of 23) in this sample at distinguishing between those with normal cognition versus mild dementia (MMSE sensitivity = .51 versus 6CIT = .79). The sensitivity of the MMSE improved to .79 when distinguishing the control group from the entire dementia group, while 6CIT sensitivity improved to .90. With superior sensitivity and shorter administration time (approximately 4–6 minutes), the 6CIT also appears to be superior to the MMSE for detecting dementia, but again it has limited empirical support at distinguishing between normal cognition and MCI.

Montreal Cognitive Assessment

The Montreal Cognitive Assessment (MoCA; Nasreddine et al., 2005) is a mental status test that was specifically designed as a screening tool for MCI, and thus it includes several test items that are intentionally more difficult than comparable test items on the MMSE. It additionally includes more items that assess executive and visuospatial functions than many of the other screening tools; these include an abbreviated version of the Trails B test (Reitan & Wolfson, 1985), a cube copy, and a clock drawing task. In addition to these items that assess combined visuospatial and executive functions, the MoCA has a two-item word similarities task that requires abstract reasoning and several items each to assess the domains of language (3-item confrontation naming, 2-item sentence repetition, and a single verbal fluency trial), attention (2-item digit span, an item assessing vigilance, and serial 7s subtraction from 100), memory (5-word list learning, free recall, and recall with semantic and multiple-choice cueing), and orientation (date, month, year, day, place, city). Similar to the MMSE, the MoCA generates a summary score ranging from 0 to 30. In contrast to the MMSE, however, the MoCA has an adjustment for lower education (an additional point is added to the total score if the examinee has 12 or fewer years of education) and a relatively higher cutoff score of 26 or greater has been recommended as a general guideline to indicate performance in the normal range. In a direct comparison of the sensitivity of both measures at distinguishing between a sample of older adults with MCI ($n = 94$) and those who were cognitively healthy (n = 90), the MoCA was found to be significantly more sensitive than the MMSE (.90 versus .18) (Nasreddine et al., 2005). Subsequently, the superiority of the MoCA to the MMSE in regards to sensitivity, specificity, positive predictive value, negative predictive value, and classification accuracy between normal cognition, MCI, and AD has been shown at different cutoffs (i.e., cutoff of 17 for MCI and 22 for AD) (Freitas et al., 2013).

Advantages of the MoCA over other screening tools include its increased sensitivity at distinguishing normal aging from MCI, the ease of obtaining test materials, its relative ease of administration, and strong evidence for its acceptance by general practitioners. It is additionally available in many different languages, and the English version is available in alternate, co-normed test forms helpful for serial evaluations. Administration time for the MoCA is estimated to be approximately 10–12 minutes, making it a slightly longer test to administer than the MMSE. The MoCA and its alternate versions in English and several languages are freely available at http://www.mocatest.org

Addenbrooke's Cognitive Examination, Revised

The original Addenbrooke's Cognitive Examination (ACE) was developed as a screening tool to detect early dementia and distinguish between AD and other forms of dementia (Mathuranath, Nestor, Berrios, Rakowicz, & Hodges, 2000). Several modifications were made in the revised version, which includes the full test items for the MMSE in addition to a number of additional items to assess attention, orientation, memory, verbal fluency, language, and visuospatial functions (Ahmed, De Jager, & Wilcock, 2012). In addition to generating an MMSE score, the Addenbrooke's Cognitive Examination, Revised (ACE-R; Mioshi, Dawson, Mitchell, Arnold, & Hodges, 2006) generates a global score ranging from 0 to 100, subscores for each of the aforementioned cognitive domains, and a formula for distinguishing between AD and frontotemporal dementia.

Using the generally recommended cutoff score of 82/100, the ACE-R has been shown to have roughly equivalent sensitivity to the MoCA (both approximately .90) at distinguishing between healthy aging and MCI (Ahmed et al., 2012). Given the MoCA is shorter in administration time (10–12 versus approximately 12–25 minutes), it can present a more attractive choice than the ACE-R for use in the primary care setting. A potential benefit of the ACE-R over the MoCA, however, is that it provides cognitive domain scores, for which normative ranges have been provided for general clinical use, thus allowing for a more detailed summary of cognitive functioning. The ACE-R has been used extensively in AD clinical trials in England and worldwide, and it is available in many languages and alternate test forms that are all freely available to the public by request to the test's authors.

Conclusion

The mental status examination can be used in a succinct form for screening for dementia or in an extended form to evaluate the type and severity of cognitive impairment or dementia. In addition to the informal and qualitative descriptions of mental status that are routinely performed by geriatricians, primary care physicians, neurologists, and psychiatrists, incorporating a standardized screening tool into routine clinical practice is recommended. The relative objectivity and consistency with which these measures are administered and interpreted reduces the subjectivity of clinical judgment and provides a quantifiable metric of a patient's current cognitive function and any change from the patient's own baseline.

References

Ahmed, S., de Jager, C., & Wilcock, G. (2012). A comparison of screening tools for the assessment of mild cognitive impairment: Preliminary findings. *Neurocase*, 18(4), 336–351.

Albert, M. S., DeKosky, S. T., Dickson, D., Dubois, B., Feldman, H. H., Fox, N. C.,...Phelps, C. H. (2011). The diagnosis of mild cognitive impairment due to alzheimer's disease: Recommendations from the national institute on aging-alzheimer's association workgroups on diagnostic guidelines for alzheimer's disease. *Alzheimers and Dementia*, 7(3), 270–279.

Alves, L., Simoes, M. R., Martins, C., Freitas, S., & Santana, I. (2013). Premorbid iq influence on screening tests' scores in healthy patients and patients with cognitive impairment. *Journal of Geriatric Psychiatry and Neurology*, 26(2), 117–126.

Barnes, D. E., Yaffe, K., Byers, A. L., McCormick, M., Schaefer, C., & Whitmer, R. A. (2012). Midlife vs late-life depressive symptoms and risk of dementia: Differential effects for alzheimer disease and vascular dementia. *Archives of General Psychiatry*, 69(5), 493–498.

Beck, A. T., Ward, C. D. H., Mendelson, M., Mock, J., & Erbaugh, J. (1961). An inventory for measuring depression. *Archives of General Psychiatry*, 4, 561–571.

Benton, A. L., Sivan, A. B., Hamsher, K. D., Varney, N. R., & Spreen, O. (1994). *Contributions to neuropsychological assessment*. New York, NY: Oxford University Press.

Blessed, G., Tomlinson, B. E., & Roth, M. (1968). The association between quantitative measures of dementia and of senile change in the cerebral grey matter of elderly subjects. *British Journal of Psychiatry*, 114, 797–811.

Borson, S., Scanlan, J., Brush, M., Vitaliano, P., & Dokmak, A. (2000). The mini-cog: A cognitive "vital signs" measure for dementia screening in multi-lingual elderly. *International Journal of Geriatric Psychiatry*, 15(11), 1021–1027.

Boustani, M., Peterson, B., Hanson, L., Harris, R., & Lohr, K. N. (2003). Screening for dementia in primary care: A summary of the evidence for the u.S. Preventive services task force. *Ann Intern Med*, 138(11), 927–937.

Brodaty, H., Pond, D., Kemp, N. M., Luscombe, G., Harding, L., Berman, K., & Huppert, F. A. (2002). The gpcog: A new screening test for dementia designed for general practice. *Journal of the American Geriatric Society*, 50(3), 530–534.

Brooke, P., & Bullock, R. (1999). Validation of a 6 item cognitive impairment test with a view to primary care usage. *International Journal of Geriatric Psychiatry*, 14(11), 936–940.

Buschke, H., Kuslansky, G., Katz, M., Stewart, W. F., Sliwinski, M. J., Eckholdt, H. M., & Lipton, R. B. (1999). Screening for dementia with the memory impairment screen. *Neurology*, 52(2), 231–238.

Cahn-Weiner, D. A., Sullivan, E. V., Shear, P. K., Fama, R., Lim, K. O., Yesavage, J. A., ... Pfefferbaum, A. (1999). Brain structural and cognitive correlates of clock drawing performance in Alzheimer's disease. *Journal of the International Neuropsychological Society*, 5(6), 502–509.

Cherrier, M. M., Mendez, M. F., Perryman, K. M., Pachana, N. A., Miller, B. L., & Cummings, J. L. (1997). Frontotemporal dementia versus vascular dementia: Differential features on mental status examination. *Journal of the American Geriatric Society*, 45(5), 579–583.

Christensen, H., & Jorm, A. F. (1992). Short report: Effect of premorbid intelligence on the mini-mental state and iqcode. *International Journal of Geriatric Psychiatry*, 7(3), 159–160.

Cordell, C. B., Borson, S., Boustani, M., Chodosh, J., Reuben, D., Verghese, J., ... Fried, L. B. (2013). Alzheimer's association recommendations for operationalizing the detection of cognitive impairment during the medicare annual wellness visit in a primary care setting. *Alzheimers Dementia*, 9(2), 141–150.

Crum, R. M., Anthony, J. C., Bassett, S. S., & Folstein, M. F. (1993). Population-based norms for the mini-mental state examination by age and educational level. *Journal of the American Medical Association*, 269(18), 2386–2391.

Cullen, B., O'Neill, B., Evans, J. J., Coen, R. F., & Lawlor, B. A. (2007). A review of screening tests for cognitive impairment. *Journal of Neurology, Neurosurgery, and Psychiatry*, 78(8), 790–799.

Edelberg, H. K., Shallenberger, E., Hausdorff, J. M., & Wei, J. Y. (2000). One-year follow-up of medication management capacity in highly functioning older adults. *Journal of Gerontology A Biological Science Medical Science*, 55(10), M550–553.

Edelberg, H. K., Shallenberger, E., & Wei, J. Y. (1999). Medication management capacity in highly functioning community-living older adults: Detection of early deficits. *Journal of the American Geriatric Society*, 47(5), 592–596.

Edelstein, B., Lichtenberg, P., Marson, D., Moye, J., Powers, D., Sabatino, C., ... Moye, J. (2008). *Assessment of older adults with dimished capacity: A handbook for psychologists*. American Bar Association and American Psychological Association. Retrieved March 2014, from http://www.apa.org/pi/aging/programs/assessment/capacity-psychologist-handbook.pdf.

Eknoyan, D., Hurley, R. A., & Taber, K. H. (2012). The clock drawing task: Common errors and functional neuroanatomy. *Journal of Neuropsychiatry and Clinical Neuroscience*, 24(3), 260–265.

Folstein, M. F., Folstein, S. E., & McHugh, P. R. (1975). "Mini-mental state". A practical method for grading the cognitive state of patients for the clinician. *Journal of Psychiatric Research*, 12(3), 189–198.

Folstein, M. F., Robins, L. N., & Helzer, J. E. (1983). The mini-mental state examination. *Archives of General Psychiatry*, 40(7), 812.

Freedman, M., Leach, L., Kaplan, E., Winocur, G., Shulman, K. I., & Delis, D. (1994). *Clock drawing: A neuropsychological analysis*. New York, NY: Oxford University Press.

Freitas, S., Simoes, M. R., Alves, L., & Santana, I. (2013). Montreal cognitive assessment: Validation study for mild cognitive impairment and alzheimer disease. *Alzheimer Disease and Associated Disorders, 27*(1), 37–43.

Galvin, J. E., Roe, C. M., Powlishta, K. K., Coats, M. A., Muich, S. J., Grant, E.,...Morris, J. C. (2005). The ad8: A brief informant interview to detect dementia. *Neurology, 65*(4), 559–564.

Galvin, J. E., Roe, C. M., Xiong, C., & Morris, J. C. (2006). Validity and reliability of the ad8 informant interview in dementia. *Neurology, 67*(11), 1942–1948.

Grober, E., & Buschke, H. (1987). Genuine memory deficits in dementia. *Developmental Neuropsychology, 3*, 13–36.

Hardy, J., Momeni, P., & Traynor, B. J. (2006). Frontal temporal dementia: Dissecting the aetiology and pathogenesis. *Brain, 129*(Pt 4), 830–831.

Hebert, L. E., Weuve, J., Scherr, P. A., & Evans, D. A. (2013). Alzheimer disease in the united states (2010-2050) estimated using the 2010 census. *Neurology, 80*(19), 1778–1783.

Hodkinson, H. M. (2012). Evaluation of a mental test score for assessment of mental impairment in the elderly. 1972. *Age and Ageing, 41*(Suppl 3), iii35–40.

James, W. (1890). *Principles of psychology*. Boston, MA: Harvard University Press.

Jost, B. C., & Grossberg, G. T. (1996). The evolution of psychiatric symptoms in alzheimer's disease: A natural history study. *Journal of the American Geriatric Society, 44*(9), 1078–1081.

Katzman, R., Brown, T., Fuld, P., Peck, A., Schechter, R., & Schimmel, H. (1983). Validation of a short orientation-memory-concentration test of cognitive impairment. *American Journal of Psychiatry, 140*(6), 734–739.

Kaufer, D. I., Cummings, J. L., Ketchel, P., Smith, V., MacMillan, A., Shelley, T.,...Dekosky, S. T. (2000). Validation of the npi-q, a brief clinical form of the neuropsychiatric inventory. *Journal of Neuropsychiatry and Clinical Neuroscience, 12*(2), 233–239.

Kitabayashi, Y., Ueda, H., Narumoto, J., Nakamura, K., Kita, H., & Fukui, K. (2001). Qualitative analyses of clock drawings in Alzheimer's disease and vascular dementia. *Psychiatry and Clinical Neuroscience, 55*(5), 485–491.

Lakhan, P., Jones, M., Wilson, A., & Gray, L. C. (2012). The decline in activities of daily living at discharge (dadld) index: Stratifying patients at lower and higher risk. *Journal of Nutrition, Health and Aging, 16*(10), 919–924.

Lawton, M. P., & Brody, E. M. (1969). Assessment of older people: Self-maintaining and instrumental activities of daily living. *Gerontologist, 9*, 179–186.

Libon, D. J., Swenson, R. A., Barnoski, E. J., & Sands, L. P. (1993). Clock drawing as an assessment tool for dementia. *Archives of Clinical Neuropsychology, 8*(5), 405–415.

Locascio, J. J., Growdon, J. H., & Corkin, S. (1995). Cognitive test performance in detecting, staging, and tracking Alzheimer's disease. *Archives of Neurology, 52*(11), 1087–1099.

Lonie, J. A., Tierney, K. M., & Ebmeier, K. P. (2009). Screening for mild cognitive impairment: A systematic review. *International Journal of Geriatric Psychiatry, 24*(9), 902–915.

Mathuranath, P. S., Nestor, P. J., Berrios, G. E., Rakowicz, W., & Hodges, J. R. (2000). A brief cognitive test battery to differentiate Alzheimer's disease and frontotemporal dementia. *Neurology, 55*(11), 1613–1620.

McKhann, G. M., Knopman, D. S., Chertkow, H., Hyman, B. T., Jack, C. R., Jr., Kawas, C. H.,...Phelps, C. H. (2011). The diagnosis of dementia due to alzheimer's disease: Recommendations from the national institute on aging-Alzheimer's association workgroups on diagnostic guidelines for Alzheimer's disease. *Alzheimers and Dementia, 7*(3), 263–269.

Mioshi, E., Dawson, K., Mitchell, J., Arnold, R., & Hodges, J. R. (2006). The Addenbrooke's cognitive examination revised (ACE-R): A brief cognitive test battery for dementia screening. *International Journal of Geriatric Psychiatry, 21*(11), 1078–1085.

Morris, J. C. (1993). The clinical dementia rating (CDR): Current version and scoring rules. *Neurology, 43*(11), 2412–2414.

Morris, J. C., Heyman, A., Mohs, R. C., Hughes, J. P., van Belle, G., Fillenbaum, G.,...Clark, C. (1989). The Consortium to Establish a Registry for Alzheimer's disease (CERAD). Part I. Clinical and neuropsychological assessment of Alzheimer's disease. *Neurology, 39*(9), 1159–1165.

Nair, A. K., Gavett, B. E., Damman, M., Dekker, W., Green, R. C., Mandel, A.,...Stern, R. A. (2010). Clock drawing test ratings by dementia specialists: Interrater reliability and diagnostic accuracy. *Journal of Neuropsychiatry and Clinical Neuroscience, 22*(1), 85–92.

Nasreddine, Z. S., Phillips, N. A., Bédirian, V., Charbonneau, S., Whitehead, V., Collin, I.,...Chertkow, H. (2005). The montreal cognitive assessment, moca: A brief screening tool for mild cognitive impairment. *Journal of the American Geriatric Society, 53*(4), 695–699.

Njegovan, V., Hing, M. M., Mitchell, S. L., & Molnar, F. J. (2001). The hierarchy of functional loss associated with cognitive decline in older persons. *Journal of Gerontology A Biological Science Medical Science, 56*(10), M638–643.

O'Brien, J. T., Wiseman, R., Burton, E. J., Barber, B., Wesnes, K., Saxby, B., & Ford, G. A. (2002). Cognitive associations of subcortical white matter lesions in older people. *Annlas of the New York Academy of Sciences, 977*, 436–444.

O'Connor, M. G., Kapust, L. R., & Hollis, A. M. (2008). Drivewise: An interdisciplinary hospital-based driving assessment program. *Gerontology and Geriatric Education, 29*(4), 351–362.

Petersen, R. C., Smith, G. E., Waring, S. C., Ivnik, R. J., Tangalos, E. G., & Kokmen, E. (1999). Mild cognitive impairment: Clinical characterization and outcome. *Archives of Neurology, 56*(3), 303–308.

Pfeffer, R. I., Kurosaki, T. T., Harrah, C. H., Jr., Chance, J. M., & Filos, S. (1982). Measurement of functional activities in older adults in the community. *Journal of Gerontology, 37*(3), 323–329.

Rascovsky, K., Hodges, J. R., Knopman, D., Mendez, M. F., Kramer, J. H., Neuhaus, J.,…Miller, B. L. (2011). Sensitivity of revised diagnostic criteria for the behavioural variant of frontotemporal dementia. *Brain, 134*(Pt 9), 2456–2477.

Raskind, M. A., Peskind, E. R., Wessel, T., & Yuan, W. (2000). Galantamine in ad: A 6-month randomized, placebo-controlled trial with a 6-month extension. The galantamine USA-1 study group. *Neurology, 54*, 2261–2268.

Reger, M. A., Welsh, R. K., Watson, G. S., Cholerton, B., Baker, L. D., & Craft, S. (2004). The relationship between neuropsychological functioning and driving ability in dementia: A meta-analysis. *Neuropsychology, 18*(1), 85–93.

Reitan, R. M., & Wolfson, D. (1985). *The halstead-reitan neuropsychological test battery* (2nd ed.). Tucson, AZ: Neuropsychology Press.

Robitaille, A., Piccinin, A. M., Muniz-Terrera, G., Hoffman, L., Johansson, B., Deeg, D. J.,…Hofer, S. M. (2013). Longitudinal mediation of processing speed on age-related change in memory and fluid intelligence. *Psychology of Aging, 28*(4), 887–901.

Rouleau, I., Salmon, D. P., Butters, N., Kennedy, C., & McGuire, K. (1992). Quantitative and qualitative analyses of clock drawings in Alzheimer's and Huntington's disease. *Brain and Cognition, 18*(1), 70–87.

Royall, D. R., Cordes, J. A., & Polk, M. (1998). Clox: An executive clock drawing task. *Journal of Neurology, Neurosurgery and Psychiatry, 64*(5), 588–594.

Rudolph, J. L., Marcantonio, E. R., Culley, D. J., Silverstein, J. H., Rasmussen, L. S., Crosby, G. J.,…Inouye, S. K. (2008). Delirium is associated with early postoperative cognitive dysfunction. *Anaesthesia, 63*(9), 941–947.

Salthouse, T. A. (2010). Selective review of cognitive aging. [Review]. *Journal of the International Neuropsychological Society, 16*(05), 754–760.

Sheikh, J. I., & Yesavage, J. A. (1986). Geriatric depression scale (GDS): Recent evidence and development of a shorter version. In Terry L. Brink (Ed.) *Clinical Gerontology: A guide to assessment and intervention* (pp. 165–173). New York: Haworth Press.

Slachevsky, A., Munoz-Neira, C., Nunez-Huasaf, J., Stern, T. A., Blesius, C. R., & Atri, A. (2011). Late-onset cinephilia and compulsive behaviors: Harbingers of frontotemporal dementia. *Primary Care Companion CNS Disorders, 13*(3). pii: PCC.10f01115.

Solomon, P. R., Hirschoff, A., Kelly, B., Relin, M., Brush, M., DeVeaux, R.D., & Pendlebury, W. W. (1998). A 7 minute neurocognitive screening battery highly sensitive to Alzheimer's disease. *Archives of Neurology, 55*(3), 349–355.

Sperling, R. A., Aisen, P. S., Beckett, L. A., Bennett, D. A., Craft, S., Fagan, A. M., et al. (2011). Toward defining the preclinical stages of Alzheimer's disease: Recommendations from the national institute on aging-Alzheimer's association workgroups on diagnostic guidelines for Alzheimer's disease. *Alzheimers and Dementia, 7*(3), 280–292.

Storey, J. E., Rowland, J. T., Basic, D., & Conforti, D. A. (2001). A comparison of five clock scoring methods using ROC (receiver operating characteristic) curve analysis. *International Journal of Geriatric Psychiatry, 16*(4), 394–399.

Stuss, D. T., & Alexander, M. P. (2000). Executive functions and the frontal lobes: A conceptual view. *Psychological Research, 63*(3–4), 289–298.

Sunderland, T., Hill, J. L., Mellow, A. M., Lawlor, B. A., Gundersheimer, J., Newhouse, P. A., & Grafman, J. H. (1989). Clock drawing in Alzheimer's disease. A novel measure of dementia severity. *Journal of the American Geriatric Society, 37*(8), 725–729.

Tangalos, E. G., Smith, G. E., Ivnik, R. J., Petersen, R. C., Kokmen, E., Kurland, L. T.,…Parisi, J. E. (1996). The mini-mental state examination in general medical practice: Clinical utility and acceptance. *Mayo Clinic Proceedings, 71*(9), 829–837.

Tariq, S. H., Tumosa, N., Chibnall, J. T., Perry, M. H., III, & Morley, J. E. (2006). Comparison of the Saint Louis University mental status examination and the mini-mental state examination for detecting dementia and mild neurocognitive disorder--a pilot study. *American Journal of Geriatric Psychiatry, 14*(11), 900–910.

Teng, E. L., & Chui, H. C. (1987). The modified mini-mental state (3MS) examination. *Journal of Clinical Psychiatry, 48*(8), 314–318.

Tombaugh, T. N., McDowell, I., Kristjansson, B., & Hubley, A. M. (1996). Mini-mental state examination (MMSE) and the modified mmse (3MS): A psychometric comparison and normative data. *Psychological Assessment*, 8(1), 48–59.

Wallin, A. K., Wattmo, C., & Minthon, L. (2011). Galantamine treatment in Alzheimer's disease: Response and long-term outcome in a routine clinical setting. *Neuropsychiatric Disease Treatment*, 7, 565–576.

Weiner, M. F., Hynan, L. S., Rossetti, H., & Falkowski, J. (2011). Luria's three-step test: What is it and what does it tell us? *International Psychogeriatrics*, 23(10), 1602–1606.

Weintraub, S. (1986). The record of independent living. An informant-completed measure of activities of daily living and behaviour in elderly patients with cognitive impairment. *American Journal of Alzheimer Care and Related Disorders, Spring*, 35–39.

Yesavage, J. A., Brink, T. L., Rolse, T. L., Lum, O., Huang, V., Adey, M., & Leirer, V. O. (1983). Development and validity of a geriatric depression scale: A preliminary report. *Journal of Psychiatric Research*, 17, 37–49.

20

Neuropsychological Assessment of Dementia
A Large-Scale Neuroanatomical Network Approach

Sandra Weintraub

This chapter presents a model for the neuropsychological assessment of dementia based on a large-scale neurocognitive network approach. For most of the last century, the neurodegenerative dementias had been clinically characterized as conditions in which cognitive deficits are widespread, and associated brain pathology diffuse. It is now understood, however, that clinical and neuropathologic changes are not widespread until the *later* stages of illness, when much of the cerebral cortex associated with cognition has been ravaged by the cellular and molecular abnormalities that mark each disease and that cause neuronal cell death and synaptic dysfunction. Most recently, revision of the criteria for the diagnosis of dementia due to Alzheimer's disease (AD) (Jack et al., 2011) has taken into consideration the notion that there are stages of disease that include a biomarker-positive but symptom-negative period, the so-called preclinical stage (Sperling et al., 2011); a period where mild symptoms are evident but not incompatible with independent living, the so-called mild cognitive impairment stage (Albert et al., 2011); and, finally, the stage of dementia marked by cognitive and disease progression as well as functional impairment (McKhann et al., 2011). Recognition of this slow evolution makes it imperative to detect disease early, at a time when the neuropathologic change is not advanced and there is the potential for treatment or prevention. In the very earliest stages of cognitive decline and dementia, deficits can be quite focal, that is, clinically restricted to a single cognitive domain or process. This "focality" of symptoms mirrors the neuroanatomical specificity of the earliest neuropathologic and physiologic changes. For reasons still not well understood, these diseases target portions of large-scale distributed neurocognitive networks, disrupting anatomical and functional connectivity, and affecting specific cognitive domains, such as episodic memory, visuospatial function, and executive function and language, which are subserved by these networks (Weintraub & Mesulam, 1996). Most recently, this principle has been further supported by the work of Seeley and colleagues (2009).

This chapter focuses on the neuropsychological evaluation of the patient with neurodegenerative dementia for purposes of differential diagnosis and also for recommending management. Vascular dementia and syndromes of progressive cognitive decline related to nonneurodegenerative etiologies (e.g., normal pressure hydrocephalus, brain tumors, toxic/metabolic encephalopathy, and others) are not covered in detail. However, the conceptual framework presented here can also be used to derive a neuropsychological profile for these disease entities, with the diagnosis resting additionally on the history, neurologic examination, and diagnostic testing. Tests and strategies for screening for dementia; gauging dementia severity; and evaluating the domains of attention, mood, language, visual perception, episodic memory, reasoning, executive functions, and social cognition are suggested. "Red flags" that should alert clinicians, especially the primary care physician, to the possibility of dementia are highlighted, with emphasis on the more atypical presentations of AD and the class of diseases under the umbrella of frontotemporal lobar degeneration (FTLD) in which language deficits, behavioral changes, and motor disorders, rather than memory loss, characterize onset. Finally, there is a brief discussion of the need to establish metrics of brain health throughout the life span for purposes of early identification and intervention.

Definitions and Diagnosis of Dementia

"Dementia" is a clinical syndrome with a differential diagnosis. Some restrict the use of this term to progressive syndromes caused by neurodegenerative disease or multiple, successive strokes, while others use this term to refer to *any type of widespread cognitive impairment*, even if static in course, such as might be seen following a single "strategic stroke" (Roman, 2003). Yet others may use the term "dementia" to refer to any syndrome in which there is progressive cognitive decline due to any cause. Some causes of cognitive decline are due to factors extrinsic to the brain that temporarily affect its ability to function normally (also called "treatable" or "reversible" dementia) and that may be reversed with treatment (Cummings, Benson, & LoVerme, 1980). Others are intrinsic to neurons (i.e., "primary" dementia) and caused by neurodegenerative brain disease. Tumors, large strokes, or strokes in "strategic areas" and traumatic brain injuries are other pathologic processes that can cause a dementia-like picture. Figure 20.1 shows classes of cognitive decline based on their mode of onset.

The *DSM-IV* (American Psychiatric Association, 1994) criteria for the diagnosis of dementia were recently revised in part because memory loss need not be the presenting, or even predominant, symptom in many forms of dementia (which was required in the *DSM-IV* criteria). The newly proposed criteria for the diagnosis of dementia due to AD also have recognized that while amnesia is a hallmark symptom of AD, other domains can be affected first (McKhann et al., 2011). This chapter uses the following definition of dementia:

> The decline and progressive worsening of one or more cognitive functions (e.g., memory, attention, language, visual perception, reasoning) and/or comportment (e.g., characteristic personality traits, insight, judgment, social cognition), from a prior, customary level of functioning, to the point where usual activities of daily living are negatively affected; caused by irreversible brain disease. (Wicklund & Weintraub, 2005, p. 568)

There is no one-to-one correspondence between the clinical symptoms of dementia and the underlying neuropathology but systematic relationships have been demonstrated (Weintraub & Mesulam, 1993, 1996, 2009). The amnestic dementia profile has a high likelihood (85% or more) of predicting AD pathology at postmortem autopsy (see Weintraub, Wicklund, & Salmon, 2012; Wicklund & Weintraub, 2005). In contrast, progressive language disorders are more often associated with one of the forms of FTLD (approximately 70%) but also can be associated with AD pathology (30%–40%) (Mesulam, 2008; Mesulam & Weintraub, 2008).

State-of-the-Art Dementia Evaluation

The neuropsychological evaluation is often conducted within the framework of a comprehensive evaluation of dementia at a specialty clinic or coordinated by the primary care physician. Information from all sources can be combined with the neuropsychological findings to

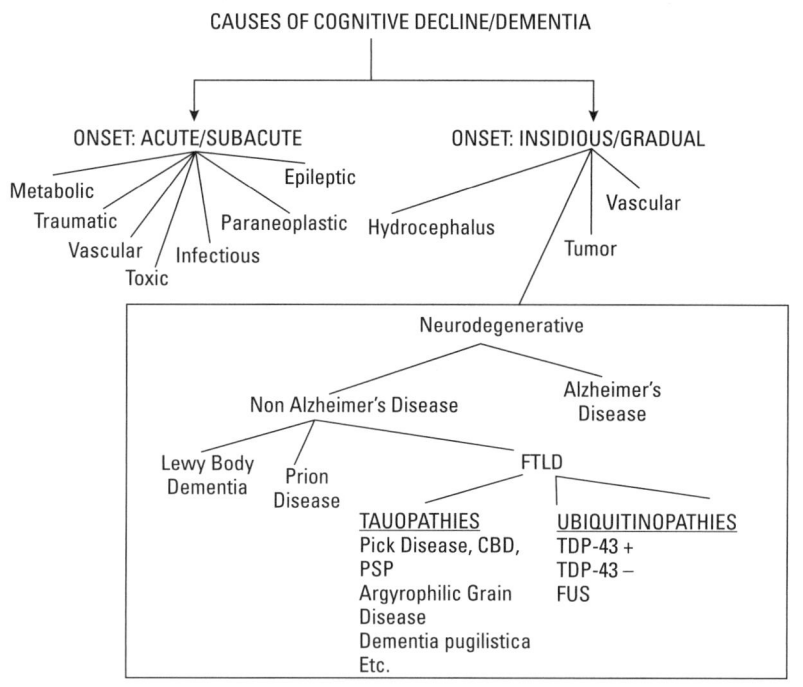

```
                    CAUSES OF COGNITIVE DECLINE/DEMENTIA
                                    │
                    ┌───────────────┴───────────────┐
                    ▼                               ▼
            ONSET: ACUTE/SUBACUTE           ONSET: INSIDIOUS/GRADUAL
```

Metabolic, Traumatic, Vascular, Toxic, Infectious, Paraneoplastic, Epileptic

Vascular, Hydrocephalus, Tumor

Neurodegenerative
- Non Alzheimer's Disease
- Alzheimer's Disease

Non Alzheimer's Disease: Lewy Body Dementia, Prion Disease, FTLD

FTLD:
- **TAUOPATHIES**: Pick Disease, CBD, PSP, Argyrophilic Grain Disease, Dementia pugilistica Etc.
- **UBIQUITINOPATHIES**: TDP-43 +, TDP-43 −, FUS

Figure 20.1 Differential diagnosis of cognitive decline and dementia. Cognitive and behavioral decline can occur acutely/subacutely or in an insidious and slowly progressive manner. This branching diagram shows some of the diseases that can be associated with each type of onset. The rectangle encircles the neurodegenerative disorders that cause a dementia syndrome and that are the main focus of this chapter. BIBID, basophilic inclusion body disease; CBD, corticobasal degeneration; FTDP-17, frontotemporal dementia with parkinsonism-17; FUS, fused in sarcoma protein; TDP-43, tar DNA binding protein 43; PSP, progressive supranuclear palsy.

predict the underlying etiology of the dementia. The state-of-the-art dementia evaluation, which may not be available in some settings, performed at major research medical centers includes a specialized clinical examination and testing often coordinated by a behavioral neurologist, geriatrician, and/or neuropsychiatrist. In the initial examination, the major clinical characteristics of the patient's syndrome are determined through history and examination and provide information about the types and severity of cognitive, affective, and motor symptoms and other clinical features that help the specialist narrow the differential diagnosis. Depending on the patient's clinical characteristics, blood tests may be obtained to evaluate for systemic illness that could be contributing to or accounting for mental state changes (e.g., thyroid dysfunction, congestive heart failure, paraneoplastic syndromes, lupus, etc.). Neuropsychological assessment is often recommended. Structural and functional neuroimaging (magnetic resonance imaging, amyloid imaging, positron emission tomography [PET], single-photon emission computed tomography [SPECT], and electroencephalography [EEG]) may be ordered to further evaluate the patient. Cerebrospinal fluid may be obtained for routine or specialized assessment, including possibly to measure levels of tau and amyloid (Jack et al., 2010) (see Chapter 22).

Screening for Dementia

Most of the current pharmacologic treatments for neurodegenerative dementia aim to treat symptoms or slow the rate of progression. Thus, early detection is essential. In some settings, however, neuropsychological assessment may not be available. In this instance, the clinician can use brief mental state screening tests to identify symptoms. The Mini Mental State Examination (MMSE) (Folstein, Folstein,

& McHugh, 1975) is commonly used in clinical practice and clinical trials but is not sensitive to very mild decline and does not cover all relevant domains. Measures such as the Montreal Cognitive Assessment (MoCA) (Nasreddine et al., 2005) and the Addenbrooke's Cognitive Examination (ACE) (Mathuranath, Nestor, Berrios, Rakowicz, & Hodges, 2000) are more sensitive to a wider range of impairment at very mild levels (Pendlebury, Mariz, Bull, Mehta, & Rothwell, 2012; Smith, Gildeh, & Holmes, 2007), although the ACE does require slightly more time than the MMSE or MoCA. It has been suggested that the MoCA should be interpreted with caution in an ethnically diverse sample where different cutoff scores may need to be employed to reflect a range of demographic variables (Rossetti, Lacritz, Cullum, & Weiner, 2011). Recent revisions of the MoCA introduce a scoring system that groups items into different domains and also that allows for more sensitive scoring of the word learning portion (Julayanont et al., 2014).

The clinician should keep in mind that some dementias do *not* affect memory in the early stages and that screening tests may miss these disorders. The group of disorders caused by FTLD presents with changes in personality, reasoning, and executive functions, or with aphasia, most of which are not suitably measured with screening tests. This class of diseases may also present with motor symptoms. Since the screening examinations have drawbacks from the standpoint of differential diagnosis and care planning, formal neuropsychological assessment is the most desirable way to demonstrate the deficits in mental state at a time when other diagnostics may be "normal" or "unremarkable."

Individuals with previously high levels of intellectual ability may subjectively experience symptoms despite normal performance on screening and other tests of mental state. The significance of subjective cognitive complaints for the subsequent diagnosis of dementia has been debated, but most recent evidence suggests that "cognitively normal" individuals with cognitive complaints show biological evidence of hippocampal volume reduction on structural neuroimaging in comparison with noncomplaining adults (Saykin et al., 2006). It is, therefore, recommended that neuropsychological evaluation be considered for patients who have subjective complaints but pass the standard screening examination. At the least, a comprehensive evaluation serves the purpose of providing a baseline against which future development of symptoms can be measured. Table 20.1 provides some rules of thumb regarding complaints that are more likely to be more representative of dementia than of "normal," age-related decline. However, these guidelines are not steadfast.

The Neuropsychological Examination of Mental State

Unlike a mental status examination in the neurologist's office, where a particular behavior may be briefly sampled, the neuropsychological assessment requires multiple items to assess each domain in order to derive a reliable score that can be compared with normative values. Thus, the full examination can take from 2–4 hours of face-to-face contact with the patient and caregiver, depending on the level of symptoms and the patient's former level of ability. More extensive testing may be necessary in the patient who is still gainfully employed, where symptoms are subtle or noncognitive in nature. The components of the comprehensive neuropsychological examination for dementia are as follows.

First, conduct a careful history. A clinical diagnostic interview should be conducted with the patient and an informant, ideally independently. Gathering information from a reliable informant is critical since many individuals with cognitive decline may not be aware of or may minimize their symptoms (Cacchione, Powlishta, Grant, Buckles, & Morris, 2003; Gavett, Stern, Cantu, Nowinski, & McKee, 2010). All of these factors will influence the clinician's interpretation of test performance and, ultimately, the differential diagnosis. As part of the history, the following information should be obtained. The nature of the onset (abrupt, subacute, insidious, and gradual), duration, and course (worsening, static, fluctuating) of symptoms is critically important. Information regarding prior medical, neurological, and psychiatric history, with special emphasis on factors that could contribute to cognitive deficits (e.g., sleep apnea, thyroid dysfunction, diabetes, history of or current substance dependency/abuse, etc.). The list of current medications should be reviewed. It is critical to obtain

TABLE 20.1 Comparison of Symptoms Consistent With "Normal Aging" Versus Dementia

Normal Age-Related Symptoms	Symptoms of Dementia
Independence in daily activities preserved	Individual becomes critically dependent on others for key independent living activities, such as check writing
Complains of memory loss but able to provide considerable detail regarding incidents of forgetfulness; this, however, should still be taken seriously since individuals may become aware of very subtle alterations at a time that functioning is still normal	May admit to "mild" memory problems only if specifically asked; unable to recall instances where memory loss was noticed; informant relays incidents of forgetfulness or other cognitive or behavioral symptoms which patient may deny or minimize
Recent memory for important events, affairs, conversations NOT impaired	Memory for recent events is impaired; repetitive questions, repetitive comments
Occasional word-finding difficulties	Frequent word finding, pauses, and substitutions
Does not get lost in familiar territory; may have to pause momentarily to remember way	Gets lost in familiar territory while walking or driving; may take hours to eventually return home
Able to operate common appliances and learn to use new ones with little difficulty	Unable to operate common appliances; unable to learn to operate even simple new appliances
Maintains prior level of interpersonal social skills	Loss of interest in social activities; exhibits socially inappropriate behavior
Character remains unchanged	Changes in character, typical ways of reacting to situations, emotional responses. Changes can be perceived by caregivers as more positive (more "laid back") or negative (obstreperous, disinhibited).

details about the patient's educational and psychosocial history and current functional status. Is there is history of pre-existing cognitive dysfunction (e.g., learning disabilities, developmental disorders, prior head trauma, etc.?). Finally, the clinician should carefully review the family history for medical, neurologic, or psychiatric disorders that might inform the differential diagnosis.

Next, the neuropsychologist should estimate the patient's premorbid level of functioning against which to compare current test scores. Some tests, for example the AMNART (Grober & Sliwinski, 1991) can be used to derive an estimated IQ since most individuals have never had detailed cognitive testing prior to the onset of dementia. Estimates also can be derived from demographic variables (Barona, Reynolds, & Chastain, 1984). The Vocabulary subtest of the Wechsler Adult Intelligence Scale-III (WAIS-IIII) (Wechsler, 1998) is robust in the face of brain damage and can be used for this purpose, especially in the absence of aphasia. The Wechsler Test of Adult Reading (Wechsler, 2001) and the reading subtest of the Wide Range Achievement Test-IV (Wilkinson & Robertson, 2006) can also yield an estimated IQ. In patients with limited levels of education, the highest level of achievement in work or civic duties may yield a better estimate of prior cognitive ability.

Next, obtain a general measure of dementia severity. The MMSE, Blessed Dementia Scale (BDS), or MOCA scores can be used for this purpose and/or to follow the patient over time. These tests are especially useful in later stages of illness when other neuropsychological tests are too difficult. Several questionnaires (e.g., the FAST (Reisberg, 1988) are also available for patients in the severe stages of illness. For patients in the milder stages of dementia, the Dementia Rating Scale (DRS) (Mattis, 2001) is more sensitive to change over time (Salmon, Thal, Butters, & Heindel, 1990) and has normative data for individuals over 89 years of age (Lucas et al., 1998; Schmidt et al., 1994). The mean score for high-school educated individuals over 70 is 27/30 on the MMSE, 34/37 on the BDS, and 137/144 on the DRS (Spreen & Strauss, 1998). These scores need to be adjusted for education and age (Tombaugh & McIntyre, 1992). The Clinical Dementia Rating (CDR) is a survey of the impact of dementia symptoms on activities of daily living and has been shown to have high reliability, validity, and association with pathologically verified AD (Morris, 1997). Caution should be exercised in examining the aphasic patient with most tests since questions require normal language for responding. Thus, the MMSE, for example, may overestimate the severity of impairment in a patient with PPA (Osher, Wicklund, Rademaker, Johnson, & Weintraub, 2007). Also, cultural and language differences can affect performance (Dodge et al., 2009).

Next, the neuropsychologist should review test performance in each of the neurocognitive domains and construct a profile of strengths and weaknesses. Tests or questionnaires should be administered to evaluate attention, mood and motivation, episodic memory (including learning and retention of information), visual perception, language, executive functions, and reasoning. Box 20.1 contains suggested tests to evaluate symptoms in each domain. These "domains" are well defined in terms of their cerebral organization and are also relevant for detecting patterns, or "profiles," that are associated with different types of dementia (Table 20.2). Thus, the amnesia of AD is a primary defect and not secondary to impairment in other processes such as poor attention, decreased motivation, or anomia. A careful examination can distinguish among these possibilities. Patients also differ with respect to specific symptoms, and knowledge of their specific deficits can lead to more personalized recommendations for management. To construct the profile of strengths and weaknesses in these domains, the patient's scores must be compared to normative values for a group of individuals of the same age, level of education, gender, and race, where available, and also to the patient's estimated premorbid level of functioning. From this information, the neuropsychologist can answer the following question: Is the patient performing as well as others in his or her own peer group? Based on this information and information from the history, the neuropsychologist can infer whether the patient is functioning at the level of her or his own peak prior ability.

"Noncognitive" behavioral symptoms, including apathy, disengagement from the environment, depression, agitation, and hallucinations can constitute the earliest symptoms of a dementia, as is often the case in Lewy body dementia or frontotemporal dementia. These are typically evaluated using interviews or questionnaires given to the informant and in some cases also the patient. The Neuropsychiatric Inventory (NPI) (Cummings et al., 1994) and the BEHAVE-AD (Reisberg, Auer, & Monteiro, 1996) provide a review of symptoms such as paranoia, depression, agitation, and hostility and the extent to which they cause distress to the caregiver. The Geriatric Depression Scale (Yesavage et al., 1983) may be useful in early stages. The Frontal Behavioral Inventory (Kertesz, Davidson, & Fox, 1997; Kertesz, Nadkarni, Davidson, & Thomas, 2000) reviews symptoms specific to frontotemporal dementia and is completed in an interview with the informant.

In addition to assessing the cognitive and affective domains described previously, the neuropsychologist needs to obtain a measure of the patient's ability to perform activities of daily living. The Activities of Daily Living Questionnaire (ADLQ) (Johnson, Barion, Rademaker, Rehkemper, & Weintraub, 2004) measures the impact of dementia on daily living activities in mildly demented, noninstitutionalized individuals. The ADLQ shows distinctive patterns of functional limitations in patients with non-Alzheimer dementia (Wicklund, Johnson, Rademaker, Weitner, & Weintraub, 2007) and may be preferable to the MMSE as a measure of dementia severity in patients with PPA (Osher et al., 2007). The ADLQ correlates with the CDR and is sensitive to change over time. Activities that may jeopardize the patient's or others' safety (e.g., driving, financial management, cooking) should be reviewed carefully. Sometimes there is a request for assistance with a determination of competency to manage finances or make health care decisions and there are neuropsychological test performance factors that can affect decision making in different realms (Marson, Cody, Ingram, & Harrell, 1995; Marson, Ingram, Cody, & Harrell, 1995; Marson et al., 2000, 2009). Assessment of safety can be accomplished with the Independent Living Scales (Loeb, 1999).

Neuropsychological tests are tools and require professional interpretation. Clinical neuropsychologists are trained in psychometric theory and measurement, psychology, brain anatomy, and physiology and on the impact of neurological, psychiatric, and medical disorders on brain functioning. The neuropsychologist interprets test findings just as the physician might interpret laboratory

BOX 20.1 Testing for Dementia

Screening and Functional Assessment

Short Mental Status Tests

Mini Mental State Examination (Folstein et al., 1975)
Blessed Dementia Scale (Blessed, Tomlinson, & Roth, 1968)
Montreal Cognitive Assessment (Nasreddine et al., 2005)

Brief Dementia Batteries

Mattis Dementia Rating Scale (Mattis, 2001)
Alzheimer's Disease Assessment Scale (Rosen et al., 1984)
CERAD Battery (Morris et al., 1993)
RBANS (Randolph, 1998)

Activities of Daily Living

Activities of Daily Living Questionnaire (ADLQ) (Johnson et al., 2004)
Functional Assessment Questionnaire (FAQ) (Galasko et al., 1997, Pfeffer, Kurosaki, Harrah, Chance, & Filos, 1982)
Independent Living Scales (ILS) (Loeb, 1999)

Behavioral Symptoms

Neuropsychiatric Inventory (NPI-Q) (Cummings et al., 1994, Kaufer et al., 2000)
Frontal Behavior Inventory (Kertesz et al., 1997)

Clinical Ratings

Clinical Dementia Rating (CDR) (Knopman, Weintraub, & Pankratz, 2011; Morris, 1993)
Functional Assessment Staging (FAST) (Reisberg, 1988)

Estimate of Premorbid IQ

Wechsler Test of Adult Reading (Wechsler, 2001)

Mood

Beck Depression Inventory-II
Geriatric Depression Scale

Tests of the Neurocognitive Domains

Attention

Concentration: Span/Vigilance/Working Memory

Digit Span, Visual Span (WMS) (Wechsler, 1998)
Number-Letter Sequences (WMS) (Wechsler, 1998)

Perseverance

Serial Recitation Tests (WMS) (Wechsler, 1998)
Word List Generation (Spreen & Strauss, 1998)

(continued)

Executive Function

Trail Making Tests (Reitan, 1958)
Motor Go- No Go (Weintraub, 2000)
Stroop Test (Golden et al., 2002)

Perceptual/Constructional Tasks

Hooper Visual Organization Test (Hooper, 1958)
Judgment of Line Orientation (Benton, Hamsher, Varney, & Spreen, 1983)
Facial Recognition (Benton et al., 1983)
Visual Target Cancellation Tasks (Weintraub, 2000)
Benson Complex Figure (Possin et al., 2011)
Copying a cube, drawing a clock

Language

Verbal Fluency Measures (Lezak, Howieson, & Loring, 2004; Spreen & Strauss, 1998)
Boston Naming Test (Kaplan, Goodglass, & Weintraub, 1983)
Boston Diagnostic Aphasia Examination (BDAE) (Goodglass et al., 2001)
Western Aphasia Battery (WAB) (Kertesz, 2006)
PALPA (Kay, Lesser, & Coltheart, 1992)
Northwestern Anagram Test (Weintraub et al., 2009)
Northwestern Naming Battery (Thompson, King, Lukic, Mesulam, & Weintraub, 2012)

Calculation Abilities

BDAE, WAB

Episodic Memory

Orientation
Wechsler Memory Scale (stories, word lists, designs) (Wechsler, 1998)
Rey Auditory Verbal Learning Test (word list) (Rey, 1941)
California Verbal Learning Test (word list) (Delis, Kramer, Kaplan, & Ober, 2000)
Rey-Osterreith Complex Figure (Rey, 1941)
Selective Reminding Procedure (Buschke, 1973)
Three Words Three Shapes Test (Weintraub, 2000; Weintraub et al., 2012, 2013)
Drilled Word Span Procedure (Weintraub, 2000)

Reasoning and Abstraction

WAIS Similarities, Matrix Reasoning (Wechsler, 1997)
Wisconsin Card Sorting Test (Heaton et al., 1993)
Visual-Verbal Test (Wicklund et al., 2004)

Planning and Sequencing

DKEFS Tower Test (Delis, Kaplan, & Kramer, 2001)

Note. This list is neither exhaustive nor exclusive. For additional instruments, consult Spreen and Strauss (1998) and Lezak and colleagues (2004).

TABLE 20.2 Neuropsychological Profiles of Mental State in Clinical Dementia Syndromes

Clinical Dementia Syndrome Defined by Prominent Symptoms	Attention	Emotions/Mood	Language	Visuospatial	Explicit Memory	Comportment Executive	Neuroanatomical Network
Primary progressive aphasia (PPA) Variants: agrammatic, semantic, logopenic	-	-	x	-	○	-	Left cerebral hemisphere
Progressive visuospatial dysfunction (posterior cortical atrophy)	*	-	*	x	*	-	Bilateral occipito-parietal regions
Primary amnestic dementia (probable Alzheimer's disease [PrAD] dementia of the Alzheimer type [DAT])	*	*	*	*	x		Limbic system
Progressive comportmental dysfunction (Behavioral variant or frontal variant FTD), BvFTD	*	-	*	○	○	x	Bilateral frontal and/or temporal
Dementia with cortical Lewy body disease (associated with extrapyramidal symptoms)	*	x	-	*	-	-	Brainstem locus coeruleus
Corticobasal degeneration syndrome†	-	-	x	x	-	-	Frontal networks (interferes with metabolic milieu)
Acute confusional state††	x	-	○	○	○	○	
Normal pressure hydrocephalus	x	-	○	○	○	○	Frontal networks (interferes with white matter connections)
Vascular dementia **	x	*	*	*	*	*	Frontal networks (multifocal cortical/subcortical lesions; also white matter lesions)

* = Impairment may be present and likely is stage or severity dependent.
** = Because of multifocal lesions typical of this disorder when it is progressive, the most common syndrome is that of frontal network dysfunction.
○ = Performance on tests of this domain may suffer *secondary* to primary deficits.
X = Most salient domain of impairment, accounting for functional daily impairments.
† = Associated with characteristic asymmetric motor symptoms that may be preceded by focal cognitive impairments (e.g., PPA, unilateral neglect).
†† = Characteristically due to toxic/metabolic encephalopathy.

values, in the context of a diagnostic hypothesis and comprehensive understanding of the history.

The examiner should have the flexibility to choose tests that are suitable for the individual patient. Thus, a patient with a third-grade education who worked as a housekeeper should be given tests that avoid floor effects, while a patient with advanced education and occupational attainment should be given tests that avoid ceiling effects. In the former example, if the tests are so hard that the patient fails everything, there is no resulting profile of strengths and weaknesses. In the latter case, if the patient performs normally for age on all tests, subtle decline could be missed.

Neuropsychologists also consider demographic variables that can alter the interpretation of test scores based on such factors as age, gender, ethnic/racial background, years of education, and quality of education (Brickman, Cabo, & Manly, 2006; Manly, 2005, 2008; Manly et al., 2011). In medical practice, there is a desire for norms, or standards, against which to measure individual patient values on laboratory tests. In neuropsychological assessment, as already noted, unlike in medical laboratory tests, there are many variables that can affect the interpretation of a score in the individual patient. In addition, the individual's test performance should be interpreted not only in comparison with age-relevant norms but also with respect to his or her own past peak level of cognitive ability. For example, if an individual would have performed in the top 2% of the population on a memory test at the age of 30, the fact that her current score at age 80 is "average for age" by normative standards alerts the neuropsychologist to the fact that there has likely been cognitive decline for that particular individual, even though the score is not abnormal. Some test scores (Vocabulary, estimated IQ) can be used to correct other obtained test scores before comparing them with normative data to obtain a measure of how much an individual has changed from her own peak performance level (Rentz et al., 2004, 2006, 2007; Rentz and Weintraub, 2000).

The comprehensive neuropsychological examination should accomplish the following goals. The first goal is to detect the presence of cognitive impairment. Most longitudinal cognitive aging studies have shown a significant decline in memory and other cognitive test scores after age 65. A decline in cognitive test scores, or the "normal aging" trajectory, however, can be identified in cross-sectional normative data even in younger individuals (Evans, Grodstein, Loewenstein, Kaye, & Weintraub, 2011). It is not known if a faster decline over early and middle adulthood presages later development of dementia. However, if detected earlier, such cognitive decline could be potentially amenable to interventions aimed at reducing risk. Second, the neuropsychological assessment should identify the overall level of cognitive impairment (i.e., absent, questionable, very mild, mild, moderate, or severe), as well as the relative level of impairment or preservation among the specific domains. Third, based on the history and functional assessment, the neuropsychologist should be able to determine the impact of cognitive dysfunction on activities of daily living. This is critical since the diagnosis of dementia requires that the cognitive changes have had an impact on functional capacity. Fourth, the results of the neuropsychological examination should help to narrow or expand the differential diagnosis. Neuropsychological reports should contain specific suggestions for further workup as needed (i.e., neurological and/or psychiatric evaluation, medical evaluation, and neuroimaging.) The examination results provide a neurocognitive profile of relative strengths and weaknesses that can be used to predict the neuroanatomical distribution of pathology and the probability of different neuropathologic (disease) diagnoses (Weintraub & Mesulam, 1993). Finally, the neuropsychological examination should contribute to management planning tailored to the patient's individual profile of strengths and weaknesses. Potential safety issues can be identified and recommendations made regarding further resources (e.g., a driving evaluation or financial supervision). Specific suggestions for practical community-based resources for assistance are also useful (e.g., Alzheimer's Association, Association for Frontotemporal Degeneration, local social service agencies, adult day health programs, geriatric care managers). Some neuropsychologists may also provide education and counseling services for patients and caregivers. While not changing the nature of the disease itself, such support and information can improve a patient's (and caregiver's) quality of life (Weintraub & Morhardt, 2005).

Neuropsychological Features of Selected Dementia and Prodromal Syndromes

Neuropsychological Features of Mild Cognitive Impairment

Some individuals experience an isolated impairment of memory or other cognitive functions but may perform relatively normally in daily living activities. This state has been referred to as "mild cognitive impairment" (Petersen, 2000a, 2000b; Petersen et al., 1997) or "age-associated memory impairment" (Crook, Bahar, & Sudilovsky, 1987-88). Petersen (2004) has proposed a classification to include nonamnestic and multidomain forms of MCI. Individuals in whom episodic memory is impaired are at elevated risk for progressing to AD dementia (Dubois & Albert, 2004; Dubois et al., 2007). The significance of other profiles of MCI, for example, isolated attention impairment, is not currently known (Luis et al., 2004; Luis, Loewenstein, Acevedo, Barker, & Duara, 2003). It is important in this population to obtain a detailed neuropsychological assessment and then to use the patient's own raw scores for comparison over time. Scores on memory and executive function tests (e.g., Trail Making Test) are particularly useful in predicting who is likely to progress to AD dementia in the future (Albert, Moss, Tanzi, & Jones, 2001). In addition, some investigators have suggested that intraindividual variability in test performance, rather than a single-point-in-time measurement, may have greater predictive value for MCI or dementia (Strauss, Bielak, Bunce, Hunter, & Hultsch, 2007). Much of the work on this topic to date has focused on groups of participants in longitudinal studies; further work in this area is required to develop prognostic models applicable to individual patients in clinical practice. See Chapter 17 for more information on MCI.

Neuropsychological Features of Alzheimer's Disease Dementia

Symptoms described in patients with AD dementia usually include a primary amnesia with forgetfulness, repetitiveness, and spatial and temporal disorientation (see Weintraub et al., 2012). The original description of the clinical syndrome of probable AD (PrAD) was marked by impairments on tests of learning and delayed recall (McKhann et al., 1984). Delayed recall shows a floor effect early in the course of AD and therefore cannot be used to track disease progression, but recognition memory performance can be used for this purpose (Locascio, Growdon, & Corkin, 1995). Although amnesia is a salient feature of AD, other cognitive deficits also emerge, including decreased verbal fluency on category list generation and reduced object naming. Impairments of attention and working memory can be seen in patients with mild to moderate dementia severity. In the most recent revision of the diagnostic criteria for AD dementia, it is also recognized that other cognitive deficits (e.g., language, visuospatial dysfunction) can lead the clinical picture in the early stages, although memory loss remains the most common presenting symptom (McKhann et al., 2011, online.). The Multilingual Aphasia Examination can screen for language deficits in adults up to 69 years of age (Benton, Hamsher, & Sivan, 1994). On average, patients with AD dementia decline annually by 3.24 points on the Information-Memory-Concentration subtest of the BDS, 2.81 points on the MMSE, and 11.38 points on the DRS (Salmon et al., 1990). The Alzheimer's Disease Assessment Scale (ADAS) (Rosen, Mohs, & Davis, 1984) has been used extensively to measure medication effects on the symptoms of AD dementia in clinical trials. The CERAD test battery focuses on the salient symptoms of AD dementia and includes tests of word list learning, category generation, naming, and constructions (Morris et al., 1989; Welsh et al., 1994). See Chapter 16 for additional information on AD.

Neuropsychological Features of Primary Progressive Aphasia

The earliest symptom of PPA is commonly word-finding difficulty in conversation. There are three major types of aphasia syndromes reported in PPA (Gorno-Tempini et al., 2011; Mesulam et al., 2009): agrammatic, semantic, and logopenic. The first type is characterized by preserved naming and single-word comprehension and impaired grammatical comprehension and/or production. The second is distinguished by impaired naming and single-word comprehension but relatively preserved grammar. The third manifests with spared comprehension but reduced verbal output due to frequent pauses for word finding in conversation and no agrammatism. Although there is no one-to-one relationship between the clinical PPA variant and the underlying disease, these clinical variants can predict the etiology with some degree of certainty. Thus, agrammatism is more likely to be associated with FTLD-tauopathy, while the logopenic variant of PPA is more likely to be associated with Alzheimer's neuropathology (Mesulam, 2008). Specialized aphasia testing is necessary to document the clinical syndromes of PPA, using such instruments as the Boston Diagnostic Aphasia Examination (Goodglass, Kaplan, & Barresi, 2001) and the Western Aphasia Battery (Kertesz, 2006). These instruments survey many language modalities, including spontaneous speech, single-word and sentence comprehension, repetition, naming, reading comprehension, and writing. The Northwestern Anagram Test (Weintraub et al., 2009) was designed to sample syntactic processing without requiring the patient to speak or rely on working memory to decode lengthy utterances. Measures that do not rely heavily on language comprehension or output are most useful for testing the integrity of reasoning (Wicklund, Johnson, & Weintraub, 2004) and episodic memory in this population (Weintraub & Mesulam, 1996; Weintraub et al., 2012). Insight is usually preserved in the early stages and patients may become depressed as a result. The Geriatric Depression Scale (Yesavage, Brooks, Taylor, & Tinklenberg, 1993) has been used to demonstrate elevated symptoms of depression in patients with PPA (Medina & Weintraub, 2007). Over time, as the pathology becomes more widespread, however, patients may develop symptoms of behavioral and other cognitive changes (Banks & Weintraub, 2004, 2008). Activities of daily living, with the exception of those dependent on normal language, are often spared for several years after onset (Wicklund et al., 2007). See Chapter 9 for more details on PPA.

Neuropsychological Features of Behavioral Variant Frontotemporal Dementia

Patients with behavioral variant frontotemporal dementia (bvFTD) experience symptoms of a change in character and/or personality (Rascovsky et al., 2007, 2011). The changes can be exaggerations of prior existing traits or a complete departure from them. Insight is typically reduced. Decreased initiative and emotional responsivity are often observed. The Frontal Behavioral Inventory (Kertesz et al., 2000) aims to provide measures of comportmental and language changes associated with FTLD. Patients may demonstrate deficits on tests of reasoning and cognitive flexibility, such as the Wisconsin Card Sorting Test (Heaton, Chelune, Talley, Kay, & Curtis, 1993) or the Visual Verbal Test (Wicklund et al., 2004). Attentional deficits can be detected with the Trail Making tests (Tombaugh, 2004), Stroop (Golden, Freshwater, & Golden, 2002) and Go No Go procedure (Weintraub, 2000). Symptoms of utilization behavior and environmental dependency syndrome (Lhermitte, Pillon, & Serdaru, 1986), whereby patients' behaviors become driven by stimuli in the environment regardless of their relevance, can also be observed. Social cognition is difficult to assess in the clinical setting, but deficits in this area are key components of bvFTD and contribute to the functional impairments prevalent in this group of patients (Rankin et al., 2008). Informant reports and observation of the patient's demeanor in the course of the evaluation can provide important clues to deficits in social cognition. Chapter 8 provides more information on bvFTD.

Neuropsychological Features of Lewy Body Dementia

Neuropsychiatric symptoms of delusions and/or hallucinations are the distinguishing early features of this form of dementia (McKeith et al., 2003). Although extrapyramidal symptoms are also usually a prominent early feature, early visual hallucinations and deficits on visuospatial constructional tasks are highly predictive of cortical Lewy body disease on autopsy examination (Tiraboschi et al., 2006). Constructions can be tested with a subtest from the CERAD battery (Morris et al., 1989) or the Benson Complex

Figure Test (Possin, Laluz, Alcantar, Miller, & Kramer, 2011). Patients are often described as fluctuating in their mental state with episodes of confusion interspersed with near normal functioning (Ferman et al., 2002; Geser, Wenning, Poewe, & McKeith, 2005; Metzler-Baddeley, Baddeley, Lovell, Laffan, & Jones, 2010; Salmon et al., 1996). Fluctuation on neuropsychological test scores from one test session to another over time is common in this syndrome. See Chapter 12 for more details on dementia with Lewy bodies.

Determination of the Clinical Neuropsychological Profile

At the completion of the neuropsychological evaluation, a clinical profile will emerge that can assist in differential diagnosis. Especially in the earliest stages of illness, it is likely that a patient will show significant impairment in one or a few domains with either normal or relatively preserved performance in others. Figure 20.2 illustrates this concept using early- and late-stage neurocognitive profiles of the progressive amnestic dementia associated with AD neuropathology and contrasts this profile with that seen in the clinical syndrome of progressive visuospatial dysfunction, also known as posterior cortical atrophy (PCA; see Chapter 10). The visuospatial profile of PCA is also associated with AD neuropathology (Renner et al., 2004), but in an unusual neuroanatomical distribution that favors the visual association cortex (Hof, Bouras, Constantinidis, & Morrison, 1990; Hof, Vogt, Bouras, & Morrison, 1997). Other pathological entities associated with PCA include cortical Lewy body disease and fatal familial insomnia (cf. Renner et al., 2004).

See Figure 20.3 for a summary of clinicopathologic relationships in AD dementia and PCA. Early in the course of the amnestic dementia of the Alzheimer type, episodic memory scores are typically impaired, while scores on tests in other domains are normal or relatively preserved. With time, however, performance on tests in other domains becomes impaired as well. In progressive visuospatial dysfunction, the earliest impairments are seen on tests of visuospatial functions, while scores on episodic memory and other tests remain normal. With time, however, these patients also develop deficits in other domains as the disease spreads to other cortical areas. The profiles of PPA and bvFTD differ from these two profiles in the early prominence of language and behavioral symptoms, respectively.

Even though the dementia may be quite selective in its behavioral and cognitive profile, however, it may be difficult to differentiate among syndromes solely on the basis of objective neuropsychological tests (Weintraub & Mesulam, 1993). The reason for this is that most neuropsychological tests are multifactorial and tend to engage more than a single cognitive process. For example, clock drawing is intended to serve as a visuospatial test. However, a primary disturbance in executive functions can lead to poor performance on this task even in the presence of preserved visuospatial functions. Similarly, word-finding difficulty may impair performance on verbal memory tests despite preserved episodic memory. Thus, the clinician needs to determine whether failure on a test is indicative of dysfunction in the targeted domain or if it is secondary to failure in another domain not targeted by the test construct. In early stages of frontotemporal dementia, all formal neuropsychological test scores may be abnormal, because impairments of motivation and executive functions may interfere with performance in a general manner. Conversely, all test scores may be normal because the primary deficit lies in social cognition and is not reflected in standard testing. Table 20.2 illustrates primary and secondary deficits on neuropsychological testing of common clinical dementia syndromes.

Neuropsychological Consultation: When and Why?

Neuropsychological consultation is not necessary in every patient with dementia. The following section provides some guidelines for identifying patients for whom a neuropsychological evaluation may be helpful.

In some patients, the detection of cognitive decline may be difficult in a routine physician's office visit. This is particularly true in mild phases of neurodegenerative dementias or in patients with high premorbid intelligence. Thus, the clinician may request neuropsychological assessment to determine whether the patient is experiencing cognitive

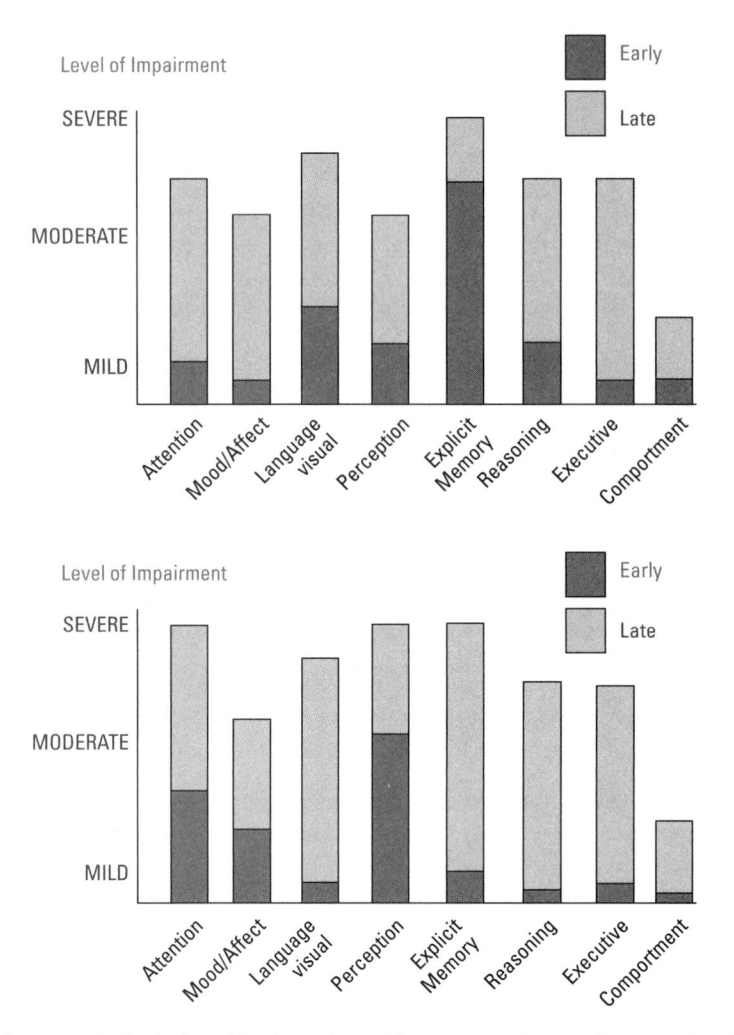

Figure 20.2 Neuropsychological profiles in early and late stages of neurodegenerative dementia. The charts display the neurocognitive profiles associated with early and late stages of the amnestic dementia of the Alzheimer type (top) and that of progressive visuospatial dysfunction, also known as posterior cortical atrophy (bottom). The early symptom profile can be clinically focal and is associated with the regional brain dysfunction. As the disease progresses, symptoms become more widespread, affecting several domains.

deficits that are abnormal for his or her age and level of education. For example, a patient may complain of, and family members may corroborate, memory difficulties in daily life, and he or she may obtain a normal score on the MMSE; neuropsychological assessment may be helpful to determine whether there is a memory deficit on more sensitive measures.

Neuropsychological testing may be useful for the *detection of atypical or early-onset (young-onset or presenile) dementias*. In a patient under 60 who presents with uncharacteristic behavior that is interfering with work, other activities, or social relationships, neuropsychological testing may help reveal evidence of early-onset dementia. With regard to atypical dementias, the early symptoms of primary progressive aphasia are often misdiagnosed as symptoms of stress or depression; formal cognitive assessment often reveals subtle but clear language abnormalities in these patients. Early symptoms of behavioral variant frontotemporal dementia are often also misdiagnosed as psychiatric in nature, and often executive dysfunction can be observed on neuropsychological testing.

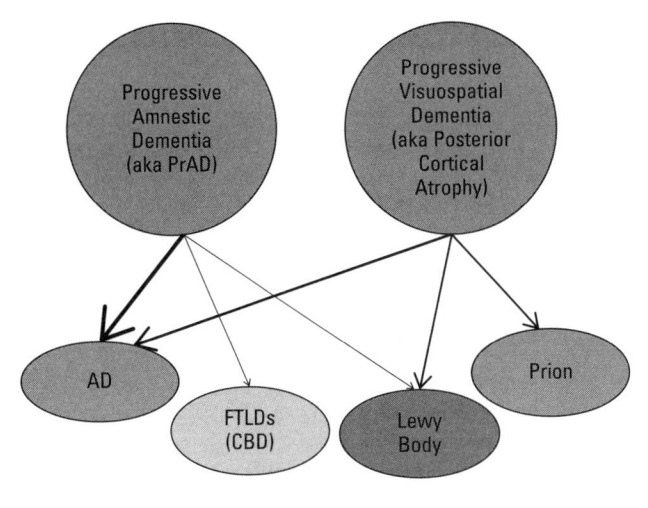

Figure 20.3 Neuropsychological profiles predict neuropathologic diagnoses with different probabilities. There is no one-to-one correspondence between clinical dementia profiles and the disease diagnosis at postmortem brain autopsy. This figure shows the association between the clinical diagnosis of dementia (circles at top, an early amnestic dementia profile and an early visuospatial dementia profile) and the neuropathologic tissue diagnoses following postmortem brain autopsy (circles at bottom). The thickness of the arrows represents the relative probability with which different types of diagnoses are associated with each profile.

Generally speaking, when a patient or family presents with cognitive-behavioral concerns and the initial physician office evaluation does not offer a clear diagnosis, neuropsychological testing can be a reasonable next step in the evaluation; results can provide not only documentation of a cognitive-behavioral deficit but also assistance in determining the likely cause of these deficits (e.g., differential diagnosis between depression, stroke, Alzheimer's, traumatic brain injury, etc.) based on the test profile.

Neuropsychological testing can also provide valuable information regarding safety, planning, and related issues. In a patient with an obvious dementia or milder cognitive impairment, the test profile can give indications of whether he or she is safe to live alone, drive, make financial decisions, or related activities.

In addition to the value of baseline testing, longitudinal neuropsychological assessment can be very important since it enables the clinician to identify changes in performance relative to the patient's own prior baseline. In a patient diagnosed with dementia, this can help to document the rate of decline and assist the patient and caregiver in planning for the future. Since dementia is progressive, regular checkups are important for altering management strategies and considering alternative living/care arrangements and safety issues. This monitoring may be possible to accomplish in the physician's office or may be augmented through longitudinal neuropsychological testing. In addition, this testing can help measure the effects of treatment, although it is always impossible to know how the patient would have performed without treatment. In addition, if a patient with a known dementia experiences an acute or subacute worsening in behavior, brief focused cognitive or neuropsychological assessment may be valuable in identifying whether there is another factor (e.g., toxic-metabolic encephalopathy) that is temporarily worsening mental state (i.e., causing a beclouded dementia?).

A Word on Brain Health Throughout the Life Span

The field of neuropsychology has highlighted the importance of brain health throughout the life span. Developmental disorders that interfere with normal acquisition of cognitive and behavioral skills can have far-ranging impact on the individual's ability to attain academic and later-life skills. Acquired injury after functions have been established, in the form of traumatic brain injury and stroke, cause cognitive and behavioral changes that may make it more difficult or impossible for an individual to resume his or her normal level of functioning. Neuropsychological science has pointed the way toward conceptualizing strategies to help restore skills or compensate for lost abilities (Wilson, 2008). In the realm of cognitive aging, it is understood that the outcome is determined by multiple factors unfolding over the life span, each of which can challenge brain plasticity and modulate risks (Mesulam, 1999). Some of the risks can occur early in life. For example, multiple traumatic brain injuries acquired in young adulthood can increase risk for late-life development of dementia (Plassman et al., 2000). Use of hormone replacement therapy at a critical point around menopause may actually decrease the risk of developing AD dementia in women later in life (Shao et al., 2012). One of the greatest challenges facing clinicians is the absence of objective cognitive measures acquired earlier in life, such as in a patient's 40s or 50s, against which to compare the scores obtained at the time of evaluation. Cognitive assessment should be incorporated into health maintenance programs that aim to prevent disease in old age, as is now mandated as part of the Medicare Annual Wellness Visit.

Conclusion

Neuropsychological assessment plays an important role in the examination of patients with suspected and known dementia. The objective neuropsychological examination addresses diagnostic, prognostic, and management issues. The search for biomarkers of dementia will no doubt ultimately provide a quick and effective method of diagnosis and point to appropriate treatments. However, neuropsychological assessment will continue to play an important role in defining the nature of deficits, their rate of progression, the impact they have on daily life, safety issues, and the ability to provide symptom-centered care for the individual patient.

References

American Pyschiatric Association. (1994). *Diagnostic and statistical manual of mental disorders* (4th ed.). Washington, DC: Author.

Albert, M. S., Dekosky, S. T., Dickson, D., Dubois, B., Feldman, H. H., Fox, N. C.,...Phelps, C. H. (2011). The diagnosis of mild cognitive impairment due to Alzheimer's disease: Recommendations from the National Institute on Aging and Alzheimer's Association workgroup. *Alzheimers and Dementia, 7*(3), 270–279.

Albert, M. S., Moss, M. B., Tanzi, R., & Jones, K. (2001). Preclinical prediction of AD using neuropsychological tests. *Journal of the International Neuropsychological Society, 7*(5), 631–639.

Banks, S., & Weintraub, S. (July 19, 2004). *Neuropsychiatric symptoms in primary progressive aphasia and the frontal variant of FTD.* Paper presented at the 9th International Conference on Alzheimer's Disease and Related Disorders Philadephia, PA.

Banks, S. J., & Weintraub, S. (2008). Cognitive deficits and reduced insight in primary progressive aphasia. *American Journal of Alzheimers Disease and Other Dementias, 23*(4), 363–371.

Barona, A., Reynolds, C. R., & Chastain, R. (1984). A demographically based index of premorbid intelligence for the WAIS-R. *Journal of Consulting and Clinical Psychology* 1984;52:885–887.

Benton, A., Hamsher, K. D., Varney, N., & Spreen, O. (1983). *Contributions to neuropsychological assessment.* New York, NY: Oxford University Press.

Benton, A., Hamsher, K. D. S., & Sivan, A. B. (1994). *Multilingual aphasia examination* (3rd ed.). Iowa City, IA: AJA Associates.

Blessed, G., Tomlinson, B. E., & Roth, M. (1968). The association between quantitative measures of dementia and of senile change in the cerebral grey matter of elderly subjects. *British Journal of Psychiatry, 114,* 797–811.

Brickman, A. M., Cabo, R., & Manly, J. J. (2006). Ethical issues in cross-cultural neuropsychology. *Applied Neuropsychology, 13*(2), 91–100.

Buschke, H. (1973). Selective reminding for analysis of memory and learning. *Journal of Verbal Learning and Verbal Behavior, 12,* 543–550.

Cacchione, P. Z., Powlishta, K. K., Grant, E. A., Buckles, V. D., & Morris, J. C. (2003). Accuracy of collateral source reports in very mild to mild dementia of the Alzheimer type. *Journal of the American Geriatric Society, 51*(6), 819–823.

Crook, T., Bahar, H., & Sudilovsky, A. (1987–1988). Age-associated memory impairment: Diagnostic criteria and treatment strategies. *International Journal of Neurology, 21-22,* 73–82.

Cummings, J., Benson, D. F., & LoVerme, S., Jr. (1980). Reversible dementia. Illustrative cases, definition, and review. *Journal of the American Medical Association, 243*(23), 2434–2439.

Cummings, J. L., Mega, M., Gray, K., Rosenberg-Thompson, S., Carusi, D. A., & Gornbein, J. (1994). The Neuropsychiatric Inventory: Comprehensive assessment of psychopathology in dementia. *Neurology, 44,* 2308–2314.

Delis, D. C., Kaplan, E., & Kramer, J. H. (2001). *Delis-Kaplan executive function system.* San Antonio, TX: The Psychological Corporation.

Delis, D. C., Kramer, J. H., Kaplan, E., & Ober, B. A. (2000). *The California Verbal Learning Test* (2nd ed.). San Antonio, TX: Psychological Corporation.

Dodge, H. H., Meguro, K., Ishii, H., Yamaguchi, S., Saxton, J. A., & Ganguli, M. (2009). Cross-cultural comparisons of the Mini-mental State Examination between Japanese and U.S. cohorts. *International Psychogeriatrics, 21*(1), 113–122.

Dubois, B., & Albert, M. L. (2004). Amnestic MCI or prodromal Alzheimer's disease? *Lancet Neurology, 3*(4), 246–248.

Dubois, B., Feldman, H. H., Jacova, C., Dekosky, S. T., Barberger-Gateau, P., Cummings, J.,...Scheltens, P. (2007). Research criteria for the diagnosis of Alzheimer's disease: Revising the NINCDS-ADRDA criteria. *Lancet Neurology, 6*(8), 734–746.

Evans, D. A., Grodstein, F., Loewenstein, D., Kaye, J., & Weintraub, S. (2011). Reducing case ascertainment costs in U.S. population studies of Alzheimer's disease, dementia, and cognitive impairment-Part 2. *Alzheimers and Dementia, 7*(1), 110–123.

Ferman, T. J., Boeve, B. F., Smith, G. E., Silber, M. H., Lucas, J. A., Graff-Radford, N. R.,...Ivnik, R. J. (2002). Dementia with Lewy bodies may present as dementia and REM sleep behavior disorder without parkinsonism or hallucinations. *Journal of the International Neuropsychological Society, 8*(7), 907–914.

Folstein, M., Folstein, S., & McHugh, P. R. (1975). Mini-mental state: A practical method for grading the cognitive state of patients for the clinician. *Journal of Psychiatric Research, 12,* 189–198.

Galasko, D., Bennett, D., Sano, M., Ernesto, C., Thomas, R., Grundman, M., & Ferris, S. (1997). An inventory to assess activities of daily living for clinical trials in Alzheimer's disease. The Alzheimer's Disease Cooperative Study. *Alzheimers Disease and Associated Disorders, 11*(Suppl 2), S33–S39.

Gavett, B. E., Stern, R. A., Cantu, R. C., Nowinski, C. J., & McKee, A. C. (2010). Mild traumatic brain injury: A risk factor for neurodegeneration. *Alzheimers Research and Therapy, 2*(3), 18.

Geser, F., Wenning, G. K., Poewe, W., & McKeith, I. (2005). How to diagnose dementia with Lewy bodies: State of the art. *Movement Disorders, 20*(Suppl 12), S11–S20.

Golden, C., Freshwater, S., & Golden, Z. (2002). *Stroop Color and Word Test.* Wood Dale, IL: Stoelting.

Goodglass, H., Kaplan, E., & Barresi, B. (2001). *Boston Diagnostic Aphasia Examination 3rd edition* (BDAE-3). Lutz, FL: Par.

Gorno-Tempini, M. L., Hillis, A., Weintraub, S., Kertesz, A., Mendez, M. F., Cappa, S. F.,...Grossman, M. (2011). Classification of primary progressive aphasia and its variants. *Neurology, 76,* 1006–1114.

Grober, E., & Sliwinski, M. (1991). Development and validation of a model for estimating premorbid verbal intelligence in the elderly. *Journal of Clinical and Experimental Neuropsychology, 13,* 933–949.

Heaton, R. K., Chelune, G. J., Talley, J. L., Kay, G. G., & Curtis, C. (1993). *Wisconsin Card Sorting Test (WCST), manual revised and expanded.* Odessa, FL: Psychological Assessment Resources.

Hof, P. R., Bouras, C., Constantinidis, J., & Morrison, J. H. (1990). Selective disconnection of specific visual association pathways in cases of Alzheimer's disease presenting with Balint's syndrome. *Journal of Neuropathology and Experimental Neurology, 49*(2), 168–184.

Hof, P. R., Vogt, B. A., Bouras, C., & Morrison, J. H. (1997). Atypical form of Alzheimer's disease with prominent posterior cortical atrophy: A review of lesion distribution and circuit disconnection in cortical visual pathways. *Vision Research, 37*(24), 3609–3625.

Hooper, H. (1958). *The Hooper visual organization test manual.* Los Angeles, CA: Western Psychological Services.

Jack, C. R., Jr., Albert, M. S., Knopman, D. S., McKhann, G. M., Sperling, R. A., Carrillo, M. C.,...Phelps, C. H. (2011). Introduction to the recommendations from the National Institute on Aging-Alzheimer's Association workgroups on diagnostic guidelines for Alzheimer's disease. *Alzheimers and Dementia, 7*(3), 257–262.

Jack, C. R., Jr., Knopman, D. S., Jagust, W. J., Shaw, L. M., Aisen, P. S., Weiner, M. W.,...Trojanowski, J. Q. (2010). Hypothetical model of dynamic biomarkers of the Alzheimer's pathological cascade. *Lancet Neurology, 9*(1), 119–128.

Johnson, N., Barion, A., Rademaker, A., Rehkemper, G., & Weintraub, S.

(2004). The Activities of Daily Living Questionnaire: A validation study in patients with dementia. *Alzheimers Disease and Associated Disorders, 18*(4), 223–230.

Julayanont, P., Brousseau, M., Chertkow, H., Phillips, N., Nasreddine, Z. S. (2014). Montreal Cognitive Assessment Memory Index Score (MoCA-MIS) as a predictor of conversion from mild cognitive impairment to Alzheimer's disease. *Journal of the American Geriatrics Society, 62*(4), 679–684.

Kaplan, E., Goodglass, H., & Weintraub, S. (1983). *The Boston Naming Test*. Philadelphia, PA: Lea and Febiger.

Kaufer, D. I., Cummings, J. L., Ketchel, P., Smith, V., MacMillan, A., Shelley, T.,...DeKosky, S. T. (2000). Validation of the NPI-Q, a brief clinical form of the neuropsychiatric inventory [In Process Citation]. *Journal of Neuropsychiatry and Clinical Neuroscience, 12*(2), 233–239.

Kay, J., Lesser, R., & Coltheart, M. (1992). *Psycholinguistic assessment of language processing in aphasia*. Hove, UK: Erlbaum.

Kertesz, A. (2006). *Western Aphasia Battery-Revised* (WAB-R). Austin, TX: Pro-Ed.

Kertesz, A., Davidson, W., & Fox, H. (1997). Frontal behavioral inventory: Diagnostic criteria for frontal lobe dementia. *Canadian Journal of Neurological Science, 24*(1), 29–36.

Kertesz, A., Nadkarni, N., Davidson, W., & Thomas, A. W. (2000). The frontal behavioral inventory in the differential diagnosis of frontotemporal dementia. *Journal of the International Neuropsychological Society, 6*(4), 460–468.

Knopman, D. S., Weintraub, S., & Pankratz, V. S. (2011). Language and behavior domains enhance the value of the clinical dementia rating scale. *Alzheimers and Dementia, 7*(3), 293–299.

Lezak, M. D., Howieson, D. B., & Loring, D. W. (2004). *Neuropsychological assessment* (5th ed.). New York, NY: Oxford University Press.

Lhermitte, F., Pillon, B., & Serdaru, M. (1986). Human autonomy and the frontal lobes. Part I: Imitation and utilization behavior: A neuropsychological study of 75 patients. *Annals of Neurology, 19*, 326–334.

Locascio, J. J., Growdon, J. H., & Corkin, S. (1995). Cognitive test performance in detecting, staging, and tracking Alzheimer's disease. *Archives of Neurology, 52*(11), 1087–1099.

Loeb, P. A. (1999). *Independent living scales*. San Antonio, TX: Pearson Assessments.

Lucas, J. A., Ivnik, R. J., Smith, G. E., Bohac, D. L., Tangalos, E. G., Kokmen, E.,...Petersen, R. C. (1998). Normative data for the Mattis Dementia Rating Scale. *Journal of Clinical and Experimental Neuropsychology, 20*(4), 536–547.

Luis, C. A., Barker, W. W., Loewenstein, D. A., Crum, T. A., Rogaeva, E., Kawarai, T.,...Duara, R. (2004). Conversion to dementia among two groups with cognitive impairment. A preliminary report. *Dementia and Geriatric Cognitive Disorders, 18*(3-4), 307–313.

Luis, C. A., Loewenstein, D. A., Acevedo, A., Barker, W. W., & Duara, R. (2003). Mild cognitive impairment: Directions for future research. *Neurology, 61*(4), 438–444.

Manly, J. J. (2005). Advantages and disadvantages of separate norms for African Americans. *Clinical Neuropsychology, 19*(2), 270–275.

Manly, J. J. (2008). Critical issues in cultural neuropsychology: Profit from diversity. *Neuropsychology Review, 18*(3), 179–183.

Manly, J. J., Smith, C., Crystal, H. A., Richardson, J., Golub, E. T., Greenblatt, R.,...Young, M. (2011). Relationship of ethnicity, age, education, and reading level to speed and executive function among HIV+ and HIV- women: The Women's Interagency HIV Study (WIHS) Neurocognitive Substudy. *Journal of Clinical and Experimental Neuropsychology, 33*(8), 853–863.

Marson, D. C., Cody, H. A., Ingram, K. K., & Harrell, L. E. (1995). Neuropsychologic predictors of competency in Alzheimer's disease using a rational reasons legal standard. *Archives of Neurology, 52*(10), 955–959.

Marson, D. C., Ingram, K. K., Cody, H. A., & Harrell, L. E. (1995). Assessing the competency of patients with Alzheimer's disease under different legal standards. A prototype instrument. *Archives of Neurology, 52*(10), 949–954.

Marson, D. C., Martin, R. C., Wadley, V., Griffith, H. R., Snyder, S., Goode, P. S.,...Harrell, L. E. (2009). Clinical interview assessment of financial capacity in older adults with mild cognitive impairment and Alzheimer's disease. *Journal of the American Geriatric Society, 57*(5), 806–814.

Marson, D. C., Sawrie, S. M., Snyder, S., McInturff, B., Stalvey, T., Boothe, A.,...Harrell, L. E. (2000). Assessing financial capacity in patients with Alzheimer disease: A conceptual model and prototype instrument. *Archives of Neurology, 57*(6), 877–884.

Mathuranath, P. S., Nestor, P. J., Berrios, G. E., Rakowicz, W., & Hodges, J. R. (2000). A brief cognitive test battery to differentiate Alzheimer's disease and frontotemporal dementia. *Neurology, 55*(11), 1613–1620.

Mattis, S. (2001). *Dementia Rating Scale-2*. Odessa, FL: Psychological Assessment Resources.

McKeith, I. G., Burn, D. J., Ballard, C. G., Collerton, D., Jaros, E., Morris, C. M.,...O'Brien, J. T. (2003). Dementia with Lewy bodies. *Seminars in Clinical Neuropsychiatry, 8*(1), 46–57.

McKhann, G., Drachman, D., Folstein, M., Katzman, R., Price, D., & Stadlan, E. (1984). Clinical diagnosis of Alzheimer's disease: Report of the NINCDS-ADRDA Work Group* under the auspices of Department of Health and Human Services Task Force on Alzheimer's Disease. *Neurology*, 34, 939–944.

McKhann, G. M., Knopman, D. S., Chertikow, H., Hyman, B. T., Jack, C. R. Jr., Kawas, C. H.,...Phelps, C. H. (2011). The diagnosis of dementia due to Alzheimer's disease: Recommendations from the National Institute on Aging and the Alzheimer's Association workgroup. *Alzheimers and Dementia*, 7(3), 263–269.

Medina, J., & Weintraub, S. (2007). Depression in primary progressive aphasia. *Journal of Geriatric Psychiatry and Neurology*, 20(3), 153–160.

Mesulam, M. (2008). Primary progressive aphasia pathology. *Annals of Neurology*, 63(1), 124–125.

Mesulam, M., & Weintraub, S. (2008). Primary progressive aphasia and kindred disorders. In C. Duyckaerts & I. Litvan (Eds.), *Handbook of clinical neurology* (pp. 573–587). New York, NY: Elsevier.

Mesulam, M., Wieneke, C., Rogalski, E., Cobia, D., Thompson, C. K., & Weintraub, S. (2009). Quantitative template for subtyping primary progressive aphasia. *Archives of Neurology*, 66(12), 1545–1551.

Mesulam, M. M. (1999). Neuroplasticity failure in Alzheimer's disease: Bridging the gap between plaques and tangles. *Neuron*, 24(3), 521–529.

Metzler-Baddeley, C., Baddeley, R. J., Lovell, P. G., Laffan, A., & Jones, R. W. (2010). Visual impairments in dementia with Lewy bodies and posterior cortical atrophy. *Neuropsychology*, 24(1), 35–48.

Morris, J. C. (1993). The Clinical Dementia Rating (CDR), Current version and scoring rules. *Neurology*, 43, 2412–2414.

Morris, J. C. (1997). Clinical dementia rating: A reliable and valid diagnostic and staging measure for dementia of the Alzheimer type. *International Psychogeriatrics*, 9(Supplement 1), 173–176; discussion 7–8.

Morris, J. C., Edland, S., Clark, C., Galasko, D., Koss, W., Mohs, R.,...Heyman, A. (1993). The Consortium to Establish a Registry for Alzheimer's Disease (CERAD). Part IV. Rates of cognitive change in the longitudinal assessment of probable Alzheimer's disease. *Neurology*, 43, 2457–2465.

Morris, J. C., Heyman, A., Mohs, R. C., Hughes, J. P., van Belle, G., Fillenbaum, G.,...Clark, C. (1989). The Consortium to Establish a Registry for Alzheimer's Disease (CERAD). Part I. Clinical and neuropsychological assessment of Alzheimer's disease. *Neurology*, 39(9), 1159–1165.

Nasreddine, Z. S., Phillips, N. A., Bedirian, V., Charbonneau, S., Whitehead, V., Collin, I.,...Chertkow, H. (2005). The Montreal Cognitive Assessment, MoCA: A brief screening tool for mild cognitive impairment. *Journal of the American Geriatric Society*, 53(4), 695–699.

Osher, J., Wicklund, A., Rademaker, A., Johnson, N., & Weintraub, S. (2007). The Mini-Mental State Examination in behavioral variant frontotemporal dementia and primary progressive aphasia. *American Journal of Alzheimer's Disease and Other Dementias*, 22, 468–473.

Pendlebury, S. T., Mariz, J., Bull, L., Mehta, Z., & Rothwell, P. M. (2012). MoCA, ACE-R, and MMSE versus the National Institute of Neurological Disorders and Stroke-Canadian Stroke Network Vascular Cognitive Impairment Harmonization Standards Neuropsychological Battery after TIA and stroke. *Stroke*, 43(2), 464–469.

Petersen, R. C. (2000). Aging, mild cognitive impairment, and Alzheimer's disease [In Process Citation]. *Neurological Clinics*, 18(4), 789–806.

Petersen, R. C. (2000b). Mild cognitive impairment: Transition between aging and Alzheimer's disease. *Neurologia*, 15(3), 93–101.

Petersen, R. C. (2004). Mild cognitive impairment as a diagnostic entity. *Journal of Internal Medicine*, 256(3), 183–194.

Petersen, R. C., Smith, G. E., Waring, S. C., Ivnik, R. J., Kokmen, E., & Tangelos, E. G. (1997). Aging, memory, and mild cognitive impairment. *International Psychogeriatrics*, 9(Supplement 1), 65–69.

Pfeffer, R. I., Kurosaki, T. T., Harrah, C. H., Jr., Chance, J. M., & Filos, S. (1982). Measurement of functional activities in older adults in the community. *Journal of Gerontology*, 37(3), 323–329.

Plassman, B. L., Havlik, R. J., Steffens, D. C., Helms, M. J., Newman, T. N., Drosdick, D.,...Breitner, J. C. (2000). Documented head injury in early adulthood and risk of Alzheimer's disease and other dementias. *Neurology*, 55(8), 1158–1166.

Possin, K. L., Laluz, V. R., Alcantar, O. Z., Miller, B. L., & Kramer, J. H. (2011). Distinct neuroanatomical substrates and cognitive mechanisms of figure copy performance in Alzheimer's disease and behavioral variant frontotemporal dementia. *Neuropsychologia*, 49(1), 43–48.

Randolph, C. (1998). *Repeatable battery for the assessment of neuropsychological status (RBANS)*. San Antonio, TX: The Psychological Corporation.

Rankin, K. P., Santos-Modesitt, W., Kramer, J. H., Pavlic, D., Beckman, V., & Miller, B. L. (2008). Spontaneous social behaviors discriminate behavioral dementias from psychiatric disorders and other dementias. *Journal of Clinical Psychiatry*, 69(1), 60–73.

Rascovsky, K., Hodges, J. R., Kipps, C. M., Johnson, J. K., Seeley, W. W., Mendez, M. F.,...Miller, B. M. (2007). Diagnostic criteria for the behavioral variant of frontotemporal dementia (bvFTD): Current limitations and future directions. *Alzheimers Disease and Associated Disorders*, 21(4), S14-S18.

Rascovsky, K., Hodges, J. R., Knopman, D., Mendez, M. F., Kramer, J. H., Neuhaus, J.,...Miller, B. L. (2011). Sensitivity of revised diagnostic criteria for the behavioural variant of frontotemporal dementia. *Brain*, 134(Pt 9), 2456–2477.

Reisberg, B. (1988). Functional assessment staging (FAST). *Psychopharmacological Bulletin*, 24(4), 653–659.

Reisberg, B., Auer, S. R., & Monteiro, I. M. (1996). Behavioral pathology in Alzheimer's disease (BEHAVE-AD) rating scale. *International Psychogeriatrics*, 8(Suppl 3), 301–308; discussion 51–54.

Reitan, R. M. (1958). Validity of the Trail-Making Test as an indication of organic brain damage. *Perceptual Motor Skills*, 8, 271–276.

Renner, J. A., Burns, J. M., Hou, C. E., McKeel, D. W., Jr., Storandt, M., & Morris, J. C. (2004). Progressive posterior cortical dysfunction: A clinicopathologic series. *Neurology*, 63(7), 1175–11880.

Rentz, D. M., Huh, T. J., Faust, R. R., Budson, A. E., Scinto, L. F., Sperling, R. A., & Daffner, K. R. (2004). Use of IQ-adjusted norms to predict progressive cognitive decline in highly intelligent older individuals. *Neuropsychology*, 18(1), 38–49.

Rentz, D. M., Huh, T. J., Sardinha, L. M., Moran, E. K., Becker, J. A., Daffner, K. R.,...Johnson, K. A. (2007). Intelligence quotient-adjusted memory impairment is associated with abnormal single photon emission computed tomography perfusion. *Journal of the International Neuropsychological Society*, 13(5), 821–831.

Rentz, D. M., & Weintraub, S. (2000). Neuropsychological detection of early probable Alzheimer's disease. In L. F. M. Scinto & K. R. Daffner (Eds.), *Early diagnosis of Alzheimer's disease* (pp. 169–189). Totowa, NJ: Humana Press.

Rentz, D. M., Sardinha, L. M., Huh, T. J., Searl, M. M., Daffner, K. R., & Sperling, R. A. (2006). IQ-based norms for highly intelligent adults. *Clinical Neuropsychology*, 20(4), 637–648.

Rey, A. (1941). L'examen psychologique dan les cas d'encephalopathie traumatique. *Archives of Psychology (Frankfurt)*, 28(112).

Roman, G. C. (2003). Vascular dementia: Distinguishing characteristics, treatment, and prevention. *Journal of the American Geriatric Society*, 51(5 Suppl Dementia), S296–304.

Rosen, W. G., Mohs, R. C., & Davis, K. L. (1984). A new rating scale for Alzheimer's disease. *American Journal of Psychiatry*, 141(11), 1356–1364.

Rossetti, H. C., Lacritz, L. H., Cullum, C. M., & Weiner, M. F. (2011). Normative data for the Montreal Cognitive Assessment (MoCA) in a population-based sample. *Neurology*, 77(13), 1272–1275.

Salmon, D. P., Galasko, D., Hansen, L. A., Masliah, E., Butters, N., Thal, L. J., & Katzman, R. (1996). Neuropsychological deficits associated with diffuse Lewy body disease. *Brain and Cognition*, 31, 148–165.

Salmon, D. P., Thal, L. J., Butters, N., & Heindel, W. C. (1990). Longitudinal evaluation of dementia of the Alzheimer type: A comparison of 3 standardized mental status examinations. *Neurology*, 40, 1225–1230.

Saykin, A. J., Wishart, H. A., Rabin, L. A., Santulli, R. B., Flashman, L. A., West, J. D.,...Mamourian, A. C. (2006). Older adults with cognitive complaints show brain atrophy similar to that of amnestic MCI. *Neurology*, 67(5), 834–842.

Schmidt, R., Freidl, W., Fazekas, F., Reinhart, B., Grieshofer, P., Koch, M.,...Lechner, H. (1994). The Mattis Dementia Rating Scale: Normative data from 1,001 healthy volunteers. *Neurology*, 44(5), 964–966.

Seeley, W. W., Crawford, R. K., Zhou, J., Miller, B. L., & Greicius, M. D. (2009). Neurodegenerative diseases target large-scale human brain networks. Neuron. 2009 Apr 16;62(1), 42–52.

Shao, H., Breitner, J. C., Whitmer, R. A., Wang, J., Hayden, K., Wengreen, H.,...Zandi, P. P. (2012). Hormone therapy and Alzheimer disease dementia: New findings from the Cache County Study. *Neurology*, 79(18), 1846–1852.

Smith, T., Gildeh, N., & Holmes, C. (2007). The Montreal Cognitive Assessment: Validity and utility in a memory clinic setting. *Canadian Journal of Psychiatry*, 52(5), 329–332.

Sperling, R. A., Aisen, P. S., Beckett, L. A., Bennett, D. A., Craft, S., Fagan, A. M.,...Phelps, C. H. (2011). Toward defining the preclinical stages of Alzheimer's disease: Recommendations from the National Institute on Aging-Alzheimer's Association workgroups on diagnostic guidelines for Alzheimer's disease. *Alzheimers and Dementia*, 7(3), 280–292.

Spreen, O., & Strauss, E. (1998). *A compendium of neuropsychological tests*. New York, NY: Oxford University Press.

Strauss, E., Bielak, A. A., Bunce, D., Hunter, M. A., & Hultsch, D. F. (2007). Within-person variability in response speed as an indicator of cognitive impairment in older adults. *Neuropsychology, Development and Cognition B: Aging, Neuropsychology and Cognition, 14*(6), 608–630.

Thompson, C. K., King, M. C., Lukic, S., Mesulam, M-M., & Weintraub, S. (2012). Noun and verb production and comprehension in stroke-induced and primary progressive aphasia: An introduction to the Northwestern Naming Battery Performance. *Aphasiology, 26*(5), 632–655.

Tiraboschi, P., Salmon, D. P., Hansen, L. A., Hofstetter, R. C., Thal, L. J., & Corey-Bloom, J. (2006). What best differentiates Lewy body from Alzheimer's disease in early-stage dementia? *Brain, 129*(Pt 3), 729–735.

Tombaugh, T. N. (2004). Trail Making Test A and B: Normative data stratified by age and education. *Archives of Clinical Neuropsychology, 19*(2), 203–224.

Tombaugh, T. N., & McIntyre, N. J. (1992). The mini-mental state examination: A comprehensive review.[see comment]. *Journal of the American Geriatric Society, 40*(9), 922–935.

Wechsler, D. (1997). *Wechsler Adult Intelligence Scale* (3rd ed.). San Antonio, TX: The Psychological Corporation.

Wechsler, D. (1998). *Wechsler Memory Scale-III*. San Antonio, TX: The Psychological Corporation.

Wechsler, D. (2001). *Wechsler Test of Adult Reading*. San Antonio, TX: Psychological Corporation.

Weintraub, S. (2000). Neuropsychological assessment of mental state. In M-M. Mesulam (Ed.), *Principles of cognitive and behavioral neurology* (pp. 121–173). New York, NY: Oxford University Press.

Weintraub, S., & Mesulam, M. (1993). Four neuropsychological profiles of dementia. In F. Boller & J. Grafman (Eds.), *Handbook of neuropsychology* (pp. 258–282). Amsterdam, The Netherlands: Elsevier.

Weintraub, S., & Mesulam M-M. (1996). From neuronal networks to dementia: Four clinical profiles. In F. Fôret, Y. Christen & F. Boller (Eds.), *La demence: Pourquoi?* (pp. 75–97). Paris, France: Foundation Nationale de Gerontologie.

Weintraub, S., & Mesulam, M. (2009). With or without FUS, it is the anatomy that dictates the dementia phenotype. *Brain, 132*(Pt 11), 2906–2908.

Weintraub, S., Mesulam, M. M, Wieneke, C., Rademaker, A., Rogalski, E. J., & Thompson, C. K. (2009). The Northwestern Anagram Test: Measuring sentence production in primary progressive aphasia. *American Journal of Alzheimer's Disease and Other Dementias, 24*(5), 408–416.

Weintraub, S., & Morhardt, D. J. (2005). Treatment, education and resources for non Alzheimer dementia: One size does not fit all. *Alzheimer's Care Quarterly, July/September*, 201–214.

Weintraub, S., Rogalski, E., Shaw, E., Salwani, S., Rademaker, A., Wieneke, C., & Mesulam, M. (2013). Verbal and nonverbal memory in primary progressive aphasia: The three words three shapes test. *Behavioral Neurology, 26*(1-2), 67–76.

Weintraub, S., Wicklund, A. H., & Salmon, D. P. (2012). *The neuropsychological profile of Alzheimer disease. Biology of Alzheimer disease*. Woodbury, NY: Cold Springs Harbor Laboratory Press

Welsh, K. A., Butters, N., Mohs, R. C., Beekly, D., Edland, S., Fillenbaum, G., & Heyman, A. (1994). The Consortium to Establish a Registry for Alzheimer's Disease (CERAD). Part V. A normative study of the neuropsychological battery. *Neurology, 44*, 609–614.

Wicklund, A. H., Johnson, N., Rademaker, A., Weitner, B. B., & Weintraub, S. (2007). Profiles of decline in activities of daily living in non-Alzheimer dementia. *Alzheimers Disease and Associated Disorders, 21*(1), 8–13.

Wicklund, A. H., Johnson, N., & Weintraub, S. (2004). Preservation of reasoning in primary progressive aphasia: Further differentiation from Alzheimer's disease and the behavioral presentation of frontotemporal dementia. *Journal of Clinical and Experimental Neuropsychology, 26*(3), 347–355.

Wicklund, A. K., & Weintraub, S. (2005). Neuropsychological features of common dementia syndromes. *Turkish Journal of Neurology, 11*, 566–588.

Wilkinson, G. S., & Robertson, G. J. (2006). *Wide range achievement test 4* (WRAT4). Lutz, FL: Psychological Assessment Resources.

Wilson, B. A. (2008). Neuropsychological rehabilitation. *Annual Review of Clinical Psychology, 4*, 141–162.

Yesavage, J. A., Brink, T. L., Rose, T. L., Lum, O., Huang, V., Adey, M.,... Leirer, V. O. (1983). Development and validation of a geriatric depression screening scale: A preliminary report. *Journal of Psychiatric Research, 17*, 37–49.

Yesavage, J. A., Brooks, J. O., III, Taylor, J., & Tinklenberg, J. (1993). Development of aphasia, apraxia, and agnosia and decline in Alzheimer's disease. *American Journal of Psychiatry, 150*(5), 742–747.

21

Neuropsychiatric Symptoms of Dementia

Haythum O. Tayeb, Evan D. Murray, and Bruce H. Price

In 1907, Alois Alzheimer described the first case study of Alzheimer's dementia (AD) (Alzheimer, Stelzmann, Schnitzlein, & Murtagh, 1995). His patient had significant and disruptive behavioral and psychiatric symptoms in addition to memory and cognitive difficulties. He reported:

> The first noticeable symptom of illness shown by this 51-year old woman was suspiciousness of her husband. Soon, a rapidly increasing memory impairment became evident; she could no longer orient herself in her own dwelling, dragged objects here and there and hid them, and at times, believing that people were out to murder her, started to scream loudly. On observation at the institution, her entire demeanor bears the stamp of utter bewilderment. She is completely disoriented to time and place. Occasionally, she remarks that she does not understand anything and is at her wits' end. Sometimes she greets the doctor as if he were a visitor and excuses herself that she has not finished with her work; on other occasions, she screams that he wants to cut her open, and on yet others, she dismisses him, full of indignation and with expressions indicating that she fears him as a threat to her honor as a woman. At times, she is totally delirious, drags her bedding around, calls for her husband or daughter and seems to have auditory hallucinations. Often, she screams for many hours in a horrible voice.

In this case, neuropsychiatric symptoms preceded and developed coincident with the onset of cognitive difficulties. Delusions of jealousy and paranoia were early manifestations. Later, her social graces deteriorated and auditory hallucinations developed along with agitation and a delirious appearance. Although AD has been viewed as predominantly a disorder of memory and cognition, the vast majority of AD patients develop neuropsychiatric symptoms during the course of the illness (Lyketsos, 2002). It has been established that AD pathology prominently disturbs cerebral networks crucial for episodic memory functioning, namely the entorhinal, hippocampal, and mesial temporal structures. Similarly, neuropsychiatric symptoms occur when AD pathology affects regions of cerebral circuitry responsible for regulating mood and affect, motivation, decision making, and higher level perceptual processing. Specific circuitry involved includes the orbitofrontal regions, the anterior cingulate, the dorsolateral prefrontal cortex, heteromodal regions of the neocortex, as well as the amygdala, periventricular and septal nuclei, and striatum.

Neuropsychiatric symptoms are not limited to AD among the dementing illnesses. Frontotemporal dementia (FTD), Lewy body dementia (DLB), vascular dementia (VaD), and other dementia subtypes all have prominent neuropsychiatric manifestations. Recognition and treatment of these features can substantially impact the clinical course of the disease and the well-being of caregivers.

In this chapter, the neuropsychiatric aspects of dementia will be reviewed focusing on the phenomenology and a clinical approach toward evaluation. Subsequent chapters will focus on management of symptoms.

Overview of the Major Neuropsychiatric Symptoms in Dementia

A variety of neuropsychiatric features are well recognized as integral aspects of dementing illnesses. These features may precede or develop concurrently with the cognitive and functional decline. Whereas cognitive and functional deficits in dementia tend to be relentlessly progressive and show relatively linear decline within different stages of the illness, neuropsychiatric symptoms may emerge more variably. They may remit, relapse, or transition from one symptom to another. The neuropathological correlates of these symptoms are only partially understood. A growing body of evidence links individual symptoms to dysfunction in discrete cerebral networks affected by neurodegenerative processes (see Table 21.1 and Table 21.2 for a synopsis of the cerebral substrates of neuropsychiatric symptoms).

Neuropsychiatric symptoms adversely impact not only patients but also their caregivers. Many symptoms have been shown to be associated with worse cognitive performance, reduced functional ability and quality of life, and increased caregiver and patient distress (D'Onofrio, 2012; Hargrave, Reed, & Mungas, 2000; Lechowski, 2009; Schneider, Murray, Banerjee, & Mann, 1999). They are a major reason for institutionalization and nursing home placement (Callahan, 2006; Rabins, 1991).

The following sections review the major neuropsychiatric manifestations of dementia, their neuroanatomical substrates, and the relative prevalence of these features in the major dementing illnesses.

Depression

Both depression and cognitive impairment occur commonly in the elderly. The relationship between the two is complex (Box 21.1). Elderly patients with depression can have associated cognitive impairments, previously referred to as pseudodementia, but now more accurately designated as depression-related cognitive impairment (DRCI). There is evidence that such depression-associated cognitive impairments may persist in a subset of elderly individuals despite resolution of their depression. Indeed, epidemiologic studies have correlated depression with an increased later risk of developing dementia (Devanand & Sano, 1996). A potential mechanism for this may be found in the excessive glucocorticoid induction associated with depression, which in turn may result in a cascade of neurotransmitter-induced excitotoxicity, leading to subsequent neuronal injury. Alternatively, late-life depression could be viewed as a prodromal symptom for a dementing illness, related to early involvement of cerebral circuits crucial for mood regulation that are damaged by the neurodegenerative or

TABLE 21.1 Synopsis of the Cerebral Localization of Neuropsychiatric Symptoms: Cortical and Subcortical Structures Implicated in Selective Psychiatric Symptoms

Depression	Hallucinations	Delusions
Orbitofrontal cortex	Orbitofrontal cortex	Orbitofrontal cortex
Striatum	Striatum	Striatum
	Thalamus	Thalamus
Dorsolateral prefrontal cortex	Paralimbic/limbic cortex	Amygdala
Anterior cingulate gyrus	Unimodal association cortex	

TABLE 21.2 Summary of the Major Imaging Studies Linking Apathy, Depression, and Psychosis in Dementia to Cerebral Substrates

Author	Imaging Modality	NP Tool	Localization
Apathy			
Ott, Noto, & Fogel, 1996	SPECT	DBDS	Right temporoparietal
Craig et al., 1996	SPECT	NPI	Prefrontal and anterior temporal
Benoit et al., 1999	SPECT	NPI	Right cingulate
Migneco et al., 2001	SPECT	NPI	Anterior cingulate bilaterally
Benoit et al., 2002	SPECT	NPI	Left ACC, right inferior and medial gyrus frontalis, the left OFC, right gyrus lingualis
Benoit et al., 2004	SPECT	AI	Bilateral superior OFC, left middle frontal gyrus, right ACC, left superior DLPFC
Robert et al., 2006	SPECT	AI	Right ACC
Lanctot et al., 2007	SPECT	NPI	Right OFC, left ACC
Holthoff et al., 2005	FDG-PET	NPI	Left OFC
Marshall et al., 2007	FDG-PET	SANS	Bilateral ACC, medial OFC, bilateral medial thalamus
Apostolova et al., 2007	MRI VBM	NPI	Right superior, bilateral middle frontal, left superior frontal, anterior cingulate correction
Bruen et al., 2008	MRI VBM	NPI	Bilateral ACC and frontal cortex, left head of caudate, bilateral putamen
Depression			
Levy-Cooperman et al., 2008	SPECT	CSDD	Right superior and bilateral middle frontal gyri, left superior frontal gyrus, AC gyrus
Akiyama H, 2008	SPECT	NPI	Left prefrontal cortex
Galynker et al., 2000	SPECT	SANS, HDS	DLPFC, AC gyrus
Liao et al., 2003	SPECT	HDS	Anterior and posterior cingulate, precuneus
Psychosis			
Kotrla et al., 1995	SPECT	HDS, BPAD	Left frontal (delusions) Parietal (hallucinations)
Staff et al., 1999	SPECT		Right hemisphere (frontal and limbic)
Mega et al., 2000	SPECT	NPI	DLPFC, left AC, dorsolateral parietal
Staff et al., 2000	SPECT	Presence of CSAD	Right frontal lobe
Fukuhara et al., 2001	SPECT	Presence of theft delusions	Right medial posterior parietal
Nakano et al., 2006	SPECT	NPI	Posterior cingulate, precunei, parietal association cortex with right-sided dominance
Starkstein et al., 1994	SPECT	PSE	Bitemporal
Metnis et al., 1995	PET	Presence of DMS	OF and cingulate and left medial temporal
Hirono et al., 2998	FDG-PET	BPAD	Left inferior temporal (hypermetabolic), left medial occipital
Lopez et al., 2001	FDG-PET		Left DLPFC, left medial temporal (delusions) Right parietal, left medial temporal, left DLPFC (hallucinations)
Sultzer et al., 2003	FDG-PET	NRS	Right superior DLPFC, right inferior frontal pole, and right lateral OF region
Geroldi et al., 2002	CT	NPI	Right temporal and left frontal

ACC, anterior cingulate cortex; CT, computerized tomography; DLPFC, dorsolateral prefrontal cortex; FDG-PET, fludeoxyglucose positron emission tomography; MRI, magnetic resonance imaging; NPI, Neuropsychiatric Inventory; OFC, orbitofrontal cortex; SPECT, single-photon emission computed tomography.

BOX 21.1 The Relationship Between Depression and Dementia

1. Depression can be associated with cognitive impairment (properly termed "depression cognitive impairment").
2. Late-life depression may be a risk factor or prodrome for dementia.
3. In dementing illnesses, depression is a common comorbidity.

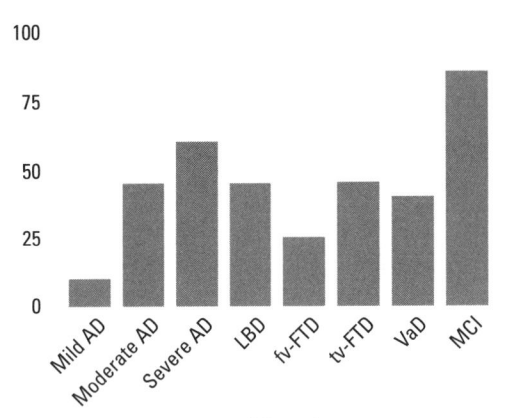

Figure 21.1 Estimates of the relative prevalence of depression in major dementia syndromes and neurodegenerative disorders. AD = alzheimer disease, LBD = Lewy body dementia, fv-FTD = frontal-variant frontotemporal dementia, tv-FTD = temporal variant FTD, VaD = vascular dementia, MCI = mild cognitive impairment.

cerebrovascular pathology. Finally, depression may result from the overwhelming stress of an evolving dementia (Geda, 2010).

Depression is prevalent in patients with established dementia, and it occurs at various stages. Figure 21.1 illustrates the average prevalence of depression in the major neurodegenerative disorders. A weakness of this data is that there is considerable variation with regard to the populations studied, stage of disease, and criteria utilized to diagnose depression. Depressive symptoms in AD have been shown to correlate with hypoperfusion or hypometabolism in the prefrontal cortical areas, including the dorsolateral prefrontal cortex (DLPFC) and the anterior cingulate cortex (ACC), presumably as a result of the neurodegenerative process (Akiyama, 2008; Butters, 2008; Galynker, 2000; Levy-Cooperman et al., 2008; Liao, 2003).

Depressive symptoms in dementia can be very similar to depressive syndromes in other contexts, especially when they occur in the mild stages of dementia (Chemerinski, Petracca, Sabe, Kremer, & Starkstein, 2001). However, the cognitive deficits in dementia, such as anosognosia and aphasia, may mask symptoms of depression by impairing the individual's ability to recognize deficits and communicate about them. Furthermore, there is a resemblance between the features of depression and those of dementia. Changes in appetite and sleep, and the presence of apathy, concentration difficulties, and slowing of psychomotor processing occur in both conditions. This superficial resemblance may lead to misdiagnosis. It is useful in such circumstances to include a caregiver's collateral history and to be vigilant while obtaining the history and performing the examination to assess for features that may indicate a primary depressive illness (Box 21.2) versus a dementing illness. Preliminary diagnostic criteria for late-life depression in AD have been proposed taking these diagnostic challenges into account (Table 21.3) (Olin, 2002).

BOX 21.2 Clinical Clues That May Improve the Detection of Depression in Patients With Dementia

Rapid uncharacteristic and unexplained deterioration of cognition
Blunted affect, decline in psychomotor reactivity
Dysthymic agitation
Disturbance in sleep/wake cycle
Food refusal, appetite decrease, and rapid weight loss
Prior history of depression
Family history of depression
Change in environment or caregiver

TABLE 21.3 Proposed Diagnostic Criteria for Depression in Alzheimer's Disease

	Major Depressive Episode	Depression of AD
Number of symptoms required	Five (or more) of the following symptoms have been present during the same 2-week period and represent a change from previous functioning	Three (or more) of the following symptoms have been present during the same 2-week period and represent a change from previous functioning
Caveat	Do not include symptoms that are clearly due to a general medical condition, or mood-incongruent delusions or hallucinations	Do not include symptoms that, in your judgment, are clearly due to a medical condition other than AD or are a direct result of non-mood-related dementia symptoms (e.g., loss of weight due to difficulties with food intake)
Symptoms	1. Depressed mood most of the day, nearly every day. as either indicated by subjective report or observation of others	1. Clinically significant depressed mood (e.g., depressed, sad, hopeless, discouraged, tearful)
	2. Markedly diminished interest or pleasure in all, or almost all, activities most the day, nearly every day (either 1 or 2 is required)	2. Decreased positive affect or pleasure in response to social contacts and usual activities (either 1 or 2 is required)
	3. Significant weight loss when not dieting or weight gain or decrease or increase in appetite nearly every day	3. Disruption in appetite
	4. Insomnia or hypersomnia nearly every day	4. Disruption in sleep
	5. Psychomotor agitation or retardation nearly every day	5. Psychomotor changes (e.g., agitation or retardation)
	6. Fatigue or loss of energy nearly every day	6. Fatigue or loss of energy
	7. Feelings of worthlessness or excessive or inappropriate guilt nearly every day	7. Feelings of worthlessness, hopelessness, or excessive or inappropriate guilt
	8. Diminished ability to think or concentrate	8. Recurrent thoughts of death, suicidal ideation, plan, attempt
	9. Recurrent thoughts of death, recurrent suicidal ideation without a specific plan, or a suicide attempt or a specific plan for committing suicide	9. Social isolation or withdrawal
		10. irritability
Other considerations	Does not meet criteria for a mixed episode	All criteria are met for dementia of the Alzheimer's type (*DSM-IV-TR*). The symptoms are not better accounted for by other conditions such as major depressive disorder, bipolar disorder, bereavement, schizophrenia, schizoaffective disorder, psychosis of AD, anxiety disorders or substance-related disorder
	The symptoms are not better accounted for by bereavement	
Physiological rule out	The symptoms are not due to the direct physiological effects or a substance (e.g., a drug of abuse or a medication) or a general medical condition (e.g., hypothyroidism)	The symptoms are not due to the direct physiological effects of substance (e.g., a drug of abuse or medication)
Functional impairment	The symptoms cause clinically significant distress or impairment in social, occupational, or other important areas of functioning	The symptoms cause clinically significant distress or disruption in functioning

AD, Alzheimer's disease; *DSM-IV-TR, Diagnostic and Statistical Manual of Mental Disorders,* fourth edition, text revision.
Source: Olin et al. (2002).

The course of depression in dementia may be mild and self-remitting over time (Devanand, 1997), but this is not uniform. A sizable proportion of patients with dementia will have a chronic major depressive illness that is resistant to treatment (Janzing, Teunisse, Bouwens, van 't. Hof, & Zitman, 2000; Starkstein et al., 1997). The recurrence rate of depression in dementia is also elevated at 85% (Levy et al., 1996). Careful monitoring of depression is a necessary component of the comprehensive care of patients with dementia. Clinical assessment tools such as the Beck Depression Inventory, the Hamilton Depression Scale, and others discussed elsewhere in this text, can be useful.

Apathy

As recently as 1990, the term *apathy* was defined as a syndrome of dysmotivation, paucity of volition, and as having a decrease in goal-directed and emotional responsiveness (Marin, 1990). Although there continues to be lingering controversy about its syndromic validity (Starkstein & Leentjens, 2008), it is now recognized as a distinct neuropsychiatric syndrome. Despite the overlap in clinical appearance between apathy and depression, they are distinct and independent syndromes with different courses. The neuropsychiatric profile of patients presenting with apathy is different from that of depression. Depression is neither necessary nor sufficient for apathy to be present (Levy et al., 1998). Proposed diagnostic criteria for the apathy syndrome delineate its most salient features (Box 21.3) (Robert et al., 2009).

Apathy is a common early feature in neurodegenerative disorders (Fig. 21.2). It is thought to result from dysfunction in frontal-subcortical neural networks affected by the neurodegenerative process (Apostolova, 2007; Benoit, 1999,

---

BOX 21.3 Diagnostic Criteria for Psychosis in Alzheimer's Disease

A. Characteristic symptoms: Presence of one (or more) of the following symptoms:
   1. Visual or auditory hallucinations
   2. Delusions
B. Primary diagnosis.
   All the criteria for dementia of the Alzheimer type are met.*
C. Chronology of the onset of symptoms of psychosis versus onset of symptoms of dementia: There is evidence from the history that the symptoms in Criterion A have not been present continuously since prior to the onset of the symptoms of dementia.
D. Duration and severity.
   The symptoms(s) in Criterion A have been present, at least intermittently, for 1 month or longer. Symptoms are severe enough to cause some disruption in the patients and/or others functioning.
E. Exclusion of schizophrenia and related psychotic disorders.
   Criteria for schizophrenia, schizoaffective disorder, delusional disorder, or mood disorder with psychotic features have never been met.
F. Relationship to delirium: The disturbance does not occur exclusively during the course of a delirium.
G. Exclusion of other causes of psychotic symptoms: The disturbance is not better accounted for by another general medical condition or direct physiological effects of a substance (e.g., a drug of abuse, a medication).
   Associated features: (Specify if associated)
   With agitation: when there is evidence, from history of examination, of prominent agitation with or without physical or verbal aggression.
   With negative symptoms: when prominent negative symptoms, such as apathy, affective flattening, avolition, or motor retardation, are present.
   With depression: when prominent depressive symptoms, such as depressed mood, insomnia or hypersomnia, feelings of worthlessness or excessive or inappropriate guilt, or recurrent thoughts of death, are present.

Source: Jeste and Finkel (2000).

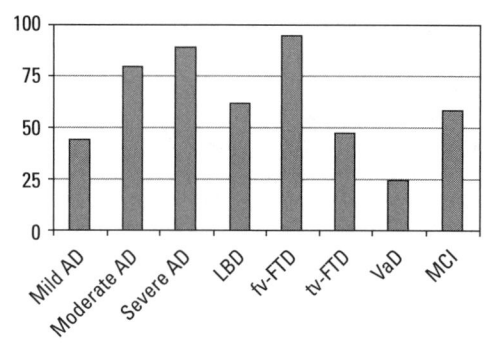

Figure 21.2 Average prevalence ranges of apathy in MCI and the major dementias. AD = alzheimer disease, LBD = Lewy body dementia, fv-FTD = frontal-variant frontotemporal dementia, tv-FTD = temporal variant FTD, VaD = vascular dementia, MCI = mild cognitive impairment.

2002; Bruen, McGeown, Shanks, & Venneri, 2008; Craig, 1996; Lanctot et al., 2007; Marshall, Fairbanks, Tekin, Vinters, & Cummings, 2006; Marshall et al., 2007; Migneco, 2001; Ott, Noto, & Fogel, 1996; Robert, 2006; Skogseth et al., 2008). Anywhere between 25% and 88% of individuals with Alzheimer's disease manifest apathy (Landes, Sperry, Strauss, & Geldmacher, 2001; Landes, Sperry, & Strauss, 2005). It is one of the early symptoms in AD, but it is also commonly seen in later disease stages. Apathy is the presenting symptom in a large percentage of patients with FTD, and it eventually develops in 62%–89% (Mendez, Lauterbach, & Sampson, 2008). The estimated prevalence of apathy in mild cognitive impairment (MCI) is as high as 59% (Apostolova & Cummings, 2008; Geda & Roberts, 2008). The presence of apathy is associated with an increased risk of conversion from MCI to dementia, as apathy was found to be present in more than 90% of MCI patients who eventually convert to AD (Robert et al., 2006).

Psychosis: Delusions and Hallucinations

Psychotic symptoms, including delusions, hallucinations, and psychotic agitation, are recognized as part of dementing illnesses. Proposed diagnostic criteria summarizing the clinical features of psychosis in dementia are provided in Box 21.3 (Jeste & Finkel, 2000). Psychosis may be accompanied by anxiety, agitation, and disruptive behavior (Flynn, Cummings, & Gornbein, 1991; Rockwell, Krull, Dimsdale, & Jeste, 1994).

Delusions, defined as fixed, false, and culturally unaccepted beliefs, occur commonly in dementing illness. There are recognized themes and patterns of paranoid delusions in dementia. Examples of these include those of theft, marital infidelity, and misidentification syndromes (Table 21.4) (Apostolova & Cummings, 2010). Bizarre delusions, such as those commonly seen in schizophrenia, are rare. Self-deprecating delusions should raise suspicion for concomitant depression. Visual hallucinations are more common than other perceptual disturbances in dementia, although all types of hallucinations can be seen, including olfactory and tactile hallucinations (Berrios, 1982; Marin et al., 1997; Simard, van Reekum, & Cohen, 2000).

Psychotic symptoms may occur during the course in all dementing illnesses. The average prevalence of psychotic symptoms in the major dementias is depicted in Figure 21.3. The time at which psychotic symptoms manifest may have diagnostic implications. Psychosis tends to occur earlier in DLB (and to a lesser extent in FTD, especially in patients with genetic *C9ORF72* repeat expansions; see Chapter 8) and comparatively later during the course of AD (Ballard et al., 1999; Marin et al., 1997; Simard et al., 2000). Patients with psychotic symptoms are more likely to have worse cognitive deficits than nonpsychotic patients (Flynn et al., 1991) and have a more rapid rate of cognitive decline (Ballard et al., 1999). Psychotic symptoms may remit in later stages of illness, when agitation and behavioral dyscontrol tend to dominate the clinical picture (Ballard et al., 2001; Lopez et al., 1991).

Anxiety

Generalized anxiety is the most common late-life psychiatric disorder, with a prevalence of close to 10% in the elderly population (de Beurs et al., 1999). This prevalence is higher in people with dementia, estimated to be between 38% and 72% (Ballard, Boyle, Bowler, & Lindesay, 1996; Ballard et al., 2000; Mega, Cummings, Fiorello, & Gornbein, 1996). The prevalence is also higher in MCI, where it ranges from 11% to 39% (Geda & Roberts, 2008; Mega et al., 1996). The

TABLE 21.4 Proposed Diagnostic Criteria for Apathy

For a diagnosis of apathy the patient should fulfil the criteria A, B, C, and D:

A—Loss of or diminished motivation in comparison to the patient's previous level of functioning and which is not consistent with his age or culture. These changes in motivation may be reported by the patient himself or by the observations of others.

B—Presence of at least one symptom in at least two of the three following domains for a period of at least 4 weeks and present most of the time.

Domain B1—Behavior

Loss of, or diminished, goal-directed behavior as evidenced by at least one of the following:

Initiation symptom: loss of self-initiated behavior (e.g., starting conversation, doing basic tasks of day-to-day living, seeking social activities, communicating choices)

Responsiveness symptom: loss of environment-stimulated behavior (e.g., responding to conversation, participating in social activities)

Domain B2—Cognition

Loss of, or diminished, goal-directed cognitive activity as evidenced by at least one of the following:

Initiation symptom: loss of spontaneous ideas and curiosity for routine and new events (i.e., challenging tasks, recent news, social opportunities, personal, family, and social affairs).

Responsiveness symptom: loss of environment-stimulated ideas and curiosity for routine and new events (i.e., in the person's residence, neighborhood, or community),

Domain B3—Emotion

Loss of, or diminished, emotion as evidenced by at least one of the following:

Initiation symptom: loss of spontaneous emotion, observed or self-reported (e.g., subjective feeling of weak or absent emotions, or observation by others of a blunted affect)

Responsiveness symptom: loss of emotional responsiveness to positive or negative stimuli or events (e.g., observer-reports of unchanging affect or of little emotional reaction to exciting events, personal loss, serious illness, emotional-laden news)

G—These symptoms (A and B) cause clinically significant impairment in personal, social, occupational, or other important areas of functioning.

0—The symptoms (A and B) are not exclusively explained or due to physical disabilities (e.g., blindness and loss of hearing), to motor disabilities, to diminished level of consciousness, or to the direct physiological effects of a substance (e.g., drug of abuse, a medication).

Source: From Robert et al. (2009).

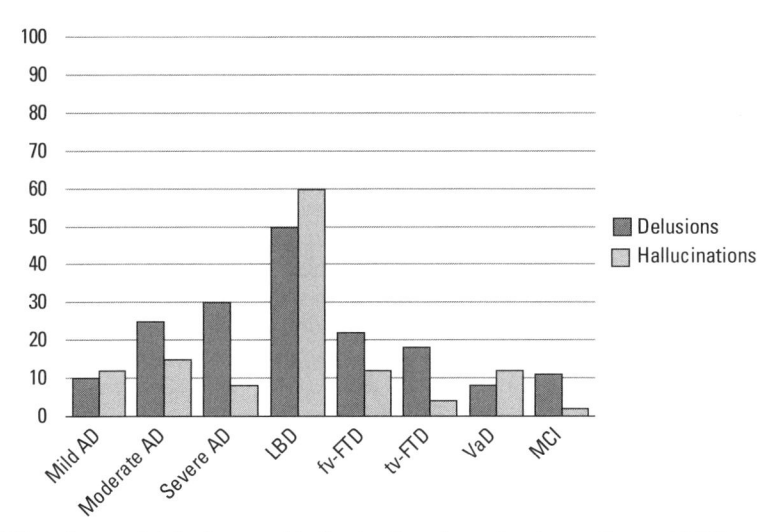

Figure 21.3 Prevalence of delusions and hallucinations in major dementias and MCI. AD = alzheimer disease, LBD = Lewy body dementia, fv-FTD = frontal-variant frontotemporal dementia, tv-FTD = temporal variant FTD, VaD = vascular dementia, MCI = mild cognitive impairment.

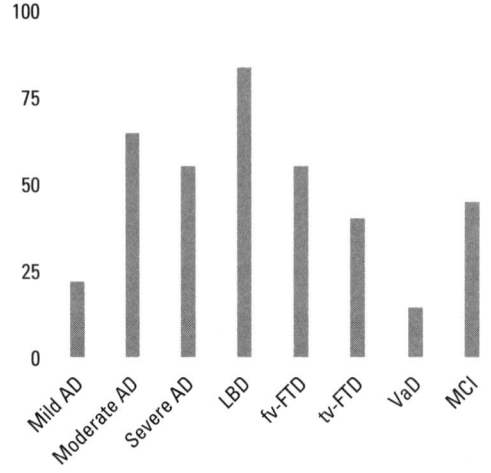

Figure 21.4 Prevalence of anxiety in major dementias and MCI. AD = alzheimer disease, LBD = Lewy body dementia, fv-FTD = frontal-variant frontotemporal dementia, tv-FTD = temporal variant FTD, VaD = vascular dementia, MCI = mild cognitive impairment.

comorbidity of anxiety with depression is high. Seventy-five percent of those who have dementia with anxiety also have depression (Starkstein, Jorge, Petracca, & Robinson, 2007). As dementia severity increases and insight deteriorates, overt anxiety becomes less prevalent (Chen, Borson, & Scanlan, 2000). Anxiety may then manifest as agitated behavior (Twelftree & Qazi, 2006). Anxiety can be a feature of all major dementia syndromes (Fig. 21.4), with some reports suggesting it is particularly common in early to moderate AD, Parkinson's disease dementia (PDD), and FTD (Aarsland et al., 2007).

Agitation, Impulsivity, and Obsessive-Compulsive Behaviors

Patients with dementia may manifest a wide range of disruptive behaviors. *Agitation* is an umbrella term that is usually defined to include motor or vocal behaviors that are disruptive or unsafe in a given environment (Rosen et al., 1994). This includes various combinations of irritability, restlessness, screaming, threatening behavior, aggressiveness, and even violence and crime. Patients with dementia may also manifest other forms of related impulsive and obsessive behaviors such as overeating, outbursts of frustration, excessive sentimentality, touching strangers, inappropriate sexual behavior, urinating in public, loss of social graces, and other changes in conduct. In FTD overeating or eating only certain foods may be present. During disease progression, the deterioration in judgment may lead to criminal behavior (such as shoplifting, indecent exposure, running stop lights) or impulsive buying. There may also be behaviors such as hoarding or repetitive rituals as seen in persons with obsessive-compulsive disorder. These changes can cause stress, frustration, and embarrassment to family and caregivers (Apostolova & Cummings, 2010).

These behaviors may occur in all the major dementias, including AD, VaD, mixed dementia, DLB, and FTD (Fig. 21.5), with some differences in the typical neuropsychiatric profile of each of these illnesses as discussed later. As many as 70% of persons with dementia manifest agitation during the course of their illness (Cohen-Mansfield, 1986). Physical injury to the patient or others may result. Agitation adversely impacts prognosis, is associated with an increase in the rate of cognitive decline, and reduces functional status. Agitated behaviors are a major precipitant of institutionalization and nursing home placement (Chen et al., 2000; D'Onofrio, 2012; Rabins, 1991).

The root causes of agitated behaviors may sometimes lie in other symptoms present in the dementia. Those who have agitation are more likely to have other neuropsychiatric symptoms (excluding apathy) (Deutsch, Bylsma, Rovner, Steele, & Folstein, 1991). The increased comorbidity of anxiety with agitation may suggest that anxiety is a contributing factor to agitation (Twelftree & Qazi, 2006). Depression may also be implicated, since 75% of those who meet criteria for dementia plus generalized anxiety disorder also fulfill diagnostic criteria for depression (Starkstein et al., 2007). Evidence points toward psychosis occurring more commonly in persons who have agitation. Furthermore, the root cause of agitated behaviors may lie in medical issues that are overlooked due to the inability of patients to fully appreciate and effectively communicate their problems. Physical discomfort and malaise due to illness may produce agitation. Infections, upper or lower gastrointestinal distress, musculoskeletal pain, headaches, neuropathic

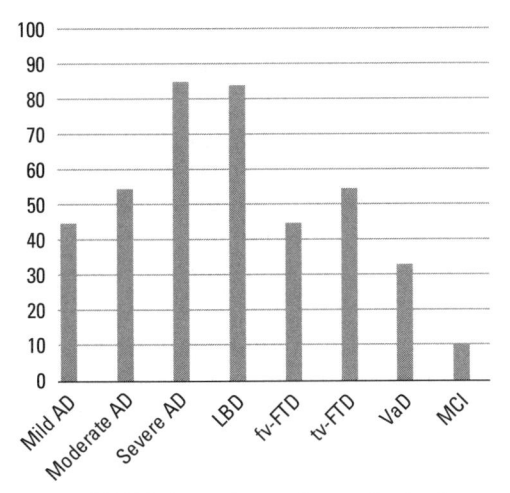

Figure 21.5 Estimated prevalence of agitation in the major neurodegenerative dementias and MCI. AD = alzheimer disease, LBD = Lewy body dementia, fv-FTD = frontal-variant frontotemporal dementia, tv-FTD = temporal variant FTD, VaD = vascular dementia, MCI = mild cognitive impairment.

pain, dystonia, medication side effects, and environmental factors may each produce agitation. Physical abuse may also result in agitated behavior.

Agitation represents a distinct and independent clinical syndrome in dementia (Senanarong et al., 2004). It is consistently found in association with increased dementia severity (Aries et al., 2010; Ballard et al., 1999). A variety of evidence supports that it is a manifestation of dysfunction in frontal cortical-subcortical circuits. Neuropsychological studies have shown an association between agitation and executive dysfunction, indicating that it might be viewed as another feature of frontal lobe dysfunction (Chen, Sultzer, Hinkin, Mahler, & Cummings, 1998). Functional imaging abnormalities in frontal lobe regions have been associated with symptoms of agitation (Hirono, Mega, Dinov, Mishkin, & Cummings, 2000; Sultzer et al., 1995). Pathological corroboration is found in the increased prevalence of neurofibrillary tangles occurring in these same areas in persons with AD who manifest agitation compared to their age-matched peers (Tekin et al., 2001).

Impairments in Insight, Judgment, and Complex Competencies

As a product of the neuropsychiatric and cognitive changes of dementia, insight, judgment, and complex reasoning are often subtly impaired during the early course of dementing illnesses. These may be present years before a clinical diagnosis is made (Sperling et al., 2011). Subtle changes occurring during early dementia may include diminished insight and concern (Starkstein, Jorge, Mizrahi, & Robinson, 2006), denial of illness, and reduced planning skills (Baddeley, Baddeley, Bucks, & Wilcock, 2001; Baudic et al., 2006; Johns et al., 2012; Leyhe, Saur, Eschweiler, & Milian, 2011). These changes may establish themselves at a stage when cognitive and behavioral abilities, and the ability to complete basic daily living activities appear grossly intact to families and health care providers. This may lead to the erroneous conclusion that complex decision-making abilities are entirely preserved (Carr, Ott, Noto, & Fogel, 2010; Tarawneh & Holtzman, 2012). This can have significant medical, financial, and legal consequences related to the patients and their families. Examples of complex competencies and social skills that can be impaired early in dementia are listed in Box 21.4. Clinicians must be prepared to assist patients and families in determining whether a patient with dementia has the capacity to make medical, legal, and financial decisions. Involving family members early during this process can be beneficial by allowing more time to make decisions. Advanced directives and a living

---

BOX 21.4 Complex Competencies That May Be Impaired Early On in the Early Course of a Dementing Illness

The ability to:

Respond to emergencies
Pilot or drive transportation vehicles
Make medical decisions
Manage complex medical treatments
Stand trial
Testify as a witness
Qualify as a juror
Handle firearms
Fulfil social and occupational roles
Engage in intimate, sexual relations
Resist undue influence over personal decisions
Execute a will and last testament

will promote the recognition and incorporation of the patients' wishes and values into their health care when they are no longer able to make these decisions for themselves. These documents may spare the family conflicts that can sometimes arise in such situations. As a general principle of care for the elderly, it is to the patient's and family's advantage for the health care provider to encourage the completion of estate planning before cognitive impairment occurs or progresses.

Sleep Disturbances

The prevalence of persistent sleep disturbances has been estimated to be 44% of patients with AD (Vitiello & Borson, 2001). Poor sleep hygiene is present in a relatively large proportion of the demented population, particularly in nursing homes (Bliwise, 2004). Circadian rhythm disturbances are a feature of dementias that can be particularly problematic during the period when daylight is lengthening (Hofman & Swaab, 2006). Damage to the suprachiasmatic hypothalamic nucleus, disturbance of melatonin secretion, optic nerve axonal degeneration, loss of retinal ganglion cells, and decreased exposure to environmental light may all be contributing factors (Ancoli-Israel et al., 2003; Blanks et al., 1996; Shochat, Martin, Marler, & Ancoli-Israel, 2000; Wu & Swaab, 2005).

Obstructive sleep apnea (OSA) is a well-known comorbidity of dementia that can potentially worsen cognition (Bedard, Montplaisir, Richer, Rouleau, & Malo, 1991; Redline et al., 2010; Young, Peppard, & Gottlieb, 2002). It also adversely impacts cardiovascular health and may increase the chance of stroke (Redline et al., 2010) and diabetes (Botros et al., 2009). Its effects on cognition may be mediated via chronic intermittent cerebral hypoxia and/or sleep deprivation with subsequent daytime sleepiness. Treatment, such as with continuous positive airway pressure (CPAP), may improve cognitive performance (Ferman et al., 2002). There is also a potential risk for irreversible executive dysfunction, most likely due to anoxic brain damage to frontal systems, highlighting the importance of early detection and treatment of OSA (Bedard et al., 1991).

REM sleep behavior disorder (RBD) occurs as a result of the loss of the normal skeletal muscle atonia during REM sleep, allowing physical enactment of dream activity. This can result in self-injury or injury to a sleeping partner. This condition is associated with neurodegenerative synucleinopathies, including Parkinson's disease (PD), DLB, and multiple system atrophy (MSA) (Boeve, Silber, & Ferman, 2003, 2004). In fact, evidence suggests that the presence of RBD may be an early manifestation of synucleinopathies, which appear to have selectivity for brain stem structures important in REM sleep regulation (Boeve et al., 2004). RBD may precede parkinsonism as may visual hallucinations in persons who later go on to develop DLB. Persons with dementia and RBD have cognitive profiles similar to those with DLB, demonstrating visuospatial and executive functional impairments in contrast to persons with AD who manifest more significant deficits in memory and language function (Boeve et al., 2004; Ferman et al., 2002).

Medications commonly used for treating dementia may also be associated with sleep disturbance. For example, the cholinesterase inhibitors, particularly donepezil, may cause insomnia in 10% of persons (Grossberg, Irwin, Satlin, Mesenbrink, & Spiegel, 2004). Galantamine and rivastigmine are less associated with this potentially troublesome side effect (Schnelle et al., 1998). Daytime dosing of the medication or switching to different members of the same class may be helpful in some cases. Antipsychotics may produce painful dystonia, akathisia and sleep disturbances.

Periodic limb movements of sleep tend to be elevated in patients with LBD and PD and may disrupt sleep architecture leading to daytime hypersomnolence (Hibi et al., 2012). Painful conditions, frequent urination due to prostatic hypertrophy or diuretic treatment of hypertension, urinary tract infections causing discomfort and polyuria, poorly regulated diabetes, consumption of caffeine or stimulants during the day or night, nighttime pill administration, and acquisition of vital signs at night may each contribute to sleep disruption.

Neuropsychiatric Symptom Profile of Main Dementia Subtypes

Alzheimer's Disease

The neuropsychiatric profile of AD encompasses the breadth of neuropsychiatric symptoms described in previous sections. These

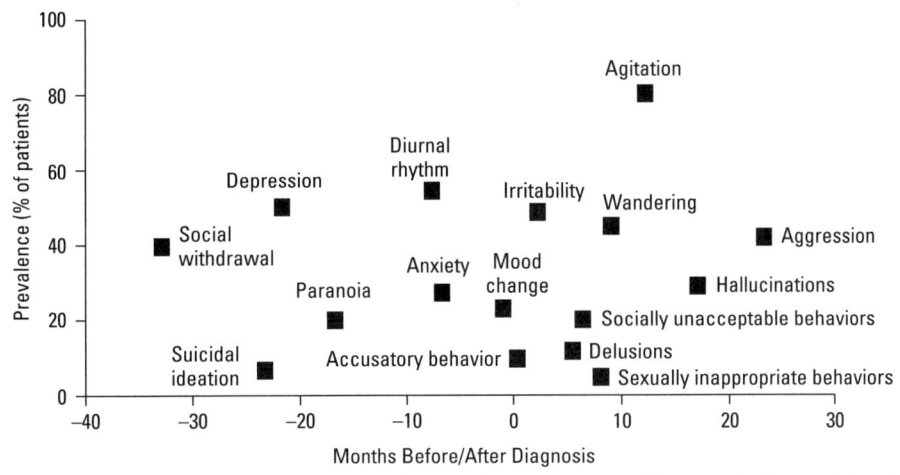

Figure 21.6 Neuropsychiatric profile depending on disease stage in Alzheimer's disease (Jost & Grossberg, 1996).

symptoms may occur at any point during the course of the illness, but certain features are more likely to appear in different disease stages (Fig. 21.6). Using the Neuropsychiatric Inventory (NPI), it has been found that up to 60% of patients with AD had at least one neuropsychiatric symptom at the time of presentation (Fig. 21.7). Apathy and depression are common early features. Apathy is present in 42% of mild AD, 80% of moderate AD, and 92% of advanced AD patients (Boyle et al., 2003; Mega et al., 1996). It is associated with a reduced quality of life. Depressive symptoms are present in about half of AD patients and are associated with diminished quality of life, functional impairment, aggression, and institutionalization as well as increased caregiver burden and depression (D'Onofrio, 2012; Hargrave, 2000; Rabins, 1991). Psychotic symptoms occur in 30% to 40% of AD patients during the course of the illness, typically in the middle to late stages (Mega et al., 1996; Wragg & Jeste, 1989). They are a common reason for early residential placement, institutionalization, increased levels of patient distress, and increased caregiver dissatisfaction (Steele, Rovner, Chase, & Folstein, 1990).

Delusions are rarely bizarre as in primary psychotic disorders. Common delusional themes include theft, infidelity, and delusional misidentification syndromes (Table 21.5). Hallucinations are less common, are typically visual, and tend to resolve over time (Marin et al., 1997). The occurrence of psychotic symptoms early in the disease course is not typical of AD and may be a clue to the diagnosis of DLB or FTD. Psychosis also occurs in the context of delirium, often driven by infections, medications, or toxic or metabolic factors. Hence, acute or subacute onset psychosis in a patient with dementia should prompt a thorough evaluation to rule out medical illness. Persons with dementia are more vulnerable to mental status changes due to illnesses, electrolyte derangements, baseline respiratory hypoxia, and medication side effects. They also recover more slowly than the cognitively normal population. Persons with AD usually have relatively intact social graces early during the disease. However, as many as 15% of AD

TABLE 21.5 Delusional Misidentification Syndromes (Apostolova and Cummings, 2010)

Capgras syndrome	Believing that familiar individuals are replaced by imposters
Fregoli syndrome	Believing strangers are familiar individuals
Foley's syndrome	Believing that images in the mirror are of other individuals or spirits
Autoscopy	Believing one's own body is a double
Doppelganger/Heautoscopy	Believing one has a double
Reduplicative paramnesia	Believing a familiar location is duplicated

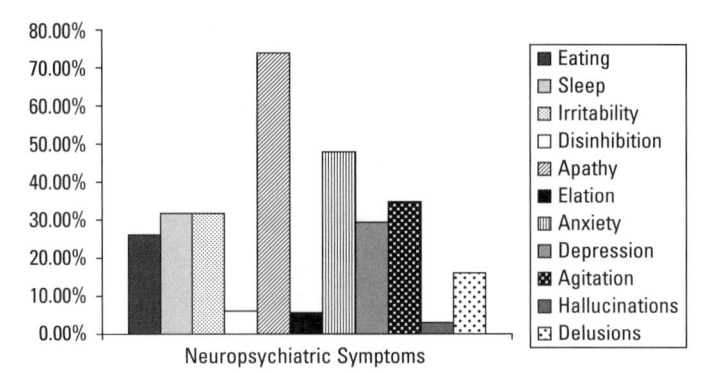

Figure 21.7 Relative prevalence of various neuropsychiatric symptoms in AD (Aarsland et al., 2007; Ballard et al., 1999; Geda & Roberts, 2008; Liu et al., 2004; Lyketsos et al., 2000; Mega et al., 1996).

patients have a frontal variant wherein they present with difficulties attributable to the frontal circuits rather than an amnesic syndrome (Balasa et al., 2011). Nonetheless, early impairment in social comportment and disinhibition should prompt consideration of other possible causes such as conditions that primarily affect the frontal lobe.

Frontotemporal Dementias

Our focus here will be on bvFTD, as opposed to the aphasic forms of FTD, in which neuropsychiatric symptoms are the sine qua non (see Chapter 2). These same features may also occur in the other FTD subtypes (Modirrousta, Price, & Dickerson, 2013). The presenting manifestation is often a personality change marked by disinhibition, impulsivity, loss of social comportment, apathy, and impairment in judgment and insight. The behavioral symptoms can be attributed to regions where the degenerative process has taken its earliest toll, in the frontal and temporal lobes. Orbitofrontal cortical dysfunction is more associated with disinhibition and impulsivity, while mesial frontal dysfunction is more associated with apathy and abulia. Patients with FTD may show obsessive-compulsive behaviors, hoarding behaviors, hyperorality, and complex ritualistic behaviors (Bathgate, Snowden, Varma, Blackshaw, & Neary, 2001; Mendez et al., 2008). Depressive symptoms in FTD have received relatively little systematic investigation and may be confused on the part of caregivers with apathy, but they may occur in as many as 30% to 40% of patients. Inappropriate sexual behaviors, agitation, delusions, and hallucinations can be seen in both early and late phases during the course of FTD (Liu et al., 2004).

Lewy Body Dementia

The neuropsychiatric profile can often be helpful for distinguishing DLB from other dementias (see Chapter 12). Visual hallucinations are common in DLB, occurring in up to 80% of those affected at some point during the course of the illness. These may be early features. More than 90% of patients who have visual hallucinations coupled with a mild dementia will be found to have DLB rather than other types of dementia. In one series, visual hallucinations were seen at onset in 65% of pathologically proven DLB, compared to only 25% in AD patients. Visual hallucinations in DLB are typically well formed and complex, and more commonly involve animate rather than inanimate objects (Ballard et al., 1996). Multimodal hallucinations occur and can be a distinguishing feature compared to AD, where they occur rarely. Auditory hallucinations occur in up to 25%, olfactory hallucinations in 5% to 10% of patients, and tactile hallucinations in up to 3% (Ballard et al., 1999; Simard et al., 2000). Delusions occur in 50% of cases and revolve around themes similar to those seen in AD (Ballard et al., 1999).

REM sleep behavior disorder is a neuropsychiatric feature that may precede the onset of extrapyramidal, cognitive, and even psychotic symptoms in up to 80% of patients with DLB (Bedard et al., 1991). Hence, its presence may herald the condition, with a positive predictive value of 92% (Wu & Swaab, 2005). Depression and anxiety are also common in DLB. The prevalence of depression in DLB is about 30% (Ballard et al., 1999). The depressed cognitively impaired patient is much more likely to have DLB than AD (Papka, Rubio, Schiffer, & Cox, 1998). Anxiety is reported in 84% of patients (Ballard et al., 1999). Although treatment issues will be discussed in further chapters, it is worth mentioning that the diagnosis of DLB has special implications for treatment of psychiatric symptoms since these patients are exquisitely sensitive to typical and atypical neuroleptics. Clozapine is the only neuroleptic that can be safely recommended for use when one is needed.

Vascular Dementias

Psychomotor slowing is often a prominent feature of vascular dementia, particularly multi-infarct dementia, with a heavy vascular disease burden in the subcortical white matter (see Chapter 13). Cognitive deficits frequently include memory retrieval, and attentional and processing speed difficulties (Schmidtke & Hull, 2002). Depression and aggression, followed by apathy, irritability, and anxiety, are commonly seen. Delusions, hallucinations, disinhibition, aberrant motor behavior, and euphoria may occur, but they are less frequent than in other dementias (Lyketsos et al., 2000).

Strategic-infarct dementia occurs when the vascular insult affects a crucial hub in cognitive and neuropsychiatric circuitry. Examples include various thalamic vascular syndromes that each have different neuropsychiatric profiles. Personality changes, apathy, and abulia are seen in the tuberothalamic artery syndrome, which involves the reticular, intralaminar, ventral anterior, rostral ventrolateral, mediodorsal, and anterior thalamic nuclei. Altered social skills, apathy, aggression, and agitation are seen in the paramedian artery thalamic syndrome, which involves the ventral internal medullary lamina, ventral amygdalofugal pathway, and mamillothalamic tract.

Poststroke dementia is another presentation of vascular dementia that is associated with neuropsychiatric symptoms related to the location of the stroke. There is a high positive association between the incidence of depression in stroke and the lesion's closer proximity to the frontal pole or its involvement of the caudate nucleus (Schmahmann, 2003), whereas mania tends to have more of an association with strokes involving right-sided basal frontotemporal regions (Starkstein et al., 1990).

Awareness, Assessment, and Intervention: General Principles

Clinicians evaluating dementia patients should routinely and regularly screen for neuropsychiatric symptoms. Initial evaluations should establish a baseline to facilitate early detection of subtle behavioral alterations and accurate monitoring of changes in preexisting ones. This is important since neuropsychiatric manifestations can change throughout the course of the illness, and they may fluctuate with medication changes, stress, or changes in the patient's living arrangements. The practitioner should educate the patient, family, and significant others about neuropsychiatric symptoms so as to improve recognition. Their observations can be vital to understanding the cause of the symptoms and to selecting the best management options (Rabins et al., 2007).

Measurement scales are important for research purposes but can also be useful in the clinic to monitor behavioral changes. Some scales focus on the assessment of a single neuropsychiatric feature, whereas others rate a number of them together. The BEHAVE-AD (Reisberg, Auer, & Monteiro, 1996) is an example of a multisymptom rating scale and is considered by some to be the gold standard. The NPI (Cummings et al., 1994), validated against BEHAVE-AD, may be easier to use within the time constraints of a clinic evaluation. Other assessment scales focus on quantifying single symptoms (see Table 21.6 for examples) and may be useful alone or in combination with a multisymptom tool.

Regular clinical assessment allows for timely implementation of intervention strategies to improve the quality of life for patients and their caregivers (see Chapters 24–26). Management strategies include pharmacological and therapeutic interventions as well as alterations in the patient's living environment. Cholinesterase inhibitors, memantine, antidepressants, anxiolytics, neuroleptics,

TABLE 21.6 Some Measurement Tools of Single-Domain Neuropsychiatric in Dementia

Symptom	Tool
Depression	The Geriatric Depression Scale (Lesher & Berryhill, 1994)
	Cornell Scale for Depression (Alexopoulos, Abrams, Young, & Shamoian, 1988)
	Dementia Mood Assessment Scale (Sunderland & Minichiello, 1997)
Agitation	Cohen-Mansfield Agitation Inventory
Apathy	Apathy Evaluation Inventory (Robert et al., 2002)
Anxiety	Worry Scale (LaBarge, 1993)
	Hospital Anxiety and Depression Scale (HADS) (Bjelland, Dahl, Haug, & Neckelmann, 2002)
	Rating of Anxiety in Dementia (RAID) (Shanka, Walker, Frost, & Orrell, 1999)

and stimulants are among the medication classes that may be helpful in managing neuropsychiatric symptoms in dementia. Electroconvulsive therapy may have a role in carefully selected cases.

Conclusion

Neuropsychiatric symptoms frequently occur during the course of dementing illnesses as a result of dysfunction in neural networks subserving mood, affect, perception, and thought processes. These features may herald the onset of the dementia and also are seen in all stages of dementia. Different dementing processes have different neuropsychiatric symptom profiles, which can aid in the differential diagnosis and have therapeutic implications. Neuropsychiatric symptoms may have an adverse impact on the quality of life and well-being of patients as well as their caregivers. Impairment of insight and judgment can lead to financial, medical, and testamentary decision-making impairments. Early recognition of neuropsychiatric changes is a crucial step towards instituting timely social and medical interventions.

References

Aarsland, D., Brønnick, K., Ehrt, U., De Deyn, P., Tekin, S., Emre, M., & Cummings, J. L. (2007). Neuropsychiatric symptoms in patients with Parkinson's disease and dementia: Frequency, profile and associated care giver stress. *Journal of Neurology, Neurosurgery and Psychiatry, 78*(1), 36–42.

Akiyama, H., Hashimoto, H., Kawabe, J., Higashiyama, S., Kai, T., Kataoka, K.,... Kiriike, N. (2008). The relationship between depressive symptoms and prefrontal hypoperfusion demonstrated by eZIS in patients with DAT. *Neuroscience Letters, 441*, 328–331.

Alexopoulos, G., Abrams, R., Young, R., & Shamoian, C. (1988). Cornell Scale for Depression in Dementia. *Biological Psychiatry, 23*(3), 271–284.

Alzheimer, A., Stelzmann, R., Schnitzlein, H., & Murtagh, F. (1995). An English translation of Alzheimer's 1907 paper, "Uber eine eigenartige Erkankung der Hirnrinde. *Clincial Anatomy, 8*(6), 429–431.

Ancoli-Israel, S., Gehrman, P., Martin, J., Shochat, T., Marler, M., Corey-Bloom, J., & Levi, L. (2003). Increased light exposure consolidates sleep and strengthens circadian rhythms in severe Alzheimer's disease patients. *Behavioral Sleep Medicine, 1*(1), 22–36.

Apostolova, L., & Cummings, J. (2008). Neuropsychiatric manifestations in mild cognitive impairment: A systematic review of the literature. *Dementia and Geriatric Cognitive Disorders, 25*(2), 115–126.

Apostolova, L., & Cummings, J. (2010). Neuropsychiatric aspects of Alzheimer's disease and other dementing illnesses. In S. C. Yudofsky (Ed.), Essentials of neuropsychiatry and behavioral neurosciences (2nd ed., pp 409). Washington, DC: American Psychiatric Publishing.

Apostolova, L. A., Akopyan, G. G., Partiali, N., Steiner, C. A., Dutton, R. A., Hayashi, K. M.,...Thompson, P. M. (2007). Structural correlates of apathy in Alzheimer's disease. *Dementia and Geriatric Cognitive Disorders, 24*(2), 91–97.

Aries, M., Le Bastard, N., Debruyne, H., Van Buggenhout, M., Nagels, G., De Deyn, P., & Engelborghs, S. (2010). Relation between frontal lobe symptoms and dementia severity within and across diagnostic dementia categories. *International Journal of Geriatric Psychiatry, 25*(11), 1186–1195.

Baddeley, A., Baddeley, H., Bucks, R., & Wilcock, G. (2001). Attentional control in Alzheimer's disease. *Brain, 124*(Pt 8), 1492–1508.

Balasa, M., Gelpi, E., Antonell, A., Rey, M. J., Sánchez-Valle, R., Molinuevo, J. L., & Lladó, A. (2011). Clinical features and APOE genotype of pathologically proven early-onset Alzheimer disease. *Neurology*, 76(20), 1720–1725.

Ballard, C., Boyle, A., Bowler, C., & Lindesay, J. (1996). Anxiety disorders in dementia sufferers. *International Journal of Geriatric Psychiatry*, 11(11), 987–990.

Ballard, C., Holmes, C., McKeith, I., Neill, D., O'Brien, J., Cairns, N.,...Perry, R. (1999). Psychiatric morbidity in dementia with Lewy bodies: A prospective clinical and neuropathological comparative study with Alzheimer's disease. *American Journal of Psychiatry*, 156(7), 1039–1045.

Ballard, C., Margallo-Lana, M., Fossey, J., Reichelt, K., Myint, P., Potkins, D., & O'Brien, J. (2001). A 1-year follow-up study of behavioral and psychological symptoms in dementia among people in care environments. *Journal of Clinical Psychiatry*, 62(8), 631–636.

Ballard, C., Neill, D., O'Brien, J., McKeith, I., Ince, P., & Perry, R. (2000). Anxiety, depression and psychosis in vascular dementia: Prevalence and associations. *Journal of Affective Disorders*, 59(2), 97–106.

Bathgate, D., Snowden, J., Varma, A., Blackshaw, A., & Neary, D. (2001). Behaviour in frontotemporal dementia, Alzheimer's disease and vascular dementia. *Acta Neurologica Scandinavica*, 103(6), 367–378.

Baudic, S., Barba, G., Thibaudet, M., Smagghe, A., Remy, P., & Traykov, L. (2006). Executive function deficits in early Alzheimer's disease and their relations with episodic memory. *Archives of Clinical Neuropsychology*, 21(1), 15–21.

Bedard, M., Montplaisir, J., Richer, F., Rouleau, I., & Malo, J (1991). Obstructive sleep apnea syndrome: Pathogenesis of neuropsychological deficits. *Journal of Clinical and Experimental Neuropsychology*, 13(6), 950–964.

Benoit, M., Dygai, I., Migneco, O., Robert, P. H., Bertogliati, C., Darcourt, J.,...Prinquey, D. (1999). Behavioral and psychological symptoms in Alzheimer's disease. Relation between apathy and regional cerebral perfusion. *Dementia and Geriatric Cognitive Disorders*, 10(6), 511–517.

Benoit, M., Koulibaly, P. M., Migneco, O., Darcourt, J., Pringuey, D. J., & Robert, P. H. (2002). Brain perfusion in Alzheimer's disease with and without apathy: A SPECT study with statistical parametric mapping analysis. *Psychiatric Research*, 114(2), 103–111.

Berrios, G. (1982). Tactile hallucinations: Conceptual and historical aspects. *Journal of Neurology, Neurosurgery and Psychiatry*, 45(4), 285–293.

Bjelland, I., Dahl, A., Haug, T., & Neckelmann, D. (2002). The validity of the Hospital Anxiety and Depression Scale - An updated literature review. *Journal of Psychosomatic Research*, 52(2), 69–77.

Blanks, J., Schmidt, S., Torigoe, Y., Porrello, K., Hinton, D., & Blanks, R. (1996). Retinal pathology in Alzheimer's disease. II. Regional neuron loss and glial changes in GCL. *Neurobiology of Aging*, 17(3), 385–395.

Bliwise, D. (2004). Sleep disorders in Alzheimer's disease and other dementias. *Clinical Cornerstone*, 6(28), S16–S28.

Boeve, B., Silber, M., & Ferman, T. (2003). Melatonin for treatment of REM sleep behavior disorder in neurologic disorders: Results in 14 patients. *Sleep Medicine*, 4(4), 281–284.

Boeve, B., Silber, M., & Ferman, T. (2004). REM sleep behavior disorder in Parkinson's disease and dementia with Lewy bodies. *Journal of Geriatric Psychiatry and Neurology*, 17(3), 146–157.

Botros, N., Concato, J., Mohsenin, V., Selim, B., Doctor, K., & Yaggi, H. (2009). Obstructive sleep apnea as a risk factor for type 2 diabetes. *American Journal of Medicine*, 122(12), 1122–1127.

Boyle, P., Malloy, P., Salloway, S., Cahn-Weiner, D., Cohen, R., & Cummings, J. (2003). Executive dysfunction and apathy predict functional impairment in Alzheimer disease. *American Journal of Geriatric Psychiatry*, 11(2), 214–221.

Bruen, P., McGeown, W., Shanks, M., & Venneri, A. (2008). Neuroanatomical correlates of neuropsychiatric symptoms in Alzheimer's disease. *Brain*, 131(Pt 9), 2455–2463.

Butters, M., Klunk,W. E., Mathis, C. A., Price, J. C., Ziolko, S. K., Hoge, J. A.,...Meltzer, C. C. (2008). Imaging Alzheimer pathology in late-life depression with PET and Pittsburgh Compound-B. *Alzheimers Disease and Associated Disorders*, 22(3), 261–268.

Callahan, C. M., Boustani, M. A., Unverzagt, F. W., Austrom, M. G., Damush, T. M., Perkins, A. J.,...Hendrie, H. C. (2006). Effectiveness of collaborative care for older adults with Alzheimer disease in primary care: A randomized controlled trial. *Journal of the American Medical Association*, 295(18), 2148–2157.

Carr, D., Ott, B., Noto, R., & Fogel, B. (2010). The older adult driver with cognitive impairment: "It's a very frustrating life". *Journal of the American Medical Association*, 303(16), 1632–1641.

Chemerinski, E., Petracca, G., Sabe, L., Kremer, J., & Starkstein, S. E. (2001). The specificity of depressive symptoms in patients with Alzheimer's disease. *American Journal of Psychiatry*, 158(1), 68–72.

Chen, J., Borson, S., & Scanlan, J. (2000). Stage-specific prevalence of behavioral symptoms in Alzheimer's disease in a multi-ethnic community sample. *American Journal of Geriatric Psychiatry, 8*(2), 123–133.

Chen, S., Sultzer, D., Hinkin, C., Mahler, M., & Cummings, J. (1998). Executive dysfunction in Alzheimer's disease: Association with neuropsychiatric symptoms and functional impairment. *Journal of Neuropsychiatry and Clinical Neuroscience, 10*(4), 426–432.

Cohen-Mansfield, J. (1986). Agitated behaviors in the elderly. II. Preliminary results in the cognitively deteriorated. *Journal of the American Geriatric Society, 34*(10), 722–727.

Craig, A. H., Cummings, J. L., Fairbanks, L., Itti, L., Miller, B. L., Li, J., & Mena, I. (1996). Cerebral blood flow correlates of apathy in Alzheimer disease. *Archives of Neurology, 53*(11), 1116–1120.

Cummings, J., Mega, M., Gray, K., Rosenberg-Thompson, S., Carusi, D., & Gornbein, J. (1994). The Neuropsychiatric Inventory. *Neurology, 44*(12), 2308.

D'Onofrio, G., Sancarlo, D., Panza, F., Copetti, M., Cascavilla, L., Paris, F.,...Pilotto, A. (2012). Neuropsychiatric symptoms and functional status in Alzheimer's disease and vascular dementia patients. *Current Alzheimer Research, 9*(6), 759–771.

de Beurs, E., Beekman, A., van Balkom, A., Deeg, D., van Dyck, R., & van Tilburg, W. (1999). Consequences of anxiety in older persons: Its effect on disability, well-being and use of health services. *Psychological Medicine, 29*(3), 583–593.

Deutsch, L., Bylsma, F., Rovner, B., Steele, C., & Folstein, M. (1991). Psychosis and physical aggression in probable Alzheimer's disease. *American Journal of Psychiatry, 148*(9), 1159–1163.

Devanand, D., Jacobs, D. M., Tang, M. X., Del Castillo-Castaneda, C., Sano, M., Marder, K.,...Stern, Y. (1997). The course of psychopathologic features in mild to moderate Alzheimer disease. *Archives of General Psychiatry, 54*(3), 257–263

Devanand, D. P., Sano, M., Tang, M. X., Taylor, S., Gurland, B., Wilder, D.,...Mayeux, R. (1996). Depressed mood and the incidence of Alzheimer's disease in the elderly living in the community. *Archives of General Psychiatry, 53*, 175–182.

Ferman, T., Boeve, B., Smith, G., Silber, M., Lucas, J., Graff-Radford, N.,...Ivnik, R. J. (2002). Dementia with Lewy bodies may present as dementia and REM sleep behavior disorder without Parkinsonism or hallucinations. *Journal of the International Neuropsychological Society, 8*(7), 907–914.

Flynn, F., Cummings, J., & Gornbein, J. (1991). Delusions in dementia syndromes: Investigation of behavioral and neuropsychological correlates. *Journal of Neuropsychiatry and Clinical Neuroscience, 3*(4), 364–370.

Galynker, I., Dutta, E., Vilkas, N., Ongseng, F., Finestone, H., Gallagher, R.,...Rosenthal, R. N. (2000) Hypofrontality and negative symptoms in patients with dementia of Alzheimer type. *Neuropsychiatry Neuropsychology and Behavioral Neurology, 13*(1), 53–59.

Geda, Y., & Roberts, R. (2008). Prevalence of neuropsychiatric symptoms in mild cognitive impairment and normal cognitive aging: Population-based study. *Archives of General Psychiatry, 65*(10), 1193–1198.

Geda, Y. E. (2010). Blowing hot and cold over depression and cognitive impairment. *Neurology, 75*, 12–14.

Grossberg, G., Irwin, P., Satlin, A., Mesenbrink, P., & Spiegel, R. (2004). Rivastigmine in Alzheimer disease: Efficacy over two years. *American Journal of Geriatric Psychiatry, 12*(4), 420–431.

Hargrave, R., Reed, B., & Mungas, D. (2000). Depressive syndromes and functional disability in dementia. *Journal of Geriatric Psychiatry and Neurology, 13*(2), 72–77.

Hibi, S., Yamaguchi, Y., Umeda-Kameyama, Y., Yamamoto, H., Iijima, K., Momose, T., Akishita, M., & Ouchi Y. (2012). The high frequency of periodic limb movements in patients with Lewy body dementia. *Journal of Psychiatric Research, 46*(12), 1590–1594.

Hirono, N., Mega, M., Dinov, I., Mishkin, F., & Cummings, J. (2000). Left frontotemporal hypoperfusion is associated with aggression in patients with dementia. *Archives of Neurology, 57*(6), 861–866.

Hofman, M., & Swaab, D. (2006). Living by the clock: The circadian pacemaker in older people. *Ageing Research Reviews, 5*(1), 33–51.

Janzing, J., Teunisse, R., Bouwens, P., van 't. Hof, M., & Zitman, F. (2000). The course of depression in elderly subjects with and without dementia. *Journal of Affective Disorders, 57*(1-3), 49–54.

Jeste, D., & Finkel, S. (2000). Psychosis of Alzheimer's disease and related dementias. Diagnostic criteria for a distinct syndrome. *American Journal of Geriatric Psychiatry, 8*(1), 29–34.

Johns, E., Phillips, N., Belleville, S., Goupil, D., Babins, L., Kelner, N.,...Chertkow, H. (2012). The profile of executive functioning in amnestic mild cognitive impairment: Disproportionate deficits in inhibitory control. *Journal of the International Neuropsychological Society, 18*(3), 541–555.

Jost, B., & Grossberg, G. (1996). The evolution of psychiatric symptoms in Alzheimer's disease: A natural history study. *Journal of the American Geriatric Society, 44*(9), 1078–1081.

LaBarge, E. (1993). A preliminary scale to measure the degree of worry among mildly demented Alzheimer disease patients. *Physical and Occupationa Therapy in Geriatrics, 11*(3), 43–57.

Lanctot, K., Moosa, S., Herrmann, N., Leibovitch, F., Rothenburg, L., Cotter, A.,...Black, S. E. (2007). A SPECT study of apathy in Alzheimer's disease. *Dementia and Geriatric Cognitive Disorders, 24*(1), 65–72.

Landes, A., Sperry, S., & Strauss, M. (2005). Prevalence of apathy, dysphoria, and depression in relation to dementia severity in Alzheimer's disease. *Journal of Neuropsychiatry and Clinical Neuroscience, 17*(3), 342–349.

Landes, A. S., Sperry, S. D., Strauss, M. E., & Geldmacher, D. S. (2001). Apathy in Alzheimer's disease. *Journal of the American Geriatrics Society, 49*(12), 1700–1707.

Lechowski, L., Benoit, M., Chassagne, P., Vedel, I., Tortrat, D., Teillet, L., & Vellas, B. (2009). Persistent apathy in Alzheimer's disease as an independent factor of rapid functional decline: The REAL longitudinal cohort study. *International Journal of Geriatric Psychiatry, 24*, 341–346.

Lesher, E., & Berryhill, J. (1994). Validation of the geriatric depression scale--short form among inpatients. *Journal of Clinical Psychology, 50*(2), 256–260.

Levy, M., Cummings, J., Fairbanks, L., Bravi, D., Calvani, M., & Carta, A. (1996). Longitudinal assessment of symptoms of depression, agitation, and psychosis in 181 patients with Alzheimer's disease. *American Journal of Psychiatry, 153*(11), 1438–1443.

Levy, M., Cummings, J., Fairbanks, L., Masterman, D., Miller, B., Craig, A.,...Litvan, I. (1998). Apathy is not depression. *Journal of Neuropsychiatry and Clinical Neuroscience, 10*(3), 314–319.

Levy-Cooperman, N., Burhan, A., Rafi-Tari, S., Kusano, M., Ramirez, J., Caldwell, C., & Black, S. E. (2008). Frontal lobe hypoperfusion and depressive symptoms in Alzheimer disease. *Journal of Psychiatry and Neuroscience, 33*(3), 218–226.

Leyhe, T., Saur, R., Eschweiler, G., & Milian, M. (2011). Impairment in proverb interpretation as an executive function deficit in patients with amnestic mild cognitive impairment and early Alzheimer's disease. *Dementia and Geriatric Cognitive Disorders Extra, 1*(1), 51–61.

Liao, Y. C., Liu, R. S., Lee, Y. C., Sun, C. M., Liu, C. Y., Wang, P. S., & Liu, H. C. (2003). Selective hypoperfusion of anterior cingulate gyrus in depressed AD patients: A brain SPECT finding by statistical parametric mapping. *Dementia and Geriatric Cognitive Disorders, 16*(4), 238–244.

Liu, W., Miller, B., Kramer, J., Rankin, K., Wyss-Coray, C., Gearhart, R.,...Rosen, H. J. (2004). Behavioral disorders in the frontal and temporal variants of frontotemporal dementia. *Neurology, 62*(5), 742–748.

Lopez, O., Becker, J., Brenner, R., Rosen, J., Bajulaiye, O., & Reynolds, C. (1991). Alzheimer's disease with delusions and hallucinations: Neuropsychological and electroencephalographic correlates. *Neurology, 41*(6), 906–912.

Lyketsos, C., Steinberg, M., Tschanz, J., Norton, M., Steffens, D., & Breitner, J. (2000). Mental and behavioral disturbances in dementia: Findings from the Cache County Study on Memory in Aging. *American Journal of Psychiatry, 157*(5), 708–714.

Lyketsos, C. G., Lopez, O., Jones, B., Fitzpatrick, A. L., Breitner, J., & DeKosky, S. (2002). Prevalence of neuropsychiatric symptoms in dementia and mild cognitive impairment: Results from the cardiovascular health study. *Journal of the American Medical Association, 288*, 1475–1483.

Marin, D., Green, C., Schmeidler, J., Harvey, P., Lawlor, B., Ryan, T.,...Mohs, R. C. (1997). Noncognitive disturbances in Alzheimer's disease: Frequency, longitudinal course, and relationship to cognitive symptoms. *Journal of the American Geriatric Society, 45*(11), 1331–1338.

Marin, R. (1990). Differential diagnosis and classification of apathy. *American Journal of Psychiatry, 147*(1), 22–30.

Marshall, G., Fairbanks, L., Tekin, S., Vinters, H., & Cummings, J. (2006). Neuropathologic correlates of apathy in Alzheimer's disease. *Dementia and Geriatric Cognitive Disorders, 21*(3), 144–147.

Marshall, G., Monserratt, L., Harwood, D., Mandelkern, M., Cummings, J., & Sultzer, D. (2007). Positron emission tomography metabolic correlates of apathy in Alzheimer disease. *Archives of Neurology, 64*(7), 1015–1020.

Mega, M., Cummings, J., Fiorello, T., & Gornbein, J. (1996). The spectrum of behavioral changes in Alzheimer's disease. *Neurology, 46*(1), 130–135.

Mendez, M., Lauterbach, E., & Sampson, S. (2008). An evidence-based review of the psychopathology of frontotemporal dementia: A report of the ANPA Committee on Research. *Journal of Neuropsychiatry and Clinical Neuroscience, 20*(2), 130–149.

Migneco, O., Benoit, M., Koulibaly, P. M., Dygai, I., BertogliatI, C., Desvignes, P.,...Darcourt, J. (2001). Perfusion brain SPECT and statistical parametric mapping analysis indicate that apathy is a cingulate syndrome: A study in Alzheimer's disease and nondemented patients. *Neuroimage, 13*(5), 896–902.

Modirrousta, M., Price, B. H., & Dickerson, B. C. (2013) Neuropsychiatric symptoms in primary progressive aphasia: Phenomenology, pathophysiology, and approach to assessment and treatment. *Neurodegenerative Disease Management, 3*(2), 133–146.

Olin, J., Schneider, L. S., Katz, I. R., Meyers, B. S., Alexopoulos, G. S., Breitner, J. C., ... Lebowitz, B. D. (2002). Provisional diagnostic criteria for depression of Alzheimer disease. *American Journal of Geriatric Psychiatry, 10*(2), 125–128.

Ott, B. R., Noto, R. B., & Fogel, B. S. (1996). Apathy and loss of insight in Alzheimer's disease: A SPECT imaging study. *Journal of Neuropsychiatry and Clinical Neuroscience, 8*(1), 41–46.

Papka, M., Rubio, A., Schiffer, R., & Cox, C. (1998). Lewy body disease: Can we diagnose it?. *Journal of Neuropsychiatry and Clinical Neuroscience, 10*(4), 405–412.

Rabins, P., Blacker, D., Rovner, B., Rummans, T., Schneider, L., Tariot, P., ... Fochtmann, L. J. (2007). American Psychiatric Association practice guideline for the treatment of patients with Alzheimer's disease and other dementias, second edition. *American Journal of Psychiatry, 164*(12 Suppl), 5–56.

Rabins, P. V., & Nicholson, M. (1991). Acute psychiatric hospitalization for patients with irreversible dementia. *International Journal of Geriatric Psychiatry, 6*(4), 209–211.

Redline, S., Yenokyan, G., Gottlieb, D., Shahar, E., O'Connor, G., Resnick, H., ... Punjabi, N. M. (2010). Obstructive sleep apnea-hypopnea and incident stroke: The sleep heart health study. *American Journal of Respiratory Critical Care Medicine, 182*(2), 269–277.

Reisberg, B., Auer, S., & Monteiro, I. (1996). Behavioral pathology in Alzheimer's disease (BEHAVE-AD) rating scale. *International Psychogeriatrics, 3*, 301–308.

Robert, P., Berr, C., Volteau, M., Bertogliati, C., Benoit, M., Sarazin, M., ... Dubois, B. (2006). Apathy in patients with mild cognitive impairment and the risk of developing dementia of Alzheimer's disease: A one-year follow-up study. *Clinical Neurology and Neurosurgery, 108*(8), 733–736.

Robert, P., Clairet, S., Benoit, M., Koutaich, J., Bertogliati, C., Tible, O., ... Bedoucha, P. (2002). The apathy inventory: Assessment of apathy and awareness in Alzheimer's disease, Parkinson's disease and mild cognitive impairment. *International Journal of Geriatric Psychiatry, 17*(12), 1099–1105.

Robert, P., Onyike, C., Leentjens, A., Dujardin, K., Aalten, P., Starkstein, S., ... Byrne, J. (2009). Proposed diagnostic criteria for apathy in Alzheimer's disease and other neuropsychiatric disorders. *European Psychiatry, 24*(2), 98–104.

Robert, P. H., Darcourt, G., Koulibaly, M. P., Clairet, S., Benoit, M., Garcia, R., ... Darcourt, J. (2006). Lack of initiative and interest in Alzheimer's disease: A single photon emission computed tomography study. *European Journal of Neurology, 13*(7), 729–735.

Rockwell, E., Krull, A., Dimsdale, J., & Jeste, D. (1994). Late-onset psychosis with somatic delusions. *Psychosomatics, 35*(1), 66–72.

Rosen, J., Burgio, L., Kollar, M., Cain, M., Allison, M., Fogleman, M., ... Zubenko, G. S. (1994). The Pittsburgh Agitation Scale: A user-friendly instrument for rating agitation in dementia patients. *American Journal of Geriatric Psychiatry, 2*, 52–59.

Schmahmann, J. (2003). Vascular syndromes of the thalamus. *Stroke, 34*(9), 2264–2278.

Schmidtke, K., & Hull, M. (2002). Neuropsychological differentiation of small vessel disease, Alzheimer's disease and mixed dementia. *Journal of Neurological Sciences, 204*, 17–22.

Schneider, J., Murray, J., Banerjee, S., & Mann, A. (1999). EUROCARE: A cross-national study of co-resident spouse carers for people with Alzheimer's disease: I--Factors associated with carer burden. *International Journal of Geriatric Psychiatry, 14*, 651–661.

Schnelle, J., Cruise, P. A., Alessi, C. A., Ludlow, K., al-Samarrai, N. R., & Ouslander, J. G. (1998). Sleep hygiene in physically dependent nursing home residents: Behavioral and environmental intervention implications. *Sleep, 21*(5), 515–523.

Senanarong, V., Cummings, J., Fairbanks, L., Mega, M., Masterman, D., O'Connor, S., & Strickland, T. L. (2004). Agitation in Alzheimer's disease is a manifestation of frontal lobe dysfunction. *Dementia and Geriatric Cognitive Disorders, 17*(1-2), 14–20.

Shanka, K., Walker, M., Frost, D., & Orrell, M. (1999). The development of a valid and reliable scale for rating anxiety in dementia (RAID). *Aging and Mental Health, 3*(1), 39–49.

Shochat, T., Martin, J., Marler, M., & Ancoli-Israel, S. (2000). Illumination levels in nursing home patients: Effects on sleep and activity rhythms. *Journal of Sleep Research, 9*(4), 373–379.

Simard, M., van Reekum, R., & Cohen, T. (2000). A review of the cognitive and behavioral symptoms in dementia with Lewy bodies. *Journal of Neuropsychiatry and Clinical Neuroscience, 12*(4), 425–450.

Skogseth, R., Mulugeta, E., Jones, E., Ballard, C., Rongve, A., Nore, S., ... Aarsland, D. (2008). Neuropsychiatric correlates of cerebrospinal fluid biomarkers in Alzheimer's disease. *Dementia and Geriatric Cognitive Disorders*, 25(6), 559–563.

Sperling, R., Aisen, P., Beckett, L., Bennett, D., Craft, S., Fagan, A., ... Phelps, C. H. (2011). Toward defining the preclinical stages of Alzheimer's disease: Recommendations from the National Institute on Aging-Alzheimer's Association workgroups on diagnostic guidelines for Alzheimer's disease. *Alzheimers and Dementia*, 7(3), 280–292.

Starkstein, S., Chemerinski, E., Sabe, L., Kuzis, G., Petracca, G., Teson, A., ... Leiguarda, R. (1997). Prospective longitudinal study of depression and anosognosia in Alzheimer's disease. *British Journal of Psychiatry*, 171, 47–52.

Starkstein, S., Jorge, R., Petracca, G., & Robinson, R. (2007). The construct of generalized anxiety disorder in Alzheimer disease. *American Journal of Geriatric Psychiatry*, 15(1), 42–49.

Starkstein, S., Jorge, R., Mizrahi, R., & Robinson, R. (2006). A diagnostic formulation for anosognosia in Alzheimer's disease. *Journal of Neurology, Neurosurgery and Psychiatry*, 77(6), 719–725.

Starkstein, S., & Leentjens, A. (2008). The nosological position of apathy in clinical practice. *Journal of Neurology, Neurosurgery and Psychiatry*, 79(10), 1088–1092.

Starkstein, S., Mayberg, H., Berthier, M., Fedoroff, P., Price, T., Dannals, R., ... Robinson, R. G. (1990). Mania after brain injury: Neuroradiological and metabolic findings. *Annals of Neurology*, 27(6), 652–659.

Steele, C., Rovner, B., Chase, G., & Folstein, M. (1990). Psychiatric symptoms and nursing home placement of patients with Alzheimer's disease. *American Journal of Psychiatry*, 147(8), 1049–1051.

Sultzer, D., Mahler, M., Mandelkern, M., Cummings, J., Van Gorp, W., Hinkin, C., & Berisford, M. A. (1995). The relationship between psychiatric symptoms and regional cortical metabolism in Alzheimer's disease. *Journal of Neuropsychiatry and Clinical Neuroscience*, 7(4), 476–484.

Sunderland, T., & Minichiello, M. (1997). Dementia mood assessment scale. *International Psychogeriatrics*, 8(Suppl S3), 329–331.

Tarawneh, R., & Holtzman, D. (2012). The clinical problem of symptomatic Alzheimer disease and mild cognitive impairment. *Cold Spring Harbor Perspectives in Medicine*, 2(5), a006148.

Tekin, S., Mega, M., Masterman, D., Chow, T., Garakian, J., Vinters, H., & Cummings, J. L. (2001). Orbitofrontal and anterior cingulate cortex neurofibrillary tangle burden is associated with agitation in Alzheimer disease. *Annals of Neurology*, 49(3), 355–361.

Twelftree, H., & Qazi, A. (2006). Relationship between anxiety and agitation in dementia. *Aging and Mental Health*, 10(4), 362–367.

Vitiello, M., & Borson, S. (2001). Sleep disturbances in patients with Alzheimer's disease: Epidemiology, pathophysiology and treatment. *CNS Drugs*, 15(10), 777–796.

Wragg, R., & Jeste, D. (1989). Overview of depression and psychosis in Alzheimer's disease. *American Journal of Psychiatry*, 146(5), 577–587.

Wu, Y., & Swaab, D. (2005). The human pineal gland and melatonin in aging and Alzheimer's disease. *Journal of Pineal Research*, 38(3), 145–152.

Young, T., Peppard, P., & Gottlieb, D. (2002). Epidemiology of obstructive sleep apnea: A population health perspective. *American Journal of Respiratory Critical Care Medicine*, 165(9), 1217–1239.

22

Neuroimaging, Cerebrospinal Fluid Markers, and Genetic Testing in Dementia

Bradford C. Dickerson

Candidate disease-modifying therapies for Alzheimer's disease (AD) have been in clinical trials for a number of years (Cummings, Doody, & Clark, 2007), with a growing list of failures. These compounds are being tested in patients with a clinical diagnosis of probable AD dementia to determine whether they will slow the inexorable course of progressive decline. Yet a clinical diagnosis of probable AD has traditionally required the determination that the patient has dementia, defined as the loss of social or occupational function due to multidomain cognitive impairment. In practice, this is often operationalized for clinical trial criteria as a Clinical Dementia Rating (CDR) of 1 (mild dementia) or in some cases CDR 0.5 (very mild dementia) and a Mini-Mental State Exam (MMSE) score less than 24 or in some cases 26 (as discussed in detail in Chapter 19). By the time this level of impairment is reached, many patients have substantial difficulties in complex activities of daily living, such as community affairs, driving, financial or household management, and planning and decision making. If efficacious disease-modifying treatments for AD are developed, it would be ideal to administer them to patients with the disease prior to the point at which impairment is this prominent (DeKosky & Marek, 2003). Partly because substantial synaptic and neuronal loss is typically present by the time patients exhibit mild AD dementia (Gomez-Isla et al., 1996; Price et al., 2001; Scheff, Price, Schmitt, & Mufson, 2005), it is possible that some disease-modifying therapies may be less efficacious if initiated at this stage than they would be if begun earlier. There has been growing consensus for over 5 years that adequate knowledge exists about the clinical and neurobiologic phenotype of typical AD that we should be attempting to make an earlier diagnosis—prior to mild dementia—particularly for the purposes of earlier clinical trial enrollment (Dubois et al., 2007, 2010). Although a careful history and examination is at the core of clinical practice and research (Chapter 9), the new diagnostic criteria that were published in April 2011 formally incorporate the use of various types of biomarkers in the diagnosis of AD at dementia and prodromal dementia stages (Albert et al., 2011; Jack et al., 2011; McKhann et al., 2011; Sperling et al., 2011). As discussed in other chapters in this book, we can now diagnose an individual with mild cognitive impairment that is highly likely to be due to AD based on a combination of clinical and biomarker data. Furthermore, we can identify individuals with preclinical AD for recruitment for research, including clinical trials of interventions aimed at delaying symptoms.

A major source of such information is neuroimaging technology. Various types of neuroimaging techniques enable elements of brain structure and function to be visualized in living people and allow quantitative measurements to be made of the anatomy, connectivity, perfusion, metabolism, and activity of various brain regions and networks. Furthermore, new molecular imaging techniques allow amyloid pathology to be identified in living individuals, and in vivo molecular imaging markers are emerging for tau. Specific abnormalities in brain structure and function, and the presence of pathologic molecular markers, have taken on prime importance in the early diagnosis and monitoring of progression of AD and related disorders. While to date many of these advanced imaging approaches have primarily been used in research and clinical trials, they are rapidly moving toward use in clinical practice. In parallel, cerebrospinal fluid (CSF) biomarkers of amyloid and tau have rapidly matured as very valuable biomarkers of AD molecular pathology and are used in both research and practice in many countries (Herskovits & Growdon, 2010).

While knowledge about imaging and CSF markers of AD is robust, such knowledge is less mature in other neurodegenerative diseases that cause dementia. Further fundamental research is needed to improve our knowledge of the anatomic, physiologic, and molecular phenotypes that can be measured using in vivo methods in patients with non-AD dementias. This chapter will provide a detailed review of imaging and fluid biomarkers with an emphasis on AD but with discussion of other dementias as well.

Biomarker Constructs

Before considering specific biomarkers, it is important to review a general framework for how they can be used. Fox et al. (2004) enumerated three aspects of disease pathophysiology in which biomarkers may play important roles: as markers of trait, state, and rate. Neuroimaging- and fluid-based measures may provide useful data in all of these situations, and other kinds of biomarkers may be valuable in this regard as well. Traits measured by biomarkers are typically thought of as risk factors for disease, which may involve genetic, anatomic, or physiologic elements. For example, a number of imaging studies of cognitively intact individuals at a younger age than the typical onset of AD have begun to investigate anatomic or physiologic differences between those at elevated genetic risk for AD and controls, and to follow these changes over time (e.g., temporoparietal hypometabolism in young APOE-ε4 carriers; Reiman et al., 2004). Ultimately, since most AD-related traits indicate risk but are not deterministic (i.e., not all APOE-ε4 carriers will manifest clinical dementia symptoms), long-term clinical follow-up coupled with the longitudinal assessment of biomarkers will be needed to determine which individuals in these risk groups develop cognitive decline and clinical AD. Thus, biomarkers of disease traits would indicate susceptibility and could potentially be combined with other risk factors to improve the accuracy of risk estimation and prediction of clinical disease, or to increase the yield of screening for preclinical AD.

A biomarker of disease state enables the detection of an abnormality associated with disease pathobiology in an individual, and it is typically thought of as a diagnostic marker. In AD, disease markers are usually considered to reflect the presence of neuropathology, and they include measures derived from neuroimaging, serum, and cerebrospinal fluid, and other biologic materials. The individual in whom a marker is "positive" is presumed to have a biological abnormality consistent with AD neuropathology, but he or she may or may not have symptoms. Studies of markers of disease state have been confounded by the notorious difficulty in correlating neuropathologic states themselves with clinical state. That is, patients with clinically probable AD who are equated on clinical metrics may exhibit marked variability in the density and distribution of senile plaques, neurofibrillary tangles, neuronal loss, and other measures of abnormal brain structure. Furthermore, postmortem studies indicate that some cognitively intact individuals and many mild cognitive impairment (MCI) patients already carry a heavy burden of AD neuropathology (Gomez-Isla et al.,

1996; Kordower et al., 2001; Price et al., 2001). Thus, it is not surprising that findings from cross-sectional studies show imaging-based markers of brain structure and function in MCI overlap substantially with both cognitively intact older control groups and with AD patient groups. These significant individual differences that confound cross-sectional studies of clinicopathologic state again reinforce the notion that detailed longitudinal investigations are needed to clarify the relationships between clinical state and measures of neuroanatomy, physiology, and pathology. These ideas have been further reinforced by recent papers proposing biomarker trajectory models of AD (Jack et al., 2010, 2013). Some of these types of measures might be useful not only to increase or reduce confidence in a particular presumed pathologic diagnosis in a symptomatic patient but also to identify asymptomatic/preclinical disease states (e.g., a cognitively normal individual with brain amyloid, similar to a neurologically intact patient with imaging evidence of prior stroke).

Finally, imaging markers of the rate of disease progression—which allow the tracking of changes over time in pathoanatomic or pathophysiologic alterations in the brain associated with AD—would be particularly useful in evaluating the efficacy of disease-modifying therapeutics. Importantly, although changes in any of these markers may represent changes in the underlying disease process, the rates of change of a marker may or may not correlate with that of other biomarkers or of clinical metrics during the time period of interest. Using imaging-based measures, it may be possible to detect the ability of a putative disease-modifying agent to impede the degenerative process of AD in a shorter period of time than would be necessary to judge slowing of cognitive decline. While validation of biomarkers against clinical outcomes is ultimately essential, as the focus of therapeutics shifts toward prevention or modulation of the neurodegenerative process prior to the presence of substantial symptoms, such validation takes longer and becomes more difficult. Therefore, the validation of new potential imaging biomarkers (e.g., amyloid imaging, functional magnetic resonance imaging [fMRI]) may be performed more efficiently in conjunction with more established imaging markers (e.g., hippocampal volume, fludeoxyglucose positron emission tomography [FDG-PET]). Finally, individual variability in rates of decline in MCI and AD and related disorders is substantial. Imaging-based biomarkers may offer an opportunity for additional power in this regard, which could be gained using a "run-in" phase to quantify subjects' individual rates of change in the imaging marker (e.g., hippocampal volume) prior to the randomization phase of the clinical trial.

However, the widely ranging initial estimates of sample sizes for clinical trials from preliminary studies have highlighted the need for further fundamental knowledge regarding the natural history of in vivo anatomic and physiologic and biofluid changes in MCI and AD, which will likely be similarly true in frontotemporal dementia (FTD), progressive supranuclear palsy with corticobasal syndrome (PSP/CBS), Lewy body dementia (DLB), and other diseases. Sample size estimates derived from power calculations are influenced primarily by the proposed size of the effect of interest (e.g., difference in rate of atrophy in treated vs. control patients) and the variance of the data derived from the particular measure used. The effect size may range from 0% (no difference) to 100% (maximum difference, which is the difference between atrophy rates in AD patients and controls). Imaging data on which to base estimates of effect sizes for putative disease-modifying therapies for AD have increasingly begun appearing in the literature. Variance of the data may be influenced by biologic variability, such as heterogeneity of atrophy rates in the sample, which may relate to age, disease severity, or individual differences in rate of disease progression. Variance is also influenced by measurement variability, which may result from differences in the data acquired between multiple time points (e.g., due to changes in instrumentation or signal acquisition) or in differences in postscan processing of the data (e.g., selection of regions of interest). Both sources of measurement variability may be compounded by differences between sites in multicenter studies. Such data may be seriously confounded if systematic bias is introduced in any of these sources of variability. Further serial imaging studies examining the natural history of changes in brain structure, function, and molecular composition in the context of detailed clinical assessments in MCI and AD has been under way as part of the American Alzheimer's Disease Neuroimaging Initiative (ADNI) (Weiner et al., 2013), as well as similar initiatives around the world. There are also similarly designed studies under way in FTD and PSP/CBS.

Traditional Role of Structural Neuroimaging in the Diagnosis of Alzheimer's Disease and Other Dementias

In the past, the major role of neuroimaging in dementia assessment has been to assist in the exclusion of nondegenerative etiologies of cognitive impairment or dementia (such as tumors, inflammatory conditions, infectious processes, etc.) or the identification of features of unusual forms of dementia (such as prion diseases) (Knopman et al., 2001). Neuroimaging can also be particularly useful for the detection of cerebrovascular contributions to cognitive impairment.

Some examples of differential diagnoses of cognitive disorders that can be informed by structural imaging include the following (see Chapter 15 for more detail on many of these conditions). In suspected cerebrovascular disease or patients with a history of stroke or significant cardiovascular risk factors, computerized tomography (CT) or magnetic resonance imaging (MRI) can be very helpful. However, it is difficult to determine to what degree cerebrovascular disease is the primary cause of a patient's dementia, as opposed to being a contributing factor along with neurodegenerative disease (see Chapter 13). "Mixed dementia" is a clinical diagnosis that is associated with structural evidence of infarction (often with cavitary or encephalomalacic change) or signal changes consistent with small vessel cerebrovascular disease, along with evidence of neurodegenerative atrophy consistent with AD or a related disorder. Neoplastic processes may include primary or metastatic brain tumors that can sometimes present with cognitive decline rather than focal sensorimotor dysfunction or other neurologic signs. Meningiomas may be possible to treat surgically. These lesions usually, but not always, present with symptoms that are atypical for a neurodegenerative disease and raise the question of a focal brain lesion. Subdural hygroma/hematomas are common in the elderly with or without other neurodegenerative diseases, but they can be easily visualized using CT or MRI. Although now thought to be relatively uncommon, normal pressure hydocephalus is a condition in which imaging has been viewed as essential: if at least part of the clinical triad of ataxia, incontinence, and dementia is associated with MR or CT evidence of ventriculomegaly, the diagnosis is strongly suggested. As described further in Chapter 15, a large volume lumbar puncture may or may not produce substantial clinical improvement, potentially predicting shunt responsiveness. Creutzfeldt-Jakob disease often has characteristic diffusion-weighted imaging (DWI) MRI abnormalities (hyperintensity of cortical ribbon and deep gray structures) (Fig. 22.1), as described in more detail in Chapter 15. A number of other rare and/or rapidly progressive dementias are associated with relatively sensitive and specific neuroimaging or CSF or other biomarker findings, as described in detail in Chapter 15.

The Neurobiologic Phenotype of Typical Amnesic Alzheimer's Disease Dementia

Research over the past two decades has led revolutionary changes in dementia research and practice, with a growing array of imaging and fluid biomarkers taking center stage in diagnostic evaluation and monitoring of progression. AD has led the way as an exemplar showing how imaging and fluid assay technology can be used to measure biomarkers of the disease and incorporate these into clinical diagnostic criteria, as described in more detail in Chapters 16–18, but nearly all other major forms of dementia have also now incorporated biomarkers into diagnostic evaluation formally or informally (see Part II of this volume).

Although a great deal of our knowledge of the neurobiologic phenotype of AD has come from postmortem studies of brain tissue, a rapidly growing body of literature includes in vivo measurements that attempt to capture elements of the biology of AD (Jack et al., 2010, 2013). While many of these studies have not followed patients to autopsy, and so we do not yet have the gold standard diagnosis of definite AD to corroborate the clinical diagnoses, there is enough consistency in some of

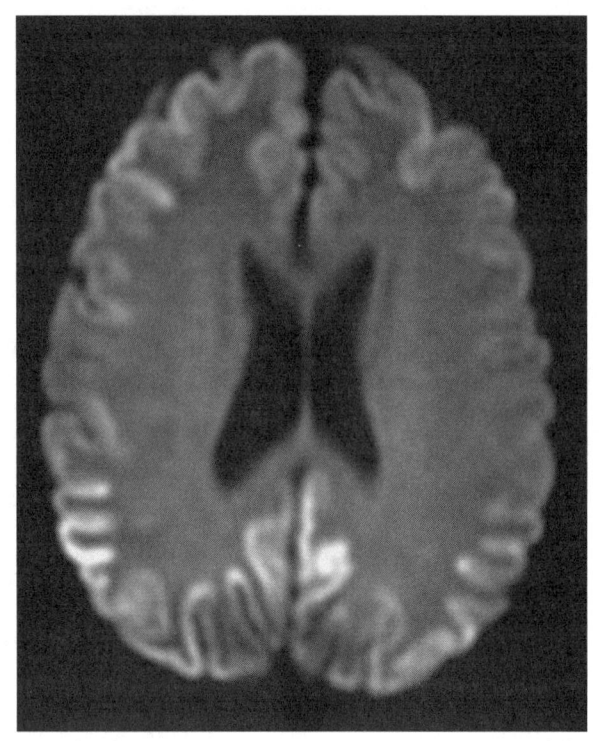

Figure 22.1 Diffusion-weighted magnetic resonance imaging (MRI, image left is patient left) from a patient who presented with progressive aphasia, which evolved over rapidly 2 years to severe dementia and death. The cortical ribbon hyperintensity shown here was localized in part to frontoparietal language regions, consistent with initial symptoms.

these measures to provide confidence that they are valid biomarkers of neurobiologic abnormalities of AD. These markers include neuroimaging measures of brain structure, function, and connectivity, all of which are able to show patterns of abnormalities characteristic of AD rather than simply excluding other possible contributors to cognitive impairment. Thus, they can provide data in support of a diagnosis of probable AD. Even more importantly, measures from molecular neuroimaging and CSF have been developed in the past decade that are sensitive and specific indicators of amyloid or tau pathology. The important advantage of such in vivo biomarkers is that they can be measured in individuals at a time when their clinical phenotype is specifically characterized, in contrast to postmortem studies in which the clinical phenotype may have less specificity due to progression to advanced disease. All of these putative biomarkers have undergone intensive longitudinal study as part of the Alzheimer's Disease Neuroimaging Initiative (Mueller et al., 2005; Weiner et al., 2011) and other large natural history studies around the world.

Imaging the Anatomic Changes of Alzheimer's Disease

Quantitative Magnetic Resonance Imaging Measurements of the Medial Temporal Lobe

In the late 1980s, the first magnetic resonance imaging (MRI) data began appearing that enabled the clear visualization of the human hippocampal formation in vivo (Jack et al., 1989; Naidich et al., 1987a, 1987b; Seab et al., 1988). Initial efforts at quantification provided data indicating that manual tracings by trained operators were valid and reliable (Jack et al., 1988, 1989). These new methods were immediately applied to visualize and quantify atrophy in patients with AD (Jack et al., 1987; Jack, Petersen, O'Brien, & Tangalos, 1992; Seab et al., 1988). As stated

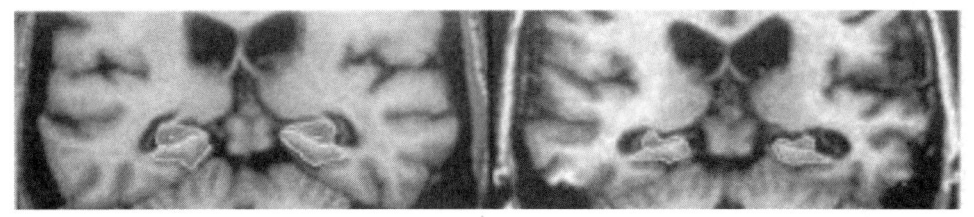

Figure 22.2 Manual tracing of the hippocampal formation and parahippocampal gyrus performed by the author in 1996. Image on left is from a cognitively intact older adult, and the image on the right is from a patient with mild Alzheimer's disease dementia.

by Jack (Jack et al., 1992), these new methods were quickly seen as having utility in the diagnostic evaluation of AD:

> The rationale for quantitative MRI of MTL atrophy in the diagnosis of AD is: (1) a memory impairment is usually the earliest and most severe clinical manifestation of AD, (2) MTL limbic structures are central to the integrity of declarative memory function, (3) MTL limbic structures are involved earliest and most extensively in the pathology of AD, and (4)several principal MTL limbic structures are amenable to accurate volumetric quantitation by MRI--the hippocampal formation, amygdala, and parahippocampal gyrus (PHG) [page 183].

During the 1990s, the scope of quantitative structural MRI efforts expanded to include more sophisticated studies of larger samples of patients with AD, in addition to investigations of normal development and aging. During those early years, quantitative MRI-based measures of brain anatomy were almost entirely obtained from manual tracings by anatomists or trained technicians. Hippocampal volume derived from MRI was shown to correlate strongly with histological HF volume and neuronal loss (Bobinski et al., 2000) and severity of AD pathology (Gosche, Mortimer, Smith, Markesbery, & Snowdon, 2002; Jack et al., 2002), as well as memory impairment (De Leon et al., 1997; de Toledo-Morrell et al., 2000). Hippocampal and entorhinal volumetric measures were also demonstrated useful for the identification of subgroups of individuals with MCI who would progress to a clinical diagnosis of AD within a few years (Convit et al., 2000; Dickerson et al., 2001; Jack et al., 1999; Killiany et al., 2000; Mungas et al., 2002; Visser et al., 1999) (Fig. 22.2). Furthermore, it was determined possible to detect atrophy of these regions up to 5 years before the expression of clinical symptoms in individuals with APP mutations (Schott et al., 2003).

As MRI and computational technologies have matured, it has become possible to perform increasingly sophisticated investigations of brain morphometry, including automated measurement of a variety of brain regions, voxel-based morphometry and related "unbiased" exploratory analyses of the whole brain or cerebral cortex, and analysis of the shape and other sophisticated measures of aspects of brain structure (Ashburner et al., 2003). In addition, new techniques for the coregistration of one scan to another improved the quantification of structural change over time within individuals (Fox & Schott, 2004). This enables individuals to be used as their own controls, which reduces the noise of individual differences in neuroanatomy that are inherently present in group-comparison studies. MRI measures of brain structure may also be confounded by within-subject variability in hydration status and probably other as yet unknown factors (Walters, Fox, Crum, Taube, & Thomas, 2001). Despite these caveats, longitudinal MRI measures of changes in brain structure have been successfully used as outcome measures in clinical trials of disease-modifying therapies for multiple sclerosis (Filippi, Dousset, McFarland, Miller, & Grossman, 2002), and they have been increasingly investigated in AD clinical trials (Fox et al., 2005).

The most intensively investigated MRI-based biomarkers include atrophy of the whole brain, hippocampal formation, and entorhinal cortex or enlargement of the temporal horn of the lateral ventricle (Dickerson & Sperling, 2005). Since it is highly reliable, whole brain atrophy (as measured using typical volumetric approaches or using longitudinal methods such as the brain boundary shift integral) may be very sensitive in the context of measuring progressive atrophy over time in patients with AD dementia (Fox, Cousens, Scahill, Harvey, & Rossor, 2000; Schott et al., 2006) or even prior to dementia (Jack et al., 2007). But because—at least in typical amnesic AD—there is early pathology in the medial temporal lobe, hippocampal and temporal horn measures are very sensitive (Schott et al., 2003). Yet they may be somewhat nonspecific because these regions can be affected by other pathologies, including frontotemporal lobar degeneration (FTLD), cerebrovascular disease, hippocampal sclerosis, and alpha-synuclein pathology (Jagust, Zheng, et al., 2007). On theoretical grounds, entorhinal measures should be both sensitive and relatively specific because this region of medial temporal cortex is affected prominently early in the course of AD, although it can also be involved in some forms of FTLD. However, there are still challenges involved in its measurement from MRI, although semiautomated entorhinal morphometric methods are improving (Dickerson et al., 2007).

Quantitative Magnetic Resonance Imaging Measurements of the Cerebral Cortex

Since AD is known to affect limbic and heteromodal regions of the neocortex, investigators have focused increasing effort on measuring atrophy in distributed cortical and limbic regions, including lateral temporoparietal and posterior cingulate cortex (Scahill, Schott, Stevens, Rossor, & Fox, 2002; Whitwell et al., 2008). Automated or semiautomated methods have been developed that provide high-throughput capacity to measure the distributed pattern ("signature") of atrophy consistent with AD in individuals with mild dementia or MCI, and to differentiate it from normal age-related atrophy (Bakkour, Morris, & Dickerson, 2009; Bakkour, Morris, Wolk, & Dickerson, 2013; Dickerson et al., 2009) (Fig. 22.3). Atrophy in AD-vulnerable brain regions can be consistently detected in individuals who do not yet have symptoms but who harbor brain amyloid (Dickerson et al., 2009) or who will eventually progress to AD dementia after longitudinal follow-up (Dickerson et al., 2011). Computational pattern-matching techniques are being developed to provide a probabilistic score to an individual person's scan as being consistent or inconsistent with AD (Davatzikos, Resnick, Wu, Parmpi, & Clark, 2008; Vemuri et al., 2008). This is an area of the research literature that is literally exploding with promising new methods, but we are still in the early phase of determining how to use these markers in clinical trials or practice.

Hippocampal Shape and Subregional Analysis

Although hippocampal volumetry has provided many scientific insights and is undoubtedly a clinically useful tool for certain conditions, the entire volume of a structure as complex as the hippocampus provides a relatively crude measure. Therefore, a number of teams have devoted effort to the analysis of the shape of the surface of the hippocampal formation. The scientific techniques involved draw from fields of geometry and topology and in their most straightforward implementation essentially determine where along the entire surface of the hippocampus there are deformations. For example, a localized inward deformation of the hippocampal surface may or may not be detectable as a reduction in overall volume but may nevertheless be an indicator of significant abnormalities in particular regions of the hippocampus. The location of such a deformation can then be used to identify, at least in probabilistic terms, the subregion(s) where the abnormality is most likely localized. Several groups have used this approach to identify localized hippocampal shape abnormalities in AD among other neuropsychiatric conditions (Boccardi et al., 2010; Cole et al., 2010; Csernansky et al., 2000, 2002; Dager et al., 2007; Hogan et al., 2004; Miller et al., 2009; Morra et al., 2008; Nicolson et al., 2006; Posener et al., 2003; Tepest, Wang, Miller, Falkai, & Csernansky, 2003; Wang et al., 2005).

In addition to inferring the hippocampal subregion-specific localization of abnormalities in the shape of the hippocampal surface, several groups have begun developing and applying protocols for the measurement of the volumes of hippocampal subregions (Kerchner et al., 2010; Mueller et al., 2007; Mueller, Schuff, Raptentsetsang, Elman, & Weiner, 2008; Mueller & Weiner, 2009; Neylan

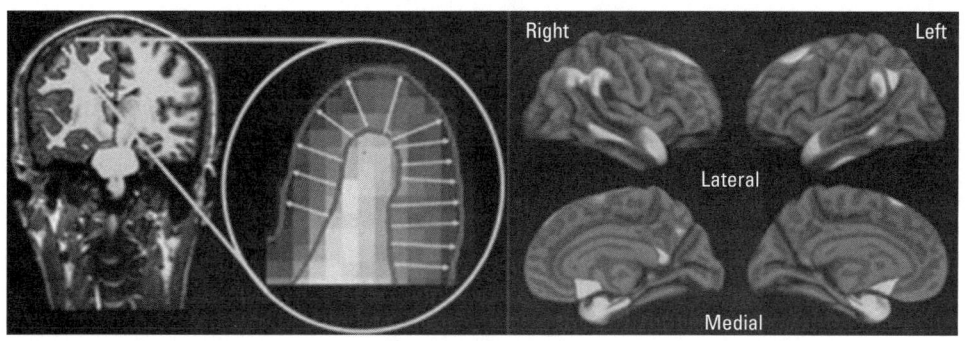

Figure 22.3 Computational neuroscience now offers methods to quantify aspects of brain structure from magnetic resonance imaging (MRI) scans. The left image depicts cortical thickness measurement from a T1-weighted MRI scan. The right image shows a map of the areas in yellow and red where the cerebral cortex is thinner in a group of mild Alzheimer's disease dementia patients compared to controls. (See color plate section)

et al.; Van Leemput et al., 2009; Wang et al., 2010; Yushkevich et al., 2008, 2009, 2010). The development of new methods for higher resolution MRI data acquisition is fueling many of these efforts, along with new computational analytic methods. Some of these methods can be used to visualize and measure detailed aspects of medial temporal lobe (MTL) atrophy in AD and other neurodegenerative diseases (Fig. 22.4).

Clinical Use of Structural Magnetic Resonance Imaging in Dementia Evaluation

The atrophy patterns typical of neurodegenerative diseases are often very difficult to visualize from relatively thick, two-dimensional axial slices that are still often the "routine" protocol in many imaging centers when a patient with suspected neurodegenerative disease is being scanned. Previously, the MRI data acquisition methodology for obtaining reasonably high-resolution images suitable for the assessment of regional atrophy existed primarily in specialized research centers. It is now commonplace on clinical scanners in routine use to obtain three-dimensional (which can be reformatted in multiple planes, as opposed to the early scans that were essentially only viewable in one orientation) MRI data with high signal-to-noise properties at resolutions of 1 mm^3 or better. Using widely available MRI technology, radiologists can set up protocols (e.g., "Dementia protocol" or "Memory Loss protocol") in which relatively high-resolution three-dimensional coronal sequences are obtained in addition to routine diagnostic images. Particularly with the use of new parallel acquisition techniques that enable faster data collection, such high-resolution sequences can be acquired

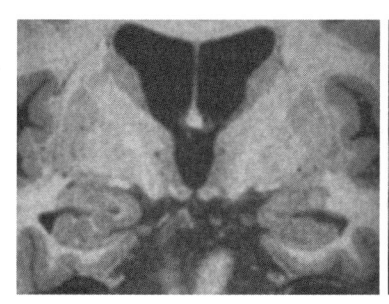

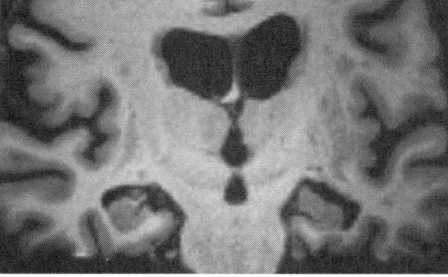

Figure 22.4 Higher resolution magnetic resonance imaging (MRI) scans offer better visualization of neuroanatomy. The left image shows a 500 micrometer resolution T1-weighted MRI scan of a cognitively intact 72-year-old adult, and the right image shows a similar image of a patient with mild Alzheimer's disease dementia, illustrating mild hippocampal atrophy.

in 5–8 minutes as part of a comprehensive multisequence MRI protocol (i.e., total time typically on the order of about ½ hour), and newer scanning technology is continuing to improve this efficiency. We routinely obtain both T1-weighted and T2-weighted scans, since T1-weighted sequences typically show many anatomic details very clearly and T2-weighted sequences demonstrate signal hyperintensities associated with cerebrovascular, gliotic/sclerotic, inflammatory, neoplastic, or other types of pathology. These images can be visually inspected for the purpose of identifying the variety of pathologic changes, including atrophy, that are associated with specific neurodegenerative diseases (Fig. 22.5). A number of efficient visual rating protocols have been described with the goal of enabling relatively standardized descriptions of the magnitude of hippocampal/MTL atrophy (Galton et al., 2001; Vermersch, Leys, Scheltens, & Barkhof, 1994) and posterior temporoparietal atrophy (Koedam et al., 2011; Lehmann et al., 2012; Likeman et al., 2005; Ryan & Fox, 2009). With these procedures now being available, it is relatively straightforward for a specialized team to be assembled for the purposes of evaluating these disorders in a comprehensive fashion using contemporary clinical and radiologic methods (typically including a radiologist or neuroradiologist; and a neurologist, psychiatrist, and/or neuropsychologist).

If a patient is not able to obtain an MRI scan due to a contraindication (e.g., pacemaker, claustrophobia), relatively high-resolution CT scans can now be acquired with multiplanar reformatting that allows for inspection of images in multiple planes, including coronal, which provides the clearest view of the MTL and many cortical regions involved in AD and other neurodegenerative diseases.

Visual inspection of MRI or CT scans for characteristic patterns of atrophy is still the most widely used approach for clinical interpretation of structural neuroimaging scans. Quantitative analysis of hippocampal volume or volumetrics of other structures is performed in some centers, but it is still not in widespread practice, partly because robust normative data are still scant and partly because a variety of analysis methods

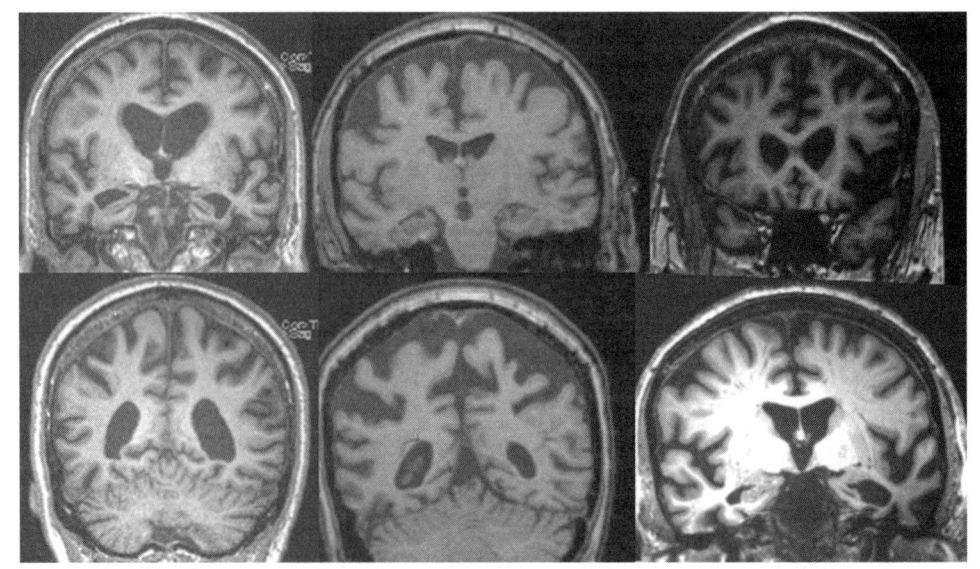

Figure 22.5 Visual inspection of magnetic resonance imaging (MRI) scans can reveal patterns of atrophy consistent with a particular type of neurodegenerative dementia. Top/bottom left images show a patient with typical amnesic Alzheimer's disease (AD) dementia, illustrating medial temporal and parietal atrophy. Middle top/bottom images show a patient with posterior cortical atrophy with cerebrospinal fluid biomarkers consistent with AD pathobiology, illustrating relative preservation of medial temporal lobe with prominent parietal atrophy. Top right image shows a patient with agrammatic primary progressive aphasia. Bottom right image shows a patient with semantic primary progressive aphasia.

are employed (and partly because of unclear reimbursement practices). Efforts are under way to try to harmonize these measurements for the purposes of clinical research and trials (Frisoni & Jack, 2011), and hopefully this will facilitate the use of quantitative MRI-based morphometry in clinical practice.

Imaging the Physiologic Changes of Alzheimer's Disease With Magnetic Resonance Imaging

Task-Related Functional Magnetic Resonance Imaging

A number of fMRI studies in patients with clinically diagnosed AD, using a variety of visually presented stimuli, have identified decreased activation in hippocampal and parahippocampal regions compared to control subjects during episodic encoding tasks (Kato, Knopman, & Liu, 2001; Machulda et al., 2003; Rombouts et al., 2000; Small, Perera, DeLaPaz, Mayeux, & Stern, 1999; Sperling et al., 2003). As for MCI, the prodromal stage of AD, studies have demonstrated conflicting results with some findings of hippocampal hypoactivation (Johnson et al., 2006; Machulda et al., 2003) similar to that seen in AD dementia and some findings of hyperactivation (Dickerson et al., 2005; Hamalainen et al., 2006; Kircher et al., 2007). Despite the inconsistencies, which we believe can be explained by a number of factors (Dickerson & Sperling, 2008), there is replicated evidence to support the hypothesis that there is a phase of increased MTL activation early in the course of prodromal AD, prior to clinical dementia.

Accumulating evidence indicates that task-related regional brain hyperactivation may be a universal neural response to insult, as it occurs in a variety of neuropsychiatric disorders and conditions, including AD/MCI, Huntington's disease (Rosas, Feigin, & Hersch, 2004), Parkinson's disease (Monchi et al., 2004), cerebrovascular disease (Carey et al., 2002; Johansen-Berg et al., 2002), multiple sclerosis (Morgen et al., 2004; Reddy et al., 2000), traumatic brain injury (McAllister et al., 1999), HIV (Ernst, Chang, Jovicich, Ames, & Arnold, 2002), alcoholism (Desmond et al., 2003), schizophrenia (Callicott et al., 2003), sleep deprivation (Drummond et al., 2000), and aging (Cabeza, Anderson, Locantore, & McIntosh, 2002). The evidence aforementioned also indicates that increased MTL activation can be seen in the absence of significant MTL atrophy, which provides in vivo support for laboratory and animal data suggesting that physiologic alterations may precede significant structural abnormalities in very early AD (Selkoe, 2002; Walsh & Selkoe, 2004) and may represent inefficient neural circuit function (Stern et al., 2004). Thus, fMRI may provide a means to detect changes in human memory circuit function that underlie the earliest symptoms of AD (Sperling et al., 2009), and it may be useful in identifying groups of subjects at high risk for future cognitive decline prior to a diagnosis of AD (Miller et al., 2006).

Recent studies are extending these initial insights using longitudinal and multimodal approaches. We recently showed that MCI subjects who declined over 2 years of clinical follow-up demonstrated an initial hippocampal hyperactivation during encoding but after 2 years a reduced level of activity, consistent with the "inverse U-shaped curve" model (O'Brien et al., 2010). Evidence of the earliest stages of this process can be seen in cognitively intact older adults with brain amyloid, who hyperactivate the hippocampus during memory encoding relative to the activation of similarly aged adults without brain amyloid (Sperling et al., 2009). Extending these approaches to genetic risk, in cognitively intact older adults (Bondi, Houston, Eyler, & Brown, 2005; Bookheimer et al., 2000; Fleisher et al., 2005; Xu et al., 2009) at elevated genetic risk for AD, hippocampal activation during memory tasks is greater than in those without such elevated risk.

Resting-State Functional Magnetic Resonance Imaging

Recent functional magnetic resonance imaging (fMRI) studies are beginning to reveal a link between disease-related hemodynamic alterations and the well-described resting perfusion/metabolic abnormalities in AD. Hypoperfusion/metabolism is typically seen with nuclear medical imaging techniques (such as FDG-PET or single-photon emission computed tomography [SPECT], as reviewed later in the chapter) in temporo-parietal/posterior cingulate cortical regions in AD patients during the "resting" state. The medial parietal/posterior cingulate cortex, along with medial frontal and lateral parietal regions, appears to compose a "default mode" network that is more active when individuals are not engaged in particular tasks, and which is thought to play a role in vigilance, readiness, or monitoring—these regions "deactivate" (BOLD signal amplitude falls below baseline) during cognitive task performance (Raichle et al., 2001). A growing number of studies in AD patients and individuals with prodromal AD as well as asymptomatic individuals with brain amyloid have demonstrated alterations in the deactivation and functional connectivity of these regions, suggesting that this default mode network is disrupted by the biology of disease early in its course (Celone et al., 2006; Greicius, Srivastava, Reiss, & Menon, 2004; Lustig et al., 2003; Rombouts, Barkhof, Goekoop, Stam, & Scheltens, 2005). Substantial overlap is present between these default mode areas and the localization of positron emission tomography (PET) amyloid tracer binding (Buckner et al., 2005). In addition to hyperactivation during task performance, MTL regions appear to have increased resting-state connectivity in MCI patients (Das et al., 2013).

Perfusion Magnetic Resonance Imaging

Another measure related to brain function is perfusion. Perfusion refers to the delivery of blood, oxygen, and nutrients to tissue, and it is tightly coupled with metabolism. Thus, although measures of perfusion are of direct relevance for clinical disorders of blood flow, such as stroke, these measures are also of value as surrogates of regional brain metabolism and function. The gold standard method for quantifying brain perfusion in vivo is PET scanning with ^{15}O-labeled water, and that for metabolism is ^{18}fluorodeoxyglucose (FDG). With regard to perfusion, water in arterial blood can also be "labeled" via magnetic resonance imaging using a technique called arterial spin labeling (ASL). This method has been developed over the last two decades but has received increasing attention in the past few years in part because it is noninvasive and relatively easy to obtain as part of a standard MRI protocol on widely available scanners.

In part because of the relatively low resolution of PET scanning technology, there has been relatively little investigation of hippocampal perfusion and metabolism. Although some studies suggest that hippocampal perfusion may be reduced in normal older adults compared with younger adults (Heo et al., 2010) while some indicate that it is preserved (Rusinek et al., 2011), analysis of hippocampal metabolism in relation to global gray matter metabolism has shown that it is relatively spared (much more so than many frontal and parietal regions) or even increased in relation to global metabolism in normal aging (Kalpouzos et al., 2009; Willis et al., 2002). One longitudinal study of older adults demonstrated that, in individuals with preserved memory over an 8-year interval, hippocampal blood flow was also preserved (relatively increased compared to global blood flow) (Beason-Held, Kraut, & Resnick, 2008). More detailed high-resolution studies suggest that particular hippocampal subregions, especially the dentate gyrus, are vulnerable to metabolic decline in normal aging while other subregions may be resilient (Small, Chawla, Buonocore, Rapp, & Barnes, 2004).

Complicating matters further, several recent reports suggest that the hippocampus and nearby MTL cortex may be hyperperfused in AD compared to controls (Alsop, Casement, de Bazelaire, Fong, & Press, 2008; Scarmeas et al., 2004). Another investigation of the relationship between hippocampal volume and perfusion in MCI and AD provided further support for these observations, indicating that MTL perfusion and atrophy were not correlated (Luckhaus et al., 2010). As expected based on prior literature, this study found that hippocampal volume was smaller in APOE ε4 carriers than in noncarriers, but that MTL perfusion was not different based on APOE genotype.

Clinical Use of Physiologic Magnetic Resonance Imaging Methods in Dementia

Despite the promising research data on physiologic measures that can be obtained from various types of MRI imaging, these techniques are not yet used in clinical practice. Most of them are being investigated as part of natural history studies such as ADNI, which will likely provide clearer data regarding their potential for use in clinical trials or practice settings.

Molecular Imaging in Alzheimer's Disease

Molecular neuroimaging techniques enable in vivo images to be obtained of radiolabeled compounds (radioligands) that are typically injected intravenously into the person undergoing imaging. A wide range of compounds can be labeled, and radiochemists regularly develop new compounds of use for neuroimaging. The two primary methods for obtaining images are PET and SPECT. In PET scanning, positrons are emitted by the radioligand, collide with electrons, and generate gamma radiation, which is ultimately detected by the sensor arrays and used to derive an image. Commonly used radioligands include carbon-11, oxygen-15, and fluorine-18 (18F). 18F is desirable because it has the longest half-life. SPECT scans work in a somewhat similar manner but employ compounds such as technetium-99 and xenon-133, which have longer half-lives than compounds used in PET scanning. For a variety of technical reasons, PET scans are able to obtain higher resolution images than SPECT scans, but they are generally less widely available. The measures commonly obtained using these tools include blood flow, glucose metabolism, and oxygen consumption. Measures of neurotransmitter function have also been developed.

It has been known for nearly 20 years that PET and SPECT imaging reveals a fairly specific pattern of lateral temporoparietal and posterior cingulate hypometabolism or hypoperfusion in AD (Herholz et al., 2002; Jagust, Friedland, Budinger, Koss, & Ober, 1988) (Fig. 22.6). The presence of such a deficit in regional brain function is useful for the prediction of AD dementia in mildly symptomatic groups of subjects (such as MCI) (Chetelat et al., 2005; Johnson et al., 1998; Mosconi et al., 2005; Minoshima et al., 1997). Furthermore, in the proper clinical context, the spatial locations of functional impairment relate to the presence of AD pathology in the same regions (Buckner et al., 2005; Mega et al., 1999).

Molecular Imaging in the Differential Diagnosis of Neurodegenerative Diseases

The early detection and differential diagnosis of neurodegenerative disorders is a promising aim for further work using molecular

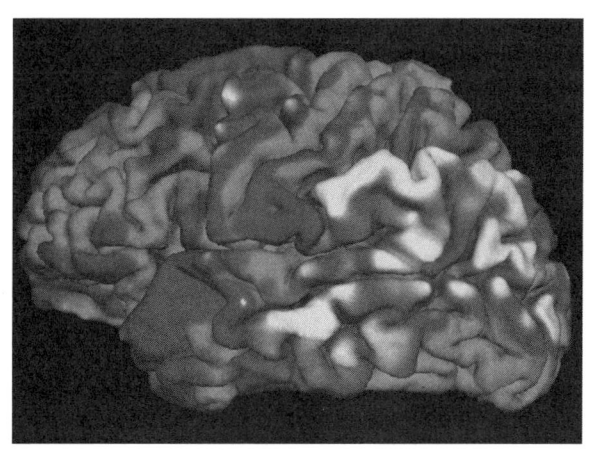

Figure 22.6 In mild Alzheimer's disease, cortical glucose metabolism is typically reduced in the temporoparietal region, as well as posterior midline and orbitofrontal regions. This now classic finding is useful clinically in differential diagnosis and may be valuable as an imaging biomarker for early detection of the metabolic signature of the disease in patients with minimal or no symptoms. This figure shows the largest reduction in metabolism in yellow, with lesser reductions in red hues from a single patient with mild AD, displayed on that patient's cortical surface as reconstructed from the anatomic magnetic resonance image. Areas without color exhibited normal metabolism compared to age-matched cognitively intact individuals. (See color plate section)

imaging. Since molecular imaging is sensitive to both the character and severity of symptoms, it seems reasonable to hope that its potential capability to detect alterations in the pattern and degree of regional brain activity may provide additional useful data to complement clinical and psychometric evaluations.

In elderly individuals with cognitive symptoms, it can be difficult to distinguish a neurodegenerative process from depression—molecular imaging may be helpful in this setting. In depression, the typical pattern of AD-related hypometabolism is not seen, but prefrontal or global hypometabolism may be seen (Guze et al., 1991). In patients with AD, those with depression have greater dorsolateral prefrontal hypometabolism, while those with apathy have greater orbitofrontal hypometabolism (Holthoff et al., 2005).

Furthermore, different forms of neurodegenerative dementias may be challenging to diagnose specifically early in their course. Molecular imaging may provide helpful data to assist in differential diagnosis of the dementias. In 2004, the US Centers for Medicare and Medicaid Services approved reimbursement of FDG-PET for the differential diagnosis of AD versus FTLD (Fig. 22.7), based largely on autopsy data relating AD pathology to FDG hypometabolism in temporoparietal association cortex (Hoffman et al., 2000; Silverman et al., 2001). In a clinicopathologic study, Jagust and colleagues (Jagust, Reed, Mungas, Ellis, & Decarli, 2007) demonstrated that FDG-PET improved upon the sensitivity and specificity of clinical diagnostic evaluation in predicting pathological diagnosis of AD. Foster and colleagues have performed a series of studies evaluating the practical value of FDG-PET in the diagnostic assessment of patients with dementia, with a particular emphasis on AD and FTLD, and also showed that FDG-PET improved upon clinical assessment with particular value in situations in which clinical diagnostic confidence was not high (Foster et al., 2007; Womack, 2011). For example, in one of these studies, six dementia experts independently reviewed the PET and clinical data and made diagnostic decisions, and the use of the PET pattern improved the accuracy of clinical diagnoses, particularly in cases in which there was uncertainty.

The differentiation of vascular dementia (VaD) from AD has been full of challenges not only in neuroimaging but also clinically and even pathologically. FDG-PET data have suggested that vascular dementia may be characterized most prominently by reductions in frontal metabolism and blood flow (Sultzer et al., 1995), but this finding has not been universal (Duara, Barker, Loewenstein, Pascal, & Bowen, 1989). And despite some of the differences that have been reported, there is significant overlap in the hypometabolic regions in AD and VaD. In the largest study to date seeking to differentiate VaD from AD using hypometabolic FDG-PET patterns,

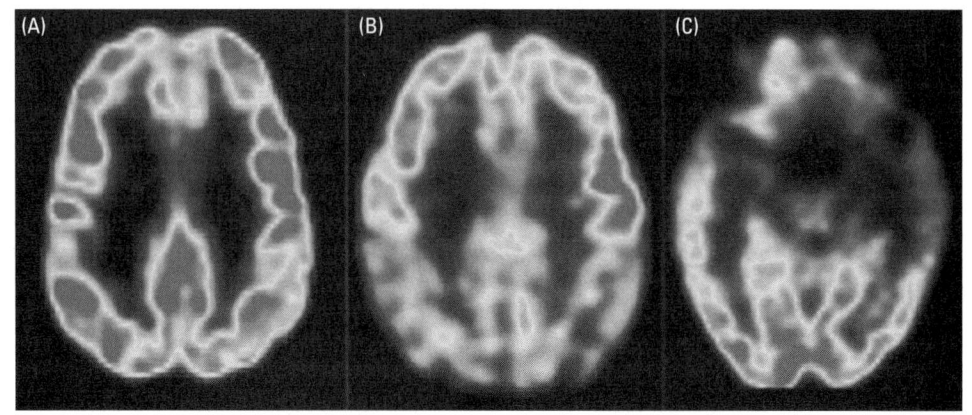

Figure 22.7 Fludeoxyglucose positron emission tomography (FDG-PET) can be very useful in the clinical evaluation of patients with dementia, particularly for the differentiation of Alzheimer's disease (AD) versus frontotemporal dementia (FTD). (A) Cognitively normal older adult; (B) mild AD dementia patient; (C) mild FTD dementia patient. (Images courtesy of Dr. Keith Johnson, Massachusetts General Hospital) (See color plate section)

principal component analysis was applied to 153 subjects and was able to differentiate the groups with 100% accuracy (Kerrouche, Herholz, Mielke, Holthoff, & Baron, 2006). The AD group showed the typical findings as described previously, but the VaD group showed hypometabolism in deep gray nuclei, cerebellum, primary cortices, middle temporal gyrus, and anterior cingulate gyrus.

Further insights into the utility of molecular imaging in assisting with differential diagnosis may potentially be gained through prospective studies of patients presenting for clinical evaluation with subtle symptoms consistent with a degenerative condition who do not yet have a clear clinical diagnosis. If such individuals are scanned and then followed clinically (and ultimately pathologically), it may be possible to learn more about the predictive power of molecular imaging in differential diagnosis (Herholz, 2003).

Molecular Imaging as a Biomarker for Monitoring or Prediction of Clinical Status

Longitudinal studies have shown that baseline PET and SPECT measures are useful for the prediction of future cognitive decline in AD patients (Jagust, Haan, Eberling, Wolfe, & Reed, 1996; Wolfe, Reed, Eberling, & Jagust, 1995) and the early detection of disease state in individuals with MCI (Arnaiz et al., 2001; Chetelat et al., 2003; Herholz et al., 1999; Johnson et al., 1998). Serial functional imaging studies have demonstrated that progressive metabolic decline correlates with cognitive decline in AD patients (Haxby et al., 1990; Jagust et al., 1988). Power calculations suggest that PET measures may be more sensitive than cognitive measures in a 1-year clinical drug trial (Alexander, Chen, Pietrini, Rapoport, & Reiman, 2002).

The Modulatory Effects of Genetic Risk Factors for Neurologic Disease on Brain Activity

In the last 15 years, there has been an explosion in literature on the basic science of genetic modulators of brain function (Hariri & Weinberger, 2003). This is an area that is ripe for study in neurologic disease, with a number of studies having been done in populations at elevated genetic risk for AD and other neurodegenerative disorders.

The *APOE* ε4 allele is a major genetic susceptibility factor associated with increased risk for AD (Saunders, 2000). A number of studies have demonstrated that cognitively intact subjects who are carriers of the *APOE* ε4 allele show evidence of temporo-parietal hypometabolism with a pattern similar to, but of milder severity, that of AD. In individuals in their 50s without cognitive decline, progressive metabolic decline has been observed in ε4 carriers after 2 years (Reiman et al., 2001). Intriguingly, this finding has been observed in carriers of the ε4 allele who are young, in their 20s and 30s (Reiman, 2007). Thus, it may be a lifelong vulnerability pattern (endophenotype) that mediates the risk effects of the gene, since it would be very unusual for young individuals to already have begun to accumulate AD pathology.

Tantalizing results are emerging from longitudinal studies with serial FDG-PET measures in subjects at elevated risk for clinical AD, but in whom symptoms are very mild or absent. Progressive metabolic abnormalities parallel cognitive decline in both older cognitively intact individuals (de Leon et al., 2001) and subjects with mild memory impairment who carry the APOE- ε4 allele (Small et al., 2000).

Uses of Molecular Imaging in Understanding and Monitoring Neurotherapeutics

Molecular imaging may be particularly valuable in evaluating acute and subacute effects of medications on neural activity. PET and SPECT measures of resting brain function appear to be sensitive to medication effects in clinical drug trials and relate to clinical measures in a manner that suggests their potential utility as surrogate markers. In four studies of cerebral metabolism or perfusion in AD patients given cholinesterase inhibitors, these functional brain measures parallel clinical measures in demonstrating stability or improvement in treated versus placebo groups or in predicting response in treated patients (Mega et al., 2001; Nakano, Asada, Matsuda, Uno, & Takasaki, 2001; Nobili et al., 2002; Tune et al., 2003).

Clinical Use of FDG-PET or SPECT in the Evaluation of Dementia Patients

Although the 2001 American Academy of Neurology practice parameter for the diagnostic evaluation of dementia did not recommend the use of FDG-PET or related techniques, citing the need for "further prospective studies... to establish the value that it brings to diagnosis over and above a competent clinical diagnosis" (Knopman et al., 2001, page 1147), a number of studies in the decade since then have provided clear evidence of added value in certain situations, as summarized previously and reviewed elsewhere in more detail (Bohnen, Djang, Herholz, Anzai, & Minoshima, 2012).

Nevertheless, FDG-PET faces several challenges in becoming more routinely used in the diagnosis of AD and related disorders. First, the clinician needs to be familiar with its utility and have access to a facility in which it is performed. Second, reimbursement for FDG-PET in the diagnostic evaluation of dementia or cognitive impairment needs to improve in the private sector; it is often particularly difficult (and sometimes impossible) to obtain authorization from private insurers for FDG-PET in patients younger than Medicare-eligible age, ironically the patients in whom it may be most useful. Finally, improved standardization of interpretation and quantification of FDG-PET scans is an important goal; a number of research groups are working on comparisons of different quantitative techniques and on comparisons of visual interpretation versus quantitative analysis, partly with the goal of incorporating FDG-PET into clinical trials.

Further research in clinical practice settings will be necessary to determine the best place for FDG-PET in relation to structural MRI, other forms of MRI, and spinal fluid markers of diseases causing cognitive impairment and dementia. Investigations of the comparative utility of FDG-PET versus amyloid PET imaging are badly needed. As these new tests become more widely available, practically oriented studies will contribute importantly to dialogue among neurologists aiming to balance diagnostic rigor with cost effectiveness.

Molecular Imaging of Pathologic Markers in Neurodegenerative Diseases

Radiochemistry research has led to the development of a class of tracers that specifically bind to amyloid plaques in mouse models of AD (Mathis et al., 2002), cross the blood–brain barrier, and label plaques in vivo in humans. The first such compound, known as Pittsburgh Compound B (PiB), was initially developed through rigorous studies in animal models of AD, human AD postmortem brain tissue, and in living healthy elderly subjects and patients with a clinical diagnosis of AD (Klunk et al., 2004).

PiB and other [18F] amyloid imaging tracers have now been tested extensively in living human subjects, including normal elderly and patients with the clinical diagnosis of mild probable AD. The absolute level of PiB retention is approximately the same in the cerebellum and white matter of AD patients and normal control subjects, brain areas known to lack substantial deposits of fibrillar amyloid. In contrast, PiB retention is very high in AD patients in frontal, temporal, and parietal neocortical regions (Klunk et al., 2004; Nordberg, 2007). As expected, PiB binding similar to AD is seen in some subjects with MCI (Forsberg et al., 2007), reflecting the presence of significant pathology even at this mild level of clinical impairment, as has also been seen in pathologic studies. However, many MCI subjects have intermediate or low levels of tracer uptake on amyloid imaging, reflecting clinical heterogeneity. PiB imaging has also confirmed what has long been known from postmortem studies (Tomlinson, Blessed, & Roth, 1968): Many elderly cognitively intact individuals carry a substantial burden of AD neuropathology (Mintun et al., 2006). Yet brain amyloid levels may plateau and remain fairly stable longitudinally in AD dementia (Engler et al., 2006). Thus, PET pathology markers may assist in diagnosis, but PET metabolic markers or MRI atrophy markers will likely be important for measuring changes in the rate of disease progression. Whether these findings will be useful in the prediction of the eventual development of AD dementia in nondemented individuals remains a topic of intense investigation. Nevertheless, amyloid imaging factors

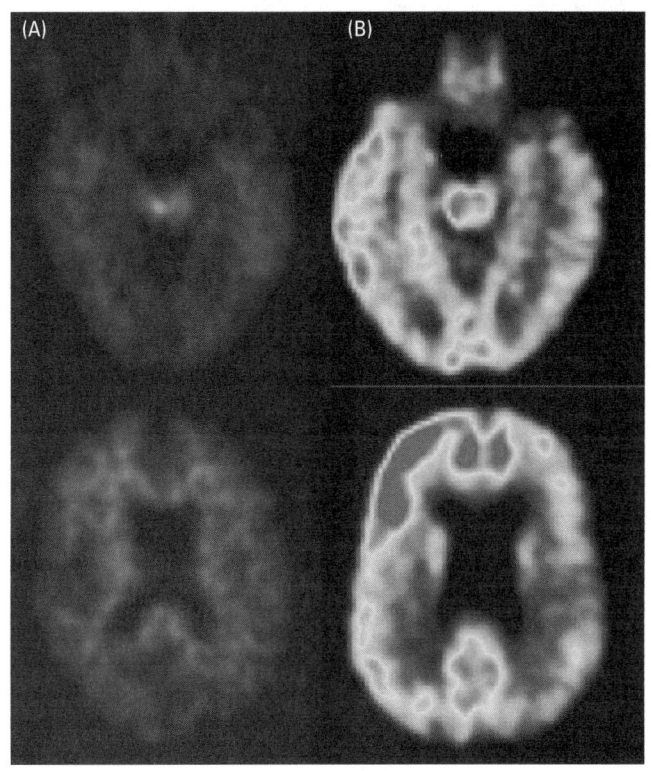

Figure 22.8 Amyloid positron emission tomography (PET) imaging is revolutionizing dementia research. Pittsburgh compound B (PiB) scan of (A) a cognitively intact 74-year-old adult demonstrates nonspecific binding ("negative"), while a scan of (B) a 73-year-old patient with mild Alzheimer's dementia shows robust signal throughout multiple cortical areas ("positive"). (Images courtesy of Dr. Keith Johnson, Massachusetts General Hospital) (See color plate section)

prominently in the revised diagnostic criteria for MCI and particularly for preclinical AD, as discussed in Chapter 2 (Fig. 22.8).

The successful visualization of direct markers of AD neuropathology in living humans is a major step forward in the field, and it suggests that more specific in vivo diagnostic and monitoring capabilities may be on the horizon. Furthermore, initial studies comparing AD and FTD patients suggest that it may be possible to differentiate neurodegenerative diseases using specific tracers that bind to pathologic proteins (Rabinovici et al., 2007), rather than indirectly through the effects of the diseases on brain function and structure.

In a recent study (Rabinovici et al., 2012), 107 patients with early-onset AD or FTLD, 12 with known histopathology, underwent both FDG-PET and amyloid PET with PiB. Images were classified as either AD-like or FTLD-like with a pair of blinded qualitative, visual reads and also with quantitative measures of tracer uptake and cut point thresholds of abnormality. Quantitatively, FDG-PET was AD-like if tracer uptake was more abnormal in temporoparietal than in either frontal or temporal FTLD-vulnerable regions and was FTLD-like if metabolism was worse in the FTLD-vulnerable areas. PiB PET was AD-like if it exceeded a threshold that was based on the mean of a PiB-negative normal control group. The authors report that PiB qualitative and quantitative readouts were virtually identical, which is consistent with the very large difference in the amount of tracer retained after 90 minutes in most amyloid-positive patients compared to most amyloid-negative patients. In contrast, FDG specificity was substantially improved by the quantitative readout compared to the visual readout, similar to a previous report (Foster, 2007).

These data are convincing that the presence or absence of AD neuropathology in these two dementias can be determined by the use of PiB, and that PiB—whether read visually or analyzed quantitatively—is also highly sensitive to the clinical diagnosis of AD. FDG, on the other hand, may still play a very important role with its ability to improve specificity of the diagnosis of AD (i.e., in this case to identify FTLD). The authors point out that the use of FDG in clinical settings is less consistent than PiB with regard to interrater reliability, especially when a quantitative comparison with a group of normal subjects is not available. One unstated conclusion is that such quantitative FDG comparisons could improve clinical practice and should be more widely adopted. For example, a recent report focused on a different regional strategy for identifying FTLD-like FDG patterns, in which greater emphasis placed on anterior cingulate and anterior temporal regions resulted in greater accuracy (Womack, 2011). Thus, it is possible that the method used here underestimated the value of FDG in differential diagnosis of AD versus FTLD since a substantial proportion of patients with FTLD exhibit temporoparietal hypometabolism.

The authors are appropriately cautious about generalizing these conclusions to situations in which other confounding features, such as older age and vascular disease comorbidity, could play an important role. They also point out that amyloid imaging will likely have less value in differentiating AD from DLB since many DLB patients have relatively high uptake consistent with amyloid pathology (Gomperts et al., 2008) and in differentiating among amyloid-negative dementias.

In addition to use in differential diagnosis, imaging molecular tracers that bind to neuropathological constituents of AD and related disorders may be very useful in the burgeoning efforts to improve translational research between animal models and humans. However, a number of issues will need to be addressed as part of the validation of these methods as surrogate markers in clinical trials or practice. While visualization of a "signal of pathology" has been demonstrated, work is still in progress to refine quantitative metrics, harmonize the reporting standards, and determine the specificity of these measures. Finally, it is not yet clear whether some prodromal or presymptomatic individuals with brain amyloid may remain relatively stable over time, which would challenge the value of these markers for prognostication at the individual level.

Further research will be necessary to determine the best place for amyloid PET in relation to FDG-PET, MRI, spinal fluid analysis, and other tests in the sequence of steps recommended for the diagnostic evaluation of patients with dementia, which will likely vary depending on the setting and the goals. An international committee of experts recently published "appropriate use" guidelines for the clinical use of amyloid PET imaging in the evaluation of patients with cognitive impairment (Johnson et al., 2013a, 2013b) (see Table 22.1). This consensus greatly restricts the recommended usage of amyloid PET imaging to specific scenarios with an emphasis on clinically uncertain dementia cases in whom AD is a possible diagnosis.

Exciting new tracers have very recently been developed for putatively measuring brain tau aggregates (Chien et al., 2013; Fodero-Tavoletti et al., 2011; Maruyama et al., 2013; Small et al., 2006). Work is currently ongoing to validate these ligands against postmortem tissue autoradiography as well as in patient populations highly likely to harbor brain tau pathology, such as *MAPT* mutation carriers or patients with a classical PSP clinical syndrome.

Clinical Use of Molecular Neuropathology Imaging in the Evaluation of Dementia Patients

The US Food and Drug Administration has approved amyloid PET imaging in the evaluation of dementia, starting with [18F] florbetapir in April 2012. The European Medicines Agency's Committee for Medicinal Products for Human Use similarly recommended approval for this ligand in October 2012. Although it remains unclear whether major reimbursement agencies will decide to pay for clinical use of amyloid imaging, it is now available and beginning to be used. As mentioned previously, the Amyloid Imaging Task (AIT) Force, a joint effort of the Society for Nuclear Medicine and Molecular Imaging and the Alzheimer's Association, has published two papers addressing the

TABLE 22.1 Appropriate Use of Amyloid Imaging in Clinical Practice

Appropriate In patients in whom (1) a cognitive complaint with objectively confirmed impairment is present; (2) AD is a possible diagnosis, but when the diagnosis is uncertain after a comprehensive evaluation by a dementia expert; and (3) when knowledge of the presence or absence of amyloid pathology is expected to increase diagnostic certainty and alter management.	Patients with persistent or progressive unexplained MCI Patients satisfying core clinical criteria for possible AD because of unclear clinical presentation, either an atypical clinical course or an etiologically mixed presentation Patients with progressive dementia and atypically early age of onset (usually defined as 65 years or less in age)
Inappropriate	Patients with core clinical criteria for probable AD with typical age of onset To determine dementia severity Based solely on a positive family history of dementia or presence of apolipoprotein E (APOE) ε4 Patients with a cognitive complaint that is unconfirmed on clinical examination In lieu of genotyping for suspected autosomal mutation carriers In asymptomatic individuals Nonmedical use (e.g., legal, insurance coverage, or employment screening)

AD, Alzheimer's disease; MCI, mild cognitive impairment.

most important issues related to the use of this class of biomarkers in clinical practice. Interested readers are encouraged to refer to those primary articles (Johnson et al., 2013a, 2013b).

In summary, the group pointed out some of the limitations of amyloid imaging, including the possibility that a "positive" scan may be purely incidental given the age-related increase in cerebral amyloid in cognitively normal older adults. In addition, they pointed out that a positive scan can be seen in conditions other than AD, including DLB and CAA. Probably most important, the group highlighted the need to consider the results of amyloid imaging in the context of the comprehensive evaluation of a patient with cognitive impairment and/or dementia, including other biomarkers and elements of the clinical profile. Questions were also raised about the potential psychological and social implications of a positive amyloid scan, which have received very little formal investigation.

Ultimately, the hope of the AIT is that amyloid imaging will be used in this context by dementia experts to achieve a number of important goals, including greater physician confidence in the diagnosis of or exclusion of AD. Hopefully, this will result in improved comprehensive management, including pharmacotherapy and education of the patient and family about prognosis. Furthermore, amyloid imaging may help to reduce the use of additional and repeated tests. Most important, the continued investigation of amyloid imaging in practice is warranted.

Cerebrospinal Fluid Biomarkers

Although major efforts are under way to explore cerebrospinal fluid (CSF) samples from patients with a variety of dementias to try to identify new biomarkers (Hu et al., 2010), one set of biomarkers is now mature enough to be relatively widely used clinically in the evaluation of dementia patients to determine whether they exhibit underlying CSF indicators of AD pathology. These measures are amyloid-β 1-42 peptide (Aβ 1-42), total tau (t-tau), and tau phosphorylated at threonine 181 (p-tau). A number of studies have demonstrated the utility of these measures for identifying patients who appear to have underlying AD pathobiology (Blennow, Hampel, Weiner, & Zetterberg, 2010). One foundational study demonstrated that, when particular cutoffs for these measures are used, Aβ 1-42 has a sensitivity of 96% and a specificity of 77% for detection of AD pathology in patients followed to autopsy. T-tau and p-tau performed with sensitivities of 70% and 69% and with specificities of 92% and 73%, respectively (Shaw et al., 2009). An assay of this type is now commercially available and CSF can be sent for analysis for clinical diagnostic purposes (Fig. 22.9). An increasing number of neurologists are now including CSF as a diagnostic test in the evaluation of dementia patients (Herskovits & Growdon, 2010).

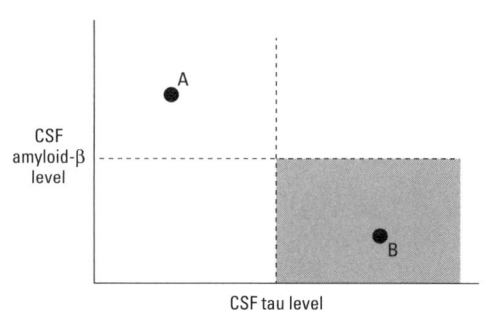

Figure 22.9 Cerebrospinal fluid (CSF) biomarkers are playing an increasing role in the evaluation of dementia patients. Currently, the primary biomarkers used in clinical practice are Alzheimer's disease (AD)-related measures of amyloid-β, total tau, and phospho-tau. This graph illustrates results from two cases. Case A has levels of both proteins that are within the normal range (relatively high amyloid-β and relatively low tau). Case B has levels of both proteins that are within the range associated with AD pathology (plaques and tangles) based on postmortem studies. The other quadrants are more difficult to interpret, although it appears that amyloid-β levels decline prior to the elevation of tau levels, at least in some cases, so an individual in the lower left quadrant may be in the early cerebral amyloidosis phase of the biological process of AD. An individual in the upper right quadrant would have elevated levels of tau with normal levels of amyloid-β, suggesting the possibility of a non-amyloid-associated tauopathy. The interpretation of data from both of these latter two quadrants is challenging and warrants further clinical investigation.

Genetic Testing

Genetic testing is often thought of as informing family members of patients with a dementia of their own potential risk for dementia. Although this is a potential goal of genetic testing in relatives of dementia patients, a much more clinically relevant goal is to assist in the diagnosis of the dementia patient. In this setting, it is typically thought of as being of potential utility in patients with strong family histories of similar dementias. For example, there are rare families with early-onset familial AD in whom multiple members of the family develop AD dementia at an early age (often 40s or 50s). The genetic mutation in these families typically involves the amyloid precursor protein (*APP*) gene on chromosome 21, or one of the presenilin (*PSEN*) genes on chromosome 1 or 14, with *PSEN1* being by far the most common.

A case example (Case 1) from my practice was a 39-year-old woman who presented with 2-year history of gradually progressive dementia primarily involving executive function with the lesser involvement of memory. Her father had been diagnosed clinically with "Pick's disease" with a dementia onset in his early 50s and death at age 57. No autopsy had been performed. Workup of the patient revealed neuropsychological evidence of executive dysfunction and an acquisition-retrieval memory deficit with a lesser effect on storage, prominent parietal atrophy with a lesser degree of medial temporal atrophy on high-resolution MRI, and temporoparietal hypometabolism on FDG-PET (Fig. 22.10). At the time she was evaluated, amyloid imaging was not yet available and we had not yet incorporated CSF analysis into our practice. Given the family history of early-onset dementia and the lack of clarity in her diagnosis, we performed genetic testing and identified a *PSEN1* mutation. Autopsy revealed AD pathology.

This case illustrates the potential diagnostic value of genetic testing, which in this case provided confirmation of my suspicion that she had early-onset AD and that her father likely had the same condition. Thus, genetic testing for diagnostic purposes provided confirmation that the molecular etiology of her dementia was highly likely to be AD, since the genetic mutation was known to be a pathogenic mutation leading to AD. This was further confirmed on pathologic analysis.

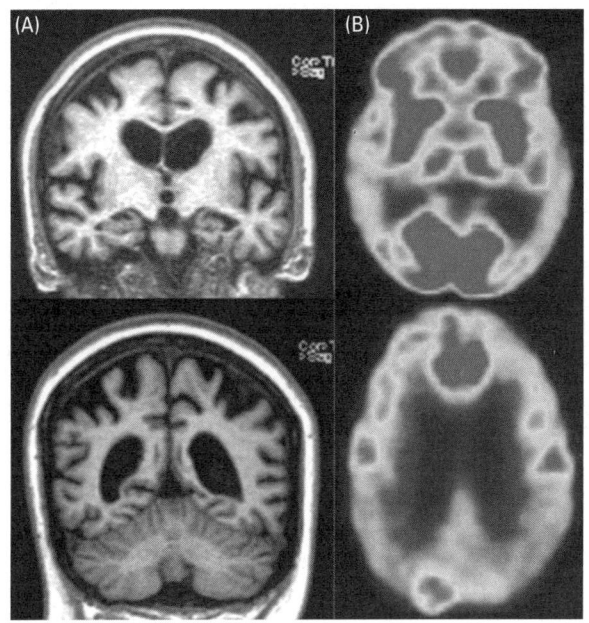

Figure 22.10 Case 1. Magnetic resonance imaging (MRI) and positron emission tomography (PET) often provide a reasonably convincing set of biomarkers in early-onset or atypical dementia patient evaluations. In this 39-year-old woman with familial dementia initially thought to be frontotemporal dementia, (A) an MRI scan showed relatively mild medial temporal lobe atrophy but prominent bilateral parietal atrophy, and (B) a fludeoxyglucose positron emission tomography (FDG-PET) scan showed prominent bilateral temporoparietal hypometabolism, supporting the diagnosis of Alzheimer's disease (AD). She was later found to carry a *PSEN1* mutation and ultimately was determined to have AD pathology at autopsy. (See color plate section)

The other genetic tests relevant at present for early-onset dementia are those for frontotemporal lobar degeneration: the microtubule associated protein tau (*MAPT*), progranulin (*GRN*), and the hexanucleotide repeat expansion on chromosome 9 (*C9ORF72*) (see Chapter 8 for more information). In some cases in which there is a clinical diagnosis of FTD and a strong family history of a similar condition, the test can be used for diagnostic purposes to confirm the molecular etiology. In other cases, there may be an unclear family history, or even the lack of a family history, and genetic testing may still reveal a pathogenic mutation. A recently published study from a large cohort at the University of Pennsylvania proposed a valuable algorithm for assigning probabilities of genetic abnormalities based on family history information (Wood et al., 2013). For example, I followed a very young man with behavioral-variant FTD—symptom onset age 28, death age 33—who lacked a family history of any form of dementia but was determined to have a *MAPT* mutation (Fig. 22.11). Our approach, similar to that described in the algorithm cited, is to perform genetic testing on any young patient with dementia regardless of family history. In the case presented here, it is thought that this mutation was possibly inherited but nonpenetrant in a parent or possibly de novo in the patient. Similar cases have been reported previously.

While the search continues for novel genes associated with AD, FTD, and other dementias, it is currently possible to test for several known genes. I typically test for these genetic mutations in patients in whom there is a family history of dementia (often unclear due to lack of precise diagnosis in prior generations) or in whom the onset is young, which is a similar approach to what others have recommended. Several articles serve as excellent references for the approach to clinical genetic testing in dementia (Goldman et al., 2004, 2011; Williamson, Goldman, & Marder, 2009). In our group, such testing is usually done

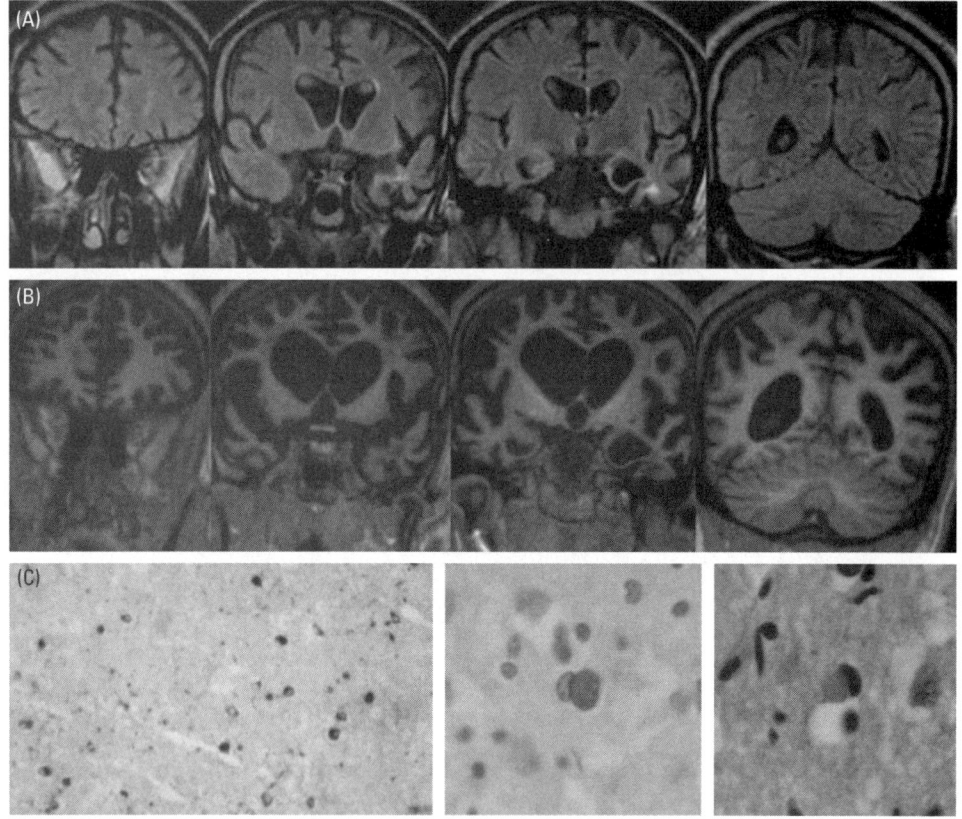

Figure 22.11 Case 2. Serial magnetic resonance imaging (MRI) scans 3 years apart show rapid progression of frontotemporal atrophy in this 31-year-old man who died of frontotemporal dementia at age 33. (A) A series of coronal FLAIR MRI images demonstrates left greater than right temporal lobe atrophy at a time when symptoms were clearly present but overall function was mildly impaired. (B) A similar series of coronal T1-weighted MRI images demonstrates marked progression of frontal, insular, and temporal atrophy with parietal involvement at a time when the patient was minimally communicative and dependent for most activities of daily living. (C) Postmortem histology demonstrated neuronal and glial cell loss with prominent tau immunohistochemical abnormalities (left), including Pick bodies (middle). The hematoxylin and eosin stained sections (right) also clearly demonstrated cellular inclusions typical of Pick-type tauopathy. (See color plate section)

after a discussion with our genetic counselor, who provides extensive education about the purpose of such testing as well as risks and benefits. Genetic testing for diagnostic purposes in symptomatic patients should be considered distinct from testing of asymptomatic individuals for the purposes of risk assessment.

Finally, apolipoprotein E (*APOE*) will be briefly discussed. The *APOE* ε4 allele has been known to be a major genetic risk factor for late-onset AD since 1993 (Saunders et al., 1993). Although expert consensus panels have recommended against testing for *APOE* genotype in asymptomatic individuals for risk assessment purposes (American College of Medical Genetics/American Society of Human Genetics, 1995; Post et al., 1997), some clinicians believe that testing of this gene has value in symptomatic patients for diagnostic purposes, since its presence or absence appears to modulate the clinical expression of AD as well as other dementias (Agosta et al., 2009; Wolk et al., 2010). Furthermore, *APOE* genotype may modulate response to or side effects from putative disease-modifying therapies, and in some clinical trials the dose is adjusted based on

APOE genotype (Salloway et al., 2009). The jury is still out on whether this information provides value in routine clinical settings, and additional study is needed.

The Combined Use of Multiple Biomarkers

The use of multiple biomarkers in combination will likely be of great value for identifying candidates for clinical trials. Nondemented mildly amnesic patients with clear abnormalities in two or more of the aforementioned biomarkers will probably be a strong candidate target population for clinical trials of disease-modifying therapies, as they will likely be at relatively high risk of progression to mild dementia within a few years. The analysis of multiple types of putative biomarkers has only recently begun, and to date it has been performed largely in patients with mild to moderate AD dementia. Several studies have been performed of brain structure and function, highlighting the brain regions in which atrophy and hypometabolism occur together as well as those in which there is a dissociation (Chetelat et al., 2008; De Santi et al., 2001; Mosconi et al., 2006). There are also data to suggest that the diagnostic utility of hippocampal volume in differentiating patients with MCI from controls is improved with the addition of CSF biomarker measures (de Leon et al., 2006), and that reduced parietal blood flow and abnormal CSF measures are useful together in predicting conversion to dementia in MCI patients (Hansson et al., 2007). Such initial forays into the territory of multibiomarker studies provides an optimistic perspective on the value of ongoing larger scale studies in which multiple data types are being collected for use in biomarker analyses, such as ADNI.

Based on results from several groups studying early-onset autosomal dominant forms of AD, it appears that combinations of biomarkers are likely going to be particularly useful for identifying and monitoring preclinical and prodromal phases of the disease. For example, results from the Dominantly Inherited Alzheimer's Initiative, while based on cross-sectional data, suggest that CSF amyloid-beta levels may begin to decrease as much as 25 years before expected onset, while cerebral amyloid can be detected by PET about 15 years prior to onset (Bateman et al., 2012). Increase CSF tau and brain atrophy could also be detected about 15 years prior to symptoms, while cerebral hypometabolism on PET could be detected about 10 years prior to symptoms. Although the precise number of years and the specific ordering of these markers will almost certainly change with continued research, our understanding of the pathophysiologic process of AD (and likely similarly for other neurodegenerative diseases) will be greatly increased through natural history studies of multimodal biomarkers. Ultimately, treatment at the preclinical stage will hinge in multiple ways on these measures (Langbaum et al., 2013).

Beyond Exclusion: The Use of Imaging and Biofluid Disease Biomarkers

At present, the potential efficacy of disease-modifying therapies for AD and other neurodegenerative diseases is evaluated primarily using clinical measures of cognition, movement, and other behaviors, but this is shifting in recent years to include increasing information from biomarkers. Although the efficacy of disease-modifying treatments for AD and other neurodegenerative diseases must ultimately be demonstrated using clinically meaningful outcome measures such as the slowing of decline in progression of symptoms or functional impairment, such trials will likely require hundreds of patients studied for a minimum of 1–2 years. Thus, surrogate markers of efficacy with less variability than clinical assessments are desperately needed to reduce the number of subjects. These markers may also prove particularly valuable in the early phases of drug development to detect a preliminary "signal of efficacy" over a shorter time period.

Since the pathophysiologic process underlying cognitive decline in AD and other neurodegenerative diseases involves the progressive degeneration of particular brain regions, repeatable in vivo neuroimaging measures of brain anatomy, chemistry, physiology, and pathology hold promise as an important class of potential biomarkers (DeKosky & Marek, 2003). A growing body of data indicates that the natural history of gradually progressive cognitive decline in AD can be reliably related to changes in such imaging measures. Furthermore, regionally specific changes in brain anatomy, chemistry, physiology, and pathology can be detected by imaging and CSF and other biomarkers prior to the point at which the disease is symptomatic enough to make a typical clinical diagnosis. Thus, potential disease-modifying therapies may act by impeding the accumulation of neuropathology, slowing the loss of neurons, altering neurochemistry, or preserving synaptic function; biomarkers exist to measure each of these putative therapeutic goals.

As advances in research provide data to support the use of specific biomarkers, it becomes apparent that these measures could be useful in diagnosis, and eventually may find applications in routine clinical practice. As neurologic diagnosis of neurodegenerative diseases moves beyond the simple use of imaging for the exclusion of mass lesions or other "potentially reversible" causes of dementia or other symptoms, these tools will become increasingly more important in routine practice (Scheltens, Fox, Barkhof, & De Carli, 2002). The American Academy of Neurology guidelines propose that a neuroimaging study should be performed in the workup of all cases of dementia (Knopman et al., 2001). An increasing number of diagnostic criteria sets, including AD, FTD, PPA, DLB, and cerebrovascular dementias, are including neuroimaging or other biomarker evidence as a core or supportive component (Albert et al., 2011; Dubois, Burn, et al., 2007; Dubois, Feldman, et al., 2007; Dubois et al., 2010; Gorno-Tempini et al., 2011; McKeith et al., 2005; McKhann et al., 2011; O'Brien et al., 2003; Rascovsky et al., 2007, 2011; Sperling et al., 2011). Thus, research motivated toward improving our understanding of the natural history of neurodegenerative diseases and toward the development of new therapies is also assisting in the translation of diagnostic tools from bench to beside.

Summarizing the Role of Biomarkers in My Current Clinical Practice

The evaluation of a patient with cognitive impairment or dementia is part of many dementia specialists' daily practice. Once it has been established that a patient has mild cognitive impairment (MCI) or dementia, our job is to determine the etiology. Why is this important? Although specific pharmacologic treatment options are still limited at present for most dementias, there are a growing number of clinical trials in which patients may participate. Furthermore, it is imperative for the specialist clinician to guide a comprehensive approach to the treatment of cognitive impairment and dementia, including management of behavioral symptoms; programs and strategies to optimize functional independence; caregiver education and support; and assistance with prognostication, planning, and connection with specific resources to assist with these issues.

All the new diagnostic criteria sets for various dementias that have recently been published—AD (McKhann et al., 2011), bvFTD (Rascovsky et al., 2011), PPA (Gorno-Tempini et al., 2011), vascular cognitive impairment (Gorelick et al., 2011)—emphasize the value of structural and functional/molecular neuroimaging, as well as CSF markers, in increasing diagnostic confidence or specificity. Although these criteria were in large part aimed at the clinical research communities studying these diseases, they also serve as guidance for practicing clinicians. These reports emphasize elements that can be summarized as the practitioner's two major goals: (1) start by establishing a diagnostic hypothesis based on a careful clinical evaluation emphasizing history and examination (including office-based cognitive testing that may be supplemented with formal neuropsychological testing); (2) perform diagnostic testing judiciously to test this hypothesis.

For most clinicians, the first diagnostic test in a patient with cognitive impairment is a brain MRI. In many patients with a presentation that is prototypical for a specific neurodegenerative disease, this test and a few other tests (e.g., thyroid testing, vitamin B12) may be all that is necessary to establish a confident diagnosis. For example, multiple studies have shown that the original 1984 diagnostic criteria for AD, which advocate essentially this approach, demonstrate a sensitivity and specificity of approximately 81% and 70%, respectively (Knopman et al., 2001).

Yet there are many patients in whom the diagnosis is still uncertain after this information has been obtained. In my opinion, the clinician faced with this situation should strongly consider using additional relatively new diagnostic testing to further evaluate

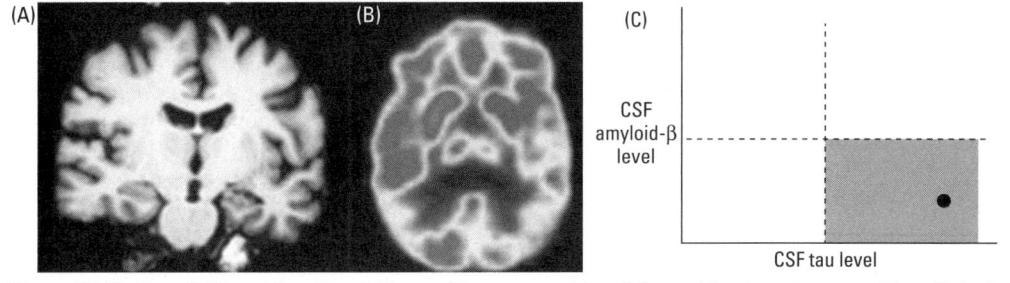

Figure 22.12 Case 3. Biomarkers in a 54-year-old woman with mild cognitive impairment with a clinical presentation suggestive of frontotemporal dementia. (A) Magnetic resonance imaging (MRI) showed a hint of hippocampal atrophy unilaterally but was otherwise normal. (B) Fludeoxyglucose positron emission tomography (FDG-PET) demonstrated bilateral (left greater than right) temporoparietal hypometabolism suggestive of Alzheimer's disease (AD) pathobiology. (C) Cerebrospinal fluid biomarkers were strongly consistent with AD pathobiology. (See color plate section)

the patient: molecular neuroimaging with FDG-PET and/or a spinal fluid examination for amyloid-β and tau proteins. For example, a patient presenting in her 50s or 60s with a syndrome of executive or language impairment and a relatively unrevealing MRI scan can be challenging to confidently diagnose. In such patients, I find FDG-PET to be an extremely valuable next step in the diagnostic evaluation, since it is minimally invasive and may provide a clear indication of whether the patient has a hypometabolic pattern consistent with atypical AD as opposed to a pattern supportive of FTD or another neurodegenerative disease. I often perform CSF analysis at this stage depending on the patient's willingness to undergo or ability to tolerate a lumbar puncture. Amyloid imaging may become a key element of this stage of the diagnostic evaluation but has largely not entered center stage due to reimbursement issues.

As a final case example (Case 3), a 54-year-old woman presented after having difficulty in her job as a psychologist and was found to have a flat affect, mild executive dysfunction, and limited insight with preserved language, memory, and visuospatial skills. At initial assessment her clinical status was consistent with MCI given relative preservation of social and occupational function, although some aspects of her job performance had begun to suffer. She was referred to me with a presumptive diagnosis of bvFTD. However, MRI was relatively unrevealing with possible subtle atrophy of the MTL and parietal cortex (Fig. 22.12). I obtained an FDG-PET to attempt to maximize my confidence given the value of a confident diagnosis for her prognosis as well as treatment considerations. Temporoparietal hypometabolism was demonstrated, suggesting an atypical form of AD. To confirm this suspicion, I obtained CSF, which demonstrated an amyloid/tau profile consistent with AD. I began treatment with donepezil and added memantine as her impairments progressed, and began discussions of AD clinical trials. She and her family were also referred to the Alzheimer's Association for assistance with planning and support. I believe that the confident diagnosis was particularly helpful for her family to proactively adapt to her gradual loss of independent function in a fashion that has continued to afford her a reasonably high quality of life, now 4 years later into the phase of mild-to-moderate AD dementia.

Acknowledgments

This chapter was written with support from the National Institute on Aging (R01-AG029411), National Institute for Neurological Disorders and Stroke (R21-NS077059, R21-NS079905, R21-NS084156), and National Institute of Mental Health (R21-MH097094).

References

Agosta, F., Vossel, K. A., Miller, B. L., Migliaccio, R., Bonasera, S. J., Filippi, M.,...Gorno-Tempini, M. L. (2009). Apolipoprotein E epsilon4 is associated with disease-specific effects on brain atrophy in Alzheimer's disease and frontotemporal dementia. *Proceedings of the National Academy of Science USA, 106,* 2018–2022.

Albert, M. S., DeKosky, S. T., Dickson, D., Dubois, B., Feldman, H. H., Fox, N. C.,...Phelps C. H. (2011). The diagnosis of mild cognitive impairment due to Alzheimer's disease: Recommendations from the National Institute on Aging-Alzheimer's Association workgroups on diagnostic guidelines for Alzheimer's disease. *Alzheimers and Dementia, 7*, 270–279.

Alexander, G. E., Chen, K., Pietrini, P., Rapoport, S. I., & Reiman, E. M. (2002). Longitudinal PET evaluation of cerebral metabolic decline in dementia: A potential outcome measure in Alzheimer's disease treatment studies. *American Journal of Psychiatry, 159*, 738–745.

Alsop, D. C., Casement, M., de Bazelaire, C., Fong, T., & Press, D. Z. (2008). Hippocampal hyperperfusion in Alzheimer's disease. *Neuroimage, 42*, 1267–1274.

American College of Medical Genetics/American Society of Human Genetics. (1995). Statement on use of apolipoprotein E testing for Alzheimer disease. American College of Medical Genetics/American Society of Human Genetics Working Group on ApoE and Alzheimer disease. *Journal of the American Medical Association, 274*, 1627–1629.

Arnaiz, E., Jelic, V., Almkvist, O., Wahlund, L. O., Winblad, B., Valind, S., & Nordberg, A. (2001). Impaired cerebral glucose metabolism and cognitive functioning predict deterioration in mild cognitive impairment. *Neuroreport, 12*, 851–855.

Ashburner, J., Csernansky, J. G., Davatzikos, C., Fox, N. C., Frisoni, G. B., & Thompson, P. M. (2003). Computer-assisted imaging to assess brain structure in healthy and diseased brains. *Lancet Neurology, 2*, 79–88.

Bakkour, A., Morris, J. C., & Dickerson, B. C. (2009). The cortical signature of prodromal AD: Regional thinning predicts mild AD dementia. *Neurology, 72*, 1048–1055.

Bakkour, A., Morris, J. C., Wolk, D. A., & Dickerson, B. C. (2013). The effects of aging and Alzheimer's disease on cerebral cortical anatomy: Specificity and differential relationships with cognition. *Neuroimage, 76*, 332–344.

Bateman, R. J., Xiong, C., Benzinger, T. L., Fagan, A. M., Goate, A., Fox, N. C.,...Morris, J. C. (2012). Clinical and biomarker changes in dominantly inherited Alzheimer's disease. *New England Journal of Medicine, 367*, 795–804.

Beason-Held, L. L., Kraut, M. A., & Resnick, S. M. (2008). I. Longitudinal changes in aging brain function. *Neurobiology of Aging, 29*, 483–496.

Blennow, K., Hampel, H., Weiner, M., & Zetterberg, H. (2010). Cerebrospinal fluid and plasma biomarkers in Alzheimer disease. *Nature Reviews Neurology, 6*, 131–144.

Bobinski, M., de Leon, M. J., Wegiel, J., Desanti, S., Convit, A., Saint Louis, L. A.,...Wisniewski, H. M. (2000). The histological validation of post mortem magnetic resonance imaging-determined hippocampal volume in Alzheimer's disease. *Neuroscience, 95*, 721–725.

Boccardi, M., Ganzola, R., Rossi, R., Sabattoli, F., Laakso, M. P., Repo-Tiihonen, E.,...Tiihonen, J. (2010). Abnormal hippocampal shape in offenders with psychopathy. *Human Brain Mapping, 31*, 438–447.

Bohnen, N. I., Djang, D. S., Herholz, K., Anzai, Y., & Minoshima, S. (2012). Effectiveness and safety of 18F-FDG PET in the evaluation of dementia: A review of the recent literature. *Journal of Nuclear Medicine, 53*, 59–71.

Bondi, M. W., Houston, W. S., Eyler, L. T., & Brown, G. G. (2005). fMRI evidence of compensatory mechanisms in older adults at genetic risk for Alzheimer disease. *Neurology, 64*, 501–508.

Bookheimer, S. Y., Strojwas, M. H., Cohen, M. S., Saunders, A. M., Pericak-Vance, M. A., Mazziotta, J. C., & Small, G. W. (2000). Patterns of brain activation in people at risk for Alzheimer's disease. *New England Journal of Medicine, 343*, 450–456.

Buckner, R. L., Snyder, A. Z., Shannon, B. J., LaRossa, G., Sachs, R., Fotenos, A. F.,...Mintun, M. A. (2005). Molecular, structural, and functional characterization of Alzheimer's disease: Evidence for a relationship between default activity, amyloid, and memory. *Journal of Neuroscience, 25*, 7709–7717.

Cabeza, R., Anderson, N. D., Locantore, J. K., & McIntosh, A. R. (2002). Aging gracefully: Compensatory brain activity in high-performing older adults. *Neuroimage, 17*, 1394–1402.

Callicott, J. H., Mattay, V. S., Verchinski, B. A., Marenco, S., Egan, M. F., & Weinberger, D. R. (2003). Complexity of prefrontal cortical dysfunction in schizophrenia: More than up or down. *American Journal of Psychiatry, 160*, 2209–2215.

Carey, J. R., Kimberley, T. J., Lewis, S. M., Auerbach, E. J., Dorsey, L., Rundquist, P., & Ugurbil, K. (2002). Analysis of fMRI and finger tracking training in subjects with chronic stroke. *Brain, 125*, 773–788.

Celone, K. A., Calhoun, V. D., Dickerson, B. C., Atri, A., Chua, E. F., Miller, S. L.,...Sperling, R. A. (2006). Alterations in memory networks in mild cognitive impairment and Alzheimer's disease: An independent component analysis. *Journal of Neuroscience, 26*, 10222–10231.

Chetelat, G., Desgranges, B., de la Sayette, V., Viader, F., Eustache, F., & Baron, J. C. (2003). Mild cognitive impairment: Can FDG-PET predict who is to rapidly convert to Alzheimer's disease? *Neurology, 60*, 1374–1377.

Chetelat, G., Desgranges, B., Landeau, B., Mezenge, F., Poline, J. B., de la Sayette, V.,...Baron, J. C. (2008). Direct voxel-based comparison between grey matter hypometabolism and atrophy in Alzheimer's disease. *Brain, 131*, 60–71.

Chetelat, G., Eustache, F., Viader, F., De La Sayette, V., Pelerin, A., Mezenge, F.,...Desgranges, B. (2005). FDG-PET measurement is more accurate than neuropsychological assessments to predict global cognitive deterioration in patients with mild cognitive impairment. *Neurocase, 11*, 14–25.

Chien, D. T., Bahri, S., Szardenings, A. K., Walsh, J. C., Mu, F., Su, M. Y.,...Kolb, H. C. (2013). Early clinical PET imaging results with the novel PHF-tau radioligand [F-18]-T807. *Journal of Alzheimers Disease, 34*, 457–468.

Cole, J., Toga, A. W., Hojatkashani, C., Thompson, P., Costafreda, S. G., Cleare, A. J.,...Fu, C. H. (2010). Subregional hippocampal deformations in major depressive disorder. *Journal of Affective Disorders, 126*, 272–277.

Convit, A., de Asis, J., de Leon, M. J., Tarshish, C. Y., De Santi, S., & Rusinek, H. (2000). Atrophy of the medial occipitotemporal, inferior, and middle temporal gyri in non-demented elderly predict decline to Alzheimer's disease. *Neurobiology of Aging, 21*, 19–26.

Csernansky, J. G., Wang, L., Jones, D., Rastogi-Cruz, D., Posener, J. A., Heydebrand, G.,...Miller, M. I. (2002). Hippocampal deformities in schizophrenia characterized by high dimensional brain mapping. *American Journal of Psychiatry, 159*, 2000–2006.

Csernansky, J. G., Wang, L., Joshi, S., Miller, J. P., Gado, M., Kido, D.,...Miller, M. I. (2000). Early DAT is distinguished from aging by high-dimensional mapping of the hippocampus. Dementia of the Alzheimer type. *Neurology, 55*, 1636–1643.

Cummings, J. L., Doody, R., & Clark, C. (2007). Disease-modifying therapies for Alzheimer disease: Challenges to early intervention. *Neurology, 69*, 1622–1634.

Dager, S. R., Wang, L., Friedman, S. D., Shaw, D. W., Constantino, J. N., Artru, A. A.,...Csernansky, J. G. (2007). Shape mapping of the hippocampus in young children with autism spectrum disorder. *American Journal of Neuroradiology, 28*, 672–677.

Das, S. R., Pluta, J., Mancuso, L., Kliot, D., Orozco, S., Dickerson, B. C.,...Wolk, D. A. (2013). Increased functional connectivity within medial temporal lobe in mild cognitive impairment. *Hippocampus, 23*, 1–6.

Davatzikos, C., Resnick, S. M., Wu, X., Parmpi, P., & Clark, C. M. (2008). Individual patient diagnosis of AD and FTD via high-dimensional pattern classification of MRI. *Neuroimage, 41*, 1220–1227.

de Leon, M. J., Convit, A., Wolf, O. T., Tarshish, C. Y., DeSanti, S., Rusinek, H.,...Fowler, J. (2001). Prediction of cognitive decline in normal elderly subjects with 2-[(18)F]fluoro-2-deoxy-D-glucose/poitron-emission tomography (FDG/PET). *Proceedings of the National Academy of Science USA, 98*, 10966–10971.

de Leon, M. J., DeSanti, S., Zinkowski, R., Mehta, P. D., Pratico, D., Segal, S.,...Davies, P. (2006). Longitudinal CSF and MRI biomarkers improve the diagnosis of mild cognitive impairment. *Neurobiology of Aging, 27*, 394–401.

de Leon, M. J., George, A. E., Golomb, J., Tarshish, C., Convit, A., Kluger, A.,...Wisniewski, H. M. (1997). Frequency of hippocampal formation atrophy in normal aging and Alzheimer's disease. *Neurobiology of Aging, 18*, 1–11.

De Santi, S., de Leon, M. J., Rusinek, H., Convit, A., Tarshish, C. Y., Roche, A.,...Fowler, J. (2001). Hippocampal formation glucose metabolism and volume losses in MCI and AD. *Neurobiology of Aging, 22*, 529–539.

de Toledo-Morrell, L., Dickerson, B., Sullivan, M. P., Spanovic, C., Wilson, R., & Bennett, D. A. (2000). Hemispheric differences in hippocampal volume predict verbal and spatial memory performance in patients with Alzheimer's disease. *Hippocampus, 10*, 136–142.

DeKosky, S. T., & Marek, K. (2003). Looking backward to move forward: Early detection of neurodegenerative disorders. *Science, 302*, 830–834.

Desmond, J. E., Chen, S. H., DeRosa, E., Pryor, M. R., Pfefferbaum, A., & Sullivan, E. V. (2003). Increased frontocerebellar activation in alcoholics during verbal working memory: An fMRI study. *Neuroimage, 19*, 1510–1520.

Dickerson, B. C., Bakkour, A., Salat, D. H., Feczko, E., Pacheco, J., Greve, D. N.,...Buckner, R. L. (2009). The cortical signature of Alzheimer's disease: Regionally specific cortical thinning relates to symptom severity in very mild to mild AD dementia and is detectable in asymptomatic amyloid-positive individuals. *Cerebral Cortex, 19*, 497–510.

Dickerson, B. C., Feczko, E., Augustinack, J. C., Pacheco, J., Morris, J. C., Fischl, B., & Buckner, R. L. (2007). Differential effects of aging and Alzheimer's disease on medial temporal lobe cortical thickness and surface area. *Neurobiology of Aging, 30*(3), 432–440.

Dickerson, B. C., Goncharova, I., Sullivan, M. P., Forchetti, C., Wilson, R. S., Bennett, D. A.,...deToledo-Morrell, L. (2001). MRI-derived entorhinal and hippocampal atrophy in incipient and very mild Alzheimer's disease. *Neurobiology of Aging, 22,* 747–754.

Dickerson, B. C., Salat, D. H., Greve, D. N., Chua, E. F., Rand-Giovannetti, E., Rentz, D. M.,...Sperling, R. A. (2005). Increased hippocampal activation in mild cognitive impairment compared to normal aging and AD. *Neurology, 65,* 404–411.

Dickerson, B. C., & Sperling, R. A. (2005). Neuroimaging biomarkers for clinical trials of disease-modifying therapies in Alzheimer's disease. *Neurorx, 2,* 348–360.

Dickerson, B. C., & Sperling, R. A. (2008). Functional abnormalities of the medial temporal lobe memory system in mild cognitive impairment and Alzheimer's disease: Insights from functional MRI studies. *Neuropsychologia, 46,* 1624–1635.

Dickerson, B. C., Stoub, T. R., Shah, R. C., Sperling, R. A., Killiany, R. J., Albert, M. S.,...Detoledo-Morrell, L. (2011). Alzheimer-signature MRI biomarker predicts AD dementia in cognitively normal adults. *Neurology, 76,* 1395–1402.

Drummond, S. P., Brown, G. G., Gillin, J. C., Stricker, J. L., Wong, E. C., & Buxton, R. B. (2000). Altered brain response to verbal learning following sleep deprivation. *Nature, 403,* 655–657.

Duara, R., Barker, W., Loewenstein, D., Pascal, S., & Bowen, B. (1989). Sensitivity and specificity of positron emission tomography and magnetic resonance imaging studies in Alzheimer's disease and multi-infarct dementia. *European Neurology, 29*(Suppl 3), 9–15.

Dubois, B., Burn, D., Goetz, C., Aarsland, D., Brown, R. G., Broe, G. A.,...Emre, M. (2007) Diagnostic procedures for Parkinson's disease dementia: Recommendations from the movement disorder society task force. *Movement Disorders, 22,* 2314–2324.

Dubois, B., Feldman, H. H., Jacova, C., Cummings, J. L., Dekosky, S. T., Barberger-Gateau, P.,...Scheltens, P. (2010). Revising the definition of Alzheimer's disease: A new lexicon. *Lancet Neurology, 9,* 1118–1127.

Dubois, B., Feldman, H. H., Jacova, C., Dekosky, S. T., Barberger-Gateau, P., Cummings, J.,...Scheltens, P. (2007). Research criteria for the diagnosis of Alzheimer's disease: Revising the NINCDS-ADRDA criteria. *Lancet Neurology, 6,* 734–746.

Engler, H., Forsberg, A., Almkvist, O., Blomquist, G., Larsson, E., Savitcheva, I.,...Nordberg, A. (2006). Two-year follow-up of amyloid deposition in patients with Alzheimer's disease. *Brain, 129,* 2856–2866.

Ernst, T., Chang, L., Jovicich, J., Ames, N., & Arnold, S. (2002). Abnormal brain activation on functional MRI in cognitively asymptomatic HIV patients. *Neurology, 59,* 1343–1349.

Filippi, M., Dousset, V., McFarland, H. F., Miller, D. H., & Grossman, R. I. (2002). Role of magnetic resonance imaging in the diagnosis and monitoring of multiple sclerosis: Consensus report of the White Matter Study Group. *Journal of Magnetic Resonance Imaging, 15,* 499–504.

Fleisher, A. S., Houston, W. S., Eyler, L. T., Frye, S., Jenkins, C., Thal, L. J., & Bondi, M. W. (2005). Identification of Alzheimer disease risk by functional magnetic resonance imaging. *Archives of Neurology, 62,* 1881–1888.

Fodero-Tavoletti, M. T., Okamura, N., Furumoto, S., Mulligan, R. S., Connor, A. R., McLean, C. A.,...Villemagne, V. L. (2011). 18F-THK523: A novel in vivo tau imaging ligand for Alzheimer's disease. *Brain, 134,* 1089–1100.

Forsberg, A., Engler, H., Almkvist, O., Blomquist, G., Hagman, G., Wall, A.,...Nordberg, A. (2007). PET imaging of amyloid deposition in patients with mild cognitive impairment. *Neurobiology of Aging, 29*(10), 1456–1465.

Foster, N. L., Heidebrink, J. L., Clark, C. M., Jagust, W. J., Arnold, S. E., Barbas, N. R.,...Minoshima, S. (2007). FDG-PET improves accuracy in distinguishing frontotemporal dementia and Alzheimer's disease. *Brain, 130,* 2616–2635.

Fox, N. C., Black, R. S., Gilman, S., Rossor, M. N., Griffith, S. G., Jenkins, L., & Koller, M. (2005). Effects of abeta immunization (AN1792) on MRI measures of cerebral volume in Alzheimer disease. *Neurology, 64,* 1563–1572.

Fox, N. C., Cousens, S., Scahill, R., Harvey, R. J., & Rossor, M. N. (2000). Using serial registered brain magnetic resonance imaging to measure disease progression in Alzheimer disease: Power calculations and estimates of sample size to detect treatment effects. *Archives of Neurology, 57,* 339–344.

Fox, N. C., & Schott, J. M. (2004). Imaging cerebral atrophy: Normal ageing to Alzheimer's disease. *Lancet, 363,* 392–394.

Frisoni, G. B., & Jack, C. R. (2011). Harmonization of magnetic resonance-based manual hippocampal segmentation: A mandatory step for wide clinical use. *Alzheimers and Dementia, 7,* 171–174.

Galton, C. J., Gomez-Anson, B., Antoun, N., Scheltens, P., Patterson, K., Graves, M.,...Hodges, J. R. (2001). Temporal lobe rating scale: Application to Alzheimer's disease and frontotemporal dementia. *Journal of Neurology, Neurosurgery and Psychiatry, 70,* 165–173.

Goldman, J. S., Farmer, J. M., Van Deerlin, V. M., Wilhelmsen, K. C., Miller, B. L., & Grossman, M. (2004). Frontotemporal dementia: Genetics and genetic counseling dilemmas. *Neurologist, 10,* 227–234.

Goldman, J. S., Rademakers, R., Huey, E. D., Boxer, A. L., Mayeux, R., Miller, B. L., & Boeve, B. F. (2011). An algorithm for genetic testing of frontotemporal lobar degeneration. *Neurology, 76,* 475–483.

Gomez-Isla, T., Price, J. L., McKeel, D. W., Jr., Morris, J. C., Growdon, J. H., & Hyman, B. T. (1996). Profound loss of layer II entorhinal cortex neurons occurs in very mild Alzheimer's disease. *Journal of Neuroscience, 16,* 4491–4500.

Gomperts, S. N., Rentz, D. M., Moran, E., Becker, J. A., Locascio, J. J., Klunk, W. E.,...Johnson, K. A. (2008). Imaging amyloid deposition in Lewy body diseases. *Neurology, 71,* 903–910.

Gorelick, P. B., Scuteri, A., Black, S. E., Decarli, C., Greenberg, S. M., Iadecola, C.,...Seshadri, S. (2011). Vascular contributions to cognitive impairment and dementia: A statement for healthcare professionals from the American Heart Association/American Stroke Association. *Stroke, 42,* 2672–2713.

Gorno-Tempini, M. L., Hillis, A. E., Weintraub, S., Kertesz, A., Mendez, M., Cappa, S. F.,...Grossman, M. (2011). Classification of primary progressive aphasia and its variants. *Neurology, 76,* 1006–1014.

Gosche, K. M., Mortimer, J. A., Smith, C. D., Markesbery, W. R., & Snowdon, D. A. (2002). Hippocampal volume as an index of Alzheimer neuropathology: Findings from the Nun Study. *Neurology, 58,* 1476–1482.

Greicius, M. D., Srivastava, G., Reiss, A. L., & Menon, V. (2004). Default-mode network activity distinguishes Alzheimer's disease from healthy aging: Evidence from functional MRI. *Proceedings of the National Academy of Science USA, 101,* 4637–4642.

Guze, B. H., Baxter, L. R., Jr., Schwartz, J. M., Szuba, M. P., Mazziotta, J. C., & Phelps, M. E. (1991). Changes in glucose metabolism in dementia of the Alzheimer type compared with depression: A preliminary report. *Psychiatry Research, 40,* 195–202.

Hamalainen, A., Pihlajamaki, M., Tanila, H., Hanninen, T., Niskanen, E., Tervo, S.,...Soininen, H. (2006). Increased fMRI responses during encoding in mild cognitive impairment. *Neurobiology of Aging, 28*(12), 1889–1903.

Hansson, O., Buchhave, P., Zetterberg, H., Blennow, K., Minthon, L., & Warkentin, S. (2007). Combined rCBF and CSF biomarkers predict progression from mild cognitive impairment to Alzheimer's disease. *Neurobiology of Aging.* Epub ahead of print.

Hariri, A. R., & Weinberger, D. R. (2003), Functional neuroimaging of genetic variation in serotonergic neurotransmission. *Genes Brain and Behavior, 2,* 341–349.

Haxby, J. V., Grady, C. L., Koss, E., Horwitz, B., Heston, L., Schapiro, M.,...Rapoport, S. I. (1990). Longitudinal study of cerebral metabolic asymmetries and associated neuropsychological patterns in early dementia of the Alzheimer type. *Archives of Neurology, 47,* 753–760.

Heo, S., Prakash, R. S., Voss, M. W., Erickson, K. I., Ouyang, C., Sutton, B. P., & Kramer, A. F. (2010). Resting hippocampal blood flow, spatial memory and aging. *Brain Research, 1315,* 119–127.

Herholz, K. (2003). PET studies in dementia. *Annals of Nuclear Medicine, 17,* 79–89.

Herholz, K., Nordberg, A., Salmon, E., Perani, D., Kessler, J., Mielke, R.,...Heiss, W. D. (1999). Impairment of neocortical metabolism predicts progression in Alzheimer's disease. *Dementia and Geriatric Cognitive Disorders, 10,* 494–504.

Herholz, K., Salmon, E., Perani, D., Baron, J. C., Holthoff, V., Frölich, L.,...Heiss, W. D. (2002). Discrimination between Alzheimer dementia and controls by automated analysis of multicenter FDG PET. *Neuroimage, 17,* 302–316.

Herskovits, A. Z., & Growdon, J. H. (2010). Sharpen that needle. *Archives of Neurology, 67,* 918–920.

Hoffman, J. M., Welsh-Bohmer, K. A., Hanson, M., Crain, B., Hulette, C., Earl, N., & Coleman, R. E. (2000). FDG PET imaging in patients with pathologically verified dementia. *Journal of Nuclear Medicine, 41,* 1920–1928.

Hogan, R. E., Wang, L., Bertrand, M. E., Willmore, L. J., Bucholz, R. D., Nassif, A. S., & Csernansky, J. G. (2004). MRI-based high-dimensional hippocampal mapping in mesial temporal lobe epilepsy. *Brain, 127,* 1731–1740.

Holthoff, V. A., Beuthien-Baumann, B., Kalbe, E., Ludecke, S., Lenz, O., Zundorf, G.,...Herholz, K. (2005). Regional cerebral metabolism in early Alzheimer's disease with clinically significant apathy or depression. *Biological Psychiatry, 57,* 412–421.

Hu, W. T., Chen-Plotkin, A., Arnold, S. E., Grossman, M., Clark, C. M., Shaw, L. M.,...Trojanowski, J. Q. (2010). Novel CSF biomarkers for Alzheimer's disease and mild cognitive impairment. *Acta Neuropathologica, 119,* 669–678.

Jack, C. R., Jr., Albert, M., Knopman, D. S., McKhann, G. M., Sperling, R. A., Carrillo, M. C.,...Phelps, C. H. (2011). Introduction to revised criteria for the diagnosis of Alzheimer's disease: National Institute on Aging and the Alzheimer's Association workgroup. *Alzheimers and Dementia, 7*(3), 257–262.

Jack, C. R., Jr., Dickson, D. W., Parisi, J. E., Xu, Y. C., Cha, R. H., O'Brien, P. C.,...Petersen, R. C. (2002). Antemortem MRI findings correlate with hippocampal neuropathology in typical aging and dementia. *Neurology, 58,* 750–757.

Jack, C. R., Jr., Gehring, D. G., Sharbrough, F. W., Felmlee, J. P., Forbes, G., Hench, V. S., & Zinsmeister, A. R. (1988). Temporal lobe volume measurement from MR images: Accuracy and left-right asymmetry in normal persons. *Journal of Computer Assisted Tomography, 12,* 21–29.

Jack, C. R., Jr., Knopman, D. S., Jagust, W. J., Petersen, R. C., Weiner, M. W., Aisen, P. S.,...Trojanowski, J. Q. (2013). Tracking pathophysiological processes in Alzheimer's disease: An updated hypothetical model of dynamic biomarkers. *Lancet Neurology, 12,* 207–216.

Jack, C. R., Jr., Knopman, D. S., Jagust, W. J., Shaw, L. M., Aisen, P. S., Weiner, M. W.,...Trojanowski, J. Q. (2010). Hypothetical model of dynamic biomarkers of the Alzheimer's pathological cascade. *Lancet Neurology, 9,* 119–128.

Jack, C. R., Jr., Mokri, B., Laws, E. R., Jr., Houser, O. W., Baker, H. L., Jr., & Petersen, R. C. (1987). MR findings in normal-pressure hydrocephalus: Significance and comparison with other forms of dementia. *Journal of Computer Assisted Tomography, 11,* 923–931.

Jack, C. R., Jr., Petersen, R. C., O'Brien, P. C., & Tangalos, E. G. (1992). MR-based hippocampal volumetry in the diagnosis of Alzheimer's disease. *Neurology, 42,* 183–188.

Jack, C. R., Jr., Petersen, R. C., Xu, Y. C., O'Brien, P. C., Smith, G. E., Ivnik, R. J.,...Kokmen, E. (1999). Prediction of AD with MRI-based hippocampal volume in mild cognitive impairment. *Neurology, 52,* 1397–1403.

Jack, C. R., Jr., Twomey, C. K., Zinsmeister, A. R., Sharbrough, F. W., Petersen, R. C., & Cascino, G. D. (1989). Anterior temporal lobes and hippocampal formations: Normative volumetric measurements from MR images in young adults. *Radiology, 172,* 549–554.

Jack, C. R., Jr., Weigand, S. D., Shiung, M. M., Przybelski, S. A., O'Brien, P. C., Gunter, J. L.,...Petersen, R. C. (2007). Atrophy rates accelerate in amnestic mild cognitive impairment. *Neurology.* Epub ahead of print.

Jagust, W. J., Friedland, R. P., Budinger, T. F., Koss, E., & Ober, B. (1988). Longitudinal studies of regional cerebral metabolism in Alzheimer's disease. *Neurology, 38,* 909–912.

Jagust, W. J., Haan, M. N., Eberling, J. L., Wolfe, N., & Reed, B. R. (1996). Functional imaging predicts cognitive decline in Alzheimer's disease. *Journal of Neuroimaging, 6,* 156–160.

Jagust, W., Reed, B., Mungas, D., Ellis, W., & Decarli, C. (2007) What does fluorodeoxyglucose PET imaging add to a clinical diagnosis of dementia? *Neurology, 69,* 871–877.

Jagust, W. J., Zheng, L., Harvey, D. J., Mack, W. J., Vinters, H. V., Weiner, M. W.,...Chui, H. C. (2007b). Neuropathological basis of magnetic resonance images in aging and dementia. *Annals of Neurology, 63*(1), 72–80.

Johansen-Berg, H., Dawes, H., Guy, C., Smith, S. M., Wade, D. T., & Matthews, P. M. (2002). Correlation between motor improvements and altered fMRI activity after rehabilitative therapy. *Brain, 125,* 2731–2742.

Johnson, K. A., Jones, K., Holman, B. L., Becker, J. A., Spiers, P. A., Satlin, A., & Albert, M. S. (1998). Preclinical prediction of Alzheimer's disease using SPECT. *Neurology, 50,* 1563-1571.

Johnson, K. A., Minoshima, S., Bohnen, N. I., Donohoe, K. J., Foster, N. L., Herscovitch, P.,...Hartley, D. M. (2013a). Update on appropriate use criteria for amyloid PET imaging: Dementia experts, mild cognitive impairment, and education. Amyloid Imaging Task Force of the Alzheimer's Association and Society for Nuclear Medicine and Molecular Imaging. *Alzheimers and Dementia, 9,* e106–e109.

Johnson, K. A., Minoshima, S., Bohnen, N. I., Donohoe, K. J., Foster, N. L., Herscovitch, P.,...Thies, W. H. (2013b). Appropriate use criteria for amyloid PET: A report of the Amyloid Imaging Task Force, the Society of Nuclear Medicine and Molecular Imaging, and the Alzheimer's Association. *Alzheimers and Dementia, 9,* e1–e16.

Johnson, S. C., Schmitz, T. W., Moritz, C. H., Meyerand, M. E., Rowley, H. A., Alexander, A. L.,...Alexander, G. E. (2006). Activation of brain regions vulnerable to Alzheimer's disease: The effect of mild cognitive impairment. *Neurobiology of Aging, 27,* 1604–1612.

Kalpouzos, G., Chetelat, G., Baron, J. C., Landeau, B., Mevel, K., Godeau, C.,...Desgranges, B.

(2009). Voxel-based mapping of brain gray matter volume and glucose metabolism profiles in normal aging. *Neurobiology of Aging*, 30, 112–124.

Kato, T., Knopman, D., & Liu, H. (2001). Dissociation of regional activation in mild AD during visual encoding: A functional MRI study. *Neurology*, 57, 812–816.

Kerchner, G. A., Hess, C. P., Hammond-Rosenbluth, K. E., Xu, D., Rabinovici, G. D., Kelley, D. A.,…Miller, B. L. (2010). Hippocampal CA1 apical neuropil atrophy in mild Alzheimer disease visualized with 7-T MRI. *Neurology*, 75, 1381–1387.

Kerrouche, N., Herholz, K., Mielke, R., Holthoff, V., & Baron, J. C. (2006). 18FDG PET in vascular dementia: Differentiation from Alzheimer's disease using voxel-based multivariate analysis. *Journal of Cerebral Blood Flow and Metabolism*, 26, 1213–1221.

Killiany, R. J., Gomez-Isla, T., Moss, M., Kikinis, R., Sandor, T., Jolesz, F.,…Albert, M. S. (2000). Use of structural magnetic resonance imaging to predict who will get Alzheimer's disease. *Annals of Neurology*, 47, 430–439.

Kircher, T., Weis, S., Freymann, K., Erb, M., Jessen, F., Grodd, W.,…Leube, D. T. (2007). Hippocampal activation in MCI patients is necessary for successful memory encoding. *Journal of Neurology, Neurosurgery and Psychiatry*, 78(8), 812–818.

Klunk, W. E., Engler, H., Nordberg, A., Wang, Y., Blomqvist, G., Holt, D. P.,…Långström, B. (2004). Imaging brain amyloid in Alzheimer's disease with Pittsburgh Compound-B. *Annals of Neurology*, 55, 306–319.

Knopman, D. S., DeKosky, S. T., Cummings, J. L., Chui, H., Corey-Bloom, J., Relkin, N.,…Stevens, J. C. (2001). Practice parameter: Diagnosis of dementia (an evidence-based review). Report of the Quality Standards Subcommittee of the American Academy of Neurology. *Neurology*, 56, 1143–1153.

Koedam, E. L., Lehmann, M., van der Flier, W. M., Scheltens, P., Pijnenburg, Y. A., Fox, N.,…Wattjes, M. P. (2011). Visual assessment of posterior atrophy development of a MRI rating scale. *European Radiology*, 21, 2618–2625.

Kordower, J. H., Chu, Y., Stebbins, G. T., DeKosky, S. T., Cochran, E. J., Bennett, D., & Mufson, E. J. (2001). Loss and atrophy of layer II entorhinal cortex neurons in elderly people with mild cognitive impairment. *Annals of Neurology*, 49, 202–213.

Langbaum, J. B., Fleisher, A. S., Chen, K., Ayutyanont, N., Lopera, F., Quiroz, Y. T.,…Reiman, E. M. (2013). Ushering in the study and treatment of preclinical Alzheimer disease. *Nature Reviews Neurology*, 9, 371–381.

Lehmann, M., Koedam, E. L., Barnes, J., Bartlett, J. W., Barkhof, F., Wattjes, M. P.,…Fox, N. C. (2012). Visual ratings of atrophy in MCI: Prediction of conversion and relationship with CSF biomarkers. *Neurobiology of Aging*, 34, 73–82.

Likeman, M., Anderson, V. M., Stevens, J. M., Waldman, A. D., Godbolt, A. K., Frost, C.,…Fox, N. C. (2005). Visual assessment of atrophy on magnetic resonance imaging in the diagnosis of pathologically confirmed young-onset dementias. *Archives of Neurology*, 62, 1410–1415.

Luckhaus, C., Cohnen, M., Fluss, M. O., Janner, M., Grass-Kapanke, B., Teipel, S. J.,…Wittsack, H. J. (2010). The relation of regional cerebral perfusion and atrophy in mild cognitive impairment (MCI) and early Alzheimer's dementia. *Psychiatry Research*, 183, 44–51.

Lustig, C., Snyder, A. Z., Bhakta, M., O'Brien, K. C., McAvoy, M., Raichle, M. E.,…Buckner, R. L. (2003). Functional deactivations: Change with age and dementia of the Alzheimer type. *Proceedings of the National Academy of Science USA*, 100, 14504–14509.

Machulda, M. M., Ward, H. A., Borowski, B., Gunter, J. L., Cha, R. H., O'Brien, P. C.,…Jack, C. R., Jr. (2003). Comparison of memory fMRI response among normal, MCI, and Alzheimer's patients. *Neurology*, 61, 500–506.

Maruyama, M., Shimada, H., Suhara, T., Shinotoh, H., Ji, B., Maeda, J.,…Higuchi, M. (2013). Imaging of tau pathology in a tauopathy mouse model and in Alzheimer patients compared to normal controls. *Neuron*, 79, 1094–1108.

Mathis, C. A., Bacskai, B. J., Kajdasz, S. T., McLellan, M. E., Frosch, M. P., Hyman, B. T.,…Klunk, W. E. (2002). A lipophilic thioflavin-T derivative for positron emission tomography (PET) imaging of amyloid in brain. *Bioorganic and Medicinal Chemistry Letters*, 12, 295–298.

McAllister, T. W., Saykin, A. J., Flashman, L. A., Sparling, M. B., Johnson, S. C., Guerin, S. J.,…Yanofsky, N. (1999). Brain activation during working memory 1 month after mild traumatic brain injury: A functional MRI study. *Neurology*, 53, 1300–1308.

McKeith, I. G., Dickson, D. W., Lowe, J., Emre, M., O'Brien, J. T., Feldman, H.,…Yamada, M. (2005). Diagnosis and management of dementia with Lewy bodies. Third report of the DLB consortium. *Neurology*, 65(12), 1863–1872.

McKhann, G. M., Knopman, D. S., Chertkow, H., Hyman, B. T., Jack, C. R., Jr., Kawas, C. H.,…Phelps, C. H. (2011). The diagnosis of dementia due to Alzheimer's disease: Recommendations from the National

Institute on Aging and the Alzheimer's Association workgroup. *Alzheimers and Dementia, 7*(3), 263–269.

Mega, M. S., Chu, T., Mazziotta, J. C., Trivedi, K. H., Thompson, P. M., Shah, A.,...Toga, A. W. (1999). Mapping biochemistry to metabolism: FDG-PET and amyloid burden in Alzheimer's disease. *Neuroreport, 10,* 2911–2917.

Mega, M. S., Cummings, J. L., O'Connor, S. M., Dinov, I. D., Reback, E., Felix, J.,...Toga, A. W. (2001). Cognitive and metabolic responses to metrifonate therapy in Alzheimer disease. *Neuropsychiatry Neuropsychology and Behavioral Neurology, 14,* 63–68.

Miller, M. I., Priebe, C. E., Qiu, A., Fischl, B., Kolasny, A., Brown, T.,...Morphometry, B. (2009). Collaborative computational anatomy: An MRI morphometry study of the human brain via diffeomorphic metric mapping. *Human Brain Mapping, 30,* 2132–2141.

Miller, S., Fenstermacher, E., Bates, J., Blacker, D., Sperling, R. A., & Dickerson, B. C. (2006). *Hippocampal activation in MCI predicts subsequent cognitive decline.* Paper presented at the International Conference on Alzheimer's Disease, Madrid, Spain.

Minoshima, S., Giordani, B., Berent, S., Frey, K. A., Foster, N. L., & Kuhl, D. E. (1997). Metabolic reduction in the posterior cingulate cortex in very early Alzheimer's disease. *Annals of Neurology, 42,* 85–94.

Mintun, M. A., Larossa, G. N., Sheline, Y. I., Dence, C. S., Lee, S. Y., Mach, R. H.,...Morris, J. C. (2006). [11C]PIB in a nondemented population: Potential antecedent marker of Alzheimer disease. *Neurology, 67,* 446–452.

Monchi, O., Petrides, M., Doyon, J., Postuma, R. B., Worsley, K., & Dagher, A. (2004). Neural bases of set-shifting deficits in Parkinson's disease. *Journal of Neuroscience, 24,* 702–710.

Morgen, K., Kadom, N., Sawaki, L., Tessitore, A., Ohayon, J., McFarland, H.,...Cohen, L. G. (2004). Training-dependent plasticity in patients with multiple sclerosis. *Brain, 127,* 2506–2517.

Morra, J. H., Tu, Z., Apostolova, L. G., Green, A. E., Avedissian, C., Madsen, S. K.,...Thompson, P. M. (2008). Validation of a fully automated 3D hippocampal segmentation method using subjects with Alzheimer's disease mild cognitive impairment, and elderly controls. *Neuroimage, 43,* 59–68.

Mosconi, L., Sorbi, S., de Leon, M. J., Li, Y., Nacmias, B., Myoung, P. S.,...Pupi, A. (2006). Hypometabolism exceeds atrophy in presymptomatic early-onset familial Alzheimer's disease. *Journal of Nuclear Medicine, 47,* 1778–1786.

Mosconi, L., Tsui, W. H., De Santi, S., Li, J., Rusinek, H., Convit, A.,...de Leon, M. J. (2005). Reduced hippocampal metabolism in MCI and AD: Automated FDG-PET image analysis. *Neurology, 64,* 1860–1867.

Mueller, S. G., Schuff, N., Raptentsetsang, S., Elman, J., & Weiner, M. W. (2008). Selective effect of Apo e4 on CA3 and dentate in normal aging and Alzheimer's disease using high resolution MRI at 4 T. *Neuroimage* 42:42–48.

Mueller, S. G., Stables, L., Du, A. T., Schuff, N., Truran, D., Cashdollar, N., & Weiner, M. W. (2007). Measurement of hippocampal subfields and age-related changes with high resolution MRI at 4T. *Neurobiology of Aging, 28,* 719–726.

Mueller, S. G., & Weiner, M. W. (2009). Selective effect of age, Apo e4, and Alzheimer's disease on hippocampal subfields. *Hippocampus, 19,* 558–564.

Mueller, S. G., Weiner, M. W., Thal, L. J., Petersen, R. C., Jack, C. R., Jagust, W.,...Beckett, L. (2005). Ways toward an early diagnosis in Alzheimer's disease: The Alzheimer's Disease Neuroimaging Initiative (ADNI). *Alzheimers and Dementia, 1,* 55–66.

Mungas, D., Reed, B. R., Jagust, W. J., DeCarli, C., Mack, W. J., Kramer, J. H.,...Chui, H. C. (2002). Volumetric MRI predicts rate of cognitive decline related to AD and cerebrovascular disease. *Neurology, 59,* 867–873.

Naidich, T. P., Daniels, D. L., Haughton, V. M., Pech, P., Williams, A., Pojunas, K., & Palacios, E. (1987b). Hippocampal formation and related structures of the limbic lobe: Anatomic-MR correlation. Part II. Sagittal sections. *Radiology, 162,* 755–761.

Naidich, T. P., Daniels, D. L., Haughton, V. M., Williams, A., Pojunas, K., & Palacios, E. (1987a). Hippocampal formation and related structures of the limbic lobe: Anatomic-MR correlation. Part I. Surface features and coronal sections. *Radiology, 162,* 747–754.

Nakano, S., Asada, T., Matsuda, H., Uno, M., & Takasaki, M. (2001). Donepezil hydrochloride preserves regional cerebral blood flow in patients with Alzheimer's disease. *Journal of Nuclear Medicine, 42,* 1441–1445.

Neylan, T. C., Mueller, S. G., Wang, Z., Metzler, T. J., Lenoci, M., Truran, D.,...Schuff, N. Insomnia severity is associated with a decreased volume of the CA3/dentate gyrus hippocampal subfield. *Biological Psychiatry, 68,* 494–496.

Nicolson, R., DeVito, T. J., Vidal, C. N., Sui, Y., Hayashi, K. M., Drost, D. J.,...Thompson, P. M. (2006). Detection and mapping of hippocampal abnormalities in autism. *Psychiatry Research, 148,* 11–21.

Nobili, F., Koulibaly, M., Vitali, P., Migneco, O., Mariani, G., Ebmeier, K., . . . Darcourt, J. (2002). Brain perfusion follow-up in Alzheimer's patients during treatment with acetylcholinesterase inhibitors. *Journal of Nuclear Medicine*, *43*, 983–990.

Nordberg, A. (2007). Amyloid imaging in Alzheimer's disease. *Current Opinion in Neurology*, *20*, 398–402.

O'Brien, J. L., O'Keefe, K. M., LaViolette, P. S., DeLuca, A. N., Blacker, D., Dickerson, B. C., & Sperling, R. A. (2010). Longitudinal fMRI in elderly reveals loss of hippocampal activation with clinical decline. *Neurology*, *74*, 1969–1976.

O'Brien, J. T., Erkinjuntti, T., Reisberg, B., Roman, G., Sawada, T., Pantoni, L., . . . DeKosky, S. T. (2003). Vascular cognitive impairment. *Lancet Neurology*, *2*, 89–98.

Posener, J. A., Wang, L., Price, J. L., Gado, M. H., Province, M. A., Miller, M. I., . . . Csernansky, J. G. (2003). High-dimensional mapping of the hippocampus in depression. *American Journal of Psychiatry*, *160*, 83–89.

Post, S. G., Whitehouse, P. J., Binstock, R. H., Bird, T. D., Eckert, S. K., Farrer, L. A., . . . Zinn, A. B. (1997). The clinical introduction of genetic testing for Alzheimer disease. An ethical perspective. *Journal of the American Medical Association*, *277*, 832–836.

Price, J. L., Ko, A. I., Wade, M. J., Tsou, S. K., McKeel, D. W., & Morris, J. C. (2001). Neuron number in the entorhinal cortex and CA1 in preclinical Alzheimer disease. *Archives of Neurology*, *58*, 1395–1402.

Rabinovici, G. D., Furst, A. J., O'Neil, J. P., Racine, C. A., Mormino, E. C., Baker, S. L., . . . Jagust, W. J. (2007). 11C-PIB PET imaging in Alzheimer disease and frontotemporal lobar degeneration. *Neurology*, *68*, 1205–1212.

Rabinovici, G. D., Rosen, H. J., Alkalay, A., Kornak, J., Furst, A. J., Agarwal, N., . . . Jagust, W. J. (2012). Amyloid vs FDG-PET in the differential diagnosis of AD and FTLD. *Neurology*, *77*, 2034–2042.

Raichle, M. E., MacLeod, A. M., Snyder, A. Z., Powers, W. J., Gusnard, D. A., & Shulman, G. L. (2001). A default mode of brain function. *Proceedings of the National Academy of Science USA*, *98*, 676–682.

Rascovsky, K., Hodges, J. R., Kipps, C. M., Johnson, J. K., Seeley, W. W., Mendez, M. F., . . . Miller, B. M. (2007). Diagnostic criteria for the behavioral variant of frontotemporal dementia (bvFTD): Current limitations and future directions. *Alzheimers Disease and Associated Disorders*, *21*, S14–S18.

Rascovsky, K., Hodges, J. R., Knopman, D., Mendez, M. F., Kramer, J. H., Neuhaus, J., . . . Miller, B. L. (2011). Sensitivity of revised diagnostic criteria for the behavioural variant of frontotemporal dementia. *Brain*, *134*, 2456–2477.

Reddy, H., Narayanan, S., Arnoutelis, R., Jenkinson, M., Antel, J., Matthews, P. M., & Arnold, D. L. (2000). Evidence for adaptive functional changes in the cerebral cortex with axonal injury from multiple sclerosis. *Brain*, *123*(Pt 11), 2314–2320.

Reiman, E. M. (2007). Linking brain imaging and genomics in the study of Alzheimer's disease and aging. *Annals of the New York Academy of Sciences*, *1097*, 94–113.

Reiman, E. M., Caselli, R. J., Chen, K., Alexander, G. E., Bandy, D., & Frost, J. (2001). Declining brain activity in cognitively normal apolipoprotein E epsilon 4 heterozygotes: A foundation for using positron emission tomography to efficiently test treatments to prevent Alzheimer's disease. *Proceedings of the National Academy of Science USA*, *98*, 3334–3339.

Reiman, E. M., Chen, K., Alexander, G. E., Caselli, R. J., Bandy, D., Osborne, D., . . . Hardy, J. (2004). Functional brain abnormalities in young adults at genetic risk for late-onset Alzheimer's dementia. *Proceedings of the National Academy of Science USA*, *101*, 284–289.

Rombouts, S. A., Barkhof, F., Goekoop, R., Stam, C. J., & Scheltens, P. (2005). Altered resting state networks in mild cognitive impairment and mild Alzheimer's disease: An fMRI study. *Human Brain Mapping*, *26*, 231–239.

Rombouts, S. A., Barkhof, F., Veltman, D. J., Machielsen, W. C., Witter, M. P., Bierlaagh, M. A., . . . Scheltens, P. (2000). Functional MR imaging in Alzheimer's disease during memory encoding. *American Journal of Neuroradiology*, *21*, 1869–1875.

Rosas, H. D., Feigin, A. S., & Hersch, S. M. (2004). Using advances in neuroimaging to detect, understand, and monitor disease progression in Huntington's disease. *NeuroRx*, *1*, 263–272.

Rusinek, H., Brys, M., Glodzik, L., Switalski, R., Tsui, W. H., Haas, F., . . . de Leon, M. J. (2011). Hippocampal blood flow in normal aging measured with arterial spin labeling at 3T. *Magnetic Resonance Medicine*, *65*, 128–137.

Ryan, N. S., & Fox, N. C. (2009). Alzheimer disease: Visual rating of atrophy aids diagnostic accuracy. *Nature Reviews Neurology*, *5*, 243–244.

Salloway, S., Sperling, R., Gilman, S., Fox, N. C., Blennow, K., Raskind, M., . . . Grundman, M. (2009). A phase 2 multiple ascending dose trial of bapineuzumab in mild to moderate Alzheimer disease. *Neurology*, *73*, 2061–2070.

Saunders, A. M. (2000). Apolipoprotein E and Alzheimer disease: An update on genetic and functional analyses. *Journal of Neuropathology and Experimental Neurology, 59,* 751–758.

Saunders, A. M., Strittmatter, W. J., Schmechel, D., George-Hyslop, P. H., Pericak-Vance, M. A., Joo, S. H.,...Alberts, M. J. (1993). Association of apolipoprotein E allele epsilon 4 with late-onset familial and sporadic Alzheimer's disease. *Neurology, 43,* 1467–1472.

Scahill, R. I., Schott, J. M., Stevens, J. M., Rossor, M. N., & Fox, N. C. (2002). Mapping the evolution of regional atrophy in Alzheimer's disease: Unbiased analysis of fluid-registered serial MRI. *Proceedings of the National Academy of Science USA, 99,* 4703–4707.

Scarmeas, N., Habeck, C. G., Zarahn, E., Anderson, K. E., Park, A., Hilton, J.,...Stern, Y. (2004). Covariance PET patterns in early Alzheimer's disease and subjects with cognitive impairment but no dementia: Utility in group discrimination and correlations with functional performance. *Neuroimage, 23,* 35–45.

Scheff, S. W., Price, D. A., Schmitt, F. A., & Mufson, E. J. (2005). Hippocampal synaptic loss in early Alzheimer's disease and mild cognitive impairment. *Neurobiology of Aging.* Epub ahead of print.

Scheltens, P., Fox, N., Barkhof, F., & De Carli, C. (2002). Structural magnetic resonance imaging in the practical assessment of dementia: Beyond exclusion. *Lancet Neurology, 1,* 13–21.

Schott, J. M., Fox, N. C., Frost, C., Scahill, R. I., Janssen, J. C., Chan, D.,...Rossor, M. N. (2003). Assessing the onset of structural change in familial Alzheimer's disease. *Annals of Neurology* 53:181–188.

Schott, J. M., Frost, C., Whitwell, J. L., Macmanus, D. G., Boyes, R. G., Rossor, M. N., & Fox, N. C. (2006). Combining short interval MRI in Alzheimer's disease: Implications for therapeutic trials. *Journal of Neurology, 253,* 1147–1153.

Seab, J. P., Jagust, W. J., Wong, S. T., Roos, M. S., Reed, B. R., & Budinger, T. F. (1988). Quantitative NMR measurements of hippocampal atrophy in Alzheimer's disease. *Magnetic Resonance Medicine, 8,* 200–208.

Selkoe, D. J. (2002). Alzheimer's disease is a synaptic failure. *Science, 298,* 789–791.

Shaw, L. M., Vanderstichele, H., Knapik-Czajka, M., Clark, C. M., Aisen, P. S., Petersen, R. C.,...Trojanowski, J. Q. (2009). Cerebrospinal fluid biomarker signature in Alzheimer's disease neuroimaging initiative subjects. *Annals of Neurology, 65,* 403–413.

Silverman, D. H., Small, G. W., Chang, C. Y., Lu, C. S., Kung De Aburto, M. A., Chen, W.,...Phelps, M. E. (2001). Positron emission tomography in evaluation of dementia: Regional brain metabolism and long-term outcome. *Journal of the American Medical Association, 286,* 2120–2127.

Small, G. W., Ercoli, L. M., Silverman, D. H., Huang, S. C., Komo, S., Bookheimer, S. Y.,...Phelps, M. E. (2000). Cerebral metabolic and cognitive decline in persons at genetic risk for Alzheimer's disease. *Proceedings of the National Academy of Science USA, 97,* 6037–6042.

Small, G. W., Kepe, V., Ercoli, L. M., Siddarth, P., Bookheimer, S. Y., Miller, K. J.,...Barrio, J. R. (2006). PET of brain amyloid and tau in mild cognitive impairment. *New England Journal of Medicine, 355,* 2652–2663.

Small, S. A., Perera, G. M., DeLaPaz, R., Mayeux, R., & Stern, Y. (1999). Differential regional dysfunction of the hippocampal formation among elderly with memory decline and Alzheimer's disease. *Annals of Neurology, 45,* 466–472.

Small, S. A., Chawla, M. K., Buonocore, M., Rapp, P. R., & Barnes, C. A. (2004) Imaging correlates of brain function in monkeys and rats isolates a hippocampal subregion differentially vulnerable to aging. *Proceedings of the National Academy of Science USA* 101:7181–7186.

Sperling, R. A., Bates, J. F., Chua, E. F., Cocchiarella, A. J., Rentz, D. M., Rosen, B. R.,...Albert, M. S. (2003). fMRI studies of associative encoding in young and elderly controls and mild Alzheimer's disease. *Journal of Neurology, Neurosurgery and Psychiatry, 74,* 44–50.

Sperling, R. A., Laviolette, P. S., O'Keefe, K., O'Brien, J., Rentz, D. M., Pihlajamaki, M.,...Johnson, K. A. (2009). Amyloid deposition is associated with impaired default network function in older persons without dementia. *Neuron, 63,* 178–188.

Sperling, R. A., Aisen, P. S., Beckett, L. A., Bennett, D. A., Craft, S., Fagan, A. M.,...Phelps, C. H. (2011). Toward defining the preclinical stages of Alzheimer's disease: Recommendations from the National Institute on Aging and the Alzheimer's Association workgroup. *Alzheimers and Dementia, 7*(3), 280–292.

Stern, E. A., Bacskai, B. J., Hickey, G. A., Attenello, F. J., Lombardo, J. A., & Hyman, B. T. (2004). Cortical synaptic integration in vivo is disrupted by amyloid-beta plaques. *Journal of Neuroscience, 24,* 4535–4540.

Sultzer, D. L., Mahler, M. E., Cummings, J. L., Van Gorp, W. G., Hinkin, C. H., & Brown, C. (1995). Cortical abnormalities associated with subcortical lesions in vascular dementia. Clinical and position emission tomographic findings. *Archives of Neurology, 52,* 773–780.

Tepest, R., Wang, L., Miller, M. I., Falkai, P., & Csernansky, J. G. (2003). Hippocampal deformities in the unaffected siblings of schizophrenia subjects. *Biological Psychiatry, 54,* 1234–1240.

Tomlinson, B. E., Blessed, G., & Roth, M. (1968). Observations on the brains of non-demented old people. *Journal of Neurological Sciences, 7,* 331–356.

Tune, L., Tiseo, P. J., Ieni, J., Perdomo, C., Pratt, R. D., Votaw, J. R.,...Hoffman, J. M. (2003). Donepezil HCl (E2020) maintains functional brain activity in patients with Alzheimer disease: Results of a 24–week, double-blind, placebo-controlled study. *American Journal of Geriatric Psychiatry, 11,* 169–177.

Van Leemput, K., Bakkour, A., Benner, T., Wiggins, G., Wald, L. L., Augustinack, J.,...Fischl, B. (2009). Automated segmentation of hippocampal subfields from ultra-high resolution in vivo MRI. *Hippocampus, 19,* 549–557.

Vemuri, P., Whitwell, J. L., Kantarci, K., Josephs, K. A., Parisi, J. E., Shiung, M. S.,...Jack, C. R., Jr. (2008). Antemortem MRI based STructural Abnormality iNDex (STAND)-scores correlate with postmortem Braak neurofibrillary tangle stage. *Neuroimage, 42,* 559–567.

Vermersch, P., Leys, D., Scheltens, P., & Barkhof, F. (1994). Visual rating of hippocampal atrophy: Correlation with volumetry. *Journal of Neurology, Neurosurgery and Psychiatry, 57,* 1015.

Visser, P. J., Scheltens, P., Verhey, F. R., Schmand, B., Launer, L. J., Jolles, J., & Jonker, C. (1999). Medial temporal lobe atrophy and memory dysfunction as predictors for dementia in subjects with mild cognitive impairment. *Journal of Neurology, 246,* 477–485.

Walsh, D. M., & Selkoe, D. J. (2004). Deciphering the molecular basis of memory failure in Alzheimer's disease. *Neuron, 44,* 181–193.

Walters, R. J., Fox, N. C., Crum, W. R., Taube, D., & Thomas, D. J. (2001). Haemodialysis and cerebral oedema. *Nephron, 87,* 143–147.

Wang, L., Miller, J. P., Gado, M. H., McKeel, D. W., Rothermich, M., Miller, M. I.,...Csernansky, J. G. (2005). Abnormalities of hippocampal surface structure in very mild dementia of the Alzheimer type. *Neuroimage.* Epub ahead of print.

Wang, Z., Neylan, T. C., Mueller, S. G., Lenoci, M., Truran, D., Marmar, C. R.,...Schuff, N. (2010). Magnetic resonance imaging of hippocampal subfields in posttraumatic stress disorder. *Archives of General Psychiatry, 67,* 296–303.

Weiner, M. W., Veitch, D. P., Aisen, P. S., Beckett, L. A., Cairns, N. J., Green, R. C.,...Trojanowski, J. Q. (2011). The Alzheimer's Disease Neuroimaging Initiative: A review of papers published since its inception. *Alzheimers and Dementia.* Epub ahead of print.

Weiner, M. W., Veitch, D. P., Aisen, P. S., Beckett, L. A., Cairns, N. J., Green, R. C.,...Trojanowski, J. Q. (2013). The Alzheimer's Disease Neuroimaging Initiative: A review of papers published since its inception. *Alzheimers and Dementia, 9,* e111–e194.

Whitwell, J. L., Shiung, M. M., Przybelski, S. A., Weigand, S. D., Knopman, D. S., Boeve, B. F.,...Jack, C. R., Jr. (2008). MRI patterns of atrophy associated with progression to AD in amnestic mild cognitive impairment. *Neurology, 70*(7), 512–520.

Williamson, J., Goldman, J., & Marder, K. S. (2009). Genetic aspects of Alzheimer disease. *Neurologist, 15,* 80–86.

Willis, M. W., Ketter, T. A., Kimbrell, T. A., George, M. S., Herscovitch, P., Danielson, A. L.,...Post, R. M. (2002). Age, sex and laterality effects on cerebral glucose metabolism in healthy adults. *Psychiatry Research, 114,* 23–37.

Wolfe, N., Reed, B. R., Eberling, J. L., & Jagust, W. J. (1995). Temporal lobe perfusion on single photon emission computed tomography predicts the rate of cognitive decline in Alzheimer's disease. *Archives of Neurology, 52,* 257–262.

Wolk, D. A., & Dickerson, B. C. (2010). Apolipoprotein E (APOE) genotype has dissociable effects on memory and attentional-executive network function in Alzheimer's disease. *Proceedings of the National Academy of Science USA, 107,* 10256–10261.

Womack, K. B., Diaz-Arrastia, R., Aizenstein, H. J., Arnold, S. E., Barbas, N. R., Boeve, B. F.,...Foster, N. L. (2011). Temporoparietal hypometabolism in frontotemporal lobar degeneration and associated imaging diagnostic errors. *Archives of Neurology, 68,* 329–337.

Wood, E. M., Falcone, D., Suh, E., Irwin, D. J., Chen-Plotkin, A. S., Lee, E. B.,...Grossman, M. (2013). Development and validation of pedigree classification criteria for frontotemporal lobar degeneration. *Journal of the American Medical Association, Neurology, 70*(11), 1411–1417.

Xu, G., McLaren, D. G., Ries, M. L., Fitzgerald, M. E., Bendlin, B. B., Rowley, H. A.,...Johnson, S. C. (2009). The influence of parental history of Alzheimer's disease and apolipoprotein E epsilon4 on the BOLD signal during recognition memory. *Brain, 132,* 383–391.

Yushkevich, P. A., Avants, B. B., Pluta, J., Das, S., Minkoff, D., Mechanic-Hamilton, D.,...Detre, J. A. (2009). A high-resolution computational atlas of the human hippocampus from postmortem magnetic resonance imaging at 9.4 T. *Neuroimage, 44,* 385–398.

Yushkevich, P. A., Avants, B. B., Pluta, J., Minkoff, D., Detre, J. A., Grossman, M., & Gee, J. C. (2008). Shape-based alignment of hippocampal subfields: Evaluation in postmortem MRI. *Medical Image Computing and Computer-Assist Intervention, 11,* 510–517.

Yushkevich, P. A., Wang, H., Pluta, J., Das, S. R., Craige, C., Avants, B. B.,...Mueller, S. (2010). Nearly automatic segmentation of hippocampal subfields in in vivo focal T2–weighted MRI. *Neuroimage, 53,* 1208–1224.

23

Pharmacological Therapies for Alzheimer's Disease
Clinical Trials and Future Directions

Michael Rafii and Paul Aisen

The neuropathology of Alzheimer's disease (AD) is characterized by degeneration and loss of basal forebrain cholinergic neurons, leading to decreased cholinergic transmission and impaired memory and cognition (Bartus, Dean, Beer, & Lippa, 1982; Whitehouse et al., 1982). The symptoms of AD dementia can be improved with acetylcholinesterase inhibitors (AChEIs) (Birks, 2006). However, such pharmacologic treatments merely afford palliative relief and do not slow or reverse the progression of the disease. Approved AChEIs include donepezil, rivastigmine, and galantamine. A dysfunction of glutamatergic neurotransmission, manifested as neuronal excitotoxicity, is also hypothesized to be involved in AD. Targeting the glutamatergic system, specifically NMDA receptors, offers a novel approach to treatment in view of the limited efficacy of existing drugs targeting the cholinergic system. Memantine is a low-affinity voltage-dependent uncompetitive antagonist at glutamatergic NMDA receptors (Chen & Lipton, 2005). Memantine is approved for treatment of moderate-to-severe AD dementia. The Food and Drug Administration (FDA) has not approved any new drugs for the treatment of AD since memantine was approved in 2003.

In 2011, the FDA approved a new formulation of Aricept (donepezil hydrochloride), a 23 mg continuous release pill and in 2012, the FDA approved a 13.3 mg formulation of the Exelon (rivastigmine) transdermal patch. In 2013 a 28 mg extended-release formulation of Namenda (memantine), Namenda XR, was introduced in the United States.

In recent years, many drug candidates have advanced into large, randomized controlled trials but have not demonstrated efficacy in treating AD dementia. In part because of these failures and in part because results from multiple longitudinal biomarker and clinicopathologic studies have shown that the AD disease process begins at least a decade before symptoms of dementia develop, the field is moving toward earlier identification and treatment of the disease (Weiner et al., 2012).

Major efforts are ongoing in academia and the pharmaceutical industry to develop drugs targeting the following mechanisms of action in AD therapeutics:

1. Reduction of beta-amyloid (known as β-amyloid, Abeta, or Aβ) production, notably secretase inhibitors

2. Reduction of beta-amyloid plaque burden via inhibition of aggregation or disruption of aggregates
3. Promotion of beta-amyloid clearance via active or passive immunotherapy
4. Prevention of tau protein phosphorylation or fibrillarization

In this chapter, we will discuss these four categories aimed at slowing the progression of the disease, as well as a category of "other therapies," which includes treatments that do not fit under a single mechanism of action but represent rational interventions for the treatment of the symptoms and, in some cases, the underlying pathology of AD.

The first three categories are motivated by the "amyloid hypothesis," which has been the focal point of research and development for the treatment of AD for the past 30 years (Selkoe, 2011). This theory is based on results from studies that indicate aberrant processing of APP in the brain leads to the production of a short fragment of APP known as beta-amyloid, which mainly consists of two peptides—one that is 40 amino acids in length (Abeta40) and the other 42 units (Abeta42).

Soluble forms of beta-amyloid 1-42 have been shown to be neuro- and synaptotoxic, and it is thought by some investigators to play an important causal role in neurodegeneration in AD (Selkoe, 2008). Beta-amyloid 1-40 is thought to be the underlying cause of amyloid angiopathy (Viswanathan & Greenberg, 2011). The insoluble deposits of beta-amyloid are known as amyloid plaques. The theory posits that there is either overproduction of beta-amyloid (i.e., in dominantly inherited forms of AD) or problems with the mechanism that usually clears it from the brain (sporadic AD), or possibly both. The excess of beta-amyloid is also thought to lead to hyperphosphorlyation of the protein tau within neurons, and this subsequently leads to neurodegeneration (Ballatore, Lee, & Trojanowski, 2007). While the sequence of events that leads to the development of AD is still ambiguous, soluble oligomers of beta-amyloid and the resulting formation of amyloid plaques are considered key features of disease pathogenesis. The tight link between all genetic determinants of AD and the generation of amyloid peptides is compelling support for the hypothesis. The majority of drug candidates that have advanced into randomized controlled trials for AD therefore target beta-amyloid. As the amyloid hypothesis represents the prevailing focus of research in AD, the majority of drug candidate failures have also been in this area. These include flurbiprofen, semagacestat, tramiprosate, ELND006, AN1792, ponezumab, bapineuzemab, and others. However, most of these failures are thought to have resulted from the disease being treated too late in its course, where significant neurodegeneration has already taken place, rather than incorrect target selection.

Drugs to Reduce Beta-Amyloid Production

Beta-Secretase Inhibitors

The beta-amyloid peptide is cut out of the amyloid beta-protein precursor (APP) by the sequential action of beta- and gamma-secretases. APP is a single-pass membrane protein that is sequentially cleaved in the luminal/extracellular region by beta-secretase and within the transmembrane domain by gamma-secretase to release beta-amyloid (Haass & Selkoe, 2007). The AD-associated missense mutations in APP are found in three different regions: (1) near the beta-secretase cleavage site, leading to elevated beta-amyloid; (2) within the beta-amyloid sequence, changing the biophysical properties of the peptide; or (3) near the gamma-secretase cleavage site, increasing the proportion of beta-amyloid that is 42 residues long (Abeta1-42) and much more prone to aggregation than the predominant 40-residue peptide (Abeta1-40) (Tanzi & Bertram, 2005). These findings have provided strong support for the amyloid hypothesis of AD pathogenesis.

Furthermore, recent genetic evidence shows that mutations near the beta-secretase cleavage site that prevent such cleavages are, in fact, protective for AD and lead to decreased production of beta-amyloid (Jonsson et al., 2012). Data on the beta-amyloid cleaving enzyme-1 (BACE1) inhibitor, MK-8931, in a once-daily oral, single and multidose Phase 1 clinical trial in healthy volunteers, reduced the cerebral spinal fluid (CSF) amyloid-beta peptide by greater than 90% without observing dose-limiting side effects. Phase II/III studies in patients with mild to moderate AD dementia began in late 2012. ACI-91 is a compound that acts indirectly on beta-secretase and is currently being studied in a Phase II multicenter double-blind, placebo-controlled trial for the treatment of mild to moderate AD dementia. The study will evaluate the compound's safety, tolerability, and efficacy of 12 months of treatment.

Gamma-Secretase Inhibitors and Modulators

Production of beta-amyloid is also regulated by gamma secretase, a protease with numerous substrates. Gamma-secretase is a membrane-embedded protease complex that cleaves the transmembrane region of APP to produce beta-amyloid. In August 2010, development of semagacestat, a gamma-secretase inhibitor, was halted when preliminary results from two ongoing long-term Phase III studies showed that it did not slow disease progression and was, in fact, associated with worsening of clinical measures of cognition and the ability to perform activities of daily living. In addition, data showed semagacestat was associated with an increased risk of skin cancer compared with those who received placebo.

Tarenflurbil (r-flurbiprofen, Flurizan) was the first gamma-secretase inhibitor that was stopped in Phase III clinical trials due to lack of efficacy. Tarenflurbil (Flurizan), the enantiomer of the nonsteroidal anti-inflammatory drug flurbiprofen, is a modulator of gamma-secretase activity, and a Phase II trial of tarenflurbil for mild to moderate AD indicated that the drug was well tolerated (Wilcock et al., 2008), while a post-hoc analysis suggested a potential signal of benefit on ADAS-Cog and the CDR-sb. However, in June 2008 a Phase III trial with over 1,700 subjects failed to show efficacy, and further development of tarenflurbil (Flurizan) for treatment of AD was discontinued.

Gamma-secretase provides additional functions, besides contributing to the production of beta-amyloid in the brain, which may explain some of the side effects experienced with semagacestat. The enzyme is also critical for the processing of Notch, a protein that controls normal cell differentiation and communication (De Strooper et al., 1999). Notch, like APP, is cleaved within its transmembrane domain, and this proteolysis is necessary for Notch signaling and cell fate determinations. These findings began to raise concerns about gamma secretase as a target for AD: Inhibition of this protease, while lowering beta-amyloid production, might cause severe toxicities due to blocking critical cell differentiation events.

A Phase II study evaluating the safety and tolerability of the investigational oral gamma secretase inhibitor avagacestat (BMS-708163) in patients with mild to moderate AD dementia failed to reach its endpoints. The compound is "Notch-sparing," and a single-ascending dose study suggested that it was tolerated at a single-dose range of 0.3 to 800 mg, raising hopes that it would be suitable for further clinical development (Tong et al., 2012). Unfortunately, when a preliminary data from a Phase II study of avagacestat in patients with prodromal AD was examined, the company announced in late 2012 that the results did not look favorable and thus development of this compound was halted.

Drugs to Prevent Beta-Amyloid Aggregation

ELND005 (scyllo-inositol) is an oral beta-amyloid antiaggregation agent. ELN005 is specifically designed to target the abnormal forms of beta-amyloid. In preclinical studies, ELND005 has been shown to slow the progression of AD pathology by neutralizing beta-amyloid oligomers, inhibiting their toxic effects on synaptic transmission, preventing the formation of beta-amyloid fibrils, and breaking down existing fibrils (Dasilva, Shaw, & McLaurin, 2010).

A Phase II placebo controlled study was completed in 351 patients with mild to moderate AD who received study drug (250 mg twice daily; 1,000 mg twice daily; 2,000 mg twice daily; or placebo) for up to 18 months (Salloway et al., 2011). The two higher dose groups were discontinued in late 2009 due to greater rates of adverse events, including nine deaths, in these dose groups. The study did not achieve significance on primary outcome measures. The 250 mg twice daily dose demonstrated a biological effect on beta-amyloid in the CSF and showed some effects on clinical endpoints in an exploratory analysis, particularly on the emergence of new neuropsychiatric symptoms. After reviewing the final safety data, it was concluded that the 250 mg twice daily dose has acceptable safety and tolerability for further study, and a Phase II study commenced in late 2012 of this compound on agitation and aggression in patients with moderate to severe AD.

Drugs to Promote Beta-Amyloid Clearance

Active Immunotherapy

The first human vaccination trial in AD, AN-1792, was discontinued over a decade ago (in 2002). The vaccine used in that study activated T cells, which led to an unacceptably high incidence of meningoencephalitis (Orgogozo et al., 2003). Interestingly, in long-term follow-up measurements, 20% of subjects had developed high levels of antibodies to beta-amyloid (Gilman et al., 2005). While placebo patients and nonantibody responders worsened, these antibody responders showed relative stability in cognitive performance as assessed by the Neuropsychological Test Battery (although not by other measures) and had lower levels of tau protein in their CSF. These results suggest reduced disease activity in the antibody-responder group. Autopsies found that immunization resulted in clearance of amyloid plaques, but it did not prevent progressive neurodegeneration (Vellas et al., 2009).

ACC-001 is a second-generation beta-amyloid vaccine intended to induce a highly specific antibody response to beta-amyloid. ACC-001, an amino-terminal immunoconjugate, was shown to be safe in a Phase I study and is currently being evaluated in ongoing Phase II clinical studies.

Another beta-amyloid vaccine clinical trial is CAD106, which is being evaluated in patients with mild AD dementia. CAD106 is also designed to induce antibodies against the beta-amyloid. Results have been published from the Phase I clinical trial looking at the safety, tolerability, and antibody response of active immunization with the CAD106 in 58 patients with AD dementia. The study participants, aged 50 to 80, had mild to moderate AD dementia and were split into two groups for a study period lasting a year. In one group of 31 patients, 24 received 50 µg of CAD106 and 7 received a placebo. In the second group of 27 patients, 22 received 150 µg of CAD106 and 5 received the placebo. In the first group, 67% of the patients receiving the vaccine developed the antibody response. In the second higher dose group, 82% of the CAD106-treated participants had the antibody response (Winblad et al., 2012). The Phase II trial, currently under way, is a randomized, double-blind, placebo-controlled, parallel group study to evaluate the safety and tolerability of CAD106 when administered as repeated subcutaneous injections in subjects with mild AD dementia.

ACI-24, an active oligo-specific amyloid vaccine, stimulates the patient's immune system to produce beta-sheet conformation-specific antibodies that prevent plaque deposition and enhance clearance of plaques (Pihlgren et al., 2012). The vaccine is designed to break immune tolerance. During preclinical development in animal models, ACI-24 has shown high efficacy in vivo by memory restoration and plaque reduction. The vaccine is also characterized by a very high specificity due to generating a conformation-specific antibody response. The favorable safety profile of ACI-24 is underlined through the absence of local inflammation in relevant models as well as its T-cell-independent mechanism shown in preclinical development.

Passive Immunotherapy

Solanezumab is a humanized monoclonal antibody that recognizes the middle region of beta-amyloid and binds soluble forms of the peptide (Farlow et al., 2012). Bapineuzumab, a humanized monoclonal antibody against the N-terminus of beta-amyloid, is designed to bind and remove insoluble beta-amyloid peptide (Salloway et al., 2009). Comparing the two monoclonal antibodies, bapineuzumab binds to aggregated beta-amyloid, which is found primarily in the brain, while solanezumab binds to monomeric beta-amyloid oligomers, found throughout the body. Solanezumab differs from bapineuzumab in several ways: It recognizes a distinct epitope in the central portion of the peptide, and whereas bapineuzumab binds amyloid plaques more strongly than soluble beta-amyloid, solanezumab selectively binds to soluble beta-amyloid with little to no affinity for the fibrillar form.

Bapineuzumab failed to meet its primary endpoints in two Phase III, multicenter, randomized, double-blind, placebo-controlled, efficacy and safety trials in patients with mild to moderate AD dementia. One of the trials was in patients who are Apolipoprotein E ε4 (*APOE* ε4) carriers and the second trial was in patients who are *APOE* ε4 noncarriers. In both trials, the primary outcome measures were cognitive and functional scales and were evaluated at 18 months. In the previous Phase II trial, bapineuzumab had not met its primary efficacy endpoint in mild to moderate AD dementia. Furthermore, amyloid-related imaging abnormalities due to vasogenic edema (ARIA-E) were observed in 0.8% of placebo and 15.8% of bapineuzumab-treated subjects overall. Risk factors for ARIA-E were dose, ApoE-ε4 allele, female gender, and baseline ARIA due to microhemorrhoage or hemosiderin deposits (ARIA-H), but not age or disease severity. Symptoms associated with ARIA-E (e.g., headache, confusion, and gait abnormalities) occurred in 2.5% of treated subjects overall but increased to 7.8% in the 2.0 mg/kg group that had led to early termination of the high-dose arm. Further development of this compound has been discontinued.

The primary endpoints, both cognitive and functional, were also not met in either of the two Phase III, double-blind, placebo-controlled solanezumab trials in patients with mild to moderate AD dementia. However, a prespecified secondary analysis of pooled data across both trials showed small but statistically significant slowing of cognitive decline in the overall study population of patients with mild to moderate AD dementia. In addition, prespecified secondary subgroup analyses of pooled data across both studies showed a statistically significant slowing of cognitive decline in patients with mild AD dementia, but not in patients with moderate AD dementia.

Adverse events with an incidence of at least 1% that occurred more frequently in the solanezumab group than in the placebo group were lethargy, rash and malaise, and angina. An independent analysis of the data from the solanezumab studies was performed by the Alzheimer's Disease Cooperative Study (ADCS), an academic national research consortium that facilitates the discovery, development, and testing of new drugs for the treatment of AD. The ADCS findings suggested that although the drug appeared to slow cognitive decline, it did not slow functional impairment. The company announced in 2013 plans to conduct a confirmatory Phase III clinical trial in patients with mild AD dementia, diagnosed using more stringent criteria, including amyloid imaging. Finally, Solanezumab is being tested in the A4 trial (Anti-Amyloid in Asymptomatic Alzheimer's Disease). The A4 trial is intended to bridge the gap between trials for autosomal-dominant and sporadic AD.

Gantenerumab is a fully human anti-beta-amyloid antibody that has a high capacity to specifically bind to cerebral amyloid plaques (Bohrmann et al., 2012). Results from Phase 1 clinical trials demonstrated that gantenerumab treatment results in a dose-dependent reduction of brain amyloid, possibly through phagocytosis via brain microglial cells, whereas amyloid load increased in patients receiving placebo treatment. A Phase II study is currently recruiting 770 patients in 15 countries to investigate the efficacy and safety of gantenerumab in subjects with prodromal AD. The Phase II study is a multicenter, randomized, double-blind, placebo-controlled, parallel-group 2-year study to evaluate the effect of subcutaneous gantenerumab on cognition and function in prodromal AD.

Crenezumab, a humanized anti-amyloid 1-40 and 1-42 antibody, is in a Phase II randomized, double-blind, parallel group, placebo-controlled study clinical trial in mild to moderate AD dementia. In the Phase I trial that concluded in 2010, crenezumab demonstrated encouraging safety data in patients with mild to moderate AD, with no signs of vasogenic edema in any of the subjects. Plasma beta-amyloid levels correlated with serum crenezumab concentration. The ongoing Phase II trial will enroll more than 370 patients in multiple centers globally. The primary outcome measures are cognitive and global function.

Finally, another passive immunotherapy approach employed intravenous immunoglobulin (IVIG). Despite suggestions of potential signals of benefit in earlier studies, the primary efficacy endpoints were not met in a 2013 report on the Phase III clinical trial in 390 patients with mild to moderate AD over an 18-month period. Investigators are continuing to analyze data from these trials, given that several post-hoc analyses in subgroups of patients suggested the possibility of cognitive benefits, at least in *APOE* ε4 carriers.

Nonimmunotherapy Clearance of Beta-Amyloid

Results of a study by researchers from Case Western Reserve University demonstrated that an oncology drug bexarotene (Targretin) reduced beta-amyloid plaques in the brains of a transgenic mouse model of AD (Cramer et al., 2012). Bexarotene activates retinoid receptors on brain cells that increase production of apolipoprotein E that helps rid excess amyloid in the fluid-filled space between neurons (Mandrekar-Colucci, Karlo, & Landret, 2012). It also appears to enhance another cleanup process, called phagocytosis. Bexarotene is FDA approved to treat cutaneous T-cell lymphoma.

After 14 days of treatment with bexarotene, beta-amyloid plaque levels decreased by 75%. In the study, transgenic mice treated with bexarotene showed an improvement in their behavior based on several different behavioral and cognitive tests, such as ability to make nests and odor discrimination. The results of this animal study lend further support for continued testing of the amyloid hypothesis as a way to address this devastating illness.

Drugs to Prevent Tau Protein Phosphorylation

The second major target being pursued in the quest for disease-modifying treatments for AD is the intracellular protein tau. Tau is a ubiquitous protein that binds to and stabilizes microtubules (MT). Hyperphosphorylation of tau disrupts its normal function in regulating axonal transport and leads to the accumulation of neurofibrillary tangles and toxic species of soluble tau (Iqbal et al., 1998). The phosphorylation state of tau plays a critical role in mediating tau mislocalization and subsequent impairment of synaptic transmission (Rapoport, Dawson, Binder, Vitek, & Ferreira, 2002). Furthermore, degradation of hyperphosphorylated tau by the proteasome is inhibited by the actions of beta-amyloid, further compounding the issue.

Beta-amyloid interacts with the signaling pathways that regulate the phosphorylation of tau. These two proteins and their associated signaling pathways therefore represent important therapeutic targets for AD. Accordingly, a possible therapeutic strategy for AD and related "tauopathies" is treatment with MT-stabilizing anticancer drugs such as paclitaxel. However, paclitaxel and related taxanes have poor blood–brain barrier permeability and thus are unsuitable for diseases of the brain. The MT-stabilizing agent, epothilone D (EpoD), is brain penetrant and has been evaluated in tau transgenic mice that develop forebrain tau inclusions, axonal degeneration, and MT deficits. In studies in aged tauopathy mice, epothilone-treated animals retained more healthy axons, lost fewer hippocampal neurons, and performed better on memory tests compared to vehicle-treated animals (Zhang et al., 2012). A Phase Ib trial of epothilone D in mild AD patients is currently enrolling patients.

Tau Immunotherapy

Tau-based immunotherapy is fairly new, but interest in the approach is growing. Boutajangout et al. demonstrate that targeting phosphorylated tau by active immunization prevents cognitive decline in the htau/PS1 mouse model. This was the third study demonstrating the efficacy of active vaccination using phosphorylated tau fragments in different animal models and confirmed previous findings (Boimel et al., 2010).

Many labs have generated antibodies specific for tau oligomers. These polyclonal and monoclonal antibodies to tau oligomers were prepared in vitro by seeding soluble tau with oligomeric Aβ (Lasagna-Reeves et al., 2010). The antibodies do not recognize tau monomers, but they do recognize both nonphosphorylated and phosphorylated tau in neurofibrillary tangles. Elevated levels of tau oligomers have been quantified in postmortem AD brains, compared to control specimens. About 10% to 20% of total tau in AD brains is oligomeric, and the few tau structures found in control brains all appeared to be neurofibrillary tangles.

Finally, another tau-modulating compound called tideglusib, an oral glycagen synthetase kinase-3 (GSK-3) inhibitor, has been evaluated for the treatment of AD. GSK-3β is the main enzyme involved in tau hyperphosphorylation (Takashima et al., 1998). Overexpression of GSK-3 leads to hyperphosphorylation of the tau protein (Sirerol-Piquer et al., 2011). Tideglusib is a member of the thiadiazolindindione family of the GSK-3 inhibitors. It is hypothesized that GSK-3 may play a key role in the pathogenesis of AD and possibly serve as the link between extracellular beta-amyloid and intracellular tau phosphorylation. Data from the Phase IIa double-blind, placebo-controlled, escalating doses trial of tideglusib in 30 mild to moderate AD patients were reported showing a trend toward cognitive benefit. A Phase IIb clinical trial of tideglusib for the treatment of AD dementia in 308 patients was reported in 2013 as not meeting primary endpoints.

Other Therapies

Alpha-7 Nicotinic Acetylcholine Receptor Agonist

EVP-6124, a selective alpha-7 nicotinic acetylcholine receptor agonist, enhances synaptic transmission and acts as a coagonist in combination with acetylcholine (ACh) to enhance cognition (Prickaerts et al., 2012). By sensitizing the alpha-7 receptor, EVP-6124 makes it possible for smaller amounts of naturally occurring ACh to be effective in activating the alpha-7 receptor. This mechanism could potentially alleviate the undesirable side effects caused by other systemic compounds, such as AChEIs, which are dose limited by toxic side effects. Additionally, beta-amyloid binds directly to alpha-7 receptors with high affinity (Wang et al., 2010). A multicenter, double-blind, placebo-controlled, 24-week Phase 2b study of EVP-6124 has been completed. In the trial of 409 people with mild to moderate AD, the drug met seven of its nine endpoints with statistical and clinical significance, with trends on the remaining two. A Phase III trial is reportedly being planned.

5-Hydroxytryptamine-6 Receptor Antagonists

In July 2013 data presented at AAIC 2013 from a 24-week Phase II randomized double-blind placebo-controlled clinical trial of 278 patients with moderate AD dementia given the serotonin/5-hydroxytryptamine-6 (5-HT_6) receptor antagonist Lu AE58054 along with the donepezil suggested that Lu AE58054 in combination with donepezil provided added cognitive benefit, measured by the ADAS-Cog, compared to placebo added to donepezil.

Activation of the 5-HT_6 receptor, a receptor primarily expressed in the cerebral cortex and hippocampus, usually represses cholinergic function (see Bentley et al., 1999), while 5-HT_6 antagonists elevate glutamatergic neurotransmission (see Dawson et al., 2003). It is posited that since Lu AE58054 selectively blocks serotonin from activating 5-HT_6 receptors, it may result in an overall enhancement of acetylcholine and glutamate levels, thereby potentially producing beneficial effects on attention, arousal, memory, learning, and cognition.

Other 5-HT6 antagonists have been previously tested in AD dementia clinical trials. Data from four Phase II clinical trials in patients with mild to moderate AD dementia treated with SB-742457 (NCT00348192, NCT00224497, NCT00708552, and NCT00710684) suggested a potential signal for modest benefit on the Clinician's Interview-Based Impression of Change with Caregiver Input (CIBIC+) (Maher-Edwards et al., 2010), and similar benefits when compared to donepezil (Maher-Edwards et al., 2011). Several other 5-HT6 antagonists have completed or are in Phase I trials. Dimebon, a drug that, among other things, antagonizes 5-HT6 receptors, showed cognitive benefits in Phase II trials, but it failed to show efficacy in larger Phase III testing. A large Phase III clinical trial program with Lu AE58054 added to background stable therapy with donepezil and other cholinesterase inhibitors in patients with mild to moderate AD dementia begins enrollment in late 2013 and early 2014.

Nerve Growth Factor

CERE-110 is a gene therapy product designed to deliver nerve growth factor (NGF). It is composed of an adeno-associated viral (AAV) vector carrying the gene for NGF and is neurosurgically injected into the nucleus basalis of Meynert (NBM). NGF is a neurotrophic protein that can enhance the function of cholinergic neurons in the NBM, prevent their death, and increase production of ACh (Hefti, 1986). The drug has the potential to induce sustained expression of NGF, which may result in a long-lasting restoration of function, protection of neurons, and slowing the progression of AD. The Phase I open label study in 10 patients with mild to moderate AD demonstrated that CERE-110 was safe and well tolerated (Rafii et al., 2014). A multicenter, placebo-controlled Phase II clinical trial in collaboration with the Alzheimer's Disease Cooperative Study (ADCS) is under way.

Insulin

Diabetes increases the risk of developing any dementia by at least 100% and of AD by about 65%, with the risk increasing the longer the patient has had diabetes. According to a current hypothesis, learning takes place as a result of changes at synapses instigated by convergent inputs from other neurons that stimulate various types of receptor on the neuron's surface. The action of the main neurotransmitter glutamate on its receptors is amplified by intracellular signaling pathways stimulated by insulin binding to the insulin receptor. An important enzyme activated by these signals is protein kinase C (PKC), which among other actions, promotes the release of calcium from intracellular stores. PKC seems to be central to the activation of synapses in the hippocampus during learning tasks, as well as stimulating the expression of genes for receptors involved in learning, including the insulin receptor. As the production of insulin receptors declines with age, or as receptors become resistant to insulin, PKC is no longer activated so strongly, weakening the increase in synaptic efficacy and the growth of new synapses thought to be essential for learning (de la Monte, 2012). Insulin stimulation also helps maintain healthy neuron infrastructure by preventing the activation of GSK3. This enzyme causes the hyperphosphorylation of the tau protein, an abnormal modification leading to the formation of neurofibrillary tangles.

A Phase II trial of intranasal insulin for AD has been completed (Craft et al., 2012). It was a double-blind, 4-month trial. Sixty-four people with mild cognitive impairment, and 40 mild to moderate AD patients, were given daily placebo or insulin (20 or 40 international units). The lower insulin dose improved delayed memory, and both doses staved off decline in general cognition (measured by ADAS-Cog) and functional abilities (measured by the Alzheimer's Disease Cooperative Study Activities of Daily Living, i.e., ADCS-ADL).

A subset of participants consented to spinal taps for measuring cerebrospinal fluid AD biomarkers and to fluorodeoxyglucose positron emission tomography (FDG-PET) scans to assess brain glucose usage. On the whole, CSF levels of $A\beta42$, $A\beta40$, tau, and phosphorylated tau stayed the same in treated participants over the 4-month study. In exploratory analyses, correlations between CSF biomarker changes and cognitive measures were observed in the treatment group (low and high doses were pooled), but not in placebo participants. On FDG-PET, metabolism decreased in AD-affected regions (bilateral frontal, right temporal, bilateral occipital, and precuneus/cuneus) in the placebo group more than in the treatment groups (Craft et al., 2012). In collaboration with the Alzheimer's Disease Cooperative Study group, a larger, 18-month Phase IIB multisite trial testing similar doses of intranasal insulin in MCI and mild AD patients is under way. The study includes cognitive and functional tests, as well as CSF biomarker and imaging endpoints.

Aerobic Physical Exercise

The putative benefits of aerobic physical exercise for maximizing cognitive function and supporting brain health have great potential for combating AD. Aerobic exercise offers a low-cost, low-risk intervention that is widely available and may have disease-modifying effects. Demonstrating that aerobic exercise alters the AD process would have enormous public health implications.

A wealth of animal research data suggest that exercise positively impacts brain health. Increased physical activity may have a trophic effect on the brain, particularly the hippocampus. Exercise appears to stimulate neurogenesis, enhance neuronal survival, increase resistance to brain insults, and increase synaptic plasticity. Exercise promotes brain vascularization, mobilizes gene expression profiles predicted to benefit brain plasticity, and maintains cognitive function. Additionally, exercise effects on the brain may reduce vascular risk factors (heart disease, atherosclerosis, stroke, and diabetes) that are believed to place an individual at risk for dementia, vascular dementia, and AD. Further, there is limited but compelling animal data suggesting that exercise may have disease-modifying benefits in AD. For instance, increased physical activity in mouse models of AD reduces neuropathological burden and may promote hippocampal neurogenesis.

In one recent study, Buchman and colleagues (2012) looked at how exercise affects cognition and risk of AD. All prior studies relied on self-reported exercise regimen. None had prospectively measured the amount of exercise or activity. In this prospective, 4-year study, 716 subjects' activity was measured using actigraphy for 10 hours per day. At the end of the observation period, a total "activity score" was calculated for each person using the information from the wrist device. During the study, each person had at least two cognitive assessments. At the beginning of the study, none of the participants had AD dementia. On average, each person wore the actigraphy monitor for just over 9 days to assess his or her activity level. Cognitive testing was done, and it was repeated each year. The group was followed for an average of 3.5 years. During that time, 9.9% of the group developed AD dementia. At the end of the observation period, a strong association was observed between exercise and the risk for developing AD. If a person had a low overall physical activity, he or she had a faster rate of cognitive decline. Subjects with the lowest activity were most likely to develop AD dementia. Compared to those with high rates of activity, the risk of developing AD dementia was two times higher.

Future Directions

The overall failure of disease-modifying drug development for AD has led to frustration and even fatalism within industry and academic research programs. Some fear that the major pharmaceutical companies will turn away from further investments in this area. But the need for therapeutic progress in the face of an exploding global epidemic is undeniable.

Despite the failures, the amyloid hypothesis has been strengthened by recent findings. While the solanezumab trials failed to meet their primary endpoints, analysis of the pooled data provides the strongest support yet for the therapeutic potential of targeting amyloid. This is further bolstered by the discovery of a rare genetic polymorphisms associated with reduced beta-secretase cleavage that affords dramatic protection against sporadic AD. So, while other targets must be vigorously pursued, anti-amyloid treatments may still hold the greatest promise in the treatment of AD.

Each of the negative pivotal trials of anti-amyloid agents has been conducted in individuals with AD dementia. As biomarker findings have been incorporated into diagnostic approaches and trial methodology, academia and pharmaceutical companies have been moving therapies into earlier interventional studies, particularly prodromal AD (mild cognitive impairment linked to AD by biomarkers). It is reasonable to anticipate that clinical benefits will be greater with earlier treatment.

But the neurobiology of the AD pathologic cascade begins many years before prodromal AD symptoms develop. So presumably disease-modifying treatment, particularly if targeting the amyloid accumulation that defines the earliest disease stage, should begin prior to the onset of cognitive symptoms. We now have diagnostic criteria for preclinical AD (see Chapter 18) based on imaging or cerebrospinal fluid biomarkers. As discussed in detail in that chapter, these ideas have now been incorporated into trial designs by several academic consortia, and trials will commence in 2013 and 2014. The ongoing ADCS Anti-Amyloid in Asymptomatic AD (A4) trial should provide the strongest evidence for or against beta-amyloid's central role in driving AD pathology during preclinical stage of the disease. Regulatory agencies have been supportive of this strategy, despite the absence of clinically relevant outcomes in such trials. The enormous need has generated effective, precompetitive collaboration that enables the launch of these studies.

Despite the lack of success to date in identifying disease-modifying drugs for AD, optimism is growing as new strategies continue to be developed.

References

Ballatore, C., Lee, V. M., & Trojanowski, J. Q. (2007). Tau-mediated neurodegeneration in Alzheimer's disease and related disorders. *Nature Reviews Neuroscience, 8*(9), 663–672.

Bartus, R. T., Dean, R. L., III, Beer, B., & Lippa, A. S. (1982). The cholinergic hypothesis of geriatric memory dysfunction. *Science, 217*(4558), 408–417.

Bentley, J. C., Bourson, A., Boess, F. G., Fone, K. C., Marsden, C. A., Petit, N., Sleight, A. J. (1999). Investigation of stretching behaviour induced by the selective 5-HT6 receptor antagonist, Ro 04-6790, in rats. *British Journal of Pharmacology, 126*(7), 1537–1542.

Birks, J. (2006). Cholinesterase inhibitors for Alzheimer's disease. *Cochrane Database of Systematic Reviews*, (1), CD005593.

Bohrmann, B., Baumann, K., Benz, J., Gerber, F., Huber, W., Knoflach, F.,...Loetscher, H. (2012). Gantenerumab: A novel human anti-Aβ antibody demonstrates sustained cerebral amyloid-β binding and elicits cell-mediated removal of human amyloid-β. *Journal of Alzheimers Disease, 28*(1), 49–69.

Boimel, M., Grigoriadis, N., Lourbopoulos, A., Haber, E., Abramsky, O., & Rosenmann, H. (2010). Efficacy and safety of immunization with phosphorylated tau against neurofibrillary tangles in mice. *Experimental Neurology, 224*(2), 472–485.

Buchman, A. S., Boyle, P. A., Yu, L., Shah, R. C., Wilson, R. S., & Bennett, D. A. (2012). Total daily physical activity and the risk of AD and cognitive decline in older adults. *Neurology, 78*(17), 1323–1329.

Chen, H. S., & Lipton, S. A. (2005). Pharmacological implications of two distinct mechanisms of interaction of memantine with N-methyl-D-aspartate-gated channels. *Journal of Pharmacology and Experimental Therapeutics, 314*(3), 961–971.

Craft, S., Baker, L. D., Montine, T. J., Minoshima, S., Watson, G. S., Claxton, A.,...Gerton, B. (2012). Intranasal insulin therapy for Alzheimer disease and amnestic mild cognitive impairment: A pilot clinical trial. *Archives of Neurology, 69*(1), 29–38

Cramer, P. E., Cirrito, J. R., Wesson, D. W., Lee, C. Y., Karlo, J. C., Zinn, A. E.,...Landreth, G. E. (2012). ApoE-directed therapeutics rapidly clear β-amyloid and reverse deficits in AD mouse models. *Science, 335*(6075), 1503–1506.

Dasilva, K. A., Shaw, J. E., & McLaurin, J. (2010). Amyloid-beta fibrillogenesis: Structural insight and therapeutic intervention. *Experimental Neurology, 223*(2), 311–321.

Dawson, L. A., Nguyen, H. Q., Li, P. (2003). Potentiation of amphetamine-induced changes in dopamine and 5-HT by a 5-HT(6) receptor antagonist. *Brain Research Bulletin 15; 59*(6), 513–521.

de la Monte, S. M. (2012). Brain insulin resistance and deficiency as therapeutic targets in Alzheimer's disease. *Current Alzheimers Research, 9*(1), 35–66.

De Strooper, B., Annaert, W., Cupers, P., Saftig, P., Craessaerts, K., Mumm, J. S.,...Kopan, R. (1999). A presenilin-1-dependent gamma-secretase-like protease mediates release of Notch intracellular domain. *Nature, 398*(6727), 518–522.

Farlow, M., Arnold, S. E., van Dyck, C. H., Aisen, P. S., Snider, B. J., Porsteinsson, A. P.,...Siemers, E. R. (2012). Safety and biomarker effects of solanezumab in patients with Alzheimer's disease. *Alzheimers and Dementia, 8*(4), 261–271.

Gilman, S., Koller, M., Black, R. S., Jenkins, L., Griffith, S. G., Fox, N. C.,...Orgogozo, J. M. (2005). Clinical effects of Abeta immunization (AN1792) in patients with AD in an interrupted trial. *Neurology, 64*(9), 1553–1562.

Haass, C., & Selkoe, D. J. (2007). Soluble protein oligomers in neurodegeneration: Lessons from the Alzheimer's amyloid beta-peptide. *Nature Reviews Molecular and Cellular Biology, 8*(2), 101–112.

Hefti, F. (1986). Nerve growth factor promotes survival of septal cholinergic neurons after fimbrial transections. *Journal of Neuroscience, 6*(8), 2155–2162.

Iqbal, K., Alonso, A. C., Gong, C. X., Khatoon, S., Pei, J. J., & Wang, J. Z. (1998). Grundke-Iqbal I. Mechanisms of neurofibrillary degeneration and the formation of neurofibrillary tangles. *Journal of Neural Transmission Supplemental, 53*, 169–180.

Jonsson, T., Atwal, J. K., Steinberg, S., Snaedal, J., Jonsson, P. V., Bjornsson, S.,...Stefansson, K. (2012). A mutation in APP protects against Alzheimer's disease and age-related cognitive decline. *Nature, 488*(7409), 96–99.

Lasagna-Reeves, C. A., Castillo-Carranza, D. L., Guerrero-Muoz, M. J., Jackson, G. R., & Kayed, R. (2010). Preparation and characterization of neurotoxic tau oligomers. *Biochemistry, 49*(47), 10039–10041.

Maher-Edwards, G., Zvartau-Hind, M., Hunter, A. J., Gold, M., Hopton, G., Jacobs, G., Davy, M., Williams, P. (2010). Double-blind, controlled phase II study of a 5-HT6 receptor antagonist, SB-742457, in Alzheimer's disease. *Current Alzheimer Research, 7*(5), 374–385.

Maher-Edwards, G., Dixon, R., Hunter, J., Gold, M., Hopton, G., Jacobs, G., Hunter, J., Williams, P. (2011). SB-742457 and donepezil in Alzheimer disease: a randomized, placebo-controlled study. *International Journal of Geriatric Psychiatry, 26*(5), 536–544.

Mandrekar-Colucci, S., Karlo, J. C., & Landreth, G. E. (2012). Mechanisms underlying the rapid peroxisome proliferator-activated receptor-γ-mediated amyloid clearance and reversal of cognitive deficits in a murine model of Alzheimer's disease. *Journal of Neuroscience, 32*(30), 10117–10128.

Orgogozo, J. M., Gilman, S., Dartigues, J. F., Laurent, B., Puel, M., Kirby, L. C., ... Hock, C. (2003). Subacute meningoencephalitis in a subset of patients with AD after Abeta42 immunization. *Neurology, 61*(1), 46–54.

Pihlgren, M., Madani, R., Hickman, D., Giriens, V., Chuard, N., ven der Auwera, I., ... Stanco-Piorko, K. (2012). The safety profile of ACI-24, an oligo-specific amyloid beta vaccine, demonstrated decrease of large microbleedings in brain of aged Alzheimer's disease mouse model. *Alzheimers and Dementia, 5*(4), Supplement, p425–p426

Prickaerts, J., van Goethem, N. P., Chesworth, R., Shapiro, G., Boess, F. G., Methfessel, C., ... König, G. (2012). EVP-6124, a novel and selective α7 nicotinic acetylcholine receptor partial agonist, improves memory performance by potentiating the acetylcholine response of α7 nicotinic acetylcholine receptors. *Neuropharmacology, 62*(2), 1099–1110.

Rafii, M. S., Baumann, T. L., Bakay, R. A., Ostrove, J. M., Siffert, J., Fleisher, A. S., ... Bartus, R. T. (2014). A phase1 study of stereotactic gene delivery of AAV2-NGF for Alzheimer's disease. *Alzheimers Dementia*, pii: S1552-5260(13)02838-0.

Rapoport, M., Dawson, H. N., Binder, L. I., Vitek, M. P., & Ferreira, A. (2002). Tau is essential to beta-amyloid-induced neurotoxicity. *Proceedings of the National Academy of Science USA, 99*(9), 6364–6369.

Salloway, S., Sperling, R., Gilman, S., Fox, N. C., Blennow, K., Raskind, M., ... Grundman, M. (2009). A phase 2 multiple ascending dose trial of bapineuzumab in mild to moderate Alzheimer disease. *Neurology, 73*(24), 2061–2070.

Salloway, S., Sperling, R., Keren, R., Porsteinsson, A. P., van Dyck, C. H., Tariot, P. N., ... Cedarbaum, J. M. (2011). A phase 2 randomized trial of ELND005, scyllo-inositol, in mild to moderate Alzheimer disease. *Neurology, 77*(13), 1253–1262.

Selkoe, D. J. (2011). Alzheimer's disease. *Cold Spring Harbor Perspectives in Biology, 3*(7), pii: a004457.

Selkoe, D. J. (2008). Soluble oligomers of the amyloid beta-protein impair synaptic plasticity and behavior. *Behavior Brain Research, 192*(1), 106–113.

Sirerol-Piquer, M., Gomez-Ramos, P., Hernández, F., Perez, M., Morán, M. A., Fuster-Matanzo, A., ... García-Verdugo, J. M. (2011). GSK3β overexpression induces neuronal death and a depletion of the neurogenic niches in the dentate gyrus. *Hippocampus, 21*(8), 910–922.

Takashima, A., Murayama, M., Murayama, O., Kohno, T., Honda, T., Yasutake, K., ... Wolozin, B. (1998). Presenilin 1 associates with glycogen synthase kinase-3beta and its substrate tau. *Proceedings of the National Academy of Science USA, 95*, 9637–9641.

Tanzi, R. E., & Bertram, L. (2005). Twenty years of the Alzheimer's disease amyloid hypothesis: A genetic perspective. *Cell, 120*(4), 545–555.

Tong, G., Wang, J. S., Sverdlov, O., Huang, S. P., Slemmon, R., Croop, R., ... Dockens, R. C. (2012). Multicenter, randomized, double-blind, placebo-controlled, single-ascending dose study of the oral γ-secretase inhibitor BMS-708163 (Avagacestat), tolerability profile, pharmacokinetic parameters, and pharmacodynamic markers. *Clinical Therapy, 34*(3), 654–667.

Vellas, B., Black, R., Thal, L. J., Fox, N. C., Daniels, M., McLennan, G., ... Grundman, M. (2009). Long-term follow-up of patients immunized with AN1792: Reduced functional decline in antibody responders. *Current Alzheimers Research, 6*(2), 144–151.

Viswanathan, A., & Greenberg, S. M. (2011). Cerebral amyloid angiopathy in the elderly. *Annals of Neurology, 70*(6), 871–880.

Wang, H. Y., Bakshi, K., Shen, C., Frankfurt, M., Trocmé-Thibierge, C., & Morain, P. (2010). S 24795 limits beta-amyloid-alpha7 nicotinic receptor interaction and reduces Alzheimer's disease-like pathologies. *Biological Psychiatry, 67*(6), 522–530

Weiner, M. W., Veitch, D. P., Aisen, P. S., Beckett, L. A., Cairns, N. J., Green, R. C., ... Trojanowski, J. Q. (2012). The Alzheimer's Disease Neuroimaging Initiative: A review of papers published since its inception. *Alzheimers and Dementia, 8*(1 Suppl), S1-68.

Whitehouse, P. J., Price, D. L., Struble, R. G., Clark, A. W., Coyle, J. T., & Delon, M. R. (1982). Alzheimer's disease and senile dementia: Loss of neurons in the basal forebrain. *Science, 215*(4537), 1237–1239.

Wilcock, G. K., Black, S. E., Hendrix, S. B., Zavitz, K. H., Swabb, E. A., & Laughlin, M. A. (2008). Efficacy and safety of tarenflurbil in mild to moderate Alzheimer's disease: A randomised phase II trial. *Lancet Neurology, 7*(6), 483–493. Erratum in *Lancet Neurology* 2008, *7*(7), 575. *Lancet Neurology* 2011, *10*(4), 297.

Winblad, B., Andreasen, N., Minthon, L., Floesser, A., Imbert, G., Dumortier, T., . . . Graf, A. (2012). Safety, tolerability, and antibody response of active Aβ immunotherapy with CAD106 in patients with Alzheimer's disease: Randomised, double-blind, placebo-controlled, first-in-human study. *Lancet Neurology, 11*(7), 597–604.

Zhang, B., Carroll, J., Trojanowski, J. Q., Yao, Y., Iba, M., Potuzak, J. S., . . . Brunden, K. R. (2012). The microtubule-stabilizing agent, epothilone D, reduces axonal dysfunction, neurotoxicity, cognitive deficits, and Alzheimer-like pathology in an interventional study with aged tau transgenic mice. *Journal of Neuroscience, 32*(11), 3601–3611.

24

Management of Agitation, Aggression, and Psychosis Associated With Alzheimer's Disease

Clive Ballard and Anne Corbett

Worldwide, 35 million people suffer from dementia (Alzheimer's Disease International, 2008), the majority of whom have Alzheimer's disease (AD). It is a devastating illness, resulting in progressive decline of cognitive ability and functional capacity and the emergence of behavioral and psychological symptoms of dementia (BPSDs). The progressive decline and the BPSDs can cause enormous distress to patients, their caregivers and families, and have a major societal impact. More than 90% of people with dementia develop at least one clinically significant behavioral or psychiatric symptom (Steinberg et al., 2008) over the course of their illness. BPSDs present as three main syndromes—agitation, psychosis, and mood disorders—although these syndromes frequently coexist. The overall frequency of BPSD, in particular agitation and aggression, increases with the severity of dementia (Aalten et al., 2003; see Chapter 21). This chapter focuses predominantly on treatment strategies for agitation, aggression, and psychosis. Common symptoms of aggression in people with AD include verbal insults and shouting, as well as physical aggression such as hitting and biting others, and throwing objects. These symptoms most commonly manifest when people with AD are being assisted with personal care. Common symptoms of agitation include restlessness and pacing, excessive fidgeting, motor activities associated with anxiety (such as hand wringing and following a caregiver around the house), and shouting/screaming. Common symptoms of psychosis include visual hallucinations (most frequently of people or animals), auditory hallucinations, delusions (most often simple nonsystematized delusions of theft, harm, or infidelity or other people living in the house) and delusional misidentification (e.g., Capgras syndrome, believing that people on TV or in photographs are real or believing that a mirror reflection is someone else (Ballard, Gauthier, et al., 2009).

Aggression and nonaggressive agitation occur in approximately 20% of people with AD in contact with clinical services (Burns, Jacoby, & Levy, 1990b) or living in the community (Lyketsos et al., 2000) and in 40%–60% of people in care facilities (Margallo-Lana et al., 2001). Delusions and hallucinations are present in 25% of people with dementia in clinical settings (Burns, Jacoby, & Levy, 1990a). Longitudinal studies indicate that hallucinations often resolve over a few months (Ballard, Patel, Solis, Lowe, & Wilcock, 1996; Haupt, Kurz, & Janner, 2000), but that delusions and agitation (Ballard et al., 2001; Haupt et al., 2000) are more likely to persist (Ballard et al., 1996).

In most individuals BPSDs have a significant impact on daily life (Lyketsos, 2007). They are often distressing for the person experiencing the symptoms (Gilley, Whalen, Wilson, & Bennett, 1991) and can lead to distress, added burden, and depression in those who care for them (Ballard, Eastwood, Gahir, & Wilcock, 1996; Rabins, Mace, & Lucas, 1982). They are also associated with a reduced quality of life (Banerjee et al., 2006) and are often the trigger for institutional care for people living in the community (Steele, Rovner, Chase, & Folstein, 1990).

Treatment

General Considerations

A broad clinical assessment is essential before specific therapies are considered (see Chapter 26). Physical health problems such as infection (including urinary tract, chest, or dental infections), pain, or dehydration are common and often precipitate BPSDs, as can visual and auditory impairment (Chapman, Dickinson, McKeith, & Ballard, 1999; Holroyd & Laurie, 1999). A comprehensive review of pharmacologic treatments may identify therapies exacerbating depression, confusion, or other BPSDs. Pain is difficult to assess in people with dementia and is underdiagnosed, but better pain management does reduce BPSDs (Cohen-Mansfield & Lipson, 2008). A recent cluster randomized trial compared stepped analgesia with usual care over 8 weeks and showed a marked and significant reduction in agitation in the group receiving analgesia, which was correlated with improvement in pain (Husebo, Ballard, Sandvik, Nilsen, & Aarsland, 2011). This perhaps indicates that treating even minor, low-level pain may confer considerable benefit as part of the management of agitation and other BPSDs.

Nonpharmacological Treatments

All best practice guides recommend nondrug approaches as the first-line treatment option for BPSDs (see Chapter 26), except in exceptional circumstances of substantial risk or extreme distress (Lyketsos et al., 2006). BPSDs that are sporadic and do not cause distress or risk may be effectively managed without a specific therapy or may respond well to simple psychological therapy or behavioral/environmental modification approaches. When symptoms are mild to moderate, valuable insights can be gained by working with relatives or care staff to monitor the symptoms and avoid the need for more intensive treatment. As an example of a practical approach to implementing nonpharmacologic interventions for BPSDs, a range of psychological intervention tools have been developed by Cohen-Mansfield. These interventions are based on activities and interactions that can be personalized within the structured framework of a care home setting, such as structured social interaction and personalized music. These approaches were rigorously evaluated in a robust, randomized controlled trial (RCT) with 167 participants, 105 of whom showed significant benefits in agitation overall. A smaller 6-week study also showed improvement in specific symptoms of agitation such as shouting (Cohen-Mansfield, Libin, & Marx, 2007; Cohen-Mansfield & Werner, 1997). RCTs of people with dementia living in their own homes have also demonstrated significant benefits in the treatment of BPSD, including agitation, with approaches focusing on promoting activities (Gitlin et al., 2008).

Despite these positive outcomes, it can be difficult to implement these individualized interventions in all clinical and care home settings because of the time constraints and level of skill required of the care staff. To try and address this issue, our group designed a simplified version of the Cohen-Mansfield intervention called the brief psychosocial therapy (BPST). The BPST involves a daily personalized social interaction for 10 to 30 minutes to be delivered by a care assistant under the supervision of a therapist who has attended a 2-day BPST training course (Ballard, Brown, et al., 2009). The BPST was evaluated in an open trial of more than 200 participants and showed a significant seven-point improvement on the Cohen-Mansfield Agitation Inventory. It should be noted that the absence of a control treatment means that it is difficult to determine the proportion of the benefit attributable to the intervention. Nevertheless, this study supports best practice guidance for BPSDs, providing professionals with options for simple, first-line nondrug interventions and highlights the finding that most individuals experience improvement without pharmacologic treatment. Reminiscence therapy also confers modest but significant benefits in BPSDs and may be valuable as part of a personalized treatment and care plan.

People experiencing more severe or challenging BPSDs still benefit from more intense individualized psychological interventions. Evidence from large case series and a couple of small but well-designed clinical trials supports the effectiveness of individualized, comprehensive interventions delivered by a clinical psychologist and designed using "antecedent, behavior, consequence" (ABC) charts.

For example, one cluster randomized trial compared a clinical psychology model based on the ABC principles with a traditional old-age psychiatry service in 55 referrals of people with BPSD. Both groups showed favorable responses to the interventions, but the model led by the clinical psychologist resulted in additional reduction of antipsychotic prescriptions and fewer hospital days (Bird, 2002).

A different but equally important approach is to improve the training and skill set of care staff to enable more effective management of BPSDs and to improve the overall quality of care. Studies evaluating this approach have reported variable results, with many shorter studies indicating that initial benefits are not sustained beyond the end of the training period. However, more recent RCTs of intensive training packages and interventions to develop practice have conferred substantial benefit over 4- to 12-month periods. One 9-month cluster RCT analyzed the effectiveness of a person-centered care training package delivered 2 days a week by a health care professional. The study was undertaken in 12 care homes with 347 residents and led to a significant reduction in antipsychotic prescriptions for people with dementia, without increasing agitation or disruptive behavior (Fossey et al., 2006). Similar benefits have also been demonstrated in a study that delivered a nursing home liaison service to nine care homes, involving a part-time old-age psychiatrist and a community psychiatric nurse. This study was based on cognitive-behavioral therapy as a first-line treatment choice (Ballard et al., 2002). Further evidence to support training approaches includes an excellent three-arm cluster RCT that demonstrated the additional value of dementia care mapping to person-centered care in 15 care homes with 289 participants with dementia. The dementia care mapping was used as a tool to improve person-centered care planning and substantially reduced agitation by more than 10 points on the Cohen-Mansfield Agitation Inventory compared with treatment as usual (standardized effect size Cohen's d > 0.5 for both treatments; Chenoweth et al., 2009).

Pharmacological Treatments—Antipsychotics

The first generation of antipsychotic drugs (usually referred to as "typical antipsychotics") was introduced as a treatment for schizophrenia in the 1950s and 1960s. By the 1970s these compounds were in frequent clinical use as an "off-license" (off-label) treatment for BPSD. In the early 1990s, a second generation of antipsychotic agents (usually referred to as atypical antipsychotics) such as risperidone, olanzapine, aripirazole, and quetiapine were introduced for the treatment of schizophrenia. The adverse effect profiles of atypical agents are generally favorable in comparison to those of typical agents in people with schizophrenia and bipolar affective disorders. Consequently, atypical antipsychotics also became the preferred option for the treatment of BPSDs in patients with AD and other dementias by the mid-1990s because of the perceived better tolerability. However, several important safety issues related to the use of these agents in patients with dementia have become apparent.

Efficacy of Antipsychotics for the Treatment of Behavioral and Psychological Symptoms of Dementia

The evidence regarding the use of antipsychotics for the treatment of BPSDs presented in the sections later in the chapter is summarized in Table 24.1.

Typical Antipsychotics

At present, there are 11 RCTs in the literature that have evaluated the efficacy of typical antipsychotics for the treatment of BPSDs. The trials have mostly involved small sample sizes and have mostly been performed over periods of between 4 and 12 weeks. A good outcome in these studies is defined by convention as a 30% improvement on standardized behavioral rating scales. Typical antipsychotics confer a significant but modest advantage compared to placebo (59% versus 41%), albeit in the context of a very high placebo response (Schneider, Pollock, & Lyness, 1990). The most comprehensive evidence base for the treatment of agitation and aggression by agents in this drug class pertains to haloperidol, for which four RCT trials (Lonergan et al., 2005) have been completed. These trials indicate a significant improvement in symptoms of aggression with haloperidol and more modest but significant benefits in the treatment of psychosis compared with placebo. There is no evidence for substantial improvement in other symptoms such as agitation. Very little clinical trial evidence is available regarding the efficacy of other typical antipsychotics for the treatment of BPSDs.

Atypical Antipsychotics

A more substantial number of trials have focused on atypical antipsychotics for the treatment of BPSDs. In total, 18 placebo-controlled RCTs have been conducted (Ballard & Howard, 2006; Schneider, Dagerman, & Insel, 2006) examining efficacy in people with AD over 6 to 12 weeks. The best evidence of efficacy for the treatment of agitation and aggression relates to risperidone. Five trials have indicated a modest but significant improvement in aggression compared to placebo, with a larger effect size conferred by a dose of 2 mg/day. In the BeHavaD (Behavioral Pathology in Alzheimer Disease) rating scale, an effect of −0.84 points (95% CI −1.28 to −0.40 points) was seen for a dose of 1 mg daily, and −1.50 points (95% CI −2.05 to −0.95 points) for a dose of 2 mg daily, over 12 weeks of treatment. This equates to a small treatment effect size (Cohen's d of 0.2 at the optimal dose). There is only limited evidence that risperidone confers benefit in the treatment of other BPSDs (Ballard & Howard, 2006; Schneider, Dagerman, & Insel, 2006). There is additional evidence from two trials that aripiprazole confers a similar magnitude of benefit to that seen with risperidone (Schneider, Dagerman, & Insel, 2006). The evidence pertaining to olanzapine is more equivocal, and there is clear evidence that quetiapine is ineffective. Beyond this there is limited evidence from published RCTs regarding other atypical antipsychotics (Ballard & Howard, 2006).

The evidence base pertaining to the treatment of psychosis in AD is more limited. A recent meta-analysis discussed seven trials that reported psychosis as an outcome (Schneider, Dagerman, & Insel, 2006). Three trials demonstrated a modest but significant improvement with risperidone compared to placebo at 1 mg/day but not at other doses (−0.8 point in BEHAV AD, Standardized effect size Cohen's d < 0.2). Two trials with olanzapine showed a nonsignificant trend toward benefit. Only two RCTs have specifically focused on people with AD with clinically significant psychosis. The first indicated that risperidone did not confer a significant benefit compared to placebo (Mintzer et al., 2006). More recently Mintzer and colleagues (2007) reported that aripiprazole conferred significant benefits for the treatment of clinically significant psychosis in more than 400 people with AD in care settings. The only published placebo-controlled RCT of quetiapine in people with AD examining psychosis as an outcome did not demonstrate any benefit compared to placebo.

Evidence for longer term efficacy (6 months or longer) of antipsychotics for the treatment of BPSDs is very limited. The AGIT and DART studies did not demonstrate any advantage for antipsychotics compared to placebo over 6 months (Ballard et al., 2005, 2008), and the

TABLE 24.1 Pharmacological Treatment of Agitation and Aggression in People With Dementia: Summary of Key Evidence

Treatment Approach	Trials Conducted	Evidence	Major Adverse Effects	Interpretation
Typical antipsychotics	11 randomized, placebo-controlled trials, mostly small sample sizes and of 4–12 weeks, one up to 16 weeks	Early meta-analysis concluded significant but modest advantage over placebo in the treatment of behavioral symptoms. Recent meta-analysis reports only one placebo-controlled trial showed significant benefit of thioridazine. Small thiothixine study suggested efficacy at low doses, but that symptoms return after discontinuation. Meta-analysis of haloperidol indicates improvement in aggression, but not in other symptoms of agitation.	Parkinsonism, dystonia, tardive dyskinesia QTc prolongation Significant increase in mortality risk compared to atypical antipsychotics (≤180 days, relative risk 1.37)	Adverse events associated with typical antipsychotics make their use inadvisable in people with Alzheimer's disease.
Atypical antipsychotics	18 placebo-controlled trials over 6–12 weeks, only three trials of 6–12 months	Significant benefit in the treatment of aggression over 12 weeks. More limited benefit for other symptoms and do not appear to be beneficial over longer treatment periods	Extrapyramidal symptoms Sedation Increased mortality (1.5–1.7-fold) Increased cerebrovascular adverse events (3-fold)	Probably still the best option for the short-term (6–12 weeks) treatment of aggression that is severe, persistent, and treatment resistant, but the serious adverse events are a major caution to long term therapy

CATIE study described no overall benefit (Schneider, Tariot, et al., 2006). However, the CATIE trial did indicate that antipsychotics were less likely to be discontinued because of perceived ineffectiveness over 9 months than placebo (Schneider, Tariot, et al., 2006).

Safety

Typical Antipsychotics

Typical antipsychotics are associated with numerous severe adverse effects in patients with AD. These include parkinsonism (Tune, Steele, & Cooper, 1991), dystonia, tardive dyskinesia, acceleration of cognitive decline, and prolongation of the QTc interval on electrocardiogram (ECG), leading to added risk of cardiac arrhythmias. Prolonged QTc has been demonstrated with several typical antipsychotics which have been widely prescribed in the past, including thioridazine and droperidol (Reilly, Ayis, Ferrier, Jones, & Thomas, 2000). Both have now either been withdrawn or are prescribed only very infrequently to people with dementia. Furthermore, there is a significant increase in mortality, which is even greater than the mortality risk associated with atypical antipsychotics (reviewed in the next section).

Until 2000, thioridazine, promazine, and haloperidol were all widely used in the clinical setting. However, prescribing practice has changed substantially in response to specific concerns related to the cardiac safety of thioridazine and general concerns regarding the side effect profile of typical antipsychotics. The potential use of haloperidol remains controversial, and it is still recommended and widely prescribed as a treatment for aggression and psychosis in some countries, despite higher risks of important side effects, including parkinsonism, gait disturbance, tardive dyskinesia, and mortality.

Atypical Antipsychotics

Widely reported side effects of atypical antipsychotics include extrapyramidal symptoms, sedation, gait disturbances, and falls. Many agents also lead to anticholinergic side effects, including delirium (Ballard & Howard, 2006; Tune et al., 1991). Tardive dyskinesia appears to be less frequent than with typical antipsychotics, but Q-Tc prolongation has also been reported as a significant problem with several atypical antipsychotics (Reilly et al., 2000). A recent meta-analysis also identified a significant increase in respiratory and urinary tract infections and peripheral edema among people treated with risperidone compared to placebo (Ballard & Howard, 2006). These are likely to be class effects for atypical antipsychotics. The limited trial data for other atypical antipsychotics precluded a comprehensive meta-analysis of adverse events.

Over the last few years, the most serious concerns regarding atypical antipsychotics have related to emergent data suggesting an increase of cerebrovascular events and increased mortality in AD patients. Observation of combined data from placebo-controlled trials shows that risperidone has been associated with a three-fold increased risk of serious cerebrovascular adverse events compared to placebo (37/1,175 vs. 8/779, OR 3.64, 95% CI 1.72 to 7.69, $p = 0.0007$; Ballard & Howard, 2006). In the Mintzer trial of aripiprazole (Mintzer et al., 2007), cerebrovascular adverse events were reported in four patients who were prescribed aripiprazole 10 mg/day but in none of the placebo-treated patients. Other sources of information, such as prescription event monitoring, would indicate that this is probably a class effect.

In 2005, the US Food and Drug Administration published a warning highlighting a significant increase in mortality risk (odds ratio [OR] = 1.7) for people with AD treated with atypical antipsychotics compared to individuals receiving placebo in RCTs. Schneider has reviewed the evidence from 15 of these trials and confirmed a significant increase in mortality (OR = 1.54) with no difference between specific agents (Schneider, Dagerman, & Insel, 2005). The recent DART-AD RCT indicated that this excess mortality risk continues over longer periods of prescribing, with an increasing impact on the absolute number of attributable deaths (Ballard, Hanney, et al., 2009). An additional important study demonstrated an even greater excess of mortality for typical antipsychotics (Wang et al., 2005).

The most common cause of death in people with dementia who are prescribed antipsychotics is pneumonia (Ballard, Creese, Corbett, & Aarsland, 2007). However thromboembolic events (including stroke, deep vein thrombosis, pulmonary embolism, and cardiac events) and an increase in sudden cardiac arrhythmias also contribute (Ballard, Creese, Corbett, & Aarsland, 2007). Oversedation, dehydration, and prolongation of QTc interval are all likely mediating factors. Importantly, many of these events may be potentially preventable by closer monitoring and early intervention.

Pharmacogenetics

In a 3-year cohort study, Angelucci et al. (2009) reported that the T allele of the 5HT2A T102C polymorphism is significantly associated with poorer response to risperidone treatment than the C allele. More recently, preliminary findings in the only genetic-association RCT study to date (Dombrovski et al., 2010) to investigate the adverse effects of atypical antipsychotic treatment in dementia indicate that the length polymorphism in the serotonin transporter gene (5-HTTLPR) is associated with a greater number of early side effects and reduced early treatment response in risperidone-treated individuals. Although this finding does require replication, it serves to highlight the importance of close monitoring in some individuals prescribed antipsychotics and shows that genetic data may assist with the initial clinical decision about prescribing.

Despite the safety concerns, the best evidence of efficacy for the pharmacological treatment of aggression relates to atypical antipsychotics, particularly risperidone. Risperidone is also the only antipsychotic specifically licensed for the treatment of aggression. In our view, their use should, however, be restricted to short-term management (6 to 12 weeks) of severe physical aggression and severe psychosis causing tangible risk or extreme distress, when non-drug treatments have not been effective. This is consistent with best practice guidelines. We would also recommend close monitoring during the period of antipsychotic prescription to reduce the risk of serious adverse outcomes. Over longer term periods of use, antipsychotics confer minimal benefit, the absolute increased mortality risk rises significantly, and the impact on cognitive decline appears to be substantial. We would therefore recommend that long-term treatment with antipsychotics should be an absolute last resort when all other treatment approaches have failed, and it should not be undertaken without regular trials of antipsychotic withdrawal. Pharmacogenetics may provide safer and more effective targeting of antipsychotic treatment in the future.

As the risks associated with antipsychotic use have become increasingly clear, there has been considerable pressure to reduce prescribing of antipsychotics to people with dementia. It is, however, imperative that this is conducted within a framework which improves the overall management of BPSD, general clinical assessment, treatment of pain, and the optimal use of nonpharmacological interventions as well as judicious short-term and well-monitored use of antipsychotics in the small number of people where their use is clinically indicated.

Best Practice Guide

To address the current priority of reducing the prescription of antipsychotics for people with dementia, a new best practice tool has been developed by Alzheimer's Society and Department of Health in the UK (n.d.). The tool builds on the best available evidence and emphasizes the importance of reducing the use of these drugs within the context of improved overall treatment and care. The tool aims to support health and social care professionals in implementing clinical practice to reduce the emergence of BPSDs in addition to providing alternative treatment options when symptoms do occur. The guide also provides a framework for monitoring and review of ongoing prescriptions, with a focus on encouraging the discontinuation of antipsychotics after 12 weeks. The key elements of the guide are framed within person-centred care, as well as introducing the concept of a period of "watchful waiting" when symptoms first emerge. This suggested strategy involves a 4-week period of ongoing assessment and simple person-centered psychological, social, and environmental interventions to be implemented as a first-line approach. The guide further highlights more specific evidence-based nondrug approaches that provide useful alternatives to pharmacological treatment. The guide provides medical care plans and assessment tools to support decisions regarding treatment, including the prescription and discontinuation of antipsychotics, and effective monitoring and review. Based upon the evidence base and current drug licenses, risperidone is highlighted as the preferred treatment if an antipsychotic is necessary. However, the guide emphasizes the importance of considering the benefit of pharmacological and nondrug treatment of other general and mental health conditions before resorting to an antipsychotic prescription. The limitations regarding the evidence base for other nonantipsychotic psychotropic drugs is also highlighted. It particularly highlights the importance of avoiding the practice of substituting antipsychotics for other drugs with an even more limited evidence base which may be equally or more harmful. The guide is available for professionals to use in clinical practice, although it is not designed for use in acute hospital settings. It is available as a download from the Alzheimer's Society (n.d.) and is endorsed and promoted by the Department of Health, Royal College of General Practitioners and Royal College of Psychiatrists as a key tool in the drive to reduce antipsychotic drugs in people with dementia.

Other Pharmacological Treatments

No pharmacological treatments other than risperidone were considered to have a sufficient evidence base to recommend for the treatment of agitation, aggression, or psychosis other than risperidone. A brief review of the emerging evidence regarding other candidate treatments is presented next.

Cholinesterase Inhibitors

A meta-analysis demonstrated a small but significant overall advantage of cholinesterase inhibitors (ChEIs) over placebo with regard to the treatment of BPSDs in AD (Trinh, Hoblyn, Mohanty, & Yaffe, 2003). Additional support for beneficial effects of ChEIs on BPSDs comes from a randomized withdrawal study, in which cessation of donepezil was associated with a significant worsening of the total Neuropsychiatric Inventory (NPI) score within 6 weeks (Holmes et al., 2004). However, there was no short-term benefit for treatment of clinically significant agitation with donepezil over 12 weeks in a large RCT (Howard et al., 2007), or over 24 weeks with rivastigmine in a smaller RCT (Ballard et al., 2005), indicating that ChEIs do not appear to be useful in the management of acute agitation. A 5-month placebo-controlled RCT of galanthamine suggested that ChEI treatment may delay the emergence of overall BPSDs (Tariot et al., 2000), and pharmacogenetic studies have suggested the possibility of a preferential response to rivastigmine in the treatment of overall BPSDs in people with the wild-type Butyrylcholinesterase genotype (Blesa et al., 2006). However, within the overall BPSD spectrum, ChEIs appear to have their greatest effects on depression and dysphoria, apathy and indifference, and anxiety (Gauthier et al., 2002).

Memantine

Individual studies, meta-analyses, and pooled analyses indicate that memantine may confer benefit in the treatment of mild to moderate irritability and lability, agitation or aggression, and psychosis over 3–6 months in patients with AD (Gauthier, Loft, & Cummings, 2008; Gauthier, Wirth, & Mobius, 2005; McShane, Areosa Sastre, & Minakaran, 2006; Wilcock, Ballard, Cooper, & Loft, 2008). Although this evidence is potentially encouraging with respect to memantine as a useful adjunct to treatment of mild BPSD, there is limited RCT evidence regarding the use of memantine in the acute treatment of clinically significant BPSD. The recent MAGD trial compared memantine and placebo over 6 and 12 weeks in 153 people with AD and clinically significant agitation. Memantine did not confer any significant benefit in the treatment of agitation over 6 or 12 weeks in compared to placebo as measured by the Cohen-Mansfield Agitation Inventory as the primary outcome measure. There was a significant benefit on the overall Neuropsychiatric Inventory score, but no advantage for memantine on the Clinical Global Impression of change as an overall clinician-measured outcome, suggesting that overall benefits were not sufficient to recommend memantine as a clinical therapy for acute agitation or aggression in people with AD (Fox et al., 2012). A post-hoc analysis (Wilcock et al., 2008), supported by a recent RCT (Howard et al., 2012), has, however, highlighted the potential contribution of memantine to the reduced emergence of overall BPSDs, with a 5.5 point significant advantage favoring memantine over placebo at 6-month follow-up on the total Neuropsychiatric Inventory in the DOMINO trial (Howard et al., 2012). It is hoped that ongoing RCTs in Canada and in the United Kingdom may clarify the role of memantine in treating agitation and aggression in patients with AD in the near future.

Antidepressants for Agitation and Aggression

In a 17-day trial in psychiatric inpatients with severe BPSDs related to AD, Pollock and colleagues (2002) reported that citalopram was superior to placebo, with the greatest efficacy for agitation or aggression, an effect not seen with perphenazine. In a later study, citalopram was found to be comparable in efficacy to risperidone, differentiated by its significant effect on agitation symptoms and its superior tolerability in the treatment of moderate to severe BPSDs (Pollock et al., 2007). RCTs of sertraline (Finkel et al., 2004) and trazadone (Teri et al., 2000) have been less promising.

Anticonvulsants

Two small parallel-group RCTs of carbamazepine for the treatment of agitation and aggression in AD, both conducted over a period of 6 weeks or less, suggested potential benefit (Olin, Fox, Pawluczyk, Taggart, & Schneider, 2001; Tariot et al., 1998). A meta-analysis of the two trials (Gauthier et al., 2002) indicates significant improvement on both the Brief Psychiatric Rating Scale (mean difference −5.5; 95% CI, −8.5 to −2.5) and on Clinical Global Improvement (OR, 10.2; 95% CI, 3.1–33.1). Both studies also suggest good tolerability. In contrast, valproate has not shown treatment benefits for BPSDs

Other Treatments

It will also be important to use our best scientific understanding of the biological basis of specific symptom clusters such as delusions, hallucinations, aggression, and agitation to develop more targeted therapies. One example is the potential use of muscarinic agonists for the treatment of delusions: A number of postmortem studies have indicated an association between altered muscarinic receptor binding and delusions in dementia patients (Konovalov, Muralee, & Tampi, 2008), and preliminary data from secondary analyses of RCTs with muscarinic agonists such as xanomeline (Ballard et al., 2000) indicate a potential treatment effect on psychosis. Another example is the relationship between altered adrenoceptors and agitation or aggression in postmortem studies in people with AD (Bodick et al., 1997); a preliminary, small RCT of the alpha-adrenoceptor blocker prazosin indicates potential benefit in the treatment of BPSDs in AD patients (Sharp, Ballard, Chen, & Francis, 2007). Targeted drug development based upon the principles of evidence-based experimental medicine is more likely to lead to the development of effective therapies.

Conclusion

Agitation, aggression, and psychosis are frequent and distressing symptoms in people with Alzheimer's disease. Implementing the best currently available evidence to optimize safe and effective management is imperative. These best practices include medical treatment of underlying conditions; treatment of pain; routinely implementing effective nonpharmacological care; and the judicious short-term use of antipschotics, when appropriate, for severe symptoms that have not responded to other approaches and pose substantial safety risk to the indiviudal or others. To move the field forward considerably, more focus is needed to evaluate potential pharmacological alternatives through adequately powered RCTs.

References

Aalten, P., de Vugt, M. E., Lousberg, R., Korten, E., Jaspers, N., Senden, B.,...Verhey, F. R. (2003). Behavioral problems in dementia: A factor analysis of the neuropsychiatric inventory. *Dementia and Geriatric Cognitive Disorders, 15,* 99–105.

Alzheimer's Disease International. (2008). *The prevalence of dementia worldwide*. Retrieved March 2014, from http://www.alz.co.uk/adi/pdf/prevalence.pdf.

Alzheimer's Society UK. (n.d.). *Optimising treatment and care for behavioural and psychological symptoms of dementia: A best practice guide*. Retrieved March 2014, from http://www.alzheimers.org.uk/site/scripts/download_info.php?downloadID=609.

Angelucci, F., Bernadini, S., Gravina, P., Bellincampi, L., Trequattrini, A., Di Iulio, F.,...Spalletta, G. (2009). Delusion symptoms and response to antipsychotic treatment are associated with the 5-HT2A receptor polymorphism (102T/C) in Alzheimer's diseases: A 3-year follow-up longitudinal study. *Journal of Alzheimers Disease, 17*, 203–211.

Ballard, C., Brown, R., Fossey, J., Douglas, S., Bradley, P., Hancock, J.,...Howard, R. (2009). Brief psychosocial therapy for the treatment of agitation in Alzheimer disease (The CALM-AD Trial). *American Journal of Geriatric Psychiatry, 17*, 726–733.

Ballard, C., Creese, B., Corbett, A., & Aarsland, D. (2011). Atypical antipsychotics for the treatment of behavioral and psychological symptoms in dementia, with a particular focus on longer term outcomes and mortality. *Expert Opinion on Drug Safety, 10*, 35–43.

Ballard, C. G., Eastwood, C., Gahir, M., & Wilcock, G. (1996). A follow up study of depression in the carers of dementia sufferers. *British Medical Journal, 312*, 947.

Ballard, C. G., Gauthier, S., & Cummings, J. L., Brodaty, H., Grossberg, G. T., Robert, P., & Lyketsos, C. G. (2009). Management of agitation and aggression associated with Alzheimer disease. *Nature Reviews Neuroscience, 5*, 245–255.

Ballard, C., Hanney, M. L., Theodoulou, M., Douglas, S., McShane, R., Kossakowski, K.,...Jacoby, R. (2009). The dementia antipsychotic withdrawal trial (DART-AD): Long-term follow-up of a randomised placebo-controlled trial. *Lancet Neurology, 8*, 151–157.

Ballard, C., & Howard, R. (2006). Neuroleptic drugs in dementia: Benefits and harm. *Nature Reviews Neuroscience, 7*, 492–500.

Ballard, C., Lana, M., Theodoulou, M., Douglas, S., McShane, R., Jacoby, R.,...Juszczak, E. (2008). A randomised, blinded, placebo-controlled trial in dementia patients continuing or stopping neuroleptics (the DART-AD trial). *PLoS Medicine, 5*, 76.

Ballard, C. G., Margallo-Lana, M., Fossey, J., Reichelt, K., Myint, P., Potkins, D., & O'Brien, J. (2001). A 1-year follow-up study of behavioral and psychological symptoms in dementia among people in care environments. *Journal of Clinical Psychiatry, 62*, 631–636.

Ballard, C., Margallo-Lana, M., Juszczak, E., Douglas, S., Swann, A., Thomas, A.,...Jacoby, R. (2005). Quetiapine and rivastigmine and cognitive decline in Alzheimer's disease: Randomised double blind placebo controlled trial. *British Medical Journal, 330*, 874.

Ballard, C. G., Patel, A., Solis, M., Lowe, K., & Wilcock, G. (1996). A one-year follow-up study of depression in dementia sufferers. *British Journal of Psychiatry, 168*, 287–291.

Ballard, C., Piggott, M., Johnson, M., Cairns, N., Perry, R., McKeith, I.,...Perry, E. (2000). Delusions associated with elevated muscarinic binding in dementia with Lewy bodies. *Annals of Neurology, 48*, 868–876.

Ballard, C., Powell, I., James, I., Reichelt, K., Myint, P., Potkins, D.,...Barber, R. (2002). Can psychiatric liaison reduce neuroleptic use and reduce health service utilization for dementia patients residing in care facilities. *International Journal of Geriatric Psychiatry, 17*, 140–145.

Banerjee, S., Smith, S. C., Lamping, D. L., Harwood, R. H., Foley, B., Smith, P.,...Knapp, M. (2006). Quality of life in dementia: More than just cognition. An analysis of associations with quality of life in dementia. *Journal of Neurology, Neurosurgery and Psychiatry, 77*, 146–148.

Bird, M. (2002). Psychosocial approaches to challenging behavior in dementia: A controlled trial. In *Report to the Commonwealth Department of Health and Ageing* (pp. 1–40). Canberra, Australia: Office for Older Australians.

Blesa, R., Bullock, R., He, Y., Gambina, G., Meyer, J., Rapatz, G.,...Lane, R. (2006). Effect of butyrylcholinesterase genotype on the response to rivastigmine or donepezil in younger patients with Alzheimer's disease. *Pharmacogenetics and Genomics, 16*, 771–774.

Bodick, N. C., Offen, W. W., Levey, A. I., Cutler, N. R., Gauthier, S. G., Satlin, A.,...Paul, S. M. (1997). Effects of xanomeline, a selective muscarinic receptor agonist, on cognitive function and behavioral symptoms in Alzheimer disease. *Archives of Neurology, 54*, 465–473.

Burns, A., Jacoby, R., & Levy, R. (1990a). Psychiatric phenomena in Alzheimer's disease. III: Disorders of mood. *British Journal of Psychiatry, 157*, 81–86, 92–94.

Burns, A., Jacoby, R., & Levy, R. (1990b). Psychiatric phenomena in Alzheimer's disease. IV: Disorders of behaviour. *British Journal of Psychiatry, 157*, 86–94.

Chapman, F. M., Dickinson, J., McKeith, I., & Ballard, C. (1999). Association among visual hallucinations, visual acuity, and specific eye pathologies in Alzheimer's disease: Treatment implications. *American Journal of Psychiatry, 156,* 1983–1985.

Chenoweth, L., King, M. T., Jeon, Y. H., Brodaty, H., Stein-Parbury, J., Norman, R., ... Luscombe, G. (2009). Caring for Aged Dementia Care Resident Study (CADRES) of person-centred care, dementia-care mapping, and usual care in dementia: A cluster-randomised trial. *Lancet Neurology, 8,* 317–325.

Cohen-Mansfield, J., Libin, A., & Marx, M. S. (2007). Nonpharmacological treatment of agitation: A controlled trial of systematic individualized intervention. *Journal of Gerontology Series A: Biological Sciences Medical Sciences, 62,* 908–916.

Cohen-Mansfield, J., & Lipson, S. (2008). The utility of pain assessment for analgesic use in persons with dementia. *Pain, 134,* 16–23.

Cohen-Mansfield, J., & Werner, P. (1997). Management of verbally disruptive behaviors in nursing home residents. *Journal of Gerontology Series A: Biological Sciences Medical Sciences, 52,* 369–377.

Dombrovski, A. Y., Mulsant, B. H., Ferrell, R. E., Lotrich, F. E., Rosen, J. I., Wallace, M., ... Pollock, B. G. (2010). Serotonin transporter triallelic genotype and response to citalopram and risperidone in dementia with behavioral symptoms. *International Clinical Psychopharmacology, 25,* 37–45.

Finkel, S. I., Mintzer, J. E., Dysken, M., Krishnan, K. R., Burt, T., & McRae, T. (2004). A randomized, placebo-controlled study of the efficacy and safety of sertraline in the treatment of the behavioral manifestations of Alzheimer's disease in outpatients treated with donepezil. *International Journal of Geriatric Psychiatry, 19,* 9–18.

Fossey, J., Ballard, C., Juszczak, E., James, I., Alder, N., Jacoby, R., & Howard, R. (2006). Effect of enhanced psychosocial care on antipsychotic use in nursing home residents with severe dementia: Cluster randomized trial. *British Medical Journal, 332,* 756–758.

Fox, C., Crugel, M., Maidment, I., Auestad, B. H., Coulton, S., Treloar, A., ... Livingston, G. (2012). Efficacy of memantine for agitation in Alzheimer's dementia: A randomised double-blind placebo controlled trial. *PLoS One, 7,* e35185.

Gauthier, S., Feldman, H., Hecker, J., Vellas, B., Ames, D., Subbiah, P., ... Emir, B. (2002). Efficacy of donepezil on behavioral symptoms in patients with moderate to severe Alzheimer's disease. *International Psychogeriatrics, 14,* 389–404.

Gauthier, S., Loft, H., & Cummings, J. (2008). Improvement in behavioural symptoms in patients with moderate to severe Alzheimer's disease by memantine: A pooled data analysis. *International Journal of Geriatric Psychiatry, 23,* 537–545.

Gauthier, S., Wirth, Y., & Mobius, H. J. (2005). Effects of memantine on behavioural symptoms in Alzheimer's disease patients: An analysis of the Neuropsychiatric Inventory (NPI) data of two randomised, controlled studies. *International Journal of Geriatric Psychiatry, 20,* 459–464.

Gilley, D. W., Whalen, M. E., Wilson, R. S., & Bennett, D. A. (1991). Hallucinations and associated factors in Alzheimer's disease. *Journal of Neuropsychiatry and Clinical Neuroscience, 3,* 371–376.

Gitlin, L. N., Winter, L., Burke, J., Chernett, N., Dennis, M. P., & Hauck, W. W. (2008). Tailored activities to manage neuropsychiatric behaviors in persons with dementia and reduce caregiver burden: A randomized pilot study. *American Journal of Geriatric Psychiatry, 16,* 229–239.

Haupt, M., Kurz, A., & Janner, M. (2000). A 2-year follow-up of behavioural and psychological symptoms in Alzheimer's disease. *Dementia and Geriatric Cognitive Disorders, 11,* 147–152.

Holmes, C., Wilkinson, D., Dean, C., Vethanayagam, S., Olivieri, S., Langley, A., ... Damms, J. (2004). The efficacy of donepezil in the treatment of neuropsychiatric symptoms in Alzheimer disease. *Neurology, 63,* 214–219.

Holroyd, S., & Laurie, S. (1999). Correlates of psychotic symptoms among elderly outpatients. *International Journal of Geriatric Psychiatry, 14,* 379–384.

Howard, R. J., Juszczak, E., Ballard, C., Bentham, P., Brown, R. G., Bullock, R., ... Rodger, M. (2007). Donepezil for the treatment of agitation in Alzheimer's disease. *New England Journal of Medicine, 357,* 1382–1392.

Howard, R., McShane, R., Lindesay, J., Ritchie, C., Baldwin, A., Barber, R., ... Phillips, P. (2012). Donepezil and memantine for moderate-to-severe Alzheimer's disease. *New England Journal of Medicine, 366,* 893–903.

Husebo, B., Ballard, C., Sandvik, R., Nilsen, O. B., & Aarsland, D. (2011). Efficacy of treating pain to reduce behavioural disturbances in residents of nursing homes with dementia: Cluster randomised clinical trial. *British Medical Journal, 343,* 4065.

Konovalov, S., Muralee, S., & Tampi, R. R. (2008). Anticonvulsants for the treatment of behavioral and psychological symptoms of dementia: A literature review. *International Psychogeriatrics, 20,* 293–308.

Lonergan, E., Luxenberg, J., Colford, J., (2005). Haloperidol for agitation in dementia.

Cochrane Database of Systematic Reviews, (4), 2005. CD002852

Lyketsos, C. G. (2007). Neuropsychiatric symptoms (behavioral and psychological symptoms of dementia) and the development of dementia treatments. International Psychogeriatrics, 19, 409–420.

Lyketsos, C. G., Colenda, C. C., Beck, C., Blank, K., Doraiswamy, M. P., Kalunian, D. A., & Yaffe, K. (2006). Position statement of the American Association for Geriatric Psychiatry regarding principles of care for patients with dementia due to Alzheimer disease. American Journal of Geriatric Psychiatry, 14, 561–572.

Lyketsos, C. G., Steinberg, M., Tschanz, J. T., Norton, M. C., Steffens, D. C., & Breitner, J. C. (2000). Mental and behavioral disturbances in dementia: Findings from the Cache County Study on Memory in Aging. American Journal of Psychiatry, 157, 708–714.

Margallo-Lana, M., Swann, A., O'Brien, J., Fairbairn, A., Reichelt, K., Potkins, D., ... Ballard, C. (2001). Prevalence and pharmacological management of behavioural and psychological symptoms amongst dementia sufferers living in care environments. International Journal of Geriatric Psychiatry, 16, 39–44.

McShane, R., Areosa Sastre, A., & Minakaran, N. (2006). Memantine for dementia. Cochrane Database Systematic Reviews, (2), CD003154.

Mintzer, J., Greenspan, A., Caers, I., Van Hove, I., Kushner, S., Weiner, M., ... Schneider, L. S. (2006). Risperidone in the treatment of psychosis of Alzheimer disease: Results from a prospective clinical trial. American Journal of Geriatric Psychiatry, 14, 280–291.

Mintzer, J. E., Tune, L. E., Breder, C. D., Swanink, R., Marcus, R. N., McQuade, R. D., & Forbes, A. (2007). Aripiprazole for the treatment of psychoses in institutionalized patients with Alzheimer dementia: A multicenter, randomized, double-blind, placebo-controlled assessment of three fixed doses. American Journal of Geriatric Psychiatry, 15, 918–931.

Olin, J. T., Fox, L. S., Pawluczyk, S., Taggart, N. A., & Schneider, L. S. (2001). A pilot randomized trial of carbamazepine for behavioral symptoms in treatment-resistant outpatients with Alzheimer disease. American Journal of Geriatric Psychiatry, 9, 400–405.

Pollock, B. G., Mulsant, B. H., Rosen, J., Mazumdar, S., Blakesley, R. E., Houck, P. R., & Huber, K. A. (2007). A doubleblind comparison of citalopram and risperidone for the treatment of behavioral and psychotic symptoms associated with dementia. American Journal of Geriatric Psychiatry, 15, 942–952.

Pollock, B. G., Mulsant, B. H., Rosen, J., Sweet, R. A., Mazumdar, S., Bharucha, A., ... Chew, M. L. (2002). Comparison of citalopram, perphenazine, and placebo for the acute treatment of psychosis and behavioral disturbances in hospitalized, demented patients. American Journal of Psychiatry, 159, 460–465.

Rabins, P. V., Mace, N. L., & Lucas, M. J. (1982). The impact of dementia on the family. Journal of the American Medical Association, 248, 333–335.

Reilly, J. G., Ayis, S. A., Ferrier, I. N., Jones, S. J., & Thomas, S. H. (2000). QTc-interval abnormalities and psychotropic drug therapy in psychiatric patients. Lancet, 355, 1048–1052.

Schneider, L. S., Dagerman, K. S., & Insel, P. (2005). Risk of death with atypical antipsychotic drug treatment for dementia: Meta-analysis of randomized placebo-controlled trials. Journal of the American Medical Association, 294, 1934–1943.

Schneider, L. S., Dagerman, K., & Insel, P. S. (2006). Efficacy and adverse effects of atypical antipsychotics for dementia: Meta-analysis of randomized, placebo-controlled trials. American Journal of Geriatric Psychiatry, 14, 191–210.

Schneider, L. S., Pollock, V. E., & Lyness, S. A. (1990). A metaanalysis of controlled trials of neuroleptic treatment in dementia. Journal of the American Geriatrics Society, 38, 553–563.

Schneider, L. S., Tariot, P. N., Dagerman, K. S., Davis, S. M., Hsiao, J. K., Ismail, M. S., ... Lieberman, J. A. (2006). Effectiveness of atypical antipsychotic drugs in patients with Alzheimer's disease. New England Journal of Medicine, 355, 1525–1538.

Sharp, S. I., Ballard, C. G., Chen, C. P., & Francis, P. T. (2007). Aggressive behavior and neuroleptic medication are associated with increased number of alpha1-adrenoceptors in patients with Alzheimer disease. American Journal of Geriatric Psychiatry, 15, 435–437.

Steele, C., Rovner, B., Chase, G. A., & Folstein, M. (1990). Psychiatric symptoms and nursing home placement of patients with Alzheimer's disease. American Journal of Psychiatry, 147, 1049–1051.

Steinberg, M., Shao, H., Zandi, P., Lyketsos, C. G., Welsh-Bohmer, K. A., Norton, M. C., ... Tschanz, J. T. (2008). Point and 5-year period prevalence of neuropsychiatric symptoms in dementia: The Cache County Study. International Journal of Geriatric Psychiatry, 23, 170–177.

Tariot, P. N., Erb, R., Podgorski, C. A., Patel, S., Jakimovich, L., & Irvine, C. (1998). Efficacy and tolerability of carbamazepine for agitation and aggression in dementia. American Journal of Psychiatry, 155, 54–61.

Tariot, P. N., Solomon, P. R., Morris, J. C., Kershaw, P., Lilienfeld, S., & Ding, C. (2000). A 5-month, randomized, placebo-controlled trial of galantamine in AD. The Galantamine USA-10 Study Group. *Neurology, 54*, 2269–2276.

Teri, L., Logsdon, R. G., Peskind, E., Raskind, M., Weiner, M. F., Tractenberg, R. E., . . . Thal, L. J. (2000). Treatment of agitation in AD: A randomized, placebo-controlled clinical trial. *Neurology, 55*, 1271–1278.

Trinh, N. H., Hoblyn, J., Mohanty, S., & Yaffe, K. (2003). Efficacy of cholinesterase inhibitors in the treatment of neuropsychiatric symptoms and functional impairment in Alzheimer disease: A meta-analysis. *Journal of the American Medical Association, 289*, 210–216.

Tune, L. E., Steele, C., & Cooper, T. (1991). Neuroleptic drugs in the management of behavioral symptoms of Alzheimer's disease. *Psychiatric Clinics of North America, 14*, 353–373.

US Food and Drug Administration. (2005). *Public Health Advisory: Deaths with antipsychotics in elderly patients with behavioral disturbances.* Retrieved March 2014, from http://www.fda.gov/drugs/drugsafety/postmarketdrugsafetyinformationforpatientsandproviders/drugsafetyinformationforheathcareprofessionals/publichealthadvisories/ucm053171.htm.

Wang, P. S., Schneeweiss, S., Avorn J., Fischer, M. A., Mogun, H., Solomon, D. H., & Brookhart, M. A. (2005). Risk of death in elderly users of conventional vs. atypical antipsychotic medications. *New England Journal of Medicine, 353*, 2335–2341.

Wilcock, G. K., Ballard, C. G., Cooper, J. A., & Loft, H. (2008). Memantine for agitation/aggression and psychosis in moderately severe to severe Alzheimer's disease: A pooled analysis of 3 studies. *Journal of Clinical Psychiatry, 69*, 341–348.

25

Management of Depression, Apathy, and Sexualized Inappropriate Behavior in Dementia

James M. Ellison and Cynthia T. Greywolf

In the care of a person with Alzheimer's disease (AD) or another dementia, management of behavioral disturbances can present even greater practical difficulties than management of diminished memory. The majority of demented individuals will at some time manifest behavioral and psychological symptoms of dementia (BPSDs), such as agitation, sometimes resulting in a crisis for caregivers (Tractenberg, Weiner, Patterson, Teri, & Thal, 2003; see Chapter 21). Depression, aggression, or sexualized inappropriate behavior can disturb and endanger not only the demented person but also others in their vicinity. BPSDs are often the source of stress that precipitates institutionalization. The diagnostic criteria for AD and other dementias have not focused on behavioral aspects of these disorders, yet BPSDs make an undeniable contribution to the morbidity of dementia. Perhaps even the hospitalization of Alzheimer's index dementia patient, Auguste D, would have been delayed had her memory difficulties not been accompanied by pathological jealousy, paranoid delusions, auditory hallucinations, screaming, and agitation (Graeber & Mehraein, 1999).

Among the BPSDs that complicate the care of demented people, whether at home or in an institutional setting, depression, apathy, and sexualized inappropriate behavior present particularly important concerns. In this chapter, we will address these behavioral syndromes. After reviewing the nature of these behaviors and the evidence-based approaches to their management, we will suggest practical management guidelines for clinicians and caregivers.

Depressive Symptoms

Depressive symptoms frequently accompany the cognitive symptoms of dementia (Jost & Grossberg, 1996). Some 30%–50% of individuals with AD display depression, though the number or severity of symptoms in about half of these falls below the threshold required for a diagnosis of major depressive disorder (Lyketsos, Steinberg, et al., 2000). The presence of depressive symptoms in AD does not depend upon the severity of cognitive symptoms, and depressive symptoms can appear even before AD is diagnosed

(Jost & Grossberg, 1996). In some cases, an individual's awareness of cognitive decline can initiate a depressive reaction; however, it is likely that the pathophysiologic changes inherent in AD, which include loss of noradrenergic and serotonergic neurons, contribute to depressive symptoms in AD (Lyketsos & Olin, 2002).

Self-assessment of depressive symptoms demands a level of cognitive and emotional awareness that may erode early in the course of dementia. Depression that is comorbid with dementia has an independently deleterious effect on functioning and quality of life, so it can be valuable to recognize its presence even when the sufferer cannot articulate an easily recognizable set of diagnostic clues. For this reason, a more lenient set of criteria has been proposed for use in diagnosing depression among AD patients (Olin et al., 2002). The suggested criteria, which are in unofficial but common clinical usage, require only three rather than five depressive symptoms to be present in order to justify the diagnosis of major depressive disorder. Depressed mood is listed among the depressive symptoms, but its presence is not a prerequisite for the diagnosis.

Masked expressions of depression in dementia are often encountered, perhaps because dysphoric feelings that cannot be put into words may find their expression in actions. The presence of delusions in a demented patient, and perhaps especially delusions with a depressive tone, should raise a clinician's suspicion that depression might be present. In one patient cohort, the presence of depression among a community-dwelling group of patients with probable AD was associated with a 1.8-fold increase in the likelihood of delusions, an increased likelihood that became even greater with control of potential confounding variables (Bassiony et al., 2002). Aggressive verbal or physical behaviors, too, may be an expression of emotional distress originating in depression (Menon et al., 2001). In some cases, patients may direct aggression toward themselves, resulting in self-destructive or suicidal behavior. Verbal outbursts or disruptive vocalizations can reflect the presence of depression that is difficult for a demented patient to describe in more understandable language (Dwyer & Byrne, 2000). Resistance to care, refusal to eat, and resulting loss of weight, too, can indicate dysphoric or depressive affect that is expressed behaviorally. In one study, the presence of depression appeared responsible for the weight loss in about one third of the 19% of nursing home residents who lost 5 pounds or more (Morley & Kraenzle, 1994).

As with depression among the cognitively intact, treatment interventions include both psychosocial and pharmacologic approaches. Early in the course of dementia, the value of insight-oriented interventions is more apparent. The progression of dementia inevitably brings with it greater need for assistance from others, and this forced increase in dependency can be very unwelcome and even quite frightening. Adults who have been especially autonomous and self-reliant may find it helpful to grieve their loss of independence. Others, who have taken pride in intellectual achievements, may be deeply pained when experiencing an increasing difficulty in cognitive performance. Inability to complete a project of personal significance, such as the writing of a book planned before significant cognitive decline had begun, may undermine self-esteem and become a focus of self-deprecation.

Later during the course of dementia, when a person's insight contributes less to the relief of distress or the production of behavioral change, behavioral interventions can still be useful for alleviating depressive symptoms. Many patients with milder depressive symptoms appear to enjoy engaging in activities such as listening to music of their choice or participating in appropriate levels of physical exercise. An important principle in such activities is to recognize the patients' limitations and avoid making functional or cognitive demands that are excessively frustrating.

Given the clinical significance of depressive symptoms in dementia, it is truly unfortunate that no specific medication has been designated by the Food and Drug Administration (FDA) as safe and effective in treating dementia-associated depression. The cognitive-enhancing cholinesterase inhibitors have not proven effective in treating established depressive symptoms in demented subjects (McDermott & Gray, 2012). Memantine, a cognitive enhancer that exerts its effects through the glutamatergic system, lacks data supporting or refuting antidepressant effects. Stimulants have not been studied in recent years as a treatment for depression associated with dementia, though an older report suggested a role for methylphenidate (Branconnier & Cole, 1980). Antipsychotic medications, considered a limited but sometimes valuable treatment for agitation in demented patients, appear not yet to have been studied as antidepressants or antidepressant augmenters in demented cohorts, perhaps in recognition of the FDA's concerns about their safety in demented, psychotic older adults. Electroconvulsive therapy (ECT), a highly effective treatment for depression in later life, has been studied only to a limited extent in the elderly. Currently available data suggest that ECT is effective in treating depression in demented patients, and that it is not expected to worsen cognitive symptoms in AD patients but might have more deleterious cognitive effects in patients with vascular or other non-AD dementia etiologies (Oudman, 2012).

A variety of antidepressant medications have been studied in cohorts of depressed and demented adults. The results of these investigations are best described as not definitive, with inconsistent indications of effectiveness. An early negative double-blind study with imipramine failed to show a significant superiority over placebo, perhaps because of the large improvement in depression ratings in both the imipramine and control groups. This was attributed by the authors to the attention that subjects received as a result of study participation (Reifler et al., 1989). Moclobemide, a selective MAO inhibitor that is not FDA approved in the United States, was compared to placebo in the treatment of depression and cognitive decline in a large international multicenter study. It was reported to be safe, effective in reducing depressive symptoms, and not associated with further cognitive decline (Roth, Mountjoy, & Amrein, 1996). Although its side effect profile might discourage use in older adults, the tricyclic antidepressant clomipramine was shown in a double-blind study to reduce depressive symptoms in depressed, demented subjects (Petracca, Teson, Chemerinski, Leiguarda, & Starkstein, 1996). A multicenter Nordic study using a combination of open and blinded treatment with citalopram, 10 to 30 mg/d for 4 weeks, versus placebo in depressed, demented patients found significant improvement in emotional symptoms, including depressed mood, emotional bluntness, anxiety, and irritability, but no improvement in cognitive symptoms was noted (Nyth & Gottfries, 1990). A small double-blind study of depression in patients with AD comparing sertraline at doses up to 150 mg/d (12 subjects) to placebo (10 subjects) demonstrated a significant benefit as measured by changes in the Cornell Scale for Depression in Dementia (Lyketsos, Sheppard, et al., 2000). Studying a group of AD patients residing in a nursing home setting, most of whom met criteria for minor rather than major depression, Magai and colleagues reported no superiority of sertraline in doses up to 100 mg/d over placebo (Magai, Kennedy, Cohen, & Gomberg, 2000). Fluoxetine in doses up to 40 mg/d, studied in another small but double-blind study, failed to show superiority over placebo in treating depressive symptoms in a group of AD subjects, though the high rate of placebo response in this study may have obfuscated a beneficial effect of the experimental medication (Petracca, Chemerinski, & Starkstein, 2001). The only controlled trial we could locate in which a serotonin-norepinephrine reuptake inhibitor (SNRI) was investigated as a treatment for major depressive disorder in demented patients showed no statistical superiority of venlafaxine over placebo (de Vasconcelos Cunha et al., 2007).

The most recent large study to address antidepressant treatment of depressive symptoms in AD, the DIADS-2, recruited a large sample of AD patients diagnosed with "depression of AD" (Olin et al., 2002) and compared sertraline (mean achieved dose of 91.1 mg/d) to placebo in a double-blind, randomized design (Weintraub et al., 2010). The majority of subjects showed improvement in depressive symptoms, and sertraline's effects failed to achieve superiority over placebo.

Some authorities, in reviewing these cited studies, have concluded that antidepressants are ineffective in treating depression in AD patients. Others have pointed out the large placebo effect that typically occurs and have noted that depressive symptoms in this population can be shifting, transient, or responsive to nonspecific factors. The use of antidepressants for behavioral symptoms other than depression, too, may in some cases be reasonable. For dementias other than AD, the effectiveness of antidepressant treatment in reducing depressive symptoms has been less thoroughly investigated, though one open study has suggested that depressive symptoms in frontotemporal dementia may benefit from treatment with a serotonin reuptake blocking antidepressant (Swartz, Miller, Lesser, & Darby, 1997). For the clinician, the choice of whether to prescribe an antidepressant to a demented person can be confusing, though the relatively good toleration of antidepressant treatment in demented patients (Nelson & Devanand, 2011), as compared to poorer tolerance of cholinesterase inhibitors or antipsychotics, encourages consideration of a potentially beneficial clinical trial despite the limited evidence supporting specific effectiveness of antidepressants in targeting AD patients' depressive symptoms. We suggest the following approach, taking into account the limitations of available data:

1. In any demented patient with behavioral disturbances, treatment interventions should be preceded by a differential diagnostic assessment process that takes into account environmental and medical factors, past psychiatric history, and family psychiatric history.
2. The more clearly the patient's symptoms resemble major depressive disorder, the more appropriate it may be to consider an antidepressant trial. Post-hoc analysis of the DIADS-2 results, for example, indicated that a subgroup of AD patients who met baseline criteria for major depressive disorder showed a noticeable trend toward achieving superior results with sertraline, although the outcome was still not statistically superior to placebo. Patients with symptoms suggesting a masked depression, too, could be considered for treatment. Along these lines, it should be noted that some antidepressants (e.g., citalopram) have demonstrated a potential signal of benefit in treating nondepressive BPSDs (see Chapter 24).
3. The serotonin reuptake inhibitors, and particularly sertraline or citalopram, may be considered first-line antidepressants in treating depression in AD patients. Caution should be exercised with citalopram dosing, given the recent FDA warning regarding prolonged QTc interval and the suggestion that older adults not be dosed higher than 20 mg/d. Clinical data have not entirely supported this level of specific caution about citalopram (Howland, 2011a, 2011b), but it is nonetheless reasonable to assess cardiac risk factors and to obtain an electrocardiogram as part of the workup of any older adult for whom antidepressant treatment is planned. Although the adverse effects of the newer antidepressants are often quite mild, appropriate psychoeducation should be given to the patient and/or authorized health care representative. The prescribing clinician should review the reasons for prescribing, the limited data supporting the use of antidepressants in demented patients, the available treatment alternatives, and the most common and most serious potential adverse effects.
4. Depressive symptoms should be measured at baseline using an appropriate instrument. For patients with higher scores on the Mini-Mental State Examination (>15/30 points), the Geriatric Depression Scale is often an efficient measure (Yesavage, 1988). For patients with greater cognitive impairment, the Cornell Scale for Depression in Dementia can be used (Alexopoulos, Abrams, Young, & Shamoian, 1988).
5. Eventual discontinuation of the pharmacotherapy should be an objective of treatment, although in some cases that will prove inadvisable. Periodic monitoring of depressive and other BPSD symptoms will inform the decision whether to taper and stop antidepressant treatment. As yet, there are no standard guidelines for antidepressant discontinuation in demented patients with depressive disorders. A reasonable standard might be to begin gradual dose reduction after 6 months of continuous depressive remission. However, a recent double-blind antidepressant discontinuation study in demented patients documented a subsequent increase in depressive symptoms supporting that clinicians who discontinue a demented patient's antidepressant should watch for subsequent re-emergence of depressive symptoms (Bergh, Selbaek, & Engedal, 2012).

Apathy

Apathy has been defined as diminished motivation not attributable to diminished level of consciousness, cognitive impairment, or emotional distress (Marin, 1991). Although dementia is not the only cause of apathy, apathy is the most frequent BPSD found in demented patients (Landes, Sperry, Strauss, & Geldmacher, 2001). Apathy may appear less debilitating, dramatic, and disruptive than depression in demented patients; nonetheless, it can undermine the cooperation of a patient with personal care or activities of daily living, participation in pleasant events, involvement in social interaction, and engagement in physical activity. Apathy easily escapes notice when lack of initiative passes for contentment or lack of distress. On the other hand, attentive caregivers may mistakenly interpret the disengagement of an apathetic person as an indication of depression. Antidepressant treatment must be undertaken with caution, however, as in some cases the serotonergic agents will increase rather than diminish the target symptoms of apathy.

In differentiating apathy from depression, it is useful to distinguish the symptoms shared by these syndromes from symptoms more characteristic of one or the other condition. Diminished interest, psychomotor retardation, fatigue, hypersomnia, and lack of insight can be found both in depression and apathy. Depression often includes dysphoria, suicidal ideation, self-criticism, guilt, pessimism, or hopelessness. Apathy's characteristic symptoms may include a blunted emotional response, low social engagement, and diminished initiation and persistence of activities (Landes et al., 2001).

Recent neuroanatomical and imaging studies have sought to understand the neurological mechanisms of apathy, although the structural lesions associated with apathy may vary among different diagnostic populations. In AD, neuropathologic studies have demonstrated loss of neurons in frontal subcortical circuits (Landes et al., 2001) and increased anterior cingulate neurofibrillary tangle count (Marshall, Fairbanks, Tekin, Vinters, & Cummings, 2006). Consistent with these findings, quantitative structural magnetic resonance imaging (MRI) has correlated apathy with changes in the anterior cingulate cortices bilaterally and in the left medial frontal cortical regions (Apostolova et al., 2007). Diminished synaptic dopamine reuptake in the right and left putamen, visualized using single-photon emission computed tomography (SPECT), was associated with apathy in AD and dementia with Lewy bodies (DLB), suggesting basal ganglia involvement in these patients (David et al., 2008). In vascular dementia and AD dementia, apathy has been correlated with increased white matter hyperintensities on MRI (Starkstein et al., 2009).

As with other BPSDs, the initial approach to management of apathy includes differential diagnosis of the target symptoms. The list of medical factors to consider is long and varied. A stroke or the sequelae of trauma from a fall or other accident may result in brain injury manifested as apathy. Hypothyroidism, if undetected, can diminish initiative. Cardiopulmonary disease, sleep disorders, and neglected nutritional needs deplete a patient of energy. It is important, too, to pare down the list of medications that can contribute to sedation. Selective serotonin reuptake inhibitor (SSRI) antidepressants, interestingly, occasionally initiate or increase apathy (Padala, Padala, Monga, Ramirez, & Sullivan, 2012). Use of alcohol or sedative hypnotics should be limited, if used at all by demented people. Prescribed medications with sedating effects should be limited to the extent possible, and their potential interactions should be reviewed.

Psychosocial factors also contribute to the development of apathy. The initiative of a bored or understimulated person who has been left unattended for long periods of time may improve once activities and interactions increase. Frustration with unsuccessful attempts to continue performing tasks that were previously manageable can lead to desperation and irritable or apathetic disengagement. Sometimes the careful matching of a demented person with a companion or caregiver with shared enthusiasms or interests can alleviate apparent apathy that was increased by a sense of alienation. When there is a clear temporal pattern of disinterest or sleepiness, the scheduling of stimulating and absorbing activities at the patient's usual time of disengagement can be helpful in diminishing apathetic withdrawal. In one 4-week controlled, randomized cross-over clinical trial, a program of music and art therapy and psychomotor activity was shown more effective than free activities in reducing apathy among demented subjects. This finding was more pronounced in those with less severe apathy (Ferrero-Arias et al., 2011).

Positive benefits from pharmacotherapy in the treatment of apathy among demented subjects have been documented for several classes of medications: cognitive enhancers, stimulants, and antidepressants (Berman, Brodaty, Withall, & Seeher, 2012). By contrast, two groups of medications often used to treat BPSD in demented patients, the antipsychotics and the anticonvulsants, have demonstrated little or no value as treatments for apathy in demented cohorts (Berman et al., 2012). The studies that have assessed pharmacotherapy of apathy in demented subjects are limited in duration and power, and focus primarily on AD. More needs to be learned about prevention of apathy, longer term pharmacologic management of apathy, and pharmacotherapy of apathy in non-AD dementias.

Based on the results of several double-blind trials, and consistent with the findings of open-label trials, cognitive enhancers appear to reduce apathy in AD patients. The cholinesterase inhibitors have been studied more extensively than memantine in this regard. Standard doses of donepezil, in two randomized controlled trials, were associated with a decreased likelihood of the emergence of apathy during the 24 weeks of assessment (Waldemar et al., 2011). In a series of other trials, mostly open-label studies in which apathy was one of multiple behaviors measured, treatment was associated with reduced behaviors in groups of patients with AD dementia (Berman et al., 2012) and also in small case series with patients with Lewy body dementia (Lanctot & Herrmann, 2000). Greater levels of apathy at study baseline were associated with a greater likelihood of response, but apathy was noted to increase in some subjects (Mega, Masterman, O'Connor, Barclay, & Cummings, 1999; Tanaka et al., 2004). While rivastigmine has been reported to reduce apathy in subjects with AD dementia and in Lewy body dementia, small and perhaps underpowered studies have failed to show significant treatment benefits in frontotemporal dementia and vascular dementia patients (Berman et al., 2012). Apathy is very common in the dementia of Parkinson's disease (Aarsland et al., 2007), and the usefulness of rivastigmine in treating this apathy was suggested in a small case series (Bullock & Cameron, 2002). Galantamine, in two double-blind studies and other open-label trials, has been associated with improvement in apathy in subjects with AD dementia and in vascular dementia (Berman et al., 2012). In one double-blind placebo-controlled trial, the emergence of apathy in subjects with AD dementia was reduced (Cummings, Schneider, Tariot, Kershaw, & Yuan, 2004). An effect on apathy with memantine treatment has been less consistently supported. Two brief, randomized, double-blind, placebo-controlled studies showed significant improvements in apathy compared to placebo in subjects with AD dementia or vascular dementia, while several other studies have supported nonsignificant a trend toward benefit (Berman et al., 2012). The data on memantine as a treatment for apathy in patients with frontotemporal dementia have produced mixed results; two small case series (Swanberg, 2007) or case reports (Links et al., 2013) suggest benefit, but a small open-label study was negative (Diehl-Schmid, Forstl, Perneczky, Pohl, & Kurz, 2008).

Dolder and colleagues recently reviewed the literature on stimulant medications in treating apathy among demented patients (Dolder, Davis, & McKinsey, 2010). While there are scarce data to reach conclusions about the potential benefits of stimulants among patients with different types of dementia or with regard to specific types of stimulants, the little available data appear to be strongest for treatment of patients with AD dementia and for the use of methylphenidate. Divided daily doses of methylphenidate between 10 and 40 mg/d have been used in the reviewed studies. Yet clinicians who prescribe stimulants in elderly patients must carefully consider and monitor cardiac effects, as the use of these medications can be associated with increases in heart rate and blood pressure.

The use of antidepressants in treating apathy has been explored to only a limited degree, and authorities have questioned whether their effects reduce or, perhaps in some cases, exacerbate apathy (Benoit et al., 2008). The SSRIs may be of particular concern as potential contributors to apathy. Yet, on the other hand, measures of psychomotor retardation were improved in a trial with demented hospitalized patients with behavioral disturbances treated with citalopram

(Nyth & Gottfries, 1990). Bupropion, which possesses stimulant properties, has also been reported to be useful in the management of apathy in patients with organic brain disease (Corcoran, Wong, & O'Keane, 2004).

Sexualized Inappropriate Behavior

Sexualized inappropriate behavior, which is estimated to occur among 7% to 25% of demented patients, is less frequent than either depression or apathy, yet it presents one of the most challenging management dilemmas (Stubbs, 2011). To begin with, many caregivers are uncomfortable with expressions of sexuality among these older and cognitively impaired individuals; this can result in a focus on the sexual content rather than the inappropriate quality of the behavior. Relabeling these behaviors as sexualized inappropriate behavior (SIB), a small semantic change that refocuses attention on disinhibition rather than sexuality as the target of our treatment interventions, can in some cases reduce caregiver shock, disgust, or aversion in the presence of behaviors that are socially unacceptable among the cognitively intact. Males are more likely than females to show this variety of BPSD, and disinhibited sexualized behavior is more characteristic of frontotemporal dementia than of AD.

SIB usually consists of masturbation in areas that lack privacy or sexualized intrusions upon others using words or actions that are unacceptable for a variety of reasons (Stubbs, 2011). Unwanted consequences can include embarrassment, disruption of a milieu or home setting, psychic or physical trauma to others, transmission of a communicable sexual disease, and reactions of various sorts that may range from inappropriate participation in sexual activity to aggressive responses. In some cases, SIB can result in legal allegations and liability. To the consternation of family caregivers, SIB can occur in public places such as health clubs or restaurants. In the home, it represents a potential hazard for children who spend time with an older, demented relative. In institutional settings, it can represent a reason for hospitalization or even expulsion. Inpatient units often encounter great difficulty finding residential placements for demented patients whose disinhibited behavior is sexualized.

Caution is warranted before labeling sexual or other behaviors as inappropriate, since in some cases the behaviors may actually be appropriate or at least acceptable. A cognitively impaired individual can remain capable of sexual interest, excitement, and activity that is appropriate within certain contexts, such as clearly consensual sexual involvement with a relationship partner. An inappropriate and apparently sexualized grab at an attendant sometimes represents a poorly modulated request for attention and affection. The engagement of the limbic system does not necessarily deteriorate in tandem with that of more recently evolved cortical areas, and there are circumstances in which offering a demented person a nonsexual hug or a relaxing hand massage is both welcome and appropriate.

Thinking beyond SIB as normal behavior or an expression of the wish for contact and affection, there are other psychosocial considerations. Our currently aging group of gay, lesbian, bisexual, and transgendered individuals may express sexuality in a way that caregivers in institutional settings will find unfamiliar (Benbow & Beeston, 2012). Cognitive impairment may modulate sexual behavior that is intended to be appropriate—for example, through misidentification of another person as a spouse—leading to behaviors that would be appropriate in the correct context. Delusional misinterpretation of another's behavior as an invitation to intimacy can lead to unwanted advances. Sexual behavior in some demented individuals may merely represent manifestation of a preexisting mental disorder such as mania or paraphilia or continuation of habitual inappropriate behavior that predated cognitive impairment.

A neurological explanation of SIB should take into account the possibilities both of decreased inhibition and increased drive. Black and colleagues, in a comprehensive review of SIB, suggest that four brain systems are potential contributors to SIB (Black, Muralee, & Tampi, 2005). Failure of inhibition and social judgment suggests impairment of the frontal executive system's restraining capacity. An increase in sexual drive, similar to the hypersexuality seen in the Kluver-Bucy syndrome, has been invoked and may be of particular importance in frontotemporal dementias. Striatal involvement is suggested by a compulsive quality to some SIBs. Finally, hypothalamic involvement, through disordered hormonal control, has also been considered a possible contributor to some cases of SIB.

As with other BPSDs, SIB should initially be addressed behaviorally. Psychoeducation of the caregiving system is an important initial step. Spouses, children of sufficient age and capacity to understand, and caregiving institutional staff may initially fail to understand that the SIB is a symptom of neurodegeneration rather than the unmasking of an evil or aggressive character. Reframing the SIB as a common symptom of dementia can diminish the moral stigmatization that might otherwise occur and can facilitate behavioral management that may include more acceptable ways of responding to whatever needs the patient is expressing through sexualized behaviors. Sex education is an important aspect of training for institutional care staff who may lack experience in distinguishing acceptable and inappropriate behaviors from those that are not tolerable within an institutional setting.

Behavioral interventions often suffice in managing SIB and should in general be employed prior to pharmacotherapeutic approaches because their effectiveness may be as great and the hazard of potential adverse medication effects can be avoided. To begin with, overstimulating external cues such as sexually exciting television shows or movies should be eliminated. Although confrontation of inappropriate behavior may fail to have lasting beneficial consequences, a sexualizing person may be responsive to distraction and redirection toward involvement in a more acceptable activity. Sexualized intrusions on a roommate or family member may necessitate a room change or avoidance of unchaperoned time together. Public masturbation or undressing can sometimes be managed by use of clothing modifications that make it more difficult to remove clothing without assistance, such as pants that fasten in the back rather than the front and do not have a zipper.

Although not yet supported by randomized, controlled, double-blind clinical trials, many different medications have been tried in the management of SIB. Clinical practice to date appears to rely primarily on the reported results of small case series or open-label trials. As with the other off-label uses described in this chapter, it is necessary that the competent patient or the authorized health care representative be informed about the use of a medication for this nonindicated purpose and be educated about the potential risks, benefits, and alternative treatment approaches. As a prelude to pharmacotherapy of SIB, it may be appropriate to discontinue medications that increase sexual drive or expression such as androgens, levodopa, or disinhibiting sedative-hypnotics. When using one of the medications suggested helpful for managing SIB, it is advisable to follow the universal guideline for geriatric pharmacotherapy, which is to start low, go slow, but do not undertreat or declare failure prematurely.

Pharmacologic management of SIB has aimed to reduce sexual drive or to diminish disinhibition. Evidence is not available to assess the effects of cognitive-enhancing cholinesterase inhibitors or memantine on sexualized behavior, though one letter describes a case in which rivastigmine alleviated sexually aggressive behavior of a demented woman (Alagiakrishnan, Sclater, & Robertson, 2003). The libido-reducing and antiorgasmic effects of serotonergic antidepressants, sometimes a cause of treatment nonadherence in younger adults, may serve advantageously in managing SIB in some demented patients. Paroxetine (Stewart & Shin, 1997), citalopram (Chen, 2010; Tosto, Talarico, Lenzi, & Bruno, 2008), and clomipramine (Leo & Kim, 1995) each have been prescribed at standard antidepressant doses and claimed to be helpful in reducing sexualized behaviors in case reports. Trazodone, though in other contexts occasionally a cause of hypersexuality, has also been used in this way. The familiar adverse effects of these antidepressants, and especially of clomipramine, can undermine their use in managing SIB. Cimetidine (Wiseman, McAuley, Freidenberg, & Freidenberg, 2000) (600 to 1,600 mg/d), perhaps through its secondary effect on testosterone levels resulting from hepatic enzyme induction, has been used to lower libido and manage SIB. As an unwanted consequence of its use, blood levels of hepatically metabolized coadministered medications may also be diminished. Nonspecific sedation or increased impulse control is a treatment objective when using antipsychotics to manage SIB, and these medications are therefore often used in an effort to affect SIB despite an evidence base apparently limited to a couple of case reports describing the use of haloperidol (Jensen, 1989) or quietiapine (MacKnight & Rojas-Fernandez, 2000) and a post-hoc analysis supporting risperidone's use at low doses in a Korean nursing home cohort (Suh, Greenspan, & Choi, 2006). The adverse effects of the antipsychotics are described in detail in Chapter 24, including the increase in overall mortality risk that is associated with their long-term use in demented older adults. Pindolol (40 mg/d), through adrenergic antagonism or perhaps through its serotonergic effects, was reported to manage SIB successfully in one patient (Jensen, 1989). There is also a case report of gabapentin's use in managing SIB (Miller, 2001).

In more severe or treatment-resistant cases, hormonal agents have been used to lower libido through effects on the hypothalamic-pituitary-gonadal hormonal circuit. Medroxyprogesterone (Light & Holroyd, 2006) (doses of 100 to 300 mg/d given as an intramuscular injection), diethylstilbesterol (Kyomen, Nobel, & Wei, 1991) (1 mg/d), or leuprolide acetate (Ott, 1995) (7.5 mg/month given as an intramuscular injection) have been reported in one or more cases to manage SIB. Estrogen (Lothstein, Fogg-Waberski, & Reynolds, 1997) (0.625 mg/d), used in a larger sample of patients, was also reported effective in managing SIB. The side effects of these hormonal agents include weight changes, dizziness, nausea, insomnia, pain, edema, and depression.

Conclusion

In the management of demented patients in home or institutional settings, BPSDs present challenges that often exceed those of reduced memory capacity. Preventive management of the environment, early recognition of BPSDs, and monitoring of the safety of patient and caregivers are important steps in providing optimal care. Behavioral interventions should generally precede pharmacologic treatment approaches, and sometimes the combination is optimal. Further research must seek a fuller understanding of BPSDs' neuropsychiatric mechanisms and explore the longer term management of these symptoms in both patients with AD dementia and in those with other neurodegenerative disorders.

References

Aarsland, D., Bronnick, K., Ehrt, U., De Deyn, P. P., Tekin, S., Emre, M., & Cummings, J. L. (2007). Neuropsychiatric symptoms in patients with Parkinson's disease and dementia: frequency, profile and associated care giver stress. *Journal of Neurology, Neurosurgery, and Psychiatry, 78*, 36–42.

Alagiakrishnan, K., Sclater, A., & Robertson, D. (2003). Role of cholinesterase inhibitor in the management of sexual aggression in an elderly demented woman. *Journal of the American Geriatrics Society, 51*, 1326.

Alexopoulos, G. S., Abrams, R. C., Young, R. C., & Shamoian, C. A. (1988). Cornell Scale for Depression in Dementia. *Biological Psychiatry, 23*, 271–284.

Apostolova, L. G., Akopyan, G. G., Partiali, N., Steiner, C. A., Dutton, R. A., Hayashi, K. M.,...Thompson, P. M. (2007). Structural correlates of apathy in Alzheimer's disease. *Dementia and Geriatric Cognitive Disorders, 24*, 91–97.

Bassiony, M. M., Warren, A., Rosenblatt, A., Baker, A., Steinberg, M., Steele, C. D.,...Lyketsos, C. G. (2002). The relationship between delusions and depression in Alzheimer's disease. *International Journal of Geriatric Psychiatry, 17*, 549–556.

Benbow, S. M., & Beeston, D. (2012). Sexuality, aging, and dementia. *International Psychogeriatrics, 24*(7), 1026–1033.

Benoit, M., Andrieu, S., Lechowski, L., Gillette-Guyonnet, S., Robert, P. H., & Vellas, B. (2008). Apathy and depression in Alzheimer's disease are associated with functional deficit and psychotropic prescription. *International Journal of Geriatric Psychiatry, 23*, 409–414.

Bergh, S., Selbaek, G., & Engedal, K. (2012). Discontinuation of antidepressants in people with dementia and neuropsychiatric symptoms (DESEP study): Double blind, randomised, parallel group, placebo controlled trial. *British Medical Journal, 344*, e1566.

Berman, K., Brodaty, H., Withall, A., & Seeher, K. (2012). Pharmacologic treatment of apathy in dementia. *American Journal of Geriatric Psychiatry, 20*, 104–122.

Black, B., Muralee, S., & Tampi, R. R. (2005). Inappropriate sexual behaviors in dementia. *Journal of Geriatric Psychiatry and Neurology, 18*, 155–162.

Branconnier, R. J., & Cole, J. O. (1980). The therapeutic role of methylphenidate in senile organic brain syndrome. *Proceedings of the Annual Meeting of the American Psychopathological Association, 69,* 183–196.

Bullock, R., & Cameron, A. (2002). Rivastigmine for the treatment of dementia and visual hallucinations associated with Parkinson's disease: A case series. *Current Medical Research and Opinion, 18,* 258–264.

Chen, S. T. (2010). Treatment of a patient with dementia and inappropriate sexual behaviors with citalopram. *Alzheimers Disease and Associated Disorders,* 24(4), 402–403.

Corcoran, C., Wong, M. L., & O'Keane, V. (2004). Bupropion in the management of apathy. *Journal of Psychopharmacology, 18,* 133–135.

Cummings, J. L., Schneider, L., Tariot, P. N., Kershaw, P. R., & Yuan, W. (2004). Reduction of behavioral disturbances and caregiver distress by galantamine in patients with Alzheimer's disease. *American Journal of Psychiatry, 161,* 532–538.

David, R., Koulibaly, M., Benoit, M., Garcia, R., Caci, H., Darcourt, J., & Robert, P. (2008). Striatal dopamine transporter levels correlate with apathy in neurodegenerative diseases A SPECT study with partial volume effect correction. *Clinical Neurology and Neurosurgery, 110,* 19–24.

de Vasconcelos Cunha, U. G., Lopes Rocha, F., Avila de Melo, R., Alves Valle, E., de Souza Neto, J. J., Mendes Brega, R.,...Sakurai, E. (2007). A placebo-controlled double-blind randomized study of venlafaxine in the treatment of depression in dementia. *Dementia and Geriatric Cognitive Disorders, 24,* 36–41.

Diehl-Schmid, J., Forstl, H., Perneczky, R., Pohl, C., & Kurz, A. (2008). A 6-month, open-label study of memantine in patients with frontotemporal dementia. *International Journal of Geriatric Psychiatry, 23,* 754–759.

Dolder, C. R., Davis, L. N., & McKinsey, J. (2010). Use of psychostimulants in patients with dementia. *Annals of Pharmacotherapy, 44,* 1624–1632.

Dwyer, M., & Byrne, G. J. (2000). Disruptive vocalization and depression in older nursing home residents. *International Psychogeriatrics, 12,* 463–471.

Ferrero-Arias, J., Goni-Imizcoz, M., Gonzalez-Bernal, J., Lara-Ortega, F., da Silva-Gonzalez, A., & Diez-Lopez, M. (2011). The efficacy of nonpharmacological treatment for dementia-related apathy. *Alzheimers Disease and Associated Disorders, 25,* 213–219.

Graeber, M. B., & Mehraein, P. (1999). Reanalysis of the first case of Alzheimer's disease. *European Archives of Psychiatry and Clinical Neuroscience,* 249(Suppl 3), 10–13.

Howland, R. H. (2011a). A critical evaluation of the cardiac toxicity of citalopram: Part 1. *Journal of Psychosocial Nursing and Mental Health Services, 49,* 13–16.

Howland, R. H. (2011b). A critical evaluation of the cardiac toxicity of citalopram: Part 2. *Journal of Psychosocial Nursing and Mental Health Services, 49,* 13–16.

Jensen, C. F. (1989). Hypersexual agitation in Alzheimer's disease. *Journal of the American Geriatrics Society, 37,* 917.

Jost, B. C., & Grossberg, G. T. (1996). The evolution of psychiatric symptoms in Alzheimer's disease: A natural history study. *Journal of the American Geriatrics Society, 44,* 1078–1081.

Kyomen, H. H., Nobel, K. W., & Wei, J. Y. (1991). The use of estrogen to decrease aggressive physical behavior in elderly men with dementia. *Journal of the American Geriatrics Society, 39,* 1110–1112.

Lanctot, K. L., & Herrmann, N. (2000). Donepezil for behavioural disorders associated with Lewy bodies: A case series. *International Journal of Geriatric Psychiatry, 15,* 338–345.

Landes, A. M., Sperry, S. D., Strauss, M. E., & Geldmacher, D. S. (2001). Apathy in Alzheimer's disease. *Journal of the American Geriatrics Society, 49,* 1700–1707.

Leo, R. J., & Kim, K. Y. (1995). Clomipramine treatment of paraphilias in elderly demented patients. *Journal of Geriatric Psychiatry and Neurology, 8,* 123–124.

Light, S. A., & Holroyd, S. (2006). The use of medroxyprogesterone acetate for the treatment of sexually inappropriate behaviour in patients with dementia. *Journal of Psychiatry and Neuroscience, 31,* 132–134.

Links, K. A., Black, S. E., Graff-Guerrero, A., Wilson, A. A., Houle, S., Pollock, B. G., & Chow, T. W. (2013). A case of apathy due to frontotemporal dementia responsive to memantine. *Neurocase,* 19(3), 256–261.

Lothstein, L. M., Fogg-Waberski, J., & Reynolds, P. (1997). Risk management and treatment of sexual disinhibition in geriatric patients. *Connecticut Medicine, 61,* 609–618.

Lyketsos, C. G., & Olin, J. (2002). Depression in Alzheimer's disease: Overview and treatment. *Biological Psychiatry, 52,* 243–252.

Lyketsos, C. G., Sheppard, J. M., Steele, C. D., Kopunek, S., Steinberg, M., Baker, A. S.,...Rabins, P. V. (2000). Randomized, placebo-controlled, double-blind clinical trial of sertraline in the treatment of depression complicating Alzheimer's disease: Initial results from the Depression in Alzheimer's Disease study. *American Journal of Psychiatry, 157,* 1686–1689.

Lyketsos, C. G., Steinberg, M., Tschanz, J. T., Norton, M. C., Steffens, D. C., & Breitner, J. C. (2000). Mental and behavioral disturbances in dementia: Findings from the Cache County

Study on Memory in Aging. *American Journal of Psychiatry, 157*, 708–714.

MacKnight, C., & Rojas-Fernandez, C. (2000). Quetiapine for sexually inappropriate behavior in dementia. *Journal of the American Geriatrics Society, 48*, 707.

Magai, C., Kennedy, G., Cohen, C. I., & Gomberg, D. (2000). A controlled clinical trial of sertraline in the treatment of depression in nursing home patients with late-stage Alzheimer's disease. *American Journal of Geriatric Psychiatry, 8*, 66–74.

Marin, R. S. (1991). Apathy: A neuropsychiatric syndrome. *Journal of Neuropsychiatry and Clinical Neurosciences, 3*, 243–254.

Marshall, G. A., Fairbanks, L. A., Tekin, S., Vinters, H. V., & Cummings, J. L. (2006). Neuropathologic correlates of apathy in Alzheimer's disease. *Dementia and Geriatric Cognitive Disorders, 21*, 144–147.

McDermott, C. L., & Gray, S. L. (2012). Cholinesterase inhibitor adjunctive therapy for cognitive impairment and depressive symptoms in older adults with depression. *Annals of Pharmacotherapy, 46*, 599–605.

Mega, M. S., Masterman, D. M., O'Connor, S. M., Barclay, T. R., & Cummings, J. L. (1999). The spectrum of behavioral responses to cholinesterase inhibitor therapy in Alzheimer disease. *Archives of Neurology, 56*, 1388–1393.

Menon, A. S., Gruber-Baldini, A. L., Hebel, J. R., Kaup, B., Loreck, D., Itkin Zimmerman, S.,...Magaziner, J. (2001). Relationship between aggressive behaviors and depression among nursing home residents with dementia. *International Journal of Geriatric Psychiatry, 16*, 139–146.

Miller, L. J. (2001). Gabapentin for treatment of behavioral and psychological symptoms of dementia. *Annals of Pharmacotherapy, 35*, 427–431.

Morley, J. E., & Kraenzle, D. (1994). Causes of weight loss in a community nursing home. *Journal of the American Geriatrics Society, 42*, 583–585.

Nelson, J. C., & Devanand, D. P. (2011). A systematic review and meta-analysis of placebo-controlled antidepressant studies in people with depression and dementia. *Journal of the American Geriatrics Society, 59*, 577–585.

Nyth, A. L., & Gottfries, C. G. (1990). The clinical efficacy of citalopram in treatment of emotional disturbances in dementia disorders. A Nordic multicentre study. *British Journal of Psychiatry, 157*, 894–901.

Olin, J. T., Schneider, L. S., Katz, I. R., Meyers, B. S., Alexopoulos, G. S.,...Lebowitz, B. D. (2002). Provisional diagnostic criteria for depression of Alzheimer disease. *American Journal of Geriatric Psychiatry, 10*, 125–128.

Ott, B. R. (1995). Leuprolide treatment of sexual aggression in a patient with Dementia and the Kluver-Bucy syndrome. *Clinical Neuropharmacology, 18*, 443–447.

Oudman, E. (2012). Is electroconvulsive therapy (ECT) effective and safe for treatment of depression in dementia? A short review. *Journal of ECT, 28*, 34–38.

Padala, P. R., Padala, K. P., Monga, V., Ramirez, D. A., & Sullivan, D. H. (2012). Reversal of SSRI-associated apathy syndrome by discontinuation of therapy. *Annals of Pharmacotherapy, 46*, e8.

Petracca, G., Teson, A., Chemerinski, E., Leiguarda, R., & Starkstein, S. E. (1996). A double-blind placebo-controlled study of clomipramine in depressed patients with Alzheimer's disease. *Journal of Neuropsychiatry and Clinical Neurosciences, 8*, 270–275.

Petracca, G. M., Chemerinski, E., & Starkstein, S. E. (2001). A double-blind, placebo-controlled study of fluoxetine in depressed patients with Alzheimer's disease. *International Psychogeriatrics, 13*, 233–240.

Reifler, B. V., Teri, L., Raskind, M., Veith, R., Barnes, R., White, E., & McLean, P. (1989). Double-blind trial of imipramine in Alzheimer's disease patients with and without depression. *American Journal of Psychiatry, 146*, 45–49.

Roth, M., Mountjoy, C. Q., & Amrein, R. (1996). Moclobemide in elderly patients with cognitive decline and depression: An international double-blind, placebo-controlled trial. *British Journal of Psychiatry, 168*, 149–157.

Starkstein, S. E., Mizrahi, R., Capizzano, A. A., Acion, L., Brockman, S., & Power, B. D. (2009). Neuroimaging correlates of apathy and depression in Alzheimer's disease. *Journal of Neuropsychiatry and Clinical Neurosciences, 21*, 259–265.

Stewart, J. T., & Shin, K. J. (1997). Paroxetine treatment of sexual disinhibition in dementia. *American Journal of Psychiatry, 154*, 1474.

Stubbs, B. (2011). Displays of inappropriate sexual behaviour by patients with progressive cognitive impairment: The forgotten form of challenging behaviour? *Journal of Psychiatric and Mental Health Nursing, 18*, 602–607.

Suh, G. H., Greenspan, A. J., & Choi, S. K. (2006). Comparative efficacy of risperidone versus haloperidol on behavioural and psychological symptoms of dementia. *International Journal of Geriatric Psychiatry, 21*, 654–660.

Swanberg, M. M. (2007). Memantine for behavioral disturbances in frontotemporal dementia: A case series. *Alzheimers Disease and Associated Disorders, 21*, 164–166.

Swartz, J. R., Miller, B. L., Lesser, I. M., & Darby, A. L. (1997). Frontotemporal dementia: Treatment response to serotonin selective reuptake inhibitors. *The Journal of clinical psychiatry, 58*, 212–216.

Tanaka, M., Namiki, C., Thuy, D. H., Yoshida, H., Kawasaki, K., Hashikawa, K.,...Kita, T. (2004). Prediction of psychiatric response to donepezil in patients with mild to moderate Alzheimer's disease. *Journal of the Neurological Sciences, 225*, 135–141.

Tosto, G., Talarico, G., Lenzi, G. L., & Bruno, G. (2008). Effect of citalopram in treating hypersexuality in an Alzheimer's disease case. *Neurological Sciences, 29.* 269–270.

Tractenberg, R. E., Weiner, M. F., Patterson, M. B., Teri, L., & Thal, L. J. (2003). Comorbidity of psychopathological domains in community-dwelling persons with Alzheimer's disease. *Journal of Geriatric Psychiatry and Neurology, 16*, 94–99.

Waldemar, G., Gauthier, S., Jones, R., Wilkinson, D., Cummings, J., Lopez, O.,...Mackell, J. (2011). Effect of donepezil on emergence of apathy in mild to moderate Alzheimer's disease. *International Journal of Geriatric Psychiatry, 26*, 150–157.

Weintraub, D., Rosenberg, P. B., Drye, L. T., Martin, B. K., Frangakis, C., Mintzer, J. E.,...Lyketsos, C. G. (2010). Sertraline for the treatment of depression in Alzheimer disease: Week-24 outcomes. *American Journal of Geriatric Psychiatry, 18*, 332–340.

Wiseman, S. V., McAuley, J. W., Freidenberg, G. R., & Freidenberg, D. L. (2000). Hypersexuality in patients with dementia: Possible response to cimetidine. *Neurology, 54*, 2024.

Yesavage, J. A. (1988). Geriatric depression scale. *Psychopharmacology Bulletin, 24*, 709–711.

26

Nonpharmacological Approaches to Managing Behavior Symptoms in Dementia

Sumer Verma

> And as with age his body uglier grows,
> So his mind cankers.
> —Shakespeare, *The Tempest* (act IV, scene 1, 213–214)

> Last scene of all,
> That ends this strange eventful history,
> Is second childishness and mere oblivion,
> Sans teeth, sans eyes, sans taste, sans everything.
> —Shakespeare, *As You Like It* (act II, scene 7, 143–170)

The contemporary history of dementia begins in 1906 with the report at a conference in Tubingen, Germany, by Alois Alzheimer "On a peculiar disease process of the cerebral cortex." However, the awareness of (senile) dementia and the cognitive and behavioral disturbances that result from this disease dates back thousands of years. Medical literature and fiction are replete with descriptions of the personal and social consequences of the illness. Older descriptions of dementia largely attributed the development of dementia to the cognitive decline that was believed to inevitably accompany old age.

It was the seminal work of Alois Alzheimer that provided the first clear understanding of a disease that is now named after him (Berchtold & Cotman, 1998).

Increase in global life expectancy and consequent aging of the population has resulted in an unprecedented increase in the incidence and prevalence of dementia. This shift will continue to pose increasing demands on global health care resources. In 2006, the worldwide prevalence of Alzheimer's disease was 26.6 million. It is projected that by 2030, the number of persons suffering from dementia worldwide will rise to nearly 1 billion. By 2050, the prevalence will quadruple, by which time 1 in 85 persons worldwide will be living with the disease. The impact of these demographic changes requires us to consider carefully the means by which we manage this epidemic while we await the discovery of an agent or agents that can effectively alter the course and outcome of dementia. Despite the very significant advances over the past 100 years in our understanding of the pathogenesis of dementia, we still lack any effective intervention that can provide any more than modest slowing of the inexorable cognitive and functional decline. We are a long way from preventing or reversing the process. It is estimated that about 43% of prevalent cases will need a high level of care, equivalent to that of a nursing home. If effective interventions could delay disease onset and progression by a modest 1 year, there could be nearly 9.2 million fewer cases of the disease by 2050, with nearly the entire decline attributable to decreases in persons needing a high level of care (Brookmeyer, Johnson, Ziegler-Graham, & Arrighi, 2007).

The appropriate management of dementia needs to focus on two main issues: slowing the deficits imposed by cognitive decline and managing the behavioral and psychological symptoms (BPSDs) that develop as the disease progresses (Cohen-Mansfield, 1994; Finkel, Costa e Silva, Cohen, Miller, & Sartorius, 1996; Tariot, 1996). Although clinicians are more knowledgeable about pharmacological interventions that treat the cognitive deficit, less is understood about the appropriate management of the BPSDs. For the most part, the dominant approach has been pharmacological, yet there are increasing questions being raised about the appropriateness of this approach. The US Department of Health and Human Services Office of the Inspector General reported that 99.5% of nursing facilities in the United States were noncompliant regarding the regulations concerning the use of antipsychotic agents in nursing homes. The Center for Medicare Services implemented an initiative to reduce the use of antipsychotic agents in nursing homes by 15% by 2013. As a result, increasing emphasis is being placed on developing and utilizing nonpharmacological interventions.

A Conceptual Overview of Behavioral and Psychological Symptoms

As detailed in Chapters 21, 24, and 25, BPSDs are a varied group of symptoms that complicate the course of dementia to varying degrees in many patients with dementia. These disturbances result in immense distress to patient and caregiver alike (Cerejeira, Lagarto, & Mukaetova-Ladinska, 2012). Symptoms such as apathy, agitation, aggressiveness, depression, and psychosis are associated with substantial personal and caregiver distress, increased health care costs both direct and indirect, and a greater risk for institutional placement. Estimates of the prevalence rates for these symptoms vary widely depending on the study population and the criteria used to ascertain symptoms (Okura et al., 2010). Between 56% and 74% of persons with moderately advanced dementia exhibit at least one BPSD (Geda et al., 2008; Lyketsos et al., 2002). Most studies show that the frequency and severity of BPSDs increase with dementia severity. For example, depression, social withdrawal, and anxiety disorders are seen more commonly in early dementia while agitation, disinhibition, and aggression are more common in advanced dementia (Jost & Grossberg, 1996). Although generalizable patterns can be seen in some aspects of behavioral symptoms across groups of patients with dementia, they may vary substantially in intensity and severity from person to person and from time to time in the same person. For the most part, these forms of variability are not well understood.

Although cognitively intact persons may respond to sources of distress in the environment (e.g., uncertainty, unpredictability) or in themselves (e.g., pain or other physical discomfort) in a variety of ways, they are generally able to communicate their distress in ways that are understandable by others and socially acceptable. In persons with dementia, however, communication abilities and insight are often impaired, which may cause forms of distress experienced by all of us to be expressed in ways we describe as BPSDs. In addition, premorbid personality traits likely color how distress is expressed as BPSDs. This may explain, in part, why one person exhibits aggressiveness and another exhibits apathy. Just as nondemented people are different, so also are people suffering from dementia. A one-size-fits-all approach to this problem fails to account for the tremendous variations seen in BPSDs.

One way to explain this behavioral variation is to draw a parallel with normal human development. Human growth and development unfolds along a predictable sequence of events from birth to adult life. The ability to manage basic and instrumental activities of daily living (ADLs and IADLs) independently is acquired hierarchically as the nervous system matures. Normal aging is often accompanied by a gradual loss of some previously acquired motor, cognitive, and psychosocial abilities. The ensuing functional decline is modulated by adaptive capacity and coping skills. When late life is complicated by prominent cognitive decline, there is also loss of previously effective adaptive and coping skills. Anxiety and depression develop with the fear of impending failure. As dementia worsens, functional communication becomes difficult and attempts at coping become less effective and more "primitive" or childlike. The difference is that in attempting to understand some of the chaotic behavior of infancy and adolescence, one has to consider "where the person is headed," whereas in late life it is useful to understand "where the person has come from." A thorough review of the life story of the individual and his or her "premorbid style" may be helpful in explaining some of the origins of and ways BPSDs are expressed, and it may also help in developing caregiving strategies.

Yet another, and perhaps complementary, conceptualization that can be used to understand BPSDs is to examine the interactions between the limbic system and the cortex. The human brain is the product of evolution. The "triune brain," as postulated by Paul MacLean in the 1960s, consists of the reptilian complex (the amygdala), the paleo-mammalian complex (the limbic system), and the neo-mammalian complex (the neocortex). Among mammals, the human brain is the largest, and the cerebral cortex is the thickest. In essence, it is what makes humans the most "evolved" species. The complex interconnections between the various parts of the brain that allow us to "seamlessly" integrate sensory inputs and organize effective responses are far from completely understood. Nevertheless, this conceptualization can serve as a useful "brain model" when conceptualizing the origins of BPSDs and behavioral/environmental strategies for intervention. The prefrontal neocortex provides us with the ability to apply reason over the more basic fight-or-flight reactions that emanate from the "reptilian" brain. The neocortex acts as a "top-down" brake applied to the "bottom-up" "reptilian" drives that originate from the amygdala and other parts of the limbic system. In this model, the "intermediary" in this process is the hippocampus. An important function of the hippocampus is to encode and retrieve a variety of types of memories. Bilateral damage to the hippocampus results in difficulty in both anterograde and, to a lesser degree, retrograde amnesia, thus making learning difficult.

George E. P. Box famously stated, "Remember that all models are wrong; the practical question is how wrong do they have to be to not be useful" (Box & Draper, 1987, p. 74). While some of the preceding discussion is clearly oversimplified, it is meant to serve as a model that can be applied to caregiving in dementia. Thus, a substantial number of BPSDs can be viewed as a consequence of the breakdown of the "communication" between amygdala, hippocampus, and prefrontal cortex. When pathology exceeds a certain threshold, the person loses the "top-down," reason-guided and learned modulation of the more primitive "bottom-up," childlike, impulsive, fight-or-flight responses. Like a young child, the cognitively impaired individual has increasing difficulty in processing change and in expressing distress appropriately. With disease progression, as impulse control and communication abilities are lost, the individual becomes progressively less able to contextualize bodily feelings (some of which may be symptoms such as pain, constipation-related discomfort, etc.), regulate emotion, and communicate needs. Unexpected environmental change may be interpreted as chaos, and without the cortical "brake" with which to modulate the associated feelings, BPSDs emerge.

Common Behavior Problems

Behavior can be defined as an action by an organism in response to its environment. Humans possess a highly evolved and complex nervous system, and they have developed the ability to acquire an extensive repertoire of responses that enable them to adapt to their environment. A corollary to this observation is that based on their different life experiences, these behaviors vary from person to person. Their acceptability or unacceptability is determined by societal norms. Barring extremes, the judgment of what makes a behavior acceptable or unacceptable can vary from culture to culture and is very much "in the eyes of the beholder."

Every species needs a system by which to quickly assess threat—real or imagined. Without this ability, survival of the species is threatened. The triune brain hypothesis proposes that this is an important ability, emanating from the amygdala and other parts of

TABLE 26.1 Disturbed or Disturbing Behaviors

Disturbed/Dangerous	Disturbing/Troubling
Assaultive	Wandering or pacing
Aggressive physically or verbally	Sleep cycle disruption
Psychosis	Inappropriate sexuality
Paranoia	Hoarding
Mood change—depression, mania	Foul language
Inappropriate or predatory sexuality	Social withdrawal
Destruction of property	Anorexia or hyperphagia
Inappropriate voiding/defecation	Resistance to care

the reptilian brain. From birth, humans learn (to varying degrees) to tolerate frustration, delay gratification, and act in accordance with social norms. This is largely a function of the prefrontal and other parts of the neocortex, and the process takes about 20 years to complete. Disruption of "higher" cortical functions can occur following cortical damage, states of intoxication, and in dementia. Depending on the degree of damage, there can be disinhibition, a disregard for social norms, disruption of language fluency, and a regression to a less developed or childlike state. The unacceptable behaviors that result can broadly be classified as either disturbed and dangerous, or disturbing and troubling (see Table 26.1).

To Medicate or Not

The management of BPSDs remains largely empiric and inconsistent. When confronted with distressing BPSDs, the clinician is confronted with the dilemma of whether to "drug or not to drug." The disruptive behaviors often exhibited by infants, children, and adolescents are tolerated as "normal" and, rightly, few would resort to the use of pharmacological agents to contain the average episode of "bad behavior." Yet, when confronted with similar behavior in demented elderly, there has often been a rush to "treatment" with psychotropics. A survey by the Office of the Inspector General in May 2011 examined the use of atypical antipsychotic drugs in nursing homes and found that off-label conditions were associated with 83% of claims for atypical antipsychotic drugs for elderly nursing home residents; 88% were associated with the condition specified in the FDA boxed warning.

There is no consensus on the most appropriate and effective way of ameliorating the BPSDs that complicate management at different stages of the illness—this is likely because there is no one-size-fits-all method that applies to each individual. General and personalized nonpharmacological approaches, sometimes combined with pharmacology, are generally recommended. While in the past, pharmacological treatment has been a mainstay of treatment efforts, there has been increasing concern raised about the efficacy and appropriateness of these interventions, especially the use of antipsychotic drugs. Nearly one in three nursing-home residents in the United States received antipsychotic drugs in 2007, which is the highest reported level of use in more than a decade (Chen et al., 2010). Twenty-eight percent of all Medicare beneficiaries in nursing homes received at least one prescription for antipsychotics during the study period: 20.3% received atypicals only; 3.7%, conventionals only; and 3.6%, both atypicals and conventionals. Less than half (41.8%) of treated residents received antipsychotic therapy in accordance with prescribing guidelines. Almost one in four (23.4%) patients had no appropriate indication for antipsychotic treatment, 17.2% had daily doses exceeding recommended levels, and 17.6% had both inappropriate indications and high dosing. Patients receiving antipsychotic therapy within guidelines were no more likely to achieve stability or improvement in behavioral symptoms than were those taking antipsychotics outside the guidelines (Briesacher et al., 2005).

Few clinicians would deny the usefulness of nonpharmacological interventions for BPSDs. However, the relative paucity of high-quality studies that demonstrate the effectiveness of many nonpharmacological treatments for BPSDs have made many clinicians reluctant to use them for all but the most trivial disturbances. Additionally, despite many nonpharmacological treatments being both effective and well tolerated, reluctance to institute them in the long-term care setting has been influenced by the fact that they often require a dedicated and trained staff with time and patience to try different modalities. Having said that, it must be added that there are situations in which patients are refractory to nonpharmacological interventions or pose serious risk to themselves and others that necessitate the acute use of pharmacological interventions. To deny a distressed patient any appropriate treatment is unacceptable and unethical. Pharmacology must be considered when the safety of the patient or others is at risk or when the benefits of pharmacology clearly outweigh the risks. Pharmacotherapy should always be employed in conjunction with nonpharmacological methods. In all such instances the drug should be used for approved indications, in the lowest possible effective dose and for a limited period of time. All interventions must be documented in terms of risk benefit and rationale, and they must be appropriately monitored.

As matters stand today, the question is not to "drug or not to drug" but rather how to use both modalities effectively in conjunction. No single modality works for all situations or persons; it is up to the treatment team to decide which modality is most effective in a particular situation. Until the advent of atypical antipsychotic drugs in the early 1990s, conventional agents were the most commonly prescribed agents for BPSDs, despite the fact that these drugs were developed and approved for the treatment of psychosis. Most cases of dementia do not exhibit frank psychosis. In addition, these conventional antipsychotic drugs were associated with serious side effects that limited their use in older patients. Concern with the overuse of these drugs led to the Omnibus Budget Reconciliation Act of 1987, which mandated that these drugs be used only as a last resort to treat BPSDs. The atypical or second-generation antipsychotic drugs were initially believed to be free of most of the side effects that limited the use of conventional antipsychotics. Two decades of clinical experience and data have proved otherwise. Unquestionably, these second-generation drugs are vastly superior in efficacy and side effect profile to the older drugs. That being said, they are not entirely free of serious cardiac, metabolic, and central nervous system effects, especially in the elderly in whom the use of these drugs, as a class, has been associated with increased risk of death, stroke, and cognitive decline (Narang et al., 2010; Vigen et al., 2011). Before utilizing these agents, a careful workup must be completed. The presence of a psychosis or serious mood disorder should be the only acceptable indication for prescribing first- and second-generation antipsychotic medications. To date, however, not one of these agents has been granted FDA approval for use in dementia and, if used, is used "off label." (In the United Kingdom, the only drug licensed for the treatment of persistent and refractory agitation and psychosis in dementia is risperidone—for short-term treatment 1–2 mg daily for only up to 6 weeks.) Suffice it to say that the prescription of antipsychotics for older demented individuals is coming under increased scrutiny and regulation in both the lay and professional press. Some have gone so far as to say that "The way antipsychotic drugs are used in nursing homes is a form of elder abuse" (as stated by Patricia McGinnis, executive director of California Advocates for Nursing Home Reform, to the Senate Special Committee on Aging in 2010) and that "Instead of providing individualized care, many homes indiscriminately use these drugs to sedate and subdue residents."

Developing Nonpharmacological Approaches

The ensuing section is based on experience gained over the past 7 years at Briarwood Nursing and Rehabilitation in Needham, Massachusetts. The program is based on the Eden Alternative model and provides care for 40 residents. Over the prior 7 years, the use of antipsychotic drugs on the dementia service has been reduced to about 5% without any noticeable increase in distress to patients or staff or increase in use of other psychotropic drugs. The process of achieving this goal is discussed in the ensuing section to provide practical suggestions on developing nonpharmacological interventions. These suggestions are offered as general guidelines with the understanding that each facility has its own patient and caregiver demographics and characteristics, as well as staff and milieu strengths and limitations.

Interdisciplinary Teamwork

Long-term care and more so, dementia care is effective when it becomes an "interdisciplinary effort." It takes a team to care for a person with dementia. Traditional hospital-based care is directed at "cure" and the lead clinician, often a physician, is the coordinator of care. On the other hand, dementia care is directed at the maintenance of function and quality of life. The most effective model is one in which the roles of nursing, social work, family, and rehabilitation services become central. The lead clinician assumes a less central role in the decision-making process. Perhaps the most important member of the team is the nursing assistant. This is the person that provides most of the care and in turn absorbs the brunt of the BPSDs. In addition to the nursing staff, social worker, and, when feasible, the nursing attendant, a nutritionist and physical therapist meet with a psychiatrist to coordinate care. The "core" team consisting of a nurse, social worker, psychiatrist, and geriatric internist meet twice a week to review problem patients. Whenever possible, the appropriate certified nursing assistant, occupational therapist, physical therapist, speech therapist, and the consulting pharmacist join the group.

Staff Education

With significant support from the facility administrator and the director of nursing, all staff in groups of three or four, attended a 6-week program (The Oasis Program) led by a nurse educator who educates all members of the team about "patient-centered care." The objective of this program is to get staff to understand how to communicate effectively with demented individuals at different stages of the illness with an emphasis on attempting to appreciate the needs of the resident. Staff learn to distinguish between "disturbed" and "disturbing" behaviors. They learn that it is often possible to redirect the behavior and remain flexible in caring for patients. This training had an immediate impact on the understanding, confidence, and ability of the staff to deal effectively with BPSDs without reflexively resorting to use of pharmacotherapy.

Modification of the Physical Environment

There is no perfect environment for patients with dementia. Unless one has the luxury of designing a facility from scratch, most facilities have to work within the limitation of the existing structure. Yet within these constraints a lot can be done to modify the environment. Color and "visuals" were extensively used. Doors to rooms were painted in different colors, and display boxes outside every room help cue patients to their own environment. Room occupancy is limited to single or double occupancy, and hallways are brightly lit. Floors are not polished to a high gloss and the area was conditioned to prevent echo and sound distortion. Most important, ambient noise is kept to a minimum.

Proposed Models of Care

No single model of care fits all situations. Staff are encouraged to attempt different models of care based on the perceived needs of the individual resident. These include the following:

1. Cognitive/emotion-oriented interventions (reminiscence and life review, simulated presence therapy, validation therapy)
2. Sensory stimulation interventions (aromatherapy, light therapy, massage/touch, music therapy)
3. Behavior management techniques
4. Psychotherapy (cognitive-behavioral therapy, psychoeducation)
5. Other psychosocial interventions such as animal-assisted therapy and exercise

Unfortunately, consistent and reliable data about the efficacy of the various psychosocial therapies are lacking. Before opting for any intervention in relation to agitation and aggressive behavior, and before opting for any intervention, it is important to carefully analyze the potential causes for the disruptive behavior (e.g., antecedents-behaviors-consequences) and to attempt to minimize the antecedent. These causes may include pain, medical illness, fatigue, depression, loneliness, under or overstimulation, and social or environmental stressors. No single intervention can work to manage the disruption caused by different types of BPSD. Our experience suggests that the key to managing disruptive behaviors using psychosocial interventions is flexibility and an institutional commitment to limiting pharmacological intervention. If the tenets of the conceptual model for BPSDs described earlier in this chapter are considered valid and are entertained, then it helps staff to understand that many disruptive behaviors are no different than those that they have experienced as parents of young children—and they did not resort to pharmacology to control them. The limbic system interprets change as chaos, and many of the symptoms of BPSDs are primitive attempts at restoring order to the environment. To this end, it helps to remember that pharmacological interventions should be resorted to only when the safety and well-being of the patient or others is at risk. Persons suffering from dementia need to feel safe and experience a sense of control. This becomes most evident when very personal activities such as bathing and toileting are met with resistance and agitation. Whenever possible, these activities should be provided by same-sex caregivers. The environment should remain constant; routine is very important. Noise should be kept to a minimum. When language is impaired and communication becomes difficult, it becomes important to be sensitive to nonverbal cues. As in communicating with nonverbal infants, touch and body language become key methods of communication. Caregivers have to appreciate that "it is not what you say but how you say it" that is most applicable to patients with dementia.

Family Involvement

A key component is the involvement of the resident's family at every stage of the resident's stay on the unit through discharge or death. Family members meet with the team at admission and provide information pertinent to the resident's care. A significant part of this discussion focuses on gathering information about the resident's premorbid personality, including likes and dislikes and responses to frustration. Another area of discussion is devoted to the family and the resident's stated desire for limitations in care and end-of-life choices. Families are encouraged to meet with members of the team informally as and when the need arises as well as formally for a monthly support group meeting.

End-of-Life Care for Severely Demented Persons

No discussion of dementia care can be considered complete without some appreciation of end-of-life care. Caring for terminally ill persons is always a complex process in which clinicians are confronted with their own religious and ethical beliefs, their clinical judgment, and their interpretation of the legal boundaries within which to practice. What defines quality of care at the end of life for persons suffering from dementia is not well understood. In 2009 Alzheimer's disease was the sixth leading cause of death in the United States. Dementia-related deaths are the most rapidly increasing cause of mortality in the United States. Despite the fact that 70% of dementia-related deaths occur in the nursing home, the provision of hospice care remains significantly limited (Kiely, Givens, Shaffer, Teno, & Mitchell, 2010). This is mainly because dementia is, erroneously, not considered by many to be a "terminal" illness, and therefore persons with advanced dementia often do not receive optimal palliative care. A review of the literature on this subject indicates that many patients with dementia die without adequate pain control, with feeding tubes in place, and without the benefits of hospice care. Only about 6% of nursing home residents are admitted to hospice (Mitchell, Kiely, & Hamel, 2004; Mitchell, Morris, Park, & Fries, 2004; Sachs, Shega, & Cox-Hayley, 2004. There are many myths that confound decision making in the ambiguity surrounding the end of life. One of the more common myths is that forgoing life-sustaining treatment and prescribing high doses of opiates to relieve pain and distress will lead to criminal prosecution (Meisel, Snyder, & Quill, 2000). Although it has been shown that the health care needs of patients dying from dementia are comparable to those of persons dying from cancer, these needs are not well articulated. Respecting patient preferences is key to quality care at the end of life, but by virtue of severe cognitive and functional deficits, these patients cannot participate in treatment decisions at late stages of illness.

As the numbers of persons dying with advanced dementia continue to increase, more attention needs to be directed to this aspect of health policy. Median survival in advanced dementia is between 3 and 6 years, during which time any number of clinical crises can complicate the clinical course of the illness. Palliative care could allow for care to be delivered according to previously stated wishes and appropriately involve family members. Hospice care can limit medical interventions that provide little or no benefit. Is it reasonable to continue therapy for issues such as hypercholesteremia and osteoporosis? Is it kind or cruel to subject a person with advanced dementia to repeated laboratory investigations, radiological procedures, and endoscopies? Is it ethical to undertreat pain to avoid "addicting" someone? Do antibiotics ameliorate distress? Or is it wiser and more humane to exercise clinical restraint, practice "masterly inactivity," and to let "thy will be done" (Meisel, Snyder, & Quill, 2000)? Can such an approach, practiced in long-term care facilities and community settings, provide a better quality of life and facilitate a "good death"?

There are no clear answers to these questions. There are moral, legal, and religious convictions that inevitably influence the clinician's consideration in end-of-life dementia care. In the final analysis every clinician has to revisit the "sacred covenant" entered into with each patient and to do no harm—*primum non nocere*.

Acknowledgments

The author wishes to acknowledge the help and cooperation of the team of care providers at the Briarwood Nursing and Rehabilitation in Needham, Massachusetts.

References

Berchtold, N. C., & Cotman, C. W. (1998). Evolution in the conceptualization of dementia and Alzheimer's disease: Greco-Roman period to the 1960s. *Neurobiology of Aging*, 19(3), 173–189.

Box, G. E. P., & Draper, N. R. (1987). *Empirical model-building and response surfaces*. New York, NY: Wiley.

Briesacher, B. A., Limcangco, M. R., Simoni-Wastila, L., Doshi, J. A., Levens, S. R., Shea, D. G., & Stuart, B. (2005). The quality of antipsychotic drug prescribing in nursing homes. *Archives of Internal Medicine*, 165(11), 1280–1285.

Brookmeyer, R., Johnson, E., Ziegler-Graham, K., & Arrighi, M. H. (2007). Forecasting the global burden of Alzheimer's disease. *Alzheimers and Dementia*, 3(3), 186–191.

Cerejeira, J., Lagarto, L., & Mukaetova-Ladinska, E. B. (2012). Behavioral and psychological symptoms of dementia. *Frontiers in Neuroscience*, 3, 73.

Chen, Y., Briesacher, B., Field, T., Tjia, J., Lau, D., & Gurwitz, J. (2010). Unexplained variation across U.S. nursing homes in antipsychotic prescribing rates. *Archives of Internal Medicine*, 170(1), 89–95.

Cohen-Mansfield, J. (1994). Reflections on the assessment of behavior in nursing home residents. *Alzheimers Disease and Associated Disorders*, 8(Suppl 1), S217–S222.

Finkel, S. I., Costa e Silva, J., Cohen, G., Miller, S., & Sartorius, N. (1996). Behavioral and psychological signs and symptoms of dementia: A consensus statement on current knowledge and implications for research and treatment. *International Psychogeriatrics*, 8(Suppl 3), 497–500.

Geda, Y. E., Roberts, R. O., Knopman, D. S., Petersen, R. C., Christianson, T. J., Pankratz, V. S., . . . Rocca, W. A. (2008). Prevalence of neuropsychiatric symptoms in mild cognitive impairment and normal cognitive aging: Population based study. *Archives of General Psychiatry*, 65(10), 1193–1198.

Jost, B. C., & Grossberg, G. T. (1996). The evolution of psychiatric symptoms in Alzheimer's disease: A natural history study. *Journal of the American Geriatric Society*, 44(9), 1078–1081.

Kiely, D. K., Givens, J. L., Shaffer, M. L., Teno, J. M., & Mitchell, S. L. (2010). Hospice utilization and outcomes among nursing home residents with advanced dementia. *Journal of the American Geriatric Society*, 58(12), 2284–2291.

Lyketsos, C. G., Lopez, O., Jones, B., Fitzpatrick, A. L., Breitner, J., & DeKosky, S. (2002). Prevalence of neuropsychiatric symptoms in dementia and mild cognitive impairment: Result from the cardiovascular health study. *Journal of the American Medical Association*, 288(12), 1475–1483.

Meisel, A., Snyder, L., & Quill, T. (2000). Seven legal barriers to end-of-life care: Myths, realities, and grains of truth. *Journal of the American Medical Association, 284*, 2495–2507.

Mitchell, S. L., Kiely, D. K., & Hamel, M. B. (2004). Dying with advanced dementia in the nursing home. *Archives of Internal Medicine, 164*(3), 321–326.

Mitchell, S. L., Morris, J. N., Park, P. S., & Fries, B. E. (2004). Terminal care for persons with advanced dementia in the nursing home and home care settings. *Journal of Palliative Medicine, 7*(6), 808–816.

Narang, P., El-Refai, M., Parlapalli, R., Danilov, L., Manda, S., Kaur, G., & Lippmann, S. (2010). Antipsychotic drugs: Sudden cardiac death among elderly patients. *Psychiatry (Edgmont), 7*(10), 25–29.

Okura, T., Plassman, B. L., Steffens, D. C., Llewellyn, D. J., Potter, G. G., & Langa, K. M. (2010). Prevalence of neuropsychiatric symptoms and their association with functional limitations in older adults in the United States: The aging, demographics and memory study. *Journal of the American Geriatric Society, 58*, 330–337.

Sachs, G. A., Shega, J. W., & Cox-Hayley, D. (2004). Barriers to excellent end-of-life care for patients with dementia. *Journal of General Internal Medicine, 19*(10), 1057–1063.

Tariot, P. N. (1996). Behavioral manifestations of dementia: A research agenda. *International Psychogeriatrics, 8*(Suppl 1), 31–38.

Vigen, C. L. P., Mack, W. J., Keefe, R., Sano, M., Sultzer, D., Stroup, S., & Schneider, L. S. (2011). Cognitive effects of atypical antipsychotic medications in patients with Alzheimer's disease: Outcomes from CATIE-AD. *American Journal of Psychiatry, 168*(8), 831–839.

27

The Role of the Family in the Care and Management of Patients With Dementia

Licet Valois and James E. Galvin

The cognitive, functional, and behavioral decline experienced by individuals diagnosed with dementia can be severe and debilitating, leading to a significant need of support from family caregivers beginning early in the course of the disease. As such, there is an increasing sense of burden, as spouses and adult children often take on a multitude of new responsibilities previously managed by the person with dementia, often beginning *prior* to when a dementia diagnosis is made. In conjunction with increasing burden, there is often an accompanying sense of grief and loss as the disease progresses.

A number of adverse outcomes for the dementia caregiver, such as stress, depression, and diminishing health status of the caregiver, directly lead to increases in (1) institutionalization of the person with dementia and (2) declines in quality of life for both the patient and the caregiver. Additional caregiver burden comes from (1) inadequate understanding of the disease for which they are providing care, and (2) a delay in recognition, diagnosis, and treatment of symptoms related to dementia (Galvin et al., 2010a, 2010b).

It is critical to increase the understanding about the dementia caregiver's stressors in order to facilitate care provision. To better address the needs of both the patient and the caregiver, the public and health care providers must recognize the caregiver–patient dyad as two distinct people, not just one. Early identification of caregiver stress, burden, and grief allows for optimum medical and psychosocial interventions, as well as access to community resources, such as caregiver support groups and online caregiving communities. The goal of this chapter is to review the nature of caregiving, identify some of its positive and negative aspects, and provide practical guidance for dementia caregivers.

What Is Caregiving?

Caregiving scenarios can be represented in many ways—for example, the wife that cares for her husband who suffered a stroke; the daughter who from a distance supervises the care of her aging parents; or the neighbor who helps the woman next door who is dealing with cancer. The definition of caregiving relates to all the activities performed by a concerned individual who contributes to the well-being of another individual. At times, this definition can be confounded with the provision of direct care or assistance with activities of daily living (ADLs); however, caregiving can be performed in different forms and at different levels. Caregiving responsibilities do not necessarily have to be fulfilled by individuals with specialized training. As long as there is a special interest or a caring attitude toward others, caregiving responsibilities can be fulfilled. A caregiver is therefore defined as an individual who oversees the welfare of another person. This individual can provide basic assistance and care for someone who is frail, disabled, ill, and/or needs help in one or more aspects of life. Caregivers perform a variety of tasks to assist someone in his or her daily life, for example, balancing a checkbook, shopping, visiting doctor's offices, giving medication reminders, or helping someone to eat, take a bath, or dress. For many caregivers, this assistance and care are not considered "caregiving." According to Carol Levine, "caregivers do not think of what they do in terms of performing tasks related to activities of daily living (ADL's) and instrumental activities of daily living (IADL's); they do whatever needs to be done. Then they watch and wait until the next thing needs to be done, and the next and the next" (Levine, 2003, p. 117). Caregivers are often ready to take care of their loved one when needed, regardless of their own circumstances. This means that, at times, caregivers can suffer or even sacrifice themselves while caring for others.

In general, caregivers are divided into "formal" or paid caregivers and "informal" or unpaid (often family) caregivers (Alzheimer's Association, 2013). All professionals who receive a financial reimbursement for directly caring or in some form supervising the care of other(s) are considered formal caregivers, including home health aides, geriatric care managers, social workers, and so on. All individuals who provide care or oversee someone's care without receiving financial reimbursement are considered informal caregivers, for instance, family members and friends. In this chapter we are specifically addressing informal, family caregivers of patients with dementia.

Considering the professional context in which formal caregivers carry out their tasks, specialized training is required. However, no experience or formalized training is necessary for the informal caregiver. Relatives and friends provide care without receiving specific training to assist their loved ones. Experience is developed over a period of years as caregivers learn from their interactions while providing care. There are many factors that exert influence during the informal caregiving process; for instance, the nature of the relation between the caregivers and their loved ones, their history, and how their interactions evolved. Caregivers usually play different roles in their families and social networks besides being caregivers. They can simultaneously be spouses, daughters, siblings, friends, neighbors, and so on. In part because of the variety of roles played at the same time, caregivers may become overwhelmed attempting to fulfill the goals of their variety of roles. In many instances, family dynamics are disturbed when the time to assume caregiving responsibilities arrives. Additionally, the caregiving process is affected by the cultural and ethnic background of the caregiver and the person receiving the care.

To fulfill their role, caregivers do not need to live in the same household as the individual for whom they are caring. They can be in the vicinity or just supervise the care of someone from a distance. A 2004 study from the Alzheimer's Association and National Alliance for Caregiving noted that only one quarter of dementia caregivers actually lived with the person for whom they were providing care (Alzheimer's Association, 2013). Other caregivers, particularly adult children and friends, can reside quite a distance from the patient with dementia. The Alzheimer's Disease Facts and Figures Report from the Alzheimer's Association reported that 10% of the nearly 10 million family and other informal caregivers lived more than 2 hours from the patient with dementia (Alzheimer's Association, 2013).

Whether it is from far away or close by, an individual can be the source of care or the focus of care. According to the Alzheimer's Association, most people will become caregivers—or need one— at some point in their lives. To foresee who will play the caregiver role or the care receiver role is not easy to determine. For example, caregiving can occur gradually over time, or it can occur overnight. In some cases, caregivers anticipate taking on the caregiving role and know in advance what is expected of them (Sheets & Mahoney-Gleason, 2011). Some relatives can see themselves performing specific tasks that they might feel comfortable doing or because it is their area of expertise. In other cases, it is more difficult to be prepared due to the unanticipated nature of caregiving. Similarly, it is difficult to think about receiving assistance from others without feeling that one's independence and dignity are jeopardized.

Caregivers may play their caregiving role on a full-time or part-time basis. Fulfilling the responsibilities of caregiving demands time, and this can constitute a job within itself for the caregiver. Whether it is full time or part time, the value of caregiving is great at all levels. The value of the services that family caregivers provide for free, while caring for older adults, is estimated at $375 billion a year. This amount is almost twice as much as what is actually spent on homecare and nursing home services combined ($158 billion) (National Alliance for Caregiving, 2009). The cost of care for patients with dementia is estimated at $172 billion annually (Alzheimer's Association, 2013).

As previously noted, caregivers can be categorized as formal or informal. Many persons with dementia have more than one caregiver at the same time: a formal caregiver, such as a home attendant or home health aide, who provides assistance with daily living activities; and an informal caregiver, such as a relative or friend, who oversees matters like mail and bills. Informal caregiving is considered the most common form of providing community care to frail older persons (Toseland, 1995). Regardless of the type of caregiving provided, self-identification as a caregiver facilitates access to services. It is important to educate and empower informal caregivers to recognize their role and the importance of this role. In the United States, there are services designed to assist caregivers specifically, but if the individual does not identify himself or herself as a caregiver, the opportunity to access such services diminishes.

The Family Caregiver

There is widespread recognition of the critical disease management and care provision tasks performed by family members of persons with dementia (Talley & Crews, 2007). Family caregivers assist older relatives in dealing with the physical and psychosocial consequences of dementia. Cognitive impairment impacts the patient's ability to live independently. The care provided by family caregivers encompasses emotional support, financial aid, and provision of services ranging from instrumental aid and personal care assistance to health care tasks and mediation with formal care providers. Dementia caregiving can involve a substantial expenditure of time over a long-lasting period (Schulz & Martire, 2004). The consequences to caregivers are widespread and include financial, health, and psychosocial burdens (Cucciare, Gray, Azar, Jimenez, & Gallagher-Thompson, 2010). Cultural beliefs and expectations may inform families' interpretation of the signs, symptoms, causes, and management of dementia and their commitment to care provision (Napoles, Chadiha, Eversley, & Moreno-John, 2010; Sayegh & Knight, 2010). For example, Hispanic cultural beliefs regarding Alzheimer's disease etiology view it as part of the normal aging process, so when behavioral and psychological symptoms emerge, their loved one is stigmatized as "gone crazy" (Gray, Jimenez, Cucciare, Tong, & Gallagher-Thompson, 2009). There is also the concept of *La Tercera Edad* (the third and final cycle of life) with a need for increased family assistance and transition of responsibilities across generations as elderly family members undergo "normal aging" (Flores, Hinton, Barker, Franz, & Velasquez, 2009). In Asian cultures, illness events are family focused, with elderly relatives trusting that family members will make the treatment decisions that are in their best interest (University of Washington Medical Center, 2007).

Personal Challenges Faced by the Family Caregiver

Caregiving is a responsibility that requires strength and support as dementia progresses, robbing the memories, energy, and freedom of loved ones. Any type of caregiving, especially for people with dementia, can have serious physical and emotional effects. Caregivers may be too overwhelmed, frustrated, or depressed to seek the help they need. It is important for caregivers to seek help to cope with the strains of caregiving as well as to make sure they attend to their own health. Caregivers play a critical role and should be empowered to speak freely to their loved ones' health care providers with any questions or concerns about caring for someone with dementia. It is essential to have open discussions to maintain the well-being of the caregiver and health of the patient. Working with a team of care providers who are connected in some way allows the provision of quality care. An alliance developed between the caregiver and patient's providers can only be advantageous.

Chronic progressive diseases such as dementia result in increasingly severe functional limitations that last indefinitely. Subsequently, these will require long-term caregiving by family members, while triggering stress reactions associated with altered relationship dynamics (Saban, Sherwood, DeVon, & Hynes, 2010), resulting in growing caregiver burden and depression (Schoenmakers, Buntinx, & DeLepeleire, 2010). Caregivers of individuals with chronic disease are at elevated risk for depression; anxiety; poor quality of life; and health problems such as heart disease (Lee, Colditz, Berkman, & Kawachi, 2003), headaches (Kreutzer et al., 2009), digestive problems (Thompson et al., 2004), and disturbed sleep (Brummett et al., 2006). Biological marker abnormalities among caregivers include increased cortisol secretion (Bremner, 2006), abnormal glucose regulation (Altuna, Lelli, San Martín de Viale, & Damasco, 2006), inflammation (Hamer, Gibson, Vuononvirta, Williams, & Steptoe, 2006), and abnormal immunologic function (Kavelaars & Heijnen, 2006). The personal implications of caregiving can involve feelings of grief and depression. Caregivers are not only responsible for supervising the care of another person but also for caring for themselves in order to be better prepared to provide care.

According to researcher and caregiver Carol Levine, "Dementia caregivers struggle with particularly difficult responsibilities and wrenching losses" (Levine, 2003, p. 116). The negative impact associated with caregiving is likely to be greater for dementia caregivers than caregivers of frail nondemented elders (Ory, Hoffman, Lee, Tennstedt, & Schulz, 1999). The dementia caregiver starts assuming more and more responsibilities as the disease progresses, from finances and legal matters to the daily household chores (Gallagher-Thompson et al., 2003). As previously mentioned, caring for a relative with dementia is linked to negative psychosocial and physical consequences for the caregiver (Pinquart & Sorensen, 2003). The negative health effects caused in some caregivers can severely diminish their quality of life and, in some cases, accelerate the need for institutionalization of the patient (Gaugler, Leitsch, Zarit, & Pearlin, 2000). Caregiving can be very difficult, full of challenges, and very taxing at the spiritual, emotional, physical, social, and economic levels (Sheets & Mahoney-Gleason, 2011).

Benefits of Caregiving

Much of the caregiving literature assumes a view of the caregiver as being burdened without consideration of the caregivers' expectations and experiences (Flores et al., 2009). Yet within the caregiving journey, individuals can experience a variety of emotions that are not solely negative. The 2009 Report of Findings on the Aging Services Network noted that while caregiving can be stressful, there are also benefits and rewards (Levine, Halper, Peist, & Gould, 2010). Caregivers have reported positive feelings about caregiving (e.g., family togetherness and the satisfaction of helping others) while simultaneously reporting high levels of stress during the care provision (Alzheimer's Association, 2013). Thus, in addition to the detrimental aspects of caregiving, there are a number of perceived benefits associated with caregiving, such as (a) the opportunity to give back; (b) improved relationships; (c) feeling good about the quality of care; (d) serving as a role model for others; (e) increased self-esteem; (f) an enhanced sense of purpose; and (g) feelings of pleasure and satisfaction (Coon et al., 2004).

Cultural Differences in Knowledge, Attitudes, and Caregiving

The older adult population in the United States is becoming more diverse. In 2006, 81% of adults age 65+ were Caucasian; by 2050 this is estimated to decrease to 61%

(Napoles et al., 2010). Given that the number of Americans from minority backgrounds is predicted to increase at a rate greater than Caucasians, studies of cross-cultural differences in caregiving experiences and outcomes are needed (Sayegh & Knight, 2010), particularly since minorities may bear a disproportionate burden of Alzheimer's disease caregiving (Napoles et al., 2010). Increased stress, strain, and burden associated with caregiving may increase risk of psychological and physical morbidities (Napoles et al., 2010). There are five important themes when considering caregiving in a multicultural community: (1) the perceived role of the family in care (a term known as familism) (Flores et al., 2009; Losada et al., 2010); (2) gender roles (Del Gaudio et al., 2012); (3) family traditions and cultural identity (Gray et al., 2009); (4) expectations about caregiving (Flores et al., 2009); and (5) role of faith and religion (Herbert et al., 2007).

Cultural beliefs and influences can shape health care choices and service use and impact the ways in which patients and their families both view and manage Alzheimer's disease (Knight & Sayegh, 2010; Livney et al., 2011). A significant challenge in establishing an Alzheimer's disease diagnosis in diverse populations is to validate and standardize assessments across different ethnic and racial groups. This includes not only differences in symptom presentation across groups but also cultural perceptions about cognitive health and attitudes and beliefs about care. For example, it is common for Korean Americans to consider themselves in good health if they are "symptom free," sometimes delaying seeking care until symptoms become severe (Han, Kang, Kim, Ryu, & Kim, 2007). Hispanic older adults are more likely to believe memory changes are part of normal aging and that Alzheimer's disease is due to experiencing a difficult life, loneliness, stress, trauma and family problems, or attribute it to external forces such as God's will or *el mal de ojo* (evil eye). Hispanics also include more emotional and behavioral symptoms as part of the spectrum of Alzheimer's disease symptoms compared with Caucasians (Hinton, Franz, Yeo, & Levkoff, 2005; Karlawish et al., 2011). Groups with high linguistic isolation have greater difficulty accessing basic health and social services, requiring outreach and services in their native language (Asian and Pacific Islander American Health Forum, 2006). It is important to consider that these groups might be deprived from accessing caregiving services because of their linguistic barriers rather than a lack of need for such services.

Family members require education and knowledge about dementia, treatment, and services to cope effectively with caregiving (Gray, 2003). Substantial evidence suggests that caregiving experiences of minority caregivers differ significantly from those of White caregivers (Aranda & Knight, 1997). To better understand caregiver help-seeking and help-accepting perspectives and actions, it is critical to learn about cultural values and expectations (Valle, 1998). Minority elders, especially Latinos, are a growing and diverse population that tends to delay entry into care until the moderate and late stages of the disease. Consequently, this makes advance care planning more challenging to implement and caregiving more stressful. Insufficient knowledge about dementia, especially prognosis and progression, obstructs efforts to plan and prepare. Ethnic minorities may lack the necessary information or hold to culturally influenced beliefs that delay accessing the help needed.

Ethnic differences at intrapersonal, interpersonal, and environmental levels are present across multiple psychosocial domains. For example, compared with non-Hispanic Caucasians, Hispanics make less use of long-term care institutions and report more positive appraisals of coping, increased spirituality, and beliefs in filial responsibility and familism, while at the same time reporting higher levels of burden and depression and diminished psychosocial health (Napoles et al., 2010). A study of African American family caregivers found that caregiving was viewed as a traditional family value (Sterritt & Pokorny, 1998). A study published by Gelman and colleagues suggests that general beliefs about aging and memory loss among Latinos are a significant barrier to early diagnostic evaluations for memory loss (Gelman et al., 2010). Minority family caregivers may feel too overwhelmed to participate in available community services and may even experience them as intrusive and unwelcome. Regardless of the perceptions minority caregivers may have about community services, if they are presented strategically with cultural sensitivity, caregivers often welcome the assistance.

Impact of Providing Caregiver Support

The stress associated with caring for an older relative suffering from Alzheimer's disease or another dementing illness is often considerable (Mittelman, Haley, Clay, & Roth, 2006; Mittelman, Roth, Clay, & Haley, 2007; Mittelman, Roth, Coon, & Haley, 2004a; Mittelman, Roth, Haley, & Zarit, 2004b). Caregivers frequently neglect their own needs as they focus on satisfying the patient's needs. Many authors have acknowledged the importance of providing encouragement to caregivers to take better care of themselves, as they can become so involved in care provision that they may delay or forget to attend to their own personal needs. According to Shaw, "caregiver support groups have been developed as a treatment response to the obvious need for relief from the stress associated with caregiving" (Shaw, 1997, p. 165).

The stress-coping paradigm (Pearlin, Mullin, Semple, & Skaff, 1990) has been adopted by many researchers to explain caregiver response to interventions (Brodaty, 2007). When caregivers feel well supported, they report reduced burden, stress, and depression. Research suggests that social support resources can reduce the consequences of stressful life experiences and contribute to preservation of psychological well-being (Fiore, Coppel, Becker, & Cox, 1986; House, Landis, & Umberson, 1988; Keyes, Shmotkin, & Ryff, 2002; Krause, 1995). Social support may be effective in part by increasing the perception that resources are available to handle stress, thereby decreasing appraisals of stressors as potentially harmful (Cohen, 2004). Individuals with greater social support report more positive affect and a greater sense of control (Ferguson & Goodwin, 2010). Regarding support groups, Toseland said: "During group meetings, caregivers can gain valuable information about the processes of aging and the progression of specific ailments. Understanding disease processes helps caregivers to anticipate and plan for future caregiving demands" (Toseland, 1995, p. 33).

The NYU Caregiver Intervention (NYUCI) was a longitudinal, controlled trial spanning more than two decades. The NYUCI demonstrated the value of social support and counseling for spouse caregivers, alleviating some deleterious effects of care provision on the spouse-caregivers' mental health, and postponing nursing home placement of their Alzheimer's disease patient spouses by 557 days compared with usual care (Mittelman et al., 2004a, 2004b, 2006, 2007). Moreover, the intervention's effects on spouse caregiver's depression were long-lasting, continuing through nursing home placement and the death of the patient (Mittelman et al., 2004a, 2004b, 2006, 2007). A mediation analysis demonstrated that a substantial proportion of effect on change in these outcomes could be attributed to intervention-induced increases in the spouse caregivers' satisfaction with their social support (Roth, Mittelman, Clay, Madan, & Haley, 2005; Roth, Perkins, Wadley, Temple, & Haley, 2009). The fundamental message underlying NYUCI was that real and perceived social support improves spouse caregivers' ability to withstand the difficulties of caregiving and defers the need for nursing home placement.

Family-Centered Care in Dementia

The family has a dual status in care of individuals with dementia. In their caregiving capacity, family members are viewed by the health care and social service system as part of the care team. In this status, family caregivers experience a variety of burdens and strains that may compromise family functioning, compete with day-to-day role responsibilities, adversely impact their health, and generate a variety of emotional sequelae. Involvement in care also negatively impacts caregivers' own health promotion activities, including delaying or canceling routine health care, screening exams, or other preventive health activities (Schulz & Martire, 2004). However, family caregivers can be further impacted by dementia, apart from the strains and burdens they experience from care provision. When learning of their relative's dementia diagnosis, family members may be simultaneously confronted by fears for their own susceptibility due to genetic risk (Raveis, 2004; Raveis, Pretter, & Carrero, 2010), particularly in families in which more than one person has developed dementia. In these situations, involvement in care provision can impose additional stress, for as caregivers, they are afforded firsthand exposure to their relative's experience. While this can serve to normalize or demystify dementia, the witnessing of their relative's difficulties may intensify caregivers' own health-related fears and concerns. It can be very challenging for caregivers to address concerns about their loved one's condition while coming to terms with their own uncertain future.

Over the last few decades, an expanding body of family-based research has documented the ramifications of illness on the family system (Bachner, Karus, & Raveis, 2009; Beard, Sakhtah, Imse, & Galvin, 2012; Galvin et al., 2010b; Raveis, 2004; Raveis et al., 2010). These efforts have informed the growing paradigm shift from a biomedical model of care to one that is patient and family centered and have led policy makers and the health professions to acknowledge that "family caregivers *must* be recognized as partners in care" (Reinhard, Brooks-Danso, Kelley, & Mason, 2008) and be supported in their care responsibilities (Raveis, 2004; Talley & Crews, 2007). Nearly half of informal family caregivers are performing medical and nursing tasks in addition to helping with activities of daily living for patients with dementia. The landmark *State of the Science Symposium: Professional Partners Supporting Family Caregivers* issued a primary recommendation to "develop and promote a patient and family-centered service paradigm" (Kelley, Reinhard, & Brooks-Danso, 2008, p. 11). Family-centered care recognizes that supporting family members in their critical role is integral to the patient's medical and psychosocial health. Although families are directly involved in health care, caregiving, treatment decision making, and health advocacy, a comprehensive attempt to attend to their concerns and information needs is not routinely targeted.

Developing an Individualized Care Plan

Although caregivers of dementia patients typically deal with a partially predictable set of issues, every caregiver, and thus every caregiving experience, is unique. For a variety of reasons, a caregiver may have particular preferences for the type of programs and services he or she would like to access. It is not always easy for caregivers to verbalize or clarify their needs, and subsequently, to identify the resources available to satisfy such needs. It is essential for the clinician to assist the caregiver in articulating needs and to respect caregiver preferences. Most caregivers benefit from discussing their needs with a social worker or a geriatric care manager.

Once the specific needs of the patient and caregiver are identified, it is imperative to facilitate the exploration of services, programs, and benefits offered in their community. It is also vital to remember that benefits are different according to location. Furthermore, availability of programs and services varies from state to state and from community to community. After the identification and exploration has taken place, a plan of action has to be implemented to satisfy caregiver and patient needs.

Assimilating and adjusting to a dementia diagnosis is a difficult task, for both the patient and the family. For most individuals affected by dementia, receiving the diagnosis is just the first step of the journey. Unfortunately, many patients and family members leave the physician's office misinformed or lacking information about the diagnosis. Assuming that a probable diagnosis has been given in a clear and informative manner, people can still use terms incorrectly and interchangeably, have misconceptions about what a dementia diagnosis means, and do not have a clear treatment plan. In addition to all the questions that might be generated after receiving a dementia diagnosis, the question of what to do next also rises.

Here we provide a practical list of activities each caregiver should consider to better prepare for his or her caregiving role:

1. After the diagnosis is given, take time to discuss what the diagnosis means to you and your loved one. Write down questions you have about the diagnosis, prognosis, treatment plan, and so on. Then make a follow-up appointment with the diagnosis provider to ask those questions.
2. Consider getting a second opinion from a specialist (neurologist, psychiatrist, geriatrician) if there are still questions about the diagnosis and treatment plan.
3. Consider any special needs of the patient. Does the patient have difficulties with walking and balance? If so, he or she may

TABLE 27.1 Family Caregiver Checklist

Although *every case is different*, here are some key points that might be helpful after a diagnosis of mild cognitive impairment or dementia is given:
1. Learn as much as possible about the diagnosis (Internet, books, or support groups)
2. Learn how to monitor the progression of symptoms and their response to therapies (see Table 27.2)
3. Identify and contact organizations associated with the diagnosis (see Table 27.3)
4. Participate in physically and mentally stimulating activities (exercising, dancing, museum visits, or computer access)
5. Join social gatherings (YMCA, local clubs, or senior groups, etc.)
6. Eat a healthy diet (consulting with a dietitian or nutritionist, if necessary)
7. Learn about the following:
   a. Transportation services (Access-A-Ride, local transit organizations, or services through Medicaid)
   b. Safety devices/alert systems at home (Comfort zone or personal response services)
   c. Meals options (home-delivered meals through Meals on Wheels or cooking assistance)
   d. Home care services or companionship services (home care agencies)
   e. Housing options:
      - Independent living
      - Senior housing
      - Naturally occurring retirement communities (NORCs)
      - Assisted living
      - Nursing homes
      - Continuum care retirement communities
8. Consider registering for the MedicAlert + SAFE Return Program (Alzheimer's Association)
9. Plan and organize legal and financial matters (using an elder law attorney, if necessary):
   - Designate a health care proxy
   - Plan to complete a living will and a durable power of attorney
   - Consider obtaining Social Security Disability, if applicable
   - Apply for early retirement if applicable
   - Add a cosigner to financial accounts

benefit from seeing a physical therapist. Does the patient need help completing activities of daily living (e.g., cooking, hygiene, dressing)? If so, he or she may benefit from meeting with an occupational therapist. Does the patient have difficulty communicating or swallowing food? If so, he or she may benefit from an evaluation by a speech therapist.
4. Create a checklist of tasks to perform (Table 27.1). This will assist the patient and caregiver in determining how to proceed according to their individual needs.
5. Build a local support system to get the help you will need. A support system can include family, friends, faith or religious groups, and local Alzheimer's organizations. Each caregiver creates a unique support system according to individualized needs.
6. Perform regular in-home evaluations of dementia symptoms to track progression of disease and response to interventions, both medicine related and behavioral/environmental. An example of a monitoring tool is the Health Brain Aging Care Monitor (Monahan et al., 2012) (Table 27.2) that can be filled out by the family caregiver and brought to the physician's office to discuss the loved one's condition. The full instrument can be viewed at the following URL: http://www.wishard.edu/our-services/senior-care/healthy-aging-brain-center/resources
7. Develop a long-range plan. Consider what resources are needed and available for care at the mild, moderate, and severe stages of dementia. Review financial resources and consider discussing estate planning with a lawyer skilled in elder care.
8. Seek additional information from reliable sources (Table 27.3) to increase your knowledge about dementia and caregiving. There are a number of organizations that deal with dementia, caregiving, or both that have a wealth of information and may also offer financial assistance or other forms of aid.
9. Consider joining a support group or obtaining other support services. Some of the programs and services that have been

TABLE 27.2 The Healthy Aging Brain Care Monitor (HABC-Monitor) Caregiver Assessment Tool

Cognitive Domain	Functional Domain	Behavioral Domain	Caregiver Domain
Judgment or decision making	Planning, preparing, or serving meals	Feeling down, depressed, or hopeless	Your quality of life
Less interest or pleasure in doing things, hobbies, or activities	Taking medications in the right dose at the right time	Being stubborn, agitated, aggressive, or resistant to help from others	Your financial future
Repeating the same things over and over such as questions or stories	Walking or physical ambulation	Feeling anxious, nervous, tense, fearful, or panicked	Your mental health
Learning how to use a tool, appliance, or gadget	Bathing	Believing others are stealing from them or planning to harm them	Your physical health
Forgetting the correct month or year	Shopping for personal items such as groceries	Hearing voices, seeing things, or talking to people who are not there	
Handling complicated financial affairs such as balancing checkbook, filing income taxes, and paying bills	Housework or household chores	Poor appetite or overeating	
Remembering appointments	Leaving her/him alone	Falling asleep, staying asleep, or sleeping too much	
Thinking or memory	Her/his safety	Acting impulsively, without thinking through the consequences of her or his actions	
	Her/his quality of life	Wandering, pacing, or doing things repeatedly	
	Falling or tripping		

Note. The Healthy Aging Brain Care Monitor is a copyrighted instrument by Drs. Malaz Boustani, James Galvin and Christopher Callahan and the Indiana University School of Medicine. The HABC-Monitor and scoring rules are available at http://www.wishard.edu/our-services/senior-care/healthy-aging-brain-center/resources

developed to assist caregivers to cope with the stress of caregiving include support groups, individual and/or family counseling, respite care, and psychoeducational programs (National Institutes of Health, 2010). A variety of interventions, including respite, financial support, and primary care interventions, have been shown to effectively improve caregiver's psychological health and well-being (Gray, 2003).

Conclusions

Caregiving is a journey, and like all journeys, there will be challenges that need to be faced and overcome. Alzheimer's disease and related dementias are complex syndromes with a spectrum of cognitive, functional, behavioral, and psychological symptoms that reduce the quality of life of both patients and their caregivers. While caregiving is often stressful, there are also potential benefits—fulfilling family obligations, feelings of self-satisfaction by giving back, and delays in nursing home placement. However, these benefits cannot be obtained if caregivers do not develop a care plan for the person with dementia, seek out available community resources, and maintain their own physical, mental, and emotional health. With public policies and practice models shifting the focus of care to outpatient settings and the

TABLE 27.3 Caregiver Resources and Useful Web Sites

Dementia-Related Sites

Alzheimer's Association	http://www.alz.org/
Alzheimer Disease Education and Referral Center	http://www.nia.nih.gov/alzheimers
Alzheimer's Foundation of America	http://www.alzfdn.org/AFAServices/tollfreehotline.html
American Parkinson's Disease Association	http://www.apdaparkinson.org/
Association for Frontotemporal Degeneration	http://www.ftd-picks.org/
Creutzfeldt-Jacob Disease Foundation	http://www.cjdfoundation.org/
Lewy Body Dementia Association	http://www.lbda.org/
US Department of Health and Human Services	http://www.alzheimers.gov

Health-Related Sites

American Heart Association	http://www.heart.org/HEARTORG/
American Stroke Association	http://www.strokeassociation.org/STROKEORG/
American Diabetes Association	http://www.diabetes.org/

General Information Sites

AARP	http://www.aarp.org/
Administration on Aging	http://www.aoa.gov/AoARoot/Elders_Families/index.aspx
Caregiver Action Network	http://caregiveraction.org/
Department of Health & Human Services: Eldercare	http://www.eldercare.gov/Eldercare.NET/Public/Index.aspx
Elder Care Lawyers	http://www.elderlawanswers.com/Default.aspx
Family Caregiver Alliance	http://www.caregiver.org/caregiver/jsp/home.jsp
Federation Employment and Guidance Services	http://www.fegs.org/fegs-services/
Healthcare Proxy	http://www.health.ny.gov/professionals/patients/health_care_proxy/index.htm
Leading Age (How to tour a Nursing Home)	http://www.leadingage.org/How_to_Tour_a_Nursing_Home.aspx
Long Term Care Information	http://longtermcare.gov/
Medicaid	http://medicaid.gov/index.html
Medicare	http://www.medicare.gov/index.html
Medline Plus	http://www.medlineplus.gov/
National Academy of Elder Law Attorney	http://www.naela.org
National Association of Geriatric Care Managers	http://www.caremanager.org/
National Institute on Aging	http://www.nia.nih.gov/
National Institutes of Health: Senior Health	http://nihseniorhealth.gov/index.html
Social Security Administration	http://www.ssa.gov/

community, there is widespread acknowledgment of the importance of disease management and care provision tasks families perform. This awareness has led policy makers and the health and social service professions to acknowledge that family caregivers must be recognized and attention devoted to promoting a family-centered service paradigm.

Acknowledgments

This work was supported by grants from the National Institutes of Health—P30 AG008051 and R01 AG040211 and the New York State Department of Health.

References

Altuna, M. E., Lelli, S. M., San Martín de Viale, L. C., & Damasco, M. C. (2006). Effect of stress on hepatic 11beta-hydroxysteroid dehydrogenase activity and its influence on carbohydrate metabolism. *Canadian Journal of Physiology and Pharmacology, 84*, 977–984.

Alzheimer' Association. (2013). *Facts and figures report, 2013*. Retrieved April 2013, from http://www.alz.org/alzheimers_disease_facts_and_figures.asp.

Asian and Pacific Islander American Health Forum. (2006). *Health brief*. Retrieved April 2013, from http://www.apiahf.org/resources/pdf/Koreans_in_the_United_States.pdf.

Aranda, M. P., & Knight, B. G. (1997). The influence of ethnicity and culture on the

caregiver stress and coping process: A sociocultural review and analysis. *Gerontologist*, 37, 342–354.
Bachner, Y., Karus, D., & Raveis, V. H. (2009). Examining the social context in the caregiving experience: Correlates of global self-esteem among adult daughter caregivers to an older parent with cancer. *Journal of Aging and Health*, 21, 1016–1039.
Beard, R. L., Sakhtah, S., Imse, V., & Galvin, J. E. (2012). Negotiating the joint career: Couples adapting to Alzheimer's and aging in place. *Journal of Aging Research*, 2012, 797023.
Bremner, J. D. (2006). Traumatic stress: Effects on the brain. *Dialogues in Clinical Neuroscience*, 8, 445–461.
Brodaty, H. (2007). Meaning and measurement of caregiver outcomes. *International Psychogeriatrics*, 19, 363–381.
Brummett, B. H., Babyak, M. A., Siegler, I. C., Vitaliano, P. P., Ballard, E. L., Gwyther, L. P., & Williams, R. B. (2006). Associations among perceptions of social support, negative affect, and quality of sleep in caregivers and noncaregivers. *Health Psychology*, 25, 220–225.
Cohen, S. (2004). Social relationships and health. *American Psychologist*, 59, 676–684.
Coon, D. W., Rubert, M., Solano, N., Mausbach, B., Kraemer, H., Arguelles, T.,...Gallagher-Thompson, D. (2004). Well-being, appraisal, and coping in Latina and Caucasian female dementia caregivers: Findings from the REACH study. *Aging and Mental Health*, 8, 330–345.
Cucciare, M. A., Gray, H., Azar, A., Jimenez, D., & Gallagher-Thompson, D. (2010). Exploring the relationship between physical health, depressive symptoms, and depression diagnoses in Hispanic dementia caregivers. *Aging and Mental Health*, 14, 274–282.
Del Gaudio, F., Hichenberg, S., Eisenberg, M., Kerr, E., Zaider, T. I., & Kissane, D. W. (2012). Latino values in the context of palliative care: Illustrative cases from the family focused grief therapy trial. *American Journal of Hospice and Palliative Care*. Epub ahead of print.
Feinberg, L., Horvath, J., Hunt, G., Plooster, L., Kaga, J., Levine, C.,...Wilkinson, A. (2003). *Family caregiving and public policy principles for change*. Retrieved March 2014, from http://www.caregiving.org/data/principles04.pdf.
Ferguson, S. J., & Goodwin, A. D. (2010). Optimism and well-being in older adults: The mediating role of social support and perceived control. *International Journal of Aging and Human Development*, 71, 43–68.
Fiore, J., Coppel, D. B., Becker, J., & Cox, G. B. (1986). Social support as a multifaceted concept: Examination of important dimensions for adjustment. *American Journal of Community Psychology*, 14, 93–111.
Flores, Y. G., Hinton, L., Barker, J. C., Franz, C. E., & Velasquez, A. (2009). Beyond familism: A case study of the ethics of care of a Latina caregiver of an elderly parent with dementia. *Health Care for Women International*, 30, 1055–1072.
Gallagher-Thompson, D., Coon, D. W., Solano, N., Ambler, C., Rabinowitz, Y., & Thompson, L. W. (2003). Change in indices of distress among Latino and Anglo female caregivers of elderly relatives with dementia: Site-specific results from the REACH national collaborative study. *Gerontologist*, 43, 580–591.
Galvin, J. E., Duda, J. E., Kaufer, D. I., Lippa, C. F., Taylor, A., & Zarit, S. H. (2010a). Lewy body dementia: Caregiver burden and unmet needs. *Alzheimers Disease and Associated Disorders*, 24, 177–181.
Galvin, J. E., Duda, J. E., Kaufer, D. I., Lippa, C. F., Taylor, A., & Zarit, S. H. (2010b). Lewy body dementia: The caregiver experience of clinical care. *Parkinson's and Related Disorders*, 16, 388–392.
Gaugler, J., Leitsch, S. A., Zarit, S. H., & Pearlin, L. (2000). Caregiver involvement following institutionalization: Effects of preplacement stress. *Research in Aging*, 22, 337–359.
Gelman, C. R. (2010). Learning from recruitment challenges: Barriers to diagnosis, treatment, and research participation for Latinos with symptoms of Alzheimer's disease. *Journal of Gerontological Social Work*, 53, 94–113.
Gray, H. L., Jimenez, D. E., Cucciare, M. A., Tong, H. Q., & Gallagher-Thompson, D. (2009). Ethnic differences in beliefs regarding Alzheimer disease among dementia family caregivers. *American Journal of Geriatric Psychiatry*, 17, 925–933.
Gray, L. (2003). *Caregiver depression: A growing mental health concern*. Policy Brief. Family Caregiver Alliance, San Francisco, CA.
Hamer, M., Gibson, E. L., Vuonovirta, R., Williams, E., & Steptoe, A. (2006). Inflammatory and hemostatic responses to repeated mental stress: Individual stability and habituation over time. *Brain Behavior and Immunity*, 20, 456–459.
Han, H. R., Kang, J., Kim, K. B., Ryu, J. P., & Kim, M. T. (2007). Barriers to and strategies for recruiting Korean Americans for community-partnered promotion research. *Journal of Immigrant and Minority Health*, 9, 137–146.
Hebert, R. S., Dang, Q., & Schulz, R. (2007). Religious beliefs and practices are associated with better mental health in family caregivers of patients with dementia: Findings from the REACH study. *American Journal of Geriatric Psychiatry*, 15, 292–300.

Hinton, L., Franz, C. E., Yeo, G., & Levkoff, S. E. (2005). Conceptions of dementia in a multiethnic sample of family caregivers. *Journal of the American Geriatric Society, 53,* 1405–1410.

House, J. S., Landis, K. R., & Umberson, D. (1988). Social relationships and health. *Science, 241,* 540–545.

Karlawish, J., Barg, F. K., Augsburger, D., Beaver, J., Ferguson, A., & Nunez, J. (2011). What Latino Puerto Ricans and non-Latinos say when they talk about Alzheimer's disease. *Alzheimers and Dementia, 7,* 161–170.

Kavelaars, A., & Heijnen, C. J. (2006). Stress, genetics, and immunity. *Brain Behavior and Immunity, 20,* 313–316.

Kelley, K., Reinhard, S. C., & Brooks-Danso, A. (2008). Executive summary: Professional partners supporting family caregivers. *American Journal of Nursing, 108*(9 Suppl), 6–12.

Keyes, C. L., Shmotkin, D., & Ryff, C. D. (2002). Optimizing well-being: The empirical encounter of two traditions. *Journal of Personal and Social Psychology, 82,* 1007–1022.

Knight, B. G., & Sayegh, P. (2010). Cultural values and caregiving: The updated sociocultural stress and coping model. *Journal of Gerontology, Psychology and Social Science, 65B,* 5–13.

Krause, N. (1995). Negative interaction and satisfaction with social support among older adults. *Journal of Gerontology, Psychology and Social Science, 50B,* 59–73.

Kreutzer, J. S., Rapport, L. J., Marwitz, J. H., Harrison-Felix, C., Hart, T., Glenn, M., & Hammond, F. (2009). Caregivers' well-being after traumatic brain injury: A multicenter prospective investigation. *Archives of Physical Medicine and Rehabilitation, 90,* 939–946.

Lee, S., Colditz, G. A., Berkman, L. F., & Kawachi, I. (2003). Caregiving and risk of coronary heart disease in U.S. women: A prospective study. *American Journal of Preventive Medicine, 24,* 113–119.

Levine, C. (2003). Family caregiving: Current challenges for a time-honored practice. *Generations, 27,* 5–8.

Levine, C., Halper, D., Peist, A., & Gould, D. A. (2010). Bridging troubled waters: Family caregivers, transitions, and long-term care. *Health Affairs, 29,* 116–124.

Livney, M. G., Clark, C. M., Karlawish, J. H., Cartmell, S., Negrón, M., Nuñez J., ... Arnold, S. E. (2011). Ethnoracial differences in the clinical characteristics of Alzheimer's disease at initial presentation at an urban Alzheimer's disease center. *American Journal of Geriatric Psychiatry, 19,* 430–439.

Losada, A., Marquez-Gonzalez, M., Knight, B. G., Yanguas, J., Sayegh, P., & Romero-Moreno, R. (2010). Psychosocial factors and caregivers distress: Effects of familism and dysfunctional thoughts *Aging and Mental Health, 14,* 193–202.

Manly, J. J., & Mayeux, R. (2004). Ethnic differences in dementia and Alzheimer's disease. In N. B. Anderson, R. A. Bulatao, & B. Cohen (Eds.), *Critical perspectives on racial and ethnic differences in health in late life* (pp. xx–xx). Washington, DC: National Research Council, the National Academies Press.

Mittelman, M. S., Haley, W. E., Clay, O. J., & Roth, D. L. (2006). Improving caregiver well-being delays nursing home placement of patients with Alzheimer disease. *Neurology, 67,* 1592–1599.

Mittelman, M. S., Roth, D. L., Clay, O. J., & Haley, W. E. (2007a). Preserving health of Alzheimer caregivers: Impact of a spouse caregiver intervention. *American Journal of Geriatric Psychiatry, 15,* 780–789.

Mittelman, M. S., Roth, D. L., Coon, D. W., & Haley, W. E. (2004a). Sustained benefit of supportive intervention for depressive symptoms in caregivers of patients with Alzheimer's disease. *American Journal of Psychiatry, 161,* 850–856.

Mittelman, M. S., Roth, D. L., Haley, W. E., & Zarit, S. H. (2004b). Effects of a caregiver intervention on negative caregiver appraisals of behavior problems in patients with Alzheimer's disease: Results of a randomized trial. *Journals of Gerontology B: Psychological Sciences Social Sciences, 59,* P27–P34.

Monahan, P. O., Boustani, M., Alder, C., Galvin, J. E., Perkins, A., Healy, P., ... Callahan, C. (2012). A practical clinical tool to monitor dementia symptoms: The HABC-Monitor. *Clinical Interventions in Aging, 7,* 143–157.

Napoles, A. M., Chadiha, L., Eversley, R., & Moreno-John, G. (2010). Developing culturally sensitive dementia caregiver interventions: Are we there yet? *American Journal of Alzheimers and Other Dementias, 25,* 389–406.

Evercare. (2009). *The Evercare Survey of the Economic Downturn and Its Impact on Family Caregiving*. National Alliance for Caregiving, Bethesda, MD

National Institutes of Health. (2010). *Caring for a person with Alzheimer's disease.* [NIH Publication # 09-6173]. March 2010. Bethesda, MD: US Department of Health and Human Services.

Ory, M., Hoffman, R., Lee, J., Tennstedt, S., & Schulz, R. (1999). Prevalence and impact of caregiving: A detailed comparison between dementia and non-dementia caregivers. *Gerontologist, 39,* 177–185.

Pearlin, L. I., Mullin, J. T., Semple, S. J., & Skaff, M. M. (1990). Caregiving and the stress process: An overview of concepts and their measures. *Gerontologist, 30,* 583–594.

Pinquart, M., & Sorensen, S. (2003). Differences between caregivers and non-caregivers in psychological health and physical health: A meta-analysis. *Psychology and Aging, 18,* 250–267.

Raveis, V. H. (2004). Psychosocial impact of spousal caregiving at the end-of-life: Challenges and consequences. *Gerontologist, 44*(Special Issue 1), 191–120.

Raveis, V. H., Pretter, S., & Carrero, M. (2010). "It should have been happening to me": The psychosocial issues older caregiving mothers experience. *Journal of Family Social Work, 13,* 131–148.

Reinhard, S. C., Brooks-Danso, A., Kelley, K., & Mason, D. J. (2008). Editorial: How are *you* doing? *American Journal of Nursing, 108*(9 Suppl), 4–5.

Roth, D. L., Mittelman, M. S., Clay, O. J., Madan, A., & Haley, W. E. (2005). Changes in social support as mediators of the impact of a psychosocial intervention for spouse caregivers of persons with Alzheimer's disease. *Psychology and Aging, 20,* 634–644.

Roth, D. L., Perkins, M., Wadley, V. G., Temple, E. M., & Haley, W. E. (2009). Family caregiving and emotional strain: Associations with quality of life in a large national sample of middle-aged and older adults. *Quality of Life Research, 18,* 679–688.

Saban, K. L., Sherwood, P. R., DeVon, H. A., & Hynes, D. M. (2010). Measures of psychological stress and physical health in family caregivers of stroke survivors: A literature review. *Journal of Neuroscience Nursing, 42,* 128–138.

Sayegh, P., & Knight, B. G. (2010). The effects of familism and cultural justification on the mental and physical health of family caregivers. *Journal of Gerontology: Psychological Sciences, 66B,* 3–14

Schoenmakers, B., Buntinx, F., & DeLepeleire, J. (2010). Supporting the dementia family caregiver: The effect of home care intervention on general well-being. *Aging and Mental Health, 14,* 44–56.

Schulz, R., & Martire, L. M. (2004). Family caregiving of persons with dementia: Prevalence, health effects, and support strategies. *American Journal of Geriatric Psychiatry, 12,* 240–249.

Shaw, S. A. (1997). Modern psychoanalytic approach to caregiver support group. *Group, 21,* 159–174.

Sheets, C., & Mahoney-Gleason, H. (2011). Caregiver support in the Veterans Health Administration: Caring for those who care. *Generations, 34,* 92–98.

Sterritt, P. F., & Pokorny, M. E. (1998). African-American caregiving for a relative with Alzheimer's disease. *Geriatric Nursing, 19,* 127–128, 133–134.

Talley, R. C., & Crews, J. E. (2007). Framing the public health of caregiving. *American Journal of Public Health, 97,* 224–228.

Thompson, R. L., Lewis, S. L., Murphy, M. R., Hale, J. M., Blackwell, P. H., Acton, G. J.,…Bonner, P. N. (2004). Are there sex differences in emotional and biological responses in spousal caregivers of patients with Alzheimer's disease? *Biological Research for Nursing, 5,* 319–330.

Toseland, R. W. (1995). *Group work with the elderly and family caregivers.* New York, NY: Springer.

University of Washington Medical Center. (2007). *Culture clues.* Retrieved April 2013, from http://depts.washington.edu/pfes/CultureClues.htm.

Valle, R. (1998). *Caregiving across cultures: Working with dementing illnesses and ethnically diverse populations.* Washington, DC: Taylor & Francis.

28

Mental Competence and Legal Issues in Dementia Care

Barry S. Fogel

Ultimately, all patients with dementing illnesses will lose their mental competence. Competence for more subtle and demanding tasks and decisions will be lost first. At the same time, patients with dementing illnesses usually will lose many elements of self-awareness, including awareness of their areas of incompetence, and will lose their ability to conform their behavior to adjust even for those deficits they acknowledge. This conflict can lead to significant challenges for physicians and other professionals involved in dementia care. Competency issues can be extremely emotional ones for patients and caregivers; clinicians must remain calm and rational in the face of families' emotions. Basing assessments and recommendations on clear principles helps; a particularly important principle is beginning the discussion of competency issues as early as possible after the diagnosis of a dementing disease—preferably before critical competencies are lost and while the patient retains sufficient metacognition, executive function, and credibility within the family to participate fully in the process. At this stage the patient may be diagnosed as having mild cognitive impairment or questionable/very mild dementia.

The lack of certainty about the underlying diagnosis and rate of progression should not deter the physician from beginning the dialogue about competency. The mere fact that there is a substantial risk of losing competency should be sufficient to raise the issue.

At the outset the physician should clarify his or her role in the process of diagnosing and managing each specific patient and should resolve any ambiguity about that role. The physician should know (1) whether the patient will authorize him or her to talk with family members, which ones he or she may talk with, and whether any subjects are off limits; (2) whether other professionals are involved, including lawyers and others who might provide counsel and advice to family members; and (3) whether there are any legal proceedings contemplated or already under way. If other professionals are involved, the physician must know whether the patient will allow all professionals involved to communicate freely with one another about the patient's case. If there are legal proceedings in the offing, the physician should know whether he or she will be expected to provide testimony, in what context, and on whose behalf.

Principles

Competency Is Specific to the Task and the Context

Competency is not an all-or-nothing determination; it depends on the task and on the context in which the task is performed. Patients can be competent to decide where they want to live but not competent in how to manage an investment portfolio or to judge whether it is safe for them to drive at night. They may be competent to choose between two reasonable alternative treatments for a medical condition but not to refuse necessary, life-saving care. They may be competent to make certain decisions when in good general health but not when suffering from a febrile illness with an associated mild delirium.

A formal determination of incompetence with designation of a legal guardian or conservator involves a global judgment about a patients' competence to manage their daily activities, their health care, or their assets. Such a determination may be appropriate for a patient with moderate to severe dementia but is likely to be inappropriate for a patient with mild dementia or mild cognitive impairment with selective and/or intermittent impairment of competence. For such patients other legal strategies or informal solutions may be better.

Executive Function and Metacognition Are Critical to Competency

Executive function is the most important cognitive factor in determining the performance of instrumental activities of daily living (IADLs) in patients with dementia (Cahn-Weiner et al., 2007; Marshall et al., 2011) and in older adults in general (Vaughan & Giovanello, 2010). Furthermore, impairment in executive function predicts further decline in IADLs, and patients with more rapid decline in executive function have more rapid decline in IADLs (Royall, Palmer, Chiodo, & Polk, 2004). While patients and families often focus on memory loss as a chief complaint, loss of declarative memory (as opposed to procedural memory or working memory) often matters less for competency than metacognition and executive function. Both of the latter are important. Patients must know they have a deficit if they are to compensate for it; such self-awareness is a form of metacognition. They must be able to keep that knowledge in mind when faced with a situation they are not competent to manage, turning to another for help rather than doing their best and failing; this requires executive functions, including working memory, inhibition of inappropriate responses, and possibly also planning to have help available when needed (see Chapter 3 for further discussion).

Patients lacking awareness of their limitations will not ask for help when they need it, may refuse help when it is offered, and may persist in dangerous behavior. Those who are aware of their deficits will modify their behavior to compensate. For example, patients with reduced insight and self-awareness are likely to be unsafe drivers even when cognitive impairment in other domains is relatively mild (Kay, Bundy, & Clemson, 2009).

Overall Cognitive Performance, Metacognition, and Executive Function Can Decline at Different Rates

Frontotemporal degeneration, especially its behavioral variant, impairs executive function and awareness of deficits long before it grossly affects memory or language. Such patients may be able to pass simple tests of orientation, memory, calculation, and language at a point in their course when they make self-destructive decisions or engage in dangerous behavior. They either do not understand that they are causing harm to themselves or others, or know they are acting badly but cannot help it at the time. In addition to frontotemporal dementia, other dementias that can show this pattern include Lewy body dementia, dementia associated with Parkinson's disease, and various forms of dementia associated with chronic psychosis. Other brain diseases with disproportionate damage to the frontal lobes and their connections can cause a similar dissociation of deficits. In Alzheimer's disease, patients with early disproportionate involvement of the nondominant hemisphere also can show disproportionate impairment of metacognition.

Criteria for Competency Should Be More Stringent When the Patient Is Making a Bad Decision

When a patient with acute appendicitis agrees to surgery, the patient's consent (or even passive assent) will be accepted as valid even if the patient suffers from delirium or dementia. In the same situation, refusal of surgery would be presumed incompetent unless it could be shown that the patient understood the proposed surgery and its alternatives, understood the potential consequences of refusing surgery, understood the implications of those consequences, and could explain how, considering the implications, his or her decision was rational. A patient giving competent refusal might point out that although untreated appendicitis could lead to life-threatening peritonitis, he or she had had severe adverse reactions to anesthesia in the past that made surgery especially dangerous, that initial treatment with antibiotics might obviate the need for surgery, and so on. The ability to assemble such facts and marshal such arguments would be unnecessary if the recommendation for surgery were accepted.

Competency Can Fluctuate

Fluctuating deficits are the rule in dementia. Drugs, acute general medical illness, pain, lack of sleep, stress, and depression all can exacerbate deficits that impair decision-making competence. Fluctuating cognitive deficits can lead to intermittent or state-dependent decision-making incompetence. When they do, the physician should seek informed consent for medical procedures during intervals of better function, designing the consent to be durable if the patient subsequently becomes delirious or otherwise incapable of making a rational decision. Soon after a diagnosis of dementia or mild cognitive impairment is made, the potential for fluctuating competency should be pointed out; it may help patients and families recognize the importance and urgency of executing a durable power of attorney and a health care proxy.

Clinical Observations and Neuropsychological Testing Have Complementary Roles in Competency Assessment

Competency is a legal judgment that is based in large part on clinical observations and their interpretation. Neuropsychological test results supplement clinical observations and aid in their interpretation, but they do not substitute for a clinical inquiry more specific to the individual patient's situation. Moreover, the context of neuropsychological testing is standardized, but the context of real-life decision making is not; real decisions are made in a context that can have more cues but also more stress and potential distraction than a neuropsychologist's office. Benefits of neuropsychological testing in assessing and managing competency issues are discussed later in the chapter.

Competency-Related Issues Should Be Addressed as Early as Possible

When a patient is diagnosed with mild cognitive impairment or mild dementia, it is likely that he or she is still competent in many areas. In particular, patients may be competent to designate who they would like to make decisions for them if they become incompetent later. Designating proxy decision makers through health care proxies, durable powers of attorney, and provisions in trust documents can avoid legal emergencies in which the medical or financial decisions are pressing and there is no one with clear authority to act on the patients' behalf. Also, as will be discussed further, patients with professional responsibilities should be advised to relinquish them before their cognitive deficits lead to expensive, embarrassing, and sometimes tragic mistakes.

Communication Should Be Clear, Redundant, and Multimodal

Issues of competency can be subtle for physicians and lawyers, even more so for lay people. Results of a competency assessment should be communicated in writing as well as explained orally, and patients and families can be directed to a range of resources, including support groups, Websites, and books. An individual practice can develop handouts customized for the specific populations served by the practice and for the approaches to testing and evaluation the practice most often uses.

Formal Legal Proceedings to Establish Incompetence Are Not Always Necessary

When medical, financial, or practical decisions can be made for the patient, the substitute decision maker is benign and trusted, the decision is a reasonable one, and the patient assents (or does not object), the patient's competency to decide or to agree is rarely challenged. When any of these factors is not present, or when the decision involves a great deal of money or substantial medical risk, a formal legal proceeding should be considered. Clinicians practicing in a hospital setting can consult the hospital's risk management department or hospital counsel for assistance with making the judgment. Greater formality and rigor in competency assessment is necessary when there is disagreement, conflict, or mistrust between concerned parties.

Executive Function and Metacognition

Adequate executive function is a prerequisite for successful goal-directed activity, for safe independent living, and for acceptable performance of complex activities like driving, managing money, or practicing a profession. Dementias of several different etiologies, including Alzheimer's disease but most consistently frontotemporal dementia, can impair executive function disproportionately early their clinical course. It is thus important to assess executive function adequately at the time dementia or mild cognitive impairment is diagnosed. If neuropsychological testing is not done, the office-based testing done by the neurologist or psychiatrist should screen for executive dysfunction using procedures like the Clock Drawing Test, the Luria hand sequence, Trail Making B, or presentation of conflicting stimuli (e.g., asking the patient to raise his or her right arm quickly if the command is given in a soft voice and slowly if the command is given in a loud voice). The Executive Interview Test (Royall, Mahurin, & Gray, 1992; Royall et al., 2004) is a concise, practical survey of executive function that is intermediate in length between a typical office examination and neuropsychological testing; it takes 10–15 minutes to do and can be administered by a nurse or technician.

Metacognition and awareness of noncognitive functional deficits involve the same brain systems. Both can be assessed by comparing the patient's self-reported performance with the performance observed on examination and the performance reported by family members or other collateral sources. A review of instrumental activities of daily living such as shopping, transportation, taking medications, keeping appointments, and managing money may yield markedly different answers when asked of the patient than when asked of a caregiver.

Metacognition has two dimensions: the "feeling of knowing" and confidence in one's knowledge. Metacognition requires functioning of the dorsomedial frontal region, especially in the right hemisphere, and the right parietal lobe. In general, metacognition is more impaired in cortical dementias than in subcortical dementias. Certainty about wrong answers and gross denial of deficits is a great threat to competent decision making; it is more likely to occur early in cases with prominent right hemisphere involvement.

Office cognitive testing affords a natural opportunity to assess the patient's awareness of his or her cognitive deficits. Comparison of directly measured and self-assessed deficits can be quantitated (Williamson et al., 2010), but a more qualitative approach provides additional information useful in competency assessment. Before testing, ask the patient how he or she thinks he or she will do on tests of memory and concentration and other cognitive abilities. Separately, ask family members whether the patient's behavior reflects any adjustment for cognitive impairments. After the test but before telling the patient the results, ask the patient again to assess his or her performance. After giving the results, ask the patient if he or she agrees or disagrees, and note whether the patient acknowledges a poor performance but excuses it or minimizes its import. If the patient does not accept the presence of a cognitive deficit during the office visit, he or she should be given a written report to review at home and be asked again about awareness of deficits on the next visit. In this way patients can be placed on a continuum of self-awareness that progresses from full appreciation of deficits to frank denial. Some points on the continuum are as follows:

1. Knowing they have cognitive deficits, appreciating their implications, and making adjustments to their behavior to account for them;
2. Knowing they have cognitive deficits, appreciating their implications, but not modifying their behavior;
3. Knowing they have cognitive deficits but not appreciating their implications;
4. Acknowledging cognitive deficits after failing a test but before being told of the test results, and then showing appreciation of their implications;
5. Acknowledging cognitive deficits after failing a test but before being told of the test results, but excusing their performance or regarding the results as insignificant or irrelevant;
6. Acknowledging cognitive deficits only after being confronted with test results and their significance by the physician;
7. Acknowledging deficits after extensive persuasion and review of a written report of performance; and
8. Completely denying deficits despite efforts at persuasion and confrontation with evidence.

Metacognition can be formally tested by neuropsychologists and by occupational therapists. Some neuropsychological tests of memory explicitly incorporate questions about how sure the patient is of his or her answer. In addition, the neuropsychologist can make and record systematic observations of the patient's comments and behavior as the testing proceeds and deficits are uncovered. Occupational therapists can perform structured assessments of performance in instrumental activities of daily living and compare them with patients' self-assessments of the same functions.

Patients with higher levels of self-awareness will be more open to memory training and other cognitive rehabilitation activities and to environmental changes and the use of cues and mnemonic aids. They also will be open to accepting help with activities and decisions they find difficult. Patients who deny deficits are at the highest risk for unsafe or self-destructive actions. These relationships apply at all levels of overall cognitive impairment, but they deserve special attention in the earlier stages of dementia, when the patient's life makes frequent demands on cognitive functions that have declined.

The Role of Neuropsychological Testing

Neuropsychological testing is not required to establish competency or lack of competency to make a specific decision in a specific context. However, results of neuropsychological testing can be useful in several important ways in managing competency-related issues in dementia care:

1. Clear-cut abnormalities on neuropsychological testing can be used in conjunction with imaging results and other biomarkers in convincing a patient or his or her family that the patient is indeed cognitively impaired, that competencies eventually will be lost, and that the problems associated with a loss of competency should be anticipated and mitigated by preventive actions.
2. Serial neuropsychological testing indicating the pace of dementia progression can aid in suggesting a time frame for action in advance of incompetence to perform a specific function or make a specific decision.
3. A neuropsychological profile suggesting disproportionate loss of executive function and/or lack of awareness of cognitive deficits can be helpful in explaining why a patient who looks relatively intact may already lack competency to make major financial decisions, to drive safely, or to validly change his or her will. Test results carry weight in legal proceedings; when conflicting opinions of experts appear to cancel one another, evidence from testing can tip the balance.
4. A neuropsychological profile can suggest specific areas of potential incompetency. Some neuropsychological tests are face valid and persuasive in this

regard: Financial incompetence would be strongly suspected in a patient unable to do simple calculations.
5. The quantitative aspect of neuropsychological tests can translate into quantitative estimates of impairment.

In addition to standard neuropsychological tests, specialized tests for decision-making competence have been devised, especially focusing on competency to consent to medical treatments and procedures. One, the MacArthur Competence Assessment Tool (MacCAT) (Grisso & Appelbaum 1998), has been most widely utilized in clinical research and in studies of the neuropsychological basis of decision-making competence and has relatively strong empirical support (Dunn, Nowrangi, Palmer, Jeste, & Saks, 2006). One version, the MacCAT-T, targets competency to consent to medical treatment; another version, the MacCAT-CR, targets competency to consent to clinical research. The MacCAT is based on presenting the patient with a vignette specifically designed for the clinical decision in question, then conducting a semi-structured interview to assess the patient's understanding of the vignette, his or her appreciation of its personal relevance and implications, his or her reasoning about risks and benefits, and his or her ability to express a decision. Each of these is rated on an ordinal scale; in the end the clinician makes a binary judgment of competence or incompetence to make the clinical decision. There are no specific cutoff scores on the ordinal items that link them to the final judgment; this allows room for consideration of contextual factors. The MacCAT requires training to administer reliably, and variability in how vignettes are related to actual clinical circumstances is a potential source of unreliability.

While research on the MacCAT-T and a few other less widely used standardized competency tests has shown acceptable psychometric properties, patients can do poorly on such tests yet make competent decisions about their own medical treatment. One reason is that real clinical decisions have a rich context of cues, motivations, and circumstances that are absent from a standardized vignette; another is that patients with impaired verbal fluency can have a hard time articulating rational reasons for their choice when they do in fact have them. Further, a patient facing a difficult decision might choose to rely on a trusted physician's advice rather than try to understand a complex medical issue at all, basing his or her reliance on the rational reason that the physician's past advice has been sound or that the issues are complex and arcane and recommendations are offered by a well-reputed specialist with extensive knowledge and experience with those issues. Or a patient may have a long-held personal belief that trumps other considerations and implies what choice should be made—for example, a belief that it is always better to live than die, regardless of the expected quality of life.

Despite their limitations, the use of a standardized assessment like the MacCAT is appropriate—and perhaps even necessary—for assessing capacity to consent to clinical trials of treatments for patients with dementia. When a patient's participation in a clinical trial is completely elective, erroneously determining that the patient is incapable of giving valid consent does no harm, and documentation of a rigorous, standardized assessment of capacity to consent protects the researcher—and the research—if there is an adverse event during the study.

Dementia and Professional Competence

As people in business and the professions retire later than they did in the past, impaired professional performance due to dementia is becoming more common. Bad judgments by lawyers, physicians, money managers, and executives (among others) can have very serious consequences, including harm to clients, financial liability, and the destruction of reputations built over lifetimes. Competent professional practice requires a high level of executive function, appropriate social behavior, working memory, and recall of many details. For this reason professional competence is lost earlier in the course of dementia than competence to make everyday decisions. At the time when professional competence first declines ordinary cognitive screening in a physician's office or at the bedside usually is above the cutoff for abnormality, because professionals are highly educated and begin with superior baseline performance.

When a physician makes the diagnosis of a dementing disease—whether the current clinical presentation is one of mild cognitive impairment or one of mild dementia—the physician should consider whether the patient is still employed and inquire in detail about the actual duties of the job. (In some family businesses and partnerships senior people may be paid but have essentially honorary roles.) Neuropsychological testing usually should be done, even if the diagnosis is not in doubt, and the neuropsychologist asked to concentrate on areas of cognitive performance essential to the patient's professional activities.

If relevant deficits are confirmed, the physician should meet with the patient and explain the risk of a costly or embarrassing professional mistake if the patient continues to work. The physician should emphasize that it is far better to retire with honor than retire in disgrace. With the patient's consent, family members or trusted professional colleagues can be included in the conversation. If the patient is under the age for full pension benefits at the time of the diagnosis, he or she should be encouraged to assert a disability claim rather than simply to retire early.

Dementia and Financial Management

Competence to manage money is a continuum ranging from management of an investment portfolio to determining whether one has received correct change at a convenience store. As dementia progresses, patients can be at risk for financial exploitation or victimization, as well as for dire consequences from unpaid bills if they have primary responsibility for paying for housing, taxes, and utilities. The consequences of financial mistakes are greater in money terms when the patient has more money; but the consequences of lost money for daily life are greater when the patient has less money. However, even moderate dementia does not necessarily imply complete loss of money-related capabilities; a patient might be unable to calculate yet still roughly understand the value of money.

Money-related behavior is of special diagnostic interest because financial transactions other than cash payments leave a documentary record. Review of credit card statements, checking account statements, and cancelled checks can show such inappropriate financial behavior as repeated payment of the same bills, failure to make necessary payments, or irrational purchases. Examination of brokerage account statements can show behavior like unexpected and unnecessary withdrawals and transfers of funds, erratic patterns of buying and selling securities, investment choices inconsistent with the patient's goals and past behavior, or activity suggesting the influence of a self-serving financial advisor. The onset and progression of signs of bad financial judgment can be used to support a diagnosis of dementia and estimate its rate of progression. Further, financial records may be useful objective evidence in legal proceedings. Review of financial records, of course, requires the patient's written permission or his or her physical delivery of the records; however, if accounts are jointly held with a caregiving spouse, it may suffice to obtain and record the patient's verbal consent to the physician's discussing financial details with the caregiver.

As an alternative to direct examination of financial records, patients' financial competency can be assessed with a structured instrument, the Financial Capacity Instrument (FCI-9) (Martin et al., 2008). The FCI-9 tests the patient on 18 financial tasks covering nine domains; they range from identifying coins and currency and making change to explaining the parts of a bank statement and comparing investment options. It has acceptable psychometric properties, and its face validity is particularly appealing.

The physician's response to dementia-related changes in money-related competency depends on the context; understanding the context may require the assistance of a social worker, a lawyer, or both. Key considerations include the following: (a) the stage of dementia; (b) the projected clinical course, including the rate of progression and expected needs for care; (c) whether there is someone trusted by the patient (and worthy of his or her trust) who can make financial decisions on the patient's behalf; (d) what must be spent on the patient's care at present and in the future; (e) the assets and income available for the patient's care; and (f) whether the patient is responsible for financial decisions and actions that affect other people's welfare.

Patients with early dementia may not yet have made any harmful financial errors but show some evidence of financial mistakes and/or deficits in calculation, memory, or executive function likely to cause them. In this situation the physician should point out that the patient has an illness that gradually will affect his or her financial ability and suggest that changes be made *before* the patient loses his or her money. The specific emphasis in the appeal to the patient can take advantage of the patient's expressed concerns; either a fear of being cheated or a concern to leave a legacy can motivate reconsideration of financial arrangements. The changes must be made while the patient is competent to make them; since the dementing illness is progressive, there is no time to lose. Competence to change financial arrangements requires a basic understanding of what one's assets are, what bills one is responsible for paying, who would control the assets following a change, and an appropriate rationale for choosing that person. A patient can retain this competence even after he or she has lost the ability to handle financial details such as paying bills on time and not paying the same bills twice.

When a reasonable prediction can be made about the needs for care in the future and what they might cost, and when the patient and family have some combination of assets and insurance that could cover the costs, they can be advised to set aside the money that will probably be needed for care and protect it from unplanned withdrawals. Legal counsel usually will be needed to do this.

As soon as possible after the dementia diagnosis, the patient should be asked whether there is someone, typically a family member, whom they would trust to handle his or her money when the patient is no longer able to do so. If the answer is other than an unqualified yes, someone—often a social worker or family therapist—should investigate the reason and determine whether the trust issue within the family is resolvable or whether an external trustee might be needed to protect the patient's assets.

When the patient has substantial assets well beyond those needed to ensure his or her own care, it is likely that there is already a lawyer, banker, and/or other professional involved in creating and implementing an estate plan. Here the physician can perform—as always with the patient's consent—a valuable service by explaining to the patient's advisers the patient's current mental capabilities, the diagnosis of a degenerative disease, the probable clinical course, and the neuropsychological deficits that might affect the patient's financial judgments, testamentary capacity, and susceptibility to undue influence. It would be within those professionals' scope to elicit and implement the patient's broader intentions for his or her assets while addressing the patient's needs to pay for his or her care and provide for dependents. If the physician suspects that the patient's advisers are not sufficiently familiar with the nuances of dementia—in particular, the potential for disproportionate impairment of executive function and metacognition, and the potential for a new onset of paranoid thinking or depression that might further impair judgment—he or she should seek an opportunity to educate the advisers.

Dementia and Driving

Patients with moderate or severe dementia cannot drive safely, and if they are currently driving, they should be unequivocally advised—both orally and in writing—to stop driving immediately. In states where reporting of such patients to the licensing authority is mandatory, this should be done without delay. When reporting the patient is not permitted without the patient's consent, the physician should ask the patient's consent to make the report and should, unless the patient objects, advise family members or other caregivers of the recommendation.

Since failing to make a required report on a driver with dementia is a major legal risk, physicians should know whether their state has mandatory reporting of dementia and, if so, what the criteria are for making the report. In some states the diagnosis of Alzheimer's disease would trigger mandatory reporting, even if the disease process were at an early stage and causing only mild cognitive impairment. The contemporary view of separating the clinical syndrome from the presumed neuropathology has not yet penetrated motor vehicle licensing agencies. For the physician's legal protection the patient's medical records must make such distinctions clearly, in the unfortunate event that a patient with mild cognitive impairment continues to drive and is involved in a crash.

Advising patients with mild cognitive impairment or mild dementia about driving is especially challenging because for many patients driving is essential to independence, activity, quality of life, and self-esteem; driving cessation for those patients can lead to an acceleration of functional decline, increased caregiver burden, earlier institutionalization, and even earlier mortality. On the other hand, the increase in crash risk associated with dementia is unequivocal. Specific errors associated with dementia in general include lower and more variable driving speed, errors at intersections with an increase in rear-end collisions, increased steering variability, less awareness of pedestrians and other drivers, worse lane control, and unexpected braking.

Even very mild dementia is associated with increased crash risk. The increase in risk is greater for mild dementia (CDR 1.0) than it is for very mild dementia (CDR 0.5). A road test study of dementia clinic patients at Washington University showed that 14% of patients with CDR 0.5 were unsafe and 42% of those with CDR 1.0 were unsafe. Half of the CDR 1.0 patients who were judged safe at baseline were unsafe when tested 6 months later; half of the CDR 0.5 patients judged safe at baseline were unsafe 1 year later (Duchek et al., 2003). Dementia patients with impairment in executive function, especially those with impaired insight, are likely to be unsafe drivers even when there is relatively mild impairment in other cognitive domains. Asimakopulos et al. (2012) comprehensively review studies of neuropsychological tests of executive function that have been correlated with driving performance, providing very strong evidence that executive function is probably the most consistent cognitive determinant of driving performance. In their review they note the criterion of driving performance used in each study—the most common being on-road tests, driving simulation, a history of crashes, and subsequent cessation of driving.

Driving impairment from early dementia can be exacerbated by the neuropsychiatric complications of dementia. Depression is associated with psychomotor slowing, increased reaction time, and lapses of attention. Patients with psychosis can misperceive their environment while driving or be distracted by internal stimuli. Aggressiveness and impulsivity associated with orbitofrontal dysfunction can manifest as aggressive driving. Apathetic patients fail to anticipate predictable road hazards, although their overall crash risk is mitigated by their decreased desire to drive.

Even when there is no legal obligation, physicians have a professional obligation to advise patients with dementia that they should not drive, and physicians are at risk legally if they do not do so and the patient subsequently causes a crash. Notice should be given both orally and in writing, and documented in the medical record. When the patient has given the physician permission to talk with a family caregiver, the caregiver should be given the same message.

The physician's task is more demanding when the patient has mild cognitive impairment and has focal or multifocal cognitive deficits that can impair driving performance but do not warrant a dementia diagnosis, or has a dementing disease but does not yet have a definitive diagnosis. In this situation the patient should be tested to quantitatively estimate the extent of driving impairment and come up with a recommendation either to cease driving immediately or to drive with restrictions that can mitigate crash risk while developing a plan to eventually cease driving. The plan should include whatever changes in living arrangements, caregiver relationships, and formal services are needed to maintain a healthy and active life without the need to drive. If the patient's prognosis is sufficiently clear, a time frame for making such changes may be suggested.

In addition to examination of the patient, there are several historical points that have a strong association with increased crash risk: recent actual at-fault crashes, getting lost while driving, falling while getting into or out of a car, and having traffic violations due to failure to heed signs or signals. The likelihood that a patient with mild cognitive impairment or mild dementia will have a second crash if he or she has a first at-fault crash is unacceptably high; an at-fault crash after the diagnosis of mild cognitive impairment is made is sufficient reason to advise immediate cessation of driving. However, fault in a crash can be ambiguous, so even with the history of a crash or a single moving violation, a patient who greatly depends on driving for mobility may appropriately insist upon being tested before giving up the car keys. Getting lost while driving in itself implies an unacceptable risk of continuing to drive, with a potential exception for getting lost while suffering from a medication side effect. In that case the patient should be advised to abstain from driving until further evaluation of his or her driving ability can be done. Falls getting into or out of a car suggest problems with weakness or coordination of the legs that could interfere with a timely response to a traffic situation.

There are several ways in which the extent of increased crash risk can be estimated:

1. *Office-based testing or neuropsychological testing of cognitive functions known to be associated with driving performance and crash risk, such as reaction time, visual perception, and ability to read and interpret road signs.* A few of the specific test performances that have been explicitly linked to increase crash risk include recalling two or fewer of four words on delayed recall, a Trails B time of greater than 180 seconds, and a time outside of normal limits for navigating a maze on a computer screen (Anderson et al., 2012; Emerson et al., 2012; Ott et al., 2008). The Clock Drawing Test, scored on a 7-point scale with a cut-off for abnormality of four or less, may be a highly specific screening test for unsafe driving (Freund, Gravenstein, Ferris, Burke, & Shaheen, 2005). In a study of 119 older drivers evaluated with a driving simulator, the test was 64.2% sensitive and 97.7% specific in identifying unsafe drivers. The interrater reliability of the 7-point scale for scoring the CDT was 0.95 in their study. The combination of low cost, brief administration time, and high reliability is impressive, but the results need to be confirmed on a larger and more diverse sample of older drivers.
2. *Testing of the Useful Field of View (UFoV), a standardized, computer-administered test of visual attention.* It measures the visual information that can be acquired in a brief glance, with or without a distracting condition. The developers of the test present evidence that a reduction of 40% or more in UFoV is associated with a seven-fold increase in crash risk. The same criterion is 89% sensitive and 81% specific in predicting that an older individual will have one or more motor vehicle crashes if he or she continues to drive. (See the developer's Web site, http://www.visualawareness.com, for a summary of research findings and bibliography.)
3. *Testing of driving performance in the virtual reality of a driving simulator.* Driving simulation can present the patient with unexpected events and emergency situations—things a patient with dementia may find difficult to manage, and things that cannot be incorporated into an on-road test. The best validated and most widely researched driving simulator is the STSIM system (see the developer's Web site, http://www.stsimdrive.com, for details). The base configuration of the system includes 80 different driving scenarios; the software counts crashes and near misses as well as driving irregularities such as lane departures.
4. *Automated analysis of "black box" (telematics) recordings of actual driving behavior.* Systems for recording and analyzing driver behavior currently are used by some automobile insurance carriers for rate setting, and by motor vehicle fleet operators to monitor their professional drivers. Current technology can detect and record several of the driving problems commonly seen in patients with dementia, including lane departures, excessive variation in speed, inappropriately slow driving, sudden stops, and abrupt turns. Units with GPS functionality can establish whether the driver got lost on a familiar route, even if the driver eventually found his or her way home. Specialized black box recording analysis for evaluating drivers with mild cognitive impairment or early dementia is not yet commercially available, but it is likely to appear given the ever-increasing scale of the issue.
5. *On-road testing by an examiner specializing in assessing the safety of older drivers and people with diseases that can affect driving ability.* A road test by a specialized examiner will be more sensitive than a road test for driver's license renewal; the former will look for *potentially* risky behavior that would not in itself cause the driver to fail the test for licensure.

In addition, the patient should have tests of hearing and vision if these were not recently done and passed. However, it has been established that poor visual acuity—the visual function tested for licensing of drivers—does not predict motor vehicle crashes in older drivers. Glare sensitivity, loss of peripheral vision, and diminished useful field of view all are associated with a significant increase in crash risk. The evidence for these relationships is direct; it comes from a study where baseline visual testing was performed in 1,801 drivers aged 65–84 years; state motor vehicle crash records were then reviewed a specific time point 2–4 years later, by which point 120 drivers had been involved in crashes (Rubin et al., 2007).

On-road testing is *not* the gold standard of driving evaluation. While failing a road test implies impaired driving performance under the conditions of the test, road test performance can be worsened by anxiety or fatigue and may not be representative of the patient's performance in the particular situations in which he or she usually drives. On the other hand, passing a road test does not imply that a patient could cope with the additional demands of night driving, bad weather, or heavy traffic, and it does not imply that the patient will respond appropriately and in time to an unexpected event like a child running across the street in front of the car. The assessment of these capabilities is better done in a driving simulator. The special value of road tests is that failing one can get the unsafe driver off the road immediately.

The expense and inconvenience of road testing or testing in a driving simulator can be avoided if the results of cognitive testing or UFoV testing are sufficiently bad to be highly specific for unsafe driving. When it becomes widely available, "black box" recording and automated analysis of actual driving behavior may be an efficient method for evaluating driving competence that offers the advantage of not requiring a *test*—a situation that may evoke the patient's anxiety or potentially his or her resistance.

In persuading a patient to discontinue driving, it is useful to identify any *noncognitive* reason why the person's driving might be unsafe. In addition to impaired hearing or vision (especially peripheral vision, glare intolerance, or UFoV), decreased neck mobility, diminished limb strength, and falls getting into and out of a car should be considered. As to the importance of leg strength and balance, patients who require more than 10 seconds to walk 10 feet, turn around, and come back have double the rate of crashes. Driving cessation for a noncognitive reason is face saving for the patient and may be more readily accepted.

For those patients who continue to drive, crash risk can be mitigated somewhat by specifying circumstances under which the patient should not drive. Also, patients should be strongly cautioned against using a mobile phone while driving. Crash risk for any driver increases with mobile phone use. The incremental risk for drivers with mild cognitive impairment or mild dementia is greater because of their difficulty dealing with distractions, redirecting attention, and processing conflicting stimuli.

Testamentary Capacity

When patients with dementia make wills that disinherit natural heirs or give large sums to unrelated caregivers, their wills are often contested. When the assets involved are substantial, the contests can lead to expensive and emotionally stressful litigation. In this litigation physicians are called to testify regarding the patient's mental state at the time of writing (or rewriting) his or her will. There are two implications for physicians treating patients with dementia. The first is that shortly after the diagnosis of dementia (or even a dementing disease with the current syndrome of mild cognitive impairment) the physician should encourage the patient to review his or her will—or to make a will if one is not on file—and make any desired changes before the disease progresses. If there already are obvious deficits in memory or judgment, special pains should be taken to establish and document the ingredients of testamentary capacity. This activity can be—and usually should be—a separately scheduled patient encounter, carried out either by the principal physician or by a neurologist or psychiatrist with an interest in dementia or experience with competency assessment. The interview should establish that the patient:

1. Knows what a will is;
2. Knows what his or her assets are;
3. Knows the people who have a reasonable claim to be beneficiaries;
4. Understands the impact of a particular distribution of assets;
5. Does not have delusions or other psychotic phenomena that would affect the decisions made; and

6. Can express his or her wishes clearly and consistently.

If the patient's decisions seem likely to evoke family conflict, video recording of the interview is advised. If the assets are modest and there is nothing unusual about the will, it is sufficient to document these basic criteria for testamentary capacity in the clinical record. As with other competencies, criteria for testamentary capacity are interpreted more liberally when less is at stake and the choices made are typical ones.

The retrospective signs of potential testamentary incapacity include the following:

1. Radical change from previous wills;
2. Changes that disinherit natural heirs such as a spouse or a child;
3. Changes made reflecting probable delusions, misperceptions, or misunderstandings;
4. Changes that disregard the testator's personal history and reflect only the person's current circumstances; and
5. Changes suggesting undue influence, such as an unusually large bequest to a recent caregiver who is not related and who was not named at all in the previous will.

When these signs are present, a judge might invalidate the will unless there is positive evidence that the testator was fully competent at the time of making the new will. If the physician learns that the patient with dementia plans to revise his or her will—or that the patient has recently done so—the physician should suggest a special interview assessing the elements of testamentary capacity, pointing out that given the diagnosis the patient's will might be challenged and that such an interview will be helpful in ensuring that the patient's valid intentions are carried out. Gutheil (2007) offers advice regarding pitfalls in the assessment of testamentary capacity, specifically emphasizing that neither a neurological or psychiatric diagnosis nor the presence of cognitive impairment is in itself evidence for testamentary incapacity.

Dementia and Voting

Participation of people with mild to moderate dementia in voting has increasing salience as the prevalence of dementia increases, reflecting changes in the age distribution of the population. A study of voting-related competency in patients with Alzheimer's disease suggested that a general understanding of the nature and effect of voting and the ability to express a choice usually are preserved in mild dementia and often are preserved in moderate dementia. However, as dementia progresses, patients are less able to reason about political issues or to understand the likely personal implications of election results (Appelbaum, Bonnie, & Karlawish, 2005). While in practice citizens' competency to vote is not verified, the issues are similar to those of testamentary capacity. One might grant a lifelong Democrat or lifelong Republican a right to vote for the party he or she has always supported. A sudden change in voting behavior inconsistent with long-held opinions would raise the issue of competency to vote (or perhaps of dyslexia or dyspraxia interfering with marking a ballot or operating a voting machine in a way consistent with the patient's intentions).

Dementia and Firearm Safety

In the United States 17 million people over the age of 65 own one or more guns (Mertens & Sorenson, 2012). Eighty percent of all homicides committed by persons over 65 are committed using guns, as are more than half of all suicides. Impairments in judgment and impulse control, mood disturbances, and paranoid thinking associated with dementia increase the risk of violence in general and gun violence in particular. For this reason patients with dementia—or even mild cognitive impairment thought to be due to a progressive degenerative brain disease—should not have access to firearms; at the very least firearms in their possession should be disabled.

A study conducted in a university hospital memory clinic found that 60% of patients with dementia had a firearm in the home. In 45% of cases the family knew that the firearm was kept loaded and in another 38% the family did not know whether the gun was loaded (Spangenberg, Wagner, Hendrix, & Bachman, 1999). These statistics do not only imply a risk of gun violence perpetrated by the patient; for example, an unlocked and loaded gun might be appropriated and misused by a visiting grandchild.

The first step in mitigating gun-related risk is recognizing the problem. Every initial evaluation of a dementia patient should include inquiry about firearms in the home. If patients are not able or willing to answer questions about firearms, they should be asked of their caregivers. Interventions to remove, disable, or securely lock up guns are more likely to succeed early in the course of illness when some insight and judgment are preserved, or late in the course where impairments in memory and praxis would make it hard for a patient to defeat simple measures like locking the weapon in a gun safe and securing the key, or removing ammunition from the home.

In situations where there is immediate danger related to guns—as when a patient with dementia has paranoid delusions and threatens to use the gun against an alleged persecutor, or when a gun-owning patient with dementia is depressed and suicidal—state mental health laws can be invoked. A physician with knowledge of the situation, not necessarily a psychiatrist, can call upon the police to remove the patient from the home for emergency psychiatric evaluation. A caregiver can remove the guns from the home and secure them while the patient is away being evaluated.

Why Assessors of Competence May Disagree

Skilled evaluators may disagree about whether a particular patient is competent to make a particular decision or undertake a specific activity. Such disagreements arise for several reasons. Competence itself is context dependent and can fluctuate over time, so two assessments at different time points may begin with different data. Context dependency is more important when there is greater impairment of executive function. Assessors may differ in the way they test competence. They may apply different thresholds for determining that a patient is competent.

Differences between assessors' conclusions usually can be resolved when the reason for them is understood. In exceptional cases disagreements are driven by conflicting motives, as when two experts are engaged by opposite sides in a legal dispute. Also, some clinicians have strongly held biases toward a more protective attitude or a more libertarian one.

Dementia and End-of-Life Planning

Ultimately patients with dementia will die, either because they develop a general medical condition such as pneumonia or because they stop eating and drinking. If patients with dementia receive aggressive treatment for general medical conditions, and receive tube feedings when they stop eating and drinking, they can live on for months or even years after they have lost the ability to participate actively in life. Many people say that if they lose their basic mental capacities, they would prefer not to live and "not to be kept alive by artificial means." However, confronted with a very specific and treatable condition like pneumonia, the patient's spouse or child may find it hard to direct that treatment be withheld, and the patient's physician may find it difficult to withhold the treatment. For such reasons patients write living wills and designate health care proxies. When a patient with mild cognitive impairment or mild dementia chooses a health care proxy, or reviews his or her choice of a health care proxy, the physician should advise the patient to choose a proxy who would feel comfortable about implementing the patient's advance directive. In some cases the spouse, who is the default substitute decision maker, would be a poor choice for health care proxy, because the spouse may know in advance that he or she would be unwilling to say no to treating an infection or to giving tube feedings even if it was the patient's expressed wish.

When implementing advance directives, it is worth considering that what patients think they would want under a given set of circumstances is not necessarily what they would want if those circumstances came to pass and they were competent to decide at the time. A health care proxy tasked with acting in the interest of the patient might in fact determine that the choices indicated in the advance directive do not accurately reflect what the patient would want at the given time if he or she were competent to say. In that case is the proxy's obligation to follow the patient's advance directive or to use his or her judgment based on full knowledge of the patient's pre-illness personality and the current medical and social circumstances? In many jurisdictions law permits a health care proxy to make decisions contrary to the patient's advance directives, i.e., the latter are not binding. One resolution is for the health care proxy to follow the advance directive unless there is a compelling reason to do otherwise, and for the proxy to discuss the deviation from the advance directive with a disinterested (and unprejudiced) third party.

Consider the following situation. A 90-year-old widower with mild dementia would prefer to die rather than live in a nursing home and no longer be able to manage his own affairs. He designates his son as his health care proxy and completes an advance directive stating he wants no "extraordinary measures" to be taken to keep him alive, specifically mentioning ventilators. Over the next year his dementing illness proceeds. He must relinquish control over his assets to a trustee. He can no longer maintain his apartment. He loses weight because he eats poorly, and he becomes incontinent and confused at night. Finally he grudgingly accepts admission to a nursing home after intensive lobbying by his children. He is admitted to a nursing home, where to his surprise he is happy: He makes a couple of friends. He likes the food and gains weight. He is relieved to be rid of oppressive responsibilities and does not care about losing control over many aspects of his life.

A few months later he develops severe pneumonia with respiratory failure. He needs intubation and ventilation along with antibiotics to have a good chance of survival. He is delirious from fever and hypoxia. Should his son honor his prior directive or contradict it by opting for aggressive treatment on the grounds that the patient was happy with his life in the nursing home immediately prior to the acute illness, and that the patient would have written a different advance directive if he knew at the time how life in the nursing home was going to turn out?

In this case the health care proxy should draw on his full knowledge of the patient and not just his expressed intentions at the time he signed the advance directive. At that time was the patient depressed and passively suicidal? Did he have a realistic idea about life in a nursing home, or was his idea based on frightening newspaper stories about neglect and abuse in long-term care institutions? Was the patient a deep thinker who was concerned about the meaning of life and would regard years spent in a nursing home as empty and meaningless even if they were pleasant? Did the patient prefer to spend his remaining assets putting his grandson through college and medical school rather than paying for long-term care in a facility? Would his view of paying for his nursing home care change if the grandson inherited money from someone else and no longer needed help with tuition?

The decision to disregard an advance directive is a weighty one. In a situation where a health care proxy thinks the patient's advance directive no longer makes sense, the physician should direct the health care proxy to a third party to help with thinking through the issues. It is always helpful, and it is essential if the health care proxy has a financial interest in the decision to be made.

The considerations just outlined can be anticipated in the design of an advance directive. The patient can state the assumptions behind the advance directive and ask the health care proxy to reconsider the directive if those assumptions are no longer true. The health care proxy can be directed to discuss any potential deviation from the directive with a disinterested third party such as a family friend or clergyman.

Finding and Developing Resources

Physicians who see a significant number of patients with dementia in their practice often will find that they need the help of other professionals with specific expertise. Developing a panel of such professionals and using them consistently makes care more efficient. Periodic conversations with them can touch on the issues of several different patients. Also, physicians can make sure that they are up to date on dementia and its care, and aware of any special features of the patient population they treat (e.g., cultural or religious issues). A physician who regularly refers patients to the same lawyer for help with estate planning can educate that lawyer about such things as executive function and metacognition, and the lawyer can educate the physician about such things as how trusts operate when a trustee or beneficiary develops impaired judgment in financial matters.

The author suggests developing the following resources:

1. A lawyer specializing in estates and trusts, with special experience in situations where the trustee, the beneficiary, or both have cognitive impairment and potential competency issues;
2. A family therapist with a special interest in family issues related to caregiving, including relationships of adult children with their parents;
3. A social worker familiar with the full range of eldercare resources in the community;
4. A psychotherapist with a special interest in caregiver stress;
5. An occupational therapist with expertise in home safety evaluations;
6. A neuropsychologist experienced in testing for purposes of establishing competency or incompetency, and in communicating results to lawyers and judges;
7. An organization or program that assesses driving safety, preferably one that uses a driving simulator; and
8. Educational programs and support groups for family caregivers.

Provide a Road Map When Possible

Patients with dementing diseases eventually will become incompetent with respect to any given task or decision if they live long enough. An accurate diagnosis of the dementing disease (as opposed to the cognitive and behavioral syndrome) and assessment of the patient's longitudinal course to date permits an estimate of when competencies will be lost. The physician should within the limits of medical certainty provide the patient and family with an assessment of what competencies are diminished and when the ones that are currently intact are likely to be lost. They should advise patients and/or their families as they make informed plans to cope with lost functioning and to mitigate the effects of incompetence on safety, health, finances, family relations, and the quality of the patient's remaining life.

References

Anderson, S. W., Aksan, N., Dawson, J. D., Uc, E. Y., Johnson, A. M., & Rizzo, M. (2012). Neuropsychological assessment of driving safety risk in older adults with and without neurologic disease. *Journal of Clinical and Experimental Neuropsychology*, 34(9), 895–905.

Appelbaum, P. S., Bonnie, R. J., & Karlawish, J. H. (2005). The capacity to vote of persons with Alzheimer's disease. *American Journal of Psychiatry*, 162, 2094–2100.

Asimakopulos, J., Boychuck, Z., Sondergaard, D., Poulin, V., Ménard, I., & Korner-Bitensky, N. (2012). Assessing executive function in relation to fitness to drive: A review of tools and their ability to predict safe driving. *Australian Occupational Therapy Journal*, 59, 402–427.

Cahn-Weiner, D. A., Farias, S. T., Julian, L., Harvey, D. J., Kramer, J. H., Reed, B. R.,...Chui, H. (2007). Cognitive and neuroimaging predictors of instrumental activities of daily living. *Journal of the International Neuropsychological Society*, 13(5), 747–757.

Duchek, J. M., Carr, D. B., Hunt, L, Roe, C. M., Xiong, C., Shah, K., & Morris, J. C. (2003). Longitudinal driving performance in early-stage dementia of the Alzheimer type. *Journal of the American Geriatric Society*, 51, 1342–1347.

Dunn, L. B., Nowrangi, M. B., Palmer, B. W., Jeste, D. V., & Saks, E. R. (2006). Assessing decisional capacity for clinical research or treatment: A review of instruments. *American Journal of Psychiatry*, 163, 1323–1334.

Emerson, J. L., Johnson, A. N., Dawson, J. D., Uc, E. Y., Anderson, S. W., & Rizzo, M. (2012). Predictors of driving outcomes in advancing age. *Psychology and Aging*, 27(3), 550–559.

Freund, B., Gravenstein, S., Ferris, B. S., Burke, B. L., & Shaheen, B. S. (2005). Drawing clocks and driving cars: Use of brief tests of cognition to screen driving competency in older adults. *Journal of General Internal Medicine*, 20, 240–244.

Grisso, T., & Appelbaum, P. S. (1998). MacArthur Competence Assessment Tool for Treatment (MacCAT- T). Sarasota, FL: Professional Resource Press.

Gutheil, T. G. (2007). Common pitfalls in the evaluation of testamentary capacity. *Journal of the American Academy of Psychiatry in Law*, 35, 514–517.

Kay, L. G., Bundy, A. C., & Clemson, L. M. (2009). Validity, reliability and predictive accuracy of the driving awareness questionnaire. *Disability and Rehabilitation*, 31, 1074–1082.

Marshall, G. A., Rentz, D. M., Frey, M. T., Locascio, J. J., Johnson, K. A., & Sperling, R. A. (2011). Executive function and instrumental activities of daily living in mild cognitive impairment and Alzheimer's disease. *Alzheimers and Dementia*, 7(3), 300–308.

Martin, R., Griffith, H. R., Belue, K., Harrell, L., Zamrini, E., Anderson, B.,...Marson, D. (2008). Declining financial capacity in patients with mild Alzheimer disease: A one year longitudinal study. *American Journal of Geriatric Psychiatry, 16*, 209–219.

Mertens, B., & Sorenson, S. B. (2012). Current considerations about the elderly and firearms. *American Journal of Public Health, 103*(3), 396–400.

Ott, B. R., Festa, E. K., Amick, M. M., Grace, J., Davis, J. D., & Heindel, W. C. (2008). Computerized maze navigation and on-road performance by drivers with dementia. *Journal of Geriatric Psychiatry Neurology, 21*(1), 18–25.

Royall, D. R., Mahurin, R. K., & Gray, K. (1992). Bedside assessment of executive dyscontrol: The Executive Interview (EXIT25). *Journal of the American Geriatric Society, 40*, 1221–1226.

Royall, D. R., Palmer, R., Chiodo, L. K., & Polk, M. J. (2004). Declining executive control in normal aging predicts change in functional status: The Freedom House study. *Journal of the American Geriatric Society, 52*, 346–352.

Rubin, G. S., Ng, E. S. W., Bandeen-Roche, K., Keyl, P. M., Freeman, E. E., & West, S. K. (2007). A prospective population-based study of the role of visual impairment in motor vehicle crashes among older drivers: The SEE study. *Investigations in Ophthalmology and Visual Science, 48*, 1483–1491.

Spangenberg, K. B., Wagner, M. T., Hendrix, S., & Bachman, D. L. (1999). Firearm presence in households of patients with Alzheimer's disease and related dementias. *Journal of the American Geriatric Society, 47*(10), 1183–1186.

Vaughan, L., & Giovanello, K. (2010). Executive function in daily life: Age-related influences of executive processes on instrumental activities of daily living. *Psychology and Aging, 25*(2), 343–355.

Williamson, C., Alcantar, O., Rothlind, J., Cahn-Weiner, D., Miller, B. L., & Rosen, H. J. (2010). Standardized measurements of self-awareness deficits in FTD and AD. *Journal of Neurology, Neurosurgery and Psychiatry, 81*(2), 140–145.

Index

Note: Page numbers followed by "f" and "t" indicate figures and tables.

abstract attitude, 72
abulia, 300, 521
acalculia, 50, 262, 345, 361
acetylcholine, 88
acquired immune deficiency syndrome (AIDS), 148, 313–314
acquired leukodystrophies, 327–331
action-intentional disorders, 126–127
activa interpolation models, 19
active immunotherapy, 566–568
Activities of Daily Living Questionnaire (ADLQ), 492
acute disseminated encephalomyelitis (ADEM), 328
acute disseminated encephalopathy, 318
acute intermittent porphyria, 306
AD8, 472–473
Adams, R.D., 145, 342–343
Addenbrooke's Cognitive Examination, Revised (ACE-R), 186, 477t, 482
AD Lewy body variant (ADLBV), 156
adult-onset leukodystrophy with neuroaxonal spheroids (AOLNAS), 331–332
aerobic exercise
 Alzheimer's Disease (AD), 570–571
 mild cognitive impairment (MCI), 443
affect, 83, 344
affective dysregulation, 58
aggression, 575–583
 about, 575–576
 antidepressants, 583
 chronic traumatic encephalopathy (CTE), 162
 frontotemporal dementia, 226

Langerhans Cell Histiocytosis (LCH), 339
Niemann-Pick Disease Type C, 340
paramedian artery infarction, 50
pharmacological treatment of, 579t
vascular dementias, 521
aging, 364
agitation, 575–583
 about, 575–576
 Alzheimer's disease and dementia, 361
 antidepressants, 583
 frontotemporal dementia, 226
 neuropsychiatric symptoms, 516–517
 Niemann-Pick Disease Type C, 340
 paramedian artery infarction, 50
 pharmacological treatment of, 579t
 prevalence of, 517f
 vascular dementias, 521
agoraphobia, 339
agraphia, 208–210, 262, 345
akinesia, 126
akinetic mutism
 delayed posthypoxic leukoencephalopathy, 328
 paramedian artery infarction, 50
alcohol, 303
alertness, variation in, 237
Alexander, G.E., 73, 74f
Alexander, M.P., 82
alexia, 208–211, 381
alien limb phenomena
 corticobasal degeneration (CBD), 225
 PSP-CBS (Progressive Supranuclear Palsy-Corticobasal Syndrome), 223

Alper, T., 320
alpha-7 nicotinic acetylcholine receptor agonist, 569
alpha-synuclein gene, 232, 236
alpha-synuclein-positive Lewy bodies (LBs), 168
Alzheimer, A., 176, 177, 508, 600
Alzheimer's Association, 191, 440, 442, 544, 610
Alzheimer's Dementia. *See* Alzheimer's disease and dementia
Alzheimer's Disease (AD)
    about, 151*f*, 448–449
    active immunotherapy, 566–568
    aerobic physical exercise, 570–571
    alpha-7 nicotinic acetylcholine receptor agonist, 569
    amygdala in, 149
    associated with cognitive disorders and ideomotor apraxia, 135
    Behavioral Variant Frontotemporal Dementia and, 90–91
    beta-secretase inhibitors, 564–565
    biomarker evidence, 452–453
    biomarker model, 450–452, 451*f*
    cholinesterase inhibitors for, 89
    chronic traumatic encephalopathy (CTE) and, 165–168
    compared with episodic memory, 115–116
    conceptual apraxia and, 129
    conceptual framework, 453–454
    detecting early, 449, 454–455
    ELND005, 565–566
    evidence-based medication therapeutics by stage of, 413–415
    5-hydroxytryptamine-6 receptor antagonists, 569
    gamma-secretase inhibitors and modulators, 565
    insulin, 570
    interaction with cerebrovascular disease, 266–267
    molecular imaging in, 539–542
    nerve growth factor, 569–570
    neuroimaging in, 531
    neuropathology of, 153
    neuropsychiatric symptoms, 518–520, 519*f*
    passive immunotherapy, 566–568
    pathophysiological sequence of, 449–450
    preclinical, 448–455
    p-tau pathology of, 166*f*
    tau immunotherapy, 568–569
Alzheimer's disease and dementia, 360–423
    about, 360–363
    Amyloid Cascade Hypothesis of Alzheimer's Disease, 366–368
    best practices and recommendations, 415–422
    biomarkers in clinical practice, 388–389
    characteristic symptoms and signs, 371, 372*t*
    clinical features, 370–375
    cognitive aging and changes in, 370–371
    cognitive testing, 390
    criteria incorporating biomarkers, 383*t*
    customizing care to the patient-caregiver dyad, 390–391
    deterministic Alzheimer's disease mutations, 369
    diagnosis, 377–384
    educational, work, and social history, 386
    environmental modification, 394–395
    epidemiology, 363–366
    etiology, 366–370, 367–368*f*
    evaluating, 384–390
    executive functions, concentration, judgment, reasoning, and insight, 373–374
    family history, 386
    genetics, 366–370
    history of present illness, 384–385
    hobbies, community activities, and health-related habits, 386
    laboratory studies, 388
    long-term treatment expectations, 391–392
    management of, 390–392, 391*t*, 395–415
    medication and supplement history, 386
    memory function, 371–373
    mild Alzheimer's disease *versus* normal cognitive aging, 370
    mortality from, 361*t*
    multitiered testing in, 389*t*
    neuropathology, 375–377
    neuropsychological features, 497
    nonpharmacological interventions and behavioral coping strategies, 392–395
    past medical history, 385–386
    personality, mood, motivation, behavior, and neuropsychiatric symptoms, 374–375
    pharmacological management, 395–415
    prevalence of, 364–365
    review of cognitive, functional, and neuropsychiatric domains, 385
    review of safety and well-being, 386–387
    review of system, 385
    risk factors, 363*t*
    Souvenaid, 416–417
    spatial and temporal orientation, 374
    susceptibility Alzheimer's disease mutations, 369–370
    2010 IWG-Dubois New Lexicon Criteria, 377, 378–379*f*
    2011 NIA-AA Criteria, 379–384, 380*t*, 381*t*
    2013 *DSM-5* Criteria, 377–379

two-hit vascular hypothesis of Alzheimer's
    Disease, 368–369
two-stage amyloid-dependent and
    amyloid-independent hypothesis of
    Alzheimer's disease, 368
visuospatial function, 374
vitamins, 416–417
word finding and language, 374
Alzheimer's Disease Cooperative Study
    (ADCS), 239
Alzheimer's Disease International (ADI), 364
Alzheimer's Disease Neuroimaging Initiative
    (ADNI), 437, 452
Alzheimer's Prevention Initiative (API), 454
amantadine, 250
American Academy of Neurology, 550
American Psychiatric Association, 177
AMNART, 491
amnesia, 48, 110, 115, 184, 248, 262, 293, 304,
    306, 332, 488, 492, 497, 602
amnestic syndrome, 50
amoxicillin, 316
amyloid beta, 236
Amyloid Cascade Hypothesis of Alzheimer's
    Disease, 366–368
amyloid hypothesis, 564
Amyloid Imaging Task (AIT) Force, 544
Amyloid PET Imaging
    as AD biomarkers, 383
    approved in evaluation of dementia, 544
    Dementia with Lewy Bodies (DLB), 236
    FDG-PET versus, 542–545, 545t
    with Pittsburg B compound, 213
    for understanding role of cerebrovascular
        disease in VCI, 265
    using for identification of AD pathology, 203
AN-1792, 566
Anderson, M.C., 83
anemia, 323
Angelucci, F., 581
anomia, 48, 60, 67, 135, 226, 492
anorexia
    dementia with Lewy bodies (DLB), 239
    Langerhans Cell Histiocytosis (LCH), 339
anoxic anoxia, 327
anterior cingulate cortex (ACC), 80–81, 86, 566
anterior commissure (AC), 39–40
anterior limb of the internal capsule (ICa), 40
anterograde amnesia, 115–116
anticonvulsants, 583
antidementia medications, 397–398
antidepressants, 387t, 583
antihistamines, 387t
antimuscarinics, 387t
antiparkinson agents, 387t

antipsychotics
    about, 396
    avoiding, 387t
    BPSDs, 578–580
    dementia with Lewy bodies (DLB), 239
    for treatment of severe and refractory
        agitation, aggression, and psychosis, 418
anxiety
    Alzheimer's disease and dementia, 361
    Creutzfeldt-Jakob Disease (CJD), 321
    dementia with Lewy bodies (DLB), 233, 239
    frontotemporal dementia, 226
    limbic encephalitis, 307
    neuropsychiatric symptoms, 514, 516
    prevalence of, 516f
    Sagging Brain Syndrome (SBS), 344
apathy, 588–596
    about, 588
    cerebellar cognitive affective syndrome
        (CCAS), 335
    dementia with Lewy bodies (DLB), 239
    depressive symptoms, 588–591
    diagnostic criteria, 515t
    frontotemporal dementia, 226
    frontotemporal lobar degeneration (FTLD),
        182
    Herpes Simplex Encephalitis, 306
    meningoencephalitis, 315
    neuropsychiatric symptoms, 513–514
    neurosyphilis, 315
    paramedian artery infarction, 50
    Parkinson's Disease Dementia (PD-D), 245
    relationship with cerebral substrate, 510t
    Sagging Brain Syndrome (SBS), 344
    Susac Syndrome, 327
    tuberothalamic artery infarction, 48, 50
    vascular dementias, 521
    Wilson's Disease, 345
Aphasia
    Frontotemporal Lobar Degeneration (FTLD),
        180, 185
    Ideomotor Apraxia, 131, 132
    polycystic lipomembranous osteodysplasia
        with sclerosing leukoencephalopathy
        (PLO-SL), 345
    posterior cortical atrophy (PCA), 208
    primary progressive aphasia (PPA), 198–204,
        536
    PSP-CBS (Corticobasal Syndrome), 223
    Sagging Brain Syndrome (SBS), 344
Aphasia Quotient, 201
APOE polymorphisms, 232
apolipoprotein E *(APOE)* gene, 170–171, 213,
    276, 548
apperceptive agnosia, 8

APP gene
   Alzheimer's disease and dementia, 375
   cerebral amyloid angiopathy (CAA), 277
apraxia
   corticobasal degeneration (CBD), 225
   defined, 471
   motor programming disorders, 126–139
   polycystic lipomembranous osteodysplasia with sclerosing leukoencephalopathy (PLO-SL), 345
   tuberothalamic artery infarction, 48, 50
   unilateral dominand hand apraxia, 190
apraxic disorders, 127–128
arcuate fasciculus (AF), 36, 37*f*
Argyll-Robertson pupil, 314, 315
Aristotle, 11
arousal
   decreased, 327
   disturbances, 50
   qualitative evaluation by, 463–464
arthralgias, 316
ascending arousal system, 84
ascending reticular activating system (ARAS), 84
aseptic meningitis, 317
Asimakopulos, J., 630
association cortex projections, 55
association fibers, 32–33, 33*f*
association fiber tracts, 35–38
Association for FTD, 191
associative agnosia, 8
associative thalamic nuclei, 47–48
asymbolia, 131
asymmetrical levodopa-nonresponsive parkinsonism, 225
asymmetrical pyramidal signs, 199
asymmetric bradykinesia, 223
ataxia
   cognition in the, 336–337
   Creutzfeldt-Jakob Disease (CJD), 320, 321
   delayed posthypoxic leukoencephalopathy, 329
   intravascular lymphoma, 323
   subacute sclerosing panencephalitis (SSPE), 323
atomoxetine, 251
Atri, A., 360–431, 461–486
attention, qualitative evaluation by, 464–465
attentional biasing, 78
attention disturbances, 60*t*, 77–78, 162, 222, 237, 339, 345
Attention-Memory-Concentration subscale, 410
Australian Imaging, Biomarker & Lifestyle Flagship Study of Ageing (AIBL), 452
autism spectrum, 60*t*

autonomic dysfunction, 60, 234, 238
autonomic features
   dementia with Lewy bodies (DLB), 233–234
   Parkinson's Disease Dementia (PD-D), 245
autonomic simple classical conditioning, 109*t*
axonal injury
   chronic traumatic encephalopathy (CTE), 167
   mild traumatic brain injury, 162

Baddeley, A.D., 72
Balint's syndrome, 208
ballooned neurons (Pick cells), 151
bapineuzumab, 566–567
barbituates, 387*t*
Barkley, R.A., 73
Barrett, A.M., 134
basal ganglia
   clinical features of basal ganglia lesions, 42–44
   connectional neuroanatomy of, 42
   thalamus and, 134–135
Basso, A., 134
Bastos-Leite, A.J., 264
Beers Criteria, 422
BEHAVE-AD, 521
behavioral and psychological symptoms of dementia (BPSDs)
   about, 575–576, 588
   anticonvulsants, 583
   antidepressants, 387*t*, 583
   antipsychotics, 578–580
   best practices, 581–582
   cholinesterase inhibitors, 582
   memantine, 582–583
   pharmacogenetics, 581
   pharmacological treatments, 577
   safety, 580–581
   treatment, 576–577
Behavioral Assessment of Dysexecutive Syndromes (BADS), 92–93
behavioral-cognitive syndromes, categories of, 42
behavioral control test, 94
behavioral disturbances, 603*t*
   Alzheimer's disease and dementia, 374–375
   delayed posthypoxic leukoencephalopathy, 328
   dementia with Lewy bodies (DLB), 233
   Frontotemporal dementia, 182–184
   metachromatic leukodystrophy (MLD), 332
   multiple sclerosis, 299
   Parkinson's Disease Dementia (PD-D), 245
   Primary progressive aphasia, 185
   PSP-RS (Richardson's Syndrome), 223
   Susac Syndrome, 327

behavioral neurology of subcortical systems, neuroanatomy and. *See* neuroanatomy and behavioral neurology of subcortical systems
behavioral variant frontotemporal dementia, 90–91, 181–184, 498
Benson, F., 208
Benson Complex Figure Test, 498–499
benzodiazepines, 387*t*
best practices
    Alzheimer's disease and dementia, 415–422
    BPSDs, 581–582
beta-amyloid, 568
beta-secretase inhibitors, 564–565
bexarotene, 568
Bianchi, L., 71–72
binding, 21–23
binge eating, 339
Binswanger disease, 148, 298
biomarkers
    Alzheimer's disease, 383, 388
    combined use of multiple, 549
    constructs, 529–531
    mild cognitive impairment (MCI), 439–440, 441*t*
    molecular imaging as, 541
    posterior cortical atrophy (PCA), 213–214
    role of, 550–551
    use of imaging and biofluid disease, 549–550
bipolar disorder, 340
Black, B., 594
Blessed Dementia Scale (BDS), 410, 491
Blessed Dementia Scale Information-Memory-Concentration (BDS-IMC), 476*t*, 481
blood oxygen level-dependent (BOLD) signal, 23–24, 55
Blumbergs, P.S.G., 162
body-part as tool errors (BPTEs), 130–131
Boston Criteria for Cerebral Amyloid Angiopathy, 277–279
Boston Diagnostic Aphasia Examination, 467, 498
Boston Naming Test (BNT), 201
bottom-up attention, 86
botulinum toxin injections, 224
Braak, H., 246
bradykinesia, 137, 328
brain, 150*f*, 152*f*, 155*f*
    biopsy of, 322
    diagram of, 117*f*
    health of during lifespan, 501–502
brain imaging
    about, 300–302
    cerebellar cognitive affective syndrome (CCAS), 337

    cerebellar related disorders with cognitive change and dementia, 333
    Dementia with Lewy Bodies (DLB), 237
    depression, 243
    focal lesions, 312
    genetic diseases, 333
    Gordon Holmes Syndrome, 338
    for initial evaluation of dementia, 388
    intravascular lymphoma, 323
    Langerhans Cell Histiocytosis, 339
    Marchiafava Bignami, 304
    mitochondrial encephalopathy with lactic acidosis and strooke-like episodes, 318–319
    normal pressure hydrocephalus, 341
    primary progressive aphasia, 198–199
    progressive multifocal leukoencephalopathy, 322
    vascular cognitive impairment, 267
    Wilson's disease, 345
brainstem, 149, 234
Brief Psychiatric Rating Scale, 583
brief psychosocial therapy (BPST), 576
Broca, P., 131
Broca's area, 28, 110
Brownwell-Oppenheimer variant, 321
buccofacial apraxia, 50
Buchman, A.S., 571
Bucks, R.S., 341
Bugiani, O., 180
bulimia, 339
Burgess, P.W., 93
butterfly gliomas, 311

C9ORF72 gene, 180–181
Cache County Study, 232
CAMCOG-R, 244
CamPaign study, 245
cardiopulmonary disease, 592
caregivers and caregiving
    about, 421
    benefits of, 612
    checklist for, 616*t*
    cultural differences, 612–614
    family, 611
    support for, 614
    time, 410, 609–611
cataplexy, 340
catatonia, 315
categories
    about, 4–5, 28n1
    differential diagnosis by , 294–295*t*
    relationship with concepts and word meanings, 10–12
    of visually presented objects, 5–12
caudate head lesions, 42

cefuroxime, 316
Center for Medicare and Medicaid Services (CMS), 437, 601
central nervous system vasculitis, 316–318
centromedian (CM) nucleus, 44
CERAD classification scheme, 376
CERE -108, 569–570
cerebellar ataxia, 339
cerebellar cognitive affective syndrome (CCAS), 60, 333–335
cerebellar infarction, 59f
cerebellar motor syndrome of gait ataxia, appendicular dysmetria, dysarthric speech, and oculomotor abnormalities, 58
cerebellar related disorders with cognitive change and dementia, 333
cerebellum
  about, 53, 55
  clinical features of cerebellar lesions, 58–61
  connectional neuroanatomy of the, 55–58
  neuropsychiatric manifestations in cerebellar disorders, 60t
  projections from, 56f
cerebral amyloid angiopathy (CAA), 274–282
  about, 274
  Boston Criteria for diagnosis of, 277t
  clinicopathologic correlation in diagnosis of, 278t
  cognitive impairment and, 279–281
  diagnosis, 277–279
  epidemiology, 274
  genetics, 276–277
  pathologic appearance of, 275f
  pathophysiology, 274–276
  potential emerging techniques for detection of, 279
  therapy considerations and future directions, 281–282
cerebral atrophy, 149
cerebral autosomal dominant arteriopathy with subcortical infarcts and leukoencephalopathy (CADASIL), 262–263, 263f
cerebral cortex
  about, 39, 41, 112f, 602
  Alzheimer's Disease, 379t, 533
  anatomic connections with, 42, 44, 55
  cerebellar cognitive affective syndrome (CCAS), 336
  cerebellar lesions, 58, 60
  cerebral amyloid angiopathy (CAA), 275
  cognitive functions and, 3–28
  connection with subcortical areas, 32, 33f
  Creutzfeldt-Jakob Disease (CJD), 322
  degeneration of, 147–148

delayed posthypoxic leukoencephalopathy, 329
Dementia with Lewy Bodies (DLB), 234
5-Hydroxytriptamine-6 Receptor Antagonists, 569
Ideomotor Apraxia (IMA), 131
mitochondrial encephalopathy with lactic acidosis and stroke-like episodes, 319
multiple sclerosis (MS), 326
Parkinson's Disease Dementia, 246
quantitative magnetic resonance imaging mewasurements of, 534
cerebral hemispheres, 32–42
cerebral white matter, 32, 147, 148, 162, 168f, 301–302t, 318, 324f, 325–330, 327f, 329f, 338, 339, 345
cerebrospinal fluid (CSF) biomarkers, 528–551, 546f
  about, 528–529, 545–546
  acute disseminated encephalopathy, 318
  cerebral amyloid angiopathy (CAA), 279
  dementia with Lewy bodies (DLB), 236–237
  frontotemporal lobar degeneration (FTLD), 187
  mild cognitive impairment (MCI), 438–439
  Parkinson's Disease Dementia (PD-D), 248
  posterior cortical atrophy (PCA), 213–214
  rapid onset of late-life neurodegenerative disorders, 346
  Sagging Brain Syndrome (SBS), 344
  subacute sclerosing panencephalitis (SSPE), 323
cerebrovascular disease, 41, 116, 137, 147, 187, 237t, 243t, 249, 260–262, 261t, 265–269, 280, 296, 316, 369, 381t, 382, 531, 534, 537
change blindness, 13
Charles Bonnet syndrome, 297
chemo-brain, 330
chemo-fog, 330
Chicago Health and Aging Project (CHAP), 364
childlike behavior, 335
chloral hydrate, 387t
cholinergic deficit, 235
cholinesterase inhibitors
  about, 249–250
  Alzheimer's Disease, 89, 541
  Alzheimer's disease (AD), 363
  BPSDs, 582
  combination therapy with memantine and, 402, 593, 595
  dementia with Lewy bodies (DLB), 239–240
  mechanisms of action, 404
  pharmacological management, 397–398, 398–400, 399t
  posterior cortical atrophy (PCA), 214

primary progressive aphasia (PPA), 204
sleep disturbances, 518
tolerance of, 591
for treating memory disortions, 116
Chong, J.Y., 310
chorea, 53
chronic traumatic encephalopathy (CTE), 160–172
  about, 160, 162–163
  acute mild traumatic brain injury, 160–162
  Alzheimer's Disease and, 167–168
  axonal injury, 162, 167
  axonal pathology of, 168f
  clinical diagnosis of, 170
  comorbidities and, 167–169
  compared with Alzheimer's Disease, 165–167
  concussion, 160–162
  criteria for pathological diagnosis of, 163–165
  frontotemporal lobar degeneration and, 168–169
  genetic risk for, 170–171
  guidelines for prevention and treatment of, 171
  hyperphosphorylated tau pathology, 164t, 165
  Lewy Body Disease and, 168
  microscopic pathology, 163–167
  motor neuron disease, 169
  neuropathology of, 163
  pathogenic mechanisms of, 169–170
  phosphorylated TDP43 pathology of, 167f
  postconcussion, 160–162
  p-tau pathology of, 166f
  stages of, 165f
  subconcussion, 160–162
  TDP-43 pathology in, 167
cingulum bundle (CB), 37, 38, 39f
citalopram, 595
claustrophobia, 339
Clinical Dementia Rating Scale (CDR), 472, 491
clinical features
  Alzheimer's disease and dementia, 370–375
  chronic traumatic encephalopathy (CTE), 170
  corticobasal degeneration (CBD), 225–226
  dementia with Lewy bodies (DLB), 233–234
  differential diagnosis, 292–293
  frontotemporal dementia (FTD), 189
  of frontotemporal lobar degeneration (FTLD), 181
  mild cognitive impairment (MCI), 433–435
  Parkinson's Disease Dementia (PD-D), 242–247, 243t
  posterior cortical atrophy (PCA), 208–212
  progressive supranuclear palsy (PSP), 221–223

vascular cognitive impairment (VCI), 262–263
vascular dementia (VaD), 262–263
Clinical Global Impression of change (CGIC), 239, 582
Clinical Global Improvement, 583
Clock Drawing Test (CDT), 475, 476t, 477, 625, 631
clomipramine, 595
clonazepam
  corticobasal degeneration (CBD), 227
  Parkinson's Disease Dementia (PD-D), 251
CNS hypomyelination, 333
cocaine use, 331
Cochrane meta-analysis, 250
cognition
  about, 15–16
  in the ataxias, 336–337
  effects on domains of, 410
  rate of decline of, 623
  See also cognitive features
  See also cognitive functions
cognitive aging, executive control and, 89–90
cognitive deficits
  Alzheimer's disease and dementia, 361
  cerebral amyloid angiopathy (CAA) and. See cerebral amyloid angiopathy (CAA)
  corticobasal degeneration (CBD), 225
  differential diagnosis, 326, 489f
  fragile X-associated tremor ataxia syndrome (FXTAS), 337
  meningoencephalitis, 315
  Niemann-Pick Disease Type C, 339–340
  vascular dementias, 521
  Whipple's Disease (WD), 325
cognitive domains, interactions of different, 15
cognitive features
  about, 79
  Alzheimer's disease (AD), 371, 450f
  cerebral amyloid angiopathy (CAA), 280
  delayed posthypoxic leukoencephalopathy, 329
  Dementia, 261t
  Dementia with Lewy Bodies (DLB), 233, 239
  late-life neurodegenerative disorders, 345
  Lyme Encephalopathy, 316
  Parkinson's Disease (PD), 243t, 250
  Parkinson's Disease Dementia (PD-D), 242–244, 243t, 244t
  primary progressive aphasia (PPA), 198
  PSP-RS (Richardson's Syndrome), 221–222
  vascular cognitive impairment, 264, 265
  white matter dementia (WMD), 326
  See also cognitive functions
cognitive flexibility disturbances, 332

cognitive functions
　about, 3–5, 87, 115, 121, 365
　Addenbrooke's Cognitive Examination, Revised (ACE-R) 482
　aerobic physical exercise for, 570–571
　age-related declines in, 371
　Blessed Dementia Scale Information-Memory-Concentration, 481
　categorization of visually presented objects, 5–12
　cerebral cortex and, 3–28
　citalopram, 418
　cognition, 15–16
　control processes, 12–15
　evaluating, 291–347
　Functional Assessment Questionnaire (FAQ), 472
　General Practitioner Assessment of Cognition, 478
　incontinence, 421
　interactions of different cognitive domains, 15
　mental status examination, 461, 469, 480
　metacognition and awareness of, 672
　mild cognitive impairment, 413, 497
　neuropsychological testing and, 434–435
　perceptual identification of visually presented objects, 5–12
　persistence in antidementia therapy and, 415
　recognition of visually presented objects, 5–12
　regional functional specialization for, 26–28
　sleep deprivation, 341
　test instruments and screening tools, 475
　See also cognitive features
cognitive neuroscience, contributions of primary progressive aphasia (PPA) to, 203–204
cognitive systems, 27, 27f
Cohen, J.D., 79
Cohen-Mansfield, J., 576
Cohen-Mansfield Agitation Inventory, 577
color constancy, 6, 6f
coma, 344
combination antoretroviral therapy (CART)
　AIDS and HIV, 313
　progressive multifocal leukoencephalopathy (PML), 322
combination treatment
　mechanisms of action, 404
　safety and tolerability of, 411–413
commissural fibers, 39–40
Committee for Medicinal Products for Human Use, 544
communication, clarity in, 624–625

comorbidities, chronic traumatic encephalopathy (CTE) and, 167–169
compensation-related utilization of neural circuits hypothesis (CRUNCH), 89–90
competency, 517–518, 624
comprehension, impaired, 48
compulsive behavior, 183
computed tomography (CT), 212
concentration disturbances
　Alzheimer's disease and dementia, 373–374
　chronic traumatic encephalopathy (CTE), 162
　Creutzfeldt-Jakob Disease (CJD), 320
　meningoencephalitis, 315
　polycystic lipomembranous osteodysplasia with sclerosing leukoencephalopathy (PLO-SL), 345
　Susac Syndrome, 327
concepts
　activation of, 24–25
　relationship with categories and word meanings, 10–12
conceptual apraxia, 128–129
conceptual priming, 109t
concomitant amyloid plaques, 235
concussion, 160–162
confusion
　delayed posthypoxic leukoencephalopathy, 328
　Herpes Simplex Encephalitis, 306
　intravascular lymphoma, 323
　limbic encephalitis, 307
　Niemann-Pick Disease Type C, 340
　in paramedian artery infarction, 50
　Sagging Brain Syndrome (SBS), 344
　sarcoidosis, 317
　Susac Syndrome, 327
　with thalamic lesions, 48
congestive attacks, 315
Connor, C.E., 17
consciousness, fluctuating levels of
　dementia with Lewy bodies (DLB), 233
　with tuberothalamic artery infarction, 48, 50
consequences, anticipating, 78–81
consolidation, 111–112
Consortium to establish a registry for Alzheimer's disease (CERAD) criteria, 235, 477
constipation
　dementia with Lewy bodies (DLB), 238
　Parkinson's Disease Dementia (PD-D), 245
continuous perseveration, 126
control processes, 12–15
convexity premotor cortex, 134
cord fiber system, 39–41
cord of fibers, 32, 33–34, 33f

Cordonnier, C., 280
corpus callosum (CC), 39–40
cortical and basal ganglia dysfunction, 225
cortical blindness
    adult-onset leukodystrophy with
        neuroaxonal spheroids (AOLNAS), 332
    delayed posthypoxic leukoencephalopathy,
        328
    subacute sclerosing panencephalitis (SSPE),
        323
    X-linked adrenoleukodystrophy, 299
cortical inputs, 73–74
cortical organization, models of, 25–26
cortical sensory deficit
    corticobasal degeneration (CBD), 225
    PSP-CBS (Corticobasal Syndrome), 223
corticobasal degeneration (CBD), 220–227
    about, 220, 225
    associated with cognitive disorders and
        ideomotor apraxia, 136
    associated with limb-kinetic apraxia
        associated with cognitive disorders, 137
    characterizations of, 297
    clinical features, 225–226
    clinical phenotypes associated with, 226t
    diagnostic criteria for, 227t
    neuropathology, 226
    therapeutics, 226–227
corticosteroids
    acute disseminated encephalopathy, 318
    MELAS, 319
corticostriatal fibers, 33
Craik O'Brien Cornsweet (COC) figure, 19, 20f
cranial irradiation, 330
cranial mononeuropathies, 316
crenezumab, 567
Creutzfeldt-Jakob Disease (CJD), 149, 152, 214,
    292, 292t, 320–322
Critchley, M., 160
Crucian, G.P., 127
cryptococcal meningitis, 315

Damasio, A.R., 25
Debette, S., 267
decision making, poor, 345
declarative learning, 337
default-mode network, 17, 85, 85f
defective response inhibition, 126–127
deficits in emotional expression, 58
degenerative diseases, 146f
Dejerine, J., 50, 198
delayed complex hyperkinetic motor syndrome
    with ataxia, 52
delayed posthypoxic leukoencephalopathy,
    327–331

Delis-Kaplan Executive Function System
    (DKEFS), 92–93
delusional misidentification syndromes, 519t
delusions
    Alzheimer's disease and dementia, 361
    dementia with Lewy bodies (DLB), 233, 239
    neuropsychiatric symptoms, 514
    Parkinson's Disease Dementia (PD-D), 245
dementia
    definitions and diagnosis of, 488
    differential diagnosis, 489f
    from diseases affecting cerebral white matter,
        325–333
    driving and, 629–632
    end-of-life planning and, 634–635
    executive control and, 90–92
    financial management and, 628–629
    firearm safety and, 633–634
    improving memory in, 120–121
    laboratory evaluations for cause of, 347t
    metachromatic leukodystrophy (MLD), 332
    "normal aging" *versus*, 491t
    testing for, 493–494
    voting and, 633
    See also specific topics
Dementia Associated with Lewy Bodies (DLB),
    231–251
    about, 91, 231
    amygdala in, 149
    autonomic features, 233–234
    behavioral features, 233
    cerebrospinal fluid biomarkers, 236–237
    clinical features, 233–234
    cognitive features, 233
    criteria for clinical diagnosis of, 237t
    definitions of, 231
    diagnosis of, 237–238
    epidemiology of, 231–232
    genetics, 232–233
    management of patients with, 238–240
    motor features, 233–234
    neuroimaging features of, 235–236
    neuropathological and biochemical correlates
        of, 234–235
    neuropathology of, 154–156
dementia of the Alzheimer-type (DAT), 198
Dementia Rating Scale (DRS), 491
demyelinating diseases, 326–327
depression, 588–596
    about, 588
    Alzheimer's disease and dementia, 361
    cerebellar cognitive affective syndrome
        (CCAS), 334–335
    chronic traumatic encephalopathy (CTE), 162
    Creutzfeldt-Jakob Disease (CJD), 320, 321

depression (*Cont.*)
  delayed posthypoxic leukoencephalopathy, 329
  dementia with Lewy bodies (DLB), 233
  depressive symptoms, 588–591
  diagnostic criteria, 512*t*
  Langerhans Cell Histiocytosis (LCH), 339
  limbic encephalitis, 307
  meningoencephalitis, 315
  multiple sclerosis, 299
  neuropsychiatric symptoms, 509, 511, 513
  neurosyphilis, 314
  Niemann-Pick Disease Type C, 340
  relationship with cerebral substrate, 510*t*
  Sagging Brain Syndrome (SBS), 344
  vascular dementias, 521
  Wilson's Disease, 345
De Renzi, E., 137
D'Esposito, M., 79
deterministic Alzheimer's disease genetic mutations, 369
de Weerd, P., 17
dexterity, 332
diagnosis
  Alzheimer's disease and dementia, 377–384
  cerebral amyloid angiopathy (CAA), 277–279
  dementia with Lewy bodies (DLB), 237–238
  frontotemporal lobar degeneration (FTLD), 186–189
  Parkinson's Disease Dementia (PD-D), 248–249
  See also differential diagnosis
Diagnostic and Statistical Manual of Mental Disorders, 177
diagnostic criteria
  about, 177, 181–182, 184, 550
  Alzheimer's Disease (AD), 448
  Alzheimer's Disease Dementia, 497, 531
  apathy, 513, 515*t*
  BPSDs, 588
  Behavioral variant Frontotemporal Dementia, 182*t*
  Cerebral Amyloid Angiopathy (CAA), 277, 277*t*
  corticobasal degeneration (CBD), 227*t*
  corticobasal syndrome (CBS), 225
  Dementia with Lewy Bodies (DLB), 231–232
  depression, 511, 512*t*, 516
  frontotemporal lobar degeneration (FTD), 185, 186
  Mild Cognitive Impairment (MCI), 441, 441*t*, 542–543
  Parkinson's Disease Dementia (PD-D), 248, 248*t*
  posterior cortical atrophy (PCA), 211*t*
  primary progressive aphasia (PPA), 185, 199, 201*f*
  progressive supranuclear palsy (PSP), 220
  psychosis, 513*t*
  Vascular Dementia (VaD), 261–262
  Vascular Mild Cognitive Impairment (VaMCI), 265
differential diagnosis, 291–347
  about, 291
  acquired leukodystrophies, 327–331
  acute confusion *versus* dementia, 291–292
  acute disseminated encephalopathy, 318
  acute intermittent porphyria, 306
  AIDS and HIV, 313–314
  alcohol, 303
  brain imaging, 300–302
  by category and disease, 294–295*t*
  central nervous system vasculitis, 316–318
  cerebellar cognitive affective syndrome (CCAS), 333–335
  cerebellar related disorders with cognitive change and dementia, 333
  cerebral white matter disorders, 301–302*t*
  clinical approach, 292–293
  cognition in the ataxias, 336–337
  cognitive decline, 489*f*
  Creutzfeldt-Jakob Disease (CJD), 320–322
  cryptococcal meningitis, 315
  delayed posthypoxic leukoencephalopathy, 327–331
  dementia, 489*f*
  dementia from diseases affecting cerebral white matter, 325–333
  demyelinating diseases, 326–327
  diseases causing dementia, 302
  elementary neurological examination, 297–300
  epilepsy and dementia, 340–341
  examination, 296–300
  focal lesions, 311–312
  fragile X-associated tremor ataxia syndrome (FXTAS), 337–338
  general medical examination, 296–297
  genetic diseases, 331–333
  Gordon Holmes syndrome, 338
  Hashimoto Encephalopathy, 309–310
  Herpes Simplex Encephalitis, 306–307
  history, 293, 296
  intravascular lymphoma, 323
  Langerhans Cell Histiocytosis (LCH), 338–339
  limbic encephalitis, 307–309
  Lyme Encephalopathy, 315–316
  medications, 303
  meningoencephalitis, 315

mental state examination, 300
metabolic disorders, 302–306
mitochondrial encephalopathy with lactic acidosis and stroke-like episodes (MELAS), 318–319
multiple sclerosis, 326
neurocysticercosis, 315
neurodegeneration with brain iron accumulation (NBIA), 345
neurosyphilis, 314–315
Niemann-Pick Disease Type C, 339–340
normal pressure hydrocephalus (NPH), 341–343
obstruction to cerebrospinal fluid flow/cerebrospinal leak, 341–344
Pellagra, 304–305
polycystic lipomembranous osteodysplasia with sclerosing leukoencephalopathy (PLO-SL), 345
Prion Disease, 319–320
progressive multifocal leukoencephalopathy (PML), 322–323
rapidly progressive dementia, 306
rapid onset of late-life neurodegenerative disorders, 345–347
Sagging Brain Syndrome (SBS), 343–344
scope of problem, 292
sleep deprivation and cognition, 341
structural disease *versus* nonfocal or multifocal brain disease, 302
subacute sclerosing panencephalitis (SSPE), 323–324
superficial siderosis, 339
Susac Syndrome, 326–327
thiamine deficiency, 303–304
thyroid disorders, 305–306
trauma, 311
vascular diseases, 310–311
vitamin B12 deficiency, 305
vitamin E deficiency, 305
Whipple's Disease (WD), 324–325
Wilson's Disease, 344–345
See also diagnosis
diffuse axonal injury (DAI), 162
diffusion tensor imaging (DTI)
    chronic traumatic encephalopathy (CTE), 161
    dementia with Lewy bodies (DLB), 236
    posterior cortical atrophy (PCA), 212
diffusion-weighted imaging (DWI), 321
diplopia
    PSP-RS (Richardson's Syndrome), 222
    Sagging Brain Syndrome (SBS), 344
direct line feedforward hierarchical processing, 26
disconnection syndromes, 24

disinhibition
    Creutzfeldt-Jakob Disease (CJD), 320
    frontotemporal dementia, 182, 226
    vascular dementias, 521
disorganization, 340
disorientation
    limbic encephalitis, 307
    neurosyphilis, 314
    paramedian artery infarction, 50
    posterior cortical atrophy (PCA), 212
    Susac Syndrome, 327
    tuberothalamic artery infarction, 48, 50
distances, misjudging, 212
dizziness, 344
DJ-1 gene, 242
Dolder, C.R., 592
domains, qualitative evaluation by, 462–472, 470–471*t*
Dominantly Inherited Alzheimer Network (DIAN), 454, 549
donepezil, 89, 214, 239–240, 249–250, 264, 363, 392, 397–399, 403, 405*t*, 407–417, 412*f*, 413*t*, 417*t*, 419, 422, 443, 518, 551, 563, 569, 582, 593
dopamine, 87, 88, 235
dopamine transporter binding, 238
doppler ultrasound (TCD), 279
dorsal and midregions of putamen, lesions of, 42
dorsal attention network, 78*f*
dorsal nucleus, 44
doxycycline, 316
Drachman, D..A., 146
driving, dementia and, 629–632
DSM-5 (Diagnostic and Statistical Manual of Mental Disorders), 365
DSM-IV, 488
Dubois, B., 186
dysarthria
    Creutzfeldt-Jakob Disease (CJD), 321
    delayed posthypoxic leukoencephalopathy, 329
    intravascular lymphoma, 323
    Niemann-Pick Disease Type C, 339
    primary progressive aphasia (PPA), 199
    Progressive Nonfluent Aphasia (PNFA), 226
    PSP-RS (Richardson's Syndrome), 222
    Sagging Brain Syndrome (SBS), 344
    tuberothalamic artery infarction, 48, 50
    X-linked adrenoleukodystrophy, 299
dyscalculia, 199
    See also acalculia
dysexecutive syndromes, 81
dysphagia
    Niemann-Pick Disease Type C, 340
    PSP-RS (Richardson's Syndrome), 222
    Sagging Brain Syndrome (SBS), 344

dysphoria, 334
dystonia
  posterior choroidal artery infarction, 52–53
  PSP-CBS (Corticobasal Syndrome), 223
dystonic posturing of the limb, 225

eating behavior changes, 183
ecologically valid neuropsychological tests, 92–93
effector thalamic nuclei, 47
electroconvulsive therapy, 522
electroencephalography (EEG)
  Creutzfeldt-Jakob Disease (CJD), 321
  dementia with Lewy bodies (DLB), 236
  frontotemporal lobar degeneration (FTLD), 187
  Hashimoto's Encephalopathy (aka. Steroid Responsive Encephalopathy associated with Autoimmune Thyroiditis (SREAT)), 310
  subacute sclerosing panencephalitis (SSPE), 323
elementary neurological examination, 297–300
Elger, C.E., 340
ELND005, 565–566
emotional control, 60t, 83
emotional liability
  frontotemporal dementia, 226
  Wilson's Disease, 345
empathy, lack of, 183, 344
encephalopathy, 326, 327
end-of-life care, 606–607, 634–635
energization, 82
enlarged inclusion-bearing astrocytes, 338
environmental dependency syndrome, 127
epidemiology
  Alzheimer's disease and dementia, 363–366
  cerebral amyloid angiopathy (CAA), 274
  dementia with Lewy bodies (DLB), 231–232
  frontal temporal lobar degeneration (FTLD), 177
  frontotemporal dementia (FTD), 177
  mild cognitive impairment (MCI), 433
  Parkinson's Disease Dementia (PD-D), 240–242
epilepsy
  dementia and, 340–341
  neurosyphilis, 315
epilepticus, 323
episodic memory, 108–117, 109t, 111f, 114f, 115–116, 115f, 201, 266
erectile dysfunction, 337
erythema, 316
erythromycin, 316
etiology
  Alzheimer's disease and dementia, 366–370
  mild cognitive impairment (MCI), 435f
euphoria
  polycystic lipomembranous osteodysplasia with sclerosing leukoencephalopathy (PLO-SL), 345
  vascular dementias, 521
European Medicines Agency, 544
examination, differential diagnosis, 296–300
executive control, 71–94
  about, 71
  Alzheimer's disease and dementia, 373–374
  CCAS, 58
  chronic traumatic encephalopathy (CTE), 162
  clinical assessment of, 92–94
  cognitive aging and, 89–90
  competency and, 623
  contributions of neurotransmitter function to, 87–89
  dementias and, 90–92
  dementia with Lewy bodies (DLB), 233
  fragile X-associated tremor ataxia syndrome (FXTAS), 337
  frontal networks and, 73–75
  frontotemporal lobar degeneration (FTLD), 183–184
  goal-directed behaviors and, 75–87
  Gordon Holmes syndrome, 336
  historical perspective, 71–73
  mental competence and legal issues, 625–626
  Niemann-Pick Disease Type C, 340
  PSP-RS (Richardson's Syndrome), 221–222
  qualitative evaluation by, 465–466
  questionnaires, 92t
  rate of decline of, 623
  Sagging Brain Syndrome (SBS), 344
  Susac Syndrome, 327
  top-down modulation and, 79
  Wilson's Disease, 345
  X-linked adrenoleukodystrophy (X-ALD), 332
Executive Control Battery (ECB), 92–93
executive control network, 75, 75f
executive deficit (frontal aging) hypothesis, 89
explosivity, 162
external capsule, 38, 39
extrapyramidal signs, 199
extreme capsule (EmC), 36, 37f
eye movement abnormalities, 53, 225

Fabry's disease, 311
face recognition, 23–24
facial emotional recognition test, 94
facial paralysis, 316
Faglioni, P., 134

falls, repeated, 222, 234, 238
family role, 609–618
　about, 609
　family caregiver, 611
　family-centered care, 614–615
　individualized care plan, 615–617
　See also caregivers and caregiving
fatal familial insomnia, 320, 321–322
fatigue, 316
Faux Pas recognition test, 94
feature bundles, 13
feature integration theory (FIT), 22
feedforward hierarchical convergence models, 22
fever
　intravascular lymphoma, 323
　Lyme Encephalopathy, 316
　Whipple's Disease (WD), 324
Financial Capacity Instrument (FCI-9), 628
financial management, dementia and, 628–629
Findings on the Aging Services Network, 612
firearm safety, dementia and, 633–634
Fisher, C.M., 48, 145
5-hydroxytriptamine-6 receptor antagonists, 569
fixation of belief, 16
FLAIR imaging
　Creutzfeldt-Jakob Disease (CJD), 321
　delayed posthypoxic leukoencephalopathy, 328
　subacute sclerosing panencephalitis (SSPE), 324
Flechsig-Meyer loop, 41
fluctuation
　in cognitive function, 233, 237
　of competency, 624
fludeoxyglucose positron emission tomography (FDG-PET), 187*f*, 189, 190*f*, 213, 236, 370, 383, 383*t*, 388, 389*t*, 414, 437*f*, 438–442, 439*f*, 451*f*, 453, 510*t*, 530, 537, 540–544, 540*f*, 546, 547*f*, 551, 551*f*, 570
fluent and meaningless discourse, 48
fluoxetine, 590
fMRI, 161–162, 537–538
focal infarction, 52*t*
focal lesions, 311–312
focal sensory/motor deficit, 323
Fodor, J., 11
Fogassi, L., 137
forces, affecting behavior, 4
forgetfulness
　delayed posthypoxic leukoencephalopathy, 328
　neurosyphilis, 314
　PSP-RS (Richardson's Syndrome), 222
　Sagging Brain Syndrome (SBS), 344

formal neuropsychological testing, of patients, 92–94
Fox, N.C., 529
fractional anisotrophy (FA), 247
fragile X-associated tremor ataxia syndrome (FXTAS), 337–338
Franceschi, F., 198
Free and Cued Selective Reminding Test, 479
FreeSurfer, 437
Freund, H.J., 134, 137
Fries, P., 23
Frontal Assessment Battery (FAB), 92–93
Frontal Behavioral Inventory, 202, 226
frontal lobe, divisions of, 73*f*
frontal lobe syndrome, 72
frontal networks, 73–75
frontoinsular cortex (FI), 86
fronto-occipital fasciculus (FOF), 36, 38*f*
frontotemporal dementia (FTD), 116–117, 176–192, 226, 520
frontotemporal lobar degeneration (FTLD)
　about, 90–91
　behavioral variant frontotemporal dementia, 181–184
　chronic traumatic encephalopathy (CTE) and, 168–169
　clinical characteristics of, 181
　diagnostic assessment of suspected, 186–189
　epidemiology, 177
　genetics of, 179–181
　neuroimaging, 186–188
　neuropathology of, 154, 177–179
　pedigree diagram, 180*f*
　progressive aphasic subtypes of, 184–185
　treatment of, 189–192
functional and structural neuroanatomy, 202
Functional Assessment Questionnaire (FAQ), 472
Funkiewiez, A., 186
fusiform face area (FFA), 23–24

gait ataxia
　fragile X-associated tremor ataxia syndrome (FXTAS), 337
　Hashimoto's Encephalopathy (aka. Steroid Responsive Encephalopathy associated with Autoimmune Thyroiditis (SREAT)), 310
gait impairment
　adult-onset leukodystrophy with neuroaxonal spheroids (AOLNAS), 332
　delayed posthypoxic leukoencephalopathy, 328
　PSP-RS (Richardson's Syndrome), 222
　Sagging Brain Syndrome (SBS), 344

galactosyl ceramidase (GLAC), 332
galantamine, 417t
    apathy, 592
    Parkinson's Disease Dementia (PD-D), 250
    relationship with sleep disturbances, 518
gamma-secretase inhibitors and modulators, 565
gantenerumab, 567
Gazzaley, A., 79
Gebhardt, A., 137
general medical examination, 296–297
general paresis of the insane (GPI), 314
General Practitioner Assessment of Cognition
        (GPCOG), 473, 476t, 478
genetic diseases, 331–333
genetics and risk factors
    Alzheimer's disease and dementia, 366–370
    cerebral amyloid angiopathy (CAA), 276–277
    chronic traumatic encephalopathy (CTE),
        170–171
    dementia with Lewy bodies (DLB), 232–233
    frontotemporal lobar degeneration (FTLD),
        179–181
    Parkinson's Disease Dementia (PD-D), 242
    posterior cortical atrophy (PCA), 213
    primary progressive aphasia (PPA), 203
    progressive supranuclear palsy (PSP), 223
genetic testing, 528–551, 546–549
geons, 6–7, 9f
Geriatric Depression Scale, Short Form
        (GDS-SF), 474, 498
Gerstmann-Straussler-Scheinker syndrome
        (GSS), 320, 322
Gerstmann syndrome
    posterior cortical atrophy (PCA), 208
    primary progressive aphasia (PPA), 199
Geschwind, N., 24, 128, 132, 133
Gestalt laws, 7f, 8f, 23
Giovannetti, T., 138
Glasgow Coma Score, 161
gliosis, 234
Global Deterioration Scale, (GDS) 432
global dysphasia, 48
globoid cell leukodystrophy (GLD), 332–333
globus pallidus (GPi), 44
glucocorticoids, 310
glucoserebrosidase (GBA) mutations, 232
glutamate, 400–401
goal-directed behaviors
    executive control and, 75–87
    how changes in salience influence, 85–87
    See also executive control
goal execution, 75–83
    about, 75–76
    outcome/reward anticipation and
        monitoring, 78–82

response/behavioral selection, 82–83
working memory, 76–78
goal selection, 83–87
    about, 83–84
    ascending arousal system, 84
    how changes in salience influence
        goal-directed behaviors, 85–87
    representation of future and past, 85
    representations of the self, 84–85
Goebel, R., 17
Goldenberg, G., 135
Goldstein, K., 72
Goodglass, H., 129–130
Gordon Holmes syndrome, 336, 338
Gorelick, P.B., 265
Gray. C.M., 23
Griffith, J.S., 320
GRN mutations, 203
Grossberg, G.T., 415
Guam Parkinsonism-dementia complex, 169
GWAS (Genome Wide Association Study), 223

Haaland, K.Y., 133, 134
hallucinations
    Alzheimer's disease and dementia, 361
    dementia with Lewy bodies (DLB), 233, 235,
        237, 238–239
    limbic encephalitis, 307
    neuropsychiatric symptoms, 514
    Niemann-Pick Disease Type C, 340
    Parkinson's Disease Dementia (PD-D), 245
    with thalamic lesions, 48
    vascular dementias, 521
haloperidol, 578, 580
Halsband, U., 133
Hanna-Pladdy, B., 134–135, 136–137
headaches
    acute disseminated encephalopathy, 318
    central nervous system vasculitis, 317
    chronic traumatic encephalopathy (CTE), 162
    Lyme Encephalopathy, 316
    Susac Syndrome, 326
    systemic lupus erythematosus (SLE), 317–318
health care costs, reduction of, 410
Healthy Aging Brain Care Monitor
        (HABC-Monitor) Caregiver Assessment
        Tool, 617t
hearing loss
    Lyme Encephalopathy, 316
    Sagging Brain Syndrome (SBS), 344
    Susac Syndrome, 327
heated heroin vapor, 330
Hebert, L., 365
Hedley-Whyte, E.T., 145
Heilman, K.M., 129, 133, 136–137, 422

Helmstaedter, C., 340
hemianopsia, 299
hemiparesis
    inferolateral artery infarction, 50–52
    intravascular lymphoma, 323
hemispatial neglect, 50
Herpes Simplex Encephalitis, 306–307, 340
heterozygote mutations, 242
hierarchical structure, of concepts, 12
hippocampal commissures, 40
hippocampal shape, 534–535
hippocampus, 22, 44, 53, 88, 110–112, 111f, 112f, 115, 146–151, 150f, 153f, 164–167, 164t, 165f, 166f, 178f, 188f, 235, 247, 266, 307, 338, 360, 436f, 534, 537–538, 569, 570, 602
Hirano bodies and granulovacuolar degeneration, 150–151
historical perspective, 71–73
Hitch, G.J., 72
HIV, 313–314
HIV-associated neurocognitive disorders (HAND), 313
Hoehn and Yahr score, 92
Holl, A.K., 136
horizontal gaze, 223
Hotel Test, 93
hubs, 26
Hull, C.L., 83
Hummelsheim, H., 134, 137
"hummingbird sign," 224
Huntington's disease, 42, 136, 156–157, 297
hyperactivity, 340
hyperbaric oxygen treatment, 328
hyperphosphyorylated tau pathology in deep nuclei, 165
hypersomnolence, 50
hypokinesia, 126, 328
hypophonia
    PSP-PAGF (Pure Akinesia with Gait Freezing), 223
    tuberothalamic artery infarction, 48, 50
hypophonic dysarthria, 42
hypothalamic involvement, 325
hypothyroidism, 592

ideational apraxia, 137–138
ideomotor apraxia (IMA), 129–136
    corticobasal degeneration (CBD), 225
    primary progressive aphasia (PPA), 199
    PSP-CBS (Corticobasal Syndrome), 223
I-Ioflupane/SPECT binding, 224
Imai, H., 223
immobility, 328
impersistence, 126
implicit memory, 244

impulsivity
    neuropsychiatric symptoms, 516–517
    Wilson's Disease, 345
inappropriate social behaviors
    cerebellar cognitive affective syndrome (CCAS), 335
    paramedian artery infarction, 48
    Sagging Brain Syndrome (SBS), 344
inattention
    delayed posthypoxic leukoencephalopathy, 328
    tuberothalamic artery infarction, 48, 50
    X-linked adrenoleukodystrophy (X-ALD), 332
incident dementia
    MRI, 267–268
    vascular risk and, 267
incompetence, establishing, 625
incontinence, 328, 421
individualized care plan, 615–617
inferior longitudinal fasciculus, 36, 38f
inferior temporal gyrus (ITG), 23
inferolateral artery infarction, 50–52, 52t
information processing, slowed, 222, 337
inhibitory control, 83
inhibitory deficit hypothesis, 89
insensitivity, 361
insight impairments
    Alzheimer's disease and dementia, 373–374
    frontotemporal lobar degeneration (FTLD), 184
    neuropsychiatric symptoms, 517–518
    polycystic lipomembranous osteodysplasia with sclerosing leukoencephalopathy (PLO-SL), 345
insulin, 570
integrative agnosia, 10f
intellectual function
    fragile X-associated tremor ataxia syndrome (FXTAS), 337
    Langerhans Cell Histiocytosis (LCH), 339
    PSP-RS (Richardson's Syndrome), 221
internal capsule, 40
internal monitoring, 78–79
internal state, control of, 79
International Working Group (IWG), 365
interscapular pain, 344
intracranial pressure (ICP) monitoring, 342
intralaminar thalamic nuclei, 44
intravascular lymphoma, 323
intrinsic factors, role of, 16
intrinsic network, 75
intrinsic properties of cells, relationship with plasticity, 28n5
in vivo neuroimaging, of neuropathologic markers, 188–189

irritability
  Alzheimer's disease and dementia, 361
  frontotemporal dementia, 226
  Herpes Simplex Encephalitis, 306
  vascular dementias, 521

Jack, C.R., 438, 440–441, 450, 532–533
Jackson, J.H., 71
Jacob-Creutzfeldt disease, 203
Jagust, W., 540
Johnson, M.K., 84–85
joint pain, 316
judgment disturbances
  Alzheimer's disease and dementia, 373–374
  neuropsychiatric symptoms, 517–518
  neurosyphilis, 314, 315
  polycystic lipomembranous osteodysplasia with sclerosing leukoencephalopathy (PLO-SL), 345
  Wilson's Disease, 345
Judgment of Line Orientation, 202

Kantarci, K., 236
Kaplan, E., 129–130
Kluver Bucy syndrome, 183, 594–595
knowledge, impaired ability to manipulate acquired, 222
Korsakoff syndrome, 303–304
Krabbe's disease, 331–332
kuru, 320
Kuypers, H.G., 137

Langerhans Cell Histiocytosis (LCH), 338–339
language
  fragile X-associated tremor ataxia syndrome (FXTAS), 337
  Progressive Nonfluent Aphasia (PNFA), 226
  qualitative evaluation by, 466–467
lateral dorsal (LD) nucleus, 44
lateral geniculate nucleus (LGN), 44, 46
lateral posterior (LP) nucleus, 47
La Tercera Edad, 611
Launer, L.J., 267
Lawrence, D.G., 137
L-dopa-responsiveness
  dementia with Lewy bodies (DLB), 238
  Parkinson's Disease Dementia (PD-D), 245
  PSP-P (Parkinsonism), 223
legal issues. *See* mental competence and legal issues
Leiguardia, R.C., 135, 136, 138
leukodystrophies, 331
Levine, C., 610, 612
levodopa, 224
Lewy body, 155*f*

Lewy Body Dementia (LBD)
  neuropsychiatric symptoms, 520–521
  neuropsychological features, 498–499
Lewy Body Disease
  characterizations of, 297
  chronic traumatic encephalopathy (CTE) and, 168
Lewy neurites, 234
Lezak, M., 72
Lhermitte, F., 127
Lichtheim, L., 132
Liepmann, H., 128, 131, 132, 137–138
limb apraxia
  corticobasal degeneration (CBD), 225
  task specific *versus* general forms of, 127–128
  tuberothalamic artery infarction, 48, 50
limbic encephalitis, 307–309
limbic thalamic nuclei, 44
limb-kinetic apraxia, 136–137
linguistic processing, deficits in, 60, 339
listeria monocytogenes, 315
local feedback, 26
Logue, M.W., 264
longer term randomized controlled trials, 408–409
Loring, D.W., 136–137
Lucchelli, F., 137
lumbar drain, 342
lumbosacral polyradiculoneuropathy, 316
Lund-Manchester criteria, 182
Luria, A.R., 127
Luria motor sequencing test, 465–466, 466*f*, 625
Lyme disease, 298
Lyme Encephalopathy, 315–316
lymphocytic meningitis, 316

Maas, O., 131
MacArthur Competence Assessment Tool (MacCAT), 627
magnetic resonance imaging (MRI)
  cerebral cortex, 534
  clinical use, 535–537, 538–539
  Creutzfeldt-Jakob Disease (CJD), 321
  delayed posthypoxic leukoencephalopathy, 328, 329, 330, 331
  dementia with Lewy bodies (DLB), 235–236
  Hashimoto's Encephalopathy (aka. Steroid Responsive Encephalopathy associated with Autoimmune Thyroiditis (SREAT)), 310
  incident dementia, 267–268
  medial temporal lobe, 532–534
  mild cognitive impairment (MCI), 436–437, 436*f*
  perfusion, 538

posterior cortical atrophy (PCA), 212
progressive multifocal leukoencephalopathy (PML), 322
progressive supranuclear palsy (PSP), 224
rapid onset of late-life neurodegenerative disorders, 346
subacute sclerosing panencephalitis (SSPE), 324
Susac Syndrome, 327
vascular cognitive impairment (VCI), 264
X-linked adrenoleukodystrophy (X-ALD), 332
malaise, 316
mammillothalamic tract (MMT), 41, 53
management
    Alzheimer's disease and dementia, 390–392, 391t
    dementia with Lewy bodies (DLB), 238–240
    Parkinson's Disease Dementia (PD-D), 249–251
    posterior cortical atrophy (PCA), 214–217
Manes, F., 186
mania
    meningoencephalitis, 315
    neurosyphilis, 314, 315
MAPT gene, 223
Marchiafava Bignami Disease, 303–304
Marcuse, H., 137–138
Marsden, C.D., 133, 134–135
Martin, A., 25
mathematical skills, 339
Mattis Dementia Rating Scale, 244
McKhann, G.M., 177, 383
McKone, E., 17, 23
Meador, K.J., 136–137
measurement tools, 522t
mechanisms, examples of, 7f, 8f
medial dorsal (MD) nucleus, 47
medial geniculate nucleus (MGN), 44
medial pulvinar (PM), 47–48
medial temporal lobe, 112f, 113f, 532–534
Medication Drift syndrome, 421–422
medications, differential diagnosis, 303
    See also specific medications
melatonin, 251
memantine, 417t
    BPSDs, 582–583
    efficacy and effectiveness of, 405–406t
    mechanisms of action, 404
    pharmacological management, 397–398, 403–408
memory deficit
    Alzheimer's disease and dementia, 371–373
    Creutzfeldt-Jakob Disease (CJD), 320
    dementia with Lewy bodies (DLB), 233

fragile X-associated tremor ataxia syndrome (FXTAS), 337
Herpes Simplex Encephalitis, 306
limbic encephalitis, 307
Niemann-Pick Disease Type C, 339–340
in paramedian artery infarction, 50
polycystic lipomembranous osteodysplasia with sclerosing leukoencephalopathy (PLO-SL), 345
PSP-RS (Richardson's Syndrome), 222
qualitative evaluation by, 468–469
sarcoidosis, 317
Susac Syndrome, 327
Wilson's Disease, 345
X-linked adrenoleukodystrophy (X-ALD), 332
Memory Impairment Screen (MIS), 476t, 477–478
memory systems, 108–121, 109t
    about, 108
    disruptions in, 110t
    episodic memory, 108–117
    improving memory in dementia, 120–121
    priming, 119
    procedural memory, 118–119
    semantic memory, 117–118
    simple classical conditioning, 118
    working memory, 119–120
meningoencephalitis, 315
meningovascular syphilis, 315
Menon, V., 90
mental activity
    inhibiting or stopping, 82–83
    initiating and sustaining, 82
mental competence and legal issues, 622–636
    about, 622
    disagreements in, 634
    driving, 629–632
    end-of-life planning, 634–635
    executive function and metacognition, 625–626
    financial management, 628–629
    firearm safety, 633–634
    neuropsychological testing, 626–627
    principles, 623–625
    professional competence and dementia, 627–628
    resources for, 635–636
    road maps for, 636
    testamentary capacity, 632–633
    voting, 633
mental status examination. *See* screening and mental status examination
meprobamate, 387t
Mesulam, M.M., 26, 84, 176–177

metabolic disorders, 302–306
metachromatic leukodystrophy (MLD), 332
metacognition
    competency and, 623
    mental competence and legal issues, 625–626
    rate of decline of, 623
methotrexate (MTX) chemotherapy, 330
microphagia, 223
microscopic pathology, 163–167
microtubule associated protein tau *(MAPT)* gene, 179
middle longitudinal fasciculus (MdLF), 37*f*, 36
Middleton, F.A., 73
migrans, 316
mild cognitive impairment (MCI), 432–443
    about, 432
    aerobic exercise, 443
    biomarkers, 439–440, 441*t*
    cerebrospinal fluid, 438–439
    clinical characterization, 433–435
    criteria for, 440–441
    diagnostic scheme for, 434*f*
    epidemiology, 433
    etiology, 435*f*
    history, 432–433
    MRI, 436–437, 436*f*
    neuropsychological features, 497
    positron emission tomography (PET), 437–438
    predictors of progression, 436–440, 436*f*
    rofecoxib, 443
    vitamin E, 443
Miller, E.K., 79
Millspaugh, J., 160
Mini-Cog, 476*t*, 477
Mini Mental State Examination (MMSE), 128, 136, 186, 201, 239, 434, 465, 476*t*, 479–480, 490
Mintzer, J.E., 578
mitochondrial encephalopathy with lactic acidosis and stroke-like episodes (MELAS), 318–319
Miyake, A., 72–73
mobility, loss of, 345
moclobemide, 590
modafinil, 251
Modofied Mini-Mental State Examination (3MS), 476*t*, 480
molecular imaging
    in Alzheimer's Disease, 539–542
    as biomarker, 541
    in neurodegenerative diseases, 539–541
    neurotherapeutics, 541
    of pathologic markers in neurodegenerative diseases, 542–545

molecular neuropathology imaging, 544–545
Molina, J.A., 236
Molinuevo, J., 414
Montreal Cognitive Assessment (MoCA), 128, 186, 244, 434, 477*t*, 481–482
Monza, D., 136
mood and psychological functioning, qualitative evaluation by, 463
mood changes
    Alzheimer's disease and dementia, 374–375
    PSP-RS (Richardson's Syndrome), 222
"morning glory sign," 224
Morvan syndrome, 309
motivation, 374–375
motor features
    control of, 79
    dementia with Lewy bodies (DLB), 233–234
    inhibiting or stopping, 82–83
    initiating and sustaining, 82
    Parkinson's Disease Dementia (PD-D), 245
    PSP-RS (Richardson's Syndrome), 222
    vascular dementias, 521
motoric simple classical conditioning, 109*t*
motor neuron disease, 169
motor perseveration, 126
motor programming disorders, 126–139
    about, 126
    action-intentional disorders, 126–127
    apraxic disorders, 127–128
    conceptual apraxia, 128–129
    ideational apraxia, 137–138
    ideomotor apraxia, 129–136
    limb-kinetic apraxia, 136–137
movement disorders, 340
Movement Disorder Society Task Force, 248–249
Moya-Moya syndrome, 311
MPFC, 84
MR spectroscopy (MRS), 236
Multilingual Aphasia Examination, 497
multimodal cognitive operations, 469, 471–472
Multiple Errands Test, 93
multiple sclerosis, 148, 326
Multiple System Atrophy, 136
multiscale spatial frequency models, 19
Mulugeta, E., 236–237
Muratoff bundle (MB), 34*f*, 38
muscle biopsy, 319
myalgias, 316
myoclonus
    corticobasal degeneration (CBD), 225
    Creutzfeldt-Jakob Disease (CJD), 320–321
    Hashimoto's Encephalopathy (aka. Steroid Responsive Encephalopathy associated with Autoimmune Thyroiditis (SREAT)), 310

posterior choroidal artery infarction, 52–53
PSP-CBS (Corticobasal Syndrome), 223
subacute sclerosing panencephalitis (SSPE), 323

narrow localization, 25–26
National Alliance for Caregiving, 610
National Institute for Health and Care Excellence (NICE), 410
National Institute on Aging (NIA), 440, 442
Natural Action Test (NAT), 138
nausea
  dementia with Lewy bodies (DLB), 239
  Sagging Brain Syndrome (SBS), 344
Neary, D., 185
neck pain, 344
neglect, 48
neocortex, 148f, 148
neologisms, 48
nerve growth factor, 569–570
neural mechanisms
  about, 16–17
  neurological correlates of aspects of visual object recognition, 17–26
  regional functional specialization for cognitive functions, 26–28
neural networks, 17
neural responses, stimuli provoking, 28n2
neuritic plaques, pathological hallmarks of, 150
neuroanatomy and behavioral neurology of subcortical systems
  about, 32
  basal ganglia, 42–44
  cerebellum, 53–61
  clinical features of white matter lesions, 41
  thalamus, 44–53
  white matter tracts of cerebral hemispheres, 32–41
neurocysticercosis, 315
neurodegeneration with brain iron accumulation (NBIA), 345
neurodegenerative dementias, neuropathology of, 145–157
  about, 145
  Alzheimer's Disease, 153
  frontotemporal lobar degeneration, 154
  Huntington's Disease, 156–157
  neurodegenerative neuropathology in cognitively normal individuals, 145–149
  neuropathy of Dementias associated with Lewy Bodies, 154–156
  pathological hallmarks of major neurodegenerative dementias, 149–152
neurodegenerative disease
  evidence of, 182t
  molecular imaging in, 539–541

neurodegenerative neuropathology, in cognitively normal individuals, 145–149
neurofibrillary changes, pathological hallmarks of, 150
neuroimaging, 528–551
  about, 528–529
  anatomic changes of Alzheimer's Disease, 532–537
  biomarker constructs, 529–531
  dementia with Lewy bodies (DLB), 235–236
  diagnosis of Alzheimer's Disease, 531
  frontotemporal lobar degeneration (FTLD), 186–188
  molecular imaging in Alzheimer's Disease, 539–542
  molecular imaging of pathologic markers in neurodegenerative diseases, 542–545
  Parkinson's Disease Dementia (PD-D), 247–248
  physiological changes of Alzheimer's Disease, 537–539
  posterior cortical atrophy (PCA), 212–213, 212f
  progressive supranuclear palsy (PSP), 224
  typical amnesic Alzheimer's Disease Dementia, 531–532
neuroleptic sensitivity, 234, 238
neurolinguistics, 203–204
neurological deficits, 316, 317
neurologic disease on brain activity, modulatory effects of genetic risk factors for, 541
neuronal loss, 234
neuropathologic markers, in vivo neuroimaging of, 188–189
neuropathology
  Alzheimer's disease and dementia, 375–377
  chronic traumatic encephalopathy (CTE), 163
  corticobasal degeneration (CBD), 226
  frontotemporal lobar degeneration (FTLD), 177–179
  primary progressive aphasia (PPA), 202–203
Neuroprotection and Natural History in Parkinson's Plus Syndromes (NNIPPS) Study Group, 221
neuropsychiatric behavior, effects on domains of, 411
Neuropsychiatric Inventory (NPI), 239, 519, 582
Neuropsychiatric Inventory Questionnaire (NPI-Q), 474
neuropsychiatric symptoms, 508–522
  about, 508–509
  agitation, 516–517
  Alzheimer's Disease, 518–520, 519f
  Alzheimer's disease and dementia, 374–375

neuropsychiatric symptoms (*Cont.*)
  anxiety, 514, 516
  apathy, 513–514
  awareness, assessment, and intervention, 521–522
  cerebral localization of, 509*t*
  delusions, 514
  depression, 509, 511, 513
  frontotemporal dementias, 520
  hallucinations, 514
  impairments in insight, judgment, and complex competencies, 517–518
  impulsivity, 516–517
  Lewy Body Dementia (LBD), 520–521
  obsessive-compulsive behaviors, 516–517
  prevalence of, 520*f*
  psychosis, 514
  sleep disturbances, 518
  vascular dementias, 521
neuropsychological assessment, 487–502
  about, 487–488, 488–489
  Alzheimer's Disease Dementia, 497
  behavioral variant frontotemporal dementia, 498
  clinical profile, 499–501
  definitions and diagnosis of dementia, 488
  Lew Body Dementia (LBD), 498–499
  mild cognitive impairment (MCI), 497
  neuropsychological examination of mental state, 490–497
  primary progressive aphasia (PPA), 497–498
  screening for dementia, 489–490
neuropsychological profiles, 200–202, 495*t*, 500*f*, 501*f*
neuropsychological testing, role of, 626–627
neurosyphilis, 314–315
neurotherapeutics, 541
NIA-AA (National Institute on Aging-Alzheimer's Association)
  clinical criteria for dementia, 380–383, 380*t*, 381*t*, 440
  diagnostic criteria for Alzheimer's disease, 365
  three-stage model for preclinical AD, 453, 453*t*
Niemann-Pick Disease Type C, 339–340
night sweats, 323
Niki, C., 138
NINDS-SPSP criteria, 221, 221*t*
Nirkko, A.C., 137
NMDA antagonists (memantine), 400–402
nonbenzodiazepine hypnotics, 387*t*
nonpharmacological approaches, 600–607
  about, 600–601
  common behavior problems, 602–603
  developing, 604–606
  end-of-life care, 606–607
  family involvement, 606
  interdisciplinary teamwork, 605
  models of care, 605–606
  modification of physical environment, 605
  overview of behavioral and psychological symptoms, 601–602
  posterior cortical atrophy (PCA), 214
  reasons for medicating, 603–604
  staff education, 605
norepinephrine, 87–88
"normal aging," dementia *versus*, 491*t*
normal pressure hydrocephalus (NPH), 341–343
Northwestern Anagram Test (NAT), 201, 498
nursing home placement, 409
nystagmus, 297
NYU Caregiver Intervention (NYUCI), 614

Oasis Program, 605
object recognition, 8–10, 10*f*, 25–26
obsessive-compulsive behavior
  cerebellar cognitive affective syndrome (CCAS), 334
  neuropsychiatric symptoms, 516–517
  Niemann-Pick Disease Type C, 340
  Sagging Brain Syndrome (SBS), 344
obstructive sleep apnea (OSA), 518
occasional paraphasias, 50
occupational therapy
  corticobasal degeneration (CBD), 227
  progressive supranuclear palsy (PSP), 224
ocular stare, 297–298
oculomasticatory myorhythmia, 325
oculomotor apraxia, 225
oculomotor palsies, 316
office cognitive testing, 625–626
Okazaki, H., 231
Olszewski, J., 220, 223
Onari, K., 176, 181
onconeuronal antibodies, 308*t*
Oppenheimer, D.R., 162
optic atrophy, 345
orbitofrontal cortex (OFC), 79–80, 86
orexin, 88
organization, as role in task setting, 77
Organization of Economic Cooperation and Development (OECD), 364
orientation, qualitative evaluation by, 463–464
orientation invariance, 9*f*
orthostatic headache, 343–344
orthostatic hypotension
  dementia with Lewy bodies (DLB), 238
  Parkinson's Disease Dementia (PD-D), 245

oscillatory synchrony models, 22–23
outcome/reward anticipation and monitoring
    about, 78–81
    anticipating consequences/outcomes, 78–81
    performance/reward monitoring, 81–82
overrecruitment, of neural activity, 89

Paget's disease, 298
pallidotomy, 43
Pandya, D.N., 61
pantothenate kinase associated neurodegeneration (PKAN), 345
Papez, J.W., 110, 113
paracentral (Pcn) nucleus, 44
parafascicular (Pf) nucleus, 44
paralimbic projections, 55
parallel processing, 222
paramedian artery infarction, 50, 52t
paraneoplastic neurological syndromes, 308t, 309t
parenchymal pallor, 338
parietal lobe, 132–133
Park, D.C., 90
parkin gene, 242
Parkinson Neuropsychometric Dementia Assessment (PANDA), 244
Parkinson Plus Syndromes
    associated with cognitive disorders and ideomotor apraxia, 136
    associated with limb-kinetic apraxia associated with cognitive disorders, 137
Parkinson's Disease (PD), 91–92
    associated with cognitive disorders and ideomotor apraxia, 135
    associated with limb-kinetic apraxia associated with cognitive disorders, 137
    basal ganglia lesions and, 42–43
    characterizations of, 297
    dopaminergic agents for, 88
    hypophonic dysarthria in, 42
Parkinson's Disease Dementia (PD-D), 231–251
    about, 231, 240
    autonomic features, 245
    behavioral features, 245
    cerebrospinal fluid (CSF) biomarkers, 248
    clinical features, 242–247, 243t
    cognitive features, 242–244, 244t
    diagnosis, 248–249
    diagnostic criteria, 248t
    epidemiology, 240–242
    genetics, 242
    management of patients, 249–251
    motor features, 245
    neuroimaging features, 247–248
    neurological and biochemical correlates of, 246–247
    risk factors, 241t
paroxetine
    Parkinson's Disease Dementia (PD-D), 250–251
    sexualized inappropriate behavior, 595
passive immunotherapy, 566–568
pathogenetic mechanisms, 169–170
pathological diagnosis, 163–165
pathology
    posterior cortical atrophy (PCA), 214
    progressive supranuclear palsy (PSP), 220–221
pathophysiology, 274–276
Paus, T., 82
Pavlov, I.P., 87
PD Cognitive Rating Scale (PD-CRS), 244
Peabody Picture Vocabulary Test (PPVT-IV), 201
Pellagra, 304–305
perceptual identification, 5–12, 25–26
perceptual priming, 109t
performance/reward monitoring, 81–82
perfusion MRI, 538
peripheral neuropathy, 298, 337
perseveration, 48, 86
personality changes
    Alzheimer's disease and dementia, 361, 374–375
    autosomal recessive metachromatic leukodystrophy, 299
    Creutzfeldt-Jakob Disease (CJD), 320
    frontotemporal dementia, 226
    frontotemporal lobar degeneration (FTLD), 184
    neurosyphilis, 315
    polycystic lipomembranous osteodysplasia with sclerosing leukoencephalopathy (PLO-SL), 345
    PSP-RS (Richardson's Syndrome), 222
    Susac Syndrome, 327
    tuberothalamic artery infarction, 48, 50
    vascular dementias, 521
Petersen, R.C., 413
pharmacogenetics, 581
pharmacological management
    agitation, aggression, and psychosis, 579t
    antidementia medications, 397–398
    antipsychotics, 396
    BPSDs, 577
    cholinesterase inhibitors, 400
    combination therapy, 402–403
    eliminating deleterious medications, 395–396
    glutamate and memantine mechanism, 400–401

pharmacological management (*Cont.*)
  identifying and treating comorbid conditions, 396
  memantine, 403–408
  NMDA antagonists (memantine), 400–402
pharmacological therapies, for Alzheimer's Disease, 563–572
  about, 563–564
  active immunotherapy, 566–568
  aerobic physical exercise, 570–571
  alpha-7 nicotinic acetylcholine receptor agonist, 569
  beta-secretase inhibitors, 564–565
  drugs to prevent tau protein phosphorylation, 568–569
  ELND005, 565–566
  future directions, 571–572
  gamma-secretase inhibitors and modulators, 565
  insulin, 570
  nerve growth factor, 569–570
  nonimmunotherapy clearance of beta-amyloid, 568
  passive immunotherapy, 566–568
  tau immunotherapy, 568–569
pharmacology, practical implementation of, 417–419
pharmacotherapy
  Alzheimer's disease and dementia, 363
  posterior cortical atrophy (PCA), 214
Pharr, V., 136
phosphorylation, drugs to prevent, 568–569
physical therapy
  corticobasal degeneration (CBD), 227
  progressive supranuclear palsy (PSP), 224
PiB-PET imaging, 279, 438
Pick, A., 137–138, 176, 177, 198, 208
Pick bodies, 151, 177
Pick cells, 177
Pick's disease, 72, 149, 154, 176, 177–178, 178*f*, 179, 181
PIGD phenotype, 241, 245
pindolol, 596
PINK1 gene, 242
planning
  management, 81
  poor, 345
  as role in task setting, 77
plasticity, relationship with intrinsic properties of cells, 28n5
Plum, F., 327
pneumonia, as cause of death, 580–581
Poeck, K., 138
Pollock, B.G., 583

polycystic lipomembranous osteodysplasia with sclerosing leukoencephalopathy (PLO-SL), 345
Porsteinsson, A.P., 407
positron emission tomography (PET)
  about, 88
  Alzheimer's disease, 265, 378*t*, 383*t*, 437–438, 450, 451*f*, 540*f*, 547*f*, 551*f*
  cerebral amyloid angiopathy (CAA), 279
  dementia with Lewy bodies (DLB), 236
  frontotemporal lobar degeneration (FTLD), 186–187
  mild cognitive impairment (MCI), 437–438
  Parkinson's Disease Dementia (PD-D), 247–248
  posterior cortical atrophy (PCA), 212, 213*f*
  primary progressive aphasia (PPA), 202
  rapid onset of late-life neurodegenerative disorders, 346
  Sagging Brain Syndrome (SBS), 344
  vascular cognitive impairment (VCI), 265
Posner, J., 327
Posner, M.I., 72
postchemotherapy cognitive impairment, 330
postconcussion, 160–162
posterior-anterior shifts in aging (PASA) hypothesis, 90
posterior choroidal artery infarction, 52–53
posterior cortical atrophy (PCA), 208–217
  about, 135, 208
  biomarkers, 213–214
  cerebrospinal fluid (CSF) biomarkers, 213–214
  clinical features, 208–212
  diagnostic criteria of, 211*t*
  genetics, 213
  home safety recommendations for, 214–217
  literature review, 209–210*t*
  management, 214–217
  neuroimaging, 212–213, 212*f*
  nonpharmacologic therapy, 214
  pathology, 214
  pharmacotherapy, 214
  safety issues, 217
posterior fossa syndrome, 60
posterior limb of the internal capsule (ICp), 40
postlesion pain, 50
postprandial hypotension, 245
poststroke dementia, 521
postural errors, 129
postural instability
  dementia with Lewy bodies (DLB), 234
  PSP-RS (Richardson's Syndrome), 222
pramipexole, 250
Pramstaller, P.P., 133, 134–135

praxicons, 132–133
predictors of progression, 436–440
prefrontal cortex (PFC), 73–75, 76
preserved syntax, 50
primary angitis of the central nervous system (PACNS), 316
primary progressive aphasia (PPA), 198–204
  about, 198–199
  contributions of to neurolinguistics and cognitive neuroscience, 203–204
  criteria for classifying, 201
  functional and structural neuroanatomy, 202
  genetics and risk factors, 203
  neuropathology, 202–203
  neuropsychological features, 497–498
  neuropsychological profiles, 200–202
  patient care, 204
  subtyping and terminology in, 199–200
priming, 119
Prion Disease, 319–320
problem-solving skills, deficits in, 332
procedural memory, 109t, 115f, 118–119
processes, 28n3
processing priorities, attentional control and, 77–78
processing speed, qualitative evaluation by, 464–465
processing speed hypothesis, 89
professional competence, dementia and, 627–628
progranulin *(GRN)* gene, 180
progressive aphasic subtypes, 184–185
progressive encephalopathy, 319
progressive multifocal leukoencephalopathy (PML), 148, 322–323
Progressive Nonfluent Aphasia (PNFA), 226
progressive pyramidal signs, 345
progressive supranuclear palsy (PSP), 220–227
  about, 220
  associated with cognitive disorders and ideomotor apraxia, 136
  associated with limb-kinetic apraxia associated with cognitive disorders, 137
  characterizations of, 297
  clinical features, 221–223
  genetics, 223
  neuroimaging, 224
  NINDS-SPSP criteria for diagnosis of, 221t
  pathology, 220–221
  therapeutics, 224–225
projection fibers, 40–41
promazine, 580
promiscuity, 345
pseudobulbar features, 345
PSP-CBS (Corticobasal Syndrome), 223

PSP-P (Parkinsonism), 223
PSP-PAGF (Pure Akinesia with Gait Freezing), 223
PSP-PNFA (Progressive Nonfluent Aphasia), 223
PSP-RS (Richardson's Syndrome), 221–223, 226
psychiatric disorders, 340
psychiatric symptoms, 314
psychomotor function
  qualitative evaluation by, 464–465
  vascular dementias, 521
  X-linked adrenoleukodystrophy (X-ALD), 332
psychosis, 575–583
  about, 575–576
  central nervous system vasculitis, 317
  Creutzfeldt-Jakob Disease (CJD), 321
  diagnostic criteria, 513t
  limbic encephalitis, 307
  meningoencephalitis, 315
  metachromatic leukodystrophy (MLD), 332
  neuropsychiatric symptoms, 514
  neurosyphilis, 314
  pharmacological treatment of, 579t
  relationship with cerebral substrate, 510t
  sarcoidosis, 317
  Susac Syndrome, 327
  systemic lupus erythematosus (SLE), 317–318
psychosis spectrum, 60t
punch drunk. *See* chronic traumatic encephalopathy (CTE)
pyramidal weakness, 315

qualitative observation, of patients, 92
Qureshi, M., 138

Rabinovici, G.D., 189
racial differences, 365
radicular upper extremity symptoms, 344
rage attacks, 339
rapid eye movement (REM) sleep behavior disorder (RBD), 241
rapidly progressive dementias. *See* differential diagnosis
rapid onset of late-life neurodegenerative disorders, 345–347
rare dementias. *See* differential diagnosis
reading difficulties, 212, 222
Reading the Mind in the Eyes Test (RMET), 94
reasoning, 373–374
recognition, of visually presented objects, 5–12
recurrent perseveration, 126
reduced heart rate variability, 245
Relevant Outcome Scale for Alzheimer's Disease (ROSA), 473–474

Religious Orders cohort Study, 280
REM sleep behavior disorder (RBD), 238, 245, 518
repetitive behavior, 183
representation, 4
response/behavioral selection
    about, 82
    inhibiting or stopping motor and mental activity, 82–83
    initiating and sustaining motor and mental activity, 82
response criteria thresholds, setting, 28n4
response maintenance, 82
resting state functional connectivity magnetic resonance imaging (rs-fcMRI), 55, 537–538
rest tremor, 223
reticular thalamic nucleus, 44
retinal degeneration, 345
retinotropic objects, 6–7
retrograde amnesia, 115–116
reversal learning and extinction test, 94
Ribot, 115–116
Richardson, E.P., 145
Richardson, J.C., 220, 223
Richardson PSP phenotype, 221
rigidity
    delayed posthypoxic leukoencephalopathy, 328
    PSP-P (Parkinsonism), 223
risk factors
    Alzheimer's disease and dementia, 363–366, 363t
    Parkinson's Disease Dementia (PD-D), 241t
ritualistic behavior, 183
rivastigmine, 417t
    apathy, 592
    dementia with Lewy bodies (DLB), 239
    Parkinson's Disease Dementia (PD-D), 249
    relationship with sleep disturbances, 518
Robot's law, 110, 110t
Roe, A.W., 19
rofecoxib, 443
Rosenfeld, M., 198
rostral head, lesions of, 42
Rothi, L.J.G., 133
Rountree, S., 415
Roussy, G., 50
rubral tremor, 53
ruminative behaviors, 334

Sabattoli, F., 235
safety issues
    BPSDs, 580–581
    posterior cortical atrophy (PCA), 217

Sagging Brain Syndrome (SBS), 343–344
sagittal stratum (SS), 40–41
salience, early, 199
salience network, 75, 75f, 86
sarcoidosis, 317
SCales for Outcomes of PArkinson's disease-cognition (SCOPA-Cog), 244
schizophrenia-like psychosis with paranoia, 340
Schmahmann, J.D., 61
scope of problem, 292
scrapie, 320
screening and mental status examination, 461–482
    about, 461–462
    appearance and indicators of functional status, 462–463
    arousal and orientation, 463–464
    attention, working memory, processing speed, and psychomotor function, 464–465
    executive function, 465–466
    functional status and dementia symptom questionnaires, 472–474
    language, 466–467
    measures of psychological function, 474–482
    memory function, 468–469
    mood and psychological functioning, 463
    multimodal cognitive operations, 469, 471–472
    qualitative evaluation by domain, 462–472
    specialized mental functions, 469, 471–472
    tools, 476–477t
    visuospatial function, 467–468
Seeley, W.W., 74–75, 90, 179, 487
seizures
    central nervous system vasculitis, 317
    epilepsy, 340
    Hashimoto's Encephalopathy (aka. Steroid Responsive Encephalopathy associated with Autoimmune Thyroiditis (SREAT)), 310
    intravascular lymphoma, 323
    limbic encephalitis, 307
    MELAS, 319
    Niemann-Pick Disease Type C, 340
    sarcoidosis, 317
    systemic lupus erythematosus (SLE), 317–318
    X-linked adrenoleukodystrophy, 299
selective regional vulnerability of the aging brain, 147
self, representations of the, 84–85
self-knowledge, 85
self-mutilation, 340
self-referential processing, 85

self-regulatory model, 73
semantic memory, 9–10, 109*t*, 115*f*, 117–118
sensation, 332
sensorineural hearing loss, 326
sensory input, control of, 79
sensory loss, 50
sensory overload, 335
sequencing, impaired, 50
Sérieux, P., 198
serotonin, 88
7-Minute Screen (7MS), 476*t*, 479
sexual dysfunction, 245
sexualized inappropriate behavior (SIB), 588–596
Shallice, T., 72, 93
short-term memory loss
    chronic traumatic encephalopathy (CTE), 162
    meningoencephalitis, 315
Short Test of Mental Status, 434
"silver tsunami," 365
Simchowicz, T., 146
simple classical conditioning, 118
Singer, W., 22
single-photon emission computed tomography (SPECT)
    clinical use, 542
    dementia with Lewy bodies (DLB), 236
    frontotemporal lobar degeneration (FTLD), 186–187
    posterior cortical atrophy (PCA), 212
    primary progressive aphasia (PPA), 202
Sjöwall, J., 316
skeletal muscle relaxants, 387*t*
sleep apnea, 341
sleep deprivation, cognition and, 341
sleep disturbances
    about, 419–420
    Alzheimer's disease and dementia, 361
    dementia with Lewy bodies (DLB), 234
    Hashimoto Encephalopathy, 310
    neuropsychiatric symptoms, 518
    Niemann-Pick Disease Type C, 340
small world organization, 26
smell, changes in, 306
social cognition, tests of, 93–94
Social Cognition and Emotional Assessment (SEA), 94
social inhibition, loss of, 345
social skills, 60*t*, 521
Society for Nuclear Medicine and Molecular Imaging, 544
solanezumab, 566–567
somnolence, 239
Souvenaid, 416–417

spasticity
    delayed posthypoxic leukoencephalopathy, 329
    subacute sclerosing panencephalitis (SSPE), 323
spatial and temporal orientation, 374
spatial cognition, 332
Spatz, H., 176, 181
specialized mental functions, 469, 471–472
specific sensory thalamic nuclei, 44, 46–47
speech patterns stereotyped, 183
speech therapy, 224
splenomegaly, 340
spongiosis, 338
spontaneous parkinsonism, 233–234, 237
Starkstein Apathy Scale, 94
State of the Science Symposium: Professional Partners Supporting Family Caregivers, 615
static objects, inability to find, 212
status spongiosus *versus* spongiform changes, pathological hallmarks of, 151–152
Steele, J.C., 220, 223
Steinthal, P., 127, 128
Stern, Y., 365
stimulants, 88
St. Louis University Mental Status Examination (SLUMS), 476*t*, 478–479
STOPIM, 346*t*, 347
stop-signal tasks, 77
strategic-infarct dementia, 521
strength, 332
stress-coping paradigm, 614
striatal fibers, 32, 33*f*, 38
Strick, P.L., 73
stroke
    central nervous system vasculitis, 317
    MELAS, 319
    probable vascular dementia diagnosis in, 262
    systemic lupus erythematosus (SLE), 317–318
    tuberothalamic artery infarction, 48, 50
Stroop Interference Task, 77, 81
Stroop Test, 92
structural descriptions, 7–8, 9*f*
structural MRI, 186–187
Stuss, D.T., 82
subacute sclerosing panencephalitis (SSPE), 323–324
subconcussion, 160–162
subcortical bundle (SB), 34
subcortical dementia, 222, 345
subcortical disease, 262–263
subcortical nuclei, 148–149
subcortical structures, 32
subregional analysis, 534–535

superficial siderosis, 339
superior longitudinal fasciculus (SLF), 35–36, 35f
supervisory attentional system (SAS), 72
supplementary motor area, 133–134
supportive therapies, 227
supranuclear vertical opthalmoplegia, 325
Susac syndrome, 298, 326–327
susceptibility Alzheimer's disease mutations, 369–370
swallow evaluations, 227
swallow therapy, 224
sweating, excessive, 245
swelling in joints, 316
sympathetic dyspraxia, 199
sympathy, loss of, 183
synchronous oscillations, 26, 28n6
syncope, 234, 238
systematized delusions, 238
systemic lupus erythematosus (SLE), 317–318

tactile defensiveness, 335
Tariot, P.N., 410, 411, 415
Task Force Movement Disorder Society, 249
task management, 81
task-related fMRI, 537
tasks, impaired, 222
task setting, 76–77
taste, changes, 306
tau *(MAPT)* gene, 242
tau immunotherapy, 568–569
TDP-43 pathology, 167
temporal-parietal junction (TPJ), 86
temporal sequencing, 337
testing
    for dementia, 493–494
    episodic memory, 201
    of social cognition, 93–94
    See also specific tests
thalamic arterial supply, 52t
thalamic peduncles, 41
thalamus
    about, 44, 45f
    anatomical features and connections, 44–48
    basal ganglia and, 134–135
    behavioral roles of thalamic nuclei, 46t
    clinical features of thalamic lesions, 48–53
    projections from, 49f, 50f
    vascular supply, 51f
Thal Phase classification, 376–377
therapeutics
    corticobasal degeneration (CBD), 226–227
    progressive supranuclear palsy (PSP), 224–225
thiamine deficiency, 303–304

thinking, slowed, 345
thioridazine, 580
three-dimensional object-centered representation, reconstruction of, 18–21
Three Words Three Shapes (3W3S) test, 201–202
thyroid disorders, 305–306
top-down attentional control, 78
top-down modulation, 78
    clinical features of enhancement, 80t
    executive control and, 79
Torralva, T., 186
Trail Making Test B, 92, 625
transcortical sensory aphasia, 208
transient aphasia, 310
transient loss of consciousness, 234, 238
transient visual loss, 323
transmissable spongiform encephalopathy (TSE), 320
trauma, 311
traumatic axonal injury (TAI), 161
traumatic brain injury, 160–162
trazodone
    Parkinson's Disease Dementia (PD-D), 251
    sexualized inappropriate behavior, 595
treatment. *See specific issues*
Treisman, A., 22
tremor, 310
Troxler fading paradigm, 19–21, 21f
Tsao, J.W., 422
tuberothalamic artery infarction, 48, 50, 52t, 53f
Tulving, E., 11
2010 IWG-Dubois New Lexicon Criteria, 377, 378–379f
2011 NIA-AA Criteria, 379–384, 380t, 381t
2013 *DSM-5* Criteria, 377–379
two-hit vascular hypothesis of Alzheimer's Disease, 368–369
two-stage amyloid-dependent and amyloid-independent hypothesis of Alzheimer's disease, 368
typical amnesic Alzheimer's Disease Dementia, 531–532

U-fibers, 32–33
Uluduz, D., 136
uncinate fascoculus (UF), 36, 37, 39f
unilateral parkinsonism, 223
urinary incontinence
    dementia with Lewy bodies (DLB), 234
    Parkinson's Disease Dementia (PD-D), 245
    Sagging Brain Syndrome (SBS), 344
urinary urgency, 337
US Census, 364
Useful Field of View (UFoV), 631
utilization behavior, 127

van der Flier, W.M., 280
vanishing white matter disease, 333
vascular cognitive impairment (VCI), 260–269
  about, 91, 260
  cerebrovascular disease, impact of, 266
  clinical components, 262–263
  future diagnostic methods, 268
  imaging, 264–265
  interaction with Alzheimer's Disease, 266–267
  MRI, 267–268
  vascular dementia (VaD), 261–262
  Vascular mild cognitive impairment (VaMCI), 265–266
  vascular risk and incident dementia, 267
vascular dementia (VaD), 116, 261–263, 521
vascular diseases
  associated with cognitive disorders and ideomotor apraxia, 135
  differential diagnosis, 310–311
Vascular mild cognitive impairment (VaMCI), 265–266
Venereal Disease Reference Laboratory (VDRL) test, 315
venlafaxine, 251
ventral anterior (VA) nucleus, 47
ventral attention network, 78f, 86–87
ventral frontal cortex (VFC), 86
ventral lateral (VL) nucleus, 47
ventral nucleus (AV), 44
ventral striatum, lesions of, 43
ventricular enlargement, pathological hallmarks of, 149
ventromedial (VM) nucleus, 47
ventroposterior nucleus, 46
verbal fluency dysfunction
  in paramedian artery infarction, 50
  PSP-PNFA (Progressive Nonfluent Aphasia), 223
  PSP-RS (Richardson's Syndrome), 222
  tuberothalamic artery infarction, 48, 50
verbal memory, 339
vertical gaze/gaze palsy
  PSP-CBS (Corticobasal Syndrome), 223
  PSP-RS (Richardson's Syndrome), 221
vertical supranuclear gaze palsy, 223
vertical supranuclear opthalmoplegia, 339
vertigo, 323
violence, 315
vision loss, 222, 233, 326
visual agnosia, 208
visual blurring
  PSP-RS (Richardson's Syndrome), 222
  Sagging Brain Syndrome, 344

visual field deficits
  focal brain lesions, 297
  in posterior choroidal artery infarction, 52–53
visually presented objects, perceptual identification, recognition, and categorization of, 5–12
visual memory, 48, 339
visual object recognition, 17–26
visual spatial disorganization
  CCAS (Cerebellar Cognitive Affective Syndrome), 58
  Gordon Holmes syndrome, 336
  X-linked adrenoleukodystrophy (X-ALD), 332
Visual Verbal Test, 202
visuospatial function, 233, 244, 337, 374, 467–468
vitamin B12 deficiency, 305
vitamin E, 305, 416, 443
vitamins, 416–417
vomiting
  dementia with Lewy bodies (DLB), 239
  Sagging Brain Syndrome (SBS), 344
Von Economo neurons, 148
voting, dementia and, 633

Wallin, A., 409
wandering, 420
Wang, J., 315
Waters, F., 341
Watson, R.T., 134
weakness, 323
Wechsler Adult Intelligence Scale-III, 491
Wegener's granulomatosis, 317
weight loss
  intravascular lymphoma, 323
  Whipple's Disease (WD), 324
Weiner, M.F., 465
Wernicke, C., 132
Wernicke area, 132
Wernicke syndrome, 303–304
Western Aphasia Battery (WAB-R), 201
Western blot analysis, 316
Whipple's Disease (WD), 297–298, 324–325
white matter dementia, 299–300
white matter fiber pathways, 33f
white matter lesions, 41
white matter tracts, 32–42
Whitmer, R.A., 267
wide-based gait, 222
Wilson's Disease
  characterizations of, 297
  differential diagnosis, 344–345
Winblad, B., 415
Wisconsin Card Sorting Task, 83, 92

word meanings, relationship with concepts and categories, 10–12
working memory, 109t, 115f, 119–120
  about, 72, 76
  attentional control and processing priorities, 77–78
  fragile X-associated tremor ataxia syndrome (FXTAS), 337
  Parkinson's Disease Dementia (PD-D), 244
  qualitative evaluation by, 464–465
  Sagging Brain Syndrome (SBS), 344
  task setting, 76–77
World Health Organization (WHO), 364

X-linked adrenoleukodystrophy (X-ALD), 332

Zlokovic, B.V., 369

About the Editors

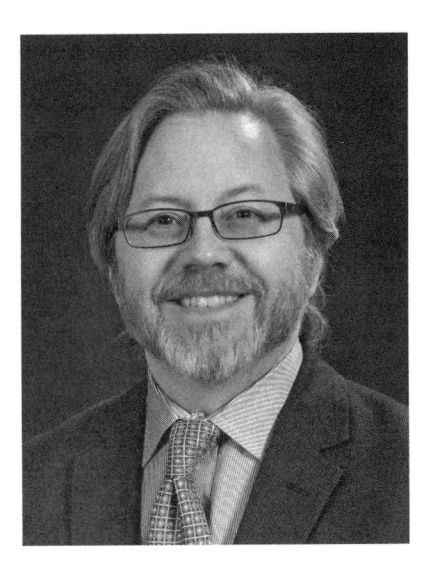

Brad C. Dickerson, MD, is a behavioral neurologist and neuroscientist at Harvard Medical School and Massachusetts General Hospital in Boston, Massachusetts. Dr. Dickerson runs a busy weekly clinic caring for patients with various forms of cognitive impairment and dementia, as well as providing training for clinical and research fellows. His research focuses primarily on the use of quantitative structural and functional neuroimaging techniques to understand the neurobiology of Alzheimer's disease, primary progressive aphasia, frontotemporal dementia, and other dementias, and on the relationships between imaging measures and behavior. He also investigates the neural substrates of changes in memory, affect, and other abilities in healthy young adults and in normal aging. He has published widely and has won a number of awards, including the prestigious American Academy of Neurology Norman Geschwind Award in Behavioral Neurology.

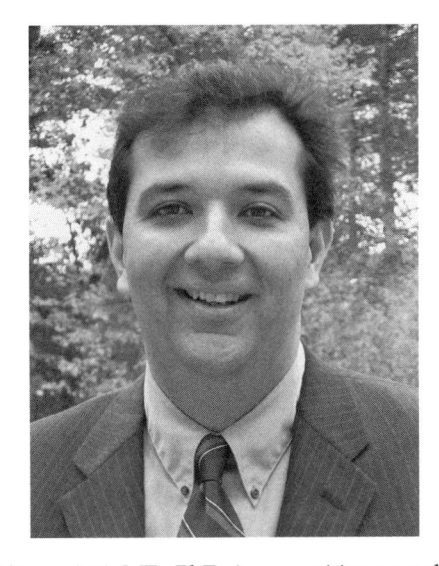

Alireza Atri, MD, PhD, is a cognitive neurologist/neuroscientist and clinical-educator at Harvard Medical School, ENRM Bedford VA Medical Center, and Massachusetts General Hospital in Boston, Massachusetts, dedicated to improving awareness, early diagnosis, treatment, and clinical practice regarding cognitive aging and dementia syndromes, particularly Alzheimer's disease (AD). Dr. Atri specializes in providing care to patients and families affected by cognitive impairment, AD, especially early-onset AD, and unusual dementias. His research involves integrating pharamacological, functional neuroimaging, mathematical, neuropsychometric, and clinical methods to improve the design, implementation, integration, and analysis of multimodal studies to better risk stratify, detect, track, and predict clinical trajectory, and to assess treatment responses in individuals along the cognitive aging–impairment–AD spectrum. Dr. Atri has published, and lectures widely, on AD-related research and clinical practice, directs integrated memory clinics and undergraduate and graduate medical courses, and teaches nationally and internationally on best evidence and practices in AD and dementia evaluation and care.